ULCERATIVE COLITIS

The Complete Guide to Medical Management

ULCERATIVE COLITIS
The Complete Guide to Medical Management

EDITED BY

GARY R. LICHTENSTEIN, MD, FACP, FACG, AGAF

PROFESSOR OF MEDICINE
UNIVERSITY OF PENNSYLVANIA SCHOOL OF MEDICINE
DIRECTOR, CENTER FOR INFLAMMATORY BOWEL DISEASE
DEPARTMENT OF MEDICINE, DIVISION OF GASTROENTEROLOGY
PHILADELPHIA, PENNSYLVANIA

ASSOCIATE EDITOR

ELLEN J. SCHERL, MD, FACP, AGAF

DIRECTOR, JILL ROBERTS CENTER FOR INFLAMMATORY BOWEL DISEASE
NEW YORK-PRESBYTERIAN HOSPITAL
JILL ROBERTS ASSOCIATE PROFESSOR OF CLINICAL MEDICINE
WEILL MEDICAL COLLEGE OF CORNELL UNIVERSITY
ADJUNCT PROFESSOR OF MEDICINE
COLUMBIA UNIVERSITY MEDICAL CENTER
NEW YORK, NEW YORK

CRC Press
Taylor & Francis Group
Boca Raton London New York

CRC Press is an imprint of the
Taylor & Francis Group, an informa business

First published 2011 by SLACK Incorporated

Published 2024 by CRC Press
2385 NW Executive Center Drive, Suite 320, Boca Raton FL 33431

and by CRC Press
4 Park Square, Milton Park, Abingdon, Oxon, OX14 4RN

CRC Press is an imprint of Taylor & Francis Group, LLC

Library of Congress Cataloging-in-Publication Data

Ulcerative colitis : the complete guide to medical management / edited by Gary R. Lichtenstein ; associate editor, Ellen J. Scherl.

p. ; cm.

Includes bibliographical references and index.

ISBN 9781556429453 (alk. paper)

1. Ulcerative colitis. I. Lichtenstein, Gary R., II. Scherl, Ellen J.

[DNLM: 1. Colitis, Ulcerative--therapy. 2. Colitis, Ulcerative--physiopathology. WI 522 U387 2010]

RC862.C63U435 2010

616.3'4473--dc22

2010007951

ISBN: 9781556429453 (hbk)
ISBN: 9781003526827 (ebk)

DOI: 10.1201/9781003526827

DEDICATION

I dedicate this book to my wife, Nancy, and my children, Danielle and Julie, whose unwavering support has permitted me the opportunity to pursue my aspirations.

I also acknowledge my patients who are victims of ulcerative colitis and Crohn's disease.

My mentors have supported me and guided me throughout my career. They have enabled me to continually learn with goals of improving the lives of patients for whom I have had the privilege of caring.

I would also like to dedicate this book to my mother, Joan Lichtenstein, and in memory of my father, Abraham Lichtenstein.

CONTENTS

ACKNOWLEDGMENTS

We would like to acknowledge many individuals who have contributed in many different ways to allow this book to become a reality.

- The contributing authors
- The staff at SLACK Incorporated (including Carrie Kotlar, Senior Acquisitions Editor and April Billick, Managing Editor) and Kristin Della Volpe, Freelance Editor. Without their dedication and tireless and endless effort, this production would not have occurred
- The Crohn's and Colitis Foundation of America
- Our respective institutions: The University of Pennsylvania School of Medicine and the University of Pennsylvania Health System and Weill Medical College of Cornell University
- Dr. Anil Rustgi, for his support and friendship

ABOUT THE EDITOR AND ASSOCIATE EDITOR

Gary R. Lichtenstein, MD, FACP, FACG, AGAF is the Director of the Inflammatory Bowel Disease Center and a Professor of Medicine in the Gastrointestinal Division of the Department of Medicine at the Hospital of the University of Pennsylvania and the University of Pennsylvania School of Medicine in Philadelphia, Pennsylvania.

Dr. Lichtenstein earned his medical degree from the Mount Sinai School of Medicine in New York, New York. He then completed his internship and residency in Internal Medicine at Duke University Medical Center in Durham, North Carolina. He also served a fellowship in Gastroenterology at the Hospital of the University of Pennsylvania of the University Of Pennsylvania School of Medicine. His current research interests encompass investigational therapies for the treatment of ulcerative colitis and Crohn's disease. Dr. Lichtenstein has received numerous research grants focusing on these areas and has served as the national/international principal investigator evaluating novel agents for therapeutic trials in the treatment of ulcerative colitis and Crohn's disease.

A Fellow of the American Gastroenterological Association, the American College of Physicians, and the American College of Gastroenterology, Dr. Lichtenstein has served as Medical Secretary for the American Board of Internal Medicine, Gastroenterology Section. He holds membership and committee positions in many professional societies at a national level, including the American Gastroenterological Association, where he has served as the vice-chair of the Clinical Practice Committee and Practice Economics Committee and where he has served as chair of the Clinical Practice Committee; the American Society for Gastrointestinal Endoscopy, where he has served on the Committee on Training; and the American College of Gastroenterology, where he has served on the Education Committee, Programs Committee, and the Nominations Committee. He recently served as a member of the Research Committee. He has been the chair of the Abstract Review Committee for Inflammatory Bowel Disease for the American College of Gastroenterology. He is also a member of the Crohn's and Colitis Foundation of America, where he serves at the national level as the chair of the Membership Committee of the Clinical Research Alliance; he has served on the National Grants Review Committee and the National Physician Education Committee as well. Additionally, Dr. Lichtenstein is a longstanding member of the American College of Physicians and the American Medical Association.

Dr. Lichtenstein has received numerous awards. including the award for the top specialist in the University of Pennsylvania Health System—the Louis A. Duhring Award. He is the recipient of the Christina and Marie Lindback award, which is the top teaching award in the entire University of Pennsylvania. He has received Penn Pearls Award for medical school teaching. He has received the Donald B. Martin Teaching Award for the Department of Medicine Housestaff. He has received the Sidney Cohen Teaching Award for the Gastroenterology Division. He is listed in "The Best Doctors in America" for Inflammatory Bowel Disease, and was listed among the Top Gastroenterologists for the Elderly in Philadelphia and Top Gastroenterologists in Philadelphia (Special Focus: Inflammatory Bowel Disease) by *Philadelphia Magazine.* He is the recipient of the CCFA Physician of the Year Award, Philadelphia and Delaware Valley Chapters.

In addition to having served on the Editorial Board of *Gastroenterology, American Journal of Gastroenterology, Inflammatory Bowel Diseases, World Journal of Gastroenterology,* and *Digestive Diseases and Sciences,* Dr. Lichtenstein is the current section editor of Selected Summaries and the section editor of Print and Media Review in *Gastroenterology.* He has served as a reviewer for such journals as *The New England Journal of Medicine, Gastroenterology, The Lancet,* the *Annals of Internal Medicine, Gut, Journal of Parenteral and Enteral Nutrition,* the *American Journal of Gastroenterology,* the *World Journal of Gastroenterology* and the *Journal of Clinical Gastroenterology.* He is the executive editor of the newly indexed journal *Gastroenterology and Hepatology,* and serves as Associate Editor of *Therapeutic Advances in Gastroenterology, The Physician and Sportsmedicine,* and *Clinical Investigation,* and is currently Assistant Editor-in-Chief of the *World Journal of Gastroenterology.* An invited lecturer at the local, national, and international levels, Dr. Lichtenstein is the author or co-author of more than 250 peer-reviewed primary articles, chapters, letters, and editorials, and he has presented over 250 abstracts and edited 18 books. He has lectured at over 300 invited conferences, symposiums, and institutional grand rounds.

Ellen J. Scherl, MD, FACP, AGAF, is the Jill Roberts Associate Professor of Clinical Medicine and Director of The Roberts Center for Inflammatory Bowel Disease at Weill Medical College of Cornell University/New York-Presbyterian Hospital. She holds a Bachelor's degree in English from Barnard College, Columbia University, and a medical degree from New York Medical College. She is a fellow of the American College of Physicians and the American Gastroenterological Association (AGA), a member of the American Society of Gastrointestinal Endoscopy, and a past president of the New York Society for Gastrointestinal Endoscopy (NYSGE). She is currently vice president of the New York Academy of Gastroenterology.

Dr. Scherl is Chairperson of the New York Chapter of the Crohn's and Colitis Foundation of America and is involved in the New York Crohn's Foundation. She received the 2008 AGA Outstanding Women in Science award, 2006 NYSGE Florence Lefcourt Distinguished Service Award, and has been awarded by the Crohn's and Colitis Foundation of America. She is an American Society of Gastrointestinal Endoscopy Circle of Life Member and a member of the AGA Legacy Society. She is board certified in medicine and gastroenterology.

Dr. Scherl is an editorial reviewer for *IBD Journal, Journal of Clinical Gastroenterology, Gastrointestinal Endoscopy, Digestive Diseases and Sciences,* and *Journal of Gastroenterology and Hepatology.* She is co-author of the chapter "Crohn's Disease of the Small Intestine" in *Gastroenterology and Hepatology: The Comprehensive Visual Reference,* associate editor of *Inflammatory Bowel Disease: The Complete Guide to Medical Management,* and coauthor of *An Interactive Dialogue on IBD.*

Dr. Scherl established the first IBD tissue bank in New York City at Weill Medical College of Cornell University/New York-Presbyterian Hospital. She has extensive experience as an investigator in clinical trials and is currently participating in national multicenter trials and in investigator-initiated trials focusing on ulcerative colitis and Crohn's disease.

CONTRIBUTING AUTHORS

Jean-Paul Achkar, MD (Chapter 31)
Department of Gastroenterology and Hepatology
Cleveland Clinic
Cleveland, Ohio

Pietro G. Andres, MD (Chapter 1)
Assistant Adjunct Professor of Medicine
Division of Gastroenterology
University of California, San Francisco
San Francisco, California

Leonard Baidoo, MD (Chapter 16)
Assistant Professor of Medicine
Subspecialty Education Coordinator
Division of Gastroenterology, Hepatology, and Nutrition
UPMC Presbyterian
Pittsburgh, Pennsylvania

Robert N. Baldassano, MD (Chapter 5)
Colman Family Chair in Pediatric Inflammatory Bowel Disease
Professor, University of Pennsylvania, School of Medicine
Director, Center for Pediatric Inflammatory Bowel Disease
The Children's Hospital of Philadelphia
Philadelphia, Pennsylvania

James M. Becker, MD, FACS (Chapter 36)
James Utley Professor and Chairman
Section of Gastrointestinal Surgery
Division of Surgery
Boston University School of Medicine
Boston, MA

Stephen J. Bickston, MD, AGAF (Chapter 33)
Professor of Internal Medicine
Director, Inflammatory Bowel Disease Center
Associate Chair for Gastroenterology
Virginia Commonwealth University Health Center
Richmond, Virginia

Wojciech Blonski, MD, PhD (Prologue, Chapter 22)
Division of Gastroenterology
University of Pennsylvania
Philadelphia, Pennsylvania
Department of Gastroenterology
Medical University
Wroclaw, Poland

Richard S. Bloomfeld, MD, MS (Chapter 33)
Associate Professor, Internal Medicine
Director, Inflammatory Bowel Disease Clinic
Wake Forest University Baptist Medical Center
Winston-Salem, North Carolina

Brian P. Bosworth, MD (Chapter 20)
Assistant Professor of Medicine
Anne and Ken Estabrook Clinical Scholar in Gastroenterology
Weill Medical College of Cornell University/New York–Presbyterian Hospital
Assistant Attending Physician
New York–Presbyterian Hospital
New York, New York

Alan L. Buchman, MD, MSPH (Chapter 38)
Division of Gastroenterology
Feinberg School of Medicine
Northwestern University
Chicago, Illinois

Anne Burke, MD (Chapter 22)
Assistant Professor of Medicine
Division of Gastroenterology
University of Pennsylvania School of Medicine
Philadelphia, Pennsylvania

Massimo Campieri, MD (Chapter 35)
Professor of Internal Medicine and Gastroenterology
University of Bologna
Bologna, Italy

Adam S. Cheifetz, MD (Chapter 3)
Clinical Director
Center for Inflammatory Bowel Disease
Beth Israel Deaconess Medical Center
Assistant Professor of Medicine
Harvard Medical School
Boston, Massachusetts

Ashish Chawla, MD (Chapter 4)
Department of Hepatology and Gastroenterology
The Cleveland Clinic
Cleveland, Ohio

Robynne Chutkan, MD (Chapter 27)
The Digestive Center for Women
Chevy Chase, Maryland

Russell D. Cohen, MD (Chapter 14)
Associate Professor of Medicine
Co-Director, Inflammatory Bowel Disease Center
Department of Medicine
Gastroenterology & Nutrition
University of Chicago Medical Center
Chicago, Illinois

Carmen Cuffari, MD (Chapter 19)
Associate Professor of Pediatrics
The Johns Hopkins University School of Medicine
Baltimore, Maryland

Eugeni Domènech, MD, PhD (Chapter 9)
Department of Gastroenterology
Hospital Universitari Germans Trias i Pujol (Badalona)
Catalonia, Spain

Marla C. Dubinsky, MD (Chapter 18)
Associate Professor of Pediatrics
Director, Pediatric IBD Center
Cedars-Sinai Medical Center
Los Angeles, California

Francis A. Farraye, MD, MSc (Chapter 7)
Section of Gastroenterology
Boston University School of Medicine
Boston, Massachusetts

Richard N. Fedorak, MD, FRCPC (Chapter 35)
Division of Gastroenterology
University of Alberta
Edmonton, Alberta, Canada

Lawrence S. Friedman, MD (Chapter 1)
Professor of Medicine, Harvard Medical School
Boston, Massachusetts
Professor of Medicine, Tufts University School of Medicine
Boston, Massachusetts
Chair, Department of Medicine, Newton-Wellesley Hospital
Newton, Massachusetts
Assistant Chief of Medicine, Massachusetts General Hospital
Boston, Massachusetts

Sonia Friedman, MD, FACP (Chapter 11)
Assistant Professor of Medicine
Harvard Medical School
Brigham and Women's Hospital
Boston, Massachusetts

Miguel Gassull, MD, PhD (Chapter 9)
Department of Gastroenterology
Hospital Universitari Germans Trias i Pujol (Badalona)
Catalonia, Spain

Louis R. Ghanem, MD, PhD (Chapter 5)
Fellow
Division of Gastroenterology, Hepatology, and Nutrition
The Children's Hospital of Philadelphia
Philadelphia, Pennsylvania

Jesse A. Green, MD, FACG (Chapter 34)
Associate Professor of Medicine
Director, Endoscopy Unit
Division of Gastroenterology
Albany Medical College
Albany, New York

Douglas B. Haghighi, DMD, MD (Chapter 29)
Gastroenterologist
Internal Medicine Associates
Anchorage, Alaska

Hans Herfarth, MD, PhD (Chapter 21)
Division of Gastroenterology and Hepatology
Department of Medicine
University of North Carolina
Chapel Hill, North Carolina

Kim L. Isaacs, MD, PhD (Chapter 15)
Professor of Medicine
University of North Carolina at Chapel Hill
Division of Gastroenterology and Hepatology
Chapel Hill, North Carolina

Vinita Elizabeth Jacob, MD (Chapters 8, 20)
Assistant Clinical Professor of Medicine
Division of Gastroenterology and Hepatology
Weill Medical College of Cornell University/New York–Presbyterian Hospital
New York, New York

Niraj Jani, MD (Chapter 26)
Chief of the Division of Gastroenterology
Greater Baltimore Medical Center
The Kroh Center for Digestive Disorders
Division of Gastroenterology
Baltimore, Maryland

Thomas A. Judge, MD (Chapter 12)
Associate Professor of Medicine
Division of Gastroenterology
Cooper University Hospital
Camden, New Jersey
Robert Wood Johnson School of Medicine/UMDNJ
Piscataway, New Jersey

Sunanda V. Kane, MD, MSPH, FACG, FACP, AGAF (Chapter 10)
Miles and Shirley Fitterman Division of Gastroenterology and Hepatology
Mayo Clinic College of Medicine
Rochester, Minnesota

Jeffry A. Katz, MD (Chapter 8)
Associate Professor of Medicine
Division of Gastroenterology
University Hospitals Case Medical Center
Cleveland, Ohio

Seymour Katz, MD, FACP, MACG (Chapter 17)
Nassau Gastroenterology Associates
Great Neck, New York

Joshua R. Korzenik, MD (Chapters 6, 23)
Gastrointestinal Unit and MGH Crohn's and Colitis Center
Massachusetts General Hospital and Harvard Medical School
Boston, Massachusetts

David Kotlyar, MD (Prologue)
Division of Gastroenterology
University of Pennsylvania
Philadelphia, Pennsylvania
Department of Medicine
Montefiore Medical Center/Albert Einstein College of Medicine
Bronx, New York

Harrison Lakehomer, BA (Chapter 20)
Amherst College
Researcher, Jill Roberts Center for Inflammatory Bowel Disease
Weill Medical College of Cornell University/New York–Presbyterian Hospital
New York, New York

Bret A. Lashner, MD, MPH (Chapter 29)
Professor of Medicine
Department of Gastroenterology and Hepatology
Cleveland Clinic
Cleveland, Ohio

James D. Lewis, MD, MSCE (Chapter 2)
Gastroenterology Division
Center for Clinical Epidemiology and Biostatistics
University of Pennsylvania
Philadelphia, PA

Ming V. Lin, MD (Prologue)
Department of Medicine
Pennsylvania Hospital
Philadelphia, Pennsylvania

Edward V. Loftus Jr, MD (Chapter 30)
Professor of Medicine
Consultant, Division of Gastroenterology and Hepatology
Chair, Inflammatory Bowel Disease Interest Group
Mayo Clinic
Rochester, Minnesota

Richard P. MacDermott, MD, FACG (Chapter 34)
The Thomas Ordway Professor of Medicine
Director, Inflammatory Bowel Disease Center
Division of Gastroenterology
Albany Medical College
Albany, New York

Karen L. Madsen, PhD (Chapter 35)
University of Alberta
Department of Medicine
Division of Gastroenterology
Edmonton, Alberta, Canada

Lloyd Mayer, MD (Chapter 32)
Professor and Co-Director of the Immunology Institute
Dorothy and David Merksamer Professor of Medicine
Mount Sinai Medical Center
New York, New York

Philip B. Miner Jr, MD (Chapter 28)
Oklahoma Foundation for Digestive Research
Oklahoma City, Oklahoma

Alan C. Moss, MD, FACG (Chapter 3)
Assistant Professor of Medicine
Harvard Medical School
Director of Translational Research
Center for Inflammatory Bowel Disease
Beth Israel Deaconess Medical Center
Boston, Massachusetts

Jeffrey W. Nathanson, MD (Chapter 14)
Clinical Instructor of Medicine
Feinberg School of Medicine
Northwestern University
Chicago, Illinois

Jaime A. Oviedo, MD (Chapter 7)
Section of Gastroenterology
Boston University School of Medicine
Boston, Massachusetts

Mansour A. Parsi, MD (Chapter 31)
Department of Gastroenterology and Hepatology
Cleveland Clinic
Cleveland, Ohio

Robert M. Penner, BSc, MD, FRCP(C), MSc (Chapter 35)
Assistant Clinical Professor
University of British Columbia
Vancouver, British Columbia, Canada
Assistant Clinical Professor
University of Alberta
Edmonton, Alberta, Canada

Robert Pittman, MD (Chapter 32)
Bergen Gastroenterology P.C.
Emerson, New Jersey

Miguel Regueiro, MD (Chapter 26)
Associate Professor of Medicine
Associate Professor of Education
Co-Director and Clinical Head, Inflammatory Bowel Disease Center
Director, GI, Hepatology, and Nutrition Fellowship
Pittsburgh, Pennsylvania

John L. Rombeau, MD (Chapter 37)
Professor of Surgery
Temple University School of Medicine
Philadelphia, Pennsylvania

Anthony L. Rosa, MD (Chapter 12)
Gastrointestinal Specialists
Bala Cynwyd, Pennsylvania

Melissa H. Rosen, MD (Chapter 30)
Gastroenterology Fellow
Department of Gastroenterology and Hepatology
Jill Roberts Center for Inflammatory Bowel Disease
Weill Medical College of Cornell University/New York–Presbyterian Hospital
New York, New York

Paul Rutgeerts, MD, PhD (Chapter 24)
Department of Internal Medicine
University Hospital, Gasthuisberg
Leuven, Belgium
Professor of Medicine
Catholic University of Leuven
Belgium

William J. Sandborn, MD (Chapter 25)
Professor of Medicine
Mayo Clinic College of Medicine
Vice Chairman
Division of Gastroenterology and Hepatology
Mayo Clinic
Rochester, Minnesota

Jürgen Schölmerich, MD, PhD (Chapter 21)
Klinik und Poliklinik für Innere Medizin I
Klinikum der Universität Regensburg
Regensburg, Germany

Kenneth W. Schroeder, MD, PhD (Chapter 39)
Division of Gastroenterology and Hepatology
Mayo Clinic
Rochester, Minnesota

Corey A. Siegel, MD (Chapter 6)
Gastrointestinal Unit and MGH Crohn's and Colitis Center
Massachusetts General Hospital and Harvard Medical School
Boston, Massachusetts

Kenneth Simpson, BVM&S, PhD (Chapter 4)
Professor of Medicine
College of Veterinary Medicine
Cornell University
Ithaca, New York

Antoni Stadnicki, MD, PhD (Chapter 22)
Associate Professor of Medicine
Department of Basic Biomedical Sciences
Medical University of Silesia
Sosnowiec, Poland

Arthur F. Stucchi, PhD (Chapter 36)
Associate Research Professor
Departments of Surgery, Pathology and Laboratory Medicine
Lab Director, Surgical Research
Boston University School of Medicine
Boston, Massachusetts

Chinyu Su, MD (Chapter 2)
Division of Gastroenterology, Department of Medicine
University of Pennsylvania School of Medicine
Philadelphia, Pennsylvania

Lloyd Sutherland, MDCM, MSc, FRCP(C), FACP (Chapter 13)
Professor of Medicine
Division of Gastroenterology
University of Calgary
Calgary, Alberta, Canada

Traci M. Temmen, MD (Chapter 37)
University of South Florida
Tampa, Florida

Nabil Toubia, MD (Chapter 27)
Roger Williams Medical Center
Department of Medicine
Providence, Rhode Island

William J. Tremaine, MD (Chapter 39)
Maxine and Jack Zarrow Professor
Division of Gastroenterology and Hepatology
Director, Mayo Clinic Office of Human Research Protection
Mayo Clinic
Rochester, Minnesota

Truc T. Trinh, MD (Chapter 33)
Gastroenterology Center of Northern Virginia
Fairfax, Virginia

Gert Van Assche, MD, PhD, FRCP (Chapter 24)
Associate Professor of Medicine
Division of Gastroenterology
University of Leuven
Belgium

Ryan Urquhart Warren, MD (Chapter 20)
Brown University
Researcher, Jill Roberts Center for Inflammatory Bowel Disease
Weill Medical College of Cornell University/New York–Presbyterian Hospital
New York, New York

INTRODUCTION

Since the historical description of Crohn's disease by Drs. Burrill Crohn, Leon Ginzburg, and Gordon Oppenheimer in 1932 and the historical description of ulcerative colitis by Dr. Samuel Wilks and Dr. Walter Moxon in 1859, much has been learned about the etiology, pathogenesis, and treatment of these two idiopathic inflammatory bowel disorders. These disorders occur at any age, spare no socioeconomic class, and have the potential to significantly impair the patient's quality of life. Significant progress has been made in the past decade related to Crohn's disease and ulcerative colitis; however, the medical therapy of inflammatory bowel disease has had the greatest impact on patients' lives. Although these disorders are remarkably similar in many ways, they have vast differences when comparing response to specific medical therapies. As a consequence, it was elected to separately focus on medical therapy of ulcerative colitis and distinguish this from medical therapy of Crohn's disease.

The authors who have contributed to this textbook are regionally and internationally recognized experts in inflammatory bowel disease. The mainstay of literature in the past decade focusing on medical therapy of inflammatory bowel disease has emanated from the work of these distinguished authors. In this book, the authors discuss the current medical therapies and review the clinical trial data that established the foundation for their use. The individual chapters in this book not only review the current medical therapy in use for treatment of patients with inflammatory bowel disease but they also review the basic pathophysiologic principles supporting the use of these and future therapeutics. Additionally, novel therapeutics that have potential impact and significance to the practicing physician are highlighted.

I am indebted to my contributors for providing superb, detailed, critical chapters amid their already busy schedules. I would also like to thank Dr. Ellen Scherl for her expertise and countless hours she has spent in making this textbook a reality. Additionally, I am appreciative and extend thanks to all my colleagues, patients, and those who have supported research in the field who have helped me uncover and extend the boundaries of my knowledge in inflammatory bowel disease. Lastly, I am most appreciative of my wife Nancy and my children Julie and Danielle for allowing me to spend countless hours doing what I thoroughly enjoy: patient care, research, and education.

Gary R. Lichtenstein, MD, FACP, FACG, AGAF

PROLOGUE
HISTORICAL PERSPECTIVE OF ULCERATIVE COLITIS

Ming V. Lin, MD; Wojciech Blonski, MD, PhD; David Kotlyar, MD; and Gary R. Lichtenstein, MD, FACP, FACG, AGAF

THE EVOLUTION OF ANCIENT DYSENTERY TO CURRENT CLINICAL ULCERATIVE COLITIS CONCEPT

The origin of ulcerative colitis can be traced back to 722 BC when China's canon of internal medicine described an illness of abdominal pain, diarrhea, and rectal bleeding. Between the years 640 BC and 170 AD, Hippocrates of Cos,[1] Aretius of Cappadocia,[2] and Soranus of Ephesus,[3] among others, referred to a type of chronic diarrhea associated with blood and ulcerations of the bowel that was different from other types of diarrhea. Knowledge was insufficient at that time to definitively diagnose these disorders but the description reasonably fit the profile of ulcerative colitis.

Multiple epidemics of dysentery occurred in colonial America in 1669-1670. "Bloody influx," described by T. Sydenham,[4] was no doubt infectious in origin but whether or not these illnesses included instances of chronic ulcerative colitis is impossible to verify. It was suggested by P.J.E. Wilson[5] that Prince Charles, the Young Pretender to the Scottish throne, suffered from ulcerative colitis and cured himself in 1745 with a milk-free diet.

In 1756 Burch et al[6] first described a 40-year-old man from Ireland suffering a persistent bloody influx and later developed episodes of fever, abdominal pain, and jaundice. These symptoms occurred intermittently for 13 additional years until the patient succumbed to the illness. Because the likelihood of a continuous infection causing episodic healing and recurrence over a period of 18 years is low, Burch proposed a link to some sort of "non-specific inflammatory bowel disease (IBD)." The jaundice described was likely to be a complication of sclerosing cholangitis.

The clinical curiosities of ulcerative colitis were translated into medical significance by Samuel Wilks in 1859.[7] He described the notorious Smethurst legal trial in London in which a 42-year-old woman died of a febrile diarrheal illness. It was first misdiagnosed as "arsenic poisoning," but the autopsy demonstrated a transmural inflammation of the entire colon and terminal ileum. Her condition was labeled as *ulcerative colitis*.

In 1862, Habershon[8] described the classic pseudopolyps of ulcerative colitis: "these ulcerations gradually extend to coalesce till at least nearly the whole of the mucous surface is destroyed, except here and there prominent isolated portions which become intensely congested, and resemble polypoid growth." Thirteen years later, Wilks and Moxon[9] were the first to define "ulcerative colitis" as a specific pathologic entity, a condition they described as "inflammation of the large intestine or idiopathic colitis." In 1881, Woodward[10] described "pseudopolyps of the colon" consistent with Habershon and Wilks/Moxon's reports. Sir William Allchin[11] in 1885 observed extensive denudation of the colonic mucosa and made a distinction between specific and non-specific colitis. He wrote: "the term dysentery is not restricted to the true tropical malady and it should not at once be applied in an adjective form to any diarrhea dependent on ulceration of the colon."

During the meeting of the Harvey Society of London in 1893, physicians from across Europe called attention to the emergence of a diarrheal disease different from the epidemic bacillary dysentery–"catarrhal ulcerative colitis." However, it was not until 1903 that Boas[12] from Berlin

Lichtenstein GR, ed.
Ulcerative Colitis: The Complete Guide to Medical Management (pp 1-10)

clinically differentiated ulcerative colitis from bacillary dysentery. He described the many points that distinguished ulcerative colitis from true dysentery.

In the late 19th century, the possible role of surgery in the management of this still-obscure disease emerged. Robson[13] performed an inguinal colostomy in a woman with ulcerative colitis in 1893, allowing for daily irrigation of the ulcerated bowel with tincture of hamamelis and boracic acid solution with later closure of colostomy. In 1902, Weir[14] from New York performed an appendicostomy in a patient with ulcerative colitis to allow irrigation of the colon with various solutions (methylene blue, silver nitrate, bismuth.) By 1909, the state-of-the-art procedures were the appendicostomy and cecostomy.

Seven London hospitals made the first cooperative efforts to correlate the clinical features. During the London Symposium on ulcerative colitis in 1909, Cammeron and Lippman[15] described the clinical findings, treatments, and various statistical data of the 317 patients seen between 1888 and 1907 with severe ulcerative colitis affecting the entire colon. Almost 50% (147 patients) died in the hospital from various complications: perforation, peritonitis, hemorrhage, septic infection, pulmonary embolism, liver disease, and exhaustion or malnutrition despite treatment. Discovery of family relatives with the same disease was considered a coincidence.

During the early 20th century, as patients with ulcerative colitis became better characterized and described, the hunt for the underlying etiology and treatment options was underway. In light of the discovery of bacteria causing enteric infections (*Entamoeba histolytica* by Losch 1873, *Salmonella typhi* by Ebarth 1880, and *Shigella dysenteriae* by Shiga 1898), the etiologic speculation focused mainly on bacteriological possibilities. In an effort to control infection, treatments included "slop diets," daily intake of 3 pints of milk soured by lactic acid ("Sydenham's remedy"), astringents, opium, tincture of hamamelis, and rectal instillations of boracic acid, silver nitrate, or creolin. The preferred operation was an appendicostomy or valvular cecostomy (if the appendix had been removed) with colonic irrigations.

In 1909, Hawkins[16] reviewed a separate group of 85 patients with ulcerative colitis, 41 of whom died. He implicated a bacterial origin and made a connection to the bloody influx of Sydenham in 1669. He also subdivided the patients into acute, chronic, dysenteric, and hemorrhagic disease. As the number of patients with ulcerative colitis increased throughout Europe during the early 1900s, it was the principal subject of discussion during the Paris Congress of Medicine in 1913. It was also when the first radiologic appearances (bismuth or barium enema) of ulcerative colitis were described by Stierlin[17] and Kienbock[18] independently.

In 1913, Brown[19] found the ileostomy advantageous based on his own experiences. He was attracted by the concept of "bowel rest," where the fecal stream would be diverted from the inflamed bowel into a temporary ileostomy. This procedure later gained popularity in 1930s and 1940s. This divided the surgical community into two camps: those who believed in irrigation with appendicostomy and those who lost faith in irrigation and favored ileostomy. The ileostomy did not provide adequate cure for the disease, however, and often turned out to be permanent, so the operation was regarded as a measure of last resort.

Bassler[20] from New York published the first American case on ulcerative colitis as a brief report in 1913. Six years later, Logan[21] from the Mayo Clinic reviewed the first clinical study of 117 patients with ulcerative colitis. In 1921, Yeomans[22] also reported a series of 65 cases.

Strauss[23] from Berlin published a brief paper in 1923 on ulcerative colitis and recommended treatment with "bland diet" and blood transfusion. In 1925, Lynch and Felsen[24] focused on bacillary dysentery as the cause for ulcerative colitis. Hurst[25] from Guy's Hospital in London also implicated an organism "closely related to B dysenteriae." He cited Mathieu and Schmidt[26] and recommended a treatment regimen consisting of daily colonic irrigation with a silver nitrate solution along with the injection of large amounts (up to 100 cc) of a polyvalent antidysenteric serum.

In 1925, Bargen et al[27] reported positive cultures from the rectal ulceration in ulcerative colitis patients and the occurrence of colonic lesions in rabbits injected with IV broth containing *diplostreptococci*. Buie[28], after reviewing 473 cases at the Mayo Clinic in 1926, accepted *Bargen diplostreptococcus* as the cause. However, this concept soon lost scientific credibility as subsequent experiments by Paulson[29] and Mones[30] failed to confirm the same finding.

In the 1920s and 1930s, reports from all over the world (United States, Canada, France, Germany, Russia, and Italy) of patients with ulcerative colitis were made. Ulcerative colitis has since been recognized as not being a rare entity. The diversity of the complications associated with ulcerative colitis steadily rose. Local and systemic complications associated with ulcerative colitis began to attract attention during the early 20th century. Sclerosing cholangitis was the first complication recorded by Burch et al[6] in 1756. Lister[31] in 1899 made an association between hepatitis and ulcerative colitis. Wilson[32] in 1904 described a simple ulcerative colitis complicated by perforation and peritonitis. In 1907, with the aid of the new electrically illuminated proctosigmoidoscope, Lockhart-Mummery[33] was the first to discover carcinoma of the colon in patients with ulcerative colitis. Hale-White[34] in 1909 described an association of ulcerative colitis with chronic interstitial nephritis, based on Richard Bright's original series of "100 cases with albuminous urine."

Crohn's[35] report in 1925 commented on an ocular complication in which he hypothesized that the two patients he treated probably suffered from keratomalacia and xerophthalmia caused by hypovitaminosis A. In 1928, Bargen[36] described cases of adenocarcinoma of the colon and rectum, lymphosarcoma, and lymphatic leukemia. In 1929, the Mayo Clinic[37] reported 268 complications seen in 693 patients with chronic ulcerative colitis, including polyposis, stricture, arteritis, skin lesions, and perirectal abscess. The latter may have represented the yet unidentified Crohn's disease of the colon.

Into the 1930s, more cases of ulcerative colitis were reported, and the search for the underlying etiologic factors continued because the proposal of bacillary dysentery was not convincing. Hern[38] in 1931 suggested bacteremia leading to secondary infections of the mucosa surface by resident colon bacilli.

In 1934, Thaysen[39] from Denmark sought to differentiate simple hemorrhagic proctitis and proctosigmoiditis from ulcerative colitis (diffuse congestion, ecchymoses of rectal mucosa, and absence of ulceration). Treatments included enemas of tannis, silver nitrate, or bismuth subnitrate, and the anti-amebic compound yatren as an anti-inflammatory agent. The International Congress of Gastroenterology in Brussels, Belgium in 1935 focused on ulcerative colitis and involved reports and discussants from various countries. Some of the issues addressed were familial ulcerative colitis (Hamburger and Bensaude) and the inconclusive evidence for pathogenic bacteria (Mones-Gallart and Sanjuan).[40]

Clinical recognition of ulcerative colitis continued to increase in the United States during the 1930s to 1950s. The reports were mainly from the Mayo Clinic,[41] Philadelphia,[42] and the University of Chicago.[43] Some of the knowledge advancement of the disease included increased age (over 50 years old),[44] arterial and venous thrombosis associated with ulcerative colitis,[45] hepatic insufficiency,[46] clubbed fingers,[47] increased frequency of nephrolithiasis,[48] iron deficiency anemia, dermatological disorders and psychogenic problems,[49] and pyoderma gangrenosum.[50] In 1946, Chisholm[51] reported an acute fulminant ulcerative colitis with multiple perforations and peritonitis that was associated with the use of opiates and anticholinergic medication in severely ill and malnourished patients with extensive disease. In 1949, Maratka and Spellberg[52] compared the cases in the US to Czech and Australian cases and confirmed a similarity in symptoms and clinical course.

Therapy during the 1930s and early 1940s had been limited to nutritional supplements, blood transfusions, "elimination diets," colonic irrigations, and occasionally fecal bacterial vaccines. With the advent of sulfanilamide[53] in 1935, and penicillin[54] and adrenocorticotropic hormone[55] in 1940, IBD therapy was changed significantly. In 1951, Kirsner et al[56] documented the clinical and radiological reversibility in 6 patients who responded promptly to medical therapy and remained in remission for many years. Jones et al[57] in 1969 also reported a similar outcome in patients with ulcerative colitis treated medically and challenged the controversial issue of early surgery in patients with severe ulcerative colitis.

The distribution of the disease has extended beyond Europe and the United States to include countries bordering the Mediterranean, Middle East, India, New Zealand, and Asia. At the Washington, DC World Congress of Gastroenterology in 1958, there were 300 cases reported in Japan.[58] In 1963 and 1964, Edwards and Truelove of Oxford[59,60] analyzed the course and prognosis of ulcerative colitis extensively. They determined that disease extent, severity, and age of onset were the principal factors affecting mortality. They also remarked on the frequency of relapses within the first year. Fourteen percent of their patients required radical surgery, and many of their patients had various local complications. Into the 1960s, colorectal carcinoma complicating chronic ulcerative colitis became a major concern.[61,62]

In 1970, Wright of Oxford[63] concluded that "... clear evidence that autoimmune or allergic mechanisms are directly concerned with ulcerative colitis pathogenesis has not been forthcoming..." Many attempts to reproduce ulcerative colitis in animals (rabbits, guinea pigs, hamsters, dogs, mice, and rats) began in the 1950s.[64] Multiple experimental methods were used to cause temporary colonic injury including nutritional depletion (vitamin A, pantothenic acid, pyridoxine), local application of Shiga and staphylococcal toxin to colonic explants, intraperitoneal adrenalin injections, intravenous injection of staphylococcus toxin, intrarectal and intra-arterial injection of collagenase and losozyme, and carrageenan orally.

Although none of these attempts adequately demonstrated a possible cause, they have significantly advanced the understanding of the interaction between T cells and proinflammatory cytokines with mucosal inflammation.[65]

ULCERATIVE COLITIS AND PREGNANCY

Ulcerative colitis and pregnancy were first mentioned during the London symposium in 1909 but the topic was not explored further for 30 years. Barnes and Hayes[66] from the United States described 3 patients with ulcerative colitis who died during pregnancy and puerperium in 1931. It was found that one of the patients had a family history of nephritis (archaically termed *Bright's disease*), and the other two had chronic nephritis. It was concluded that pregnancy with ulcerative colitis was associated with advanced renal insufficiency, called *azotemic colitis*. In 1951, Abramson et al[67] from the United States described a mortality rate of 80% and 75%, respectively, during pregnancy and puerperium in patients with an acute exacerbation of ulcerative colitis. MacDougall[68] reported in 1955 that ulcerative colitis did not adversely affect the pregnancy in his review of 64 patients with 100 pregnancies. In Crohn et al,[69] a retrospective study of 110 patients with 150 pregnancies during 1956, it was noted that the onset or recurrence of ulcerative colitis was most frequent during the first trimester and puerperium. Therapeutic abortion in the first trimester was then recommended in patients with severe ulcerative colitis. It was not until 1985 that Korelitz[70] from the United States published authoritative information on pregnancy, fertility, and IBD. In his opinion, ulcerative colitis and pregnancy appeared to be independent processes, and therapeutic abortion had not been shown to affect the course of ulcerative colitis. He recommended that one should become pregnant during a quiescent stage and emphasized the need to increase nutritional intake and continue medical treatment with sulfasalazine and steroids during a flare.

ULCERATIVE COLITIS IN CHILDREN

Helmholz[71] from the Mayo Clinic (1923) was the first to describe ulcerative colitis in children with 5 case series. In 1926, Bourne[72] from London reviewed 10 cases and described one child with ulcerative colitis. By 1940, the Mayo clinic[73] had reported 95 children with ulcerative colitis. Bargen and Kennedy,[74] in 1955, after reporting an additional 139 pediatric patients with ulcerative colitis, concluded that children with ulcerative colitis shared a similar disease course to adults with the same condition, and it was not as uncommon as previously thought. The youngest recorded patient was a newborn male infant at the age of 21 days, who died shortly after an operation for rapidly deteriorating ulcerative colitis in 1952.[75] Lagercrantz,[76] Kirsner et al,[77] Hijmans and Enzer,[78] Durham and Korelitz,[79] and Davidson et al[80] all have contributed toward literature on IBD in children.

The nutritional impact on growth and sexual development of children with ulcerative colitis caught attention around the 1930s.[81] Severe growth retardation and delayed sexual maturation secondary to multiple nutritional deficiencies, so called "infantilism," was described by Ricketts, Benditt and Palmer[82] from the University of Chicago in 1945. The nutritional impact was also explained by substantial fecal losses of proteins and electrolytes in these patients, demonstrated by Welch et al[83] from the Mayo Clinic in 1937, confirmed by Sappington and Bockus[84] in 1949 and further detailed with protein balance studies by Kirsner and Sheffner[85] in 1950.

ETIOLOGY OF ULCERATIVE COLITIS

While clinical experience with the disease was increasing, its etiology and pathogenesis remained obscure. Multiple attempts have been made to unravel this complicated problem, which have resulted in several theories.

MICROBES AND INFECTIONS

Ulcerative colitis was differentiated from bacillary dysentery by its prolonged and intermittent course. Even though it had clearly been separated from the contagious form of diarrhea by the middle of 19th century, it was still hard to convince many physicians of its non-infectious nature. With the identification of the different intestinal bacteria (*Entamoeba*, *Salmonella typhi*, and *Shigella* dysentery) causing diarrheal illness, bacterial causes of ulcerative colitis had influenced the treatment for many years. *Bacillus coli* (1909), *Streptococci* (1911), and *B. coli* communis (1913) were some of the implicated pathogens.

In 1921, Hurst[25] implicated an organism "closely related to *B. dysenteriae*" and advocated polyvalent anti-dysenteric serum intravenously. Focal infections such as dental abscesses were cited as a popular cause of disease in the United States during the 1920s, and removal of teeth, gall bladders, and appendices was encouraged.[86] In 1925, Bargen[27] reported *diplostreptococci* as a cause, after finding positive cultures from the rectal ulcerations. Autologous vaccine of *diplostreptococci* was a treatment option, but with limited success. This concept soon lost scientific credibility. Since then, many studies have been conducted but have failed to identify any offending agents causing ulcerative colitis.

PSYCHOGENIC FACTORS

Psychogenic factors were implicated in ulcerative colitis by Murray[87] and Sullivan,[88] who found a chronological association between the outbreak of an emotional disturbance and the onset of bowel symptoms. "Typical ulcerative colitis personality" was observed in patients with ulcerative colitis, which included immaturity, indecisiveness, overdependence, sensitivity, and inhibited interpersonal relationships and critical emotional events. Psychotherapy was reported to have a positive influence on the outcome of the disease with lower operation, complication, and mortality rates.

In seeking a physiologic explanation for the psychogenic hypothesis, Almy et al[89] demonstrated the effects of emotional stress upon the colonic mucosa of patients with ulcerative colitis, manifesting as increased hyperemia, vascular engorgement, increased secretion of mucous, and augmented colonic motor activities. Kern et al[90] of Cornell University studied the motility of distal colon in nonspecific ulcerative colitis using a balloon technique. He found a decrease or absence of phasic activity correlated with severe diarrhea and attributed to psychogenic-induced autonomic bombardment of the colon.

It was noted by Meyer et al[91] that there was an increased production of an enzyme, lysozyme (mucinase), in patients with active ulcerative colitis during emotional stress. It was believed that lysozyme destroyed the colonic mucous lining and increased vulnerability of the colon to invasive pathogens and other cytolytic agents. This theory lost credibility when it was shown in vitro that lysozyme was incapable of dissolving or digesting human mucous.[92] With little evidence to suggest that the majority of patients suffering from ulcerative colitis have an inherently different emotional makeup from the rest of the population, it was concluded that emotional disturbances play a role in the exacerbation, chronicity, and severity of the disease, but are not the cause of ulcerative colitis.[93]

Immune Mechanisms

In the late 1940s, immune mechanisms were implicated in various diseases of unknown etiology (eg, rheumatoid arthritis). Kirsner et al[94] described a series of clinical experiences, occurring during the 1930s and 1940s, which suggested the possible involvement of immune factors in ulcerative colitis. The events included an abrupt onset of severe ulcerative colitis in patients who had acute food poisoning, an association with allergy (hay fever or asthma) or other immune diseases (autoimmune hemolytic anemia), familial occurrences of IBD, and the beneficial effects of corticosteroids. Kirsner[95] in 1954 suggested sensitization of the bowel via early microbial infection as in an antigen-antibody reaction occurring among hyper-reactive people.

Broberger and Perlmann[96] in 1959 demonstrated hemagglutinin antibodies to the colonic mucosa in 20 out of 30 children with ulcerative colitis. This was in support of the "autoimmunity" concept. However, in 1966, Wright and Truelove[97] showed the presence of autoantibodies to colonic mucosa in only 15% to 20% of patients with ulcerative colitis, and there was little correlation between the clinical course of colitis and incidence of circulating antibodies to colon. Thus, it seemed clear that some patients do certainly develop circulating antibodies but it was not known whether these arise as a cause or effect of the pathology. By the 1970s, the immune mechanisms in ulcerative colitis and Crohn's disease became the most active area of IBD research, and until recently, immunologic research has focused on gut mucosal immune system and proinflammatory cytokines.

Genetic

Familial cases of IBD were first described at the London symposium[16] on ulcerative colitis in 1909. Family members with IBD were considered coincidences. This view prevailed for more than 50 years until the 1960s when reports of familial IBD were again described. With the increasing incidence, implications were made to a genetic relationship. Moltke[98] in 1936 described families with ulcerative colitis (mother and daughter, brother and sister, father and daughter). Many similar reports followed. In 1954, Kirsner and Palmer[95] introduced the concept of an "individual vulnerability," which later was revised to a genetically influenced individual with disease susceptibility.[99] Schlesinger and Platt[100] in 1958 obtained a family history in 17% of 60 children with ulcerative colitis, and it was noted that those with Ashkenazi Jewish origin were at a 4 times higher risk of acquiring ulcerative colitis than other ethnicities.

TREATMENT OF ULCERATIVE COLITIS FROM A HISTORICAL PERSPECTIVE

Corticosteroids

Studies evaluating the use of corticotropin and corticosteroids as a therapy of ulcerative colitis were initiated in the 1950s. Kirsner et al compared the clinical effects of corticotropin and cortisone in chronic ulcerative colitis in an open study.[101] Two subsequent open studies by Kirsner and Palmer observed beneficial therapeutic effects of corticotropin on the course of ulcerative colitis.[102,103] In 1954, Truelove and Witts published a preliminary report on the treatment of ulcerative colitis with cortisone.[104,105] In 1955, the seminal placebo-controlled study by Truelove and Witts on the treatment of ulcerative colitis with cortisone (100 mg daily for 6 weeks) was published in the *British Medical Journal*.[106] Since then, corticosteroids have become the mainstay therapy for IBD. The safety issue of corticosteroid use was raised in 1967 by Goldstein et al.[107] In 1983, Meyers et al recommended that corticosteroid-naïve patients with severe ulcerative colitis should be treated with intravenous corticotropin, whereas those with a prior history of corticosteroid use should be treated with intravenous hydrocortisone.[108] In 1985, Auphan et al in the journal *Science* described the major anti-inflammatory mechanism of corticosteroids through inhibition of nuclear factor kappa B activation in mice and cultured cells.[109]

Aminosalicylates

In 1941, Dr. Nana Svartz from the Karolinska Hospital in Stockholm, Sweden introduced sulfasalazine (5-aminosalicylic acid [5-ASA] and sulfapyridine joined by a chemical azo-bond) for the treatment of rheumatoid arthritis and ulcerative colitis.[110] The initial name of the drug was salicylazosulfapyridine, which was later abbreviated to salazopyrin, and finally to azulfidine or sulfasalazine.[111] Her uncontrolled observations of patients with ulcerative colitis treated with sulfasalazine demonstrated the great efficacy of this new drug,[112] with 75% to 80% improvement rates.[111] The first placebo-controlled trial that demonstrated the efficacy of oral sulfasalazine in the treatment of ulcerative colitis was published in 1962 by Baron et al.[113] In 1965, Misiewicz et al reported for the first time that oral sulfasalazine reduced the relapse rate of ulcerative colitis.[114] In 1977, Azad Khan et al determined that 5-ASA was the active therapeutic moiety of sulfasalazine, whereas sulfapyridine was considered the carrier that cleaved 5-ASA within the colon.[115] In 1980, Klotz et al showed that 5-ASA could be used as an alternative to sulfasalazine in the treatment of IBD.[116] It was also shown that 5-ASA suppositories had comparable efficacy to oral sulfasalazine and were superior over oral sulfapyridine.[116] In 1982, Rasmussen et al described the pharmacokinetics of a 5-ASA tablet with sustained release in humans.[117] In 1983, Chan et al published a study presenting two novel sulfasalazine analogs, ipsalazide and balsalazide (diazo bond of 5-ASA + 4-aminobenzoyl-B-alanine carrier).[118] In 1985, Klotz et al presented pharmacokinetic data on an enteric-coated form of 5-ASA in patients with IBD.[119] At the same time, Selby et al published preliminary results indicating acceptable efficacy of a new oral formulation—olsalazine (azodisalicylate)—in which two molecules of 5-ASA are connected by an azo bond.[120] In 1988, Riley et al published the results of a double-blind and double-dummy trial in which they observed the superiority of enteric-coated 5-ASA over sulfasalazine in patients with ulcerative colitis.[121] Delayed-release 5-ASA was also considered an effective treatment for maintaining remissions of ulcerative colitis and was associated with fewer side effects than enteric-coated sulfasalazine.[122] At the same time, the first randomized, double-blind trial with balsalazide was published.[123] In the 21st century, the novel and high-strength formulation of 5-ASA using a Multi Matrix System technology designed to release 5-ASA throughout the colon was developed. Clinical trials have demonstrated possible superiority over placebo in inducing remission of ulcerative colitis.[124-127]

Immune Modulators

The use of immune modulators was initiated after observations indicating the role of immune mechanisms in the pathophysiology of ulcerative colitis were published. Bean introduced 6-mercaptopurine (6-MP) in the treatment of ulcerative colitis in 1962[128] and 1966.[129] An initial case report published in 1962 described a patient with rapid improvement and long-term remission after 6-MP was added to an existing unsuccessful treatment.[128] In 1966, Bowen et al reported severe toxic effects of azathioprine administered at a daily dose of 6 mg/kg to 10 patients with IBD, which were eliminated after decreasing the daily dose to 2 to 3 mg/kg.[130] The first interim report of a controlled trial of azathioprine in ulcerative colitis was published in 1972 by Jewell and Truelove[131] and was followed by a final report in 1974.[132] The authors concluded that azathioprine should be used in patients with ulcerative colitis who have failed maintenance treatment with corticosteroids and sulfasalazine, and in whom surgery should be postponed or avoided.[132]

Cyclosporine, an immunosuppressive agent with a rapid onset of action, was evaluated and found to be effective in intravenous form in several uncontrolled trials[133-136] and one controlled randomized trial of patients with severe steroid-refractory ulcerative colitis in the 1980s and 1990s.[137]

Biologic Therapy

Studies performed in the 1990s found increased concentrations of tumor necrosis factor alpha (TNFα), a proinflammatory cytokine, in the blood, colonic tissue, and stools of patients with ulcerative colitis.[138-140] The first 3 pilot studies evaluating the use of intravenous infusions of infliximab, a chimeric monoclonal anti-TNFα antibody in patients with steroid-refractory ulcerative colitis, were performed in 2001.[141-143] In 2005, the results of the first multicenter randomized placebo-controlled trial of infliximab induction and maintenance therapy for ulcerative colitis (ACT 1 and ACT 2 trials) were published and showed the beneficial effect of this biologic agent on the course of ulcerative colitis.[144] In light of the data from ACT 1 and ACT 2 trials, infliximab was approved in 2005 by the US Food and Drug Administration (FDA) for the treatment of ulcerative colitis to reduce signs and symptoms, to induce clinical remission and healing of the intestinal mucosa, and to eliminate the use of corticosteroids in patients with moderately to severely active ulcerative colitis who have had an inadequate response, who are intolerant, or have medical contraindications to therapy with corticosteroids or immunosuppressive agents. So far, this is the only FDA-approved biologic agent for the treatment of ulcerative colitis.

The first promising results of treatment of ulcerative colitis with the fully human monoclonal antibody adalimumab have just been published.[145] Other biologic agents targeting various proinflammatory cytokines and chemokines involved in inflammatory processes in ulcerative colitis have been studied. These include visilizumab (humanized anti-CD3 monoclonal antibody binding the

CD3 chain of the T-cell receptor expressed on activated T cells),[146] interferon-α-2a,[147,148] pegylated interferon-α,[149] RDP-58 (an anti-inflammatory D-amino acid decapeptide),[150] epidermal growth factor,[151] keratinocyte growth factor-2,[152] basiliximab,[153] and daclizumab[154] (anti-interleukin-2 receptor antibodies).

CONCLUSION

Ulcerative colitis has been observed since the beginning of recorded human history. Paralleling the increased scientific nature of medicine, the trajectory of understanding ulcerative colitis in the past century, with an explosion of knowledge and treatments, is increasing exponentially. It remains to be seen what possible treatments and eventual cure of ulcerative colitis may be achieved by humanity, but it is likely such discoveries will occur sooner rather than later.

REFERENCES

1. Hippocrates. The genuine works of Hippocrates. Sydenham Society, London, 2 Volumes cited by Guthrie- A History of Medicine. Philadelphia, PA: JB Lippincott Co. (2 Volumes); 1946, 1849.
2. Aretius. On the causes and symptoms chronic diseases. cited by de Dombal FT. Ulcerative colitis: definition, historical background, aetiology, diagnosis, natural history, and local complciations. *Postgrad Med J.* 1968;44:684-692.
3. Ephesus. So. Cited by Mettler CC. *History of Medicine.* Philadephia, PA: Blakiston, 1947, 1947.
4. Sydenham T. *Medical Observations concerning history and cure of acute diseases.* London: Greenhill, 1898.
5. Wilson P. The young pretender. *Br Med J.* 1961;ii:1226.
6. Burch W, Gump DW, Krawitt EL, Burch W, Gump DW, Krawitt EL. Historical case report of Sir William Johnson, the Mohawk Baronet. *Am J Gastroenterol.* 1992;87:1023-1025.
7. Wilks S. Morbid appearances in the intestine of Miss Bankes. *London Medical Times and Gazette.* 1859;2:264-268.
8. Habershon S. *Diseases of the abdomen.* London: J Churchill, 1862.
9. Wilks S, Moxon W. *Lectures on pathological anatomy.* London: Lindsay and Blackiston, 1875:408.
10. Woodward J. Pseudopolyps of the colon: An anomalous result of follicular ulceration (of the colon). *Am J Med Sci.* 1881;81:142-145.
11. Allchin W. A case of extensive ulceration of the colon. *Trans Path Soc London.* 1885;36:199-202.
12. Lups S. Vaccine therapy in ulcerative colitis. *Am J Dig Dis.* 1935;2:65-90;139-160.
13. Robson M. Case of colitis with ulceration. Treated by inguinal colostomy and local treatment of the ulcerated surfaces with subsequent closure of the artificial anus. *Trans Clin Soc London.* 1893.
14. Weir R. A new use for the useless appendix in the surgical treatment of obstinate colitis. *Med Record.* 1902;62:201-202.
15. Cammeron HC, Lippman RC. Statistics of ulcerative colitis from London hospitals. *Prc Roy Soc Med* 1909;2:100-106.
16. Hawkins H. An address on the natural history of ulcerative colitis and its bearing upon treatment. *Br Med J.* 1909;1:765-770.
17. Stierlin E. Zur rontgen diagnostic der colitis ulcerosa. *Z Klin Med.* 1913;75:486-493.
18. Kienbock R. Zur rontgendiagnose der colitis ulcerosa. *Fortschr Geb Rontgenstrahlen.* 1913;20:231-239.
19. Brown J. The value of complete physiological rest of the large bowel in the treatment of certain ulcerative and obstructive lesions of this organ. *Surg Gynecol Obstet.* 1913;16:610-613.
20. Bassler A. Ulcerative colitis. *Interstate Med J.* 1913;20:705-706.
21. Logan A. Chronic ulcerative colitis: a review of one hundred and seventeen cases. *Northwest Med.* 1919;18:1-9.
22. Yeomans F. Chronic ulcerative colitis. *JAMA.* 1921;77:2043-2048.
23. Strauss H. Ueber colitis-probleme. *Dtsch Med Wochschr.* 1923;49:1568-1570.
24. Lynch JM, Felsen FJ. Nonspecific ulcerative colitis. *Arch Intern Med.* 1925;35:433-456.
25. Hurst A. Ulceative colitis. *Guy's Hosp Rep.* 1921;71:26-41.
26. Mathieu A, Schmidt RJ. Pathologie gastrointerstinale. A Schmidt. VII Colitis chronica mucosa et membranacea VIII Colitis chronica suppurativa (Colitis Gravis, Colitis Ulcerosa). Darmkrankheiten Wiesbaden, Clinique et Therapeutique. Paris: O'Dorn; 1909;325:486-494.
27. Bargen JA. The etiology of chronic ulcerative colitis: experimental studies with suggestions for a more rational form of treatment. *Arch Intern Med.* 1925;36:818-829.
28. Buie L. Chronic ulcerative colitis. *JAMA.* 1926;87:1271-1214.
29. Paulson M. Chronic ulcerative colitis with reference to a bacterial etiology. Experimental Studies. *Arch Intern Med.* 1928;41:75.
30. Mones PG. Colitis ulcerosa graves non amibianas:etiologic diagnostico and tratamiento medico. Salvat Editores SA, Barcelona, 41 calle de Mallaraca. 1935;49.
31. Lister T. A specimen of diffuse ulcerative colitis with secondary acute interstitial hepatitis. *Trans Path Soc London.* 1899;50:130-131.
32. Wilson A. A case of ulcerative colitis with multiple perforations. *Lancet.* 1904;2:1208-1209.
33. Lockhart-Mummery J. The causes of colitis: with special reference to its surgical treatment, with an account of 36 cases. *Lancet.* 1907;1:1638-1643.
34. Hale-White W. Discussion—1909 London Symposium on ulcerative colitis. *Proc Roy Soc Med.*1909;2:59-156.
35. Crohn B. Ocular lesions complicating ulcerative colitis. *Am J Med Sci.* 1925;169:260-267.
36. Bargen JA. Chronic ulcerative colitis associated with carcinoma. *Arch Surg.* 1928;17:561-576.
37. Bargen J. Complications and sequelae of ulcerative colitis. *Ann Intern Med.* 1929;3:335-352.
38. Hern J. Ulcerative colitis. *Guy's Hosp Rep.* 1931;81:322-374.
39. Thaysen T. Simple haemorrhagic proctitis and proctosigmoiditis. *Acta Med Scand.* 1934;84:1-24.
40. Mones-Gallart E. Colitis ulcerosa graves non amibianas-etiologia, diagnostica, y tratamiento. Salvat. Barcelona: LA Barcelone; 1935.
41. Sloan WP Jr., Bargen JA, Gage RP. Life histories of patients with chronic ulcerative colitis: a review of 2,000 cases. *Gastroenterology.* 1950;16:25-38.
42. Bockus HL, Roth JL, Buchman E, et al. Life history of nonspecific ulcerative colitis: relation of prognosis to anatomical and clinical varieties. *Gastroenterologia.* 1956;86:549-581.
43. Ricketts WE, Kirsner JB, Palmer WL. Chronic non-specific ulcerative colitis; a roentgenologic study of its course. *Gastroenterology.* 1948;10:1-15.
44. Brust JCM, Bargen BJ. Chronic ulcerative colitis among elderly persons. *Minnesota Med.* 1935;18:583-585.
45. Bargen JA, Barker BN. Extensive arterial and venous thrombosis complicating ulcerative colitis. *Arch Intern Med.* 1936;58:17-31.

46. Comfort MW, Morlock CG. The association of chronic ulcerative colitis (colitis gravis) with hepatic insufficiency. *Med Clin North Am.* 1938;22:1089-1097.
47. Schlicke CP, Bargen BJ. Clubbed fingers and ulcerative colitis. *Am J Dig Dis.* 1940;7:17-22.
48. Lindahl WW, Bargen BJ. Nephrolithiasis complicating chronic ulcerative colitis after ileostomy. A report of six cases. *J Urol.* 1941;46:183-192.
49. Jankelson IR, Sweetsir FN. Chronic ulcerative colitis II. Complications outside the digestive tract. *Review Gastroenterology.* 1942;9:99-104.
50. Ricketts WE, Kirsner JB, Rothman S. Pyoderma gangrenosum in chronic non-specific ulcerative colitis; a report of three cases. *Am J Med.* 1948;5:69-75.
51. Chisholm T. Acute fulminating ulcerative colitis with massive perforation and peritonitis– report of a case. *Arch Surg.* 1946;53:362-376.
52. Maratka Z, Spellberg MA. Observations on the clinical course of non-specific ulcerative colitis. *Gastroenterology.* 1949;12:79-86.
53. Domagk G. Ein beitrag zur chemotherapie der bakteriellen infektione. *Dtsch Med Wochschr.* 1935;61:250-253.
54. Fleming A. The 1928 discovery of penicillin. *Br Med Bull.* 1944;2:4-5.
55. Hench PS, Kendall EC, et al. The effect of a hormone of the adrenal cortex (17-hydroxy-11-dehydrocorticosterone; compound E) and of pituitary adrenocorticotropic hormone on rheumatoid arthritis. *Mayo Clin Proc.* 1949;24:181-197.
56. Kirsner JB, Palmer WL, Klotz A. Reversibility in ulcerative colitis; clinical and roentgenologic observations. *Radiology.* 1951;57:1-14.
57. Jones JH, Lennard-Jones JE, Young AC. Reversibility of radiological appearances during clinical improvement in colonic Crohn's disease. *Gut.* 1969;10:738-743.
58. Matsunaga F. Clinical studies in ulcerative colitis and its related increase in Japan. *Proc World Congress of Gastroenterol Washington.* Vol. 2. Baltimore: Williams and Wilkins;1958:955-960.
59. Edwards FC, Truelove SC. The course and prognosis of ulcerative colitis. *Gut.* 1963;4:299-315.
60. Edwards FC, Truelove SC. The course and prognosis of ulcerative colitis. III. Complications. *Gut.* 1964;5:1-22.
61. Dawson IM, Pryse-Davies J. The development of carcinoma of the large intestine in ulcerative colitis. *Br J Surg.* 1959;47:113-128.
62. Goldgraber MB, Kirsner JB. Carcinoma of the colon in ulcerative colitis. *Cancer.* 1964;17:657-665.
63. Wright R. Ulcerative colitis. *Gastroenterology.* 1970;58:875-897.
64. Cave DR. Animal models of inflammatory bowel disease. *Ztschr F gastroenterology.* 1979;17(suppl):125.
65. Strober W, Fuss IJ, Ehrhardt RO, Neurath M, Boirivant M, Ludviksson BR. Mucosal immunoregulation and inflammatory bowel disease: new insights from murine models of inflammation. *Scand J Immunol.* 1998;48:453-458.
66. Barnes CS, Hayes HH. Ulcerative colitis complicating pregnancy and the puerperium. *Am J Obstet Gynecol.* 1931;22:907-912.
67. Abramson D, Jankelson IR, Milner LR. Pregnancy in idiopathic ulcerative colitis. *Am J Obstet Gynecol.* 1951;61:121-129.
68. MacDougall I. Ulcerative colitis and pregnancy. *Lancet.* 1956;271:641-643.
69. Crohn BB, Yarnis H, Crohn EB, Walter RI, Gabrilove LJ. Ulcerative colitis and pregnancy. *Gastroenterology.* 1956;30:391-403.
70. Korelitz BI. Pregnancy, fertility, and inflammatory bowel disease. *Am J Gastroenterol.* 1985;80:365-370.
71. Helmholz H. Chronic ulcerative colitis in childhood. *Am J Dis Child.* 1923;26:418-430.
72. Bourne G. Chronic ulcerative colitis in children. *Arch Dis Children.* 1926;1:175-181.
73. Jackman RP, Helmholz HF. Life histories of ninety-five children with chronic ulcerative colitis: A statistical study based on comparison with a whole group of eight hundred and seventy-one patients. *Am J Dis Children.* 1940;59:459-467.
74. Bargen JA, Kennedy RL. Chronic ulcerative colitis in children. *Postgrad Med.* 1955;17:127-131.
75. Beranbaum SL, Waldron RJ. Chronic ulcerative colitis; case report in a newborn infant. *Pediatrics.* 1952;9:773-778.
76. Lagercrantz R. [Ulcerative colitis in children]. *Nord Med.* 1949;41:258-262.
77. Kirsner JB, Raskin HF, Palmer WL. Ulcerative colitis in children; observations in selected patients. *AMA Am J Dis Child.* 1955;90:141-152.
78. Hijmans JC, Enzer NB. Ulcerative colitis in childhood. A study of 43 cases. *Pediatrics.* 1962;29:389-403.
79. Korelitz BI, Gribetz D, Danziger I. The prognosis of ulcerative colitis with onset in childhood. I. The presteroid era. *Ann Intern Med.* 1962;57:582-591.
80. Davidson M, Bloom AA, Kugler MM. Chronic ulcerative colitis of childhood: an evaluative review. *J Pediatr.* 1965;67:471-490.
81. Davidson M. Juvenile ulcerative colitis. *Arch Intern Med.* 1939;64:1187-1195.
82. Ricketts WE, Palmer WL. Chronic ulcerative colitis with infantilism and carcinoma of the colon. *Gastroenterology.* 1945;5:272-280.
83. Welch C, Wakefield EG. Metabolic studies in ulcerative colitis. *J Clin Invest.* 1937;16:161-168.
84. Sappington TS, Bockus HL. Nitrogen metabolism in chronic idiopathic ulcerative colitis and its therapeutic significance. *Ann Intern Med.* 1949;31:282-302.
85. Kirsner JB, Sheffner AL. Studies on amino acid excretion in man; effect of various protein supplements in a normal man, two patients with benign gastric ulcer and two patients with chronic ulcerative colitis. *J Clin Invest.* 1950;29:828.
86. Bargen J. Experimental studies on the etiology of chronic ulcerative colitis (preliminary report). *JAMA.* 1924;83:332.
87. Murray C. Psychogenic factors in the etiology of ulcerative colitis. *Am J Dig Dis.* 1930;180:239.
88. Sullivan A. Psychogenic factors and ulcerative colitis. *Am J Dig Dis.* 1935;2:651.
89. Almy TP, Kern F Jr, Tulin M. Alterations in colonic function in man under stress; experimental production of sigmoid spasm in healthy persons. *Gastroenterology.* 1949;12:425-436.
90. Kern F Jr, Almy TP, Abbot FK, Bogdonoff MD. The motility of the distal colon in nonspecific ulcerative colitis. *Gastroenterology.* 1951;19:492-503.
91. Meyer K, Gellhorn A, Prudden JF, et al. Lysozyme in chronic ulcerative colitis. *Proc Soc Exp Biol.* 1947;65:221-222.
92. Glass GB, Pugh BL, et al. Observations on the treatment of human gastric and colonic mucus with lysozyme. *J Clin Invest.* 1950;29:12-19.
93. Karush A, Daniels GE, O'Connor JF, et al. The response to psychotherapy in chronic ulcerative colitis. I. Pretreatment factors. *Psychosom Med.* 1968;30:255-276.
94. Kirsner JB, Goldgraber MB. Hypersensitivity, autoimmunity, and the digestive tract. *Gastroenterology.* 1960;38:536-562.
95. Kirsner JB, Palmer WL. Ulcerative colitis: considerations of its etiology and treatment. *J Am Med Assoc.* 1954;155:341-346.
96. Broberger O, Perlmann P. Autoantibodies in human ulcerative colitis. *J Exp Med.* 1959;110:657-674.
97. Wright R, Truelove SC. Auto-immune reactions in ulcerative colitis. *Gut.* 1966;7:32-40.
98. Moltke O. Familial occurrence of non specific ulcerative colitis. *Acta Med Scand.* 1936;78 (suppl 72):426.

99. Kirsner JB, Spencer JA. Family occurrences of ulcerative colitis, regional enteritis, and ileocolitis. *Ann Intern Med.* 1963;59:133-144.
100. Schlesinger B, Platt J. Ulcerative colitis in childhood and a follow-up study. *Proc R Soc Med.* 1958;51:733-735.
101. Kirsner JB, Palmer WL, Klotz AP. ACTH and cortisone in chronic ulcerative colitis: a comparison of clinical effects. *J Lab Clin Med.* 1950;36:846.
102. Kirsner JB, Palmer WL. ACTH in ulcerative colitis; report of progress. *Gastroenterology.* 1951;18:143-144.
103. Kirsner JB, Palmer WL. Effect of corticotropin (ACTH) in chronic ulcerative colitis; observations in forty patients. *J Am Med Assoc.* 1951;147:541-549.
104. Witts L. A therapeutic trial of cortisone in chronic ulcerative colitis. *Acta Gastroenterol Belg.* 1954;17:653-659.
105. Truelove SC, Witts LJ. Cortisone in ulcerative colitis; preliminary report on a therapeutic trial. *Br Med J.* 1954;2:375-378.
106. Truelove SC, Witts LJ. Cortisone in ulcerative colitis; final report on a therapeutic trial. *Br Med J.* 1955;2:1041-1048.
107. Goldstein MJ, Gelzayd EA, Kirsner JB. Some observations on the hazards of corticosteroid therapy in patients with inflammatory bowel disease. *Trans Am Acad Ophthalmol Otolaryngol.* 1967;71:254-261.
108. Meyers S, Sachar DB, Goldberg JD, Janowitz HD. Corticotropin versus hydrocortisone in the intravenous treatment of ulcerative colitis. A prospective, randomized, double-blind clinical trial. *Gastroenterology.* 1983;85:351-357.
109. Auphan N, DiDonato JA, Rosette C, Helmberg A, Karin M. Immunosuppression by glucocorticoids: inhibition of NF-kappa B activity through induction of I kappa B synthesis. *Science.* 1995;270:286-290.
110. Svartz N. Salazopyrin—a new sulfanilamide preparation. A. Therapeutic results in rheumatoid arthritis. B. Therapeutic results in ulcerative colitis. C. Toxic manifestations on treatment with sulfanilamide preparations. *Acta Med Scand.* 1942;110:577-590.
111. Svartz N. Sulfasalazine: II. Some notes on the discovery and development of salazopyrin. *Am J Gastroenterol.* 1988;83:497-503.
112. Svartz N. The treatment of 124 cases of ulcerative colitis with salazopyrine and attempts of desensitization in cases of hypersensitivness to sulfa. *Acta Med Scand.* 1948;139 (suppl 206):465-472.
113. Baron JH, Connell AM, Lennard-Jones JE, Jones FA. Sulphasalazine and salicylazosulphadimidine in ulcerative colitis. *Lancet.* 1962;1:1094-1096.
114. Misiewicz JJ, Lennard-Jones JE, Connell AM, Baron JH, Jones FA. Controlled trial of sulphasalazine in maintenance therapy for ulcerative colitis. *Lancet.* 1965;1:185-188.
115. Azad Khan AK, Piris J, Truelove SC. An experiment to determine the active therapeutic moiety of sulphasalazine. *Lancet.* 1977;2:892-895.
116. Klotz U, Maier K, Fischer C, Heinkel K. Therapeutic efficacy of sulfasalazine and its metabolites in patients with ulcerative colitis and Crohn's disease. *N Engl J Med.* 1980;303:1499-1502.
117. Rasmussen SN, Bondesen S, Hvidberg EF, et al. 5-aminosalicylic acid in a slow-release preparation: bioavailability, plasma level, and excretion in humans. *Gastroenterology.* 1982;83:1062-1070.
118. Chan RP, Pope DJ, Gilbert AP, Sacra PJ, Baron JH, Lennard-Jones JE. Studies of two novel sulfasalazine analogs, ipsalazide and balsalazide. *Dig Dis Sci.* 1983;28:609-615.
119. Klotz U, Maier KE, Fischer C, Bauer KH. A new slow-release form of 5-aminosalicylic acid for the oral treatment of inflammatory bowel disease. Biopharmaceutic and clinical pharmacokinetic characteristics. *Arzneimittelforschung.* 1985;35:636-639.
120. Selby WS, Barr GD, Ireland A, Mason CH, Jewell DP. Olsalazine in active ulcerative colitis. *Br Med J.* 1985;291:1373-1375.
121. Riley SA, Mani V, Goodman MJ, Herd ME, Dutt S, Turnberg LA. Comparison of delayed release 5 aminosalicylic acid (mesalazine) and sulphasalazine in the treatment of mild to moderate ulcerative colitis relapse. *Gut.* 1988;29:669-674.
122. Riley SA, Mani V, Goodman MJ, Herd ME, Dutt S, Turnberg LA. Comparison of delayed-release 5-aminosalicylic acid (mesalazine) and sulfasalazine as maintenance treatment for patients with ulcerative colitis. *Gastroenterology.* 1988;94:1383-1389.
123. McIntyre PB, Rodrigues CA, Lennard-Jones JE, et al. Balsalazide in the maintenance treatment of patients with ulcerative colitis, a double-blind comparison with sulphasalazine. *Aliment Pharmacol Ther.* 1988;2:237-243.
124. D'Haens G, Hommes D, Engels L, et al. Once daily MMX mesalazine for the treatment of mild-to-moderate ulcerative colitis: a phase II, dose-ranging study. *Aliment Pharmacol Ther.* 2006;24:1087-1097.
125. Sandborn WJ, Kamm MA, Lichtenstein GR, Lyne A, Butler T, Joseph RE. MMX Multi Matrix System mesalazine for the induction of remission in patients with mild-to-moderate ulcerative colitis: a combined analysis of two randomized, double-blind, placebo-controlled trials. *Aliment Pharmacol Ther.* 2007;26:205-215.
126. Kamm MA, Sandborn WJ, et al. Once-daily, high-concentration MMX mesalamine in active ulcerative colitis. *Gastroenterology.* 2007;132:66-75; quiz 432-433.
127. Lichtenstein GR, Kamm MA, Boddu P, et al. Effect of once- or twice-daily MMX mesalamine (SPD476) for the induction of remission of mild to moderately active ulcerative colitis. *Clin Gastroenterol Hepatol.* 2007;5:95-102.
128. Bean RH. The treatment of chronic ulcerative colitis with 6-mercaptopurine. *Med J Aust.* 1962;49:592-593.
129. Bean RH. Treatment of ulcerative colitis with anti-metabolites. *Br Med J.* 1966;1.
130. Bowen GE, Irons GV Jr, Rhodes JB, Kirsner JB. Early experiences with azathioprine in ulcerative colitis; a note of caution. *JAMA.* 1966;195:460-464.
131. Jewell DP, Truelove SC. Azathioprine in ulcerative colitis: an interim report on a controlled therapeutic trial. *Br Med J.* 1972;1:709-712.
132. Jewell DP, Truelove SC. Azathioprine in ulcerative colitis: final report on controlled therapeutic trial. *Br Med J.* 1974;4:627-630.
133. Gupta S, Keshavarzian A, Hodgson HJ. Cyclosporin in ulcerative colitis. *Lancet.* 1984;2:1277-1278.
134. Lichtiger S, Present DH. Preliminary report: cyclosporin in treatment of severe active ulcerative colitis. *Lancet.* 1990;336:16-19.
135. Bianchi Porro G, Petrillo M, Ardizzone S. Cyclosporin treatment for severe active ulcerative colitis. *Lancet.* 1990;336:439.
136. Treem WR, Davis PM, Hyams JS. Cyclosporine treatment of severe ulcerative colitis in children. *J Pediatr.* 1991;119:994-997.
137. Lichtiger S, Present DH, Kornbluth A, et al. Cyclosporine in severe ulcerative colitis refractory to steroid therapy. *N Engl J Med.* 1994;330:1841-1845.
138. Braegger CP, Nicholls S, Murch SH, Stephens S, MacDonald TT. Tumour necrosis factor alpha in stool as a marker of intestinal inflammation. *Lancet.* 1992;339:89-91.
139. Murch SH, Braegger CP, Walker-Smith JA, MacDonald TT. Location of tumour necrosis factor alpha by immunohistochemistry in chronic inflammatory bowel disease. *Gut.* 1993;34:1705-1709.
140. Murch SH, Lamkin VA, Savage MO, Walker-Smith JA, MacDonald TT. Serum concentrations of tumour necrosis factor alpha in childhood chronic inflammatory bowel disease. *Gut.* 1991;32:913-917.
141. Chey WY. Infliximab for patients with refractory ulcerative colitis. *Inflamm Bowel Dis.* 2001;7(suppl 1):S30-S33.

142. Chey WY, Hussain A, Ryan C, Potter GD, Shah A. Infliximab for refractory ulcerative colitis. *Am J Gastroenterol.* 2001;96:2373-2381.

143. Sands BE, Tremaine WJ, Sandborn WJ, et al. Infliximab in the treatment of severe, steroid-refractory ulcerative colitis: a pilot study. *Inflamm Bowel Dis.* 2001;7:83-88.

144. Rutgeerts P, Sandborn WJ, Feagan BG, et al. Infliximab for induction and maintenance therapy for ulcerative colitis. *N Engl J Med.* 2005;353:2462-2476.

145. Afif W, Leighton JA, Hanauer SB, et al. Open-label study of adalimumab in patients with ulcerative colitis including those with prior loss of response or intolerance to infliximab. *Inflamm Bowel Dis.* 2009;15(9):1302-1307.

146. Plevy S, Salzberg B, Van Assche G, et al. A phase I study of visilizumab, a humanized anti-CD3 monoclonal antibody, in severe steroid-refractory ulcerative colitis. *Gastroenterology.* 2007;133:1414-1422.

147. Sumer N, Palabiyikoglu M. Induction of remission by interferon-alpha in patients with chronic active ulcerative colitis. *Eur J Gastroenterol Hepatol.* 1995;7:597-602.

148. Madsen SM, Schlichting P, Davidsen B, et al. An open-labeled, randomized study comparing systemic interferon-alpha-2A and prednisolone enemas in the treatment of left-sided ulcerative colitis. *Am J Gastroenterol.* 2001;96:1807-1815.

149. Tilg H, Vogelsang H, Ludwiczek O, et al. A randomised placebo controlled trial of pegylated interferon alpha in active ulcerative colitis. *Gut.* 2003;52:1728-1733.

150. Travis S, Yap LM, Hawkey C, et al. RDP58 is a novel and potentially effective oral therapy for ulcerative colitis. *Inflamm Bowel Dis.* 2005;11:713-719.Sinha A, Nightingale J, West KP, Berlanga-Acosta J, Playford RJ. Epidermal growth factor enemas with oral mesalamine for mild-to-moderate left-sided ulcerative colitis or proctitis. *N Engl J Med.* 2003;349:350-357.

151. Sandborn WJ, Sands BE, Wolf DC, et al. Repifermin (keratinocyte growth factor-2) for the treatment of active ulcerative colitis: a randomized, double-blind, placebo-controlled, dose-escalation trial. *Aliment Pharmacol Ther.* 2003;17:1355-1364.

152. Creed TJ, Norman MR, Probert CS, et al. Basiliximab (anti-CD25) in combination with steroids may be an effective new treatment for steroid-resistant ulcerative colitis. *Aliment Pharmacol Ther.* 2003;18:65-75.

153. Van Assche G, Dalle I, Noman M, et al. A pilot study on the use of the humanized anti-interleukin-2 receptor antibody daclizumab in active ulcerative colitis. *Am J Gastroenterol.* 2003;98:369-376.

154. Van Assche G, Dalle I, Noman M, et al. A pilot study on the use of the humanized anti-interleukin-2 receptor antibody daclizumab in active ulcerative colitis. *Am J Gastroenterol.* 2003;98:369-376.

SECTION I

GENERAL

The Natural History of Inflammatory Bowel Disease

Pietro G. Andres, MD and Lawrence S. Friedman, MD

Inflammatory bowel disease (IBD) encompasses at least two forms of idiopathic intestinal inflammation: ulcerative colitis (UC) and Crohn's disease (CD). The latter is also called *regional enteritis, regional ileitis, Crohn's ileitis,* and *granulomatous colitis.* Although other inflammatory disorders affect the gastrointestinal tract, they can be distinguished from IBD by the presence of a specific underlying agent or by the character and manifestations of the inflammatory activity. In contrast, the causes of IBD are unknown.

UC and CD are at least partially distinct in their initial pathogenic events, but they may have key pathophysiologic processes in common. Moreover, UC and CD each may encompass several variants, which are at least partially distinct. For example, patients with CD may manifest different complications (fistulas or stenoses) and may express different inflammatory mediators, perhaps due to underlying genetic differences or environmental exposures between the two groups. Thus, patient subgroups defined by disease location, specific pathologic findings (the presence or absence of granulomas in patients with CD), or disease complications may reflect a multiplicity of diseases with some shared features. In the absence of identifiable causative agents, UC and CD are defined by their typical clinical, pathologic, endoscopic, and laboratory features. In some patients, it is impossible to distinguish with confidence UC from CD affecting the colon using any of the conventional diagnostic criteria. Such cases are labeled *indeterminate colitis.*

Study of the natural history of UC and CD is challenging, in part because of the intrinsic nature of the disorders.[1,2] The clinical presentation of IBD may be insidious, and the time interval between the initial etiologic event and diagnosis of the disease may be quite long, thereby making it difficult to identify and study the inciting events. Because IBD is relatively uncommon, it is also difficult to find a population of adequate size from which deductions about natural history can be drawn.[2] Moreover, many affected people may be asymptomatic or have only mild symptoms and may either not seek medical attention or escape detection.[3]

Performance of natural history studies of IBD that are similar and easily compared has been hampered by the lack of universally adopted diagnostic criteria for these disorders. Published diagnostic criteria[4-6] have been difficult to apply in many studies, because the criteria include endoscopic and radiologic techniques that require skill and expertise and that are not easily performed on a large scale. To compensate, investigators have often selected patients from specialized medical centers, a practice associated with a risk of bias toward more severely ill patients.[1] The problems created by a lack of universally adopted diagnostic criteria are further compounded by a high rate of misdiagnosis in patients with inflammatory colitis. Not only are infectious processes often difficult to differentiate from idiopathic IBD, but (as noted previously) in up to 10% of patients it may also be impossible to distinguish UC from CD at the time of initial presentation.[7]

Lichtenstein GR, ed.
Ulcerative Colitis: The Complete Guide to Medical Management (pp. 13-26)

ULCERATIVE COLITIS

EXTENT AND SEVERITY OF DISEASE

At the time of diagnosis, a majority of patients with UC have disease limited to the rectum, rectosigmoid, or left colon (ie, from the rectum to the splenic flexure). Assessing the precise frequencies of the extent of colonic involvement is difficult to determine from the literature, because different investigators have not used the same definitions of disease extent consistently. Various studies have found that 14% to 36.7% of patients have pancolitis, 36% to 41% have disease extending beyond the rectum (but not to the cecum), and 44% to 49% have proctitis (defined as mucosal changes in the rectum on sigmoidoscopy with a normal colonic appearance) in more proximal segments as determined by barium enema (BE).[8-11] Because the extent of disease in these studies was determined by flexible sigmoidoscopy and BE, rather than colonoscopy, the extent of involvement was probably underestimated.

In general, the clinical severity of disease at presentation correlates with the extent of colonic involvement. Patients with pancolitis tend to have more severe clinical symptoms than do those with disease limited to the rectum. In a population-based study from Copenhagen, Langholz et al found that of all patients diagnosed with UC between 1962 and 1987, 20.2% experienced mild symptoms (defined as less than 4 stools per day, no systemic disturbances, and a normal erythrocyte sedimentation rate [ESR]); 70.7% had moderate disease (defined as more than 4 stools per day but minimal systemic effects); and 9.1% had severe disease (defined as 6 or more bowel movements per day with bloody stools, fever, tachycardia, anemia, or an ESR >30 mm/h).[12]

DISEASE COURSE

Most patients with UC experience a chronic, intermittent clinical course. Less commonly, patients have either continuous, unrelenting symptoms or a single episode of colitis. Among 1161 patients with UC from Copenhagen who did not require colectomy and were followed for up to 25 years by Langholz et al, the cumulative probability of a relapsing course (defined as "clinical remission longer than one month without corticosteroid or immunosuppressive therapy within one year *or* years without disease activity in between years with disease activity") was 90%.[9] The probability of a completely relapse-free course was 10.6% at 25 years, whereas that of a continuously active course was only 0.1%. By using a Markov chain analysis, the authors calculated that the probability that a patient with clinically inactive disease would remain in remission the following year was 80% to 90%, whereas the risk of relapse in the following year was only 10% to 20%. In contrast, those patients with clinically active disease had a 70% probability of having a relapse during the following year. Overall, as the number of years in which a patient had active disease increased, so did the probability of relapse during the following year. However, the probability of having active disease every year after a relapse fell from 50% at 2 years to 10% to 15% at 10 years.

In this study,[9] the clinical course over the 25-year follow-up was not influenced by the age or gender of the patient, anatomic extent of disease at the time of diagnosis, presenting symptoms, length of time between onset of symptoms and diagnosis, initial treatment, use of systemic corticosteroids, or occurrence of extraintestinal manifestations. Only three factors influenced the course of the disease in these patients. First, the number of years in relapse since diagnosis correlated directly with the subsequent chance of disease flares. Second, the occurrence of systemic symptoms (fever and weight loss) at diagnosis correlated inversely with subsequent disease activity. (That is, patients presenting initially with severe disease that subsequently responded to medical therapy, and thus did not require surgery, had a high probability of a subsequent long-term remission.) Lastly, development of disease later in the study period correlated with a greater chance of a prolonged remission, an indication that medical management had improved over the 25 years of the study.[9]

When patients who require colectomy are included in the analysis of disease course, investigators have found that, at least in the short term, the extent of colonic involvement at the time of diagnosis influences both the frequency of subsequent anatomic extension and the clinical severity of the disease.[13,14] For example, patients with proctitis are unlikely to develop extension past the splenic flexure. In two case-control studies by Meucci et al[13] and Powell-Tuck et al,[14] 60% to 70% of patients who presented with proctitis continued to have disease limited to the rectosigmoid colon after 20 years. Moreover, the majority of patients who developed more extensive disease did so within the first 5 years. The overall prognosis of patients diagnosed with proctitis is good, with only 4% to 5% requiring surgery for their disease within 20 years of diagnosis.[14]

In contrast, Langholz et al found that patients with proctosigmoiditis had a greater than 50% chance of developing more extensive disease and a 12% frequency of colectomy within 25 years of diagnosis. Similarly, these investigators observed that patients with radiological evidence of colitis proximal to the rectum had a 9% chance of progression to pancolitis and a 23% frequency of colectomy. As one would expect, the probability of colectomy was highest in patients with pancolitis (40%)[8] (Figure 1-1). Hendriksen et al also found that one-third of patients with pancolitis required colectomy within the first year of diagnosis, compared with less than 8% of those with more limited disease.[10]

Patients with total colonic involvement are more likely to experience complications of UC than are patients with more limited disease. In a cohort study of 1116 patients

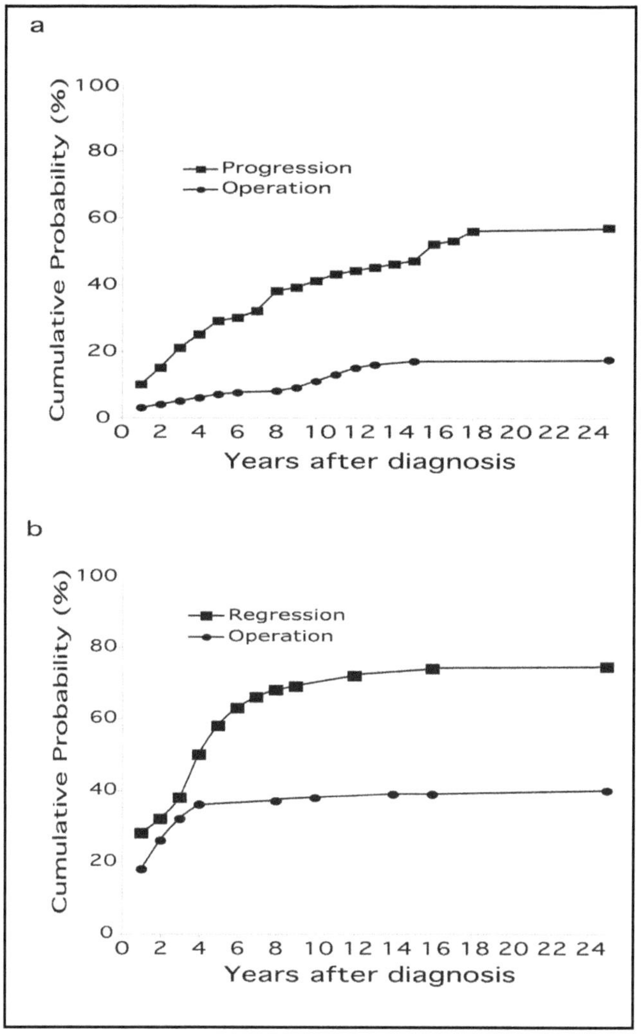

FIGURE 1-1. (A) Cumulative probability of progression and colectomy in patients with UC who present with proctosigmoiditis. (B) Cumulative probability of regression and colectomy in patients with UC who present with pancolitis. (Reprinted with permission from Langholz E, Munkholm P, Davidsen M, Nielsen OH, Binder V. Changes in extent of ulcerative colitis: a study on the course and prognostic factors. *Scand J Gastroenterol.* 1996;31:260-266.)

diagnosed with UC at the Cleveland Clinic Foundation between 1960 and 1983, Farmer et al found that in patients with pancolitis, toxic dilatation developed in 21%, bleeding developed in 25%, and surgery was required in 60%.[11] In contrast, in patients with proctitis, the frequency of toxic dilatation and bleeding was 3% and 9.5%, respectively, and only 14% required surgery. However, once the first year after diagnosis had passed, the clinical course of the disease became similar for all patients regardless of initial extent at the time of presentation. Thus, after the first year, the annual colectomy rate was 1% for all patients.[11]

Complications

Acute Local Complications

As discussed above, the frequency of acute colonic complications of UC is generally related to the anatomic extent and clinical severity of the disease. Massive hemorrhage occurs in up to 3.5% of patients and may be an indication for colectomy if bleeding persists despite blood transfusions and immunosuppressive therapy. Acute colonic dilatation can occur in up to 5% of patients with severe attacks of UC. Half of these patients may respond to medical therapy alone, whereas those who fail to respond to therapy or show signs of deterioration require colectomy.[15] Colonic perforation is the most dangerous local complication and is an indication for urgent colectomy. Greenstein and Aufses reported a mortality rate of 16% in UC patients with colonic perforation,[16] a finding that underscores the need for aggressive medical and surgical management in these patients.

Extraintestinal Complications

Many extraintestinal manifestations are associated with UC (Table 1-1). The most common is an acute arthropathy, which can affect up to 20% of patients[17] and can present as either a large joint pauciarticular arthritis or a small joint symmetrical polyarthropathy reminiscent of rheumatoid arthritis. Orchard et al found pauciarticular arthritis in 3.6% of patients with UC and observed that the clinical flares of arthritis generally paralleled the activity of the bowel disease. In contrast, the vast majority of the 2.5% of UC patients with small joint polyarthropathy experienced persistent articular symptoms independent of the clinical activity of colitis.[18]

Sacroiliitis and ankylosing spondylitis are less common than peripheral arthropathy, with frequencies of 11% to 15% and 1% to 2% of UC patients, respectively. The frequency is higher if asymptomatic patients with radiologic evidence of axial arthropathy are included in the analysis. For example, 11% of patients with UC have evidence of sacroiliitis by plain radiography, but 70% have evidence of the disease by technetium bone scan.[17] The majority of patients with sacroiliitis are HLA-B27-negative and do not progress to ankylosing spondylitis. In contrast, 80% of UC patients with ankylosing spondylitis are HLA-B27-positive. The course of the spondylitis is independent of the activity of the bowel disease; in fact, spinal symptoms may develop prior to the onset of colitis.[15]

Ocular complications of UC include anterior uveitis and episcleritis and occur in 5% to 15% of patients with UC. The course of these complications tends to parallel that of the underlying bowel disease.[19]

TABLE 1-1

EXTRAINTESTINAL COMPLICATION OF INFLAMMATORY BOWEL DISEASE

Complication	Ulcerative Colitis (%)	Crohn's Disease (%)
Acute arthropathy	10 to 20	15 to 20
Sacroiliitis	9 to 11	9 to 11
Ankylosing spondylitis	1 to 3	3 to 5
Ocular complications	5 to 15	5 to 15
Erythema nodosum	10 to 15	15
Pyoderma gangrenosum	1 to 2	1 to 2
Primary sclerosing cholangitis	2 to 7.6	1
Choledocholithiasis	–	15 to 30 (patients with small bowel disease)
Nephrolithiasis	–	5 to 10
Amyloidosis	–	Rare

The most common dermatologic complication of UC is erythema nodosum, occurring in up to 15% of UC patients, often in association with peripheral arthropathy or ankylosing spondylitis.[17,20] Both uveitis and erythema nodosum are associated with HLA-B27, -B58, and -DRB1*0103.[20] Other less common cutaneous manifestations of UC include pyoderma gangrenosum (1% to 2% of patients with UC) and Sweet's syndrome, or neutrophilic dermatosis (rare).[21] The activity of these dermatologic complications tends to parallel the activity of the bowel disease,[15] although pyoderma gangrenosum may persist despite resolution of colitis or even colectomy.

Hepatobiliary disease is common in patients with UC. Elevations of serum aminotransferase levels may be found in more than 50% of patients with active colitis,[22] usually as a consequence of malnutrition, sepsis, fatty liver, or administration of total parenteral nutrition. The elevated enzyme levels usually return to normal with treatment of the underlying colitis. Primary sclerosing cholangitis (PSC) is a chronic hepatobiliary disease found in 2% to 7.6% of patients with UC. The converse association is stronger, with 70% of patients with PSC having IBD, usually UC. In most of these patients (60%), the diagnosis of IBD is made before that of PSC.[23] People with PSC are usually diagnosed in the fourth decade of life, although liver biochemical abnormalities may be noted up to 10 years earlier.[24-26] Two-thirds of patients are men. The disease is progressive, eventually causing cirrhosis and liver failure. Five- and 10-year survival rates are 85% and 75%, respectively. The 5-year survival rate after liver transplantation for PSC has been reported to be 85%.[27-30] PSC is also associated with a risk of cholangiocarcinoma, with a frequency of 8% to 10% over 6 years, although the risk is much lower in patients with the intrahepatic small-duct variant of PSC.[31]

Several reports have linked UC with an increased risk of lymphoma[32]; however, a large population-based cohort study did not confirm this association.[33]

Colon Cancer

The association between UC and colon cancer is well-established. The exact risk of colon cancer associated with UC has varied among epidemiologic studies, but most indicate that the risk is highest in patients with extensive colonic involvement and a duration of disease of more than 10 years.[15] Other risk factors for colon cancer include a family history of colon cancer and possibly young age at diagnosis of UC and presence of backwash ileitis.[34]

For unclear reasons, the risk of colon cancer in patients with UC has declined, and in some populations an elevated risk of colon cancer relative to the general population can no longer be demonstrated.[34] Possible reasons for the decline in incidence of colon cancer in this population are widespread use of surveillance colonoscopy and maintenance drug therapy.

Ekbom et al followed a cohort of 3117 patients with UC for up to 35 years and found that the incidence of colorectal cancer was 5.7 times the expected rate for an age-matched cohort.[35] The risk was proportional to the extent of colonic disease: patients with proctitis had a standardized incidence ratio of 1.7 (95% confidence interval [CI] 0.8 to 3.2), those with left-sided colitis had a ratio of 2.8 (95% CI 1.6 to 4.4), and those with pancolitis had a ratio of 14.8 (95% CI 11.4 to 18.9). The cumulative incidence of colorectal cancer was also found to depend on the age at diagnosis (Figure 1-2). Patients with pancolitis diagnosed after age 40 had a 20-year frequency of colon cancer of 16%, compared to 5% in those diagnosed before age 14. With longer

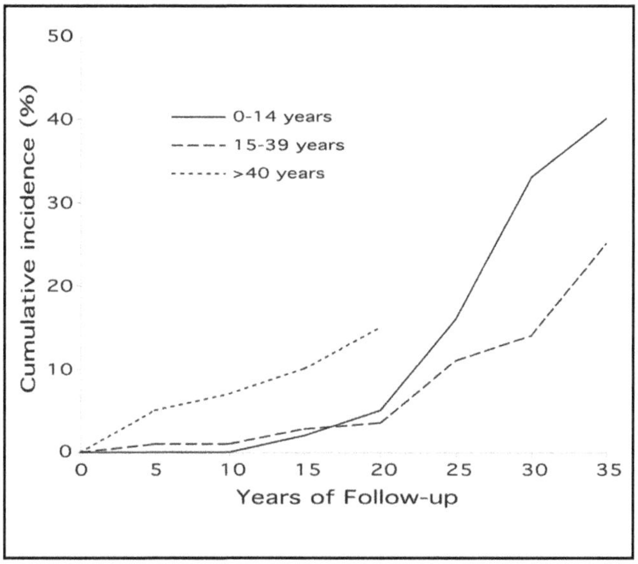

FIGURE 1-2. Cumulative incidence of colorectal cancer for patients with pancolitis according to age at diagnosis. (Reprinted with permission from Ekbom A, Helmick C, Zack M, Adami HO. Ulcerative colitis and colorectal cancer: a population-based study. *N Engl J Med.* 1990;323(18):1228-1233. Copyright © 1990 Massachusetts Medical Society. All rights reserved, used with permission.)

follow-up, however, those with pancolitis diagnosed at a younger age were found to have a higher absolute risk of colon cancer than patients who were older at the time of diagnosis.[35] In contrast, Jess et al found that in Olmsted County, Minnesota, the risk of colon cancer was increased among patients with extensive UC but not among UC patients overall.[36] Although greater clinical severity and frequency of attacks of colitis do not seem to increase the risk of colorectal cancer,[37] there is a direct correlation with the severity of colonic inflammation.[38]

Overall, the annual incidence of colon cancer in patients with UC of more than 10 years' duration may be as low as 1 in 500 to 1 in 1600.[34] The prognosis of colon cancer is poorer in patients with UC than in those without UC, despite a similar distribution of stages at diagnosis.[39]

It has been recognized that colonic malignancies in patients with IBD originate from mucosal dysplasia. Up to 19% of patients with low-grade dysplasia (LGD) have associated cancer found on examination of colectomy specimens.[40] Moreover, in patients who initially had a negative colonoscopy and were later diagnosed with LGD, 16% to 53% progressed to high-grade dysplasia (HGD), dysplasia-associated lesion or mass (DALM), or cancer.[40-42] However, because 50% of patients with LGD do not have dysplasia on follow-up surveillance,[43] optimal therapy for LGD remains controversial. Because HGD and DALM are associated with the presence of cancer in 32% to 53% of cases,[40,44] colectomy rather than continued surveillance is recommended for these lesions.

The risk of colorectal cancer appears to be especially high in patients with both UC and PSC. Several population and cohort studies have estimated that these patients have a 3- to 10-fold increased risk for developing colonic neoplasia as compared to patients with UC alone.[45-48] The cancers in these patients tend to occur in the right colon, supporting the concept that secondary bile acids are carcinogenic and increase the likelihood of cancer in the proximal colon.[47] Further support for this hypothesis comes from data demonstrating that oral administration of ursodeoxycholic acid (UDCA), which decreases fecal levels of deoxycholic acid,[49,50] significantly reduces the risk of colonic neoplasia (risk ratio [RR] = 0.26; CI 0.07 to 0.99).[51]

Retrospective matched case-control studies have generated optimism that mesalamine (5-aminosalicylic acid, 5-ASA) therapy may protect against the development of colonic neoplasia in patients with UC.[52-54] Using a conditional logistic regression analysis, Eaden et al found that regular use of these agents has a profound protective effect (up to a 91% risk reduction with mesalamine use).[52] Prospective trials designed to confirm this effect are ongoing.[55,56] A meta-analysis has suggested that use of mesalamine reduces the risk of colorectal carcinoma by 50%.[56] A case-control study suggested that the risk of colorectal carcinoma is higher in patients who have pseudopolyps and lower in those who take anti-inflammatory medications.[57]

Mortality

Mortality as a consequence of UC has decreased dramatically since the introduction of corticosteroids, and studies indicate that long-term survival rates for patients with UC do not differ from that of the general population.[6,19,58,59] Ekbom et al, however, found that the 10-year survival rate of patients with UC was slightly (but significantly) less than that of the general Swedish population. The slightly increased mortality rate in patients with UC was attributable to patients with extensive colonic involvement. The prognosis was slightly worse in patients with pancolitis than in those with left-sided colitis, with 10-year survival rates of 92.8% and 96.0%, respectively. Moreover, patients with ulcerative proctitis had a 10-year survival rate of 97.9%, which was not significantly lower than that of the control population.[60]

In a large, population-based cohort study, Persson et al found a similar pattern, with a standardized 15-year mortality ratio of 1.37 for patients with UC.[61] The increase in mortality may be most prominent in patients in whom colitis develops after age 60: Persson et al found the 15-year relative survival rate for this cohort was 24%; however, this rate was not significantly different from that of the general population.[61] Using a similar study design, Winther et al found a significantly increased mortality risk in men and women diagnosed with extensive ulcerative colitis after age 50 (Figure 1-3).[59] Jess et al found that in Olmsted County, Minnesota, overall survival in patients with UC was actually slightly greater than expected because of decreased mortality from cardiovascular disease.[62] Sonnenberg has

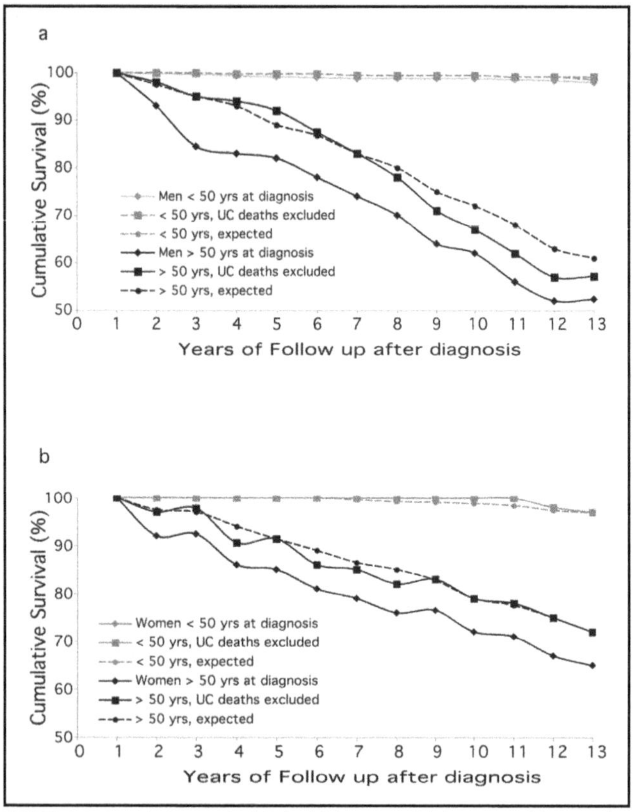

FIGURE 1-3. Cumulative survival (%) of (A) men and (B) women with extensive colitis at diagnosis and aged <50 years and >50 years at diagnosis, respectively. (Reprinted with permission from Winther KV, Jess T, Langholz E, Munkholm P, Binder V. Survival and cause-specific mortality in ulcerative colitis: follow-up of a population-based cohort in Copenhagen County. *Gastroenterology.* 2003;125:1576-1582.)

cautioned that data from cohort studies may underestimate the actual mortality risk from UC, which generally affects populations of higher socioeconomic strata, a subgroup characterized by low death rates for other diagnoses.[63]

As discussed earlier, the occurrence of acute, local complications of UC is associated with a significant increase in 1-year mortality rates in patients with newly diagnosed UC. In this group of patients, the mortality rate is 2.4- to 2.78-fold higher than that of age-matched controls.[59,64] The mortality rate for patients with complications in the setting of pancolitis is greater than that for patients with complications in the setting of less extensive disease.[59,60]

Quality of Life

UC is a chronic disease with a significant lifelong impact on a patient's quality of life. Nevertheless, many studies have demonstrated that more than 90% of affected people are fully capable of working effectively after successful treatment of an initial attack of UC.[9,10] Despite the tendency for intermittent disease activity, UC does not appear to affect the capacity of patients in the workplace substantially. These data do not, however, provide information about the impact of UC on other aspects of a patient's lifestyle.

Several questionnaire-based tools designed to determine health-related quality of life (HRQOL) have been developed and applied to IBD.[65] The results suggest that patients with UC experience moderate impairment in social and emotional functioning and that these impairments are more severe than the cumulative physical obstacles patients endure. This impairment may be more pronounced in women than men.[66,67] The emotional concerns of patients with IBD were examined by Hjortswang et al, who found that patients with UC worried most frequently about the impact that an ostomy bag would have on their lives. Their other concerns (in order of decreasing frequency) were having surgery, cancer, losing bowel control, uncertainty about the course of the disease, and effects of medication.[68] The degree of a patient's concerns correlates inversely with his or her knowledge of the disease.[69] This observation underscores the important role of the physician in not only treating a patient's medical symptoms but also instructing the patient about the natural history of the disease to alleviate some of the associated emotional concerns.

CROHN'S DISEASE

Extent and Severity of Disease

Unlike UC, CD can involve any or multiple segments of the gastrointestinal tract. Of 615 new patients diagnosed consecutively at the Cleveland Clinic, Farmer et al found that 40.9% had ileocolonic disease, 28.6% had disease limited to the small intestine, and 30.4% had disease involving only the colon or anorectal area.[70] Of patients with disease limited to the colon, only 25% have inflammation affecting the entire colon. In the remaining 75%, any area of the colon may be affected, with the distal colon affected most commonly. In the vast majority of patients with small intestinal disease, the terminal ileum is involved.[71]

Because of the variable nature of CD, the severity of disease does not correlate directly with the extent of bowel involvement. Instead, patients generally present with one of three patterns of disease: predominantly inflammatory, stricturing, or fistulizing. These disease patterns, rather than the extent of inflammation, determine the disease course and the nature of associated complications.

Disease Course

The clinical course of CD is often erratic. Years of frequent relapses may be followed by years of virtually complete remission. Munkholm et al followed 373 patients with CD in Copenhagen for a mean of 8.5 years and found that the number of patients with a relapse-free course decreased

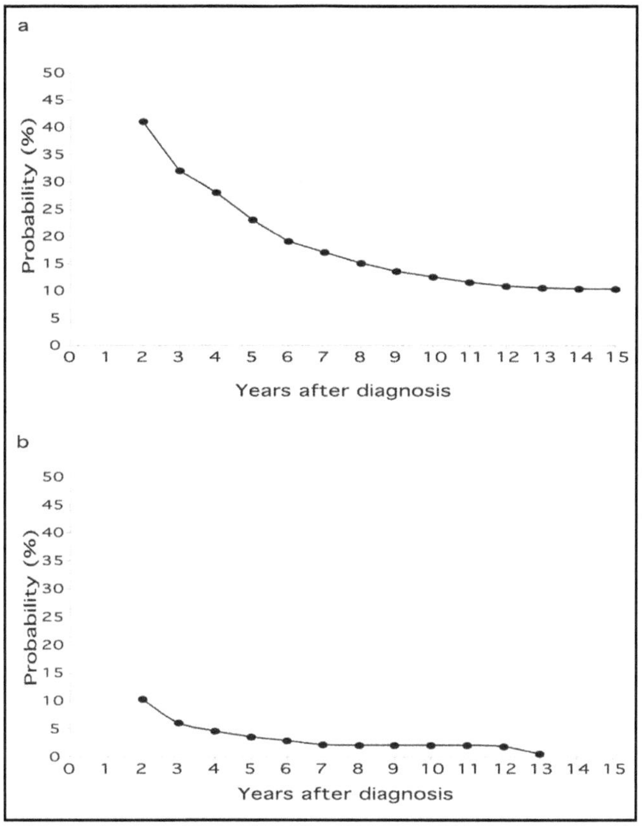

FIGURE 1-4. Cumulative probability of patients experiencing (A) only one attack of CD and (B) a chronic persistent course of CD over a 15-year period. (Reprinted with permission from Munkholm P, Langholz E, Davidsen M, Binder V. Disease activity courses in a regional cohort of Crohn's disease patients. *Scand J Gastroenterol.* 1995;30:699-706.)

rapidly, from 42% at 2 years to 12% after 10 years.[72] The probability of a continuously active course was also low, declining from 10% at 2 years to 1% after 10 years (Figure 1-4). By Markov chain analysis, the investigators determined that a patient with clinically active disease has a 70% to 80% chance of having clinically active disease the following year. Similarly, 80% of patients in remission will remain so the following year. Over a 4-year period, 25% of patients had persistently active disease, 22% were in remission, and 53% had a course that fluctuated between years of remission and years with clinically active disease. The disease course was not affected by the patient's age, gender, time between onset of symptoms and diagnosis, anatomic location of disease, nature of the symptoms at the time of diagnosis, or initial mode of treatment (medical vs surgical).[72]

Although the clinical activity of CD is independent of the anatomic location and extent of the disease, the clinical manifestations and need for surgery are not. Several studies have shown that patients with small intestinal disease are more likely to have an obstructive disease pattern characterized by symptomatic fixed narrowing (fibrostenosis) of the bowel.[70,73,74] In contrast, those with colonic disease are more likely to have symptoms resulting from inflammation, including bleeding.[73] In addition, 16% to 35% of all patients with CD develop fistulas or abscesses regardless of the anatomic location of the intestinal inflammation.[70,73,75] In one population-based study, 46% of patients with fistulizing disease developed a fistula before or at the time of diagnosis.[75]

The frequency of indications for surgery parallels the frequency of local intestinal complications of CD. Up to 74% of all patients will eventually require surgical intervention for their disease,[70,76] and more than 80% of patients with fistulizing disease will require an operation.[75] In 50% of patients, surgery is required within 6 months of diagnosis.[76] Not surprisingly, surgery to relieve obstruction is required most often in patients with small bowel disease, whereas surgery for toxic dilatation and perineal disease is required most often in those with colonic disease (Table 1-2).[70] As observed by Polito et al, patients diagnosed before age 20 are at higher risk of small bowel disease than are patients diagnosed after age 20 and have an almost two-fold relative risk of requiring surgery. Moreover, patients diagnosed before age 20 have a nearly two-fold relative risk of requiring surgery for intractable disease. Because younger patients are more likely to have a positive family history of CD, Polito et al speculated that an inherited form of CD may exist that has a younger age of onset and is associated with a more severe course than later-onset CD.[73] An association between mutations in the NOD2/CARD15 gene and ileal and fibrostenotic disease is consistent with this observation.[77,78] An association between the TC haplotype of the organic cation transporter genes (OCTN1 and OCTN2) and nonfistulizing, nonfibrostenotic colonic disease has been suggested.[79]

One of the greatest challenges in managing patients with CD is the high frequency of recurrent disease following surgery. The anatomic distribution of recurrent disease correlates with the original pattern of disease: patients who undergo ileal resection typically develop recurrent disease just proximal to the ileocolonic anastomosis, whereas in those with colonic disease, the site of recurrence can be on either or both sides of the anastomosis.[71] Ascertaining the exact frequency of recurrence after surgical resection depends on how recurrence is defined. If recurrence is defined as the need for another surgical intervention, 25% to 38% of CD patients treated surgically will have a recurrence by 5 years, and 40% to 70% will have a recurrence by 15 years.[80,81] Of those who undergo a second operation, 37% will require a third operation.[80] In contrast, endoscopic evidence of recurrence can be found in up to 93% of patients 1 year after surgery.[82] Overall, the data suggest that patients should be advised that disease recurrence following surgery for CD is likely. Nevertheless, surgery is an important therapeutic modality that, at least in the short term, can provide substantial improvement in clinical symptoms and quality of life.

TABLE 1-2

INDICATION FOR INITIAL SURGERY IN PATIENTS WITH CROHN'S DISEASE, WITH RESPECT TO CLINICAL PATTERN OF PRESENTATION*

	Clinical Pattern		
Indication for Surgery*	**Ileocolonic (N = 199)**	**Colonic or Anorectal (N = 97)**	**Small Intestinal (N = 100)**
Intestinal obstruction	96 (48.2%)	21 (22.3%)	56 (61.1%)
Internal fistula	53 (26.8%)	16 (17.0%)	21 (22.1%)
Toxic dilatation	10 (5%)	25 (26.6%)	2 (2.1%)
Perianal disease	63 (31.7%)	36 (37.9%)	15 (15.8%)
Perforation or abscess	43 (21.6%)	13 (13.8%)	15 (15.8%)

*At times, more than one indication was present (internal fistula and perforation with abscess was the most frequent combination).

Reprinted from Farmer RG, Whelan G, Fazio VW. Long-term follow-up of patients with Crohn's disease. *Gastroenterology.* 1985;88(6):1818-1825 with permission from American Gastroenterological Association.

Treatment with biologic agents, such as infliximab, a chimeric monoclonal antibody against tumor necrosis factor-alpha, may alter the natural history of CD. Within 2 weeks of starting therapy, nearly 60% of patients have a clinical response, and, of these, approximately 40% can be maintained in remission for 54 weeks with infusions of the drug every 8 weeks, as compared to 21% of those receiving infusions of placebo.[83] Similarly, maintenance therapy with infliximab maintains closure of fistulas in 36% of treated patients compared to 19% of those treated with placebo.[84] Although more than 50% of patients treated with infliximab for fistulas will still require surgery,[85] the ability of this agent to promote endoscopic healing in parallel with clinical improvement suggests that the drug has the potential to alter the natural history of the disease.[86]

Extraintestinal Manifestations

Patients with CD are at risk of developing many of the same extraintestinal complications seen in patients with UC (see Table 1-2). Indeed, the frequencies of dermatologic, arthritic, and ocular complications are similar in both forms of IBD,[21] although the frequency of erythema nodosum is slightly higher in patients with CD than in those with UC.[71] Several additional complications are unique to CD patients as a consequence of either the ulcerating nature of CD or involvement of the small intestine.

Although patients with either UC or CD are at risk of osteoporosis as a consequence of corticosteroid use, patients with CD and extensive small bowel involvement are at additional risk of vitamin D and calcium malabsorption.[87] As a result, these patients have an excess risk of fracture of both vertebra and hip (odds ratio [OR] of 2.5 and 1.8, respectively), and the risk is proportional to the severity of the bowel disease, as assessed by the number of symptoms.[88] Therefore, these patients should start on a medical regimen to preserve bone density, including combined calcium and vitamin D and possibly estrogen therapy for women. Perhaps most effective are bisphosphonates, which can increase bone density in patients with IBD.[89]

Patients with terminal ileal disease or resection are also at risk of bile acid malabsorption that may result in formation of gallstones. In addition, interruption of the enterohepatic circulation may lead to oxalate kidney stones because of both an increase in oxalate absorption in the colon as a result of increased mucosal permeability and a reduction in luminal calcium concentrations as a result of increased binding to long-chain free fatty acids. Gallstones develop in 15% to 30% of patients with small bowel CD, whereas oxalate nephrolithiasis occurs in 5% to 10%.[71] Folate absorption may also be reduced because of small bowel disease as well as treatment with sulfasalazine, and folate supplementation should be considered.

Less frequent complications of CD include amyloidosis and hepatobiliary dysfunction. Amyloidosis is rare in patients with CD. Farmer et al found only one case of amyloidosis in 615 CD patients followed prospectively.[70] This complication generally presents several years after the diagnosis of CD has been made, most frequently in patients with longstanding fistulizing disease, and may involve almost any organ, most often the kidneys.[71] As in UC, abnormal liver biochemical tests are common in patients with CD, occurring in up to 30% of patients.[90] However, PSC is less common in CD than in UC. PSC has been reported as a complication in 1% to 2% of CD cases, and of the 70% of patients with PSC who have IBD, only 6% have CD.[91]

Intestinal and Extraintestinal Cancer

Patients with CD are at increased risk of cancer of both the small and large intestines. Compared to sporadic small intestinal adenocarcinomas, small bowel adenocarcinomas in patients with CD tend to occur at a younger age and have a different anatomic distribution. The mean age at diagnosis in patients with CD is 46, compared to 64 in the general population.[92] Whereas sporadic small intestinal carcinomas occur most commonly in the duodenum and proximal jejunum, those in patients with CD tend to arise in areas of longstanding inflammation, often the distal jejunum and ileum.[93] Although patients with CD are up to 40 times as likely as the general population to develop small bowel carcinoma,[36,94,95] the absolute risk is exceedingly small.

It is now clear that patients with CD, like those with UC, are at increased risk of colon cancer.[95-97] The risk is especially high in patients with extensive colonic involvement. In this group, the overall risk of colorectal cancer is increased as much as 18-fold, and the cumulative risk is 8% at 22 years. The relative risk is especially high in patients in whom CD is diagnosed before age 25. The risk of colon cancer in patients with extensive colonic CD is equal to that of patients with ulcerative pancolitis,[95,96] a finding that suggests that the extent and duration of the inflammation, not the form of IBD, predisposes to cancer.

The risk of colon cancer in CD patients with less extensive colonic inflammation is not well-defined but appears to be small.[94,95] For patients with ileal disease, the risk of colon cancer does not appear to be increased above that of the general population.[94] Perhaps because the symptoms of CD may resemble those of rectal cancer, rectal tumors tend to be diagnosed at a later stage than those in patients without CD and thus have a poorer prognosis.[98]

There is evidence that patients with CD have a higher relative risk of developing certain extraintestinal malignancies. Both Hodgkin's and non-Hodgkin's lymphomas have been reported to occur with increased frequency in patients with CD,[95,99,100] although this association has been put into question by results of a large population-based cohort study.[33] In addition, squamous cell cancer of the anus and vulva occur with a frequency up to five-fold that of the general population.[101] The risk is especially high in patients with longstanding perineal disease.[102,103]

Mortality

Crohn's disease is associated with an increased mortality rate relative to the general population and independent of whether the small intestine, large intestine, or both are affected.[19,60-62,70] The excess mortality is most notable in the first few years after diagnosis and is most often attributable to complications of CD, including gastrointestinal cancer,[60-62] as well as a number of comorbid conditions or complications, such as shock, volume depletion, protein/calorie malnutrition, and anemia.[104] Most population-based studies have found an overall standardized mortality ratio (SMR) of 1.3 to 1.5 for patients with CD.[61,105] In a population-based study from Copenhagen, Jess et al found that the highest mortality risk was in women younger than 50 years of age at diagnosis (SMR 3.42; 95% CI 2.21 to 5.04). In this study, the higher mortality risk in women with disease onset before age 50 was attributed to a more aggressive disease course[105]; other studies have found a similar association between female gender and increased mortality.[60,61,106] On the other hand, a population-based study from 7 European countries and Israel reported an increased overall mortality risk in patients with CD 10 years after diagnosis, with an age older than 40 years at diagnosis as the sole factor associated with increased mortality.[107] Which concurrent medications patients were using in many of these studies is uncertain. Certain medications (ie, corticosteroids) have been recognized to augment the risk of severe infectious complications and even the risk of mortality in this patient population.[108]

Quality of Life

Like UC, CD is a lifelong disease that causes symptoms that may interfere with social activities, interpersonal relationships, and employment. Several questionnaire-based studies have found that patients with CD have worse HRQOL scores than healthy controls or patients with UC (standardized IBD questionnaire [IBDQ] scores of 6.66 for healthy subjects, 5.90 for inactive UC, and 5.25 for patients with stable CD; range: 1 = poor to 7 = optimum).[69,109-111] Not surprisingly, patients with active ileocolonic disease and ileocecal disease have an even worse quality of life than the overall CD population (HRQOL scores of 4.09 and 3.97, respectively).[65] The reduction in quality of life is attributable, in part, to stress that patients experience because of concerns about their disease. Blondel-Kucharski et al found that patients' principal concern was having an ostomy bag, followed in frequency by the uncertain prognosis associated with their disease, reduced energy level, and possibility of needing surgery. Factors associated with a reduced HRQOL include female gender, tobacco use, involvement of the colon, hospitalization, corticosteroid treatment, and recent surgery.[112] Use of immunomodulators,[112] including infliximab,[113,114] was associated with a better HRQOL. As in patients with UC, patients' concerns were best allayed when physicians instructed them about what to expect from their disease.[69]

Despite an impaired quality of life, several studies have found that patients with CD can lead lives that are as productive as those of healthy subjects. Although younger patients with CD miss more school days than healthy controls, they achieve similar academic success.[115] Similarly, unemployment rates are not higher among patients with CD than among age-matched controls.[71]

SPECIAL POPULATIONS

IBD in the Pediatric Population

IBD often has its onset in adolescence; however, the incidence of IBD in children remains lower than in adults. Langholz et al found the incidence of UC in children below age 15 to be 2.0 per 10^5 and that for CD to be 0.2 per 10^5.[116] In this age group, up to 15% of patients change diagnosis from UC to CD or CD to UC during the course of the illness,[117] and 23% to 50% may be diagnosed with indeterminate colitis at initial presentation.[117-119] In the pediatric population, however, the incidence of CD has increased since the 1950s, whereas that of UC has remained relatively constant.[120] In fact, the incidence of CD in children is approaching, and in some areas has overtaken, that of UC.

Ulcerative Colitis

Although the clinical features and natural history of IBD in children are similar to those of adults, several important differences exist. In a study comparing the natural history of UC in adults and children, Langholz et al found that children tended to have more extensive disease (29% had pancolitis and 25% had proctitis, compared to 14% and 46% in adults, respectively). In addition, pediatric patients presented more frequently with abdominal pain as a chief complaint.[116] In another series of 171 children with UC, 22% had proctosigmoiditis, 36% left-sided colitis, and 43% pancolitis. Forty-three percent were initially diagnosed with mild disease. Of these, more than 90% had their symptoms resolve after 6 months. After 1 year of follow-up, 55% were symptom free, 38% had intermittent symptoms, and 7% had persistent symptoms. Of the 57% initially diagnosed with moderate to severe disease, 81% were symptom free at 6 months. The outcome was independent of the disease extent, and the overall 5-year rate of surgery was 19%.[121]

Crohn's Disease

Comprehensive studies of the natural history of Crohn's disease in children are lacking.[119] Growth retardation has been found to be an important clue to the diagnosis of CD in children, and growth rates are less than expected in up to 40% of children with CD.[122] In a study of 100 consecutive pediatric patients with CD, Griffiths et al found that 33% had mild disease and never required corticosteroids, whereas 33% had at least one flare that required the use of these agents. In addition, 19% had chronically active disease that required immunomodulatory or surgical therapy to induce remission, and 10% had corticosteroid-dependent or refractory disease.[122] The use of infliximab has been shown, at least in the short term, to be safe in children with CD.[123] It is not yet clear how this agent will alter the natural history of the disease in this population.

IBD in the Elderly

Ulcerative Colitis

The clinical features of UC in the elderly are generally similar to those in younger patients. However, at the time of presentation, patients over age 60 tend to have less extensive, predominantly distal disease. Watts et al found that 42% of older patients presented with proctitis, and 12% presented with pancolitis; the corresponding rates for patients younger than age 60 were 33% and 26.5%, respectively.[124] Surprisingly, the higher frequency of distal colonic disease in the older group does not translate into less clinical severity. In a retrospective population-based study of patients from Scotland, Sinclair et al found that 14% of patients presenting after age 70 had a severe initial attack, compared to only 7% of those under age 30 and 3% of those between ages 30 and 69. Severe attacks carried a mortality rate of 23%, and in this study, the overall mortality rate was higher in elderly patients than in younger patients.[125]

Not all studies have demonstrated a worse prognosis for elderly patients. In fact, most have shown that patients over age 60 respond well to medical management, have lower rates of relapse than younger patients, and have mortality rates that are comparable to that of age-matched controls.[126] Hendriksen et al followed 783 Dutch patients with UC over an 18-year period and found only a slight increase in mortality in patients diagnosed after age 40. The increase in mortality was confined to the first 2 years after presentation; the subsequent survival rate was equal to that of the younger population.[10]

Crohn's Disease

Compared to younger populations, older patients with CD tend to develop disease involving the colon and obstructive and inflammatory (rather than fistulizing) complications. Despite these differences, young and elderly patients present with similar symptoms, although on initial presentation, elderly patients are more likely to be misdiagnosed as having diverticulitis or colon cancer.[127] Elderly patients respond as well as younger patients to medical and surgical therapy.[126,128] Moreover, postoperative recurrence rates are up to 5 times higher in younger patients.[126,129] In fact, the onset of CD later in life does not appear to affect mortality adversely, and mortality rates for elderly patients with CD are no different from those for the general population.[72]

REFERENCES

1. Sandler R, Loftus EV Jr. The epidemiology of idiopathic inflammatory bowel disease. In: Sartor R, Sanborn W, eds. *Kirsner's Inflammatory Bowel Disease.* Baltimore, MD: Saunders; 2004:259-268.

2. Panaccione R, Sutherland L. Clinical course and complications of ulcerative colitis. In: Targan S, Sharahan F, Karp L, eds. *Inflammatory Bowel Disease: From Bench to Bedside.* Baltimore, MD: Kluwer Academic Publishers; 2003:269-290.
3. Mayberry JF, Ballantyne KC, Hardcastle JD, Mangham C, Pye G. Epidemiological study of asymptomatic inflammatory bowel disease: the identification of cases during a screening programme for colorectal cancer. *Gut.* 1989;30:481-483.
4. Garland CF, Lilienfeld AM, Mendeloff AI, Markowitz JA, Terrell KB, Garland FC. Incidence rates of ulcerative colitis and Crohn's disease in fifteen areas of the United States. *Gastroenterology.* 1981;81:1115-1124.
5. Stowe SP, Redmond SR, Stormont JM, et al. An epidemiologic study of inflammatory bowel disease in Rochester, New York. Hospital incidence. *Gastroenterology.* 1990;98:104-110.
6. Hiatt RA, Kaufman L. Epidemiology of inflammatory bowel disease in a defined Northern California population. *West J Med.* 1988;149:541-546.
7. Podolsky DK. Inflammatory bowel disease. *N Engl J Med.* 2002; 347:417-429.
8. Langholz E, Munkholm P, Davidsen M, Nielsen OH, Binder V. Changes in extent of ulcerative colitis: a study on the course and prognostic factors. *Scand J Gastroenterol.* 1996;31:260-266.
9. Langholz E, Munkholm P, Davidsen M, Binder V. Course of ulcerative colitis: analysis of changes in disease activity over years. *Gastroenterology.* 1994;107:3-11.
10. Hendriksen C, Kreiner S, Binder V. Long term prognosis in ulcerative colitis—based on results from a regional patient group from the county of Copenhagen. *Gut.* 1985;26:158-163.
11. Farmer RG, Easley KA, Rankin GB. Clinical patterns, natural history, and progression of ulcerative colitis. A long-term follow-up of 1116 patients. *Dig Dis Sci.* 1993;38:1137-1146.
12. Langholz E, Munkholm P, Nielsen OH, Kreiner S, Binder V. Incidence and prevalence of ulcerative colitis in Copenhagen county from 1962 to 1987. *Scand J Gastroenterol.* 1991;26:1247-1256.
13. Meucci G, Vecchi M, Astegiano M, et al. The natural history of ulcerative proctitis: a multicenter, retrospective study. Gruppo di Studio per le Malattie Infiammatorie Intestinali (GSMII). *Am J Gastroenterol.* 2000;95:469-473.
14. Powell-Tuck J, Ritchie JK, Lennard-Jones JE. The prognosis of idiopathic proctitis. *Scand J Gastroenterol.* 1977;12:727-732.
15. Jewell D. Ulcerative colitis. In: Feldman M, Friedman LS, Sleisenger MH, eds. *Sleisenger and Fordtran's Gastrointestinal and Liver Disease.* Vol. 2. Philadelphia, PA: WB Saunders; 2002:2039-2067.
16. Greenstein AJ, Aufses AH Jr. Differences in pathogenesis, incidence and outcome of perforation in inflammatory bowel disease. *Surg Gynecol Obstet.* 1985;160:63-69.
17. Levine JB, Lukawski-Trubish D. Extraintestinal considerations in inflammatory bowel disease. *Gastroenterol Clin North Am.* 1995;24:633-646.
18. Orchard TR, Wordsworth BP, Jewell DP. Peripheral arthropathies in inflammatory bowel disease: their articular distribution and natural history. *Gut.* 1998;42:387-391.
19. Palli D, Trallori G, Saieva C, et al. General and cancer specific mortality of a population based cohort of patients with inflammatory bowel disease: the Florence Study. *Gut.* 1998;42:175-179.
20. Orchard TR, Chua CN, Ahmad T, Cheng H, Welsh KI, Jewell DP. Uveitis and erythema nodosum in inflammatory bowel disease: clinical features and the role of HLA genes. *Gastroenterology.* 2002;123:714-718.
21. Bernstein CN. Extraintestinal manifestations of inflammatory bowel disease. *Curr Gastroenterol Rep.* 2001;3:477-483.
22. Raj V, Lichtenstein DR. Hepatobiliary manifestations of inflammatory bowel disease. *Gastroenterol Clin North Am.* 1999;28:491-513.
23. MacLean AR, Lilly L, Cohen Z, O'Connor B, McLeod RS. Outcome of patients undergoing liver transplantation for primary sclerosing cholangitis. *Dis Colon Rectum.* 2003;46:1124-1128.
24. Chapman RW, Arborgh BA, Rhodes JM, et al. Primary sclerosing cholangitis: a review of its clinical features, cholangiography, and hepatic histology. *Gut.* 1980;21:870-877.
25. Wiesner RH, LaRusso NF. Clinicopathologic features of the syndrome of primary sclerosing cholangitis. *Gastroenterology.* 1980; 79:200-206.
26. Lee YM, Kaplan MM. Primary sclerosing cholangitis. *N Engl J Med.* 1995;332:924-933.
27. Gow PJ, Chapman RW. Liver transplantation for primary sclerosing cholangitis. *Liver.* 2000;20:97-103.
28. Feith MP, Klompmaker IJ, Maring JK, et al. Biliary reconstruction during liver transplantation in patients with primary sclerosing cholangitis. *Transplant Proc.* 1997;29:560-561.
29. Harrison RF, Davies MH, Neuberger JM, Hubscher SG. Fibrous and obliterative cholangitis in liver allografts: evidence of recurrent primary sclerosing cholangitis? *Hepatology.* 1994;20:356-361.
30. Abu-Elmagd KM, Malinchoc M, Dickson ER, et al. Efficacy of hepatic transplantation in patients with primary sclerosing cholangitis. *Surg Gynecol Obstet.* 1993;177:335-344.
31. Broome U, Glaumann H, Lindstom E, et al. Natural history and outcome in 32 Swedish patients with small duct primary sclerosing cholangitis (PSC). *J Hepatol.* 2002;36:586-589.
32. Loftus EV Jr, Sandborn WJ. Lymphoma risk in inflammatory bowel disease: influences of referral bias and therapy. *Gastroenterology.* 2001;121:1239-1242.
33. Lewis JD, Bilker WB, Brensinger C, Deren JJ, Vaughn DJ, Strom BL. Inflammatory bowel disease is not associated with an increased risk of lymphoma. *Gastroenterology.* 2001;121:1080-1087.
34. Loftus EV Jr. Epidemiology and risk factors for colorectal dysplasia and cancer in ulcerative colitis. *Gastroenterol Clin North Am.* 2006:517-531.
35. Ekbom A, Helmick C, Zack M, Adami HO. Ulcerative colitis and colorectal cancer. A population-based study. *N Engl J Med.* 1990; 323:1228-1233.
36. Jess T, Loftus EV Jr, Velayos FS, et al. Risk of intestinal cancer in inflammatory bowel disease: a population-based study from Olmsted County, Minnesota. *Gastroenterology.* 2006:1039-1046.
37. Choi PM, Kim WH. Colon cancer surveillance. *Gastroenterol Clin North Am.* 1995;24:671-687.
38. Rutter M, Saunders B, Wilkinson K, et al. Severity of inflammation is a risk factor for colorectal neoplasia in ulcerative colitis. *Gastroenterology.* 2004;126:451-459.
39. Jensen AB, Larsen M, Gislum M, et al. Survival after colorectal cancer in patients with ulcerative colitis: a nationwide population-based Danish study. *Am J Gastroenterol.* 2006;1283-1287.
40. Bernstein CN, Shanahan F, Weinstein WM. Are we telling patients the truth about surveillance colonoscopy in ulcerative colitis? *Lancet.* 1994;343:71-74.
41. Ullman TA, Loftus EV Jr, Kakar S, Burgart LJ, Sandborn WJ, Tremaine WJ. The fate of low grade dysplasia in ulcerative colitis. *Am J Gastroenterol.* 2002;97:922-927.
42. Ullman T, Croog V, Harpaz N, Sachar D, Itzkowitz S. Progression of flat low-grade dysplasia to advanced neoplasia in patients with ulcerative colitis. *Gastroenterology.* 2003;125:1311-1319.
43. Lynch DA, Lobo AJ, Sobala GM, Dixon MF, Axon AT. Failure of colonoscopic surveillance in ulcerative colitis. *Gut.* 1993;34:1075-1080.
44. Blackstone MO, Riddell RH, Rogers BH, Levin B. Dysplasia-associated lesion or mass (DALM) detected by colonoscopy in long-standing ulcerative colitis: an indication for colectomy. *Gastroenterology.* 1981;80:366-374.

45. Broome U, Lofberg R, Veress B, Eriksson LS. Primary sclerosing cholangitis and ulcerative colitis: evidence for increased neoplastic potential. *Hepatology.* 1995;22:1404-1408.
46. Kornfeld D, Ekbom A, Ihre T. Is there an excess risk for colorectal cancer in patients with ulcerative colitis and concomitant primary sclerosing cholangitis? A population based study. *Gut.* 1997;41:522-525.
47. Marchesa P, Lashner BA, Lavery IC, et al. The risk of cancer and dysplasia among ulcerative colitis patients with primary sclerosing cholangitis. *Am J Gastroenterol.* 1997;92:1285-1288.
48. Leidenius MH, Farkkila MA, Karkkainen P, Taskinen EI, Kellokumpu IH, Hockerstedt KA. Colorectal dysplasia and carcinoma in patients with ulcerative colitis and primary sclerosing cholangitis. *Scand J Gastroenterol.* 1997;32:706-711.
49. Rodrigues CM, Kren BT, Steer CJ, Setchell KD. The site-specific delivery of ursodeoxycholic acid to the rat colon by sulfate conjugation. *Gastroenterology.* 1995;109:1835-1844.
50. Batta AK, Salen G, Holubec H, Brasitus TA, Alberts D, Earnest DL. Enrichment of the more hydrophilic bile acid ursodeoxycholic acid in the fecal water-soluble fraction after feeding to rats with colon polyps. *Cancer Res.* 1998;58:1684-1687.
51. Pardi DS, Loftus EV Jr, Kremers WK, Keach J, Lindor KD. Ursodeoxycholic acid as a chemopreventive agent in patients with ulcerative colitis and primary sclerosing cholangitis. *Gastroenterology.* 2003;124:889-893.
52. Eaden J, Abrams K, Ekbom A, Jackson E, Mayberry J. Colorectal cancer prevention in ulcerative colitis: a case-control study. *Aliment Pharmacol Ther.* 2000;14:145-153.
53. van Staa TP, Card T, Logan RF, Leufkens HGM. 5-Aminosalicylate use and colorectal cancer risk in inflammatory bowel disease: a large epidemiologic study. *Gut.* 2005:1573-1578.
54. Rubin DT, LoSavio A, Yadron N, et al. Aminosalicylate therapy in the prevention of dysplasia and colorectal cancer in ulcerative colitis. *Clin Gastroenterol Hepatol.* 2006:1346-1350.
55. Bernstein CN, Eaden J, Steinhart AH, Munkholm P, Gordon PH. Cancer prevention in inflammatory bowel disease and the chemoprophylactic potential of 5-aminosalicylic acid. *Inflamm Bowel Dis.* 2002;8:356-361.
56. Velayos FS, Terdiman JP, Walsh JM. Effect of 5-aminosalicylate use on colorectal cancer and dysplasia risk: a systematic review and metaanalysis of observational studies. *Am J Gastroenterol.* 2005; 100:1345-1353.
57. Velayos FS, Loftus EV Jr, Jess T, et al. Predictive and protective factors associated with colorectal cancer in ulcerative colitis: a case-control study. *Gastroenterology.* 2006;130:1941-1949.
58. Selby W. The natural history of ulcerative colitis. *Baillieres Clin Gastroenterol.* 1997;11:53-64.
59. Winther KV, Jess T, Langholz E, Munkholm P, Binder V. Survival and cause-specific mortality in ulcerative colitis: follow-up of a population-based cohort in Copenhagen County. *Gastroenterology.* 2003;125:1576-1582.
60. Ekbom A, Helmick CG, Zack M, Holmberg L, Adami HO. Survival and causes of death in patients with inflammatory bowel disease: a population-based study. *Gastroenterology.* 1992;103:954-960.
61. Persson PG, Bernell O, Leijonmarck CE, Farahmand BY, Hellers G, Ahlbom A. Survival and cause-specific mortality in inflammatory bowel disease: a population-based cohort study. *Gastroenterology.* 1996;110:1339-1345.
62. Jess T, Loftus EV Jr, Harmsen WS, et al. Survival and cause specific mortality in patients with inflammatory bowel disease: a long term outcome study in Olmsted County, Minnesota, 1940-2004. *Gut.* 2006;55:1248-1254.
63. Sonnenberg A. Deadly IBD. *Inflammatory Bowel Diseases.* 2006;3:246.
64. Langholz E, Munkholm P, Davidsen M, Binder V. Colorectal cancer risk and mortality in patients with ulcerative colitis. *Gastroenterology.* 1992;103:1444-1451.
65. Irvine EJ. Quality of life issues in patients with inflammatory bowel disease. *Am J Gastroenterol.* 1997;92(12 suppl):18S-24S.
66. Hjortswang H, Jarnerot G, Curman B, et al. The influence of demographic and disease-related factors on health-related quality of life in patients with ulcerative colitis. *Eur J Gastroenterol Hepatol.* 2003;15:1011-1020.
67. Rubin GP, Hungin AP, Chinn DJ, Dwarakanath D. Quality of life in patients with established inflammatory bowel disease: a UK general practice survey. *Aliment Pharmacol Ther.* 2004;19:529-535.
68. Hjortswang H, Strom M, Almer S. Health-related quality of life in Swedish patients with ulcerative colitis. *Am J Gastroenterol.* 1998; 93:2203-2211.
69. Drossman DA, Patrick DL, Mitchell CM, Zagami EA, Appelbaum MI. Health-related quality of life in inflammatory bowel disease. Functional status and patient worries and concerns. *Dig Dis Sci.* 1989;34:1379-1386.
70. Farmer RG, Whelan G, Fazio VW. Long-term follow-up of patients with Crohn's disease. Relationship between the clinical pattern and prognosis. *Gastroenterology.* 1985;88:1818-1825.
71. Sands BE. Crohn's disease. In: Feldman M, Friedman LS, Sleisenger MH, eds. *Sleisenger and Fordtran's Gastrointestinal and Liver Disease.* Vol. 2. Philadelphia, PA: WB Saunders; 2002:2005-2038.
72. Munkholm P, Langholz E, Davidsen M, Binder V. Disease activity courses in a regional cohort of Crohn's disease patients. *Scand J Gastroenterol.* 1995;30:699-706.
73. Polito JM II, Childs B, Mellits ED, Tokayer AZ, Harris ML, Bayless TM. Crohn's disease: influence of age at diagnosis on site and clinical type of disease. *Gastroenterology.* 1996;111:580-586.
74. Lichtenstein GR, Olson A, Travers S, et al. Factors associated with the development of intestinal strictures or obstructions in patients with Crohn's disease. *Am J Gastroenterol.* 2006:1030-1038.
75. Schwartz DA, Loftus EV Jr, Tremaine WJ, et al. The natural history of fistulizing Crohn's disease in Olmsted County, Minnesota. *Gastroenterology.* 2002;122:875-880.
76. Sands BE, Arsenault JE, Rosen MJ, et al. Risk of early surgery for Crohn's disease: implications for early treatment strategies. *Am J Gastroenterol.* 2003;98:2712-2718.
77. Cuthbert AP, Fisher SA, Mirza MM, et al. The contribution of NOD2 gene mutations to the risk and site of disease in inflammatory bowel disease. *Gastroenterology.* 2002;122:867-874.
78. Abreu MT, Taylor KD, Lin YC, et al. Mutations in NOD2 are associated with fibrostenosing disease in patients with Crohn's disease. *Gastroenterology.* 2002;123:679-688.
79. Torok HP, Glas J, Tonenchi L, et al. Polymorphisms in the DLG5 and OCTN cation transporter genes in Crohn's disease. *Gut.* 2005;54:1421-1427.
80. Whelan G, Farmer RG, Fazio VW, Goormastic M. Recurrence after surgery in Crohn's disease. Relationship to location of disease (clinical pattern) and surgical indication. *Gastroenterology.* 1985;88:1826-1833.
81. Sachar DB. The problem of postoperative recurrence of Crohn's disease. *Med Clin North Am.* 1990;74:183-188.
82. Olaison G, Smedh K, Sjodahl R. Natural course of Crohn's disease after ileocolic resection: endoscopically visualised ileal ulcers preceding symptoms. *Gut.* 1992;33:331-335.

83. Hanauer SB, Feagan BG, Lichtenstein GR, et al. Maintenance infliximab for Crohn's disease: the ACCENT I randomised trial. *Lancet.* 2002;359:1541-1549.

84. Sands BE, Anderson FH, Bernstein CN, et al. Infliximab maintenance therapy for fistulizing Crohn's disease. *N Engl J Med.* 2004; 350:876-885.

85. Poritz LS, Rowe WA, Koltun WA. Remicade does not abolish the need for surgery in fistulizing Crohn's disease. *Dis Colon Rectum.* 2002;45:771-775.

86. Sninsky CA. Altering the natural history of Crohn's disease? *Inflamm Bowel Dis.* 2001;7(suppl 1):S34-S39.

87. Vestergaard P, Krogh K, Rejnmark L, Laurberg S, Mosekilde L. Fracture risk is increased in Crohn's disease, but not in ulcerative colitis. *Gut.* 2000;46:176-181.

88. van Staa TP, Cooper C, Brusse LS, Leufkens H, Javaid MK, Arden NK. Inflammatory bowel disease and the risk of fracture. *Gastroenterology.* 2003;125:1591-1597.

89. Haderslev KV, Tjellesen L, Sorensen HA, Staun M. Alendronate increases lumbar spine bone mineral density in patients with Crohn's disease. *Gastroenterology.* 2000;119:639-646.

90. Heikius B, Niemela S, Lehtola J, Karttunen T, Lahde S. Hepatobiliary and coexisting pancreatic duct abnormalities in patients with inflammatory bowel disease. *Scand J Gastroenterol.* 1997;32:153-161.

91. Rasmussen HH, Fallingborg JF, Mortensen PB, Vyberg M, Tage-Jensen U, Rasmussen SN. Hepatobiliary dysfunction and primary sclerosing cholangitis in patients with Crohn's disease. *Scand J Gastroenterol.* 1997;32:604-610.

92. Collier PE, Turowski P, Diamond DL. Small intestinal adenocarcinoma complicating regional enteritis. *Cancer.* 1985;55:516-521.

93. Bernstein D, Rogers A. Malignancy in Crohn's disease. *Am J Gastroenterol.* 1996;91:434-440.

94. Canavan C, Abrams KR, Mayberry J. Meta-analysis: colorectal and small bowel cancer risk in patients with Crohn's disease. *Aliment Pharmacol Ther.* 2006;23:1097-1104.

95. Bernstein CN, Blanchard JF, Kliewer E, Wajda A. Cancer risk in patients with inflammatory bowel disease: a population-based study. *Cancer.* 2001;91:854-862.

96. Gillen CD, Walmsley RS, Prior P, Andrews HA, Allan RN. Ulcerative colitis and Crohn's disease: a comparison of the colorectal cancer risk in extensive colitis. *Gut.* 1994;35:1590-1592.

97. Gillen CD, Andrews HA, Prior P, Allan RN. Crohn's disease and colorectal cancer. *Gut.* 1994;35:651-655.

98. Sjodahl RI, Myrelid P, Soderholm JD. Anal and rectal cancer in Crohn's disease. *Colorectal Dis.* 2003;5:490-495.

99. Loftus EV Jr, Tremaine WJ, Habermann TM, Harmsen WS, Zinsmeister AR, Sandborn WJ. Risk of lymphoma in inflammatory bowel disease. *Am J Gastroenterol.* 2000;95:2308-2312.

100. Greenstein AJ, Mullin GE, Strauchen JA, et al. Lymphoma in inflammatory bowel disease. *Cancer.* 1992;69:1119-1123.

101. Ekbom A, Helmick C, Zack M, Adami HO. Extracolonic malignancies in inflammatory bowel disease. *Cancer.* 1991;67:2015-2019.

102. Ky A, Sohn N, Weinstein MA, Korelitz BI. Carcinoma arising in anorectal fistulas of Crohn's disease. *Dis Colon Rectum.* 1998; 41:992-996.

103. Buchman AL, Ament ME, Doty J. Development of squamous cell carcinoma in chronic perineal sinus and wounds in Crohn's disease. *Am J Gastroenterol.* 1991;86:1829-1832.

104. Cucino C, Sonnenberg A. Cause of death in patients with inflammatory bowel disease. *Inflamm Bowel Dis.* 2001;7:250-255.

105. Jess T, Winther KV, Munkholm P, Langholz E, Binder V. Mortality and causes of death in Crohn's disease: follow-up of a population-based cohort in Copenhagen County, Denmark. *Gastroenterology.* 2002;122:1808-1814.

106. Card T, Hubbard R, Logan RF. Mortality in inflammatory bowel disease: a population-based cohort study. *Gastroenterology.* 2003;125:1583-1590.

107. Wolters FL, Russel MG, Sijbrandij J, et al. Crohn's disease: increased mortality 10 years after diagnosis in a Europe-wide population based cohort. *Gut.* 2006;55:510-518.

108. Lichtenstein GR, Feagan BG, Cohen RD, et al. Serious infections and mortality in association with therapies for Crohn's disease: TREAT registry. *Clin Gastroenterol Hepatol.* 2006;4:621-630.

109. Farmer RG, Easley KA, Farmer JM. Quality of life assessment by patients with inflammatory bowel disease. *Cleve Clin J Med.* 1992; 59:35-42.

110. Drossman DA, Leserman J, Li ZM, Mitchell CM, Zagami EA, Patrick DL. The rating form of IBD patient concerns: a new measure of health status. *Psychosom Med.* 1991;53:701-712.

111. Cohen RD. The quality of life in patients with Crohn's disease. *Aliment Pharmacol Ther.* 2002;16:1603-1609.

112. Blondel-Kucharski F, Chircop C, Marquis P, et al. Health-related quality of life in Crohn's disease: a prospective longitudinal study in 231 patients. *Am J Gastroenterol.* 2001;96:2915-2920.

113. Lichtenstein GR, Yan S, Bala M, Hanauer S. Remission in patients with Crohn's disease is associated with improvement in employment and quality of life and a decrease in hospitalizations and surgeries. *Am J Gastroenterol.* 2004;99:91-96.

114. Feagan BG, Yan S, Bala M, Bao W, Lichtenstein GR. The effects of infliximab maintenance therapy on health-related quality of life. *Am J Gastroenterol.* 2003;98:2232-2238.

115. Mayberry MK, Probert C, Srivastava E, Rhodes J, Mayberry JF. Perceived discrimination in education and employment by people with Crohn's disease: a case control study of educational achievement and employment. *Gut.* 1992;33:312-314.

116. Langholz E, Munkholm P, Krasilnikoff PA, Binder V. Inflammatory bowel diseases with onset in childhood. Clinical features, morbidity, and mortality in a regional cohort. *Scand J Gastroenterol.* 1997; 32:139-147.

117. Mamula P, Telega GW, Markowitz JE, et al. Inflammatory bowel disease in children 5 years of age and younger. *Am J Gastroenterol.* 2002;97:2005-2010.

118. Lindberg E, Lindquist B, Holmquist L, Hildebrand H. Inflammatory bowel disease in children and adolescents in Sweden, 1984-1995. *J Pediatr Gastroenterol Nutr.* 2000;30:259-264.

119. Mamula P, Markowitz JE, Baldassano RN. Inflammatory bowel disease in early childhood and adolescence: special considerations. *Gastroenterol Clin North Am.* 2003;32:967-995, viii.

120. Kirschner BS. Ulcerative colitis in children. *Pediatr Clin North Am.* 1996;43:235-254.

121. Hyams JS, Davis P, Grancher K, Lerer T, Justinich CJ, Markowitz J. Clinical outcome of ulcerative colitis in children. *J Pediatr.* 1996; 129:81-88.

122. Griffiths AM, Nguyen P, Smith C, MacMillan JH, Sherman PM. Growth and clinical course of children with Crohn's disease. *Gut.* 1993;34:939-943.

123. Stephens MC, Shepanski MA, Mamula P, Markowitz JE, Brown KA, Baldassano RN. Safety and steroid-sparing experience using infliximab for Crohn's disease at a pediatric inflammatory bowel disease center. *Am J Gastroenterol.* 2003;98:104-111.

124. Watts JM, De Dombal FT, Watkinson G, Goligher JC. Long-term prognosis of ulcerative colitis. *Br Med J.* 1966;5501:1447-1453.

125. Sinclair TS, Brunt PW, Mowat NA. Nonspecific proctocolitis in northeastern Scotland: a community study. *Gastroenterology.* 1983; 85:1-11.

126. Fleischer DE, Grimm IS, Friedman LS. Inflammatory bowel disease in older patients. *Med Clin North Am.* 1994;78:1303-1319.

127. Wagtmans MJ, Verspaget HW, Lamers CB, van Hogezand RA. Crohn's disease in the elderly: a comparison with young adults. *J Clin Gastroenterol.* 1998;27:129-133.
128. Shivananda S, Lennard-Jones J, Logan R, et al. Incidence of inflammatory bowel disease across Europe: is there a difference between north and south? Results of the European Collaborative Study on Inflammatory Bowel Disease (EC-IBD). *Gut.* 1996;39:690-697.
129. Softley A, Myren J, Clamp SE, Bouchier IA, Watkinson G, de Dombal FT. Inflammatory bowel disease in the elderly patient. *Scand J Gastroenterol Suppl.* 1988;144:27-30.

2

Clinical Research in Inflammatory Bowel Disease

Placebo Response in Clinical Trials

Chinyu Su, MD and James D. Lewis, MD, MSCE

A major goal of clinical research is to identify new therapies for the treatment of disease. In addition, research is used to define the potential risks of therapeutic interventions. In the realm of inflammatory bowel disease (IBD), there has been an enormous explosion in our knowledge of the underlying cause of these diseases and in development of therapeutic interventions. This chapter will provide a brief overview of the design and interpretation of clinical trials, with a focus on the role of placebo.

Overview of Clinical Research Designs

Clinical research can be divided into descriptive and analytic studies. Descriptive studies include case reports, case series, and analyses of secular trends. The feature that most distinguishes descriptive studies from analytic studies is the lack of a control group. Because there is no control group for comparison, descriptive studies are generally viewed as useful for hypothesis generation but play a small role in proving causality. As will be discussed later in this chapter, uncontrolled studies of drug therapies for IBD (ie, case series) play an important role in selecting medications for further investigation. By themselves, however, these studies cannot be used to determine efficacy.

In contrast to descriptive studies, analytic studies are characterized by the inclusion of a control group, thereby allowing the investigator to test a hypothesis. Analytic studies can be further divided into observational studies and experimental studies. The prototypical classification of observational analytic studies includes case-control studies and cohort studies. In case-control studies, the investigator identifies subjects with the outcome of interest and control subjects without the outcome. One then examines the subjects' prior exposures to determine whether there is an association between the outcome and the exposure. An example would include studies comparing patients with ulcerative colitis and colon cancer to others with ulcerative colitis and no colon cancer to determine whether prior use of mesalamine is associated with a reduced risk of colon cancer.

Cohort studies use the opposite design, starting with subjects who are exposed to medication and others who are not. These subjects are then followed over time to determine which subjects develop the outcome of interest. For example, one could follow a group of patients with ulcerative colitis, some of whom are receiving mesalamine therapy and others who are not. The investigator could then determine whether the incidence of colon cancer differed between these two groups.

In broad terms, major potential limitations of observational analytic studies include information bias, selection bias, and confounding. Information bias (ie, bias resulting from inaccurate or incomplete data collection) can often be prevented or minimized through appropriate design of the study. Selection bias can lead to incorrect conclusions from observational studies when the probability of selection is related to both the exposure under study and the outcome of interest. Appropriate measures can minimize the probability of selection bias, although in practical terms, it is often difficult to know for certain how well this has been

Lichtenstein GR, ed.
Ulcerative Colitis: The Complete Guide to Medical Management (pp. 27-32)

accomplished. *Confounding* refers to a mixing of effects. If the exposure of interest is associated with a third factor that is also associated with the outcome of interest, failure to account for this third factor in the design or analysis of the study can lead to a biased result. Unfortunately, one can only account for confounding factors that are known or suspected prior to the start of the study. Thus, all observational analytic studies have the potential limitation of bias from unknown (and/or unmeasured) confounders.

Experimental analytic studies include clinical trials. The key feature that distinguishes experimental studies from observational studies is that the investigator assigns the treatment to subjects. The randomized clinical trial design is considered the gold standard for proving efficacy of an intervention. In the case of IBD, the intervention is typically medical therapy. Nearly all clinical trials use random allocation to assign the treatment categories. In the prototypical randomized clinical trial, patients are randomly assigned to receive one of the two or more exposures or interventions to be tested. They are then followed over a predetermined study period to measure the incidence of the outcome of interest. The main reason that the randomized clinical trial is afforded such accolades is that with a large enough sample size, the use of randomization prevents bias from unequal distribution of known and unknown confounders. In addition, because assignment of exposure status is random, selection bias is not a problem. For these reasons, the randomized clinical trial usually provides the strongest evidence of efficacy of any of the analytic designs.

Not all clinical trials are randomized controlled trials. Phase I drug studies are used to examine the safety of compounds that have not been previously given to humans. These studies typically treat a small number of subjects with the new medication. The study begins with very low doses and gradually increases the dose either between subjects or within subjects to establish a maximum tolerated dose. There is no control group in phase I studies. Phase II studies are designed to gain additional safety data, to begin to collect evidence of efficacy, and to select the optimal dose for use in phase III studies. Phase II studies will often include several different doses of the medications. While traditionally phase II studies did not include a placebo arm, in recent years it has been common to see placebo arms in phase II trials. Phase III trials are designed to prove efficacy. These are generally large randomized controlled trials that typically include a placebo arm but could also compare the new therapy to an existing alternative.

INTERPRETATION OF CLINICAL TRIAL RESULTS

Clinical trials generally report their results as incidence rates in the different treatment arms, relative risks, risk differences, and/or the number needed to treat. For studies with two treatment arms, the investigators may report relative risks (or relative rates for longer studies). Relative risks are a proportion of incidence rates. Thus, a relative risk of 2 implies that the exposed group is twice as likely as the control group to experience the outcome of interest. Results may also be reported as risk differences. This is the absolute difference in the incidence rates between the two groups. For example, if the incidence of remission in the group treated with mesalamine was 50% and it was 10% in the control group, the risk difference would be 40%. This provides a measure of the absolute benefit one might expect from the therapy. It is important to realize that two interventions can have the same relative risk and yet have very different risk differences, or vice versa. For example, if arm A had a 20% remission rate and arm B had a 40% remission rate, the relative risk of arm B versus arm A would be 2 with a risk difference of 20%. In contrast, if arm A had a 10% remission rate and arm B had a 20% remission rate, the relative risk of arm B versus arm A would again be 2, but with a risk difference of only 10%. To help place these into context, investigators often report the number needed to treat in order to achieve one additional outcome with one therapy versus the alternative. This is calculated as the inverse of the risk difference. Thus, in these examples, in the first study, the number needed to treat with B compared to A to achieve one additional remission would be 5, whereas in the second study it would be 10. Thus, for a fixed relative risk, one must look at the risk difference to understand the number needed to treat.

CHOICE OF CONTROL GROUPS FOR RANDOMIZED CLINICAL TRIALS

When designing a randomized clinical trial, investigators must choose between an active control or a placebo (ie, an inert substance). There are several advantages and disadvantages to each option. Let's consider an example of a new therapy for severe steroid refractory ulcerative colitis. If one compares the new therapy to placebo therapy, the results will provide strong evidence of whether the new therapy is biologically active. It will not provide information on whether the intervention is as good or better than the currently available therapies, however. In addition, patients with severe disease may be reluctant to enroll in a study where they may receive a placebo. Finally, some people might argue that enrolling patients into a trial with a placebo arm when there are known efficacious alternatives is unethical. Though discussion of the ethics of the use of placebo is beyond the scope of this chapter, there are nearly always at least some subgroups of patients for whom no reasonable alternative therapy exists, thus making placebo an option.

It is this concern over the ethics of the use of placebo that often leads people to suggest the use of an active comparator arm. Use of active comparator arms is also fraught with problems of interpretation, particularly if studies do not prove superior or equivalent efficacy of the new therapy. When designing a study using an active comparator, it is critical that the active comparator be proven to be efficacious. Even if this criterion is met, use of an active comparator can still result in difficulties with interpretation. Imagine a scenario where the standard therapy is known to induce remission in 60% of patients. In a clinical trial of a new therapy versus the standard therapy, the remission rates are 40% and 60%, respectively. After the study, one concludes that the new therapy is not superior or even equivalent to the standard therapy. However, it is still possible that the new therapy is efficacious, albeit less so than the standard therapy. Without a placebo control arm, this cannot be known. As such, a potentially beneficial therapy may be wrongly discarded. Patients who do not respond to the standard therapy or who have a contraindication to the standard therapy may have been wrongly deprived of potentially helpful therapy because no placebo arm was used. Thus, even in the 21st century, the use of placebo in randomized controlled trials remains important and often preferred to active comparators for initial studies of efficacy. Once an intervention is proven efficacious, head-to-head comparisons to alternative therapies are incredibly helpful in designing appropriate treatment algorithms. Bypassing the placebo controlled studies is, however, potentially fraught with error. Placebo control is particularly important in diseases such as IBD that are characterized by spontaneous periods of acute exacerbation and quiescence.

PLACEBO VERSUS BLINDING

One might ask whether it is necessary to use a placebo versus randomizing patients to no therapy. To understand this, one must understand the concept of *blinding* (also referred to as *masking*). Blinding refers to concealing the treatment assignment in such a manner that the subject and/or the investigator do not know who is receiving which treatment. The importance of blinding is to prevent detection bias. From the perspective of the patient, he or she may be more likely to report a side effect or to report improvement in symptoms if he or she knows that he or she is receiving the active therapy. Likewise, the investigator may be biased in his or her assessment of efficacy or adverse events if he or she knows which patients are receiving which therapy. Blinding can prevent such bias. One role of placebo is to facilitate blinding in medication studies. By using an inactive substance designed to be indistinguishable from the active therapy, one can achieve blinding of both patients and physicians.

Not all placebos are able to achieve blinding. Many medications have known side effect profiles or other characteristics that can result in unblinding. For example, if a medication has a unique taste or odor, this may be difficult to mimic in the placebo. Thus, use of a placebo does not assure effective blinding of subjects or investigators.

IS THE USE OF PLACEBO REALLY INERT?

Although the goal of a placebo-controlled trial is to determine whether a new therapy is better than no therapy, one might suspect that the use of placebo is not entirely inert. In fact, placebo can be defined as "any therapeutic procedure, without any specific activity, given deliberately to have an effect, or unknowingly has an effect on a patient, symptom, syndrome or disease, but which is objectively without specific activity for the condition being treated."[1] There is ample evidence in the medical literature that placebo therapy may not be inert. A systematic review of clinical trials comparing placebo to no treatment documented superiority of placebo in several conditions.[2] In general, placebo appeared superior to no treatment when the outcome was subjective and was measured on a continuous scale.[2]

Better outcomes with placebo compared to no treatment could occur for several reasons. First, the magnitude of the "placebo effect" may depend on the type of patient, the personality of the physician and health-care providers involved in the care, and their interactions. Patients who enroll in a clinical trial do not receive standard care. Rather, they usually receive much closer follow-up and frequent questioning about their medication adherence and are asked to pay closer attention to their symptoms, etc. All of these could potentially affect the outcome of the disease. For these reasons, the outcomes observed in clinical trials do not always mirror those observed in actual practice (ie, efficacy does not always equate to effectiveness). Another important factor is the patient's expectation regarding the therapy. Placebo effect is unlikely to be present if the patient knows that the treatment is ineffective. In addition, it is possible that there are true biological effects resulting from treatment with a substance that the patient believes to be effective, even if it is not. Thus, the placebo effect likely has no single specific mechanism of action whereby clinical and/or physiological changes take place.

It is also important to note that response or improvement observed in placebo-treated patients is in reality the result of the sum of the true placebo effect and the natural history of the disease. Importantly, patients tend to enroll in clinical trials when their disease is near its worst. In this case, there is greater opportunity for improvement than for further worsening. This is often referred to as *regression to the mean.*

TABLE 2-1

FACTORS ASSOCIATED WITH REMISSION OUTCOMES IN PLACEBO-TREATED GROUPS IN SYSTEMATIC REVIEWS OF CLINICAL TRIALS FOR ACTIVE CROHN'S DISEASE*

Positive Association	Negative Association
Study duration	Baseline CDAI scores
Number of study visits	Baseline CRP levels

* CDAI indicates Crohn's Disease Activity Index; CRP, c-reactive protein.

Adapted from Su C, Lichtenstein GR, Krok K, Brensinger CM, Lewis JD. A meta-analysis of the placebo rates of remission and response in clinical trials of active Crohn's disease. *Gastroenterology.* 2004;126:1257-1269 and Will M, Nikolaus S, Freitag S, Arpe N, Krawczak M, Schreiber S. Placebo response in the therapy of Crohn's disease: A comprehensive analysis of primary data from 733 patients from 13 randomized controlled trials. *Gastroenterology.* 2005;128:A-48.

WHAT FACTORS INFLUENCE THE OUTCOMES IN THE PLACEBO GROUP

Several studies have examined the outcomes of patients treated with placebo in both ulcerative colitis and Crohn's disease trials. Systematic reviews of the literature in this regard have generally focused on patients with active disease. Much less is known about patients who receive placebo in maintenance trials. Furthermore, these trials are more difficult to interpret because many studies allowed all patients to be on some form of therapy with or without the medication under study. The discussion in this chapter will therefore focus predominantly on trials of therapies for active IBD.

Crohn's Disease

One major difficulty in interpreting the placebo outcomes in randomized controlled trials for IBD is the variability in the definition of outcomes among studies. In trials for Crohn's disease, the Crohn's Disease Activity Index (CDAI) is the most commonly employed disease activity measure.[3] This measure incorporates both objective and subjective measures of disease activity. The summary score can range from 0 to approximately 600 with higher scores reflecting more severe disease. A CDAI of less than 150 is generally used to define remission, and a decrease of more than 70 or 100 points is often used to define a clinical response.

Meyers and Janowitz reviewed the outcomes of patients receiving placebo for active Crohn's disease in 3 early clinical trials.[4] Their qualitative review highlighted several important observations. First, some patients treated with placebo will enter clinical remission. They noted that remission rates were relatively similar in the National Cooperative Crohn's Disease Study (NCCDS; 26% at 17 weeks)[5] and the European Cooperative Crohn's Disease Study (ECCDS; 42% at 100 days).[6] In addition, Meyers and Janowitz noted that there were a few features that seemed to identify which patients treated with placebo were more likely to improve. In the NCCDS study, patients not previously treated with steroids, with lower initial CDAI scores, with postsurgical recurrence, and without perianal disease appeared to fare better.[5] In the ECCDS, patients treated with placebo were more likely to enter remission if they had not received prior therapy for Crohn's disease or if they had small bowel disease.[6]

More recently, we examined the outcome of patients randomized to placebo in a systematic review and meta-analysis.[7] Our meta-analysis included 23 studies that used the CDAI to measure disease activity. All studies were randomized controlled trials of therapies for active Crohn's disease. We observed a pooled estimate of remission among placebo-treated patients of 18%, although there was wide variability between studies. The median remission rate was 19% with a range from 0% to 50%. The pooled estimate of placebo response was 19%, with similarly wide variability among studies (range, 0%-46%).

Several factors were identified that appeared to contribute to the remission rate among placebo-treated patients (Table 2-1). The most important factor appeared to be the study duration. The pooled estimate of the remission rate was 12% for studies less than 2 months in duration, 19% for studies 2 to 4 months in duration, and 32% for studies more than 4 months in duration. Other factors that were also positively associated with remission included increasing number of study visits and lower CDAI scores at entry into the study. The positive association between the placebo remission rate and duration of follow-up was unlikely a sustaining phenomenon over time. Few placebo, randomized controlled trials provided outcomes at multiple time points beyond 4 months. In the NCCDS, 18% and 12% of

TABLE 2-2

SUMMARY OF PLACEBO OUTCOMES IN PUBLISHED META-ANALYSES OF CLINICAL TRIALS FOR ACTIVE ULCERATIVE COLITIS

Studies	Remission			Response		
	Clinical	Endoscopic	Histologic	Clinical	Endoscopic	Histologic
Su[7]	13%	18%	8%	28%	–	–
Sutherland[15]	–	–	–	21.6%	–	–
Kornbluth[16]	–	–	–	31.4%	–	–
Ilnyckyj[18]	9.1%	13.5%	8.6%	26.7%	30.3%	25.2%

patients remained in remission on placebo therapy at 1 year and 2 years, respectively.[5] Similar findings were reported in ECCDS, where the remission rates among placebo-treated patients were 18% at 300 days and 9% at 700 days.[6]

We also examined factors associated with a clinical response among the placebo-treated patients. In general, the relationship between factors present at randomization and the probability of response were the same as those that were associated with remission. The major exception was that patients with a higher CDAI score at entry appeared more likely to have a response and less likely to achieve remission.

Both of the systematic reviews described above focused on clinical factors. Several investigators have also looked at biochemical predictors of outcome among placebo-treated patients. C-reactive protein (CRP) levels have been the most widely studied. Will and colleagues performed a pooled analysis of response to placebo therapy using primary data from 13 clinical trials.[8] In both acute disease and maintenance trials, mean CRP levels at randomization were lower in placebo responders than non-responders. In another trial, Schreiber et al demonstrated a strongly negative correlation between baseline CRP levels and the placebo response rate, providing further evidence that CRP levels are related to outcomes among placebo-treated patients.[9]

There are several potential explanations for the relation between CRP levels and outcomes among placebo-treated patients. Despite symptoms suggestive of active Crohn's disease, some patients with low CRP likely do not have active disease despite an elevated CDAI score. For example, some patients may have concomitant irritable bowel syndrome (IBS). The natural history of IBS would project that some patients would have improved symptoms over the time course of a study.[10,11] Alternatively, patients with a low CRP may represent those with milder Crohn's disease.[12-14] This population may be more likely to experience spontaneous improvement in their disease.

Ulcerative Colitis

A few investigators have also explored the outcomes of patients treated with placebo in ulcerative colitis trials (Table 2-2). Sutherland and colleagues performed a meta-analysis of randomized clinical trials of sulfasalazine and mesalamine for ulcerative colitis. From among 8 clinical trials for active disease, the median placebo response rate was 21.6%.[15] In reviews of the early literature on placebo-controlled trials for active ulcerative colitis, clinical response was reported in a mean of approximately 32% of patients.[16,17] Ilnyckyj et al subsequently performed a systematic review of placebo-controlled trials for active ulcerative colitis that included 38 studies.[18] In these studies, the pooled estimates of response were 9.1% for clinical remission, 26.7% for clinical response, 13.5% for endoscopic remission, 30.3% for endoscopic response, 8.6% for histological remission, and 25.2% for histological improvement. These investigators noted that placebo-treated patients with 3 or more study visits had higher rates of clinical response, endoscopic remission, and histological remission, but not clinical remission. They did not observe differences in remission or response rates according to the route of administration of the drug, type of drug, or duration of treatment.

We have also examined this question by performing a meta-analysis of 22 studies that examined the remission rate in active treatment studies.[19] In our analysis, the pooled estimate of remission rate was 13%. Secondary analyses were also performed limiting the studies using a common metric, the Disease Activity Index[20] or slight modifications of this index. This 12-point scale is widely used in ulcerative colitis clinical trials, although no consensus exists for defining remission. Six studies used a definition of remission of a score less than 3 and 6 used a score of 0 to define remission. The pooled estimate of the placebo remission rate in these studies was 17% and 5%, respectively. Both follow-up duration and number of study visits were positively associated with a final Disease Activity Index score of 0 in the placebo-treated patients, whereas the baseline Disease Activity Index score was negatively associated with the placebo remission rate. The estimated rates of endoscopic and histological remission in placebo-treated patients were 18% and 8%, respectively.

CONCLUSION

There are a wide range of clinical research studies, each bearing respective advantages and limitations. Randomized placebo-controlled trials remain the gold standard for proving efficacy of a new or existing therapy in IBD. Placebo outcomes in published clinical trials for active Crohn's disease varied among studies, with an estimated remission rate of 18%. Study duration and number of study visits appeared to be positively associated with achieving remission in placebo-treated patients, whereas the CDAI scores and CRP levels at study entry were inversely associated with such an outcome. Systematic reviews of placebo outcomes in clinical trials for active ulcerative colitis were hampered by the inconsistency of definition of outcomes. Similar to clinical trials for active Crohn's disease, the number of study visits, study duration, and baseline disease severity have all been identified to influence the remission rate in placebo-treated groups. Further studies are clearly necessary to examine factors, both clinical and biochemical, influencing the placebo outcomes in clinical trials for active and quiescent IBD.

REFERENCES

1. Shapiro AK. Factors contributing to the placebo effect. *Am J Psychother.* 1961;18:73-88.
2. Hrobjartsson A, Gotzsche PC. Is the placebo powerless? An analysis of clinical trials comparing placebo with no treatment. [erratum appears in *N Engl J Med.* 2001;345(4):304]. *N Engl J Med.* 2001;344:1594-1602.
3. Best WR, Becktel JM, Singleton JW, Kern F Jr. Development of a Crohn's disease activity index. National Cooperative Crohn's Disease Study. *Gastroenterology.* 1976;70:439-444.
4. Meyers S, Janowitz HD. "Natural history" of Crohn's disease. An analytic review of the placebo lesson. *Gastroenterology.* 1984;87:1189-1192.
5. Summers RW, Switz DM, Sessions JT Jr, et al. National Cooperative Crohn's Disease Study: results of drug treatment. *Gastroenterology.* 1979;77:847-869.
6. Malchow H, Ewe K, Brandes JW, et al. European Cooperative Crohn's Disease Study (ECCDS): results of drug treatment. *Gastroenterology.* 1984;86:249-266.
7. Su C, Lichtenstein GR, Krok K, Brensinger CM, Lewis JD. A meta-analysis of the placebo rates of remission and response in clinical trials of active Crohn's disease. *Gastroenterology.* 2004;126:1257-1269.
8. Will M, Nikolaus S, Freitag S, Arpe N, Krawczak M, Schreiber S. Placebo response in the therapy of Crohn's disease: A comprehensive analysis of primary data from 733 patients from 13 randomized controlled trials. *Gastroenterology.* 2005;128:A-48.
9. Schreiber S, Rutgeerts P, Fedorak RN, et al. Certolizumab pegol (CDP870) appears effective and is well tolerated in Crohn's disease: A randomized, placebo-controlled trial. *Gastroenterology.* 2005;129:807-818.
10. Camilleri M, Northcutt AR, Kong S, Dukes GE, McSorley D, Mangel AW. Efficacy and safety of alosetron in women with irritable bowel syndrome: A randomised, placebo-controlled trial. *Lancet.* 2000;355:1035-1040.
11. Camilleri M, Chey WY, Mayer EA, et al. A randomized controlled clinical trial of the serotonin type 3 receptor antagonist alosetron in women with diarrhea-predominant irritable bowel syndrome. *Arch Intern Med.* 2001;161:1733-1740.
12. Fagan EA, Dyck RF, Maton PN, et al. Serum levels of C-reactive protein in Crohn's disease and ulcerative colitis. *Eur J Clin Invest.* 1982;12:351-359.
13. Chambers RE, Stross P, Barry RE, Whicher JT. Serum amyloid A protein compared with C-reactive protein, alpha 1-antichymotrypsin and alpha 1-acid glycoprotein as a monitor of inflammatory bowel disease. *Eur J Clin Invest.* 1987;17:460-467.
14. Solem CA, Loftus EV, Tremaine WJ, Harmsen S, Zinsmeister AR, Sandborn WJ. Correlation of C-reactive protein (CRP) with clinical, radiographic, and endoscopic activity in inflammatory bowel disease. *Gastroenterology.* 2004;126:A-477.
15. Sutherland LR, May GR, Shaffer EA. Sulfasalazine revisited: a meta-analysis of 5-aminosalicylic acid in the treatment of ulcerative colitis. *Ann Intern Med.* 1993;118:540-549.
16. Kornbluth AA, Salomon P, Sacks HS, Mitty R, Janowitz HD. Meta-analysis of the effectiveness of current drug therapy of ulcerative colitis. *J Clin Gastroenterol.* 1993;16:215-218.
17. Meyers S, Janowitz HD. The "natural history" of ulcerative colitis: an analysis of the placebo response. *J Clin Gastroenterol.* 1989;11:33-37.
18. Ilnyckyj A, Shanahan F, Anton PA, Cheang M, Bernstein CN. Quantification of the placebo response in ulcerative colitis. *Gastroenterology.* 1997;112:1854-1858.
19. Su C, Lewis J, Goldberg B, Brensinger C, Lichtenstein G. A meta-analysis of the placebo rates of remission and response in clinical trials of active ulcerative colitis. *Gastroenterology.* 2007;132(2):516-526.
20. Sutherland LR, Martin F. 5-Aminosalicylic acid enemas in treatment of distal ulcerative colitis and proctitis in Canada. *Dig Dis Sci.* 1987;32:64S-66S.

3

The Role of the FDA in Drug Development in Inflammatory Bowel Disease

Alan C. Moss, MD, FACG and Adam S. Cheifetz, MD

Inflammatory bowel disease (IBD) affects approximately 1 million individuals in the United States and 4 million people worldwide, the majority of whom are prescribed medication for induction or maintenance of remission. At any point in time, more than 75% of patients with IBD are taking prescription medication, which is 3 times higher than the non-IBD population.[1] In addition to standard therapies, developments in molecular biology have identified many novel therapeutic targets that will add to the patient's options. Currently, 24 new drugs are registered in development for ulcerative colitis and 36 for Crohn's disease, in the United States.[2] As a consequence, the market for drugs for IBD patients is valued at $1 to $2 billion in the United States, a number that is expected to rise with increasing use of biologics.[3] The Food and Drug Administration (FDA) has the responsibility to ensure the safety and efficacy of all drugs used in the "cure, mitigation, treatment, or prevention of disease in man." In IBD, a major role for the FDA is its assessment of new therapeutic agents as they navigate the drug development pipeline.

A Brief History of the FDA

The FDA has the broad oversight responsibility for all medical products in the United States.[4] Its legislative basis originated in the Federal Food, Drug and Cosmetic Act of 1938, which required that new drugs be tested for safety before they could be marketed and the results submitted to the FDA. This act arose out of the sulfanilamide elixir disaster of 1937, when more than 100 people died from poisoning by diethylene glycol contained in the elixir. The FDA's role was further expanded with the Kefauver-Harris Amendments in 1962, after the harmful effects of thalidomide on the fetus became known. These amendments required drug manufacturers to prove to the FDA that their products were both safe *and* effective prior to marketing. They also included control over prescription drug advertising and the requirement of informed consent for clinical trials. Biologic agents, medical products derived from living sources, came under the FDA's control in 1972 and later the Center for Biologics Evaluation and Research (CBER).

The Prescription Drug User Fee Act (PDUFA) of 1992 authorized the FDA to levy user fees on manufacturers who submit applications to the agency. This is a method of funding additional staff positions from fees collected directly from drug companies, in order to reduce new drug approval times. The Food and Drug Administration Modernization Act of 1997 expanded the legislation to include accelerated review of drugs and medical devices, as well as regulation of advertising of unapproved uses (off-label) of approved drugs. In 2003, the FDA transferred jurisdiction of many biologics, including monoclonal antibodies, cytokines, novel proteins, immunomodulators, and growth factors, to the Center for Drug Evaluation and Research (CDER), which regulates the approval process for most drugs. CBER maintained jurisdiction over other biologics, such as vaccines, blood products, and gene therapy.

Lichtenstein GR, ed.
Ulcerative Colitis: The Complete Guide to Medical Management (pp. 33-40)

TABLE 3-1

CENTERS OF THE FOOD AND DRUG ADMINISTRATION PERTINENT TO MEDICAL THERAPY

	Center	Responsible For
CDER	Center for Drug Evaluation & Research	Drugs, biologics
CBER	Center for Biologics Evaluation & Research	Vaccines, blood, gene therapy
CDRH	Center for Devices & Radiological Health	Medical devices
NCTR	National Center for Toxicological Research	Toxicology research
ORA	Office of Regulatory Affairs	Enforcement

FDA ORGANIZATION

The FDA is supervised by the Commissioner of Food and Drugs, who is appointed by the president of the United States. The Office of the Commissioner (OC) oversees all the agency's workings and is responsible for implementing the FDA's mission. There are 7 centers within the FDA, each with a different product responsibility (Table 3-1). The CDER has oversight for all drugs and most biologic therapeutic products. CDER is responsible for regulating the manufacturing, labeling, and advertising of drug products. Its main objective is to ensure "safe and effective agents are available to improve the health of consumers."[4] The CDER has 4 functional areas: new drug development and review, post-market drug surveillance, generic drug review, and over-the-counter drug review. New drug development constitutes a major function of the CDER, as it takes approximately 8 years to study and test a new drug before it is approved for use by the public.

FDA PROCESS OF DRUG APPROVAL

The Code of Federal Regulations governs the supervision of new drug development by the FDA. There are 3 key stages: an investigational new drug application, a new drug application, and postmarketing surveillance. This process (Figure 3-1) starts with the filing of an Investigational New Drug (IND) application, a requirement before any clinical trials can take place in humans.[5] The IND is not an application for marketing approval but actually a request for an exemption from the federal statute that prohibits an unapproved drug from being shipped in interstate commerce. Commercial INDs are applications that are submitted primarily by companies whose ultimate goal is to obtain marketing approval for a new product. However, the vast majority of INDs are in fact filed for noncommercial research, including Investigator INDs for research proposals and Emergency Use INDs and Treatment INDs in cases where no other treatments are available for a condition. Once the IND application has been approved, the drug sponsor can undertake clinical trials in humans. This clinical studies process typically takes months to years to complete and involves hundreds to thousands of patients (Table 3-2). At its completion, the drug sponsor can submit a New Drug Application (NDA) to the FDA. Once the division director for that therapeutic area signs an approval action letter, the product can be legally marketed starting that day in the United States.

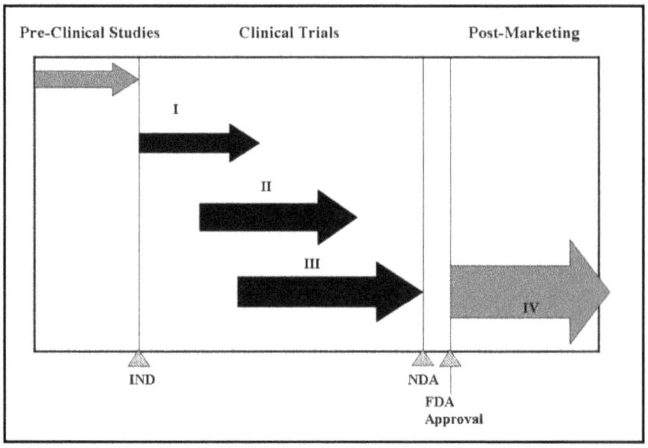

FIGURE 3-1. Overview of drug development process in relation to Food and Drug Administration (FDA) requirements.

PRECLINICAL TESTING

Prior to submission of a commercial IND, the sponsor will have compiled evidence of extensive preclinical testing in vitro and in vivo in animals to test the safety of any potential therapeutic agent. The FDA requires a minimum information profile on the drug's pharmacological profile (pharmacokinetics and pharmacodynamics), acute toxicity in at least 2 animal species, and short-term toxicity studies from 2 weeks to 3 months' duration.[6] Genotoxicity (DNA mutations) screening is performed, as well as investigations

TABLE 3-2

PHASES OF DRUG TESTING REQUIRED FOR FOOD AND DRUG ADMINISTRATION ASSESSMENT

PHASE	PARTICIPANTS	PURPOSE	TIMELINE (APPROX)
Preclinical	Cell lines ≥2 Animal models	Pharmacokinetics Pharmacodynamics Toxicology	18 months (1 to 3 years)
I	<100 healthy volunteers	Safety Dose escalation Pharmacokinetics	12 to 18 months
II	<500 affected patients and controls in trial setting	Safety Effectiveness	1 to 2 years
III	100s to 1000s of affected patients and controls in trial setting	Safety Effectiveness Dosing	~3 years
IV	1000s of affected patients in actual practice setting (after FDA approval)	Safety Long-term effects Expanded variety of recipients	Indefinite

on drug absorption and metabolism, the toxicity of the drug's metabolites, and the speed with which the drug and its metabolites are excreted from the body.[7] This process can take up to 3 years, but in most cases, it can be completed in 18 months. With some agents, long-term animal studies may continue in parallel with human clinical trials, particularly if the drug is to be used for chronic or recurrent conditions. A sponsor can also demonstrate that a drug is safe by providing data from previous clinical testing or marketing of the drug in the United States or another country. The FDA encourages meetings with the sponsor at this stage to review plans for further testing.

Comprehensive preclinical testing alone does not entirely predict safety of new agents in humans. The starkest example of this was with the drug TGN1412, a monoclonal antibody against the CD28 receptor in T-cells approved by the European Medicines Agency in 2005. TGN1412's role as an activator of regulatory T-cells would have made it attractive for IBD studies. Although preclinical testing in macaques caused mild lymphadenopathy, phase I studies in healthy human volunteers caused multi-organ failure in 4 subjects within hours of receiving the drug by infusion.[8] Systemic allergic reactions such as these are difficult to predict in preclinical models. A study of more than 400 new drugs identified 14 that elicited systemic hypersensitivity in guinea pigs in preclinical testing, of which only 3 caused immune-related adverse reactions in humans.[9] Similarly, preclinical studies of immunosuppressive effects are limited to conventional measurements of myelosuppression, or increased incidence of tumors or infections in animal models.[6] These studies may not detect functional alterations in immune function not apparent in morphological testing, which involves immune function testing as required by European regulators.[10]

Investigational New Drug Application

Once the preclinical data collection is completed, the sponsor submits an IND application, which includes manufacturing information, pharmacological data, and toxicology results. The manufacturing data details production processes to ensure consistent and untainted drug product. The sponsor also provides names of the principal investigators (PIs) who will undertake the clinical trials if the IND is approved. Once the IND is received by the FDA, it has 30 days in which to notify the sponsor of concerns that may lead it to place a "hold" on the process or permit the sponsor to proceed with clinical trials while addressing deficiencies in the IND. If the sponsor receives no communication from the FDA, it can proceed with the proposed clinical trials at the end of the 30-day period.

Clinical Trials

The process of organizing clinical trials, recruiting healthy volunteers and patients, and compiling outcomes constitutes the most expensive and time-consuming component of the

FDA approval process. Each center that intends to recruit participants will be headed by a PI, who has responsibility for ensuring that the study has local institutional review board (IRB) approval and that the safety and rights of participants are protected during the clinical trial.[11] The PIs must maintain adequate records and submit timely reports that contain relevant features of enrolled patients, outcomes, and adverse events during the study process. The local IRB is mandated by the federal Office of Human Research Protection to oversee the implementation of the trial in a manner that protects the safety, rights, and privacy of participants. The IRB reviews reports of adverse events, as well as reports from the data and safety monitoring committee for each study to decide whether the study may continue based on interim safety reports. Once the IRB approves the design and implementation of a study and its consent form, the investigator may recruit patients. In practice, industry-sponsored trials for new agents, such as biologics, will often involve contract research organizations to assist the investigator in compliance with local and federal regulations pertinent to clinical trials.

Phase I Studies

The purpose of phase I studies is to determine a drug's safety and side effects at different doses. This involves pharmacokinetics, metabolism and excretion, and toxicity by administering the agent starting at subclinical doses in healthy human volunteers. Typically, up to 100 volunteers are recruited over 6 to 18 months until sufficient pharmacologic data are available to plan valid phase II studies. Occasionally, phase I studies may involve those with advanced malignancies for whom no other therapies are available. Only about 70% of all INDs proceed from phase I to phase II studies.[12]

Phase II Studies

The next step in the development process assesses the drug's efficacy and safety in a well-defined cohort of patients with the disease of interest. This may include open trials (IIA) followed by randomized controlled trials (IIB) or randomized trials alone. The primary aim here is proof-of-concept that the drug is effective in treating a specific illness. A few hundred patients with strict eligibility criteria are enrolled and followed over a few years, usually at least 2 years. Further evidence of safety is also obtained from these studies, as a larger number of participants are involved, and adverse events particular to patients with the disease of interest may be highlighted. If the efficacy and safety data from a phase II trial are positive and robust, the next step is a large, expensive phase III study. Examples of phase II trials include the original infliximab trial in Crohn's disease, the CLASSIC trial of adalimumab, and the anti-interleukin-12 and ustekinumab trials.[13,14]

Phase III Studies

These are the pivotal, large randomized controlled trials that validate the results of phase II studies and further assess safety and dosing schedules in a defined population with the disease and controls. Most such studies include hundreds or thousands of patients over a number of years and contain sufficient statistical power to detect differences between the agent and placebo. The results from phase III studies are the cornerstone of a sponsor's NDA to the FDA and are the basis of the prescribing and package insert information if the drug is approved for marketing. Only about 30% of INDs submitted will complete phase III studies.[12] Examples of phase III include the ACCENT, CHARM, PRECISE, ENACT-1, and ENACT-2 trials.[15-18]

New Drug Application

The endpoint of this massive undertaking is the accumulation of sufficient data to submit an application to the FDA for approval to market the drug. The NDA includes a comprehensive evaluation of the drug's characteristics, including physical composition, manufacturing process, pharmacological effects, toxicology, clinical efficacy, and case report data. Such case reports are required for all study participants. The NDA is reviewed by CDER expert panels in each of the areas of interest, and external advisory committees (FDA Advisory Committees) provide further input. In recent years, the composition and potential conflicts of interest of these committees has been the subject of scrutiny, particularly in light of cardiovascular safety concerns with the coxibs.[19]

The key questions the FDA has to answer are as follows:

1. Is this drug effective in treating the condition it purports to treat?
2. Do the results support an acceptable benefit-to-risk ratio?

The FDA's evaluation may include inspection of the manufacturing facilities and clinical trial sites to verify the details in the submitted application. If the information supplied by the sponsor is insufficient to answer these questions, then further data are sought. The FDA is required to provide an interim evaluation within 6 months, and the average time to final decision is around 24 months. During this time, the FDA is in regular contact with the drug's sponsor to ensure that all additional information or data required by the expert panels is provided. The final decision of the CDER panel is either "approval," "approvable with minor changes," or "not approvable." The majority of NDAs are approved, allowing the sponsor to begin manufacturing and distribution. Those considered not approvable can request an appeal hearing or retract the application and reapply with adjustments.

Postmarketing Surveillance

Once an agent is approved for general use, it is really the first time it is tested in individuals who were ineligible for controlled trials, which may include women of child-bearing age, children, the elderly, and patients with comorbid conditions. Ironically, the elderly, who constitute about 70% of medication recipients, only make up about 30% of clinical trial participants. In addition, the numbers of people exposed to the drug expands significantly beyond the confines of clinical studies to general practice. As a consequence, rare side effects or adverse events in special situations and long-term morbidity may only become apparent at this point. The CDER's Office of Drug Safety (ODS) thus monitors a drug's safety profile even after it has been approved for use. This is undertaken via a requirement of pharmaceutical companies to report all adverse events associated with a new drug and the voluntary system of reporting by health-care workers (MedWatch). The ODS is responsible for updating labeling, public notification of new risks, implementing risk management programs, and (rarely) drug withdrawal. So-called phase IV studies incorporate such postmarketing surveillance. For example, the risk of progressive multifocal leukoencephalopathy (PML) was detected during postmarketing surveillance of natalizumab in 1 patient with Crohn's disease and 2 with multiple sclerosis.[20] This led the sponsors to voluntarily withdraw the drug for a period of time, although it was eventually brought back to the market for multiple sclerosis with certain stipulations.

Similarly, an increased number of cases of tuberculosis (TB) were identified with early use of infliximab through MedWatch.[21] More recently, histoplasmosis and lymphomas have been recognized with both infliximab and adalimumab.[22,23] Such instances may lead the FDA to revise a drug's package inserts, warn the public and health-care providers, or (rarely) withdraw approval of a drug. The postmarketing surveillance "net" has its flaws also, as it is dependent on either health-care providers or pharmaceutical companies to notify the FDA of adverse events.

Though the Prescription Drug User Fee Act (PDUFA) deadlines have favorably changed approval decisions of the FDA, discovery of unanticipated postmarketing safety problems is more likely to occur among drugs approved immediately before a deadline. Relying more on increased staffing and less on deadlines may result in greater efficiency without increasing cost and the risk of postmarketing drug safety problems.[24] The renewal and reauthorization of PDUFA may improve the way FDA regulation responds to the risk and benefits of drugs and may allow Congress to provide increased funding for postapproval drug safety.[25]

ALTERNATIVE PATHWAYS

The process outlined above is obviously time-consuming and expensive; the estimated time for development of a new drug is 15 years and $900 million from drug discovery to market launch.[26] There are many cases where such an undertaking may impede access to potential therapy for life-threatening conditions or be commercially unattractive for rare diseases. A number of pathways exist in such circumstances, but those that are relevant to IBD include the following.

Orphan Drugs

A condition that affects fewer than 200,000 patients in the United States, or one whose prevalence exceeds 200,000 but there is "no reasonable expectation" that the costs of developing and making the drug available will be recovered from sales in the United States is considered a rare disease.[27] In these circumstances, drugs used to treat these diseases are called *orphan drugs*, and their development is promoted by tax incentives, FDA assistance in study design, phase I/II funding, and 7 years of marketing exclusivity. More than 200 such agents have been approved, and a number of agents used in IBD have received FDA grant funding from this program, including infliximab, rifabutin, and 4-aminosalicylic acid.[28] A number of biotech companies have specialized in such markets.

Treatment IND

A treatment IND allows expanded access to promising drugs in serious or life-threatening diseases where there is preliminary evidence of efficacy or diseases where no comparable treatment exists. This was originally developed for new cancer agents in the 1970s but later became prominent in the treatment of acquired immune deficiency syndrome (AIDS) in the 1980s. The sponsor still has to seek IRB approval, and the recipient may be charged by the sponsor for the costs of the agent with the FDA's knowledge.

Accelerated Review

Accelerated review process was introduced in 1992 to expedite development of promising agents for serious or life-threatening diseases without existing treatments. In this situation, the FDA can grant approval of a drug based on a surrogate endpoint that predicted therapeutic benefit, rather than "hard" endpoints such as survival. Once approved, the sponsor must continue postmarketing studies to confirm the safety and efficacy using clinical endpoints. An example would be reduction in c-reactive protein (CRP) or improved endoscopic appearance, rather than long-term remission rates. Natalizumab was initially approved for multiple sclerosis in this manner in 2004.

CURRENT ISSUES IN DRUG DEVELOPMENT IN IBD

The drug development process is a major undertaking for any drug sponsor. Challenges exist in providing safe, effective, and affordable therapies to patients with IBD in a timely manner, as the regulatory and clinical research environment becomes more complex.[29] For clinicians and hospitals enrolling patients, and their IRBs, the increasing emphasis on training and regulatory compliance places a significant time burden on research-associated staff.[30] The FDA expects principal investigators to personally supervise the trials for which they are responsible, in addition to their other clinical and research responsibilities. The increasing number of trainees opting for private practice rather than academic medicine has limited the number of gastroenterologists willing or able to undertake the mantle of PI for clinical trials.[31] For the FDA, there are opposing pressures to approve therapies as rapidly as possible, while comprehensively assessing for potential adverse effects and protecting the public.

In IBD, there are a number of issues in the drug development process that present challenges. We have yet to see agents that incorporate advances in genomic medicine into effective therapies for CD or UC. The majority of agents in development target late events in the inflammatory cascade, as a consequence of our lack of understanding of the key factors that "trigger" the process in susceptible individuals. A number of disease phenotypes, such as pouchitis, irritable pouch syndrome, prevention of postoperative CD, perianal disease, and structuring disease would benefit from targeted therapies beyond conventional agents. The heterogeneous nature of patients with IBD, and the wide variation of some clinical markers such as the Crohn's Disease Activity Index (CDAI), has invariably produced high placebo response rates in clinical trials in CD. More objective, minimally invasive markers of disease activity would strengthen the statistical analysis in phase II and III trials in patients with IBD. Finally, the many exclusion criteria of sponsored trials have limited the numbers of eligible patients, leading to increased recruitment in South America and Eastern Europe for these studies. The ethical issues arising from clinical trials in settings where other therapeutic options are limited for financial or supply reasons are complex.

The past 10 years have seen a major expansion in the available biologic agents to treat active IBD, agents whose mechanism of action we still, in some cases, do not understand and that have been associated with rare but serious adverse effects. The current FDA system is effective at requiring sponsors to provide evidence of safety in a contained setting and superiority to placebo but has limitations in terms of rare side effects and the effects in a variety of patient phenotypes. This knowledge should encourage physicians treating patients with IBD to be vigilant as these agents reach their patient population, while taking advantage of their efficacy.

REFERENCES

1. Longobardi T, Jacobs P, Bernstein CN. Utilization of health care resources by individuals with inflammatory bowel disease in the United States: a profile of time since diagnosis. *Am J Gastroenterol.* 2004;99:650-655.
2. The Pharmaceutical Research and Manufacturers of America. New medicines database. 2007. Available at: http://newmeds.phrma.org/results.php?drug=&indication=332&company=&status=. Accessed February 12, 2010.
3. Lead Discovery. Emerging treatments for inflammatory bowel disease (IBD). 2005. Available at: http://www.leaddiscovery.co.uk/PharmaReport%20Alert-Emerging%20treatments%20for%20inflammatory%20bowel%20disease%20(IBD).html#feature. Accessed May 21, 2007.
4. Center for Drug Evaluation and Research. A brief history of the Center for Drug Evaluation and Research. 2007. Available at: http://www.fda.gov/cder/about/history/default.htm. Accessed February 12, 2010.
5. Meadows M. The FDA's drug review process: Ensuring drugs are safe and effective. *FDA Consum.* 2002;36:19-24.
6. Center for Drug Evaluation and Research. *Immunotoxicology Evaluation of Investigational New Drugs.* Washington, DC: US Department of Health and Human Services, Food and Drug Administration; 2002.
7. Lesko LJ, Salerno RA, Spear BB, et al. Pharmacogenetics and pharmacogenomics in drug development and regulatory decision making: report of the first FDA-PWG-PhRMA-DruSafe Workshop. *J Clin Pharmacol.* 2003; 43:342-358.
8. Suntharalingam G, Perry MR, Ward S, et al. Cytokine storm in a phase 1 trial of the anti-CD28 monoclonal antibody TGN1412. *N Engl J Med.* 2006;355:1018-1028.
9. Weaver JL, Staten D, Swann J, Armstrong G, Bates M, Hastings KL. Detection of systemic hypersensitivity to drugs using standard guinea pig assays. *Toxicology.* 2003;193:203-217.
10. Vos JG, Van Loveren H. Markers for immunotoxic effects in rodents and man. *Toxicol Lett.* 1995;82-83:385-394.
11. Department of Health and Human Services. *The CDER Handbook.* Available at: http://www.fda.gov/downloads/AboutFDA/CentersOffices/CDER/UCM198415.pdf/. Accessed December 1, 2010.
12. Flieger K. FDA finds new ways to speed treatment to patients. *FDA Consum.* 1993;27:14-18.
13. Mannon PJ, Fuss IJ, Mayer L, et al. Anti-interleukin-12 antibody for active Crohn's disease. *N Engl J Med.* 2004;351:2069-2079.
14. Sandborn WJ, Feagan BG, Fedorak RN, et al. A randomized trial of ustekinumab, a human interleukin-12/23 monoclonal antibody, in patients with moderate-to-severe Crohn's disease. *Gastroenterology.* 2008;135:1130-1141.
15. Hanauer SB, Feagan BG, Lichtenstein GR, et al. Maintenance infliximab for Crohn's disease: the ACCENT I randomised trial. *Lancet.* 2002;359:1541-1549.
16. Colombel JF, Sandborn WJ, Rutgeerts P, et al. Adalimumab for maintenance of clinical response and remission in patients with Crohn's disease: the CHARM trial. *Gastroenterology.* 2007; 132(1):52-65.
17. Schreiber S, Khaliq-Kareemi M, Lawrance IC, et al. Maintenance therapy with certolizumab pegol for Crohn's disease. *N Engl J Med.* 2007;357:239-250.

18. Sandborn WJ, Colombel JF, Enns R, et al. Natalizumab induction and maintenance therapy for Crohn's disease. *N Engl J Med.* 2005;353:1912-1925.
19. Okie S. Raising the safety bar—the FDA's coxib meeting. *N Engl J Med.* 2005;352:1283-1285.
20. Van Assche G, Van Ranst M, Sciot R, et al. Progressive multifocal leukoencephalopathy after natalizumab therapy for Crohn's disease. *N Engl J Med.* 2005;353:362-368.
21. Keane J, Gershon S, Wise RP, et al. Tuberculosis associated with infliximab, a tumor necrosis factor alpha-neutralizing agent. *N Engl J Med.* 2001;345:1098-1104.
22. Infliximab [package insert]. Malvern, PA: Centocor, Inc; 2008.
23. Adalimumab [package insert]. Abbott Park, IL: Abbott Laboratories; 2008.
24. Carpenter D, Zucker EJ, Avorn J. Drug-review deadlines and safety problems. *N Engl J Med.* 2008;358:1354-1361.
25. Hennessy S, Strom BL. PDUFA reauthorization—drug safety's golden moment of opportunity? *N Engl J Med.* 2007;356:1703-1704.
26. DiMasi JA, Hansen RW, Grabowski HG. The price of innovation: new estimates of drug development costs. *J Health Econ.* 2003; 22:151-185.
27. Department of Health and Human Services. Orphan drugs. 2007. Available at: http://www.fda.gov/cder/handbook/orphan.htm. Accessed June 25, 2008.
28. Office of Orphan Products Development. Orphan Products Grants Program. 2007. Available at: http://www.fda.gov/ForIndustry/DevelopingProductsforRareDiseasesConditions/WhomtoContactaboutOrphanProductDevelopment/ucm134580.htm. Accessed December 1, 2010.
29. DeMets D, Califf R, Dixon D, et al. Issues in regulatory guidelines for data monitoring committees. *Clin Trials.* 2004;1:162-169.
30. Department of Health and Human Services. Institutional Review Boards: A Time for Reform. Washington, DC: Author; 1998.
31. Hanauer SB. Another one bites the dust. *Nat Clin Pract Gastroenterol Hepatol.* 2005;2:435.

4 Utility of Animal Models for the Study and Treatment of Inflammatory Bowel Disease

Ashish Chawla, MD and Kenneth Simpson, BVM&S, PhD

Inflammatory bowel disease (IBD) is a chronic inflammatory disorder of the intestine that is characterized by exaggerated adaptive and acquired immune responses. Because the exact pathogenesis of IBD is unknown, murine models of colitis have been developed to investigate disease pathogenesis and novel treatment modalities. These model systems suggest that either an excessive Th1 or Th2 T cell response mediates mucosal inflammation. This dysregulated cytokine response results from defects in peripheral T cell responses and plays a critical role in colitis. The models of murine colitis can be divided up into five categories: chemically induced models, immune cell transfer models, colitis due to gene knockout, colitis via introduction of a transgene, and spontaneous colitis models. Each model has unique advantages for studying the pathway of mucosal inflammation. The spontaneous colitis models and gene knockout models have been particularly influential in current human immune therapies. The objective of this review is to give an overview of the colitis models and to highlight potential novel therapies based on specific models. Limitations of each model and applicability toward human disease are also discussed.

IBD develops in approximately 0.1% of the Western population, but the etiology and pathogenesis of the disease is unknown. During the past decade, UC and CD have gained increased importance because of increased incidence and prevalence. Older treatment modalities are largely nonspecific and just alleviate the symptoms without altering the natural history of the disease. Therefore, murine models of colitis have been developed to study the pathogenesis, genetics, and treatment of colitis. These models have increased our knowledge of mucosal inflammation and have led to the development of alternative therapies. In order to better understand murine colitis models, it is first important to understand the key players in the intestinal immune response.

T Cell Differentiation and the Intestinal Immune System

The intestinal mucosa serves as an interface for the interaction of the host with its environment. Due to its large surface area, the intestinal mucosa is constantly exposed to bacterial flora and exogenous antigens. In general, the intestinal immune system displays a state of hyporesponsiveness and "tolerance" toward commensal bacteria and some foreign antigens. Oral tolerance results from a complex interplay between the intestinal immune system and the mucosal flora, such that most mucosal responses are self-limited and do not result in inflammation. This homeostatic balance is functionally disturbed in human IBD. Many components in the intestinal immune response have been evaluated as a source for human IBD. These include T cells, antigen presenting cells (APCs), epithelial cells, and cytokines. Though distinct alterations in these components have been noted in human CD and ulcerative colitis, most evidence suggests that mucosal inflammation is almost always mediated by exaggeration of one of two pathways: either an excessive T helper 1 (Th1) T cell response or an excessive T helper 2 (Th2) T cell response.

Lichtenstein GR, ed.
Ulcerative Colitis: The Complete Guide to Medical Management (pp. 41-52)

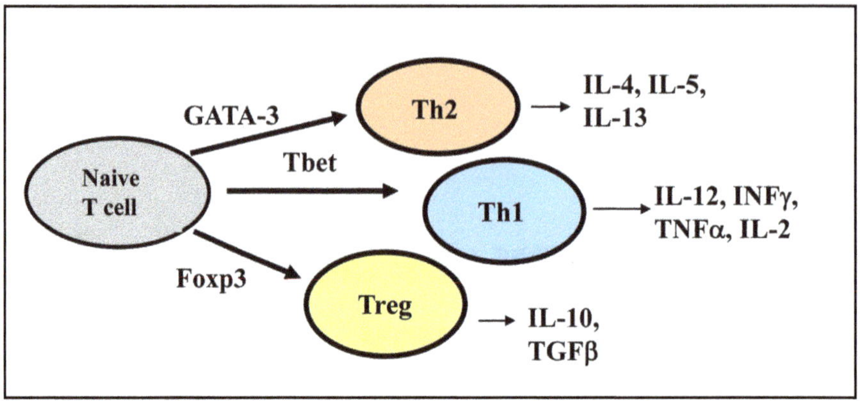

FIGURE 4-1. Peripheral T cell differentiation. Upon antigen exposure, naïve T cells can differentiate into three functionally distinct subsets: T helper 1 (Th1), T helper 2 (Th2), and T regulatory cells. Differentiation to a specific effector type is based on the stimulus and cytokine milieu. The specific cell fate is driven by transcription factors (Tbet, GATA-3, and Foxp3), which serve as master regulators of lineage commitment. Th1 type T cells secrete IL-12, interferon gamma (INFγ), tumor necrosis factor alpha (TNFα), and IL-2, whereas Th2 cells secrete IL-4, IL-5, and IL-13. T regulatory cells can secrete transforming growth factor (TGF)-β and/or IL-10.

CD4+ T cells are pivotal in mediating and controlling mucosal immune responses. Upon exposure to an antigen, naïve CD4+ T cells can differentiate into three distinct subsets of T cells: Th1, Th2, and T regulatory cells (Tr1, Th3, and $CD^{4+}CD^{25+}$) (Figure 4-1). These cells can be distinguished from each other based on functional cytokine production, cell surface phenotypes, and survival requirements.[1] The Th1 cells are critical for macrophage activation and help secrete IL-2, IL-12, interferon gamma (Infγ), and tumor necrosis factor (TNFα). Unlike the Th1 response, Th2-mediated inflammation occurs secondary to IL-4, IL-5, and IL-13. In addition, Th2 responses aid in the production of antibodies. In recent years, it has become evident that there is another set of effector cells involved in post-thymic tolerance. These regulatory T cells are able to suppress responder T cells via the production of transforming growth factor (TGF)-β, IL-10, or both.[2] One such T regulatory subset ($CD4^+$ $CD25^+$) is present in 5% to 10% of peripheral $CD4^+$ T cells, and elimination of this subset leads to autoimmune diseases in mice (eg, gastritis, colitis, orchitis, and thyroiditis).[3] This balance between Th1/Th2 effector versus T regulatory cell responses plays a key role in the production of mucosal inflammation.

ANIMAL MODELS OF COLITIS

Despite the varying nature and source of inflammation in these models, most murine models of colitis support the notion that IBD results from an inappropriate and exaggerated immune response to normal constituents of intestinal microflora in genetically susceptible hosts. These models can be broadly characterized into 5 groups: chemically induced models, immune cell transfer models, colitis due to gene knockout, colitis via introduction of a transgene, and spontaneous colitis models (Table 4-1).

CHEMICALLY INDUCED COLITIS

Several important murine models utilize the exposure of exogenous chemical (haptenizing) agents in order to instigate colitis. Chemically induced models of colitis are produced by either rectal installation or oral consumption of different agents including trinitrobenzene sulphonic acid (TNBS), oxazolone, and dextran sodium sulfate (DSS).

TNBS Colitis

Murine colitis due to TNBS installation occurs after destruction of the mucosal barrier with an ethanol enema. The extent of colitis can vary with mouse strain, but some strains develop an acute colitis, which eventually leads to a Th1-mediated chronic colitis. There is transmural inflammation present in the intestine often associated with granulomas, thus mimicking CD. Exposure to TNBS leads to a hapten-induced delayed hypersensitivity reaction with production of IL-12 by macrophages and Inf-γ and IL-2 by lymphocytes.[4] This simple model has been particularly useful in the development and testing of novel therapeutic molecules (including antibodies to IL-12 that abrogate the colitis). Monoclonal antibody neutralization of IL-12/23 via the shared p40 subunit has reversed active colitis in T cell–mediated mouse models.[5] Recently, genome-wide association studies have identified genes that encode a subunit for the receptor of IL-23 in CD.[6] Ustekinumab is a monoclonal antibody against the p40 subunit of IL-12/23 and has induced clinical response in a subgroup of patients with moderate-to-severe CD who are nonresponsive to infliximab.[7]

Oxazolone Colitis

Similar to TNBS colitis, the rectal installation of oxazolone with ethanol has been shown to induce murine colitis.[8] Unlike the TNBS colitis, the colitis induced by

TABLE 4-1

MOUSE MODELS OF INFLAMMATORY BOWEL DISEASE

Animal Models	Type of Inflammation	Utility Toward IBD
Chemically Induced		
TNBS colitis	Chronic Th1 type	Models identify the role of Th1 (Crohn's) versus Th2 (UC) responses in IBD. Useful models for investigation for potential therapies for IBD.
Oxazolone colitis	Chronic Th2 type	
DSS colitis	Superficial acute, Th1/Th2 (chronic)	
Immune Transfer		
Adoptive transfer colitis	Chronic Th1 type	Stress the importance of T regulatory cells in prevention and amelioration of IBD. Suggest a role for TGFβ and IL-10 for inhibition of Th1 cytokine response.
Gene Knockout		
IL-2 KO	Th1/Th2	Gene KO models have identified the specific cytokines important in pathogenesis of IBD. Proof of concept for anti-TNF therapy for CD. Suggest possible roles for other therapy (anti-IL-6).
IL-10 KO	Th1 early/Th2 late	
TNF ΔARE mice	Th1, ileocolitis/granulomas	
TCRα KO	Th2 colitis	
Trefoil factor KO	Th1	
Transgenic Models		
IL-7 Transgenic	Th2 colitis	Demonstrate role of specific bacteria in development/treatment of colitis. Role of defects in innate immunity (APCs, macrophages, NK cells) in IBD. Exciting as no exogenous manipulation required for development of colitis.
HLA-B27	Th1 colitis	
Myeloid-specific STAT3 deficiency	Th1 colitis due to loss of IL-10 signaling	
Spontaneous Colitis		
C3H/HejBir mice	Th1 colitis	These models have been described to develop colitis and are also prone to developing colonic carcinoma and sclerosing cholangitis.
Cotton top tamarins	Colitis	Histiocytic ulcerative/granulomatous colitis in the Boxer dogs represents an overly aggressive inflammatory response to a subset of resident *Escherichia coli*.
Boxer dogs	Histiocytic granulomatous colitis	First mouse model to demonstrate ileitis with perianal disease and fistulas.
Spontaneous Ileitis		
SAMP1/Yit	Th1 ileitis	
SAMP1/YitFc	Perianal disease (fistulas)	

IBD indicates inflammatory bowel disease; TNBS, trinitrobenzene sulfuric acid; TH1, T helper 1; Th2, T helper 2; DSS, dextransodium sulfate; TFG, transforming growth factor; KO, knockout; TNF, tumor necrosis factor; ARE, AU=rich element; TCR, T-cell receptor; APC, antigen presenting cells; NK, natural killer.

oxazolone occurs earlier and is characterized by superficial ulceration and inflammation predominantly localized to the distal colon, features that mimic human ulcerative colitis. Recent studies have shown that oxazolone-induced colitis results from the induction of natural killer T cells (NKT) that produce IL-13 and subsequently IL-4 (Th2-mediated cytokines). In fact, elimination of NKT cells or suppression of IL-13 can prevent the development of colitis. These data suggest that oxazolone colitis is mediated by an excessive Th2 effector response.[9]

FIGURE 4-2. Adoptive transfer colitis model.

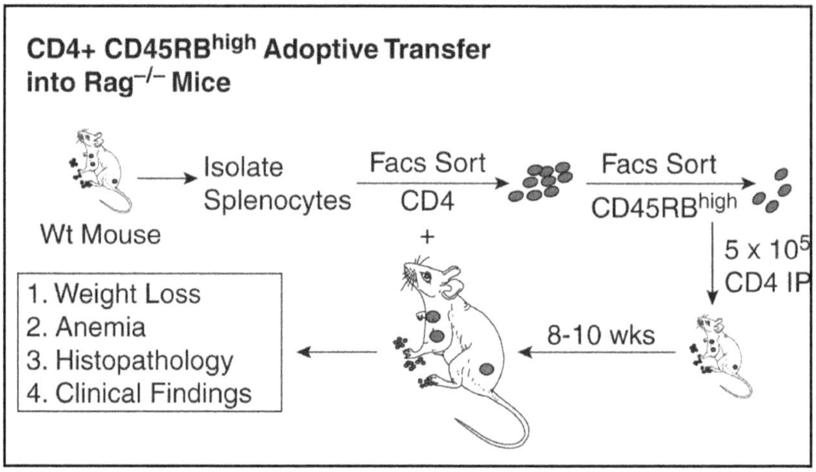

The dichotomy of mucosal inflammation (Th1 or Th2) by TNBS and oxazolone-mediated colitis is also suggested in human IBD. There is considerable evidence that T cells derived from ulcerations in human CD produce IFN-γ and IL-12 (Th1 cytokines) but little evidence exists that T cells from UC lesions produce excess IL-4. However, recent findings support the role of Th2-mediated inflammation in the pathogenesis of ulcerative colitis. The presence of increased levels of autoantibodies and increased secretion of IL-5 and IL-13 seen in UC are both features of Th2-mediated response.[10] Through the development of these 2 mouse models, we have been able to elucidate the inflammatory mediators (lymphocytes, macrophages, and cytokines) important in chronic colitis. The use of these models also helps demonstrate the differential cytokine response that can be seen in human CD and ulcerative colitis.

DSS Colitis

Colitis occurs after DSS is dissolved in the water given to mice or rats and leads to progressive weight loss, diarrhea, hematochezia, and shortening of the intestine in a few weeks. The acute colitis results from epithelial disruption, which results in luminal bacterial translocation and subsequent infiltration of neutrophils. This response is induced by the innate immune system because severe combined immunodeficiency mice (SCID mice, who lack B and T cells) also develop acute colitis upon exposure to DSS.[11] Unlike acute colitis, the chronic colitis seen with DSS is caused by the activation of lymphocytes and release of cytokines (both Th1 and Th2).[12] The DSS colitis model has led to increased understanding in the pathogenic role of activated lymphocytes and the secreted cytokines. Others have used this model to evaluate the role of leukocyte adhesion molecules in the prevention of colitis. Soriano et al demonstrated that blockade of adhesion molecules that prevent leukocyte adhesion and migration on endothelial cells could represent a novel approach to treatment of IBD. This study demonstrated that immunoneutralization of VCAM-1 can lead to amelioration of DSS colitis and possible treatment of human IBD.[13]

Limitations

Although the chemical colitis models help us understand the pathways of inflammation, a major limitation is that they do not represent the initiating events in human IBD. The models rely on the chemical destruction of the epithelial barrier. This allows for evaluation of the acute colitic process but makes it difficult to analyze chronic colitis. For example, acute DSS colitis occurs in the absence of the acquired immune system (SCID mice that lack lymphocytes). Unlike DSS colitis, human IBD clearly involves a complex interplay between defective T cell and innate immune response to host mucosal antigens.

IMMUNE TRANSFER MODEL OF COLITIS

The adoptive transfer model of colitis results from a change in the number of naïve versus regulatory T cells that are usually required to maintain oral tolerance. This model involves the transfer of $CD4^+$ T cells expressing $CD45RB^{high}$ (naïve) from immunocompetent mice into immunodeficient SCID or $Rag^{-/-}$ mice, resulting in Th1-mediated colitis.[14] The recipient mice develop a chronic and terminal wasting disease, accompanied by anemia and diarrhea within 6 to 8 weeks. The mice generally die after 16 weeks (Figure 4-2). On histopathology, the entire colon is involved with almost complete sparing of the small intestine. During the course of 6 to 8 weeks, the $CD4^+$ $CD45RB^{high}$ T cells expand and proliferate in the peripheral compartment of the recipient mice. These naïve cells are primed and develop into Th1 effector cells via exposure to commensal bacteria in the recipient mice. The pathogenic potential of these cells, which is normally controlled by $CD4^+$ $CD45RB^{low}$ T regulatory lymphocytes, is left unchecked. This allows for T effector cells to proliferate and secrete TNFα and IFN-γ in the lamina propria of the intestine.[15]

The $CD4^+$ $CD45RB^{low}$ T cell pool is composed of T regulatory cells ($CD4^+$ $CD25^+$) and recent thymic emigrants. Transfer of the $CD4^+$ $CD45RB^{low}$ T lymphocytes into immunodeficient mice does not lead to the induction of colitis. In fact, cotransfer of $CD4^+$ $CD45RB^{low}$ with the $CD45RB^{high}$ cells inhibits the development of colitis.[16,17] Recent data also indicate that transfer of $CD45RB^{low}$ cells ($CD4^+$ $CD25^+$) into a mouse with pre-existing colitis leads to resolution of both the colitis and the terminal wasting.[18] Interestingly, control of the immune pathology is regulated by the expression of TGF-β. This observation is based on experiments where cotransfer of both $CD4^+$ CD45RB subsets along with intraperineal (IP) injection of anti-TGF-β antibody resulted in the development of colitis.[19] These findings suggest that deficiencies in regulatory T cell responses play a critical role in mucosal inflammation. Whether patients with IBD have underlying defects in regulatory T cells has not been clearly determined. It is known that T cells isolated from patients with IBD can proliferate and produce cytokines in vitro in response to their own microflora (whereas cells from control patients do not). These findings suggest either an excessive effector or defective regulatory T cell response. At present, it is not possible to measure human regulatory T cell response with any degree of confidence. Despite these limitations, it is clear that activation of T regulatory cells could serve as novel therapy for IBD.

Limitations

The adoptive transfer colitis model highlights the importance of T regulatory cells in the prevention of murine colitis. This model also emphasizes the role of IL-10 and TGF-β for the amelioration of already developed colitis. However, the profound immune abnormalities in the recipient mice (lack of B and T cells) make this model unsuitable for investigating the complex interplay of the acquired immune response in human IBD.

GENE KNOCKOUT MOUSE MODELS OF COLITIS

Gene knockout models of colitis have increased our understanding of IBD and have led to the development of novel therapies (anti-TNFα therapy). Through the deletion of genes critically involved in the inflammatory cascade, researchers have been able to dissect the sequence and pathogenesis of chronic intestinal inflammation.

Interleukin-2 Knockout/IL-2 Receptor (R) a Knockout Mice

IL-2 is an indispensable cytokine that is important in the regulation and activation of T cells, macrophages, natural killer cells, and NKT cells. It also plays a key role in B cell differentiation and in the induction of apoptosis of T cells (activation-induced cell death). In 1993, Sadlack et al[20] demonstrated that mice with a disrupted IL-2 gene developed autoimmune hemolytic anemia, lymphadenopathy, and splenomegaly. Half of these mice died at 4 to 9 weeks of age, whereas the rest of the animals developed chronic colitis with inflammation, ulcers, and wall thickening from cecum to the rectum. The colitis occurred between 6 and 15 weeks and seemed to spare the small intestine. Histology confirmed crypt abscesses, mucin depletion, and dysplasia of epithelial cells, features that are consistent with human IBD.[20] Other studies crossbred the IL-2 knockout mice with deletion of other genes including $RAG\text{-}2^{-/-}$, $JH^{-/-}$, and β2 microglobulin$^{-/}$. These studies confirmed that $CD4^+$ T cells but not B cells or $CD8^+$ T cells were essential for the activation of colitis. Colitis in the IL-2 knockout model is considered secondary to lack of T cell apoptosis and thymic agenesis, which leads to incomplete depletion of activated T cells.[21] Loss of activation-induced cell death may explain the presence of pathogenic T effector cells found in human chronic colitis. In fact, evidence suggests that human IBD is caused by a loss of oral tolerance, which could be caused by defective deletion of pathogenic T cells.

IL-10 Knockout Mice

IL-10, which is produced by T cells, B cells, macrophages, thymic cells, and keratinocytes, plays a critical role in down-regulating the function of Th1 cells and macrophages. IL-10 knockout mice develop colitis in the entire intestine with significant inflammation in the duodenum, jejunum, and ascending colon. As with the IL-2 knockout mice, the source of inflammation is felt to be secondary to the presence of activated $CD4^+$ Th1 cells and depletion of regulatory T cells.[22] IL-10 knockout mice have also been used to evaluate the role of anti-TNFα antibodies in treatment of murine colitis. IL-10 knockout mice injected intraperitoneally with anti-TNFα antibodies showed significant improvement in inflammation with resolution of diarrhea and bleeding.[23] However, treatment of patients with CD with IL-10 has been more variable. Patients with mild to moderate colitis (not on steroids) had a beneficial effect with subcutaneous IL-10. However, patients with severe CD had clinical improvement in Crohn's disease activity index (CDAI) (decrease to 100 or less) but remission was not seen. A major problem of human IL-10 therapy has been its side effects, including fever, arthralgias, headaches, lymphopenia, and thrombocytopenia.[24] Also, discontinuation of IL-10 therapy results in recurrence of disease.

TNF ΔARE Mice

A large body of data is emerging in regard to the role of TNFα in the pathogenesis of CD. TNFα is an inflammatory cytokine produced by T cells and macrophages. It is secreted in an inactive form and is activated by a metalloproteinase, TNFα-activating enzyme. The TNFα mRNA contains a repeated AU-rich element (ARE) consisting of AUUUA repeats in its 3′ untranslated region that is implicated in post-transcriptional and translational regulation of TNF synthesis. Mice that have a 69 bp deletion of the ARE region (ΔARE) have high circulating levels of TNFα and develop severe wasting syndrome, chronic inflammatory arthritis, and inflammation of the terminal ileum and proximal colon. This phenotype is similar to CD and occurs between 2 and 4 weeks of age.[25] Studies have demonstrated that intestinal inflammation in the ΔARE mouse depends on Th1- type cytokines, IL-12, and IFN-γ, and requires the function of $CD8^+$ T cells.[26] Although no mutation in the 3′ AU-rich region of the TNF gene has been isolated in patients with CD, anti-TNFα therapy has become the mainstay in the treatment of CD. Infliximab, a monoclonal mouse human chimeric antibody against TNFα, has been shown to improve moderate to severe CD in several randomized control studies. There is a marked improvement in the CDAI and in the endoscopic/histologic appearance in the colitis.[27] This treatment also seems to be effective in patients who have abdominal or perianal fistulas, with 55% of patients having complete closure of the fistula, compared to 13% in the placebo group.[28] In vitro and in vivo, infliximab seems to bind to activated lymphocytes and induce apoptosis, resulting in a decrease of pathogenic T cells.[29] Other treatments used in IBD may also act through this mechanism. Sulfasalazine, azathioprine, and thalidomide also induce T cell apoptosis. Thalidomide may reduce chronic inflammation by modifying the intestinal immune response in human IBD. The TNF ΔARE model of murine colitis has been important in dissecting the pathophysiology of CD and in developing novel therapies.

TCRα Knockout Mice

Upon deletion of the alpha subunit of the T cell receptor, colitis develops in these mice at 16 weeks. TCRα knockout mice develop hypertrophy and inflammation of the colon from the rectum to cecum, with sparing of the small intestine. The histology of the large intestine demonstrates crypt abscesses with goblet cell depletion and infiltration of plasma cells, lymphocytes, and neutrophils. Interestingly, the mice develop autoantibodies due to polyclonal B cell activation.[30] As colitis is worse in double knockout mice deficient in TCRα and B cells (Igμ-/-), these autoantibodies are presumed to prevent inflammation and promote healing. The inflammation in this model is driven by Th2 immune response due to predominance of IL-4 and IL-5.[31] The pathologic lesions, autoantibodies, and Th2 immune response reflect a UC model. Recent studies suggest that anti-IL-4 antibody inhibits the activation of colitis in TCRα knockout mice, suggesting a possible novel agent for human ulcerative colitis.

Trefoil Factor-Deficient Mice

Intestinal trefoil factors (ITFs) are peptides secreted by mucus cells of the colon and small intestine after inflammation occurs. Mice deficient in ITF develop impaired wound healing and decreased epithelial regeneration. After induction of colitis by addition of DSS, ITF-deficient mice develop severe colitis and die. Addition of ITF has been shown to improve mucosal repair in chemical models of colitis.[32]

Limitations

Collectively, gene knockout models of murine colitis have helped identify the key components of immune regulation and oral tolerance in the gut. It is unlikely, however, that a single genetic mutation in key cytokines represents the underlying defect in IBD. No single gene defect in key molecules has been observed in the pathogenesis of human IBD. In fact, the most compelling evidence that genetic factors play a key role in the development of IBD comes from the identification of the NOD2 gene, which codes for a protein involved in the recognition of bacteria.[33] Data from two separate studies suggest that NOD2 mutations occur exclusively in patients with CD and not in patients with ulcerative colitis. Patients with heterozygous and homozygous NOD2 gene mutations have an increased relative risk for the development of CD (3-fold versus 38-fold).[34] Mutations in the NOD2 gene do not account for all cases of CD, however, suggesting the complex interplay of genetic predisposition and the mucosal microenvironment in the pathogenesis of IBD. In fact, studies have shown that normal individuals occasionally have NOD2 mutations on both chromosomes in the absence of disease. Also, none of the known mutations have been seen in 483 Japanese patients with CD.[35] These findings support the notion that single gene knockout models are important but do not represent the causative factors in the development of human IBD.

TRANSGENIC MODELS OF COLITIS

Like knockout models, transgenic murine models result in colitis after genetic manipulation leads to either overexpression of proteins or loss of proteins in specific tissues. These models stress the importance of the loss of homeostasis in the mucosal immune system for the development of colitis. Three models will be discussed in detail, including IL-7 transgenic mice, HLA-B27 transgenic rats, and mice with myeloid-specific STAT 3 deficiency.

IL-7 Transgenic Mice

IL-7 is derived from epithelial cells in the colon (along with thymic stromal cells and bone marrow cells) and plays a critical role in the regulation and proliferation of intraepithelial lymphocytes, intramucosal lymphocytes, and epithelial cells.[36] Studies with transgenic IL-7 mice, which overexpress IL-7, demonstrate increased incidence of acute colitis at 1 to 3 weeks of age. The mucosa of the large intestine has high levels of IL-7 with predominance of neutrophils, CD4+ T cells, and γδT cells. At 8 to 12 weeks of age, proctoptosis with anal bleeding and formation of crypt abscesses with monocyte infiltration occurs, resembling ulcerative colitis. Interestingly, IL-7 levels decrease at this stage, due to a decrease in goblet cells that are rich in IL-7.[37] UC patients have also been noted to have high serum levels of IL-7 during times of an acute flare. These findings demonstrate that IL-7 and IL-7 receptor-dependent signaling is important in the development of chronic colitis, suggesting a possible therapeutic target in human IBD.

HLA-B27 Transgenic Rats

The class I MHC allele HLA-B27 is highly associated with the human spondyloarthropathies, but the basis for this is poorly understood. Rats transgenic for human HLA-B27 and β2-microglobulin genes spontaneously develop colitis, gastritis, arthritis, dermatitis, alopecia, and nail changes. The disease susceptibility correlates with HLA-B27 expression in the bone marrow–derived cells and is influenced by the genetic background. The mechanism of colitis in this model is still not completely understood. The entire colon is affected with crypt hyperplasia, mononuclear infiltration, and increased number of activated Th1 cells.[38] There is evidence that normal luminal bacteria play an essential role in initiating and perpetuating chronic colitis and gastritis in this system. Transgenic rats raised under germ-free conditions do not develop gastrointestinal disease, whereas littermates exposed to specific pathogen-free bacteria (*Bacteroides* spp.) develop colitis and gastritis within 2 to 4 weeks.[39] Similar to human IBD, antibiotic therapy and, recently, probiotics have been shown to decrease recurrence of colitis in this model.

Myeloid Specific STAT-3–Deficient Mice

The STAT family of transcription factors, consisting of 7 members, is critically involved in cytokine signaling. The knockout of each member of the STAT family in mice has resulted in impaired responses to corresponding cytokines. Unlike other STAT knockout models, the knockout of STAT-3 results in early death in embryogenesis. Therefore, STAT-3 has been deleted in a cell- or tissue-specific manner via the Cre-loxP recombination system in myeloid cells (macrophages, neutrophils, and dendritic cells). These mice develop chronic enterocolitis due to an impaired response in IL-10 signaling and have increased secretion of IL-12, IL-6, and TNF. Macrophages from the STAT-3 mutant mice do not show any anti-inflammatory response to IL-10 and produce increased levels of inflammatory cytokines in response to bacterial LPS.[40] These findings suggest that abnormal activation of myeloid cells is involved in the pathogenesis of chronic colitis via stimulation of effector T cells and disruption of homeostatic balance. This scenario may also be seen in CD, which is associated with mutations in NOD2 protein—a protein that senses bacterial peptidoglycans. Absence of NOD2 activity in myeloid cells may result in activated macrophages, which induce a strong effector T cell response and a weak regulatory T cell response.

Limitations

The transgenic mouse models have helped reveal other important pathways in mucosal inflammation. The myeloid-specific STAT-3 mouse model has identified the importance of the innate immune response in IBD. However, like knockout models, they represent genetic manipulation with artificial increases in cytokines or loss of signaling in certain cells. These changes may represent a final common pathway of mucosal inflammation in human IBD but are not the instigating factors.

SPONTANEOUS MODELS OF COLITIS

Spontaneous colitis models offer an exciting way to study human IBD because inflammation in the intestines occurs without direct exogenous manipulation. There are 3 important models of spontaneous colitis that will be discussed: C3H/HejBir mice, cotton top tamarins, and Boxer dogs.

C3H/HejBir Mice

Colitis and perianal ulcers have been occasionally seen in the C3H/Hej strain of mice. Selective interbreeding of the C3H/Hej mice with colitis resulted in the substrain of C3H/HejBir mice. These mice develop colitis limited to the ileocecal region and the right side of the colon at 3 to 4 weeks of life. The colitis develops spontaneously and usually regresses after 10 to 12 weeks of life. Ulcers, crypt abscesses, and regeneration of epithelium are noted, but granulomas and mucosal hypertrophy are not seen. Increased levels of IFN-γ and IL-2 suggest a Th1-mediated immune response.[41] Similar to SCID mice and some knockout mice models, there seems to be a correlation between *Helicobacter* infection and the onset of colitis. These findings stress the importance of gut flora in the development of IBD. When mice are kept in a germ-free environment, colitis does not occur. Even though no specific microorganisms have been associated with murine colitis or human disease, it is clear that normal mucosal microflora is required to initiate or maintain the inflammatory process in genetically susceptible hosts.

Colitis in the Cotton Top Tamarin (*Saguinus oedipus*)

Colitis is an important health problem in cotton top tamarins (*Saguinus oedipus*) housed in biomedical research institutes.[42-44] A prospective study in one research colony documented colitis in 24% of animals at 4 months of age and 52% at 48 months of age.[45] Clinical signs include weight loss, diarrhea, and rectal bleeding. The colitis is diffuse and characterized histologically by an inflammatory cell infiltrate in the lamina propria, hyperplasia of the colonic epithelium, decreased numbers of goblet cells, and crypt abscesses. Increased amounts of TNF have been detected in feces of tamarins with colitis.[45] Treatment with sulfasalazine[46,47] or anti-TNF antibody ameliorates colitis in affected tamarins.[48]

As tamarins in their native habitat are free of the disease,[49] tamarins housed in isolation are less frequently affected than colony-housed animals (56% versus 93%),[46] and diversion of the fecal stream ameliorates inflammation.[50] Environmental factors such as diet and infectious agents are suspected to play a major role in the etiopathogenesis of colitis in cotton top tamarins.

Prospective evaluation of diets showed no effect on acute colitis, but chronic mucosal changes were significantly higher in animals fed a standard diet than semipurified diets.[46] *Campylobacter*, *Helicobacter*, and *Escherichia coli* have been variously implicated as infectious agents involved in the development of colitis. *Campylobacter* infection was not associated with colitis or diarrhea in colony-housed animals[46,51] but was related to colitis in tamarins housed in isolation.[46] A novel group of *Helicobacter* resembling *Flexispira rappini* and *Helicobacter fenelliae* has been isolated from affected individuals,[52] and spiral bacteria resembling *Helicobacter* were observed to invade colonic mucosa after re-introduction of the fecal stream.[50] Luminal bacteria on their own are not considered sufficient to induce colitis, however, and both an adverse environment and the fecal contents appear to be required for expression of the disease.[50] A role for *E coli* is suggested by the finding that tamarins with fecal cultures positive for enteropathogenic *E coli* containing intimin sequences have a higher frequency of active colitis (75.0% versus 27.2%; $P < 0.005$) and higher histological scores of colonic inflammation (0.875 versus 0.455, respectively; $P < 0.05$).[53]

Cotton top tamarins with colitis are prone to developing colonic carcinoma and sclerosing cholangitis.[42,43] Approximately 25% to 40% of tamarins with active colitis progress to colonic adenocarcinoma.[51] In a prospective study, 7 of 212 animals in the study groups developed adenocarcinoma of the colon at 4 or more years of age.[46] Colonic adenocarcinoma arises spontaneously (ie, is not preceded by dysplasia) in areas of colonic inflammation, is multifocal, and shares lectin staining with UeA-1.[54]

Histiocytic/Granulomatous Colitis of Boxer Dogs

Histiocytic UC (HUC; also known as granulomatous colitis) is a severe inflammatory disease of unknown etiology that typically affects Boxer dogs younger than 4 years of age.[55-57] Others breeds such as Mastiff, Alaskan Malamute, Doberman Pinscher, and French Bulldogs are sporadically affected.

Dogs are usually presented for the investigation of frequent bloody mucoid stools and weight loss. Clinicopathological abnormalities are generally limited to anemia and hypoalbuminemia. Abdominal ultrasonography may show thickening of the colon and regional lymphadenopathy. Lymph node aspirates may contain histiocytes. Colonoscopy is frequently characterized by thickening and ulceration of the colon.

The dominant histological features of colonic biopsies are loss of colonic epithelium and goblet cells and the accumulation of large numbers of PAS-positive macrophages. The PAS-positive material is thought to be derived from remnants of bacterial cell wall glycoprotein, and the accumulation of PAS-positive material in macrophages may be due to defective phagocytosis. Immunopathological studies describe an increase in immunoglobulin (Ig) G_3 and IgG_4 plasma cells, CD_3 T cells, L1, and MHCII-positive cells.[56]

Several studies have described bacteria within the mucosa of affected dogs, but known enteropathogens such as *Salmonella, Campylobacter yersinia,* and *Shigella* have not been isolated. Ultrastructural studies suggest active phagocytosis of bacteria that in some instances resemble *Chlamydia*.[55] An attempt to reproduce colitis in Boxer dogs with *Mycoplasma* isolated from the colon and regional lymph nodes of 4 affected dogs was unsuccessful. The predilection for Boxer dogs, with only sporadic cases of this type of colitis reported in non-Boxer dogs, and absence of a causal infectious agent has led to HUC being considered a breed-specific, immune-mediated disease of unknown etiology.

In contrast to the widely accepted view that HUC is an incurable immune-mediated disease, the original description by Van Kruningen[55] describes a favorable outcome in 6 of 9 dogs treated with chloramphenicol. The results of 3 recent studies provide clear evidence of clinical and histological remission in 12 Boxer dogs and 1 English Bulldog treated with antibiotic regimens containing fluoroquinolones.[57-59] Treatment with enrofloxacin, alone or in combination with metronidazole, and/or amoxicillin was generally reported to induce resolution of clinical signs within

2 weeks. Approximately one-third of dogs remained free of clinical signs during a 5- to 14-month follow-up after discontinuation of treatment. In the remaining dogs, clinical remission was maintained by continuing enrofloxacin at doses ranging from 68 mg orally every 24 hours to 68 mg orally every 72 hours for 2 to 21 months. A few dogs relapsed, and remission was achieved by re-treatment with enrofloxacin. Repeated biopsy specimens were obtained from 8 dogs after treatment, and all showed marked histologic improvement.

From a comparative perspective, it is clear that HUC in dogs has features in common with spontaneous idiopathic inflammatory bowel diseases in people such as UC (macroscopic appearance, regional distribution, immunopathology), CD (granulomatous inflammation, bacteria within macrophages, response to fluoroquinolones), and Whipple's disease (PAS-positive macrophages, bacteria within macrophages), but it is not identical to any one of these diseases.

Evidence is mounting that inflammatory bowel disease in people is a consequence of an abnormal host response to the enteric bacteria that can be viewed as normal flora or opportunistic pathogens.[60] With this thought in mind, 2 studies have recently explored the possibility that an uncharacterized infectious agent such as *Trophyrema whippelii* (the causative agent of Whipple's disease)[61] or an abnormal mucosa-associated flora are involved in the etiopathogenesis of HUC in Boxer dogs. One of these studies used a combination of culture-independent molecular techniques (16srDNA sequencing and fluorescence in situ hybridization) to examine the mucosa-associated bacterial flora of colonic biopsies from healthy dogs, dogs with lymphoplasmacytic colitis, and Boxer dogs with HUC.[59] Those investigators demonstrated selective intramucosal colonization of HUC biopsies by *E coli*. Another study described the immunolocalization of *E coli*, *Lawsonia intracellularis*, *Campylobacter*, and *Salmonella* to macrophages in the colon of 10/10, 3/10, 2/10, and 1/10 Boxer dogs with granulomatous colitis, respectively (dogs without colitis or other forms of colitis were not examined).[62] These findings strongly suggest that HUC is a consequence of mucosal colonization by luminal *E coli* in a susceptible individual (ie, an undefined breed-specific abnormality in Boxer dogs).

Interestingly, the *E coli* strains isolated from the colonic mucosa of dogs with HUC adhered to, invaded, and persisted in cultured epithelial cells to the same degree as *E coli* strains associated with CD.[63,64] Initial investigations of HUC and Crohn's-associated *E coli* indicate that they are more similar in phylogeny and virulence gene profiles to extraintestinal pathogenic *E coli* (eg, uropathogenic *E coli*) than diarrheogenic *E coli* and point to the associations of *E coli* that resemble extraintestinal pathogenic strains in genotype with chronic intestinal inflammation.[64]

Taken as a whole, histiocytic ulcerative/granulomatous colitis in the Boxer dogs represents an overly aggressive inflammatory response to a subset of resident *E coli* in a genetically susceptible individual. Identification of the genetic basis of susceptibility in Boxer dogs and virulence determinants of opportunistic pathogenic adherent and invasive *E coli* could provide useful insights into IBD in people.

SPONTANEOUS MODELS OF ILEITIS

In SAMP1/Yit and the SAMP1/YitFc mouse models, the mice develop ileitis and colitis, skin lesions, and perianal disease with fistula (findings that mimic CD).

SAMP1/Yit Mice

The SAMP1/Yit model, which was generated by >20 generations of brother-sister mating of a senescence-accelerated mouse line, develops spontaneous ileitis at 20 weeks of age. The ileitis develops without genetic or immunologic manipulation with almost 100% penetrance. These mice have segmental inflammation of the terminal ileum with transmural involvement, presence of granulomas, architectural distortion of the mucosa, and muscular hypertrophy. This chronic ileitis resembles human CD.[65] The ileitis can also be adoptively transferred to immunodeficient mice via $CD4^+$ T cells isolated from SAMP1/Yit mice, again mediated by a Th1-induced immune response.[66]

SAMP1/YitFc Mice

Recent studies using this strain of mice after an additional >20 generations of brother-sister matings have revealed new phenotypic features. The SAMP1/YitFc substrain develops ileitis as early as 10 weeks of age. These mice also have high levels of intestinal IFN-γ by 4 weeks of age, preceding the onset of ileitis. The mesenteric lymph node lymphocytes develop an activated phenotype coincident with the development of ileitis. Finally, approximately 5% of the mice develop perianal disease with ulceration and fistulas. The emergence of perianal disease is the first report of such an occurrence in an animal model of IBD.[67] The ileitis noted in this model is driven by Th1-mediated cytokines. Administration of anti-TNFα and anti-IL-12 antibodies can improve the colitis by induction of apoptosis in lamina propria mononuclear cells.[68] In addition to the benefit of anti-TNFα antibodies, the role of antibiotics has been tested in the SAMP1/YitFc model. The use of ciprofloxacin and metronidazole antibiotic therapy has been shown to prevent and treat colitis, by decreasing the number of activated gut lymphocytes. As a consequence, there is a decrease in the characteristic Th1 cytokine production.[69] Finally, this mouse model has also been used to investigate the role of adhesion molecules such as integrins (VCAM-1 and ICAM-1) in the role of colitis. These adhesion molecules have been implicated in T cell homing and neutrophil trafficking during an inflammatory response. Blockade of ICAM-1 and α_4 integrins or a combination of ICAM-1 and VCAM-1 leads to a 70% improvement in the severity of inflammation in SAMP1/YitFc colitis.[70] Similar studies in human CD have been encouraging using an antibody to α_4 integrins. The recombinant antibody natalizumab, with specificity to $\alpha_4\beta_1$ and $\alpha_4\beta_7$ integrins, has been used in a small trial involving 30 patients with CD. A single infusion of this drug resulted in a 39% remission rate in treated group versus 8% in placebo. Taken together, studies using the SAMP1/YitFc mice have had significant therapeutic implications in the management of IBD.

LIMITATIONS

Spontaneous colitis models mimic CD in many pathogenic features. Apart from ileal inflammation, the SAMP1/YitFc model is the first animal model to develop fistulizing disease with perianal ulcers. This model has increased our knowledge in the pathogenesis and treatment of CD. It may also help identify other genes that may be involved in the development of CD. Unlike monogenic disorders, the identification of mutated genes in complex genetic disorders (like IBD) is quite difficult. Generally, the whole genome of affected families is probed using polymorphic microsatellite markers. The whole genome screens are based on the principle that a marker that is located close to a disease gene is less likely to be separated during meiosis and can be co-inherited with the disease gene. Using cohorts of Crohn's patients, the NOD2 gene was recently identified in this manner. This approach can also be used to study an inbred stain of rodents in a controlled environment. The SAMP1/YitFc model develops colitis with a 100% penetrance, without exogenous environmental influence. The genetic analysis of this animal model of colitis may help identify disease susceptibility genes that are orthologues of human disease.

CONCLUSION

Animal models of colitis have increased our knowledge in understanding the pathogenesis and treatment of IBD. Immune therapies (anti-TNF therapy) derived from colitis models have become the mainstay of disease management. It has become clear that CD results from a Th1-mediated immune response. New therapies that target the resultant cytokines may further add to the current arsenal (including anti-IL-12 and anti-IL-6). Because UC is influenced by a Th2-mediated immune response, antibody therapy that reduces this response may be useful in the treatment of UC (including anti-IL-13). In addition to limiting effector T cell response, augmenting the T regulatory response in human disease will serve as another avenue of novel treatments (TGF-β). Recognizing that results from four-legged animals (ie, mice) do not always predict results in two-legged animals (ie, humans), identification of disease susceptibility genes using murine colitis models holds great promise for the future.

REFERENCES

1. Croft M. Activation of naïve, memory and effector T cells. *Curr Opin Immunol.* 1994;6:431-437.
2. Shevach EM, McHugh RS, Piccirillo CA, Thornton AM. Control of T-cell activation by CD4+ CD25+ suppressor T cells. *Immunol Rev.* 2001;182:58-67.
3. McHugh RS, Shevach EM, et al. Cutting edge: depletion of CD4+CD25+ regulatory T cells is necessary, but not sufficient, for induction of organ-specific autoimmune disease. *J Immunol.* 2002;168:5979-5983.
4. Neurath MF, Fuss I, Kelsall BL, et al. Antibodies to interleukin 12 abrogate established experimental colitis in mice. *J Exp Med.* 1995;182:1281-1290.
5. Elson CO, Cong Y, Weaver CT, et al. Monoclonal anti-interleukin 23 reverses active colitis in a T cell-mediated model in mice. *Gastroenterology.* 2007;132:2359-2370.
6. Duerr RH, Taylor KD, Brant SR, et al. A genome-wide association study identifies IL23R as an inflammatory bowel disease gene. *Science.* 2006;314:1461-1463.
7. Sandborn WJ, Feagan BG, Fedorak RN, et al. A randomized trial of ustekinumab, a human interleukin-12/23 monoclonal antibody, in patients with moderate-to-severe Crohn's disease. *Gastroenterology.* 2008;135:1130-1141.
8. Boirivant M, Fuss IJ, Chu A, et al. Oxazolone colitis: a murine model of T helper cell type 2 colitis treatable by antibodies to interleukin-4. *J Exp Med.* 1998;188:1929-1939.
9. Heller F, Fuss IJ, Nieuwenhuis EE. Oxazolone colitis, a Th2 colitis model resembling ulcerative colitis, is mediated by IL-13 producing NK-T cells. *Immunity.* 2002;17:629-638.
10. Bouma G, Strober W, Bouma G, et al. The immunological and genetic basis of inflammatory bowel disease. *Nat Rev Immunol.* 2003;3:521-533.
11. Okayasu I, Hatakeyama S, Yamada M, et al. A novel method in the induction of reliable experimental acute and chronic ulcerative colitis in mice. *Gastroenterology.* 1990;98:694-702.
12. Dieleman LA, Palmen MJ, Akol H, et al. Chronic experimental colitis induced by dextran sulphate sodium (DSS) is characterized by Th1 and Th2 cytokines. *Clin Exp Immunol.* 1998;114:385-391.
13. Soriano A, Salas A, Salas A, et al. VCAM-1, but no ICAM-1 or MadCAM-1 immunoblockade ameliorated DSS induced colitis in mice. *Lab Invest.* 2000;80:1541-1551.
14. Powrie F, Correa-Oliveira R, Mauze S, Coffman RL. Regulatory interactions between C D45RBhigh and CD45RBlow CD4+ T cells are important for the balance between protective and pathogenic cell-mediated immunity. *J Exp Med.* 1994;179:589-600.
15. Neurath MF, Weigmann B, Finotto S, et al. The transcription factor T-beta regulates mucosal T cell activation in experimental colitis and Crohn's disease. *J Exp Med.* 2002;195:1129-1143.
16. Powrie F. T cells in inflammatory bowel disease: protective and pathogenic roles. *Immunity.* 1991;3:171-174.
17. Asseman C, Powrie F. Interleukin 10 is a growth factor for a population of regulatory T cells. *Gut.* 1998;42;157-158.
18. Mottet C, Uhlig HH, Powrie F. Cutting edge: cure of colitis by CD4+CD25+ regulatory T cells. *J Immunol.* 2003;170:3939-3943.
19. Fuss IJ, Boirivant M, Lacy B, Strober W. The interrelated roles of TGF-beta and IL-10 in the regulation of experimental colitis. *J Immunol.* 2002;168:900-908.

20. Sadlack B, Merz H, Schorle H, Schimpl A, Feller AC, Horak I. Ulcerative colitis-like disease in mice with a disrupted IL-2 gene. *Cell.* 1993;75:253-261.
21. Boone DL, Dassopoulos T, Lodolce JP, et al. Interleukin deficient mice develop colitis in the absence of CD28 costimulation. *Inflamm Bowel Dis.* 2002;8:35-42.
22. Kühn R, Löhler J, Rennick D, Rajewsky K, Müller W. Interleukin-10 deficient mice develop chronic enterocolitis. *Cell.* 1993;75:263-274.
23. Gratz R, Becker S, Sokolowski N, et al. Murine monoclonal anti–TNF antibody administration has a beneficial effect on IBD that develops in IL-10 knockout mice. *Dig Dis Sci.* 2002;47:1723-1727.
24. Schreiber S, Fedorak RN, Nielsen OH. Safety and efficacy of recombinant human IL-10 in chronic active Crohn's disease. Crohn's disease IL-10 cooperative study group. *Gastroenterology.* 2000;119:1461-1472.
25. Kontoyiannis D, Pasparakis M, Pizarro TT, Cominelli F, Kollias G. Impaired on/off regulation of TNF biosynthesis in mice lacking TNF AU-rich elements: implications for joint and gut-associated immunopathologies. *Immunity.* 1999;10:387-398.
26. Kontoyiannis D, Boulougouris G, Manoloukos M, et al. Genetics of dissection of the cellular pathways and signaling mechanisms in modeled TNF tumor necrosis factor-induced Crohn's-like IBD. *J Exp Med.* 2002;196:1563-1574.
27. Targan SR, Hanauer SB, van Deventer SJ. A short-term study of chimeric monoclonal antibody cA2 to TNF alpha for Crohn's disease. Crohn's Disease cA2 study group. *N Engl J Med.* 1997;337:1029-1035.
28. Present DH, Rutgeerts P, Targan S, et al. Infliximab for the treatment of fistulas in patient with Crohn's disease. *N Engl J Med.* 1999;340:1398-1405.
29. Di Sabatino A, Ciccocioppo R, Cinque B, et al. Defective mucosal T cell death is reverted by infliximab in Crohn's disease. *Gut.* 2004;53:70-77.
30. Mombaerts P, Mizoguchi E, Grusby MJ, Glimcher LH, Bhan AK, Tonegawa S. Spontaneous development of IBD in T cell receptor mutant mice. *Cell.* 1993;75:1-20.
31. Bhan AK, Mizoguchi E, Smith RN, Mizoguchi A. Colitis in transgenic and knockout animals as models of human IBD. *Immunol Rev.* 1999;169:195-207.
32. Mashimo H, Wu DC, Podolsky DK, Fishman MC. Impaired defense of intestinal mucosa in mice lacking intestinal trefoil factor. *Science.* 1996;272:262-265.
33. Ogura Y, Bonen DK, Inohara N, et al. A frameshift mutation in NOD2 associated with susceptibility to Crohn's disease. *Nature.* 2001;411:603-606.
34. Hugot JP, Chamaillard M, Zouali H, et al. Association of NOD2 leucine-rich repeat variants with susceptibility to Crohn's disease. *Nature.* 2001;411:599-603.
35. Yamazaki K, Takazoe M, Tanaka T, Kazumori T, Nakamura Y. Absence of mutation in the NOD2.Card15 gene among 483 Japanese patients with Crohn's disease. *J Hum Genet.* 2002;47:469-472.
36. Watanabe M, Watanabe N, Iwao Y, et al. The serum factor from patients with ulcerative colitis induces T cell proliferation in the mouse thymus is IL-7. *J Clin Immunol.* 1997;17:282-292.
37. Watanabe M, Yamazaki M, Kanai T. Mucosal T cells as a target for treatment of IBD. *J Gastroenterol.* 2003;38:48-50.
38. Rath HC, Ikeda JS, Linde HJ, Schölmerich J, Wilson KH, Sartor RB. Varying cecal bacterial loads influences colitis and gastritis in HLA-B27 transgenic rats. *Gastroenterology.* 1999;116:310-319.
39. Rath HC. Role of commensal bacteria in chronic experimental colitis: lessons from the HLA-B27 transgenic rat. *Pathobiology.* 2003;70:130-138.
40. Takeda K, Clausen BE, Kaisho T, et al. Enhanced Th1 activity and development of chronic enterocolitis in mice devoid of Stat3 in macrophages and neutrophils. *Immunity.* 1999;10:39-49.
41. Cong Y, Brandwein SL, McCabe RP, et al. CD4+ T cells reactive to enteric bacterial antigens in spontaneously colitic C3H/HejBir mice: increased T helper cell type 1 response and ability to transfer disease. *J Exp Med.* 1998;187:855-864.
42. Kirkwood JK, Pearson GR, Epstein MA. Adenocarcinoma of the large bowel and colitis in cottontop tamarins. *J Comp Pathol.* 1986;96:507-515.
43. Warren BF, Henke M, Clapp N. Extra-intestinal manifestations of cottontop tamarin colitis. In: Clapp N, ed. *A Primate Model for the Study of Colitis and Colonic Carcinoma.* Boca Raton, FL: CRC Press; 1993:127-132.
44. Leong KM, Terrell SP, Savage A. Causes of mortality in captive cotton-top tamarins (*Saguinus oedipus*). *Zoo Biol.* 2004;23:127-137.
45. Watkins PE, Foulkes R, Ward P, Stephens S, Warren BF. Faecal tumour necrosis factor alpha in cotton-top tamarin colitis [abstract]. *J Pathol.* 1993;170:364A.
46. Johnson LD, Ausman LM, Sehgal PK, King NW. A prospective study of the epidemiology of colitis and colon cancer in cotton-top tamarins (*Saguinus oedipus*). *Gastroenterology.* 1996;110:102-115.
47. Madara JL, Podolsky DK, King NW, Sehgal PK, Moore R, Winter HS. Characterization of spontaneous colitis in cotton-top tamarins (*Saguinus oedipus*) and its response to sulfasalazine. *Gastroenterology.* 1985;88(1 Pt 1):13-19.
48. Watkins PE, Warren BF, Stephens S, Ward P, Foulkes R. Treatment of ulcerative colitis in the cottontop tamarin using antibody to tumour necrosis factor alpha. *Gut.* 1997;40:628-633.
49. Wood JD, Peck OC, Tefend KS, et al. Colitis and colon cancer in cotton-top tamarins (*Saguinus oedipus oedipus*) living wild in their natural habitat. *Dig Dis Sci.* 1998;43:1443-1453.
50. Wood JD, Peck OC, Tefend KS, et al. Evidence that colitis is initiated by environmental stress and sustained by fecal factors in the cotton-top tamarin (*Saguinus oedipus*). *Dig Dis Sci.* 2000;45:385-393.
51. Johnson LD, Ausman LM, Rolland RM, Chalifoux LV, Russell RG. *Campylobacter*-induced enteritis and diarrhea in captive cotton-top tamarins (*Saguinus oedipus*) during the first year of life. *Comp Med.* 2001;51:257-261.
52. Saunders KE, Shen Z, Dewhirst FE, Paster BJ, Dangler CA, Fox JG. Novel intestinal *Helicobacter* species isolated from cotton-top tamarins (Saguinus oedipus) with chronic colitis. *J Clin Microbiol.* 1999;37:146-151.
53. Mansfield KG, Lin KC, Xia D, et al. Enteropathogenic *E. coli* and ulcerative colitis in cotton-top tamarins (Saguinus oedipus). *J Infect Dis.* 2001;184:803-807.
54. Moore R, King N, Alroy J. Differences in cellular glycoconjugates of quiescent, inflamed, and neoplastic colonic epithelium in colitis and cancer-prone tamarins. *Am J Pathol.* 1988;131(3):484-489.
55. Van Kruiningen HJ, Montali RJ, Strandberg JD, Kirk RW. A granulomatous colitis of dogs with histologic resemblance to Whipple's disease. *Pathol Vet.* 1965;2:521-544.
56. German AJ, Hall EJ, Kelly DF, Watson AD, Day MJ. An immunohistochemical study of histiocytic ulcerative colitis in boxer dogs. *J Comp Pathol.* 2000;122(2-3):163-175.
57. Hostutler RA, Luria BJ, Johnson SE, et al. Antibiotic-responsive histiocytic ulcerative colitis in 9 dogs. *J Vet Intern Med.* 2004;18:499-504.
58. Davies DR, O'Hara AJ, Irwin PJ, Guilford WG. Successful management of histiocytic ulcerative colitis with enrofloxacin in two boxer dogs. *Aust Vet J.* 2004;82:58-61.
59. Baumgart M, Dogan B, Rishniw M, et al. Adherent and invasive *Escherichia coli* is associated with granulomatous colitis in boxer dogs. *Infect Immun.* 2006;74:4778-4792.

60. Hanauer SB. Inflammatory bowel disease: epidemiology, pathogenesis, and therapeutic opportunities. *Inflamm Bowel Dis.* 2006;12(suppl 1):S3-S9.
61. Relman DA, Schmidt TM, MacDermott RP, Falkow S. Identification of the uncultured bacillus of Whipple's disease. *N Engl J Med.* 1992;327:293-301.
62. Van Kruiningen HJ, Civco IC, Cartun RW. The comparative importance of *E. coli* antigen in granulomatous colitis of Boxer dogs. *APMIS.* 2005;113:420-425.
63. Darfeuille-Michaud A, Boudeau J, Bulois P, et al. High prevalence of adherent-invasive *Escherichia coli* associated with ileal mucosa in Crohn's disease. *Gastroenterology.* 2004;127:412-421.
64. Baumgart M, Dogan B, Rishniw M, et al. Culture independent analysis of ileal mucosa reveals a selective increase in invasive *Escherichia coli* of novel phylogeny relative to depletion of Clostridiales in Crohn's disease involving the ileum. *ISME J.* 2007;1(5):403-418.
65. Matsumoto S, Okabe Y, Setoyama H, et al. Inflammatory bowel disease-like enteritis and caecitis in a senescence accelerated mouse P1/Yit strain. *Gut.* 1998;43;71-78.
66. Kosiewicz MM, Nast CC, Krishnan A, et al. Th1 type responses mediate spontaneous ileitis in a novel murine model of Crohn's disease. *J Clin Invest.* 2001;107:695-702.
67. Rivera-Nieves J, Bamias G, Vidrich A, et al. Emergence of perianal fistualizing disease in the SAMP1/YitFc mouse, a spontaneous model of chronic ileitis. *Gastroenterology.* 2003;124;972-982.
68. Marini M, Bamias G, Rivera-Nieves J, et al. TNF-α neutralization ameliorated the severity of murine Crohn's like ileitis by abrogation of intestinal cell apoptosis. *Proc Natl Acad Sci U S A.* 2003;100:8366-8371.
69. Bamias G, Marini M, Moskaluk CA, et al. Down regulation of intestinal lymphocyte activation and Th1 cytokine production by antibiotic therapy in a murine model of Crohn's disease. *J Immunology.* 2002;169:5308-5314.
70. Burns RC, Rivera-Nieves J, Moskaluk CA, Matsumoto S, Cominelli F, Ley K. Antibody blockade of ICAM-1 and VCAM-1 ameliorates inflammation in the SAMP1/Yit adoptive transfer model of Crohn's disease in mice. *Gastroenterology.* 2001;121:1428-1436.

5

Pediatric Considerations in Medical Therapy in Patients With Inflammatory Bowel Disease

Louis R. Ghanem, MD, PhD and Robert N. Baldassano, MD

Once considered rare in pediatric practice, chronic inflammatory bowel disease (IBD) is now being recognized with increasing frequency in children of all ages. In fact, 25% to 30% of all patients with Crohn's disease (CD) and 20% of those with ulcerative colitis present before the age of 20 years.[1] Four percent of pediatric IBD occurs before the age of 5 years, with a peak age of onset in the late adolescent years. With the increasing recognition of IBD among pediatric patients, it has become one of the most significant chronic diseases afflicting children and adolescents.[2]

Although the similarities between adult and pediatric patients diagnosed with IBD are numerous, several important differences should be emphasized. In addition to the usual gastrointestinal symptoms of diarrhea, abdominal pain, and rectal bleeding, children may exhibit prominent extraintestinal manifestations, such as growth failure, weight loss, anemia, delayed puberty, and joint symptoms. Other problems unique to pediatrics include the lack of appropriate numbers of controlled clinical trials and the psychological issues that occur in children and adolescents with IBD. These unique problems encountered in the pediatric population necessitate a different medical approach than is used for adult-onset IBD. This chapter reviews aspects in the management of pediatric inflammatory bowel disease that merit special consideration.

EPIDEMIOLOGY

Since the 1930s, the incidence of IBD has greatly increased. In the 1950s, ulcerative colitis was twice as prevalent as Crohn's disease, but recent studies in the United States show that CD has been steadily increasing.[3] IBD is now recognized as one of the most significant chronic diseases to affect children and adolescents.[4] Pediatric IBD population-based epidemiological studies are sparse. They are difficult to perform because of the large number of patients needed, high cost, and potential for surveillance error, and they are difficult to compare due to different criteria and design.[5,6] Analysis of time trends indicates a rapid rise in incidence of Crohn's from the 1960s to 1980s with subsequent stabilization,[7] although some studies indicate a continuing rise in recent years.[5,8,9] The incidence of UC showed a more stable pattern, although again with a tendency for an increase over the years.[8,9] The incidence rates for pediatric IBD range from 0.2 to 8.5 per 100,000 for CD and 0.5 to 4.3 per 100,000 for UC.

The gender distribution of IBD among children indicates slightly increased preponderance of CD in boys,[2] whereas UC affects both genders equally. At the author's institution, there is a 2:1 male to female ratio for CD. A recent hypothesis regarding the etiology of IBD supports the multifactorial theory encompassing genetic predisposition, internal and external environmental influences, and immune system disorder.[10] Genetic factors are well-recognized, with a high rate of concordance between monozygotic twins (44.4%) compared to dizygotic twins (3.8%).[11] Though there is no simple Mendelian genetic mechanism at work in the transmission of IBD, multiple familial occurrences are well-documented in 30% of patients diagnosed with CD under 20 years of age compared to only 13% in patients diagnosed later. Familial IBD is particularly common with early-onset IBD; in our institution, the incidence of IBD in first-degree relatives among the patients who present before 5 years of age is 56%. It is imperative that large, prospective genetic studies as well as studies of environmental expo-

Lichtenstein GR, ed.
Ulcerative Colitis: The Complete Guide to Medical Management (pp. 53-70)

TABLE 5-1

FREQUENCY OF COMMON PRESENTING SYMPTOMS

Symptom	Crohn's Disease (%)	Ulcerative Colitis (%)
Abdominal pain	62 to 95	54 to 76
Diarrhea	52 to 78	67 to 93
Hematochezia	14 to 60	52 to 97
Weight loss	43 to 92	22 to 55
Fever	11 to 48	4 to 34

Reprinted with permissino from Mamula P, Markowitz J, Baldassano RN. Clinical features and natural history of pediatric inflammatory bowel disease. In: Sartor RB, Sandborn WJ, eds. *Kirsner's Inflammatory Bowel Diseases.* 6th ed. Philadelphia, PA: Saunders Company; 2004:301-315.

sures to infections and living conditions are performed in children. The pediatric population is ideal for this type of research for various reasons. Environmental factors potentially leading to IBD may occur early in life; modification of early environment may be attempted. Patients with early-onset disease tend to show more aggressive disease with a stronger genetic influence. Access to patients' relatives is easier when the diagnosis is made in childhood than in adult populations.[4,10] Recent genomic-wide association studies have identified multiple genes that are associated with pediatric-onset IBD.

CLINICAL FEATURES

Crohn's Disease

Unlike the findings in UC, the intestinal involvement in CD may occur in any portion of the gastrointestinal tract. The presentation is determined primarily by the location and extent of disease involvement. The majority of children have disease involving the terminal ileum (50% to 70%), with more than half of these patients also having inflammation in variable segments of the colon, usually the ascending colon.[12-14] Ten percent to 20% of children have isolated colonic disease, and 10% to 15% have diffuse small bowel disease of the more proximal ileum or jejunum. Isolated gastroduodenal disease is uncommon (fewer than 5% of patients), but there may be endoscopic and histologic evidence of gastroduodenal inflammation in up to 30% to 40% of children with CD.[15] CD involving the small intestine usually presents with evidence of malabsorption including diarrhea, abdominal pain, growth deceleration, weight loss, and anorexia. Initially, these symptoms may be quite subtle, and any one may predominate the clinical picture. The onset of growth failure is usually insidious, and any child or adolescent with persistent alterations in growth should have an appropriate diagnostic evaluation for IBD. Growth failure may precede the onset of intestinal symptoms by years.[16] There are multiple causes of growth failure in patients with CD, but inadequate nutrient intake is usually present. Anorexia, reduced intake, malabsorption, increased losses, and increased metabolic demands all contribute to poor growth. Small bowel mucosal disease may result in malabsorption of iron, zinc, folate, or vitamin B_{12} deficiency. CD involving the colon may be clinically indistinguishable from UC, with symptoms of bloody mucopurulent diarrhea, crampy abdominal pain, and urgency to defecate. Table 5-1 summarizes common presenting symptoms in patients with CD and UC. Symptoms of painful defecation, bright red rectal bleeding, and perirectal pain may signal perianal disease, which may occur without symptomatic involvement in any other area of the intestinal tract. Perianal involvement includes simple skin tags, fissures, abscesses, and fistulae. The perineum should be inspected in all patients presenting with signs and symptoms of CD because abnormalities detectable in this region will substantially increase the clinical suspicion of IBD.

Delay in diagnosis of IBD in the pediatric population continues to be a concern, even with increasing incidence and heightened awareness of IBD. Mean delay for CD in children is reported to be between 7 and 11 months, in UC between 5 and 8 months, and in indeterminate colitis 14 months.[17-19] At the same time, the delay in the adult population is even longer and is measured in years.[20] The time lag between onset of symptoms and correct diagnosis of CD appears to be prolonged if the disease affects more proximal bowel and if presenting symptoms do not include diarrhea. The diagnosis is particularly difficult when the presenting symptoms are uncharacteristic and consist mainly of extraintestinal manifestations.

Ulcerative Colitis

UC is a diffuse mucosal inflammation limited to the colon; it invariably affects the rectum and may extend proximally in a symmetrical uninterrupted pattern to involve parts or all of the large intestine. Because UC is a mucosal disease limited to the colon, the most common presenting symptoms are rectal bleeding, diarrhea, and abdominal pain. Langholz et al reported that, at diagnosis, children with UC had more extensive disease than did adults.[12] Abdominal pain was also more common. The cumulative colectomy probability was 6% after 1 year and 29% after 20 years, not different from that of adults. They also reported that when a child presents with a proctitis at diagnosis, there is a 65% chance of further spread of the disease to other parts of the large intestine during the course of the disease. This compares to a 39% chance of progression among adult-onset patients (not significant).[12] There are multiple patterns of presentation of UC in the pediatric age group, and 50% to 60% have mild disease. The diarrhea is insidious in onset and later associated with hematochezia. There are no systemic signs of fever, weight loss, or hypoalbuminemia. The disease is usually confined to the distal colon and responds well to therapy. Thirty percent of pediatric patients present with moderate disease characterized by bloody diarrhea, cramps, urgency to defecate, and abdominal tenderness according to population-based data. These patients have associated systemic signs, such as anorexia, weight loss, low-grade fever, and mild anemia. Severe colitis occurs in approximately 10% of patients. This presentation is characterized by more than 6 bloody stools per day, abdominal tenderness, fever, anemia, leukocytosis, and hypoalbuminemia. Severe hemorrhage, toxic megacolon, and perforation are serious complications in this group of patients.[21-23] Occasionally, children with UC may have a presentation dominated by extraintestinal manifestations, such as growth failure, arthropathy, skin manifestations, or liver disease. This is uncommon in adults and accounts for less than 5% of the pediatric disease.[13] Delay in diagnosis in UC is between 5 and 8 months.

Complications

CD and UC are both associated with significant gastrointestinal complications. The major intestinal complications of UC are massive bleeding, toxic megacolon, and carcinoma.

GASTROINTESTINAL COMPLICATIONS

CD is associated with significant gastrointestinal complications. The major intestinal complications of CD are due to the transmural nature of the disease. This leads to the formation of abscesses, fistulae, strictures, and adhesions, which may also contribute to the development of obstruction or bacterial overgrowth.

Colonic malignancy is a significant complication in both UC and CD in patients with pancolitis beginning in childhood.[24] Duration of disease and pancolitis are well-recognized as risk factors for the development of malignancy, with the risk of cancer increasing over that of the general population after 10 years of disease.[25] Other less well-characterized risk factors include concomitant sclerosing cholangitis; an excluded, defunctionalized, or bypassed segment; and depressed red blood cell folate levels. Although the risk of malignancy in CD is not as high as in UC, the risk of adenocarcinoma of the colon for Crohn's colitis is 4 to 20 times that of the general population. Patients with small intestinal disease are 50 to 100 times more likely to develop small intestinal carcinoma. Because small intestinal carcinoma is a rare event in the general population, it is also uncommon in CD.

Perforation is one of the more serious complications of IBD and is less common in CD than UC. Colonic perforation in UC usually occurs in association with toxic megacolon or severe fulminant disease. Perforation in CD usually occurs in the ileum and is not correlated with disease activity.[27] The presenting features of perforation are those of classic peritonitis, although these features may be masked by high-dose corticosteroid therapy.

Fistula and abscess formation is common in CD due to transmural bowel inflammation. Perianal and perirectal fistulization is the most common, with the most common enteroenteric fistula being between the ileum and sigmoid colon. Perianal disease occurs in 15% of pediatric patients with CD.[28] Perianal disease may precede the appearance of the intestinal manifestations of CD by several years and is seen most commonly in patients with colitis. Perianal disease may not respond to medical therapy, and surgical management would be necessary.

EXTRAINTESTINAL MANIFESTATIONS

Up to 35% of pediatric IBD patients in some series have at least one extraintestinal manifestation as a presenting sign.[29,30] Common symptoms in a series of pediatric IBD patients from Israel included anorexia, joint complaints, and anemia.[31] Table 5-2 lists extraintestinal manifestations commonly seen in children with IBD. These manifestations may also be noted concurrently or after the diagnosis of IBD is made.[29]

Skin manifestations include erythema nodosum and pyoderma gangrenosum. Erythema nodosum is more common in CD and affects 3% of pediatric patients with CD.[32] It is estimated that 75% of the patients with erythema nodosum ultimately develop arthritis.[33]

Mouth ulceration is the most common oral manifestation of IBD. It is more common in CD, frequently associated with skin and joint lesions, and together with skin and eye manifestations often parallels the activity of disease.[34]

TABLE 5-2

EXTRAINTESTINAL MANIFESTATIONS OF INFLAMMATORY BOWEL DISEASE

Skin	**Eye**
Erythema nodosum	Uveitis
Pyoderma gangrenosum	Episcleritis
Perianal disease	Conjunctivitis
Metastatic Crohn's disease	
	Lungs
Mouth	Pulmonary vasculitis
Cheilitis	Fibrosing alveolitis
Stomatitis	
Aphthae	**Vascular**
	Vasculitis
Liver	Thrombosis (pulmonary, limb, cerebrovascular)
Primary sclerosing cholangitis	
Hepatitis	**Joints**
Cholelithiasis	Arthralgia
	Arthritis
Pancreas	Ankylosing spondylitis
Pancreatitis	
	Blood
Kidney	Iron deficiency anemia
Nephrolithiasis	Anemia of chronic disease
Obstructive hydronephrosis	Thrombocytosis
Enterovesical fistula	Autoimmune hemolytic anemia
Urinary tract infection	Vitamin B_{12} deficiency
Amyloidosis	
	General
Growth	Fever
Delayed growth	Fatigue
Delayed puberty	Weight loss
	Anorexia
Bone	
Osteoporosis	
Osteopenia	

Courtesy of Mamula P, Markowitz J, Baldassano RN. Clinical features and natural history of pediatric inflammatory bowel disease. In: Sartor RB, Sandborn WJ, eds. *Kirsner's Inflammatory Bowel Diseases.* 6th ed. Philadelphia, PA: Saunders Company: 2004:301-315.

Ophthalmologic manifestations occur in about 4% of the adult population with IBD but less frequently in children and adolescents with UC and CD.[35] The most common ocular findings are episcleritis and anterior uveitis.

Arthritis is the most common extraintestinal manifestation in children and adolescents, occurring in 7% to 25% of pediatric IBD patients.[36] The arthritis is usually transient, nondeforming synovitis, asymmetric in distribution, and involves the large joints of the lower extremities. In adults, the arthritis occurs when the disease is active, but in children the arthritis may occur years before any gastrointestinal symptoms develop.[37] Ankylosing spondylitis occurs in 2% to 6% of patients and is more common in males. It is associated with HLA-B27. Though not truly an arthritis, clubbing is common in children with CD involving the small intestine.[34]

Hepatobiliary manifestations in children may precede the onset of IBD, accompany active disease, or develop after surgical resection of all diseased bowel.[38] Hepatic manifestations include elevation of aminotransferases, chronic active hepatitis, granulomatous hepatitis, amyloidosis, fatty liver, and sclerosing cholangitis. Abnormal serum aminotransferases are commonly transient and appear to relate to medications or disease activity. If elevation persists, patients should be evaluated for the etiology of viral hepatitis. Chronic active hepatitis develops in less than 1% of children with IBD.[39] Colitis at the time may be relatively asymptomatic, although the hepatitis may proceed to cirrhosis. Sclerosing cholangitis develops in 3.5% of pediatric patients with UC, usually with extensive disease, and less than 1% of pediatric patients with CD.[39] It is not related to disease activity and may appear years before any gastrointestinal disease develops or even years after a colectomy for UC. In a series of 36 pediatric patients with IBD who developed sclerosing cholangitis, only 4 had CD and 32 had UC.[40] The authors suggested heightened endoscopic surveillance once the diagnosis of IBD is made in the setting of sclerosing cholangitis because the time to dysplasia may be accelerated, as noted in 3 pediatric patients who underwent proctocolectomy due to dysplasia. Endoscopic retrograde cholangiopancreatography and magnetic resonance cholangiopancreatography have significantly improved the ability to diagnose this disease in the pediatric population. Cholelithiasis has been described in both UC and CD but more frequently in CD, especially after ileal resection.

The common urologic manifestations of IBD include nephrolithiasis, hydronephrosis, and enterovesicular fistulae. Nephrolithiasis is a common renal complication in pediatrics and occurs in approximately 5% of the children with IBD.[4] It usually is the result of fat malabsorption that occurs with small bowel CD. Dietary calcium binds to malabsorbed fatty acids in the colonic lumen, and free oxalate is absorbed. This results in hyperoxaluria and oxalate stones.[41] In patients with an ileostomy, increased fluid and electrolyte losses may lead to a concentrated, acidic urine and the formation of uric acid stones. External compression of the ureter by an inflammatory mass or abscess may lead to hydronephrosis. Enterovesical fistulae, which are more common in males, may present with recurrent urinary tract infections or pneumaturia.

Thromboembolic disease is a rare but severe complication of IBD. Both UC and CD are thought to be associated with a prothrombotic state with enhanced parameters of coagulation.[42] Several different coagulation abnormalities have been reported in patients with IBD, imparting an increased risk of thrombotic vascular disease over the general population: increased fibrinogen, thrombocytosis and abnormal platelet activation, accelerated thromboplastin generation, elevation of factors V and VIII, decreased antithrombin III, protein S and C deficiency, elevated anticardiolipin antibodies, high plasma factor VII coagulant activity, resistance to activated protein C, and prothrombin gene mutation (G20210).[43-45] Thromboembolic complications are reported in 1.3% to 6.4% of pediatric patients with IBD.[42,44] In the adult population, pulmonary, abdominal, and peripheral veins and arteries are more commonly involved than cerebral or retinal vessels. In pediatric IBD patients, cerebral and retinal vessels seem to be affected more frequently than other sites; thrombosis in these sites carries a better prognosis than in adults.[44,46] The majority of patients have active disease at the time of the thromboembolic event, more so in children than in the adult population.

Other extraintestinal manifestations may develop due to side effects of treatment. Those include pancreatitis, pericarditis, alopecia, osteoporosis, cataracts, acne, hepatitis, anemia, neutropenia, fibrosing alveolitis, interstitial pneumonitis, and peripheral neuropathy. For example, pancreatitis may result from therapy with 5-aminosalicylic acid, 6-mercaptopurine (6-MP), corticosteroids, and methotrexate; peripheral neuropathy may occur with metronidazole therapy; and corticosteroid therapy is associated with acne, cataracts, and osteoporosis.

GROWTH AND NUTRITION

Growth failure is a common problem in pediatric and adolescent patients with IBD. Abnormal nutritional status in IBD is now universally acknowledged. Poor growth in IBD is often attributed to chronic malnutrition related to decreased intake, as well as increased intestinal losses and metabolic demands, which if present concurrently produce a situation almost impossible to compensate for by oral intake alone.[47-49]

Growth failure may be the earliest sign of IBD in children and adolescents. Up to 85% of children with CD, and as many as 65% of those with UC, will demonstrate growth failure at the time of diagnosis.[50] A decreased rate of height accrual (growth velocity) may also precede diagnosis. In a review of 50 children and prepubescent adolescents with CD, 88% showed a decrease in height velocity before diagnosis.[51] Perhaps more importantly, 46% revealed evidence of decreased height velocity prior to the development of symptoms attributable to CD. Surprisingly, 34 of the 44 patients with decreased linear growth were still above the 5th percentile for height based on age. This fact may have contributed to further delay in diagnosis, as the time between onset of growth failure and diagnosis was more than twice as long in the group with heights above the 5th percentile. Accordingly, growth velocity (rather than height for age percentile) has been incorporated into the scoring system of the Pediatric Crohn's Disease Activity Index (PCDAI). This index was developed and validated by a group of senior pediatric gastroenterologists in 1991[52] and correlates well with the original Crohn's Disease Activity Index (CDAI) developed for adult patients.[53]

Because decreasing height velocity is evident in the majority of CD patients several months or years before they develop symptoms attributable to the disease, there is a high likelihood they already demonstrate signs of chronic malnutrition at the time of diagnosis. Therefore, management of these patients should incorporate a plan for nutritional rehabilitation.

Poor intake is commonly felt to be the most important etiology of malnutrition in IBD.[4,54,55] Several studies have documented that dietary intake is chronically deficient in the majority of growth-retarded children with CD.[49,56,57] The causes of decreased food intake are multifactorial. Children and adolescents with IBD may limit their diet because eating exacerbates abdominal symptoms, including pain, nausea and bloating from partial obstruction, or diarrhea. Additionally, they may suffer from anorexia related to depression or increased inflammatory mediators such as tumor necrosis factor alpha (TNFα) and interleukin-1 (IL-1).[58] These repeated symptoms after eating lead to behavioral conditioning.[59] The impact of nutritional status is perhaps most significant during adolescence as the pubertal growth spurt accounts for about 16% of the adult height. Also, delays in skeletal maturation, onset of menarche, and epiphyseal fusion in long bones occur with undernutrition.

Several studies of patients with IBD demonstrate significant weight gain when calories are supplemented by a variety of means. Intravenous nutrition administered during acute exacerbations has been demonstrated to maintain fluid and electrolyte status and to arrest some of the early catabolism of protein stores.[58,60] Therapy for children with growth failure and IBD must initially be directed toward achieving remission and maximizing nutritional support. Kirschner et al demonstrated in a small series of children with CD that growth retardation responded to enterally administered calories, as measured by height velocity and height percentile.[61] To achieve these results, caloric intake was increased from 56% to 91% of the recommended goal for a period of 12 months. Improved linear growth rates and growth percentiles were seen in all patients. This study was among the first that was able to show that nutritional therapy was a useful adjunct to medical therapy of CD and suggested that enteral nutrition should be employed before more invasive therapies such as surgery or parenteral nutrition. The ability of enteral feeding to reverse malnutrition was also demonstrated by Motil et al.[56] In a series of 6 adolescents with active CD, caloric intake was increased by more than 40% (from 67 to 96 kcal/kg/day), with protein intake increasing from 2.3 to 3.2 g/kg/day for a period of 3 weeks. Patients gained an average of 3.3 kg over the study period, with a resultant increase in newly synthesized body protein stores as measured by radiolabeled leucine metabolism. The authors concluded that significant weight gain is achievable with short-term enteral nutritional supplementation and that the weight gain resulted largely from lean body mass accretion.

Despite the ability to induce both weight and height acquisition through calorie and nutrient supplementation, it is also clear that some effects of malnutrition are irreversible. When adjusting height for genetic potential based on parental height, many patients with CD never achieve expected levels, as demonstrated by measuring body composition in 132 subjects with CD and 66 controls aged 5 to 25 years.[55] In this population, adjusted height *z* scores (which compare a pediatric patient in standard deviations from the mean for that age) were significantly lower than predicted heights. These findings were most pronounced in male patients, in whom the average adjusted height *z* score was a full standard deviation below expected.

ASSESSMENT OF GROWTH AND NUTRITION

Accurately assessing growth and nutritional status is the first step in successfully addressing these issues in IBD. Growth irregularities in children with IBD have been measured in various ways, including weight for age, height for age, height and weight adjusted *z* score, height velocity, and various anthropometric measures such as head circumference, midarm circumference, and triceps skinfold thickness.[50,62] When assessing a patient with IBD for growth failure, one must first use accurate measurements. Weight measurement should be performed on the same scale, with the patient wearing similar amounts of clothing each time. Height measurement should be obtained using a stadiometer, and the patient should be measured without shoes.

Accurate assessment of nutritional status, however, relies on more than just height and weight at a given time. Genetic height potential, determined by mid-parental height, should be calculated.[63] Previous height and weight points should be considered, with calculation of growth velocity. Height and weight deficit calculations expressed as a ratio of the actual height or weight divided by the expected value based on the 50th percentile for age can give insight into the duration of malnutrition. In cases of short-term deficiencies, one can expect weight deficit (wasting), whereas long-term malnutrition often results in height deficit (stunting).[62]

Stage of sexual maturation is an important reflection of nutritional status, with significant implications for the patient. Adolescents with CD often have delay in the onset of pubertal development, and active disease could potentially delay the onset of puberty indefinitely with a deleterious effect on growth.[64] Duration of puberty can also be affected in children with IBD, as active or relapsing disease during the years after puberty may slow down or even arrest the progression of puberty.

Patients who are in remission by the time they reach puberty may experience good catch-up growth with improved height velocity.[65] However, the persistence of growth deficits after the development of secondary sexual characteristics may signify irreversible loss of growth potential. Therefore, accurate staging of sexual development, using the parameters described by Tanner,[66] should be a routine component of the ongoing evaluation and care of any young patient with IBD.

Nutritional assessment should also include evaluation for macro- and micronutrient deficiencies. Overall caloric intake should be assessed using diet diaries, recorded for at least 3 consecutive days. This type of assessment allows accurate calculation of not just overall calories but the breakdown of fat, protein, and carbohydrate intake, as well as the amount of various micronutrients in the diet.

Iron intake is important in the diet of all children and adolescents, especially those with IBD, with more than 70% of patients manifesting iron deficiency.[67] Small bowel disease, a history of small bowel resection, and increased intestinal transit time may result in poor absorption of iron. Iron supplementation may cause frequent adverse side effects including indigestion and diarrhea, resulting in poor patient compliance.[68] Diet diaries may suggest that one is at risk of iron deficiency, with confirmation from objective measures such as hemoglobin, mean corpuscular volume, reticulocyte count, and levels of iron, ferritin, and transferrin saturation. Absorption of other micronutrients, in particular vitamin B_{12}, folic acid, vitamin D, and calcium, may also be impaired under various conditions in IBD. For example, extensive ileal disease or resection may result in B_{12} deficiency, whereas sulfasalazine administration can interfere with folate metabolism, resulting in megaloblastic anemia. Of all the micronutrients, calcium and vitamin D have received the greatest attention because of their role in bone disease.

BONE DISEASE AND OSTEOPOROSIS

Calcium homeostasis and bone growth are important aspects of malnutrition in pediatric IBD. Bone disease suffered by patients with IBD can be a combination of *osteomalacia*, defined as abnormal bone mineralization, and *osteoporosis*, defined as reduced bone mass.[69] *Osteopenia* is the general term used for any abnormality of bone density and may occur in the context of either osteomalacia or osteoporosis.

Osteoporosis can be reliably detected by measurement of bone mineral density, of which dual energy x-ray absorptiometry (DEXA) is the favored approach.[70] When measured by DEXA, bone mineral density is expressed as the number of standard deviations above or below the mean for age-matched controls (*z* score). One must be careful in interpreting bone density under circumstances of abnormal growth, however. For example, a patient with significant stunting may exhibit an abnormal *z* score for age but may in turn have a normal *z* score for height. Under these circumstances, the bone density changes over time have more clinical significance than any individual *z* score. One should also be aware of the use of T scores in the expression of bone density. These scores express bone density as compared to other young adults and have little interpretive value for pediatric patients with IBD.

It is now believed that osteoporosis in the elderly has its roots in childhood. Adult levels of bone mineralization are predominantly achieved during childhood and adolescence,[71] and there remains no definitive treatment for significant osteoporosis. Therefore, derangements in calcium intake and bone growth early in life, such as those that occur with early-onset IBD, may have profound permanent results on bone density. One of the serious consequences of osteoporosis is bone fracture, with vertebral compression fracture representing a frequent complication.[72] The health-care costs of disability from osteoporosis-related fractures are considerable.[73] As a result, childhood prevention of adult bone disease takes on a high level of significance. Effective prevention of osteoporosis and its consequences must occur during childhood, and identifying those patients at risk of abnormal bones is the cornerstone of successful prevention.

Rates of bone turnover are higher in children and adolescents than in adults. In a study of bone mass and biochemical markers of bone turnover in children at various stages of sexual development, bone formation markers were found to be highest at mid-puberty with reduction in late puberty.[74] Measures of bone formation correlated most highly with bone density, emphasizing the importance of this period of development on final bone composition.

The skeletal complications of IBD are in large part related to poor nutrition. Vitamin D deficiency is common among patients with IBD, and CD in particular, with more than 50% of patients demonstrating abnormal levels.[75] This deficiency could relate to decreased intake of dairy products, which may exacerbate abdominal symptoms in patients with lactose intolerance. Alternatively, patients with a history of ileal resection or active ileal disease may undergo treatment with cholestyramine, which binds vitamin D in addition to binding bile acids. Other disordered mechanisms of

TABLE 5-3

PHARMACOLOGIC THERAPY FOR INFLAMMATORY BOWEL DISEASE IN PEDIATRICS

	Ulcerative Colitis	Crohn's Disease
Mild Disease and Remission	Sulfasalazine (Azulfidine) 50 to 75 mg/kg/day divided bid to qid (max. 5 g/day)	
	Mesalamine (Asacol, Pentasa) 50 to 75 mg/kg/day divided tid to qid (max. Asacol 4.8 g/day, Pentasa 4.0 g/day)	
	Mesalamine enema (Rowasa) 4 g qhs	
	Mesalamine suppository (Canasa) 500 mg qhs or bid	
	Hydrocortisone enema (Cortenema) qd to bid	
	Budesonide enema (Entocort enema 2 g/100 mL qd)	
Moderate Disease		Metronidazole (Flagyl) 15 mg/kg/d divided tid (max. 1 g/day)
		Nutritional therapy
	Continue the above therapies with the addition of prednisone, to be tapered to every other day over a 4- to 6-week period, depending on clinical remission. 1 to 2 mg/kg/daily qid (maximum oral dose of 40 mg/day)	
	Budesonide (Entocort) (controlled ileal release) 9 mg qd, may replace prednisone for acute flare	
Refractory Disease	Azathioprine (Imuran) 2.0 to 2.5 mg/kg/day qd	
	6-Mercaptopurine (Purinethol) 1.0 to 1.5 mg/kg/day qd	
	Cyclosporine A (Sandimmune IV or PO) 4 to 6 mg/kg continuous infusion or bid	
	Infliximab (Remicade) 5-10 mg/kg/dose IV	

bid indicates twice a day; qid, 4 times a day; tid, 3 times a day; qhs, every hour of sleep; qd, every day; IV, intravenously; PO, orally.

Adapted from Baldassano RN, Piccoli DA. Inflammatory bowel disease in pediatric and adolescent patients. *Gastroenterol Clin North Am.* 1999;28:445-458.

vitamin D homeostasis may be present in IBD patients, such as changes in the metabolic clearance of vitamin D related to calcium deficiency,[76,77] and could explain why ultraviolet light is not adequate to overcome dietary deficiencies. This would be of particular importance in IBD as, once established, a derangement in vitamin D or calcium homeostasis could become a self-perpetuating problem.[69]

Calcium homeostasis is another important factor in bone mineralization and density in IBD patients. As with vitamin D, decreased intake coupled with avoidance of dairy products may lead to inadequate dietary calcium. In contrast to vitamin D, however, calcium cannot be synthesized de novo. Furthermore, calcium deficiency may be exacerbated by fat malabsorption, which is present in patients with CD-related small bowel disease. The most important effects on calcium homeostasis may be secondary to the use of corticosteroids, as long-term corticosteroid therapy has been shown to inhibit intestinal calcium absorption and tubular resorption of calcium in the kidney.[78,79]

Beyond calcium malabsorption, corticosteroids may have a negative impact on bone remodeling in IBD patients. This includes the inhibition of osteoblastic activity, which limits bone formation, while osteoblastic activity continues unabated.[80,81] Corticosteroids also depress calcitonin levels, resulting in further bone resorption.[82] The clinician treating IBD is often faced with a double-edged sword when considering treatment with corticosteroids. Disease activity may be improved by treatment with corticosteroids, resulting in improved intake and absorption of vital nutrients. The use of corticosteroids may also undermine the development of adequate linear growth and bone density, however. It is unclear which situation is less desirable, but neither one is optimal. It is still debated whether the short-term benefits that corticosteroids offer for control of symptoms offset the long-term effects on bones. This dilemma may be resolved by rapidly metabolized corticosteroids such as budesonide or avoidance of corticosteroids by using alternatives such as anti-TNFα agents.

Various inflammatory cytokines also impact calcium homeostasis. IBD patients who have increased secretion of the proinflammatory cytokine IL-1β on a genetic basis are at increased risk of developing osteopenia.[83] In a study of 83 patients with IBD, it was shown that noncarriage of the allele for normal IL-1ra expression was independently associated with the development of increased bone loss.[84] In this same study, carrying an allele for increased expression of IL-6 was correlated with bone loss. Bone loss in this study was not, however, related to disease severity or use of corticosteroids. Based on these results, it was felt that genetic variation in the genes responsible for cytokine expression has a significant role in whether patients with IBD develop metabolic bone disease.

DELAYED PUBERTY

Children with Crohn's disease often have delay in the onset of pubertal development, and careful evaluation of pubertal staging should be part of their routine evaluation. Active disease uncontrolled by medical therapy could potentially delay the onset of puberty indefinitely with a deleterious effect on pubertal growth.[85] The duration of puberty could also be affected in children with CD. Active or relapsing disease during the years following the onset of puberty may slow down or even arrest the progression of puberty. Arrest of pubertal development in children with CD may be an early indication of disease relapse, and in the same way delay in pubertal onset may indicate persistent occult disease. Inducing disease remission before the onset of puberty and maintaining it during the pubertal years is crucial in order to avoid losing valuable height as a consequence of a missed pubertal growth spurt. Patients who are in remission by the time they go into puberty can experience good catch-up growth with peak height velocities greater than 12 cm/year.[65] The potential for catch-up growth may be severely compromised in those children who suffered relapse or whose disease activity is not controlled in the peripubertal years. Differing from healthy children, delayed puberty in CD may not allow future prolonged and/or greater linear growth.[55]

Factors affecting pubertal development in children with CD include nutritional deprivation, the inflammatory process, hormonal disturbances, and the effects of therapy. Severe protein-calorie malnutrition and weight loss can be associated with prepubertal levels of sex steroids, despite previous evidence of pubertal progression. Secondary amenorrhea is also observed following severe weight loss in these patients, similar to patients with anorexia nervosa where there is suppression of gonadotrophin secretion.[86]

Delayed puberty in patients with CD may affect the normal bone mineral accumulation peak that follows the pubertal growth spurt[87-89] and is another factor contributing to osteoporosis. Estrogen and testosterone are important for normal bone mineralization, as shown by the osteopenia found in estrogen-[90] and androgen-resistant[91] syndromes.

THERAPEUTIC OPTIONS

The physician or nurse practitioner caring for the pediatric patient with IBD faces many difficult challenges when considering the approach to treatment. Issues including growth, bone development, and sexual maturation should be considered when selecting therapies. General goals for optimizing outcome should achieve the best clinical and laboratory control of disease with the fewest side effects, promote growth through adequate nutrition, and permit the patient to function as normally as possible with consideration for school attendance and participation in activities. Table 5-3 summarizes current treatment options available. Because few randomized controlled drug trials have been performed in children, the gastroenterologist caring for a pediatric patient with IBD is often forced to use adult data or extrapolate success from anecdotal experiences. This section will provide treatment options that currently exist with a focus on the available pediatric literature.

NUTRITIONAL THERAPIES

Nutritional therapy in IBD is still underused, although it is gaining wider acceptance. One of the most appealing aspects of nutritional therapy is that it addresses the well-known effects of malnutrition, while providing a therapeutic option as well. Although parental nutrition is traditionally reserved for the sickest pediatric patients, enteral nutrition provides needed calories and eliminates dietary antigens that may trigger the immune system.

Perhaps the most basic form of nutritional therapy in IBD is the use of bowel rest and parenteral nutrition. In 1977, it was suggested that home total parenteral nutrition (TPN) be employed for the treatment of severe small bowel CD in children.[60] This study demonstrated that home TPN was safe and effective at promoting growth, while allowing the slow reintroduction of oral alimentation. Subsequently, trials of TPN and bowel rest have resulted in clinical remission of CD in adolescents and adults. Response rates as high as 90% have been reported with the use of exclusive TPN, even in steroid-refractory disease.[92] A study comparing TPN with a specified liquid diet and combined oral and parenteral nutrition showed that 71% of patients solely receiving TPN achieved remission after 21 days.[93] The other forms of nutritional support resulted in remission rates of 58% and 60%, respectively, with 1-year remission rates decreasing to 42% in the TPN group and 55% in the other groups. A subsequent study similarly demonstrated superior response rates in a group receiving TPN, when compared to elemental diet and polymeric diet.[94]

Despite the reported success with TPN, enteral nutrition represents a more physiologic and safer delivery system and therefore would be preferable if similar results could be achieved. In 1995, Griffiths et al[95] reviewed 37 pediatric and adult trials of enteral nutrition as primary therapy for active CD. Thirteen trials met the inclusion criteria for meta-analysis, with 8 trials comprising 413 patients comparing liquid diet and corticosteroids. In this analysis, the pooled odds ratio for the likelihood of clinical remission with liquid diet therapy versus corticosteroids was 0.35, demonstrating that diet therapy alone was inferior to corticosteroid therapy for the induction of remission. Various sensitivity analyses did not significantly change the results. Approximately 20% of patients randomized to receive nutritional therapy failed to complete the trials due to intolerance to the formulas. The likelihood of intolerance was lower (8%) when the formula was administered strictly via nasogastric tube. The remaining 5 studies in the meta-analysis compared efficacy between polymeric and elemental diets. Out of 134 patients, tolerance for the liquid diets was quite high, with 94% completing the trials. In this analysis, there was no demonstrable difference in efficacy between the 2 types of diets. A subsequent meta-analysis demonstrated similar findings.[96] When including 10 studies comparing elemental diet with polymeric diet, no significant difference was found in efficacy of inducing remission. It should be noted that both TPN and enteral feeding are more effective for CD than for UC, where these interventions should be reserved for repletion of malnutrition rather than treatment of active disease.

AMINOSALICYLATES

The aminosalicylates, including sulfasalazine and the newer 5-aminosalicylic acid (5-ASA) compounds mesalamine and mesalazine, are first-line drugs with limited anti-inflammatory properties. They are felt to act locally with limited systemic absorption. The primary mechanism of action appears to be the drug's inhibition of the lipoxygenase pathway of arachidonic acid metabolism.[97]

There are limited pediatric data that evaluates the use of aminosalicylates in pediatric patients with IBD. Though there have been many studies evaluating the efficacy of these agents in adults with IBD, only a few randomized trials have been carried out in children. Based on findings from a large clinical trial, balsalazide is now one of two FDA-approved agents for treatment of UC in pediatric patients.[98] In a double-blind, placebo-controlled trial carried out by Griffiths et al, a small clinical and dose-related benefit was seen among the 6 patients treated with slow-release 5-ASA who completed the 20-week trial. A high drop-out rate among the placebo group and low recruitment rate led to termination of the study prior to its completion.[99] A novel high-strength formulation of 5-ASA—the multimatrix mesalamine—is now available as 2.4 g and 4.8 g once daily (2 to 4 tablets at 1.2 g each tablet).[100,101] Although this formulation is not approved for children, because of the lower pill volume, it is an attractive option for use in the pediatric population.

Mesalamine (in Europe mesalazine) appears to be better tolerated than sulfasalazine among children.[102] Nausea and vomiting were more common with sulfasalazine. Other side effects including pancreatitis, hepatotoxicity, interstitial nephritis, and pericarditis have been described with the use of mesalamine. Rash and fever secondary to hypersensitivity can occur and are often linked to the sulfa moiety in sulfasalazine.[97]

Because of the limited number of controlled trials among children, dosing guidelines have not clearly been established for the use of the aminosalicylates. There is a trend toward using mesalamine in doses between 50 and 75 mg/kg/d, and doses as high as 100 mg/kg/d have been used. Limited availability of liquid preparations (Azulfidine) of this class of drugs complicates its use among young patients who have difficulties swallowing pills or capsules, although patients are sometimes instructed to open Pentasa or Colazal capsules and place the microbeads or capsule contents in pudding, applesauce, or yogurt.

CORTICOSTEROIDS

Corticosteroids continue to be a mainstay of therapy for acute exacerbations of pediatric inflammatory bowel disease. Despite the known long list of side effects, no drug to date has shown a better ability to provide symptomatic relief. Previous studies have shown a 20% to 36% dependence rate among Crohn's patients, and 20% of patients are steroid-resistant.[97] There have been no controlled trials using corticosteroids versus placebo among pediatric patients. Previous studies have, however, evaluated enteral nutrition and corticosteroids. A recent meta-analysis found similar remission rates, close to 85%, among patients using corticosteroids and those treated with enteral nutrition.[103]

Budesonide, a newer steroid formulation with extensive first-pass hepatic metabolism, has been reported to reduce the unwanted side effects of corticosteroids. Although no placebo-controlled trials have been carried out using this drug in pediatrics, several studies comparing budesonide and prednisolone have been conducted recently. Levine et al performed an age-matched retrospective study using budesonide and prednisone in pediatric CD patients with mild to moderate disease.[104] Remission was achieved in 48% of patients in the budesonide group versus 77% of patients who received prednisone. They also demonstrated that budesonide was more effective than mesalamine and antibiotics at inducing remission. The authors concluded that budesonide should be considered a first-line agent in mild-to-moderate CD to induce remission. In 2004, Escher and the European Collaborative Research Group on Budesonide in Pediatric IBD conducted a prospective, double-blind trial comparing budesonide and prednisolone in active pediatric CD involving the ileum and/or the ascending colon. The study showed that both medications achieved some remission (55% among budesonide users versus 71% among prednisolone users). Though the prednisolone group showed a trend towards being more effective at inducing remission, budesonide demonstrated a better side effect profile with less adrenal suppression measured by mean cortisol levels and fewer cosmetic side effects.[105]

A prospective study of 128 children with severe UC identified several predictors of steroid unresponsiveness. Pediatric UC Activity Index (PUCAI) measures at days 3 and 5 after initiation of IV corticosteroid therapy were found to be strong predictors of treatment failure and an indication for salvage therapy.[106]

Although corticosteroids offer an effective short-term remediation of symptoms for active CD and UC, the side effect profiles prohibit long-term use. Side effects including fluid retention, fat redistribution, hypertension, hyperglycemia, cataracts, and weight gain are well-known and appear to be related to dose and duration of therapy.[97] As discussed previously, bone demineralization and linear growth retardation that also occur with corticosteroid use are more damaging and often more difficult to correct. In the MATRIX study, budesonide was associated with a significantly smaller reduction in bone mass compared with prednisolone in corticosteroid-naïve patients with active ileocecal CD.[107]

IMMUNOMODULATORS

6-Mercaptopurine and Azathioprine

Used for more than 50 years in oncology patients, 6-MP and its predrug azathioprine (AZA) are being used with increasing frequency in pediatric patients with IBD. Markowitz et al conducted a survey among 718 pediatric gastroenterologists in North America that compared attitudes towards the use of immunomodulatory therapy in 1990 and 2000. His group found significant increases in physicians' willingness to prescribe these agents and an expansion in physicians' indications for prescribing this drug. Among the immunomodulators mentioned in this study, AZA and 6-MP were prescribed by the greatest number of responders.[108]

Among pediatric IBD patients, clinical evidence supporting the use of AZA and 6-MP was limited to retrospective studies until the last few years. In 1990, Verhave et al showed partial or complete clinical remission in 75% of patients with CD or UC who took AZA. Additionally, most of the patients who responded to the medication were able to discontinue corticosteroids within 6 months of starting AZA.[97,109] Markowitz et al also demonstrated a significant reduction in steroid use for patients who received 6-MP. They reported that 57% were able to discontinue corticosteroids within 6 months and 80% within 1 year of the initiation of 6-MP.[110]

In 2000, Markowitz et al published the first randomized, placebo-controlled trial evaluating the early use of 6-MP in newly diagnosed pediatric patients with moderate to severe Crohn's. His group found a significantly shorter duration of steroid use and lower cumulative steroid dose at 6, 12, and 18 months among patients who received 6-MP versus placebo. And though remission was initially induced in 89% of both groups, only 9% of patients who were maintained on 6-MP relapsed versus 47% of controls. Long-term remission at 18 months was 89% in the 6-MP group versus 39% in the placebo group.[111]

Given the known side effects of the use of this class of medications including both allergic (pancreatitis, arthralgias, rash, and fever) and nonallergic reactions (leukopenia, thrombocytopenia, infection, hepatitis, and malignancy), safety remains a concern when prescribing this drug to pediatric patients. Kirschner reported that 28% of 95 pediatric patients who received 6-MP or AZA had some side effects (most commonly elevated aminotransferase levels) and that cessation of the drug occurred in 18% of patients because of drug hypersensitivity or infection.[112] Other retrospective studies showed mild side effects including leukopenia and elevated aminotransferases in almost 40% of pediatric patients.[97] Immunomodulators are generally well-tolerated, although the potential for long-term exposure and the possibility of malignancy are a concern.[113] The risks of immunomodulators are contrasted with the benefits of steroid sparing in vulnerable pediatric patients.[114]

Though the Markowitz study recommended the early use of 6-MP or AZA for all newly diagnosed pediatric patients with moderate to severe CD, clearer guidelines for selected use have not been reported. A study conducted at our institution found that patients with lower serum albumin at diagnosis (3.1 g/dL versus 3.75 g/dL) and higher PCDAI at diagnosis (40 versus 24) were significantly more likely to be started on immunomodulators. In addition, all patients with serum albumin of 2.8 g/dL or less were placed on immunomodulators within 6 months of diagnosis versus only 45% of patients with serum albumin of 2.9 g/dL or greater.[115]

No studies to date have been performed with regard to appropriate pediatric dosing. Accepted practice among clinicians is to start with doses of 1 to 1.5 mg/kg when using 6-MP and 2.0 to 2.5 mg/kg when using AZA.

Methotrexate

Limited studies exist evaluating the use of methotrexate in pediatric IBD. In the only published full study to date assessing clinical outcomes with subcutaneous methotrexate, Mack et al established clinical efficacy with this medication. In a study of 14 patients with steroid-dependent CD who failed or did not tolerate 6-MP, 9 (64%) showed improvement within 4 weeks of initiation of therapy.[116]

Side effects including gastrointestinal problems (nausea, anorexia, and diarrhea), headaches, dizziness, fatigue, and mood changes have been reported. Additionally, leukopenia, thrombocytopenia, pulmonary toxicity, and opportunistic infections are also possible. Hepatotoxicity, although still a concern, is less common than once thought.[97] Recent data in pediatrics suggest that oral methotrexate may be better tolerated and has similar bioavailability to the subcutaneous form.[117]

Cyclosporine

Cyclosporine, developed initially for the prevention of organ rejection, has a role in the treatment of patients with IBD and in particular those patients with refractory, severe UC.[118-121] To date, no controlled trials have been conducted using cyclosporine in refractory UC in a pediatric population.

ANTIBIOTICS

Although bacteria flora has been given a central role in the development of IBD, the role of antibiotics in the treatment of pediatric IBD has only been studied on a limited basis. No randomized trials using antibiotics have been published in a pediatric population to date. In one pediatric reference, Hildebrand et al showed clinical efficacy of metronidazole among 20 children with CD with perianal involvement. Of the 20 patients, more than half showed some clinical improvement during 6 months of treatment. After discontinuation of therapy in 9 patients, 5 had a relapse within 1 month of discontinuation.[122]

Side effects with the use of metronidazole have been reported in children. Duffy et al documented peripheral neuropathies in 11 of 13 patients treated with metronidazole.[123] Other antibiotics including the fluoroquinolones, which have demonstrated some efficacy among adult patients with perianal and fistulous CD,[124] have been linked to cartilage damage in laboratory animals. Safety data for this class of drug have been published after studies in children in Great Britain and Japan; however, no safety data exist for pediatric IBD patients.[97] Fluoroquinolones and cephalosporins are strongly associated with the increasing incidence of *Clostridium difficile*-associated diarrhea (CDAD), which parallels the incidence of CDAD in patients with IBD.[125] Nitazoxanide 500 mg twice daily for 7 to 10 days is effective against *C difficile*. A recent study demonstrated the noninferiority of nitazoxanide compared with metronidazole in treating *C difficile* colitis.[126]

INFLIXIMAB

Infliximab, a humanized, chimeric, monoclonal anti-TNFα antibody, is approved by the Food and Drug Administration (FDA) for use in children with CD and represents the first biologic agent approved for use in children. In fact, the agent was first used in a 13-year-old girl with refractory Crohn's colitis. The first published controlled trial in children was carried out in a joint European–American trial. In this study, patients with severe refractory CD were randomized to receive either 1, 5, or 10 mg/kg of infliximab. The medication demonstrated clinical efficacy in the 5 and 10 mg/kg groups at 4, 12, and 20 weeks with better outcome at 20 weeks among the 5 mg/kg group versus the 10 mg/kg (50% versus 33%) in achieving clinical remission.[127] A retrospective study conducted by Stephens et al reviewed the experience with infliximab at a large pediatric institution. A total of 432 infusions were given to 82 patients with severe refractory Crohn's disease. Of 33 patients who were using corticosteroids at the initiation of infliximab, almost 60% were able to discontinue their use. The study also showed significant decreases between steroid doses at 0 and 4 weeks and 0 and 8 weeks.[128] Several other open-label trials using infliximab have demonstrated clinical efficacy.[97] The REACH study evaluated the safety and efficacy of infliximab in children with moderately to severely active CD. After 1 year of treatment, 63.5% and 55.8% of patients who received infliximab every 8 weeks achieved clinical response and were in clinical remission, respectively, and did not require dose adjustment. Most importantly, at the end of 1 year, almost 50% of children receiving infliximab every 8 weeks were in remission and no longer required steroids, compared with only 17% of children receiving infliximab every 12 weeks.[129] Rare postmarketing cases of hepatosplenic T cell lymphoma have been reported; all of the cases occurred in patients on concomitant treatment with 6-MP or AZA. The role of early top-down infliximab or immunomodulators in steroid-naïve children with CD[130] or infliximab monotherapy in children with CD exposed to steroids[131] needs to be evaluated in light of the recent adult trials showing treatment efficacy and a reduced need for steroids in patients taking these agents.

Infliximab has also been used with some success in pediatric patients with UC.[132,133] Mamula et al demonstrated clinical efficacy with this medication among 9 patients consecutively treated with doses of infliximab at 0 and 2 weeks. Seven of 9 patients had a decrease of disease activity based on lowering of the Physician Global Assessment, and corticosteroids were discontinued in 6 of the 11 patients who received infliximab.[120] While this study showed some success in the short term, questions remain about the role of infliximab in the long-term management of pediatric UC.

Side effects of the medication, including opportunistic infections, tuberculosis and herpes zoster, systemic lupus, erythematosus drug-induced reaction serum sickness, and malignancies, although rare, have been reported. More common side effects from the medication are infusion reactions. Thought to occur in about 6% of patients who receive infliximab, reactions including diaphoresis, shortness of breath, blood pressure changes, and tachycardia are well-documented.[97,127] Recent studies in pediatrics have focused on the role that human anti-chimeric antibodies (HACA, otherwise known as antibodies to infliximab or ATI) play in infusion reactions and efficacy of the medication. Miele et al evaluated the role that HACA plays in infusion reactions and found that they occurred in higher proportions in patients who were HACA-positive than in those who were HACA-negative. In addition, they found that patients with HACA levels above 8.0 μg/mL were more likely to have infusion reactions, and concomitant immunomodulator use was associated with a lower risk of developing HACA.[134]

TRANSITION OF THE PATIENT WITH INFLAMMATORY BOWEL DISEASE FROM PEDIATRIC TO ADULT CARE

Children with IBD should be cared for by a physician trained to manage issues unique to pediatric patients.[135] Pediatric gastroenterologists have the expertise to address a multitude of important problems that uniquely occur during childhood, particularly growth and development. Internist gastroenterologists have a different set of skills that are necessary to provide optimal care to adult patients with IBD.

The passage from adolescence to adulthood is a time of internal turmoil and intense examination of personal goals and wishes. Being ill during this time of growing and changing may cause frustration about the present and anxiety about the future. The growing adolescent must be able to progressively shed the sheltered environment of childhood and achieve self-reliance and independent living as a decision maker. Under normal circumstances, this process is painful for the healthiest of individuals. For the chronically ill adolescent, this period of transition can be stressful not only for the patient but for their families and health-care providers.[136-140]

During the transition to an internist-gastroenterologist, patients, parents, and other family members may feel threatened by changes in the pattern of care and resentful of the effort required to adjust to a new setting and different staff. They have weathered many crises and made vital decisions with the support of the pediatric team and frequently regard this strong source of advocacy as a permanent arrangement. In contrast, they may perceive the internist who expects to care for an independent individual as less involved or less sensitive to the developmental and social aspects of his or her medical condition.

Health-care providers may also feel ambivalent during this period of change. The pediatrician may view the maturation of the child as a professional and personal achievement and find difficulty in relinquishing the patient to others whose style of practice he or she may not know well.

The process of transition should begin when a patient enters early to middle adolescence. The pediatric gastroenterologist should begin seeing adolescent patients without their parents in order to build a relationship that promotes independence and self-reliance. It is important to discuss with the patient and the family that in the future they will need to transition to a gastroenterologist who is also trained in internal medicine with expertise in dealing with medical problems that occur during adulthood, including pregnancy, fertility, and cancer surveillance.

Once the decision to pursue a transition program has been made, the next step is to identify a skilled gastroenterologist who cares for young adults. This individual must realize that a young adult with childhood-onset IBD may have a different set of expectations than the young adult with a recent onset of IBD. These young adults also have a heightened risk for the development of cancer and will require an increased need for cancer surveillance. The pediatrician needs to provide all of the necessary medical records and medical summaries so that all providers are working together to deliver excellent care.

Timing for transition will require some flexibility, because many patients have special circumstances. Any adolescent who has additional growth potential as a result of delayed puberty should be followed by a pediatric gastroenterologist. Also, children with neurologic delay should be transitioned to an adult gastroenterologist who has the expertise and the support necessary to provide comprehensive care.

CONCLUSION

Due to the complex nature of issues surrounding the care of a child or adolescent with IBD, it is necessary to adopt a multidisciplinary approach and devise an individual plan for therapy. Pediatric patients with IBD are not "little" adults, and the specific set of problems that they face including issues around growth, sexual development and puberty, and osteoporosis should be thought about when caring for these individuals. Though many of the same medications are available for pediatric patients that exist in the management of adult IBD, the judicious use of corticosteroids should be remembered as it has demonstrated such profound deleterious effects on bone density and final height outcomes. Adopting a team approach that includes physicians, nurses and nurse practitioners, nutritionists, social workers, and psychologists is necessary to ensure comprehensive care that will allow pediatric IBD patients to achieve appropriate levels of physical, mental, and social well-being.

REFERENCES

1. Mendelhoff AI, Calkins BM. The epidemiology of idiopathic inflammatory bowel disease. In: Kirsner JB, Shorter RG, eds. *Inflammatory Bowel Disease*. Philadelphia, PA: Lea & Febiger; 1988:3-34.
2. Farmer RG, Michener WM. Prognosis of Crohn's disease with onset in childhood or adolescence. *Dig Dis Sci*. 1979;24:752-757.
3. Garland CF, Lilienfield AM, Mendelhoff AI, et al. Incidence rates of ulcerative colitis and Crohn's disease in 15 areas of the United States. *Gastroenterology*. 1981;81:1115.
4. Baldassano RN, Piccoli DA. Inflammatory bowel disease in pediatric and adolescent patients. *Gastroenterol Clin North Am*. 1999;28:445-458.
5. Fonager K, Sorensen HT, Olsen J. Change in incidence of Crohn's disease and ulcerative colitis in Denmark. A study based on the National Registry of Patients, 1981-1992. *Int J Epidemiol*. 1997; 26:1003-1008.
6. Lindberg E, Lindquist B, Holmquist L, et al. Inflammatory bowel disease in children and adolescents in Sweden, 1984-1995. *J Pediatr Gastroenterol Nutr*. 2000;30:259-264.
7. Russel MG, Stockbrugger RW. Epidemiology of inflammatory bowel disease: an update. *Scand J Gastroenterol*. 1996;31:417-427.
8. Logan RF. Inflammatory bowel disease incidence: Up, down or unchanged? *Gut*. 1998;42:309-311.
9. Bjornsson S, Johannsson JH, Oddsson E. Inflammatory bowel disease in Iceland, 1980-89. A retrospective nationwide epidemiologic study. *Scand J Gastroenterol*. 1998;33:71-77.
10. Oliva-Hemker M, Fiocchi C. Etiopathogenesis of inflammatory bowel disease: the importance of the pediatric perspective. *Inflamm Bowel Dis*. 2002;8:112-128.
11. Tysk C, Lindberg E, Jarnerot G, et al. Ulcerative colitis and Crohn's disease in an unselected population of monozygotic and dizygotic twins. A study of heritability and the influence of smoking. *Gut*. 1988;29:990-996.
12. Langholz E, Munkholm P, Krasilnikoff PA. Inflammatory bowel disease with onset in childhood. *Scand J Gastroenterol*. 1997;32: 139-147.
13. Grand RJ, Homer DR. Inflammatory bowel disease in childhood and adolescence. *Pediatr Clin North Am*. 1975;22:835.
14. Griffiths AM. Crohn's disease. *Rec Adv Pediatr*. 1992;10:145.
15. Lenaerts C, Roy CC, Vaillancourt M, et al. High incidence of upper gastrointestinal tract involvement in children with Crohn's disease. *Pediatrics*. 1989;83:777.
16. Hildebrand H, Karlberg J, Kristiansson B. Longitudinal growth in children and adolescents with inflammatory bowel disease. *J Pediatr Gastroenterol Nutr*. 1994;18:165-173.
17. Tourtelier Y, Dabadie A, Tron I, et al. Incidence of inflammatory bowel disease in children in Brittany (1994-1997). Breton Association of Study and Research on Digestive System Diseases (Abermad). *Arch Pediatr*. 2000;7:377-384.
18. Heikenen JB, Werlin SL, Brown CW, et al. Presenting symptoms and diagnostic lag in children with inflammatory bowel disease. *Inflamm Bowel Dis*. 1999;5:158-160.
19. Spray C, Debelle GD, Murphy MS. Current diagnosis, management and morbidity in paediatric inflammatory bowel disease. *Acta Paediatr*. 2001;90:400-405.
20. Wagtmans MJ, Verspaget HW, Lamers CB, et al. Crohn's disease in the elderly: a comparison with young adults. *J Clin Gastroenterol*. 1998;27:129-133.
21. Fazio VW. Toxic megacolon in ulcerative colitis and Crohn's colitis. *Clin Gastroenterol*. 1980;9:271.
22. Huizenga KA, Schroeder KW. *Gastrointestinal Complications of Ulcerative Colitis and Crohn's Disease*. 3rd ed. Philadelphia, PA: Lea and Febiger; 1988.
23. Binder SC, Patterson JF, Glotzer DJ. Toxic megacolon in ulcerative colitis. *Gastroenterology*. 1974;66:1088.
24. Devroede GJ, Taylor WF, Sauer J, et al. Cancer risk and life expectancy of children with ulcerative colitis. *N Engl J Med*. 1973; 289:491.
25. Ekbom A, Melmick C, Zack M, et al. Ulcerative colitis and colorectal cancer: a population based study. *N Engl J Med*. 1990;323:1228-1233.
26. Griffiths AM, Sherman PM. Colonscopic surveillance for cancer in ulcerative colitis: a critical review. *J Pediatr Gastoenterol Nutr*. 1997;24:202-210.
27. Hoffley PM, Piccoli DA. Inflammatory bowel disease in children. *Med Clin North Am*. 1994;78:1281-1302.
28. Markowitz J, Daum F, Algar M, et al. Perianal disease in children and adolescents with Crohn's disease. *Gastroenterology*. 1984; 86:829.
29. Danzi JT. Extraintestinal manifestations of idiopathic inflammatory bowel disease. *Arch Intern Med*. 1988;148:297-302.
30. Hyams JS. Crohn's disease in children. *Pediatr Clin North Am*. 1996;43:255-277.
31. Menachem Y, Weizman Z, Locker C, et al. Clinical characteristics of Crohn's disease in children and adults. *Harefuah*. 1998;134:173-175, 247.
32. Gryboski JD, Spiro HM. Prognosis in children with Crohn's disease. *Gastroenterology*. 1978;74:807-817.
33. Winesett M. Inflammatory bowel disease in children and adolescents. *Pediatr Ann*. 1997;26:227-234.
34. Hyams JS. Extraintestinal manifestations of inflammatory bowel disease in children. *J Pediatr Gastroenterol Nutr*. 1994;19:7-21.
35. Hofley P, Roarty J, McGinnity G, et al. Asymptomatic uveitis in children with chronic inflammatory bowel diseases. *J Pediatr Gastroenterol Nutr*. 1993;17:397-400.
36. Burbige EJ, Huang SH, Bayless TM. Clinical manifestations of Crohn's disease in children and adolescents. *Pediatrics*. 1975; 55:866-871.
37. Lindsley C, Schaller JG. Arthritis associated with inflammatory bowel disease in children. *J Pediatr*. 1974;86:76.
38. Kane W, Miller K, Sharp HL. Inflammatory bowel disease presenting as liver disease during childhood. *J Pediatr*. 1980;97:775-778.
39. Hyams J, Markowitz J, Treem W, et al. Characterization of hepatic abnormalities in children with inflammatory bowel disease. *Inflamm Bowel Dis*. 1995;1:27-33.
40. Faubion WA Jr, Loftus EV, Sandborn WJ, et al. Pediatric "PSC-IBD": a descriptive report of associated inflammatory bowel disease among pediatric patients with PSC. *J Pediatr Gastroenterol Nutr*. 2001;33:296-300.
41. McLeod RS, Churchill DN. Urolithiasis complicating inflammatory bowel disease. *J Urol*. 1992;148:974-978.
42. Lloyd-Still JD, Tomasi L. Neurovascular and thromboembolic complications of inflammatory bowel disease in childhood. *J Pediatr Gastroenterol Nutr*. 1989;9:461-466.
43. Hudson M, Chitolie A, Hutton RA, et al. Thrombotic vascular risk factors in inflammatory bowel disease. *Gut*. 1996;38:733-737.
44. Markowitz RL, Ment LR, Gryboski JD. Cerebral thromboembolic disease in pediatric and adult inflammatory bowel disease: case report and review of the literature. *J Pediatr Gastroenterol Nutr*. 1989;8:413-420.
45. Reuner KH, Ruf A, Grau A, et al. Prothrombin gene G20210—a transition is a risk factor for cerebral venous thrombosis. *Stroke*. 1998;29:1765-1769.

46. Harper PH, Fazio VW, Lavery IC, et al. The long-term outcome in Crohn's disease. *Dis Colon Rectum.* 1987;30:174-179.
47. Motil KJ, Grand RJ, Maletskos CJ, et al. The effect of disease, drug, and diet on whole body protein metabolism in adolescents with Crohn disease and growth failure. *J Pediatr.* 1982;101:345-351.
48. Grill BB, Hillemeier AC, Gryboski JD. Fecal alpha 1-antitrypsin clearance in patients with inflammatory bowel disease. *J Pediatr Gastroenterol Nutr.* 1984;3:56-61.
49. Kelts D, Grand R, Shen G, et al. Nutritional basis of growth failure in children and adolescents with Crohn's disease. *Gastroenterology.* 1979;76:720-727.
50. Seidman E, LeLeiko N, Ament M, et al. Nutritional issues in pediatric inflammatory bowel disease. *J Pediatr Gastroenterol Nutr.* 1991;12:424-438.
51. Kanof ME, Lake AM, Bayless TM. Decreased height velocity in children and adolescents before the diagnosis of Crohn's disease. *Gastroenterology.* 1988;95:1523-1527.
52. Hyams JS, Ferry GD, Mandel FS, et al. Development and validation of pediatric Crohn's Disease Activity Index. *J Pediatr Gastroenterol Nutr.* 1991;12:439-447.
53. Otley A, Loonen H, Parekh N, et al. Assessing activity of pediatric Crohn's disease: which index to use? *Gastroenterology.* 1999; 116:527-531.
54. Rigaud D, Cosnes J, Le Quintrec Y, et al. Controlled trial comparing two types of enteral nutrition in treatment of active Crohn's disease: elemental versus polymeric diet. *Gut.* 1991;32:1492-1497.
55. Sentongo T, Semeao E, Piccoli D, et al. Growth, body composition, and nutritional status in children and adolescents with Crohn's disease. *J Pediatr Gastroenterol Nutr.* 2000;31:33-40.
56. Motil K, Grand R, Matthews D, et al. Whole body leucine metabolism in adolescents with Crohn's disease and growth failure during nutritional supplementation. *Gastroenterology.* 1982;82:1361-1368.
57. Layden T, Rosenberg F, Nemchausky G, et al. Reversal of growth arrest in adolescents with Crohn's disease after parenteral alimentation. *Gastroenterology.* 1976;70:1017-1021.
58. Christie P, Hill G. Effect of intravenous nutrition on nutrition and function in acute attacks of inflammatory bowel disease. *Gastroenterology.* 1990;99:730-736.
59. Ferguson A, Glen M, Ghosh S. Crohn's disease: nutrition and nutritional therapy. *Bailliere's Clin Gastroenterol.* 1998;12:93-114.
60. Byrne W, Halpin T, Asch M, et al. Home total parenteral nutrition: an alternative approach to the management of children with severe chronic small bowel disease. *J Ped Surg.* 1977;12:359-366.
61. Kirschner B, Klich J, Kalman S, et al. Reversal of growth retardation in Crohn's disease with therapy emphasizing oral nutritional restitution. *Gastroenterology.* 1980;80:10-15.
62. Motil K. Aggressive nutritional therapy in growth retardation. *Clin Nutr.* 1985;4:75-84.
63. Himes JH, Roche AF, Thissen D, et al. Parent-specific adjustments for evaluation of recumbent length and stature of children. *Pediatrics.* 1985;75:304-313.
64. Rosen DS. Pubertal growth and sexual maturation for adolescents with chronic illness or disability. *Pediatrician.* 1991;18:105-120.
65. Brain CE, Savage MO. Growth and puberty in chronic inflammatory bowel disease. *Bailliere's Clin Gastroenterol.* 1994;8:83-100.
66. Tanner JM. *Growth at Adolescence.* Oxford: Blackwell Scientific; 1972.
67. de Vizia B, Poggi V, Conenna R, et al. Iron absorption and iron deficiency in infants and children with gastrointestinal diseases. *J Pediatr Gastroenterol Nutr.* 1992;14:21-26.
68. Galloway R, McGuire J. Determinants of compliance with iron supplementation: supplies, side effects, or psychology? *Soc Sci Med.* 1994;39:381-390.
69. Mailloux R, Sitrin M. The skeletal complications of inflammatory bowel disease and their treatment. *Prog Inflamm Bowel Dis.* 1994;15:1-21.
70. Scott EM, Gaywood I, Scott BB. Guidelines for osteoporosis in coeliac disease and inflammatory bowel disease. British Society of Gastroenterology. *Gut.* 2000;46(suppl 1):1-8.
71. Caulfield L, Himes J, Rivera J. Nutritional supplementation during early childhood and bone mineralization during adolescence. *J Nutr.* 1995;125:1104-1110.
72. Kanis JA, Pitt FA. Epidemiology of osteoporosis. *Bone.* 1992; 13(suppl 1):S7-15.
73. Kanis JA, McCloskey EV. Epidemiology of vertebral osteoporosis. *Bone.* 1992;13(suppl 2):S1-S10.
74. Mora S, Pitukcheewanont P, Kaufman F, et al. Biochemical markers of bone turnover and the volume and the density of bone in children at different stages of sexual development. *J Bone Miner Res.* 1999;14:1664-1671.
75. Compston JE, Creamer B. Plasma levels and intestinal absorption of 25-hydroxyvitamin D in patients with small bowel resection. *Gut.* 1977;18:171-175.
76. Bell NH, Shaw S, Turner RT. Evidence that calcium modulates circulating 25-hydroxyvitamin D in man. *J Bone Miner Res.* 1987;2: 211-214.
77. Clements MR, Johnson L, Fraser DR. A new mechanism for induced vitamin D deficiency in calcium deprivation. *Nature.* 1987;325:62-65.
78. Caniggia A, Nuti R, Lore F, et al. Pathophysiology of the adverse effects of glucoactive corticosteroids on calcium metabolism in man. *J Steroid Biochem.* 1981;15:153-161.
79. Suzuki Y, Ichikawa Y, Saito E, et al. Importance of increased urinary calcium excretion in the development of secondary hyperparathyroidism of patients under glucocorticoid therapy. *Metabolism.* 1983;32:151-156.
80. Lukert BP, Raisz LG. Glucocorticoid-induced osteoporosis: pathogenesis and management. *Ann Intern Med.* 1990;112:352-364.
81. Schoon EJ, Geerling BG, Van Dooren IM, et al. Abnormal bone turnover in long-standing Crohn's disease in remission. *Aliment Pharmacol Ther.* 2001;15:783-792.
82. LoCascio V, Adami S, Avioli LV, et al. Suppressive effect of chronic glucocorticoid treatment on circulating calcitonin in man. *Calcif Tissue Int.* 1982;34:309-310.
83. Nemetz A, Toth M, Garcia-Gonzalez MA, et al. Allelic variation at the interleukin 1 beta gene is associated with decreased bone mass in patients with inflammatory bowel diseases. *Gut.* 2001;49:644-649.
84. Schulte CM, Dignass AU, Goebell H, et al. Genetic factors determine extent of bone loss in inflammatory bowel disease. *Gastroenterology.* 2000;119:909-920.
85. Brain C, Savage M, Leonard J, et al. Characteristics of pubertal development in inflammatory bowel disease (IBD). *Pediatr Res.* 1993;33(Suppl):S86.
86. Kirschner BS. Growth and development in chronic inflammatory bowel disease. *Acta Paediatr Scand Suppl.* 1990;366:98-104.
87. Molgaard C, Thomsen BL, Michaelsen KF. Influence of weight, age and puberty on bone size and bone mineral content in healthy children and adolescents. *Acta Paediatr.* 1998;87:494-499.
88. Bonjour JP, Theintz G, Buchs B, et al. Critical years and stages of puberty for spinal and femoral bone mass accumulation during adolescence. *J Clin Endocrinol Metab.* 1991;73:555-563.
89. Bailey DA, Martin AD, McKay HA, et al. Calcium accretion in girls and boys during puberty: A longitudinal analysis. *J Bone Miner Res.* 2000;15:2245-2250.

90. Smith EP, Boyd J, Frank GR, et al. Estrogen resistance caused by a mutation in the estrogen-receptor gene in a man. *N Engl J Med.* 1994;331:1056-1061.
91. Bertolloni S, Cappa M, Lala R, et al. Altered bone mineralization in complete androgen insensitivity syndrome [abstract]. *Horm Res.* 1997;48(suppl):811A.
92. Forbes A. Crohn's disease: the role of nutritional therapy. *Aliment Pharmacol Ther.* 2002;16(suppl 4):48-52.
93. Greenberg G, Fleming C, Jeejeebhoy K, et al. Controlled trial of bowel rest and nutritional support in the management of Crohn's disease. *Gut.* 1988;29:1309-1315.
94. Kobayashi K, Katsumata T, Yokoyama K, et al. A randomized controlled study of total parenteral nutrition and enteral nutrition by elemental and polymeric diet as primary therapy in active phase of Crohn's disease. *Nippon Shokakibyo Gakkai Zasshi.* 1998;95:1212-1221.
95. Griffiths AM, Ohlsson A, Sherman PM, et al. Meta-analysis of enteral nutrition as a primary treatment of active Crohn's disease. *Gastroenterology.* 1995;108:1056-1067.
96. Zachos M, Tondeur M, Griffiths AM. Enteral nutritional therapy for inducing remission of Crohn's disease. *Cochrane Database Syst Rev.* 2001:CD000542.
97. Escher JC, Taminiau JA, Nieuwenhuis EE, et al. Treatment of inflammatory bowel disease in childhood: best available evidence. *Inflamm Bowel Dis.* 2003;9:34-38.
98. Bosworth BP, Pruitt RE, Gordon GL, et al. Balsalazide tablets 3.3 g twice daily improves signs and symptoms of mild-to-moderate ulcerative colitis [abstract T1152]. *Gastroenterology.* 2008;134: A-495.
99. Griffiths A, Koletzko S, Sylvester F, et al. Slow release 5-aminosalicylic acid therapy in children with small intestinal Crohn's disease. *J Pediatr Gastroenterol Nutr.* 1993;17:186-192.
100. Lichtenstein GR, Kamm MA, Boddu P, et al. Effect of once or twice-daily MMX mesalamine (SPD476) for the induction of remission of mild to moderately active ulcerative colitis. *Clin Gastroenterol Hepatol.* 2007;5:95-102.
101. Kamm MA, Sandborn WJ, Gassull M, et al. Once-daily, high concentration MMX mesalamine in active ulcerative colitis. *Gastroenterology.* 2007;132:66-73.
102. Ferry GD, Kirschner BS, Grand RJ, et al. Olsalazine versus sulfasalazine in mild to moderate childhood ulcerative colitis: results of the Pediatric Gastroenterology Collaborative Research Group Clinical Trial. *J Pediatr Gastroenterol Nutr.* 1993;17:32-38.
103. Heuschkel RB, Menache CC, Megerian JT, et al. Enteral nutrition and corticosteroids in the treatment of acute Crohn's disease in children. *J Pediatr Gastroenterol Nutr.* 2000;31:8-15.
104. Levine A, Broide E, Stein M, et al. Evaluation of oral budesonide for treatment of mild and moderate exacerbations of Crohn's disease in children. *J Pediatr.* 2002;140:75-80.
105. Escher JC and the European Collaborative Research Group on Budesonide in Pediatric IBD. Budesonide versus prednisolone for the treatment of active Crohn's disease in children: a randomized, double-blind, controlled, multi-centre trial. *Eur J Gastroenterol Hepatol.* 2004;16:47-54.
106. Turner D, Mack D, Leleiko N, et al. Severe pediatric ulcerative colitis: a prospective multicenter study of outcomes and predictors of response. *Gastroenterology.* In press.
107. Schoon EJ, Bollani S, Mills PR, et al. Bone mineral density in relation to efficacy and side effects of budesonide and prednisolone in Crohn's disease. *Clin Gastroenterol Hepatol.* 2005;3:113-121.
108. Markowitz J, Grancher K, Kohn N, et al. Immunomodulatory therapy for pediatric inflammatory bowel disease: changing patterns of use, 1990-2000. *Am J Gastroenterol.* 2002;97:928-932.
109. Verhave M, Winter HS, Grand RJ. Azathioprine in the treatment of children with inflammatory bowel disease. *J Pediatr.* 1990;117:809-814.
110. Markowitz J, Rosa J, Grancher K, et al. Long-term 6-mercaptopurine treatment in adolescents with Crohn's disease. *Gastroenterology.* 1990;99:1347-1351.
111. Markowitz J, Grancher K, Kohn N, et al. A multicenter trial of 6-mercaptopurine and prednisone in children with newly diagnosed Crohn's disease. *Gastroenterology.* 2000;119:895-902.
112. Kirschner BS. Safety of azathiprine and 6-mercaptopurine in pediatric patients with inflammatory bowel disease. *Gastroenterology.* 1998;115:813-821.
113. Beaugerie L, Carrat F, Bouvier AM, et al, for the CESAME Study Group. Excess risk of lymphoproliferative disorders (LPD) in inflammatory bowel diseases (IBD): interim results of the CESAME cohort [abstract 818]. *Gastroenterology.* 2008;134(4 suppl 1):A116.
114. Griffiths AM. Specificities of inflammatory bowel disease in childhood. *Best Pract Res Clin Gastroenterol.* 2004;18:509-523.
115. Jacobstein D, Mamula P, Markowitz JE, et al. Predictors of immunomodulator use as early therapy in pediatric Crohn's disease (abstract). *J Pediatr Gastroenterol Nutr.* 2004;39:A678.
116. Mack DR, Young R, Kaufman SS, et al. Methotrexate in patients with Crohn's disease after 6-mercaptopurine. *J Pediatr.* 1998;132:830-835.
117. Stephens MC, Baldassano RN, York A, et al. The oral bioavailability of methotrexate in pediatric patients with inflammatory bowel disease [abstract]. *J Pediatr Gastroenterol Nutr.* 2004;39:A287.
118. Treem WR, Cohen J, Davis PM, et al. Cyclosporine for the treatment of fulminant ulcerative colitis in children. Immediate response, long-term results, and impact on surgery. *Dis Colon Rectum.* 1995;38:474-479.
119. Nicholls SW, Domizio P, Williams CB, et al. Cyclosporin as initial treatment of Crohn's disease. *Arch Dis Child.* 1994;71:243-247.
120. Turner D, Walsh CM, Benchimol EI, et al. Severe paediatric ulcerative colitis: incidence, outcomes and optimal timing for second-line therapy. *Gut.* 2008;57:331-338.
121. Sandborn WJ. A critical review of cyclosporine therapy in inflammatory bowel disease. *Inflamm Bowel Dis.* 1995;1:48-63.
122. Hildebrand H, Berg NO, Hoevels J, et al. Treatment of Crohn's disease with metronidazole in childhood and adolescence. Evaluation of a six months trial. *Gastroenterol Clin Biol.* 1980;4:19-25.
123. Duffy LF, Daum F, Fisher SE, et al. Peripheral neuropathy in Crohn's disease patients treated with metronidazole. *Gastroenterology.* 1985;88:681-684.
124. Turunen U, Farkkila V, Valtonen V, et al. Long-term outcome of ciprofloxacin treatment in sever perianal of fistulous Crohn's disease [abstract]. *Gastroenterology.* 1993;104:A793.
125. Issa M, Ananthakrishnan AN, Binion DG. *Clostridium difficile* and inflammatory bowel disease. *Inflamm Bowel Dis.* 2008;14:1432-1442.
126. Musher DM, Logan N, Hamill RJ, et al. Nitazoxanide for the treatment of *Clostridium difficile* colitis. *Clin Infect Dis.* 2006;43:421-427.
127. Baldassano RN, Braegger CP, Escher JC, et al. Infliximab (REMICADE) therapy in the treatment of pediatric Crohn's disease. *Am J Gastroenterol.* 2003;98:833-838.
128. Stephens MC, Shepanski MA, Mamula P, et al. Safety and steroid-sparing experience using infliximab for Crohn's disease at a pediatric inflammatory bowel disease center. *Am J Gastroenterol.* 2003;98:104-111.

129. Hyams J, Crandall W, Kugathasan S, et al. Induction and maintenance infliximab therapy for the treatment of moderate-to severe Crohn's disease in children. *Gastroenterology.* 2007;132:863-873.

130. D'Haens G, Baert F, van Assche G, et al, and the Belgian Inflammatory Bowel Disease Research Group and North-Holland Gut Club. Early combined immunosuppression or conventional management in patients with newly diagnosed Crohn's disease: An open randomised trial. *Lancet.* 2008;371:660-667.

131. Sandborn W, Rutgeerts P, Reinisch W, et al. SONIC: A randomized, double-blind, controlled trial comparing infliximab and infliximab and azathioprine to azathioprine in patients with Crohn's disease naïve to immunomodulators and biologic therapy. Paper presented at the American College of Gastroenterology 2008 Annual Scientific Meeting; Orlando, FL; October 7, 2008.

132. Mamula P, Markowitz JE, Brown, KA, et al. Infliximab as a novel therapy for pediatric ulcerative colitis. *J Pediatr Gastroenterol Nutr.* 2002;34:307-311.

133. Cucchiara S, Romeo E, Viola F, et al. Infliximab for pediatric ulcerative colitis: a retrospective Italian multicenter study. *Dig Liver Dis.* 2008;40(suppl 2):S260-S264.

134. Miele E, Markowitz JE, Mamula P, et al. Human antichimeric antibody in children and young adults with inflammatory bowel disease receiving infliximab. *J Pediatr Gastroenterol Nutr.* 2004;38:502-508.

135. Baldassano R, Ferry G, Griffiths A, et al. Transition of the patient with inflammatory bowel disease from pediatric to adult care: recommendations of the North American Society for Pediatric Gastroenterology, Hepatology and Nutrition. *J Pediatr Gastroenterol Nutr.* 2002;34:245-248.

136. Betz CL. Facilitating the transition of adolescents with chronic conditions from pediatric to adult health care and community settings. *Issues Compr Pediatr Nurs.* 1998;21:97-115.

137. Blum RW, Garell D, Hodgman CH, et al. Transition from child-centered to adult health-care systems for adolescents with chronic conditions. A position paper of the Society for Adolescent Medicine. *J Adolesc Health.* 1993;14:570-576.

138. Rosen D. Between two worlds: bridging the cultures of child health and adult medicine. *J Adolesc Health.* 1995;17:10-16.

139. Sawyer SM, Blair S, Bowes G. Chronic illness in adolescents: transfer or transition to adult services? *J Pediatr Child Health.* 1997;33:88-90.

140. American Academy of Pediatrics Committee on Children With Disabilities and Committee on Adolescence. Transition of care provided for adolescents with special health care needs. *Pediatrics.* 1996;98:1203-1206.

The Limitations of Applying Evidence-Based Medicine to Inflammatory Bowel Disease

What We Do Not Learn From Clinical Trials

Joshua R. Korzenik, MD and Corey A. Siegel, MD

The support and enthusiasm for evidence-based medicine emerged from the hope that utilizing data from the best-performed studies would minimize the biases and inaccuracies inherent in relying heavily on personal experience to guide patient care. Though invaluable, clinical practice can present a random set of occurrences that alter the approach to particular patient circumstances. Evidence-based medicine aims to minimize those biases by grounding decision-making in the data generated by studies conducted according to the highest standards. Randomized controlled trials have evolved to be conducted according to a rigorous set of criteria to provide evidence to direct clinical care. However, these trials have their weaknesses as well. This chapter aims to examine the limitations of the evidence we rely on to guide our clinical practice.

APPLICABILITY

The protean nature of inflammatory bowel disease (IBD) complicates the process of determining the applicability of trial results to an individual patient. The peculiarities of a particular study often are not generalizable to broader situations. The specific question that a study is designed to answer may not be applicable to the immediate dilemma facing the clinician. The inclusion and exclusion criteria for a study referred to for guidance may have excluded the patient that the physician is assessing for treatment. For instance, the medications a patient is taking or his or her level of disease activity may have prevented the patient from enrolling in the study, limiting the applicability of the results to that individual.

Often, a study is reduced to its bottom line result: Is the study drug effective or not effective in treating the disease? However, a positive trial does not imply that this drug is appropriate for any patient with the diagnosis. The specifics of the trial must be reviewed: What was the severity of patients enrolled—mild, moderate, or severe? What concomitant medications were permitted? What was the distribution of disease in patients? What was the duration of the study? Was this a maintenance study or evaluation of short-term efficacy? Were there subgroups that responded or failed to respond?

A central issue is whether the population studied resembles the individual being considered for therapy. Patients enrolled in clinical trials often have a disproportionate recruitment from academic centers, which by their nature differ from a typical community practice. An academic center will have a group of patients referred due to refractory disease, having failed numerous other agents. In addition, patients enrolled in a study may have fewer options for care as they may not have health insurance and are turning to a study as an opportunity to obtain medications. This population may have socioeconomic characteristics different from a typical community practice, as well as other associated complications such as nutritional deficits. In addition, as IBD management has changed in recent years, a shifting population may be enrolled in current trials compared to even just several years ago. As a variety of centers and countries are being brought in to enhance recruitment in the competitive proliferation of trials, there may be a shift in the nature of patients enrolled, making the applicability of the findings to an individual patient more in question. Placebo remission rates have had a significant amount of variability,[1] ranging from 4%[2] to as high as 27%,[3] reflect-

Lichtenstein GR, ed.
Ulcerative Colitis: The Complete Guide to Medical Management (pp. 71-78)

ing the heterogeneity of patients included in studies, which further complicates the interpretation of trial results.

TRIAL DESIGN

The conduct of trials has changed over the years. Comparisons across trials are always dubious at best given different entry criteria, patient populations, and endpoints. In addition, trial methodology in IBD has evolved considerably over the years. The current standard assessment for clinical improvement in Crohn's trials—the Crohn's Disease Activity Index (CDAI)—is an imperfect tool developed in 1976.[4] However, some landmark studies did not use this and may not be appropriately compared to other studies.[5] Even in recent studies of CD, the standard for assessment of improvement is shifting. A 50-point decrease was used as a minimal response in earlier studies.[6] A 70-point decrease in CDAI was then considered a minimal criteria for clinical response. Due to an increase in placebo response as well as other factors, a 100-point decrement is increasingly considered as the minimum decrease required to be categorized as a response to therapy, which will make comparisons across trials increasingly difficult. The common acceptance and use of standard evaluation tools in UC trials is even more recent.

The use of the CDAI as an evaluative tool presents its own problems. The index, utilizing a composite score of 8 different factors, is heavily weighted to reflect a subjective assessment of disease activity. As this may be in part appropriate, it also suggests that it is more susceptible to influence by factors other than an improvement in the inflammation responsible for disease activity. Furthermore, a recent publication suggests that even skilled clinicians interpret the CDAI differently.[7] Few, if any, use the CDAI as a clinical tool. When considering a specific treatment, the patient may have a CDAI above or below the entry criteria of the reference trial. The relevance of the study findings to that patient would be in question. Furthermore, the expectations of a patient and treating physician for a response to a particular therapy may be misled by CDAI endpoints. A remission in a trial, defined as a CDAI below 150 points, can still reflect considerable disease activity that patients would not consider a clinical remission.

PATIENT SUBGROUPS

The broad brush of diagnosis in IBD, dividing patients into 2 basic categories, UC and CD, likely subsumes a number of subtypes of disease that may have a different pathophysiology, clinical behavior, and response to medications. Many of these subcategories of disease have been suggested but are poorly defined and even less well-assessed in association with study results. The clinical relevance of these subgroups remains unclear but it is worth considering some potential subgroups of patients and trying to assess applicability.

Subgroups can be considered in terms of demographic characteristics, clinical behavior, biologic markers, genetic associations, or a more detailed microarray fingerprint. The patient characteristics and clinical behaviors suggested in the Vienna classification include age at diagnosis above or below 40 years, disease location, and disease behavior (nonstricturing/nonpenetrating, stricturing, penetrating).[8] Genetic subtypes are being increasingly well-identified, though the clinical relevance remains incompletely defined. At least in a broader category, however, familial versus sporadic Crohn's may be important in disease behavior. More specific genotypes, such as NOD2/CARD15 genotypes, may predict behavior and identify distinct subgroups.[9] Biomarkers such as pANCA, ASCA, OmpC, I2, and anti-flagellin likely identify subgroups of patients[10] and may be useful to predict disease aggressiveness.[11] A distinct subpopulation is characterized by those with an elevated C-reactive protein (CRP), though its clinical significance remains uncertain.

The relevance and appropriate use of these markers are undefined. We are perhaps emerging into an era where microarray profiles hold a promise to identify patients more distinctly and allow for the identification of distinct pathophysiologic subgroups that have a common biologic behavior and response to therapy. The increasing number of agents available makes selection of the appropriate medication more challenging. In the future, the ability to identify which subgroups have an increased likelihood of response to a drug will hopefully allow for more targeted therapy. The size of most studies limits the close assessment of disease subtypes. It is possible, if not likely, that useful therapeutic agents have been discarded as ineffective because of the failure to determine a subgroup for which that medication might be highly beneficial.

ADVERSE EVENTS

In assessing the results of a clinical study, an additional issue involves understanding the risks associated with the study medication. Common events are likely to be identified in a large clinical trial. Less common side effects, however, are poorly defined even in relatively large studies. Most individual studies provide inadequate information to make clinical decisions and to explain risk to patients. Two cases in point are the assessment of lymphoma in relation to infliximab and the identification of progressive multifocal leukoencephalopathy (PML) in studies of natalizumab (Tysabri).

The association of infliximab and adalimumab with lymphoma is likely a rare event but how uncommon remains in dispute. Though one of the better studies based on a primary care database suggests that lymphoma is not increased in the Crohn's population,[12] this issue remains controversial. Best evidence suggests that lymphoma may occur in one or 2 per 1000 individuals treated with infliximab, information that has emerged after several other randomized controlled trials and observational studies have been completed.[13-18] Initial individual randomized trials were too inadequate to provide these data. Further data, which have emerged since the completion of randomized controlled trials, suggests an associated mortality with infliximab as high as 1% to 2%.[13,15] Though such observational studies must be taken with appropriate weight, the relevance to a community practice is in question—as are the results of the randomized clinical trials for reasons detailed previously. Additionally, it is typical to normalize the mortality to patient years of follow-up. Thus, the generally accepted number of 1% mortality per patient year of follow-up is often quoted. This also needs to be looked at in the context question of does this augment baseline risk for lymphoma? The available published data suggest that similar rates of mortality in IBD population cohorts were observed prior to the introduction of infliximab to general use. Recently, a large retrospective analysis of more than 20,000 CD and UC patients recruited into a French registry confirmed an increased risk of non-Hodgkin's lymphoma and Epstein-Barr virus (EBV)-associated lymphoma in patients treated with azathioprine and 6-mercaptopurine (6-MP).[19] A meta-analysis of 26 studies of anti-TNFα therapy with infliximab, adalimumab, and certolizumab showed an elevated incidence rate ratio of non-Hodgkin's lymphoma compared to the general population.[20] Identification of subgroups experiencing significant morbidity and mortality is critical but not yet possible on the basis of available data. In addition, a broader issue that remains poorly defined is the natural history of IBD itself.

The dilemmas raised by natalizumab involve a different set of issues. The recent information presented in part in the media has described 6 cases of progressive PML in patients treated with natalizumab, 5 with multiple sclerosis (MS) and one with Crohn's disease.[21] Only 2 cases have been fatal—one patient with MS and one patient with CD in the controlled trials—and both patients were on combined immunosuppression. Some uncommon side effects not seen in clinical trials may emerge after Food and Drug Administration (FDA) approval in postmarketing surveillance, as was the case for use of natalizumab in MS. The relevance of the findings in MS to Crohn's was uncertain when the first 2 cases of PML were identified in patients with MS. The concern was whether these cases resulted from the concomitant use of natalizumab with interferon or whether there was a unique or particular risk of PML in MS. Until the third case was identified (in a patient with Crohn's disease), the medication was speculated as possibly safe or at least potentially safer in Crohn's patients than MS—though such an assessment was made on inadequate data. The risks involved in the use of this medication remain uncertain, as further evaluations of patients who have received this drug are underway. How to apply this developing information to an individual will remain a challenge if this drug is reintroduced into the market.

CLINICAL APPLICATION OF STUDIES

Translating the results of clinical trials into practice requires a detailed knowledge of the clinical data. But even then, for reasons detailed previously, clinical trials have significant limitations in guiding the care of patients. Many of our decisions, even when informed by the best research available, are based on inferences and suppositions one step removed from the data because of the differences between the individual patient being treated and the study population. In addition, conflicting data may further complicate an already difficult clinical decision. As examples of the difficulty of applying research results to an individual patient, we discuss 2 publications in the following paragraphs, one that changed clinical practice and another that has led us to question a long-time standard of care.

ACCENT 1, published by Hanauer et al in the *Lancet* in 2002,[14] changed the clinical practice of treating patients with Crohn's disease. ACCENT 1 studied 573 patients with moderate to severely active luminal Crohn's disease. All patients received an initial intravenous infusion of 5 mg/kg of infliximab. Two weeks later, patients were assessed for a clinical response. Responders, based on a drop in CDAI of 70 points, were randomized to receive repeat infusions of either infliximab or placebo at weeks 2 and 6 and then every 8 weeks thereafter until week 46. The primary endpoint of the study was the time to loss of response (up to 1 year). The results show that, among initial responders, patients who received repeated infliximab infusions had a significantly longer time to loss of response when compared to the placebo group (46 weeks compared with 19 weeks, $P < 0.0002$). Furthermore, about 3 times as many patients in the treatment groups had discontinued corticosteroids, and significantly more patients maintained a remission ($P < 0.007$) and/or response ($P < 0.0001$) at the end of 1 year. Serious adverse events were infrequent (4% had serious infections, one death was attributable to infliximab), and most patients (90%) were able to continue receiving infusions for the 1-year study period. Based on these results, the use of infliximab for induction and maintenance of moderate to severely active CD has become standard of care.

What doesn't this study show us? Figure 6-1 shows us that the median age was 35 years old, the median disease duration was 7.9 years, and 51% of patients had already had a segmental bowel resection. Although we do see these

	All patients (n=573)	Week-2 responders (n=335)	Week-2 non-responders (n=238)
Sex			
Male	239 (42%)	130 (39%)	109 (46%)
Female	334 (58%)	205 (61%)	129 (54%)
Race			
White	549 (96%)	315 (94%)	234 (98%)
Black	12 (2%)	10 (3%)	2 (1%)
Asian	5 (1%)	4 (1%)	1
Other	7 (1%)	6 (2%)	1
Age (years), median (IQR)	35 (28–46)	35 (27–46)	37 (30–46)
Disease duration (years), median (range)	7·9 (3·9–14·7)	7·5 (3·7–14·2)	9·3 (4·6–15·3)
Involved intestinal area			
Ileum	137/568 (24%)	74/331 (22%)	63/237 (27%)
Colon	109/568 (19%)	74/331 (22%)	35/237 (15%)
Ileum and colon	322/568 (57%)	183/331 (55%)	139/237 (59%)
Gastroduodenum	43/573 (8%)	24/335 (7%)	19/238 (7%)
Previous segmental resection(s)	291/573 (51%)	148/335 (44%)	143/238 (60%)
CDAI*, median (IQR)	297 (260–342)	299 (264–342)	291 (249–340)
IBDQ, median (IQR)	127 (110–147)	129 (114–147)	125 (106–145)
C-reactive protein concentration (mg/dL), median (IQR)	0·8 (0·4–2·3)	1·1 (0·4–2·8)	0·6 (0·4–1·5)
Patients with concomitant medication			
5-aminosalicylates	288 (50%)	159 (47%)	129 (54%)
6-mercaptopurine and azathioprine	144 (25%)	81 (24%)	63 (27%)
Methotrexate	23 (4%)	10 (3%)	13 (6%)
Patients with concomitant corticosteroids			
Any	293 (51%)	175 (52%)	118 (50%)
>20 mg per day	93 (16%)	61 (18%)	32 (13%)

IBDQ=inflammatory bowel disease questionnaire (values can range from 32 to 224). *On final clinical data review, 13 enrolled patients had baseline Crohn's disease activity index (CDAI) <220. For nine of these patients, CDAI as calculated by investigator was ≥220. Remaining four patients were protocol violators.

FIGURE 6-1. Baseline patient characteristics from ACCENT 1. (Reproduced with permission from Hanauer SB, Feagan BG, Lichtenstein GR, et al. Maintenance infliximab for Crohn's disease: the ACCENT I randomised trial. *Lancet.* 2002;359:1541-1549.)

characteristics in many patients with Crohn's disease, there is a large cohort of patients routinely receiving infliximab who differ significantly from this population. For example, younger patients with early aggressive disease in whom we are trying to prevent surgery may benefit most from infliximab, but we do not get an indication of how these patients responded in ACCENT 1 (or whether they were adequately represented). Furthermore, only 25% of all patients were on 6-MP or azathioprine. In general, unless there is a contraindication, our practice is to maintain all patients on concomitant immunomodulators. Now, a few years later, the question of the clinical utility of this tactic is still controversial. We also do not know how concomitant medications (ie, immunomodulators, 5-aminosalicylic acid [5-ASA], steroids, antibiotics) influenced response. This becomes very important when our patients ask us whether they need to continue their cocktail of drugs, and, unfortunately, we are not armed with an evidence-based answer. Patients also ask us how long they need to continue infliximab once started. The answer "until you lose a benefit or have an adverse event" is far from optimal. Although ACCENT 1 shows us the course of patients over a 1-year period, we still lack good data for long-term efficacy, expanding the dosing interval, or withdrawal studies.

When discussing risks of infliximab with patients, good evidence-based data are also inadequate. ACCENT 1 had limited severe toxicity, but adverse event reporting included only 385 patients and also did not have a complete placebo group as a comparison for safety (as all patients received at least one dose of the medication). What if severe, life-threatening toxicity were 1/500, 1/1000, 1/10,000, or even less common? Unfortunately, this is a question that can never be answered in trials like ACCENT 1 but waits for postmarketing analysis and future trials, which may be reported years later.

The role of a study like ACCENT 1 is to define efficacy in a homogeneous population, not explore alternative indications, long-term results, and adverse effects, or to characterize subpopulations of patients most likely to benefit from therapy. A single study can answer a limited set of questions. Once a landmark study like ACCENT 1 is presented, we are required to evaluate data critically and to heed further publications and our own clinical experience to guide our day-to-day management of patients. To that end, the follow-up REACH study confirmed safety and efficacy of infliximab in children with moderate to severely active Crohn's disease and confirms that infliximab every 8 weeks is more effective in maintaining remission than infliximab every 12 weeks.[22] An open randomized trial evaluating patients with Crohn's disease of short duration was recently performed. This study compared early use of combination therapy with infliximab and azathioprine and compared this to conventional step-up therapy where steroids are used initially and then after 2 courses of steroids, azathioprine is initiated. The early use of combination therapy with infliximab and azathioprine demonstrated a steroid-avoiding effect and significant mucosal healing (more so than with the corticosteroid step-up approach) after 2 years of early combined therapy.[23]

SONIC is a large definitive randomized double-blind controlled trial comparing early intervention with infliximab/azathioprine combination therapy, infliximab monotherapy, and azathioprine monotherapy for 1 year in patients with moderate-to-severe Crohn's disease of short duration. Patients in the trial were steroid exposed but naïve to biologics or immunomodulators. SONIC showed that patients with evidence of inflammation (elevated CRP level and endoscopic lesions at baseline colonoscopy) achieved superior steroid-free clinical remission (50%, 42%, and 23%, respectively) associated with mucosal healing from early infliximab combination therapy or monotherapy.[24] These infliximab treatments were superior to azathioprine alone with similar safety outcome in all 3 arms. Just as ACCENT 1 was a pivotal study in establishing the role of maintenance therapy in Crohn's disease, SONIC is a landmark study supporting the tectonic shift toward early intervention with anti-tumor necrosis factor alpha (TNFα) therapy and away from unlimited steroid and azathioprine therapy.

A review of studies of 5-ASAs in Crohn's disease makes a different point about using evidence-based medicine to guide our medical decision-making. Over time, new data may emerge, and on some occasions, old data may materialize that change the way we interpret the literature. In 1993, Singleton et al published a manuscript on the use of slow-release mesalamine capsules (Pentasa, Ferring, Van Lowes, Denmark) for the treatment of active Crohn's disease.[6] This was a double-blind, randomized, placebo-controlled trial that included 310 patients with Crohn's disease. The primary endpoint was a change in the CDAI from baseline. Patients taking 4 g/day of mesalamine had a mean decrease of 72 points in the CDAI compared with 21 points in the placebo group ($P < 0.01$). At the end of 16 weeks, 43% of patients in the 4 g/day mesalamine group were in remission compared to 18% in the placebo group. There was no significant toxicity related to mesalamine. The authors concluded that controlled-release mesalamine at 4 g/day was safe and effective in the treatment of Crohn's disease of the ileum and colon. This study changed clinical practice and went unchallenged by further published placebo-controlled trials. It is worth noting that, to date, none of the 5-ASA agents have been approved by the FDA for the treatment of Crohn's disease.

It was not until 2004 that additional data became available that questioned standard clinical practice. Hanauer's meta-analysis of double-blind, placebo-controlled trials of Pentasa in the treatment of active Crohn's disease[25] added 2 previously unpublished studies to the Singleton data for this analysis.[26,27] Although the authors confirmed that there was a statistically significant improvement of CDAI in Pentasa-treated patients as compared to controls, the net difference was a clinically insignificant 18 points in the CDAI. These results, as argued by some experts,[28] should change our clinical practice by abandoning the use of newer 5-ASA agents for Crohn's disease.

Should new data like these cause us to change clinical practice? Certainly, such studies should motivate more critical thinking about the utility of these agents, but we do not want to make the same mistake twice and too quickly rely on a single publication. The studies of 5-ASA agents in Crohn's disease overall present relatively limited support for a benefit, but it may be inappropriate to jettison the use of these medications in all Crohn's patients. For instance, what was not addressed in this meta-analysis was an evaluation of subgroups of patients with different clinical behaviors of Crohn's disease. Certain subgroups of patients may benefit from mesalamine, and it would be beneficial to treat them with this safe medication. Furthermore, perhaps other formulations or alternative dosing would make a difference. Is there a clinical benefit of 5-ASAs when used in combination with other agents? Are 5-ASAs protective against colorectal cancer in Crohn's disease, as they appear to be in ulcerative colitis?

This scenario also exposes the impact of publication bias. Publication bias refers to the fact that positive studies are more likely to be published than those that are negative. The two sets of data added to the meta-analysis were both from internal industry sources and not previously released publicly. Recent awareness of the gravity of this problem had led to a call from the International Committee of Medical Journal Editors to register all clinical trials in a public trial registry.[29]

Evidence guiding clinical practice evolves over time. A single "landmark" publication may tempt a change in the standard of care, but skepticism is healthy. A single study represents a reference point, or a guide. However, as above, it may not be entirely applicable to the patient sitting in front of us in clinic and may be one report in a large body of potentially conflicting data. These examples point out the limitations of even the best data from well-done randomized clinical trials.

COMMON CLINICAL DECISIONS

Numerous commonly faced clinical dilemmas underscore the fact that many of the decisions we make every day in clinical practice are guided by minimal or weak data at best. It may be fair to say that more clinical scenarios are without guiding evidence or with conflicting evidence than with a clear-cut answer. What is the optimal dose of steroids for a flare? How should steroids be tapered? Who is the appropriate patient for 6-MP or infliximab? How should 6-

MP be initiated and monitored? Can we stop 5-ASAs once on an effective dose of 6-MP or infliximab? Should we premedicate patients with steroids prior to infliximab infusions? How do concomitant medications or environmental exposures impact efficacy of drugs? Questions regarding practical and common circumstances are frequently without solid guiding evidence. In these cases, we must abandon dependence on evidence-based medicine, extrapolate from the literature, and rely on clinical experience.

CONCLUSION

The explosion of IBD publications in recent years will require that we become even more astute in interpreting results and their applicability to our patients. The limitations of current clinical trials remain considerable, and a variety of changes in the conduct of clinical trials could be hoped for to help enhance their utility. Over the next decade, an accepted set of biomarkers will hopefully be identified to assess biologic improvement in inflammation as well as to characterize distinct subsets of disease. It may be that trials have rejected a particular medication as being ineffective in a broad population of UC or Crohn's patients, while it may be highly useful in a particular subset of either disease. Though most authors identify biologic and environmental factors, such as the recent use of CRP and the characterization of disease location or smoking, those involved in the conduct of a trial should be encouraged to assess patients with other available markers such as pANCA, ASCA, as well as genetic markers and microarrays. This information will be critical to allow identification of subgroups of patients who may respond optimally to certain medications as well as others with a low likelihood of response. The blunt tools currently used for disease characterization cause a fundamental weakness in the data derived from clinical trials. As the knowledge of genetic and environmental factors in IBD develops further, it can be hoped that controlled trials will increase in sophistication to provide guidance in our clinical decision-making and improve the care of patients with IBD.

REFERENCES

1. Su C, Lichtenstein GR, Krok K, Brensinger CM, Lewis JD. A meta-analysis of the placebo rates of remission and response in clinical trials of active Crohn's disease. *Gastroenterology.* 2004;126:1257-1269.
2. Targan SR, Hanauer SB, van Deventer SJ, et al. A short-term study of chimeric monoclonal antibody cA2 to tumor necrosis factor alpha for Crohn's disease. Crohn's Disease cA2 Study Group. *N Engl J Med.* 1997;337:1029-1035.
3. Ghosh S, Goldin E, Gordon FH, et al. Natalizumab for active Crohn's disease. *N Engl J Med.* 2003;348:24-32.
4. Best WR, Becktel JM, Singleton JW, Kern F Jr. Development of a Crohn's disease activity index. National Cooperative Crohn's Disease Study. *Gastroenterology.* 1976;70:439-444.
5. Present DH, Korelitz BI, Wisch N, Glass JL, Sachar DB, Pasternack BS. Treatment of Crohn's disease with 6-mercaptopurine. A long-term, randomized, double-blind study. *N Engl J Med.* 1980;302:981-987.
6. Singleton JW, Hanauer SB, Gitnick GL, et al. Mesalamine capsules for the treatment of active Crohn's disease: results of a 16-week trial. Pentasa Crohn's Disease Study Group. *Gastroenterology.* 1993;104:1293-1301.
7. Sands BE, Ooi CJ. A survey of methodological variation in the Crohn's disease activity index. *Inflamm Bowel Dis.* 2005;11:133-138.
8. Gasche C, Scholmerich J, Brynskov J, et al. A simple classification of Crohn's disease: report of the Working Party for the World Congresses of Gastroenterology, Vienna 1998. *Inflamm Bowel Dis.* 2000;6:8-15.
9. Abreu MT, Taylor KD, Lin YC, et al. Mutations in NOD2 are associated with fibrostenosing disease in patients with Crohn's disease. *Gastroenterology.* 2002;123:679-688.
10. Mow WS, Vasiliauskas EA, Lin YC, et al. Association of antibody responses to microbial antigens and complications of small bowel Crohn's disease. *Gastroenterology.* 2004;126:414-424.
11. Forcione DG, Rosen MJ, Kisiel JB, Sands BE. Anti-*Saccharomyces cerevisiae* antibody (ASCA) positivity is associated with increased risk for early surgery in Crohn's disease. *Gut.* 2004;53:1117-1122.
12. Lewis JD, Bilker WB, Brensinger C, et al. Inflammatory bowel disease is not associated with an increased risk of lymphoma. *Gastroenterology.* 2001;121:1080-1087.
13. Colombel JF, Loftus EV Jr, Tremaine WJ, et al. The safety profile of infliximab in patients with Crohn's disease: the Mayo clinic experience in 500 patients. *Gastroenterology.* 2004;126:19-31.
14. Hanauer SB, Feagan BG, Lichtenstein GR, et al. Maintenance infliximab for Crohn's disease: the ACCENT I randomised trial. *Lancet.* 2002;359:1541-1549.
15. Ljung T, Karlen P, Schmidt D, et al. Infliximab in inflammatory bowel disease: clinical outcome in a population based cohort from Stockholm County. *Gut.* 2004;53:849-853.
16. Rutgeerts P, D'Haens G, Targan S, et al. Efficacy and safety of retreatment with anti-tumor necrosis factor antibody (infliximab) to maintain remission in Crohn's disease. *Gastroenterology.* 1999;117:761-769.
17. Sands BE, Anderson FH, Bernstein CN, et al. Infliximab maintenance therapy for fistulizing Crohn's disease. *N Engl J Med.* 2004; 350:876-885.
18. Seiderer J, Goke B, Ochsenkuhn T. Safety aspects of infliximab in inflammatory bowel disease patients. A retrospective cohort study in 100 patients of a German University Hospital. *Digestion.* 2004;70:3-9.
19. Beaugerie L, Carrat F, Bouvier A-M, et al. Excess risk of lymphoproliferative disorders in inflammatory bowel disease: Interim results of the Cesame cohort [abstract 818]. *Gastroenterology.* 2008;134(suppl 1):A116-A117.
20. Siegel C, Sadie M, Marden S, Persing SM, Larson RJ, Sands BE. Risk of lymphoma associated with anti-TNF agents for the treatment of Crohn's disease: a meta-analysis [abstract 970]. *Gastroenterology.* 2008;134(suppl 1):A144.
21. Van Assche G, Van Ranst M, Sciot R, et al. Progressive multifocal leukoencephalopathy after natalizumab therapy for Crohn's disease. *N Engl J Med.* 2005;353:362-368.
22. Hyams J, Crandall W, Kugathasan S, et al. Induction and maintenance infliximab therapy for the treatment of moderate-to severe Crohn's disease in children. *Gastroenterology.* 2007;132:863-873.
23. D'Haens G, Baert F, van Assche G, et al. Early combined immunosuppression or conventional management in patients with newly diagnosed Crohn's disease: an open randomised trial. *Lancet.* 2008;371:660-667.

24. Lichtenstein GR, Hanauer SB, Sandborn WJ, and the Practice Parameters Committee of the American College of Gastroenterology. Management of Crohn's disease in adults. *Am J Gastroenterol.* 2009;104(2):465-483.
25. Hanauer SB, Stromberg U. Oral Pentasa in the treatment of active Crohn's disease: a meta-analysis of double-blind, placebo-controlled trials. *Clin Gastroenterol Hepatol.* 2004;2:379-388.
26. Nordic, Research Inc. Clinical research report: Efficacy and safety of oral Pentasa in the treatment of active Crohn's disease. October 23, 1991.
27. Hoechst, Marion Roussel Inc. Clinical study report: efficacy and safety of oral Pentasa in the treatment of active Crohn's disease. January 28, 1997.
28. Feagan BG. 5-ASA therapy for active Crohn's disease: old friends, old data, and a new conclusion. *Clin Gastroenterol Hepatol.* 2004;2:376-378.
29. DeAngelis CD, Drazen JM, Frizelle FA, et al. Clinical trial registration: A statement from the International Committee of Medical Journal Editors. *JAMA.* 2004;292:1363-1364.

7

Disease Modifiers in Inflammatory Bowel Disease

Jaime A. Oviedo, MD and Francis A. Farraye, MD, MSc, FACP, FACG

Although the individual susceptibility to develop inflammatory bowel disease (IBD) appears to be genetically determined, the actual occurrence of the disease is largely influenced by environmental factors. Though extraordinary advances have been made in our understanding of the genetics, pathogenesis, diagnosis, and medical management of patients with IBD, our emphasis on environmental modifiers, health maintenance, and lifestyle factors that can affect the course, complications, and severity of the disease has not been nearly as significant. Several modifying factors have been identified and are becoming increasingly relevant for physicians and patients alike. This chapter summarizes the available evidence surrounding the influence of disease modifiers on the natural history and course of IBD.

Perinatal and Childhood Factors

The first year of life is considered a crucial period for immune system maturation and development of tolerance. Exposure to specific antigens during early childhood is likely to lead to immune tolerance and might, at least in part, dictate the responses to antigens that are presumably involved in the pathogenesis of IBD.[1]

Based on these concepts, the influence of early life events such as mode of feeding, household hygiene, and perinatal infections on the development of IBD has been examined.

Breastfeeding

Evidence of a possible inverse association between breastfeeding and IBD remains controversial. Although several studies suggested a protective effect of breastfeeding against the development of IBD,[2-6] in some cases, the association did not reach statistical significance and in others was not apparent at all.[7-10] In general, the association appears to be stronger for Crohn's disease (CD) than for ulcerative colitis (UC), but as mentioned, the evidence is controversial at best, and no firm conclusions can be made.

Early weaning has also been implicated as a risk factor for both UC and CD.[9] Though the notion that early weaning has an impact on both immune system and bacterial colonization of the gut is appealing, a case-control study did not confirm an association between early formula feeding and IBD.[8] It is thus possible that in studies showing a positive association, early weaning may be a surrogate marker for higher socioeconomic status. In addition, long recall intervals and the potential for introduction of recall bias may also render studies on infant feeding unreliable.

Socioeconomic and Hygienic Factors

Although in early reports, high socioeconomic status was postulated as a risk factor for both UC and CD,[11,12] subsequent studies have not confirmed this observation.[8,13] The contradicting results over time may be explained by

Lichtenstein GR, ed.
Ulcerative Colitis: The Complete Guide to Medical Management (pp. 79-92)

the reduction or disappearance of differences in living conditions between socioeconomic groups following World War II.

Improvements in hygiene and living conditions during the 20th century have been associated with an increased risk of development of CD. Hygiene, especially early in life, appears to have an impact on the bacterial colonization of the gut and other infectious exposures that determine the development of the immune system.[14] In epidemiological studies, patients with CD were more likely to have running hot water, separate bathroom, less bed and bedroom sharing, and central heating compared to controls.[15,16]

Some authors advocate that the use of domestic refrigeration has contributed to the increasing incidence of CD during the 20th century. The hypothesis is based on the assumption that bacteria such as *Yersinia* spp. and *Listeria*, which can grow at cold temperatures, play a role in the pathogenesis of CD.[17]

Use of toothpaste in Western societies has also been implicated as a possible risk factor for IBD.[18] Dietary microparticles present in toothpaste are the theoretical culprit; however, no observational studies have corroborated this association.[14,19]

In an isolated report, exposure to soft toys during childhood was found to be protective against the development of IBD.[19] This finding has not been validated or reproduced in other studies.[14]

In summary, these reports suggest that strict attention to hygiene and environmental exposure during infancy might prevent the development of tolerance to many bacteria commonly found in the environment and perhaps predispose the individual to active immune-mediated events when the exposure occurs later in life. Although interesting from an epidemiological perspective, these findings are unlikely to lead to any specific recommendations to prevent IBD.

INFECTIONS AND IBD

In addition to the capacity to respond to sporadic challenges from pathogens, the mucosal immune system has the ability to recognize, tolerate, and avoid reacting against nonpathogenic intestinal bacteria. Available evidence from clinical observations and animal studies suggests that intestinal bacteria may play a role in triggering and perpetuating chronic bowel inflammation. IBD appears to result from the interaction of three essential cofactors: host susceptibility, enteric microflora, and mucosal immunity. In susceptible individuals, a breakdown in the regulatory constraints of the mucosal immune response to enteric bacteria may result in the development of IBD.[20]

Since the 1950s, infectious agents have been proposed to be causally related to the occurrence of IBD.[13] A wide range of different microorganisms including *Mycobacterium paratuberculosis* (MAP),[21] *Listeria*,[22] unspecified childhood gastroenteritis, and viral infections such as measles,[23] influenza, and varicella[24] have been linked with either UC, CD, or both (Table 7-1).

TABLE 7-1

INFECTIOUS AGENTS POSSIBLY LINKED TO THE OCCURRENCE OF INFLAMMATORY BOWEL DISEASE

BACTERIAL
Mycobacterium paratuberculosis[21]
Listeria[22]
Pharyngitis and otitis[49]
VIRAL
Unspecified childhood gastroenteritis
Measles and measles vaccination[23]
Mumps[38]
Influenza[24]
Varicella[24]
PARASITES
Helminthic parasites[20]

M. PARATUBERCULOSIS

M paratuberculosis, a subspecies of *Mycobacterium avium*, known to cause Johne's disease (a granulomatous enterocolitis that resembles Crohn's disease in sheep and cattle), has been widely studied for its possible role in the development of CD. DNA from this organism has been detected by culture and molecular techniques in intestinal tissue of patients with CD.[1,25] In a recent study,[26] investigators detected viable MAP in peripheral blood in a higher proportion of patients with CD (13 out of 28) than in individuals without inflammatory bowel disease (0 out of 15). This evidence has, however, not been confirmed by other investigators, as atypical mycobacteria have also been recovered from intestinal tissue of unaffected individuals.[27,28]

Recent microbiological studies have renewed the controversy by showing increased rates of detection of MAP in subepithelial Crohn's-related granulomas when compared to granulomas from other conditions such as foreign-body reaction or sarcoidosis.[28,29] In addition, several open-label studies that evaluated antibiotic regimens with antimycobacterial activity have shown clinical improvement in affected patients.[30-32] However, the results of randomized studies are not nearly as impressive, with a meta-analysis yielding conflicting results.[33] Furthermore, a recent study by Toracchio et al does not support MAP as a primary cause of Crohn's disease. The researchers examined ileal or colonic tissue from 29 patients with Crohn's disease and found MAP DNA in granuloma tissue from only one patient (5%); MAP DNA was not found in non-granuloma tissue samples.[34] Thus, although the hypothesis involving mycobacteria in the pathogenesis of CD is intriguing, the theory has not been unequivocally proven, and antimycobacterial therapy cannot be recommended in the management of affected patients.[35]

Listeria monocytogenes

Early reports suggested that *Listeria monocytogenes* may have the potential to cause IBD.[22,36] Recently, this theory has lost strength when studies utilizing tissue culture and polymerase chain reaction (PCR) have not found the bacteria in biopsy specimens from IBD patients.[37]

Measles Infection or Vaccination

A chronic granulomatous vasculitis of the mesenteric endothelium has been postulated as the mechanism to explain a possible association between exposure to measles and other viruses and the onset of IBD.[38] Although the possibility of this association was described as early as 1950, the supporting data have become increasingly controversial.

In a British cohort study,[39] mumps infection before age 2 was found to be a risk for UC (odds ratio [OR] 25.12; 95% confidence interval [CI] 6.35 to 99.36). Similarly, measles and mumps infections in the same year of life were significantly associated with UC and CD (OR 7.47, 95% CI 2.42 to 23.06 and 4.27; 95% CI 1.24 to 14.46, respectively). These relationships were reported to be independent of each other as well as of gender, social class at birth, household crowding in childhood, and family history of IBD. No significant relationship between measles infection or vaccination at a young age and subsequent IBD was found in this cohort. An increased incidence of IBD following concurrent epidemics of mumps and measles has also been reported in other parts of the world.[40] Similarly, the use of attenuated live measles vaccine was implicated as a possible cause of CD when the prevalence of the disease in a group of people who received the vaccine was 2 to 3 times higher than in the group that did not. However, the findings from the population, as well as microbiologic studies, do not support the relationship between viral infections or vaccinations and IBD.[41-44] A recent study showed no significant differences in the titers of serum anti-mumps immunoglobulin (IgG) in IBD patients when compared to healthy controls.[45,46] Similarly, studies using amplification techniques found no evidence of mumps viral genome in intestinal mucosa or peripheral lymphocytes of patients with IBD.[47-49]

In general, the available evidence does not support the theory that measles infection or vaccination leads to IBD.

Other Infections

Childhood infections have also been postulated as a potential factor associated with the development of IBD. In a population study, patients with CD were more likely to report an increased frequency of childhood infections in general (OR 4.67, 95% CI 2.65 to 8.23) and pharyngitis specifically (OR 2.14, 95% CI 1.30 to 3.51) than healthy counterparts. Treatment with antibiotics for both otitis media (OR 2.07, 95% CI 1.03 to 4.14) and pharyngitis (OR 2.14, 95% CI 1.20 to 3.84) was also more common in the group with CD. Patients with UC also reported an excess of infections in general (OR 2.37, 95% CI 1.19 to 4.71), but not an excess of specific infections or treatments with antibiotics. People who reported an increased frequency of infections tended to have an earlier onset of CD ($P<0.0001$) and ulcerative colitis ($P=0.04$).[50]

Several studies have reported a higher frequency of gastroenteritis or diarrheal illness during infancy among future IBD patients.[3,9,13] As noted earlier, recall bias may affect the validity of the conclusions obtained from these studies.

An adhesive strain of *Escherichia coli* has been implicated in the pathogenesis of UC.[51] Adherent-invasive *E coli* (AIEC) strains have been described in patients with ileal CD.[52] A selective increase in a number of invasive *E coli* of novel phylogeny has been described in patients with ileal CD.[53] AIEC strains have been associated with Crohn's colitis and colonic cancer.[54] Many other agents including *Clostridium*, *Campylobacter*, *Pseudomonas*, *Mycoplasma*, *Cytomegalovirus*, herpes, and rotaviruses have been considered but not proven to have a role in IBD.[1]

Reduced immunologic exposure to helminthic parasites has also been proposed as a potential factor to explain the increased incidence of CD in industrialized societies when compared to developing countries.[20] Colonization with pathogenically attenuated helminths has been used to switch the mucosal cytokine profile in patients with CD. In a small open-label trial, the administration of porcine whipworm eggs was safe and resulted in improvement of CDAI scores for both CD and UC.[55]

In summary, although the bulk of evidence does not suggest that IBD is an infectious or a self-antigen-specific autoimmune disease, recent findings suggest that mucosal damage might be initiated and driven by common, ubiquitous microbial agents derived from the normal bacterial flora in the intestinal lumen.[56]

The role of the normal intestinal flora in the development and progression of IBD has thus generated considerable interest. Products of the commensal flora may promote inflammation in the presence of an impaired mucosal barrier or injury to the mucosa. There is also growing evidence suggesting that a change in the quantity or quality of bacterial luminal content may lead to induction or persistence of mucosal inflammation.[57] Conversely, the manipulation of the normal intestinal flora with antibiotics, or with other nonpathogenic organisms (probiotics), appears to be a promising method to modify mucosal cytokine balance and inflammatory response.

ANTIBIOTICS

Because the increasing exposure to antibiotics experienced after World War II coincided with an increase in the incidence of IBD, some investigators speculate that antibiotics may cause IBD.[58] However, the evidence supporting this hypothesis is limited, based on retrospective studies,[7,50] and likely influenced by indication bias (ie, patients receiving antibiotics for insidious symptoms not yet diagnosed as IBD) or by the increased susceptibility to other infections occasionally seen in patients with IBD. In addition, the prevalence of antibiotic use varies significantly between countries and does not appear to correlate well with the incidence of IBD.[14]

Antibiotics are widely used in patients with IBD and have been shown to be beneficial in the treatment of perianal and colonic CD and pouchitis.[20] Trials in both human IBD and experimental colitis have demonstrated that broad-spectrum antibiotics may influence the course of UC and CD. Antibiotics with narrow anaerobic coverage are effective for preventing relapse in CD after surgically induced remission.[59,60] The use of antibiotics in the management of IBD is reviewed in detail in Chapters 15 and 41.

PROBIOTICS

Probiotics are live, nonpathogenic microbial food ingredients, usually of the genera *Bifidobacterium* or *Lactobacillus,* that alter the enteric flora and have been associated with beneficial effects on human health. Some noninvasive coliforms and nonbacterial organisms such as *Saccharomyces boulardii* are also categorized as probiotics.[20] Based on their ability to prevent the overgrowth of potentially pathogenic organisms and stimulate the intestinal immune defense system,[61] probiotics are being increasingly used as an adjuvant or alternative therapy for IBD. In 2 controlled studies,[62,63] a nonpathogenic strain of *E coli* was as effective as a 5-aminosalicylic acid (5-ASA) preparation in maintaining remission in patients with UC. Probiotic combinations have also shown impressive results in the treatment of chronic pouchitis, reducing the relapse rate by up to 85% when compared to placebo.[64] VSL#3 900, a probiotic with 450 billion live bacteria per packet, has been studied in 2 randomized, placebo-controlled trials evaluating 147 adult patients and 29 children with mild to moderate UC. Both studies suggested an induction and maintenance response. Further studies evaluating VSL#3 in UC are warranted.[65,66] In CD, an open-label study of approximately 20 patients with mild to moderately active disease showed that probiotics reduced the need for corticosteroid therapy in more than 75% of the cases and were safe and well-tolerated.[67] The use of probiotics in IBD is discussed in chapters 36 and 59.

APPENDECTOMY/APPENDICITIS

Appendectomy has been consistently found to be protective against the development of UC.[7,15,68,69] A meta-analysis of 17 case-control studies including more than 3600 cases and more than 4600 controls showed that appendectomy was associated with a 69% reduction in the subsequent risk of UC.[34,70] The results of cohort studies have been less consistent, with 2 large series producing conflicting results. A Swedish inpatient register of 212,963 patients with more than 5 million person-years of follow-up showed that patients who underwent appendectomy for appendicitis and mesenteric lymphadenitis had a 25% reduction of the risk of developing UC. The protective effect was only seen if the appendectomy was performed before the age of 20 years. Appendectomy for noninflammatory conditions such as nonspecific abdominal pain did not appear to confer protection against UC.[71] In another large cohort from Denmark, 154,000 patients who had undergone appendectomy were followed for more than 1 million person-years. Although the cohort was found to be 13% less likely to be diagnosed with UC than previously documented national averages, the difference was not statistically significant.[71] Despite these somewhat conflicting results, most evidence from case-control and cohort studies suggests that appendectomy is a protective factor against UC.[34]

The influence of appendicitis and appendectomy on UC is not limited to the onset of the disease. Appendectomy also appears to influence the clinical course of UC. When compared to patients with UC and an intact appendix, patients who have undergone appendectomy and develop UC are diagnosed at an older age,[72,73] develop fewer recurrent symptoms,[72] require colectomy less frequently,[69,74] and require less immunosuppressive therapy to control the disease.[69] The effect of appendectomy on the clinical course of patients with known UC is limited to case reports and small case series, and results are conflicting.[34]

The relationship between appendectomy and CD is less clear. Appendectomy has been associated with an increased risk of developing CD[75]; however, in many of the published studies, the results did not reach statistical significance. Appendicitis may mimic CD, and ileo-colonic involvement by CD is frequently misdiagnosed as appendicitis, which may overestimate the strength of the association.[69,76]

The mechanism by which appendectomy protects against UC and increases the risk of CD is unknown. The appendix is part of the mucosa-associated lymphoid tissue system and is involved in B lymphocyte–mediated immune responses and extrathymic T lymphocytes. Because of its role as a reservoir for enteric bacteria, removal of the appendix may influence the mucosal immune system and the antigenic exposure in the bowel lumen.[1]

DIET

Various dietary exposures have been proposed as causative factors in IBD. Based on population and immigration studies, and considering the increase in the incidence of CD and UC in countries like Japan and South Korea during the 1990s, a Westernized diet has been implicated in the development of IBD.[14,77-79] Studies examining associations between diet and disease are difficult to perform because of recall bias and the possibility that the diet was modified before the formal diagnosis of IBD as a result of chronic gastrointestinal symptoms. Early dietary studies have been found to be poorly conducted and fraught with methodological deficiencies, making it impossible to draw any meaningful conclusion.[80]

The following dietary components are consistently cited in epidemiological studies.

Refined Sugar

Consumption of refined sugar has been consistently found to be associated with CD in several retrospective case-control studies.[19,81,82] It is possible, however, that the increase in dietary sugar consumption may be driven by symptoms, as patients with CD tend to prefer easily digested foods.[14] Trials that have aimed to minimize difficulties with dietary recall bias by studying patients diagnosed within 1 year have shown contradictory results, with some[83-85] but not all studies showing an association.[82,86]

Because smoking is positively associated with sugar consumption, the interpretation of data derived from dietary studies is complicated. When analyzed separately, sugar intake and smoking have been shown to be independent risk factors; however, combined exposure did not result in a further increased risk.[87,88]

Although a positive association between consumption of refined sugar and the risk of UC has been proposed,[85] the studies are also affected by methodological problems and low statistical power.[14] The results of studies evaluating the effects of a low sugar diet on CD were disappointing.[89]

Protein and Fat

Although the results are inconsistent, and the studies may also be affected by methodological problems, a positive association has been demonstrated for both protein and fat consumption with UC and CD.[71,85,90] In a recently published prospective study,[91] dietary factors such as a high intake of red and processed meat, protein, and alcohol were associated with an increased likelihood of relapse in patients with UC.

Fruit and Vegetables

High intake of dietary fiber, fruit, or vegetables may be protective against the development of IBD, but results vary among studies.[78,85,92] It is unclear whether this finding is the result of decreased fiber intake in response to symptoms of stricturing CD.[34]

Fast Food and Cola Drinks

Both fast food and cola drinks have been implicated as risk factors for UC and CD.[19,92] As mentioned earlier, the retrospective nature of the studies limits the validity of the association.

Many more foods have been implicated in the development or worsening of IBD, including margarine,[93] dairy products,[94] baker's yeast,[95,96] coffee,[92,97] alcohol,[97,98] cornflakes,[99,100] and curry,[101] among others. Lactase or other enzymatic deficiencies secondary to extensive mucosal involvement may be involved in specific food intolerance in patients with CD. In general, none of these associations has been irrefutably proven, and no firm clinical recommendations can be made in this regard.

The low incidence of IBD in populations with high consumption of curried and highly spiced food is intriguing. It has been postulated that curcumin, a major component of curry, has antioxidant and anti-inflammatory activity and acts as a protective factor against the development of IBD.[101]

Because dietary antigens may act as immunoregulators, it has been proposed that food allergies may play a role in the pathogenesis of IBD.[102,103] Small studies have shown that patients with CD feature a stronger response to food antigens than healthy individuals.[103] The success of treatment with elemental or exclusion diets would support food allergy as a biological pathway in patients with CD. Similarly, food additives present in modern urban diets may be involved in immune reactions both locally and systemically and have been proposed as an etiological factor in IBD, especially CD.[104,105] The role of elemental and exclusion diets and other dietary manipulations in IBD is discussed in chapters 37 and 38.

ORAL CONTRACEPTIVES

Since the 1970s, several case reports, as well as case-control and cohort studies, have described an increased risk of

IBD in women who use oral contraceptives (OCPs).[106-108] Although cohort studies compiling more than 80,000 women reported increases in IBD risk ranging from 40% to three-fold, the results were not statistically significant, especially after adjusting for cigarette smoking.[34,107-109] In a meta-analysis of 2 cohort studies and 7 case-control studies, the pooled OR for CD among users of OCPs, after adjusting for smoking, was 1.4 (95% CI 1.1 to 1.9). OR for UC among OCP users was 1.29 but did not reach statistical significance (95% CI 0.9 to 1.8).[110] The association was thus found to be weak and not necessarily causal, as confounding factors could not be ruled out.[14]

Other case-control studies have also suggested an association between OCP use and IBD, and especially with CD.[111,112] The risk appears to be higher among longtime users[111,113,114] and among users of high-dose estrogen preparations.[111]

Although a single study reported an increased incidence of relapse among OCP users,[115] OCPs do not appear to increase the risk of relapse or modify the course of CD.[116]

In summary, available evidence supports a weak association between OCP use and IBD. The thrombogenic potential of OCPs, leading to multifocal gastrointestinal infarctions mediated by chronic mesenteric vasculitis, similar to those of smoking, are the proposed mechanism underlying the effect of OCPs on CD.[34,117]

ENVIRONMENTAL FACTORS

Smoking

Smoking is the best characterized of the environmental factors that can affect the severity and natural history of IBD. Smoking cigarettes is associated with an increased prevalence of CD, and nonsmoking is associated with UC.[118] There is also strong evidence suggesting that smoking cigarettes has a negative effect on the course of CD and that smoking cigarettes may improve the disease severity or have a "protective" effect in some patients with UC.[119]

Smoking and UC

UC is predominately a disease of nonsmokers. Several meta-analyses as well as observational and case-control studies have confirmed that the relative risk of colitis is reduced in smokers when compared to people who have never smoked and to individuals who have quit smoking.[120,121] The incidence of UC in the Mormon community where smoking is discouraged is five-fold higher than the general population.[122,123] Lifetime nonsmokers are almost 3 times more likely to have UC than current smokers.[124] Furthermore, approximately two-thirds of former smokers with UC develop the disease after quitting smoking, with a particularly high incidence in the first few years.[125-127]

Smokers have also been noted to have a reduced incidence of conditions such as primary sclerosing cholangitis (PSC), with or without associated IBD[128-130] and pouchitis.[131] The protective effect against PSC suggests a systemic effect rather than a local effect on the colon.[34]

Smoking also appears to have an effect on the clinical course of UC. A significant proportion of patients report that their colitis improves while smoking ~20 cigarettes daily. Similarly, smokers with UC report fewer bowel complaints than their nonsmoking counterparts.[132] Most of the available evidence supports the contention that smoking is a significant disease modifier in UC. Several studies have reported lower hospitalization rates in smokers with UC, higher colectomy rates in ex-smokers who quit smoking before the onset of their colitis,[133] reduced rates of clinical relapse in patients who began smoking after diagnosis,[134] and reduced incidence of pouchitis in smokers following proctocolectomy.[131] Conversely, smoking cessation is usually followed by a statistically significant increase in disease severity, hospitalization rate, and a need for major medical therapy, when compared to continuing smoking.[135]

Smoking and CD

Smoking is a well-recognized risk factor for CD,[124] and patients with CD have higher rates of tobacco use than the general population.[124,136] Compared with non-smokers, patients with CD who smoke suffer more clinical relapses,[116,132,137] develop more complications,[138] require surgery more often,[119,139] and need more immunosuppressive therapy.[140,141]

There is also evidence suggesting that the detrimental effect of smoking on CD subsides after smoking cessation. Patients who quit smoking have a reduced risk of relapse[115,142] and postoperative recurrence when compared to current smokers.[139] On the basis of these associations, smoking cessation is a potential therapy for CD. However, many patients are unaware of the risk of worsening their CD by smoking and do not recall their physician ever informing them about these risks.[143]

Although it has been suggested that CD patients are poorly receptive to smoking cessation counseling,[144] which may explain why more efforts are not made to get these patients to quit, the percentages of people considering and attempting to quit are similar to those reported in other groups of smokers in the general population. Therefore, there is no evidence to conclude that patients with CD are any more refractory to smoking cessation than smokers in the general population.

Though remaining abstinent is as difficult for people with CD as it is for the smokers in the general population, the benefits of discontinuing smoking in patients with CD justify all the effort involved in achieving smoking cessa-

TABLE 7-2

EFFECTS OF SMOKING AND SMOKING CESSATION ON INFLAMMATORY BOWEL DISEASE

	Crohn's Disease	Ulcerative Colitis
Smoking	Increased prevalence	Decreased prevalence
	Negative effect on course	"Protective" effect
	• More relapses	• Fewer flares
	• Increased complications	• Reduced hospitalizations
	• More surgeries	• Reduced colectomy rates
	• Increased need for use of immunomodulators	• Reduced incidence of pouchitis
Smoking cessation	Decreased risk of relapse and postoperative recurrence	Increased disease activity
	Decreased risk for steroids and immunomodulators	Increased need for hospitalization, steroids, and immunomodulators
		• Increased need for colectomy

tion. Patients who successfully quit smoking for more than 1 year appear to significantly reduce their risk of experiencing a flare, as well as reduce the need for the use of steroids or immunomodulators when compared to continuing smokers.[145]

Passive smoking has also been linked to increased IBD risk. In one study, passive smoking at birth was significantly associated with the development of either subtype of IBD.[146] The effect of passive smoking in childhood appears to be similar to that of active smoking in adults, as demonstrated by a study following children exposed to cigarette smoke at home who were found to be half as likely to develop UC.[147] In another study, exposure to cigarette smoke during childhood increased the risk of CD but not UC.[138]

Despite these well-described associations, the mechanism by which cigarette smoking affects UC and CD in opposite ways is not fully understood. In addition to nicotine, tobacco smoke contains hundreds of substances including free radicals and carbon monoxide (CO).[148] Several effects of nicotine are likely contributors to the role of smoking as a disease modifier in IBD. Nicotine modifies the thickness of mucus and abolishes the synthesis of inflammatory cytokines in the colonic mucosa in animal models.[58,112] In humans, nicotine is known to decrease the production of mucosal eicosanoids and some cytokines, such as IL-2, IL-8, and tumor necrosis factor alpha (TNFα).[148-150] Nicotine also reduces smooth muscle tone and contractile activity as a result of CO release, changes in the microcirculation, and transient ischemia.[13,16] Cigarette smoke, in turn, increases lipid peroxidation and modifies the mucosal immune response.[151] Smoking increases CO concentration, which might amplify the impairment in vasodilation capacity in chronically inflamed microvessels, resulting in ischemia and perpetuating ulceration and fibrosis.[148,152]

Patient-related factors have also been found to play a role in the type and magnitude of the effects of smoking in IBD. The effects of nicotine on IBD appear to be dose-related, with significant changes seen with 15 or more cigarettes per day. Women appear to be more susceptible than men to the harmful effect of smoking on CD, and as seen in patients with UC the protective effect of nicotine is more efficient in the distal intestine.[148] Table 7-2 summarizes the effects of smoking and smoking cessation on IBD.

Based on the known effects of cigarette smoking in the incidence and course of UC, nicotine has been studied as a potential therapeutic alternative. The role of nicotine therapy in the management of UC is discussed in chapter 34.

SMOKING AND IBD IN CLINICAL PRACTICE

Individuals with CD should be strongly encouraged to quit smoking. Like any other smokers, Crohn's patients will have low abstinence rates without additional support. Counseling, smoking cessation groups, and pharmacotherapy should be offered by providers treating these patients.

Although most evidence supports a beneficial effect of cigarette smoking on the course of UC, these patients should not be encouraged to smoke and should, as any other smoker, receive education about the health risks of nicotine use. Patients with UC should be educated about the relationship between smoking and their disease and should be allowed to make their own decisions based on the facts. Smokers with UC who plan to stop smoking should be informed of the potential risk of increase in disease activity, and, accordingly, therapy should be adjusted to prevent a flare of their colitis.

NONSTEROIDAL ANTI-INFLAMMATORY DRUGS

Nonsteroidal anti-inflammatory drugs (NSAIDs) are one of the most commonly used medications worldwide. In the United States alone, more than 70 million NSAID prescriptions and 30 billion over-the-counter preparations are sold every year.[153] Although NSAID use has typically been associated with the development of gastroduodenal injury, evidence implicating these agents in inducing and exacerbating damage in the distal gastrointestinal tract is also mounting. Colonic injury ranging from colitis resembling inflammatory bowel disease to colonic perforation and bleeding has been described.[154-156] NSAIDs have been associated with the onset of acute IBD lesions, as well as exacerbation of pre-existing disease.[157] A relationship between NSAID use and the development of collagenous colitis has also been postulated.[158,159]

More than 80% of patients with IBD interviewed for one study reported use of NSAIDs within the previous month, and approximately one-third of these patients thought that there was an association between their IBD symptoms and NSAID use. In contrast, only 2% of the IBS population used as control reported worsening symptoms following NSAID use.[160,161]

Although most of the available clinical evidence points toward an adverse influence of NSAIDs on the course of IBD, the exact mechanism by which NSAIDs can lead to exacerbations of the disease is not fully understood. Inhibition of colonic prostaglandin (PG) synthesis is likely a contributing factor.[162] The key enzyme in this pathway is cyclooxygenase (COX), which exists in 2 isoforms: COX-1, the constitutive enzyme involved in maintaining mucosal integrity in the gastrointestinal (GI) tract, and COX-2, an inducible enzyme that is expressed at sites of inflammation. COX-2 expression is significantly increased in the colonic mucosa of patients with active IBD when compared to inactive disease or healthy controls.[163] COX-2 appears to have a beneficial effect in healing experimental colitis, and, in theory, COX-2 inhibition might impair colitis healing.[162]

Because of the evidence suggesting that COX-2–specific inhibitors are less toxic to the gastrointestinal tract than traditional NSAIDs, patients and physicians have assumed that coxibs would not increase the risk of exacerbation of IBD. However, cases of flares of IBD associated with use of COX-2 inhibitors have been reported in the literature.[164-166] In two case series of IBD patients who were prescribed COX-2 inhibitors, the risk of disease exacerbation was reported at 7%[167] and 13%,[168] respectively. In a recent series of 33 patients with IBD who were prescribed celecoxib or rofecoxib, 39% experienced exacerbation of their disease.[169] A recent randomized, placebo-controlled trial found no difference in relapse rate among 222 patients with ulcerative colitis in remission who were given oral celecoxib 200 mg or placebo twice daily for 14 days.[170] Until more information is available, however, the general expert consensus is that the use of COX-2-specific inhibitors in patients with IBD should be viewed with the same caution as the use of traditional NSAIDs.[171]

There is no simple solution for the small number of patients who require NSAIDs and have significant IBD activity. When patients are using NSAIDs to control the pain from IBD-related arthritis, the intestinal disease should be treated aggressively, in the hopes that the severity of the arthritis will decrease as the intestinal inflammatory activity resolves. Non-NSAID analgesics can be prescribed in the interim to control joint pain. In rheumatoid arthritis or other arthritides, this strategy may not be as successful because the course of the arthritis is independent of the activity of the intestinal disease.[172] Non-NSAID analgesics and local measures can be used for the treatment of trauma-related pain and inflammation in patients with IBD. If these fail, a short course of NSAIDs or COX-2–selective inhibitors may be prescribed with close monitoring of symptoms and side effects.

EXERCISE

Sedentary and physically less-demanding occupations have been associated with a higher incidence of IBD.[173-175] Regular exercise, in contrast, has been associated with significant improvements in quality of life and activity index scores, as well as with a reduction in the frequency of flares in patients with CD.[176]

Though GI symptoms such as nausea, heartburn, diarrhea, and occasionally GI bleeding are common during intense sports,[177-180] physical activity has also been associated with long-term benefits in the GI tract, especially a consistent reduction in colon cancer risk, which (although documented in non-IBD patients) is likely to also extend to individuals with IBD.[181,182]

Although the preventive effect of exercise remains inconclusive, it seems clear that physical activity is not harmful for patients with IBD. Another important reason to recommend regular physical activity is that IBD patients, especially those on chronic steroids, are at risk for osteoporosis and osteopenia.[182,183] A low-impact exercise program can potentially increase bone density in these patients.[184] Exercise may also alleviate stress and allow people to deal with stressful events more effectively, increasing the sense of general well-being and quality of life.[176] Physical activity

TABLE 7-3

POSSIBLE EFFECTS OF EXERCISE IN INFLAMMATORY BOWEL DISEASE

- Decreased incidence of CD and UC
- Possible reduction in incidence of colon cancer
- Increased bone density
- Improvement in quality of life in CD
- Reduction in flares and activity index in CD

should be recommended, keeping in mind that there are limited data regarding exactly how much exercise is appropriate[171] (Table 7-3).

SEASONAL VARIATION

Whether the natural history of IBD follows a seasonal pattern remains controversial. Some patients report disease relapses at similar times during the year, and available evidence suggests that seasonal variation may occur, especially for UC. Study results are conflicting and difficult to reproduce, however. Though some studies demonstrated increased rates of UC flares in the spring,[185,186] others reported more flares in the fall and winter,[187,188] and a few others found no association at all.[189,190]

The results for CD are equally conflicting.[186,187,189,190] A seasonal increase in the incidence of upper respiratory infections has been implicated as a potential mechanism to explain flares that occur at similar times every year.[191,192] Most studies are limited by small sample size and difficulties determining exact temporal relationships between infections and IBD relapses, which makes any conclusions drawn from the data controversial at best. A recent retrospective study of more than 1500 patients with CD and more than 2700 patients with UC, evaluated a population-based cohort of patients. The study reported a slight increase of UC exacerbations during the spring and no association between seasons and flares of CD.[193]

The potential variability of the natural history of IBD during different seasons of the year, although intriguing, is a factor that will be very difficult to completely elucidate and, if present, impossible to modify.

STRESS

Patients with IBD can experience considerable psychological stress. Factors such as potential disability caused by the symptoms of IBD and the uncertainty regarding disease outcomes can produce significant stress, anxiety, and depression.[194] Stress and emotional issues appear to play a significant role in increasing disease activity and frequency of relapses, as well as use of medical services in patients with IBD.[194-198] Whether stress contributes to the onset or precipitates exacerbations of CD remains controversial. Although many patients and family members are convinced that stress is an essential factor in the onset and course of IBD, it has not been possible to correlate the development of disease with any psychological issues or disease exacerbations with stressful life events.[199] Though short-term stress does not appear to trigger disease flares in patients with UC in remission, perceived long-term stress has been associated with an increased risk of exacerbation.[200] A recent study found no evidence of an association between psychological stress, as measured by the death of a child, and the development of IBD.[201]

The possibility of concurrent IBS-related symptoms and their relation to stressful events should also be recognized to minimize the use of potent anti-inflammatory or disease-modifying therapies in the absence of a documented inflammatory component.

Strategies that improve social support, including local groups where individuals can share their experiences, can have a favorable impact on psychological distress and ultimately can improve health outcomes in patients with IBD.[198] Empathy, understanding, positive regard, and psychological support can improve the patient-physician relationship and lead to better quality of life for the patients.[202]

CONCLUSION

The role of certain environmental and lifestyle factors in the onset, severity, and course of IBD is significant. An approach that involves patients in the self-care of their condition includes open discussion, and (when possible) modifications of these factors should be part of the integral care provided to patients with IBD. Smoking is the best studied of the so-called disease-modifiers in IBD. Smoking cessation is of proven benefit for CD patients and is known to exert a negative impact on the course and severity of UC. Although achieving long-term smoking cessation is difficult, IBD patients, including those with UC, should be encouraged to quit smoking. The benefits of smoking cessation outweigh the risk of aggravating UC, and providers caring for these patients should be prepared to adjust the medical regimen to mitigate the adverse effects of nicotine discontinuation.

Though appendectomy appears to be protective against UC, the use of both traditional NSAIDs and selective COX-2 inhibitors appears to exert a negative effect on the onset and course of IBD. The influence of other factors such as diet, childhood infections, socioeconomic factors, psychological stress, and oral contraceptives is less clear, and specific recommendations cannot be generalized to all patients.

REFERENCES

1. Howlett M, Gibson P. Environmental influences on IBD. *IBD Monitor.* 2004;5:74-83.
2. Bergstrand O, Hellers G. Breast-feeding during infancy in patients who later develop Crohn's disease. *Scand J Gastroenterol.* 1983; 18:903-906.
3. Koletzko S, Sherman P, Corey M, Griffiths A, Smith C. Role of infant feeding practices in development of Crohn's disease in childhood. *BMJ.* 1989;298:1617-1618.
4. Rigas A, Rigas B, Glassman M, et al. Breast-feeding and maternal smoking in the etiology of Crohn's disease and ulcerative colitis in childhood. *Ann Epidemiol.* 1993;3:387-392.
5. Gruber M, Marshall JR, Zielezny M, Lance P. A case-control study to examine the influence of maternal perinatal behaviors on the incidence of Crohn's disease. *Gastroenterol Nurs.* 1996;19:53-59.
6. Thompson NP, Montgomery SM, Wadsworth ME, Pounder RE, Wakefield AJ. Early determinants of inflammatory bowel disease: use of two national longitudinal birth cohorts. *Eur J Gastroenterol Hepatol.* 2000;12:25-30.
7. Gilat T, Hacohen D, Lilos P, Langman MJ. Childhood factors in ulcerative colitis and Crohn's disease. An international cooperative study. *Scand J Gastroenterol.* 1987;22:1009-1024.
8. Ekbom A, Adami HO, Helmick CG, Jonzon A, Zack MM. Perinatal risk factors for inflammatory bowel disease: a case-control study. *Am J Epidemiol.* 1990;132:1111-1119.
9. Koletzko S, Griffiths A, Corey M, Smith C, Sherman P. Infant feeding practices and ulcerative colitis in childhood. *BMJ.* 1991;302:1580-1581.
10. Thompson NP, Pounder RE, Wakefield AJ. Perinatal and childhood risk factors for inflammatory bowel disease: a case-control study. *Eur J Gastroenterol Hepatol.* 1995;7:385-390.
11. Acheson ED, Nefzger MD. Ulcerative colitis in the United States Army in 1944. Epidemiology: comparisons between patients and controls. *Gastroenterology.* 1963;44:7-19.
12. Sonnenberg A. Disability from inflammatory bowel disease among employees in West Germany. *Gut.* 1989;30:367-370.
13. Whorwell PJ, Holdstock G, Whorwell GM, Wright R. Bottle feeding, early gastroenteritis, and inflammatory bowel disease. *Br Med J.* 1979;1:382.
14. Ekbom A, Montgomery SM. Environmental risk factors (excluding tobacco and microorganisms): critical analysis of old and new hypotheses. *Best Pract Res Clin Gastroenterol.* 2004;18:497-508.
15. Duggan AE, Usmani I, Neal KR, Logan RF. Appendicectomy, childhood hygiene, *Helicobacter pylori* status, and risk of inflammatory bowel disease: A case control study. *Gut.* 1998;43:494-498.
16. Gent AE, Hellier MD, Grace RH, Swarbrick ET, Coggon D. Inflammatory bowel disease and domestic hygiene in infancy. *Lancet.* 1994;343:766-767.
17. Hugot JP, Alberti C, Berrebi D, Bingen E, Cezard JP. Crohn's disease: the cold chain hypothesis. *Lancet.* 2003;362:2012-2015.
18. Sullivan SN. Hypothesis revisited: toothpaste and the cause of Crohn's disease. *Lancet.* 1990;336:1096-1097.
19. Russel MG, Engels LG, Muris JW, et al. Modern life in the epidemiology of inflammatory bowel disease: a case-control study with special emphasis on nutritional factors. *Eur J Gastroenterol Hepatol.* 1998;10:243-249.
20. Shanahan F. Inflammatory bowel disease: immunodiagnostics, immunotherapeutics, and ecotherapeutics. *Gastroenterology.* 2001; 120:622-635.
21. Morgan KL. Johne's and Crohn's. Chronic inflammatory bowel diseases of infectious aetiology? *Lancet.* 1987;1:1017-1019.
22. Van Kruiningen HJ, Colombel JF, Cartun RW, et al. An in-depth study of Crohn's disease in two French families. *Gastroenterology.* 1993;104:351-360.
23. Pardi DS, Tremaine WJ, Sandborn WJ, et al. Early measles virus infection is associated with the development of inflammatory bowel disease. *Am J Gastroenterol.* 2000;95:1480-1485.
24. Ekbom A, Adami HO, Helmick CG, Jonzon A, Zack MM. Perinatal risk factors for inflammatory bowel disease: a case-control study. *Am J Epidemiol.* 1990;132:1111-1119.
25. Greenstein RJ. Is Crohn's disease caused by a mycobacterium? Comparisons with leprosy, tuberculosis, and Johne's disease. *Lancet Infect Dis.* 2003;3:507-514.
26. Naser SA, Ghobrial G, Romero C, Valentine JF. Culture of *Mycobacterium avium* subspecies *paratuberculosis* from the blood of patients with Crohn's disease. *Lancet.* 2004;364:1039-1044.
27. Van Kruiningen HJ. Lack of support for a common etiology in Johne's disease of animals and Crohn's disease in humans. *Inflamm Bowel Dis.* 1999;5:183-191.
28. Ryan P, Kelly RG, Lee G, et al. Bacterial DNA within granulomas of patients with Crohn's disease-detection by laser capture microdissection and PCR. *Am J Gastroenterol.* 2004;99:1539-1543.
29. Ryan P, Bennett MW, Aarons S, et al. PCR detection of *Mycobacterium paratuberculosis* in Crohn's disease granulomas isolated by laser capture microdissection. *Gut.* 2002;51:665-670.
30. Gui GP, Thomas PR, Tizard ML, Lake J, Sanderson JD, Hermon-Taylor J. Two-year-outcomes analysis of Crohn's disease treated with rifabutin and macrolide antibiotics. *J Antimicrob Chemother.* 1997;39:393-400.
31. Shafran I, Kugler L, El-Zaatari FA, Naser SA, Sandoval J. Open clinical trial of rifabutin and clarithromycin therapy in Crohn's disease. *Dig Liver Dis.* 2002;34:22-28.
32. Borody TJ, Leis S, Warren EF, Surace R. Treatment of severe Crohn's disease using antimycobacterial triple therapy—approaching a cure? *Dig Liver Dis.* 2002;34:29-38.
33. Borgaonkar MR, MacIntosh DG, Fardy JM. A meta-analysis of antimycobacterial therapy for Crohn's disease. *Am J Gastroenterol.* 2000;95:725-729.
34. Toracchio S, El-Zimaity HM, Urmacher C, Katz S, Graham DY. *Mycobacterium avium* subspecies *paratuberculosis* and Crohn's disease granulomas. *Scand J Gastroenterol.* 2008;43:1108-1111.
35. Loftus EV Jr. Clinical epidemiology of inflammatory bowel disease: incidence, prevalence, and environmental influences. *Gastroenterology.* 2004;126:1504-1517.
36. Liu Y, van Kruiningen HJ, West AB, Cartun RW, Cortot A, Colombel JF. Immunocytochemical evidence of *Listeria, Escherichia coli,* and *Streptococcus* antigens in Crohn's disease. *Gastroenterology.* 1995;108:1396-1404.
37. Swidsinski A, Ladhoff A, Pernthaler A, et al. Mucosal flora in inflammatory bowel disease. *Gastroenterology.* 2002;122:44-54.
38. Wakefield AJ, Ekbom A, Dhillon AP, Pittilo RM, Pounder RE. Crohn's disease: pathogenesis and persistent measles virus infection. *Gastroenterology.* 1995;108:911-916.
39. Montgomery SM, Morris DL, Pounder RE, Wakefield AJ. Paramyxovirus infections in childhood and subsequent inflammatory bowel disease. *Gastroenterology.* 1999;116:796-803.
40. Montgomery SM, Bjornsson S, Johannsson JH, Thjodleifsson B, Pounder RE, Wakefield AJ. Concurrent measles and mumps epidemics in Iceland are a risk factor for later inflammatory bowel disease. *Gut.* 1998;42:A41.
41. Anonymous. Case control study finds no link between measles vaccine and inflammatory bowel disease. *Commun Dis Rep CDR Wkly.* 1997;7:339.

42. Feeney M, Ciegg A, Winwood P, Snook J. A case-control study of measles vaccination and inflammatory bowel disease. The East Dorset Gastroenterology Group. *Lancet.* 1997;350:764-766.
43. Morris DL, Montgomery SM, Thompson NP, Ebrahim S, Pounder RE, Wakefield AJ. Measles vaccination and inflammatory bowel disease: a national British Cohort Study. *Am J Gastroenterol.* 2000;95:3507-3512.
44. Davis RL, Kramarz P, Bohlke K, et al. Measles-mumps-rubella and other measles-containing vaccines do not increase the risk for inflammatory bowel disease: a case-control study from the Vaccine Safety Datalink project. *Arch Pediatr Adolesc Med.* 2001; 155:354-359.
45. Iizuka M, Saito H, Yukawa M, et al. No evidence of persistent mumps virus infection in inflammatory bowel disease. *Gut.* 2001; 48:637-641.
46. Peltola H, Patja A, Leinikki P, Valle M, Davidkin I, Paunio M. No evidence for measles, mumps, and rubella vaccine-associated inflammatory bowel disease or autism in a 14-year prospective study. *Lancet.* 1998;351:1327-1328.
47. Haga Y, Funakoshi O, Kuroe K, et al. Absence of measles viral genomic sequence in intestinal tissues from Crohn's disease by nested polymerase chain reaction. *Gut.* 1996;38:211-215.
48. Afzal MA, Armitage E, Begley J, et al. Absence of detectable measles virus genome sequence in inflammatory bowel disease tissues and peripheral blood lymphocytes. *J Med Virol.* 1998;55:243-249.
49. Folwaczny C, Jager G, Schnettler D, Wiebecke B, Loeschke K. Search for mumps virus genome in intestinal biopsy specimens of patients with IBD. *Gastroenterology.* 1999;117:1253-1255.
50. Wurzelmann JI, Lyles CM, Sandler RS. Childhood infections and the risk of inflammatory bowel disease. *Dig Dis Sci.* 1994;39:555-560.
51. Burke DA, Axon AT. Adhesive *Escherichia coli* in inflammatory bowel disease and infective diarrhoea. *BMJ.* 1988;297:102-104.
52. Darfeuille-Michaud A, Boudeau J, Bulois P, et al. High prevalence of adherent-invasive *Escherichia coli* associated with ileal mucosa in Crohn's disease. *Gastroenterology.* 2004;127:412-421.
53. Baumgart M, Dogan B, Rishniw M, et al. Culture independent analysis of ileal mucosa reveals a selective increase in invasive *Escherichia coli* of novel phylogeny relative to depletion of *Clostridiales* in Crohn's disease involving the ileum. *ISME J.* 2007;1:403-418.
54. Martin HM, Campbell BJ, Hart CA, et al. Enhanced *Escherichia coli* adherence and invasion in Crohn's disease and colon cancer. *Gastroenterology.* 2004;127:80-93.
55. Summers RW, Elliott DE, Qadir K, Urban JF Jr, Thompson R, Weinstock JV. *Trichuris suis* seems to be safe and possibly effective in the treatment of inflammatory bowel disease. *Am J Gastroenterol.* 2003;98:2034-2041.
56. Merger M, Croitoru K. Infections in the immunopathogenesis of chronic inflammatory bowel disease. *Semin Immunol.* 1998; 10:69-78.
57. Fiocchi C. Inflammatory bowel disease: etiology and pathogenesis. *Gastroenterology.* 1998;115:182-205.
58. Demling L. Is Crohn's disease caused by antibiotics? *Hepatogastroenterology.* 1994;41:549-551.
59. Schultz M, Scholmerich J, Rath HC. Rationale for probiotic and antibiotic treatment strategies in inflammatory bowel diseases. *Dig Dis.* 2003;21:105-128.
60. D'Haens GR, Vermeire S, Van Assche G, et al. Therapy of metronidazole with azathioprine to prevent postoperative recurrence of Crohn's disease: a controlled randomized trial. *Gastroenterology.* 2008;135:1123-1129.
61. Bengmark S. Colonic food: pre- and probiotics. *Am J Gastroenterol.* 2000;95(1 Suppl):S5-S7.
62. Kruis W, Schulz T, Fric P, et al. Double blind comparison of an oral *Eschericia coli* preparation and mesalazine in maintaining remission of ulcerative colitis. *Aliment Pharmacol Ther.* 1997;11:853-858.
63. Rembacken BJ, Snelling AM, Hawkey PM, et al. Non-pathogenic *Escherichia coli* versus mesalazine for the treatment of ulcerative colitis: A randomized trial. *Lancet.* 1999;354:635-639.
64. Gionchetti P, Rizzello F, Venturi A, Campieri M. Probiotics in infective diarrhoea and inflammatory bowel diseases. *J Gastroenterol Hepatol.* 2000;15:489-493.
65. Makharia GK, Sood A, Midha V. A randomized, controlled trial of probiotic preperation VSL#3 for the treatment of mild to moderate ulcerative colitis [abstract]. *Gastroenterology.* 2008;134(suppl 1): A701.
66. Miele E, Baldessano R, Pascarella S. The effect of a probiotic preparation VSL#3 on induction and remission in mild UC [abstract]. *Gastroenterology.* 2008;134(suppl 1):1013.
67. Shanahan F. Probiotics: science or snake oil. *Clin Persp Gastroenterol.* 2001;4:47-50.
68. Rutgeerts P, D'Haens G, Hiele M, Geboes K, Vantrappen G. Appendectomy protects against ulcerative colitis. *Gastroenterology.* 1994;106:1251-1253.
69. Radford-Smith GL, Edwards JE, Purdie DM, et al. Protective role of appendicectomy on onset and severity of ulcerative colitis and Crohn's disease. *Gut.* 2002;51:808-813.
70. Koutroubakis IE, Vlachonikolis IG, Kouroumalis EA. Role of appendicitis and appendectomy in the pathogenesis of ulcerative colitis: a critical review. *Inflamm Bowel Dis.* 2002;8:277-286.
71. Andersson RE, Olaison G, Tysk C, Ekbom A. Appendectomy and protection against ulcerative colitis. *N Engl J Med.* 2001;344:808-814.
72. Naganuma M, Iizuka B, Torii A, et al. Appendectomy protects against the development of ulcerative colitis and reduces its recurrence: results of a multicenter case-controlled study in Japan. *Am J Gastroenterol.* 2001;96:1123-1126.
73. Selby WS, Griffin S, Abraham N, Solomon MJ. Appendectomy protects against the development of ulcerative colitis but does not affect its course. *Am J Gastroenterol.* 2002;97:2834-2838.
74. Cosnes J, Carbonnel F, Beaugerie L, Blain A, Reijasse D, Gendre JP. Effects of appendicectomy on the course of ulcerative colitis. *Gut.* 2002;51:803-807.
75. Andersson RE, Olaison G, Tysk C, Ekbom A. Appendectomy is followed by increased risk of Crohn's disease. *Gastroenterology.* 2003;124:40-46.
76. Kurina LM, Goldacre MJ, Yeates D, Seagroatt V. Appendicectomy, tonsillectomy, and inflammatory bowel disease: a case-control record linkage study. *J Epidemiol Community Health.* 2002;56:551-554.
77. Probert CS, Jayanthi V, Pinder D, Wicks AC, Mayberry JF. Epidemiological study of ulcerative proctocolitis in Indian migrants and the indigenous population of Leicestershire. *Gut.* 1992;33:687-693.
78. Shoda R, Matsueda K, Yamato S, Umeda N. Epidemiologic analysis of Crohn disease in Japan: increased dietary intake of n-6 polyunsaturated fatty acids and animal protein relates to the increased incidence of Crohn disease in Japan. *Am J Clin Nutr.* 1996;63:741-745.
79. Yang SK, Hong WS, Min YI, et al. Incidence and prevalence of ulcerative colitis in the Songpa-Kangdong District, Seoul, Korea, 1986-1997. *J Gastroenterol Hepatol.* 2000;15:1037-1042.
80. Persson PG, Ahlbom A, Hellers G. Crohn's disease and ulcerative colitis: a review of dietary studies with emphasis on methodologic aspects. *Scand J Gastroenterol.* 1987;22:385-389.
81. Mayberry JF, Rhodes J, Newcombe RG. Increased sugar consumption in Crohn's disease. *Digestion.* 1980;20:323-326.

82. Jarnerot G, Jarnmark I, Nilsson K. Consumption of refined sugar by patients with Crohn's disease, ulcerative colitis, or irritable bowel syndrome. *Scand J Gastroenterol.* 1983;18:999-1002.
83. Mayberry JF, Rhodes J, Allan R, et al. Diet in Crohn's disease: two studies of current and previous habits in newly diagnosed patients. *Dig Dis Sci.* 1981;26:444-448.
84. Tragnone A, Valpiani D, Miglio F, et al. Dietary habits as risk factors for inflammatory bowel disease. *Eur J Gastroenterol Hepatol.* 1995;7:47-51.
85. Reif S, Klein I, Lubin F, Farbstein M, Hallak A, Gilat T. Pre-illness dietary factors in inflammatory bowel disease. *Gut.* 1997;40:754-760.
86. Brauer PM, Gee MI, Grace M, Thomson AB. Diet of women with Crohn's and other gastrointestinal diseases. *J Am Diet Assoc.* 1983; 82:659-664.
87. Katschinski B, Logan RF, Edmond M, Langman MJ. Smoking and sugar intake are separate but interactive risk factors in Crohn's disease. *Gut.* 1988;29:1202-1206.
88. Thornton JR, Emmett PM, Heaton KW. Smoking, sugar, and inflammatory bowel disease. *Br Med J (Clin Res Ed).* 1985;290:1786-1787.
89. Riordan AM, Ruxton CH, Hunter JO. A review of associations between Crohn's disease and consumption of sugars. *Eur J Clin Nutr.* 1998;52:229-238.
90. Geerling BJ, Dagnelie PC, Badart-Smook A, Russel MG, Stockbrugger RW, Brummer RJ. Diet as a risk factor for the development of ulcerative colitis. *Am J Gastroenterol.* 2000;95:1008-1013.
91. Jowett SL, Seal CJ, Pearce MS, et al. Influence of dietary factors on the clinical course of ulcerative colitis: a prospective cohort study. *Gut.* 2004;53:1479-1484.
92. Persson PG, Ahlbom A, Hellers G. Diet and inflammatory bowel disease: a case-control study. *Epidemiology.* 1992;3:47-52.
93. Sonnenberg A. Geographic and temporal variations of sugar and margarine consumption in relation to Crohn's disease. *Digestion.* 1988;41:161-171.
94. Millar D, Ford J, Sanderson J, et al. IS900 PCR to detect *Mycobacterium paratuberculosis* in retail supplies of whole pasteurized cows' milk in England and Wales. *Appl Environ Microbiol.* 1996;62:3446-3452.
95. Main J, McKenzie H, Yeaman GR, et al. Antibody to *Saccharomyces cerevisiae* (bakers' yeast) in Crohn's disease. *BMJ.* 1988;297:1105-1106.
96. Barclay GR, McKenzie H, Pennington J, Parratt D, Pennington CR. The effect of dietary yeast on the activity of stable chronic Crohn's disease. *Scand J Gastroenterol.* 1992;27:196-200.
97. Boyko EJ, Perera DR, Koepsell TD, Keane EM, Inui TS. Coffee and alcohol use and the risk of ulcerative colitis. *Am J Gastroenterol.* 1989;84:530-534.
98. Hendriksen C, Binder V. Social prognosis in patients with ulcerative colitis. *BMJ.* 1980;281:581-583.
99. James AH. Breakfast and Crohn's disease. *BMJ.* 1977;1:943-945.
100. Mayberry JF, Rhodes J, Newcombe RG. Breakfast and dietary aspects of Crohn's disease. *BMJ.* 1978;2:1401.
101. Ukil A, Maity S, Karmakar S, Datta N, Vedasiromoni JR, Das PK. Curcumin, the major component of food flavour turmeric, reduces mucosal injury in trinitrobenzene sulphonic acid-induced colitis. *Br J Pharmacol.* 2003;139:209-218.
102. Suchner U, Kuhn KS, Furst P. The scientific basis of immunonutrition. *Proc Nutr Soc.* 2000;59:553-563.
103. Van Den Bogaerde J, Cahill J, Emmanuel AV, et al. Gut mucosal response to food antigens in Crohn's disease. *Aliment Pharmacol Ther.* 2002;16:1903-1915.
104. Lomer MC, Thompson RP, Powell JJ. Fine and ultrafine particles of the diet: influence on the mucosal immune response and association with Crohn's disease. *Proc Nutr Soc.* 2002;61:123-130.
105. Lomer MC, Harvey RS, Evans SM, Thompson RP, Powell JJ. Efficacy and tolerability of a low microparticle diet in a double blind, randomized, pilot study in Crohn's disease. *Eur J Gastroenterol Hepatol.* 2001;13:101-106.
106. Rhodes JM, Cockel R, Allan RN, Hawker PC, Dawson J, Elias E. Colonic Crohn's disease and use of oral contraception. *Br Med J (Clin Res Ed).* 1984;288:595-596.
107. Ramcharan S, Pellegrin FA, Ray RM, Hsu JP. The Walnut Creek Contraceptive Drug Study. A prospective study of the side effects of oral contraceptives. Volume III, an interim report: a comparison of disease occurrence leading to hospitalization or death in users and nonusers of oral contraceptives. *J Reprod Med.* 1980;25(6 Suppl):345-372.
108. Logan RF, Kay CR. Oral contraception, smoking and inflammatory bowel disease—findings in the Royal College of General Practitioners Oral Contraception Study. *Int J Epidemiol.* 1989; 18:105-107.
109. Vessey M, Jewell D, Smith A, Yeates D, McPherson K. Chronic inflammatory bowel disease, cigarette smoking, and use of oral contraceptives: findings in a large cohort study of women of childbearing age. *Br Med J (Clin Res Ed).* 1986;292:1101-1103.
110. Godet PG, May GR, Sutherland LR. Meta-analysis of the role of oral contraceptive agents in inflammatory bowel disease. *Gut.* 1995;37:668-673.
111. Boyko EJ, Theis MK, Vaughan TL, Nicol-Blades B. Increased risk of inflammatory bowel disease associated with oral contraceptive use. *Am J Epidemiol.* 1994;140:268-278.
112. Corrao G, Tragnone A, Caprilli R, et al. Risk of inflammatory bowel disease attributable to smoking, oral contraception and breastfeeding in Italy: a nationwide case-control study. Cooperative Investigators of the Italian Group for the Study of the Colon and the Rectum (GISC). *Int J Epidemiol.* 1998;27:397-404.
113. Lesko SM, Kaufman DW, Rosenberg L, et al. Evidence for an increased risk of Crohn's disease in oral contraceptive users. *Gastroenterology.* 1985;89:1046-1049.
114. Katschinski B, Fingerle D, Scherbaum B, Goebell H. Oral contraceptive use and cigarette smoking in Crohn's disease. *Dig Dis Sci.* 1993;38:1596-1600.
115. Timmer A, Sutherland LR, Martin F. Oral contraceptive use and smoking are risk factors for relapse in Crohn's disease. The Canadian Mesalamine for Remission of Crohn's Disease Study Group. *Gastroenterology.* 1998;114:1143-1150.
116. Cosnes J, Carbonnel F, Carrat F, Beaugerie L, Gendre JP. Oral contraceptive use and the clinical course of Crohn's disease: a prospective cohort study. *Gut.* 1999;45:218-222.
117. Wakefield AJ, Sawyer AM, Hudson M, Dhillon AP, Pounder RE. Smoking, the oral contraceptive pill, and Crohn's disease. *Dig Dis Sci.* 1991;36:1147-1150.
118. Harries AD, Baird A, Rhodes J. Non-smoking: a feature of ulcerative colitis. *BMJ.* 1982;284:706.
119. Sutherland LR, Ramcharan S, Bryant H, Fick G. Effect of cigarette smoking on recurrence of Crohn's disease. *Gastroenterology.* 1990;98:1123-1128.
120. Gareth AO, Thomas BS, Rhodes J, Green JT. Inflammatory bowel disease and smoking—a review. *Am J Gastroenterol.* 1998;93:144-149.
121. Reif S, Lavy A, Keter D, et al. Lack of association between smoking and Crohn's disease but the usual association with ulcerative colitis in Jewish patients in Israel: a multicenter study. *Am J Gastroenterol.* 2000;95:474-478.

122. Penny WJ, Penny E, Mayberry JF, Rhodes J. Mormons, smoking and ulcerative colitis. *Lancet.* 1983;2:1315.
123. Penny WJ, Penny E, Mayberry JF, et al. Prevalence of inflammatory bowel disease amongst mormoms in Britain and Ireland. *Soc Sci Med.* 1985;21:287-290.
124. Calkins BM. A meta-analysis of the role of smoking in inflammatory bowel disease. *Dig Dis Sci.* 1989;34:1841-1854.
125. Motley RJ, Rhodes J, Ford GA, et al. Time relationship between cessation of smoking and onset of ulcerative colitis. *Digestion.* 1987;37:125-127.
126. Doyko EJ, Koepsell TD, Perera DR, et al. Risk of ulcerative colitis among former and current cigarette smokers. *N Engl J Med.* 1987;316:707-710.
127. Lindberg E, Tysk C, Anderson K, et al. Smoking and inflammatory bowel disease: a case-control study. *Gut.* 1988;29:352-357.
128. Loftus EV Jr, Sandborn WJ, Tremaine WJ, et al. Primary sclerosing cholangitis is associated with nonsmoking: a case-control study. *Gastroenterology.* 1996;110:1496-1502.
129. van Erpecum KJ, Smits SJ, van de Meeberg PC, et al. Risk of primary sclerosing cholangitis is associated with nonsmoking behavior. *Gastroenterology.* 1996;110:1503-1506.
130. Mitchell SA, Thyssen M, Orchard TR, Jewell DP, Fleming KA, Chapman RW. Cigarette smoking, appendectomy, and tonsillectomy as risk factors for the development of primary sclerosing cholangitis: a case-control study. *Gut.* 2002;51:567-573.
131. Merrett MN, Mortensen N, Kettlewell M, Jewell DO. Smoking may prevent pouchitis in patients with restorative proctocolectomy for ulcerative colitis. *Gut.* 1996;38:362-364.
132. Russel MG, Nieman FH, Bergers JM, Stockbrugger RW. Cigarette smoking and quality of life in patients with inflammatory bowel disease. South Limburg IBD Study Group. *Eur J Gastroenterol Hepatol.* 1996;8:1075-1081.
133. Boyko EJ, Perera DR, Koepsell TD, et al. Effects of cigarrette smoking on the clinical course of ulcerative colitis. *Scand J Gastroenterol.* 1988;23:1147-1152.
134. Fraga XF, Vergara M, Medina C, Casellas F, Bermejo B, Malagelada JR. Effects of smoking on the presentation and clinical course of inflammatory bowel disease. *Eur J Gastroenterol Hepatol.* 1997; 9:683-687.
135. Beaugerie L, Massot N, Carbonnel F, et al. Impact of cessation of smoking on the course of ulcerative colitis. *Am J Gastroenterol.* 2001;96:2113-2116.
136. Hilsden RJ, Hodgins D, Czechowsky D, Verhoef MJ, Sutherland LR. Attitudes toward smoking and smoking behaviors of patients with Crohn's disease. *Am J Gastroenterol.* 2001;96:1849-1853.
137. Breuer-Katschinski BD, Hollander N, Goebell H. Effect of cigarette smoking on the course of Crohn's disease. *Eur J Gastroenterol Hepatol.* 1996;8:225-228.
138. Lindberg E, Jarnerot G, Huitfeldt B. Smoking in Crohn's disease: effect on localization and clinical course. *Gut.* 1992;33:779-782.
139. Cottone M, Rosselli M, Orlando A, et al. Smoking habits and recurrence in Crohn's disease. *Gastroenterology.* 1994;106:643-648.
140. Cosnes J, Carbonnel F, Beaugerie L, Le Quintrec Y, Gendre JP. Effects of cigarette smoking on the long-term course of Crohn's disease. *Gastroenterology.* 1996;110:424-431.
141. Russel MG, Volovics A, Schoon EJ, et al. Inflammatory bowel disease: is there any relation between smoking status and disease presentation? European Collaborative IBD Study Group. *Inflamm Bowel Dis.* 1998;4:182-186.
142. Cosnes J, Carbonnel F, Carrat F, Beaugerie L, Cattan S, Gendre J. Effects of current and former cigarette smoking on the clinical course of Crohn's disease. *Aliment Pharmacol Ther.* 1999;13:1403-1411.
143. Shields PL, Low-Beer TS. Patients' awareness of adverse relation between Crohn's disease and their smoking: questionnaire survey. *BMJ.* 1996;313:265-266.
144. Cosnes J, Beaugerie L, Carbonnel F, Gendre JP. Decreased severity of Crohn's disease after smoking cessation, preliminary results of a prospective intervention study. *Gastroenterology.* 2000;118(4):A870.
145. Cosnes J, Beaugerie L, Carbonnel F, Gendre JP. Smoking cessation and the course of Crohn's disease: an intervention study. *Gastroenterology.* 2001;120(5):1093-1099.
146. Lashner BA, Shaheen NJ, Hanauer SB, et al. Passive smoking is associated with an increased risk of developing inflammatory bowel disease in children. *Am J Gastroenterol.* 1993;88:356-359.
147. Sandler RS, Sandler DP, McDonnell CW, Wurzelmann JI. Childhood exposure to environmental tobacco smoke and the risk of ulcerative colitis. *Am J Epidemiol.* 1992;135:603-608.
148. Cosnes J. Tobacco and IBD: Relevance in the understanding of disease mechanisms and clinical practice. *Best Pract Res Clin Gastroenterol.* 2004;18:481-496.
149. Motley RJ, Rhodes J, Williams G, et al. Smoking, eicosanoids and ulcerative colitis. *J Pharm Pharmacol.* 1990;42:288-289.
150. Madretsma S, Wolters LM, van Dijk JP, et al. In-vivo effect of nicotine on cytokine production by human non-adherent mononuclear cells. *Eur J Gastroenterol Hepatol.* 1996;8:1017-1020.
151. Euler DE, Dave SJ, Guo H. Effect of cigarette smoking on pentane excretion in alveolar breath. *Clin Chem.* 1996;42:303-308.
152. Hatoum OA, Binion DG, Otterson MF, Gutterman DD. Acquired microvascular dysfunction in inflammatory bowel disease: loss of nitric oxide-mediated vasodilation. *Gastroenterology.* 2003; 125:58-69.
153. Wolfe MM, Lichtenstein DR, Singh G. Gastrointestinal toxicity of nonsteroidal antiinflamatory drugs. *N Engl J Med.* 1999;340: 1888-1899.
154. Katsinelos P, Christodoulou K, Pilpilidis I, et al. Colopathy associated with the systemic use of nonsteroidal antiinflammatory medications: an underestimated entity. *Hepatogastroenterology.* 2002;49:345-348.
155. Oren R, Ligumsky M. Indomethacin-induced colonic ulceration and bleeding. *Ann Pharmacother.* 1994;28:883-885.
156. Gibson GR, Whitacre EB, Ricotti CA. Colitis induced by nonsteroidal anti-inflammatory drugs: report of four cases and review of the literature. *Arch Intern Med.* 1992;152:625-632.
157. O'Brien J. Nonsteroidal anti-inflammatory drugs in patients with inflammatory bowel disease. *Am J Gastroenterol.* 2000;95:1859-1861.
158. Kakar S, Pardi DS, Burgart LJ. Colonic ulcers accompanying collagenous colitis: implication of nonsteroidal anti-inflammatory drugs. *Am J Gastroenterol.* 2003;98:1834-1837.
159. Al-Ghamdi MY, Malatjalian DA, Veldhuyzen van Zanten S. Causation: recurrent collagenous colitis following repeated use of NSAIDs. *Can J Gastroenterol.* 2002;16:861-862.
160. Felder JB, Korelitz BI, Rajapakse R, Schwarz S, Horatagis AP, Gleim G. Effects of nonsteroidal antiinflammatory drugs on inflammatory bowel disease: a case-control study. *Am J Gastroenterol.* 2000;95:1949-1954.
161. Bonner GF, Walczak M, Kitchen L, Bayona M. Tolerance of nonsteroidal antiinflammatory drugs in patients with inflammatory bowel disease. *Am J Gastroenterol.* 2000;95:1946-1948.
162. Wallace JL. Nonsteroidal anti-inflammatory drugs and gastroenteropathy: the second hundred years. *Gastroenterology.* 1997; 112:1000-1016.
163. Hendel J, Nielsen OH. Expression of cyclooxygenase-2 mRNA in active inflammatory bowel disease. *Am J Gastroenterol.* 1997; 92:1170-1173.

164. Bonner GF. Exacerbation of inflammatory bowel disease associated with use of celecoxib. *Am J Gastroenterol.* 2001;96:1306-1308.
165. Goh J, Wight D, Parkes M, Middleton SJ, Hunter JO. Rofecoxib and cytomegalovirus in acute flare-up of ulcerative colitis: coprecipitants or coincidence? *Am J Gastroenterol.* 2002;97:1061-1062.
166. Gornet JM, Hassani Z, Modiglian R, Lemann M. Exacerbation of Crohn's colitis with severe colonic hemorrhage in a patient on rofecoxib. *Am J Gastroenterol.* 2002;97(12):3209-3210.
167. Mahadevan U, Loftus EV Jr, Tremaine WJ, Sandborn WJ. Safety of selective cyclooxygenase-2 inhibitors in inflammatory bowel disease. *Am J Gastroenterol.* 2002;97:910-914.
168. Reinisch W, Miehsler W, Dejaco C, et al. An open-label trial of the selective cyclo-oxygenase-2 inhibitor, rofecoxib, in inflammatory bowel disease-associated peripheral arthritis and arthralgia. *Aliment Pharmacol Ther.* 2003;17:1371-1380.
169. Matuk R, Crawford J, Abreu M, Targan S, Vasiliauskas E, Papadakis K. The spectrum of gastrointestinal toxicity and effect on disease activity of selective COX-2 inhibitors in patients with inflammatory bowel disease. *Inflamm Bowel Dis.* 2004;10:352-356.
170. Sandborn WJ, Stenson WF, Brynskov J, et al. Safety of celecoxib in patients with ulcerative colitis in remission: a randomized, placebo-controlled, pilot study. *Clin Gastroenterol Hepatol.* 2006; 4:203-211.
171. Oviedo J, Farraye FA. Self-care for the inflammatory bowel disease patient: what can the professional recommend? *Semin Gastrointest Dis.* 2001;12:223-236.
172. Smale S, Bjarnason I. Nonsteroidal anti-inflammatory drugs, enterocolonic ulceration and inflammatory bowel disease. In: Bayless-Hanauer, ed. *Advance Therapy of Inflammatory Bowel Disease.* London: B.C Decker; 2001:625-627.
173. Sonnenberg A. Occupational distribution of inflammatory bowel disease among German employees. *Gut.* 1990;31:1037-1040.
174. Persson PG, Leijonmarck CE, Bernell O, Hellers G, Ahlbom A. Risk indicators for inflammatory bowel disease. *Int J Epidemiol.* 1993;22:268-272.
175. Klein I, Reif S, Farbstein H, Halak A, Gilat T. Preillness nondietary factors and habits in inflammatory bowel disease. *Ital J Gastroenterol Hepatol.* 1998;30:247-251.
176. Loudon CP, Corroll V, Butcher J, Rawsthorne P, Bernstein CN. The effects of physical exercise on patients with Crohn's disease. *Am J Gastroenterol.* 1999;94:697-703.
177. Oktedalen O, Lunde OC, Opstad PK, et al. Changes in the gastrointestinal mucosa after long-distance running. *Scand J Gastroenterol.* 1992;27:270-274.
178. Peters HP, Bos M, Seebregts L, et al. Gastrointestinal symptoms in long-distance runners, cyclists and triathletes: prevalence, medication, and etiology. *Am J Gastroenterol.* 1999;94:1570-1581.
179. Peters HP, Zweers M, Backx FJ, et al. Gastrointestinal symptoms during long-distance walking. *Med Sci Sports Exerc.* 1999;31:767-773.
180. Lucas W, Schroy PC. Reversible ischemic colitis in a high endurance athlete. *Am J Gastroenterol.* 1998;93:2231-2234.
181. Oliveria SA, Christos PJ. The epidemiology of physical activity and cancer. *Ann N Y Acad Sci.* 1997;833:79-90.
182. Peters HP, De Vries WR, Vanberge-Henegouwen GP, Akkermans LM. Potential benefits and hazards of physical activity and exercise on the gastrointestinal tract. *Gut.* 2001;48:435-439.
183. Robinson RJ, al-Azzawi F, Iqbal SJ, et al. Osteoporosis and determinants of bone density in patients with Crohn's disease. *Dig Dis Sci.* 1998;43:2500-2506.
184. Robinson RJ, Krzywicki T, Almond L, et al. Effect of a low-impact exercise program on bone mineral density in Crohn's disease: a randomized controlled trial. *Gastroenterology.* 1998;115:36-41.
185. Tysk C, Jarnerot G. Seasonal variation in exacerbations of ulcerative colitis. *Scand J Gastroenterol.* 1993;28:95-96.
186. Kangro HO, Chong SK, Hardiman A, Heath RB, Walker-Smith JA. A prospective study of viral and mycoplasma infections in chronic inflammatory bowel disease. *Gastroenterology.* 1990;98:549-553.
187. Myszor M, Calam J. Seasonality of ulcerative colitis. *Lancet.* 1984;2:522-523.
188. Sellu DP. Seasonal variation in onset of exacerbations of ulcerative proctocolitis. *J R Coll Surg Edinb.* 1986;31:158-160.
189. Don BA, Goldacre MJ. Absence of seasonality in emergency hospital admissions for inflammatory bowel disease. *Lancet.* 1984; 2:1156-1157.
190. Sonnenberg A, Jacobsen SJ, Wasserman IH. Periodicity of hospital admissions for inflammatory bowel disease. *Am J Gastroenterol.* 1994;89:847-851.
191. Dowell SF. Seasonal variation in host susceptibility and cycles of certain infectious diseases. *Emerg Infect Dis.* 2001;7:369-374.
192. Noah ND. Cyclical patterns and predictability in infection. *Epidemiol Infect.* 1989;102:175-190.
193. Lewis JD, Aberra FN, Lichtenstein GR, Bilker WB, Brensinger C, Strom BL. Seasonal variation in flares of inflammatory bowel disease. *Gastroenterology.* 2004;126:665-673.
194. Drossman DA, Leserman J, Mitchell M, et al. Health status and healthcare use in persons with inflammatory bowel disease: a national sample. *Dig Dis Sci.* 1991;36:1746-1755.
195. Porcelli P, Zaka S, Centonze S, Sisto G. Psychological distress and levels of disease activity in inflammatory bowel disease. *Ital J Gastroenterol.* 1994;26:111-115.
196. Porcelli P, Leoci C, Guerra V. A prospective study of the relationship between disease activity and psychologic distress in patients with inflammatory bowel disease. *Scand J Gastroenterol.* 1996;31:792-796.
197. North CS, Alpers DH, Helzer JE, et al. Do life events or depression exacerbate inflammatory bowel disease? A prospective study. *Ann Intern Med.* 1991;114:381-386.
198. Sewitch MJ, Abrahamowicz M, Bitton A, et al. Psychological distress, social support, and disease activity in patients with inflammatory bowel disease. *Am J Gastroenterol.* 2001;96:1470-1479.
199. Hanauer SB, Sandborn WJ; Practice Parameters Committee of the American College of Gastroenterology. Management of Crohn's disease in adults. *Am J Gastroenterol.* 2001;96:635-643.
200. Levenstein S, Prantera C, Varvo V, et al. Stress and exacerbation in ulcerative colitis: a prospective study of patients enrolled in remission. *Am J Gastroenterol.* 2000;95:1213-1220.
201. Li J, Norgard B, Precht DH, Olsen J. Psychological stress and inflammatory bowel disease: a follow-up study in parents who lost a child in Denmark. *Am J Gastroenterol.* 2004;99:1129-1133.
202. Moser G, Drossman DA. Managing patients' concerns. In: Bayless-Hanauer, ed. *Advanced Therapy of Inflammatory Bowel Disease.* London: BC Decker Inc; 2001:527-529.

8

Fertility and Pregnancy in Inflammatory Bowel Disease

Jeffry A. Katz, MD and Vinita Elizabeth Jacob, MD

The incidence of inflammatory bowel disease (IBD) appears to be increasing worldwide, even in areas not previously described as having an increased prevalence of the disease. Given the bimodal age distribution of the onset of symptoms, the issue of inflammatory bowel disease during peak reproductive years is an important one to deal with. In this chapter, we discuss several relevant topics including fertility, the natural impact of pregnancy on the course of IBD, obstetric complications from IBD, and the effect of IBD medications on pregnancy outcomes.

IBD often presents before or during childbearing years, and young women with IBD are likely to become pregnant at some point. Patients with IBD naturally are concerned about the potential effects of their chronic illness on sexuality, fertility, pregnancy, and the fetus. Most evidence suggests that women with IBD can expect a normal pregnancy and delivery, provided their disease is inactive. Although Crohn's disease appears to be associated with an increased risk of premature delivery and low birthweight (LBW), children born to women with IBD are typically healthy. Neither ulcerative colitis nor Crohn's disease causes an increase in congenital abnormalities, and most of the usual medical therapies for IBD appear to be safe and well tolerated during pregnancy. Major concerns of the gastroenterologist and obstetrician should be the optimal timing of the pregnancy, the potential for symptomatic recurrence of IBD during pregnancy and after delivery, and the safety of and need for medical or surgical treatment during pregnancy. A clear understanding of the issues surrounding fertility and pregnancy in IBD help the physician better care for these patients. Although at times challenging, guiding a young person with IBD through conception and pregnancy to the delivery of a healthy child can be a tremendously rewarding experience for the treating physician.

Fertility

Little information exists exploring the factors that influence an IBD patient's decision to have children,[1] but difficulties with intimacy, body image problems, disease activity, surgery, chronic pain, fear of pregnancy, and inaccurate medical advice may all affect this decision. Older studies suggest that patients with IBD have fewer children than expected for the population.[2] Women with IBD whose first pregnancy occurred after disease onset have been reported to have fewer pregnancies than controls, whereas women whose first pregnancies occurred before the disease onset had the same average number of pregnancies as controls.[3] This decrease may, however, represent voluntary childlessness rather than a disease-related decrease in fertility. Newer data show normal female fecundity among 343 women with ulcerative colitis before and after their diagnosis.[4]

Fertility in women with Crohn's disease may be decreased compared to the normal population, though some of this is perceived to be voluntary.[5] A study by Khosla showed a 12% rate of infertility among women with Crohn's disease who were younger than age 45 years, a rate that is similar to that found among women without inflammatory bowel disease.[5] A study by Baird et al showed that measures of childlessness, infertility, and fecundability were mainly a consequence of the patient's choice rather than a disease-mediated process.[3] In an often-quoted study by Hudson et

Lichtenstein GR, ed.
Ulcerative Colitis: The Complete Guide to Medical Management (pp. 93-108)

al, women with both ulcerative colitis and Crohn's disease had normal fertility (~14%), a percentage similar to the general population of northeast Scotland.[6] In regard to ulcerative colitis, the Baird and Hudson studies all showed that women with ulcerative colitis all had normal fertility when compared to the general population as well.

The study by Hudson et al suggested that infertility issues were more frequent in women who had undergone surgery for inflammatory bowel disease when compared to IBD pregnant women who had not, leading many to speculate that significant pelvic inflammation may scar and block fallopian tubes.[6] In addition, the inflammation that is present in patients with Crohn's disease occasionally affects the ovaries and the fallopian tubes, especially on the right side because of proximity to the terminal ileum, explaining some reduced fertility.[7] Additionally, Crohn's disease patients with perianal disease may have secondary dyspareunia and decreased libido contributing to lower fertility rates.[7] Fever, pain, diarrhea, and malnutrition have also been implicated in causing decreased fertility.[5,8] In large part, fertility is reduced in Crohn's disease in proportion to the disease activity, and IBD patients in general are less likely to conceive successfully while their disease is active.[6,9] Normal fertility can be restored when drug therapy achieves disease remission.[8] Patients with inactive Crohn's disease have normal fertility.

Although most data suggest that inactive IBD is associated with normal fecundity, it is becoming increasingly evident that surgical intervention is associated with decreased fertility, particularly in ulcerative colitis when a total proctocolectomy with an ileal pouch anal anastomosis is created.[4,6] A recent historical case-control study of 343 Scandinavian women with ulcerative colitis found an 80% reduction in fecundity after proctocolectomy and ileal pouch-anal anastomosis (IPAA) but not before diagnosis or before surgery. This observation persisted when examined by the length of time after surgery, as well as when analyzed only for women desiring conception. A second recent study of 153 Canadian women reported a 98% reduction in fertility after IPAA.[10] No difference in fertility rates was found before or after the diagnosis of ulcerative colitis. Pelvic adhesions are believed to play a role in decreased fertility after IPAA. Women with ulcerative colitis who wish to conceive should attempt to delay surgery until after having children. When this is not possible, early referral for in vitro fertilization should be considered.[4] Alternatively, the creation of an ileostomy with a Hartmann's pouch or the creation of an ileorectal anastomosis has also been demonstrated to decrease the probability of infertility.

Infertility in male patients with IBD caused by sulfasalazine has been well-documented.[11,12] Within 2 months of starting therapy, the density of the patient's semen decreases, abnormal forms of spermatozoa increase, and sperm motility is reduced.[11,13,14] These events are dose-related and do not respond to supplemental folate.[13] Two to 3 months after withdrawal of the sulfasalazine, semen quality returns to normal.[15] A male patient who is trying to conceive should be switched to another oral mesalamine preparation. The overall reproductive capacity of men with IBD is not markedly diminished,[16] although male patients with Crohn's disease have been noted to have small families.[2,17]

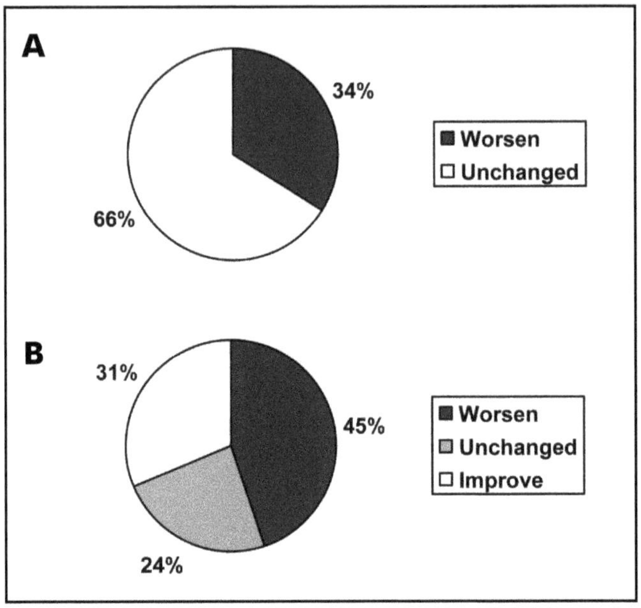

FIGURE 8-1. Effect of pregnancy on the activity of ulcerative colitis. (A) Ulcerative colitis inactive at time of conception. (B) Ulcerative colitis active at time of conception.

PREGNANCY AND DISEASE ACTIVITY

Active IBD makes conception more difficult and a healthy pregnancy less certain. In pregnancy, the course of ulcerative colitis correlates with disease activity at the time of conception (Figure 8-1). A review of more than 500 pregnancies occurring in patients with inactive ulcerative colitis showed that approximately 34% relapsed during gestation, similar to the relapse rate in the nonpregnant ulcerative colitis patients.[18] Most relapses occur during the first trimester,[9,19] which may be partially related to patients stopping maintenance medications. Approximately two-thirds of pregnant ulcerative colitis patients will have quiescent disease throughout the pregnancy.[18,19] Without drug therapy, active ulcerative colitis at conception is at risk of worsening during pregnancy.[20] In women with active ulcerative colitis at the time of conception, the disease activity worsens in 45%, remains unchanged in 24%, and decreases in 27%.[18] Nearly one-third of the time, however, pregnancy will induce an improvement in disease activity or clini-

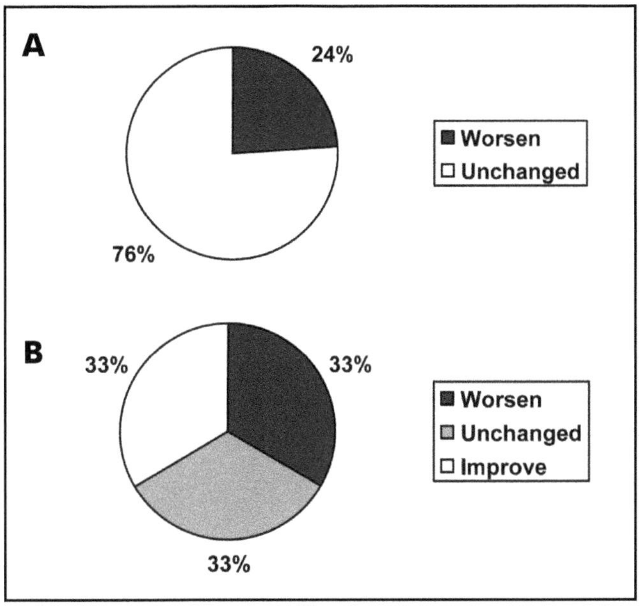

FIGURE 8-2. Effect of pregnancy on the activity of Crohn's disease. (A) Crohn's disease inactive at time of conception. (B) Crohn's disease active at time of conception.

cal remission, usually during the first trimester.[9] In about 5% of patients, the first presentation of ulcerative colitis will coincide with pregnancy. Additionally, some patients will have symptomatic disease only when pregnant, with quiescence between pregnancies and exacerbations during subsequent pregnancies.[9]

The course of Crohn's disease during pregnancy is similar to that of ulcerative colitis (Figure 8-2). Patients with quiescent disease at conception will typically remain in remission. In a study of 186 women with Crohn's disease, 27% of those with inactive disease at conception experienced a relapse.[18] Patients with active Crohn's disease during conception had an approximately 33% chance of worsened activity, continued activity, or decreased activity.[18] Khosla et al reported that 85% (44/52) of women with inactive Crohn's disease at conception remained well during the pregnancy, with almost all relapses occurring during the first trimester.[5] In contrast, active disease at conception is likely to remain active. Women who have active disease at conception remain active one-third of the time and worsen one-third of the time.[5] Additionally, patients with active Crohn's disease during pregnancy are at greater risk for spontaneous abortions[5,21] and preterm delivery.[22] A study by Beaulieau et al reviewed 51 pregnancies in 37 women (81% had Crohn's disease and 19% had ulcerative colitis).[23] The IBD flares mainly occurred in the first trimester (63.6%) and 1 month postpartum (13.7%) and were seen in 12.2% of patients. In the first-trimester and postpartum flares, 43% and 28.6% of patients discontinued their maintenance medications, respectively. No data exist on the optimal duration of remission before conception that will ensure a good outcome for both mother and fetus; however, in general, the longer the remission, the better the outcome.

The clinical course or outcome of previous pregnancies can predict neither the clinical course of IBD nor the outcome of pregnancy. The activity of IBD remains the primary predictor of the course of pregnancy. Interestingly, there has been one report suggesting that patients with distal ileal and colonic Crohn's disease who had been pregnant in the past subsequently need fewer surgical resections.[24] The authors hypothesized that pregnancy could influence the natural history of Crohn's disease by decreasing immune responsiveness or retarding fibrous stricture formation.

PREGNANCY OUTCOME

Retrospective studies have suggested no significant impact of ulcerative colitis on pregnancy outcome, including miscarriage, stillbirth, or fetal demise, when compared to non-IBD controls.[7,25] Rates of healthy offspring of 76% to 97%, spontaneous abortions of 5% to 13%, stillbirths of 1% to 3%, and congenital abnormalities of 1% to 3% do not differ significantly from those expected in the normal population.[7,25] Several large, controlled, population-based studies showed an increased risk of preterm delivery (before 37 weeks gestation) and LBW infants (less than 2500 g) in women with ulcerative colitis,[26-29] although not all population-based studies have confirmed LBW among the offspring of mothers with ulcerative colitis (Table 8-1).[28] The risk of preterm birth appears particularly increased when the first hospitalization for ulcerative colitis occurred during pregnancy.[28] Kornfeld et al evaluated the effect of IBD on birth outcomes in Sweden from 1991 to 1992.[27] The study involved 756 women with IBD and 239,000 controls. The adverse outcomes that carried higher risks for women with IBD were LBW infants, preterm births, and infants who were small for gestational age. The authors also found that the likelihood of delivery by cesarean section was higher for women with IBD than controls. These risks were overall low and not alarming to the newborn offspring of women with IBD. Kornfeld's findings were corroborated by Fonager et al[26] and Nørgård et al[28] in later studies in 1998 and 2000.

Most data support the position that Crohn's disease has a generally greater impact on fetal outcome than ulcerative colitis. Retrospective studies suggest that the rates of prematurity, fetal loss, and congenital anomalies in Crohn's disease approximate the incidence of these findings in the normal population.[25] Among IBD patients who experience stillbirths, spontaneous abortions, or children with birth defects, however, the majority of these women have Crohn's disease.[7] Recent population-based cohort studies have found children born to mothers with Crohn's disease to have LBW and be small for gestational age (see

TABLE 8-1

OUTCOME OF PREGNANCY IN INFLAMMATORY BOWEL DISEASE: SUMMARY OF POPULATION-BASED STUDIES

Reference	Year	Study Population	LBW (Odds Ratio; 95% CI)	SGA (Odds Ratio; 95% CI)	Preterm Birth Odds Ratio; (95% CI)	Comments
Crohn's Disease						
Fonager[26]	1998	Denmark	2.4 (1.6 to 3.7)	NR	1.6 (1.1 to 2.3)	510 Crohn's births
Dominitz[30]	2002	Washington	3.6 (2.2 to 5.9)	2.3 (1.3 to 3.9)	2.3 (1.4 to 3.8)	155 mothers with Crohn's disease
Ludvigsson[29]	2002	Southeast Sweden	ND	NR	ND	13 mothers with Crohn's disease
Ulcerative Colitis						
Nørgård[28]	2000	Denmark	ND	NR	1.4 (1.1 to 1.9)	1531 ulcerative colitis births
Dominitz[30]	2002	Washington	ND	ND	ND	107 ulcerative colitis births
Ludvigsson[29]	2002	Southeast Sweden	Adjusted diff –330 g (–509 to –150 g)	NR	ND	26 ulcerative colitis births
IBD						
Kornfeld[27]	1997	Sweden	2.15 (1.11 to 4.15)	1.4 (0.97 to 2.02)	1.81 (1.06 to 3.07)	756 IBD births

CI indicates confidence interval; ND, no difference; NR, not reported; LBW, low birthweight; SGA, small for gestational age.

Table 8-1).[26,27,30] Patients who have ileal disease or have undergone previous surgery may be particularly at risk for these events.[31]

Understanding the cause of LBW in IBD is important because LBW predisposes to future diseases, like diabetes.[29] The etiology of LBW infants in IBD remains unknown but may be related to the underlying disease itself, disease activity, or medication use. Unfortunately, none of the available analyses directly assesses the suspected critical impact of disease activity and medication history on fetal outcome.

Although several studies have shown no increase in congenital malformations among infants born to women with IBD,[8,9,19,32] a recent large population-based cohort study by Dominitz et al reported a four-fold increased risk of fetal malformations in ulcerative colitis, but not Crohn's disease, as compared to the control population. In all, there were 8 malformations in 107 exposed ulcerative colitis pregnancies, although no malformation occurred more than once and no clear pattern of malformation was evident.[30] The pregnancy outcome of greatest concern was the rate of congenital malformations of 7.9% in the ulcerative colitis group versus 1.7% in the general population. Other listed malformations, such as hip dislocation, are common, mild, and probably clinically unimportant. It is difficult to put these data into perspective for several reasons: the number of congenital malformations was small and it was difficult to identify any patterns, several of the malformations were of minor importance such as pilonidal cysts and congenital subluxation of the hip, and the medical histories of the mothers were not known (eg, nutritional status, disease activity, IBD medications, and possible effects of treatment). A second case-control population study by Nørgård et al has reported no significantly increased overall risk of congenital abnormalities in 22,000 children born to women with ulcerative colitis compared with 38,000 children born to controls.[33] The large size of this study allowed independent analysis of the risk for selected individual congenital abnormalities, and an increased risk of some selected congenital abnormalities was detected, including limb deficiencies, obstructive urinary complications, and multiple simultaneous congenital abnormalities.[33] Although both the studies by Dominitz et al[30] and Nørgård et al[33] seem to show a small increased risk of congenital abnormalities in ulcerative colitis, it remains unclear whether this risk is directly associated with the disease, its treatment, or some other bias. Certainly, the available data suggest that the risk of a woman with ulcerative colitis giving birth to a child with a congenital abnormality appears to be low. Women with ulcerative colitis who wish to have children should be encouraged to do so, ideally conceiving when their disease is quiescent and they are receiving appropriately attentive prenatal care.

A community-based study by Mahadevan et al in 2007 examined pregnancy outcomes in 461 pregnant women with a prebirth diagnosis of IBD (300 UC patients, 154 Crohn's patients, 7 indeterminate colitis) matched to 493 controls.[34] Adverse neonatal outcomes and congenital anomalies were not significantly increased in infants born to women with inflammatory bowel disease. Disease activity was not associated with any adverse outcomes; however, it is important to point out that the majority of both UC and CD patients had inactive or mild disease throughout the pregnancy.

Recently, Nørgård et al found an increased relative risk of 18.5% for preterm births in patients exposed to 6-mercaptopurine (6-MP) and azathioprine during pregnancy.[35] These findings were based on combined national data registries and national prescription databases. Most of the small number of patients on 6-MP and azathioprine were hospitalized, suggesting that disease activity rates rather than 6-MP/azathioprine were likely to be associated with adverse pregnancy outcomes. The effect of disease activity and immunomodulators or biologics on birth outcomes in pregnant IBD patients will best be assessed by a prospective pregnancy registry.

Retrospective analyses of pregnancy outcome in IBD have documented a higher rate of cesarean section for patients with Crohn's disease and ulcerative colitis versus controls (26% versus 13%, $P<0.0001$).[9,30,36] In 2007, Cornish et al published a meta-analysis on the influence of IBD on pregnancy including at least 12 different studies.[37] The results suggest that women with IBD are more likely to experience adverse pregnancy outcomes than the general population. A greater risk of LBW babies and cesarean section birth was significant only in Crohn's disease patients; the rationale behind this increased mode of delivery was not discussed in the studies. IBD has also been associated with an increased risk for labor induction and chorioamnionitis.[22] Population studies have confirmed these findings.[27] The explanation for this finding is uncertain, though it may relate to concerns over the potential risk of perineal trauma causing postpartum complications. In a survey of Crohn's disease patients, the overall rate of developing perineal involvement after vaginal delivery, with or without episiotomy, in patients with no pre-existing perineal involvement was 17.9%.[38] Others, however, have not reproduced these results.[39] Among 54 patients, 27/39 Crohn's disease patients without a history of perianal disease had an episiotomy at delivery. Of these, only one patient developed perianal disease after delivery, and this one patient had a third-degree laceration and an episiotomy. Ten of 15 Crohn's disease patients with inactive perianal disease had an episiotomy at delivery, and none of these patients progressed to develop recurrent perineal disease during a 2-year follow-up period.[39] Thus, women with Crohn's disease and either no perianal disease or inactive perianal disease at term do not require a cesarean section solely because of a concern about the integrity of the perineum. If an episiotomy is needed, a mediolateral episiotomy should be done to avoid trauma to the rectal sphincter.

EVALUATING INFLAMMATORY BOWEL DISEASE ACTIVITY DURING PREGNANCY

An accurate assessment of disease activity in the pregnant patient may be challenging. Many pregnant women will have intermittent abdominal discomfort related to changes in bowel habits or increased gastroesophageal reflux. In addition, abdominal pain in the pregnant IBD patient need not be due to ulcerative colitis or Crohn's disease but rather may be related to pregnancy-related disorders such as cholelithiasis, pancreatitis, toxemia, or a problem with the pregnancy itself. Despite these challenges, these acute processes can usually be distinguished from an IBD flare with a careful history, examination, and appropriate laboratory and diagnostic studies.

During pregnancy, a number of physiologically normal changes occur in routine laboratory parameters that should not be attributed to worsening IBD activity. These include a normal 1 g/dL fall in the hemoglobin due to dilution from an increased blood volume and reduced iron stores, a two- to threefold increase in the erythrocyte sedimentation rate, a 1 g/dL fall in the serum albumin, and a 1.5-fold rise in the serum alkaline phosphatase.

When necessary in the evaluation of the pregnant patient with possible new-onset IBD or the IBD patient with worsening symptoms, flexible sigmoidoscopy can be safely used.[40,41] Although colonoscopy has been reported

TABLE 8-2

SAFETY OF DRUGS IN PREGNANCY

Safe	Probably Safe	Not Safe
Loperamide	Azathioprine	Diphenoxylate
Sulfasalazine	6-Mercaptopurine	Methotrexate
Mesalamine	Ciprofloxacin	Thalidomide
Corticosteroids	Metronidazole	
Total parenteral nutrition	Cyclosporine	
	Infliximab	

to be safe in pregnancy,[42] its use should probably be restricted to those patients where the information gained is critical to patient care. Colonoscopy is safest during the second trimester, and close fetal monitoring is indicated for the procedure.

Both ultrasound and magnetic resonance imaging can be safely used in pregnancy.[43] Clearly, it is best to avoid exposure of the fetus to radiation from abdominal x-rays, especially early in the pregnancy. The absolute risk to the fetus of abdominal radiography is minimal, however, and clinical necessity should guide the decision-making.[44]

MEDICAL THERAPY

Two significant questions frame the issue of medical therapy for IBD in the pregnant patient: First, does the outcome of the pregnancy differ among pregnant IBD patients on drug therapy when compared to those not on treatment? And second, are medications used to treat the pregnant IBD patient safe and effective? Although some studies suggest an increase in the frequency of prematurity, spontaneous abortion, and fetal malformations among mothers with IBD undergoing medical treatment,[7,45] most investigations show that medical therapy, when analyzed as an independent variable, has no effect on pregnancy outcome.[5,9,21,37,46-48] As discussed previously, it is quite evident that disease activity, not medication, most strongly affects pregnancy outcome. In fact, although Baiocco and Korelitz[8] reported that their patients who received drug therapy during pregnancy had an increased complication rate compared to the general population, 50% of patients who had complications also had active disease. In addition, 50% of complications in untreated Crohn's disease patients occurred in the setting of active disease. Thus, there is at present little evidence that drug therapy increases the risk of pregnancy-related complications in the IBD patient.

The decision to stop or continue drug therapy during pregnancy needs to be carefully addressed with each individual couple prior to any decision to conceive. Most pregnant women are concerned about the risks of drugs to the fetus. Decisions surrounding continued medical therapy during pregnancy may be particularly difficult for the woman with IBD, who must balance concerns for the developing fetus against fears of increased disease activity. Counseling should stress the importance of controlling disease activity prior to an attempt at conception. Discussions with patients and their partners need to take into account the specific natural history of the individual patient's disease. Thus, patients with difficult-to-control disease may require continuation of multi-drug therapy during pregnancy and consequently have potentially greater risk, whereas patients with stable quiescent disease may be able to discontinue maintenance therapy before or shortly after conception. An open dialogue between patient and physician facilitates the formulation of a prepregnancy management plan incorporating both the available data and the patient's wishes. Fortunately, much information exists on the safety of medical therapy for IBD during pregnancy, allowing for thorough and thoughtful counseling of the patient (Table 8-2).

5-Aminosalicylates

Sulfasalazine

Both sulfasalazine and sulfapyridine cross the placenta, with fetal serum levels equivalent to maternal levels.[49] Although sulfasalazine and sulfapyridine are excreted in breast milk, the levels are lower than in serum, and sulfasalazine is only occasionally detected in the serum of breast-fed infants whose mothers were taking the drug.[49] Because sulfa drugs can displace bilirubin bound to albumin, there has been concern that circulating fetal sulfasalazine and sulfapyridine could put newborns at risk for jaundice and kernicterus. The fetal levels of these drugs are low, however, and have minimal effect on displacing bilirubin from albumin.[49] Multiple studies have shown that there is no increased incidence of neonatal jaundice or kernicterus in the term infant associated with the use of sulfasalazine by pregnant women.[5,7,19,37,50]

Sulfasalazine has been used safely in many pregnant IBD patients. Although there are occasional case reports of congenital abnormalities associated with its use during pregnancy,[51-53] larger case series have proved sulfasalazine to be safe.[5,9,19,21,38] A recent population-based case-control study showed no increase in congenital abnormalities among Hungarian women taking sulfasalazine while pregnant, although the total number of women exposed was small.[53] Although a survey study of 1400 patients from the United Kingdom did report a statistically significant association between congenital abnormalities and sulfasalazine, the rate of congenital abnormalities was nearly identical to that in the general population.[54]

Sulfasalazine interferes with normal folate metabolism, and folate is critical to normal fetal development. Pregnant women are recommended to take 0.4 mg of supplemental folate daily; pregnant IBD patients on sulfasalazine should receive 2 mg of supplemental folate daily.[40]

MESALAMINE

Mesalamine remains a category B medication for pregnancy. 5-aminosalicylic acid (5-ASA) and its metabolite acetyl-5-aminosalicylic acid (Ac-5-ASA) are found in both maternal and fetal plasma in women taking mesalamine, and the concentrations are comparable to those found in women taking equivalent doses of sulfasalazine.[55] Mesalamine and its metabolites are also present at low levels in the breast milk of lactating women. Although these drugs have only been in clinical use for a little over a decade, information on their safety during pregnancy is gradually increasing.[56-58]

Diav-Citrin and colleagues conducted a prospective controlled cohort study of 165 women exposed to mesalamine during pregnancy; 146 women had first-trimester exposure.[59] Pregnancy outcome was compared to a matched control group counseled for nonteratogenic medication exposure. The mean daily mesalamine dose was 2 g, with 20% of women taking between 2.4 g and 3.2 g, and another 20% taking 3.2 g or more per day. No increase in major malformations or significant difference in the rates of live births, miscarriages, pregnancy termination, delivery method, or fetal distress was detected between the mesalamine-treated women compared to controls.[59] However, a statistically significant increase in preterm deliveries (13% versus 5%), a decrease in mean maternal weight gain (13 kg versus 15 kg), and a decrease in mean birth weight (3253 g versus 3461 g) occurred. Women with IBD who had active disease during pregnancy had babies with significantly lower birthweight compared to women with inactive disease, and women who were treated with polytherapy had babies with significantly lower birthweight and lower gestational ages compared to those women on monotherapy, suggesting a significant effect of disease activity on pregnancy outcome.

A new large epidemiological cohort study provides further evidence supporting the overall safety of 5-ASA during pregnancy.[60] Analyzing registry data over 10 years, the authors were able to identify all prescriptions for 5-ASA provided in either the 3 months prior to conception or throughout the pregnancy (n = 148) and a control group of women not prescribed medications during pregnancy (n = 19,418), including untreated pregnant women with IBD. No significant increase of congenital malformations or LBW infants was found. Although an increased risk of stillbirth and preterm birth was noted, this increased risk was restricted to women with UC. This risk remained elevated even when pregnant women with IBD using no medication were included as the control group. Interestingly, the odds ratio of stillbirth was highest in women using both 5-ASA and steroids, and the risk of preterm birth was highest in women treated with 5-ASA alone. Unfortunately, the authors were unable to adequately assess the precise relationship of disease activity, 5-ASA use, and birth outcome. Taken together, the smaller case series[56-58] and the larger studies[59,60] suggest that mesalamine is safe during pregnancy.

ANTIBIOTICS

For the treatment of IBD, metronidazole and ciprofloxacin are the most widely used antibiotics. Animal studies have not shown evidence of teratogenicity or increased fetal loss with metronidazole.[61] Although there have been reports of fetal malformation, particularly cleft lip, with use of metronidazole early in pregnancy,[62,63] 2 meta-analyses have found no relationship between metronidazole exposure during pregnancy and birth defects.[64,65]

In animal studies, no teratogenicity has been observed with ciprofloxacin, although arthropathy has been identified in immature animals.[66] This has led to restricted use of ciprofloxacin during pregnancy. A report of 35 women who received short-term ciprofloxacin during the first trimester for treatment of infections showed no association with fetal malformations or musculoskeletal problems, however.[67] A larger prospective controlled trial confirmed these preliminary results.[68] However, a higher rate of therapeutic abortions was observed in the quinolone-exposed women when compared to their controls (women treated with nonembryotoxic antimicrobials for similar indications).[68] The explanation for this observation remains uncertain.

Review of the non-IBD literature suggests that it is safe to use short courses of both metronidazole and ciprofloxacin during pregnancy. These agents are more commonly used for longer duration in IBD, however, and there currently exist no direct safety data on prolonged therapeutic use of these agents during pregnancy.

CORTICOSTEROIDS

Corticosteroids have been used to treat a variety of illnesses during pregnancy. Case series examining corticosteroid therapy in asthma,[69] systemic lupus

TABLE 8-3

FOOD AND DRUG ADMINISTRATION CLASSIFICATION OF DRUGS IN PREGNANCY

CATEGORY A

Controlled studies in women fail to demonstrate a risk to the fetus and the possibility of fetal harm appears remote.

CATEGORY B

Either animal reproduction studies have not demonstrated fetal risk but there are no controlled studies in pregnant women or animal reproduction studies have shown an adverse effect that was not confirmed in controlled studies in women.

CATEGORY C

Either studies in animals have revealed adverse effects on the fetus and there are no controlled studies in women or studies in women and animals are not available. Drugs should be given only if the potential benefits justify the potential risk to the fetus.

CATEGORY D

There is positive evidence of human fetal risk, but the benefits from use in pregnant women may be acceptable despite the risk.

CATEGORY X

Studies in animals or human beings have demonstrated fetal abnormalities. The risk of use of the drug in pregnant women clearly outweighs any possible benefit. The drug is contraindicated in women who are or may become pregnant.

erythematosus,[70] and rheumatoid arthritis[71] have not revealed an increased risk of fetal malformation. Older animal studies in pregnant mice have shown an increase in cleft palate,[72] however, and similar concerns have been raised for the human fetus.[73,74] A recent case-control study reviewing data on 1184 live births with nonsyndromic oral clefts showed a relationship between first trimester exposure to corticosteroids and an increase in cleft lip among newborns (odds ratio [OR] = 6.55; confidence interval [CI] +1.44 to 29.76; P=0.015).[73] Corticosteroids cross the placenta and are transferred into breast milk, but the ratio of maternal to fetal serum concentration depends upon the choice of corticosteroid used. Prednisolone is more efficiently metabolized compared to dexamethasone, and fetal levels are only approximately 10% of maternal levels.[75] Although there is a concern regarding possible adrenal suppression among the neonates of mothers taking corticosteroids, in practice, this has rarely occurred.[74] If steroids must be used during pregnancy, it makes sense to use one more extensively metabolized by the placenta, such as prednisone or prednisolone.

Among patients with IBD, corticosteroid therapy has not been found to be harmful to the fetus.[19,50] In a study of 531 pregnant women, 168 received corticosteroids for an extended period of time, mostly during the second and third trimesters.[50] No increased incidence of prematurity, spontaneous abortion, stillbirth, or developmental defects was noted. When necessary, corticosteroids can be safely used to control active disease during pregnancy. They are considered category C in pregnancy, given an association with cleft lip and cleft palate; however, the impact of the deformity they are associated with is usually more a cosmetic issue.

IMMUNOMODULATORS

AZATHIOPRINE/6-MERCAPTOPURINE

Azathioprine/6-mercaptopurine (AZA/6-MP) has been shown to be teratogenic in mice and rabbits but not in rats.[76] Given these known teratogenic effects, AZA/6-MP have been labeled as class D medication during pregnancy. This rating means that there is positive evidence of human fetal risk but that the benefits from use in pregnant women may be acceptable despite the risk (Table 8-3). These differences among species suggest that variable metabolism may play a role in potential drug toxicity and make extrapolation of animal data to pregnant humans difficult. In addition, allelic variance for AZA/6-MP metabolism may make some people more susceptible than others to adverse drug effects.[77] AZA crosses the placenta, but the fetal liver lacks the enzyme inosinate pyrophosphorylase, which converts AZA to its active metabolite, and, as expected, only trace amounts of its metabolites are detected in fetal serum.[78]

Both AZA/6-MP are excreted in low amounts in breast milk and rarely have immunosuppressant effects on the fetus.

The majority of the available published literature for IBD suggests that AZA/6-MP is safe and well-tolerated during pregnancy. A retrospective analysis of 16 pregnancies among 14 women with IBD being treated with AZA found no increase in spontaneous abortion, fetal abnormalities, prematurity, or LBW.[76] Seven women continued AZA throughout the pregnancy, 5 stopped before week 16, and 2 had elective termination of pregnancy. One mother did contract hepatitis B infection during pregnancy. All pregnancies went to term, except for the voluntary termination and an elective cesarean section at 32 weeks gestation. No congenital anomalies or subsequent health problems occurred among 15 children. All neonates weighed 2.5 kg or greater. The authors recommended continuing AZA therapy throughout pregnancy if the drug is considered to play an important part in the control of the disease.

In contrast, small retrospective studies of the use of 6-MP during pregnancy have found an increased incidence of fetal demise[79] and an increase in fetal complications when fathers used 6-MP within 3 months of conception.[80] These studies were not carefully controlled, however, bringing into question their generalizability. The recent publication of a large retrospective analysis of the use of 6-MP during pregnancy provides much-needed additional safety information. Francella et al[81] evaluated drug treatment and pregnancy outcome among 155 IBD patients exposed to 6-MP. Compared to IBD patients not exposed to 6-MP, patients treated with 6-MP—prior to conception (40 women/44 men), at the time of conception (24 women/37 men), or throughout pregnancy (15 women)—showed no increased incidence of spontaneous abortion, major congenital abnormalities, neoplasia, or fetal infections.[81] It is important to keep in mind that most of these patients had quiescent disease. These results were further confirmed by a 2007 study by Mahadevan et al showing that "disease activity and medical treatment did not predict adverse outcomes in a large, nonreferral population."[34]

Data obtained from analysis of a Danish population database in 2003 contradict these findings, with Nørgård et al reporting increased risk of congenital malformations (OR 6.7, 95% CI 1.4 to 32.4), perinatal mortality (OR 20, 95% CI 2.5 to 161.4), and preterm birth (OR 3.8, 95% CI 0.4 to 33.3) in women exposed to AZA or 6-MP. Although the control group for this study included more than 19,000 pregnancies, only 11 women had exposure to AZA/6-MP, of whom only 6 had IBD.[82] The authors were unable to separate the effects of disease activity from drug effects and could not determine whether the observed associations are causal or occur through confounding. As already discussed, 2007 data from the Nørgård group showed an increased relative risk of 18.5% for preterm birth and 9.7% for congenital anomalies in patients exposed to these drugs during pregnancy.[35] This study impressively combined national data registries with a national prescription database. It is difficult to interpret these results, however, as disease activity was not measured by a review of the outpatient charts but determined by hospitalizations.

In 2008, Jharap et al looked at the effect of thiopurine metabolites during pregnancy in mother and child.[83] This study was a prospective study of 10 IBD patients who were on azathioprine for at least 8 weeks before getting pregnant. 6-methylmercaptopurine (6-MMP) and 6-thioguanine (6-TG) levels were drawn from the mothers before, during, and after pregnancy. These measurements were drawn in the infants from the umbilical cord directly after birth to test for intrauterine exposure. The metabolite levels varied highly during pregnancy in the mothers: 8/10 had decreased 6-TG levels, 3/8 had increased 6-MMP levels compared to prepregnancy baseline (1 with elevated aspartate aminotransferase/alanine aminotransferase that normalized after delivery), and 1/10 with increased 6-TG level and mild leukopenia that normalized after delivery. In the infants, the median 6-TG levels were significantly lower compared to the mothers at time of delivery. No 6-MMP was detected in the infants. There were no premature babies or congenital anomalies. The placenta appears to form a relative barrier to AZA. Where, then, are we with regard to AZA/6-MP use during pregnancy? The effects of disease activity and medication use on birth outcomes in pregnant inflammatory bowel disease patients will be best assessed by a prospective pregnancy registry. For now, given the years of experience in IBD, transplantation, and other autoimmune diseases (eg, rheumatoid arthritis), there has been no direct and clear association with immunomodulator therapy and congenital malformations. What needs to be assessed by the clinician is the risk of the medications versus the risk of uncontrolled symptomatic disease. The days of recommending voluntary termination following any fetal exposure to AZA/6-MP have passed. Because a flare of ulcerative colitis or Crohn's disease can result in significant fetal risk, patients taking AZA/6-MP should not unilaterally discontinue these medications when trying to conceive. All IBD couples considering conception should be carefully counseled regarding the limits of our knowledge regarding the safety of immunomodulator therapy during pregnancy but also reassured that most data support their safe use. Remembering that active disease represents the greatest difficulty to conception and pregnancy for the IBD patient, if AZA/6-MP is critical to maintain the health of the mother, then therapy with these drugs should be continued. For a couple who feels strongly that they do not wish to conceive while continuing AZA/6-MP, the drug should be stopped for at least 3 months before proceeding with attempts at conception. It must be emphasized to this group that should the disease flare during pregnancy, corticosteroid therapy would likely be recommended.

METHOTREXATE

Methotrexate (MTX) is increasingly used for the therapy of resistant Crohn's disease.[84] In a variety of animals, including chicks, rats, and mice, embryonic exposure to MTX has been associated with fetal loss and congenital anomalies, including neural tube and craniofacial defects.[78] In humans, high-dose MTX is an abortifacient.[85] Spontaneous abortions as high as 40% have been reported after MTX exposure, as have frequent neural tube defects, such as spina bifida.[86] Among 10 patients exposed to methotrexate during the first trimester, 30% resulted in malformed fetuses.[87] It is not surprising, therefore, that MTX is contraindicated before conception and during pregnancy. With increasing use among IBD patients, however, inadvertent pregnancies are bound to occur. What advice should be given to a couple in this situation? Clearly, the risks of fetal loss and congenital malformation are high. Although some congenital abnormalities, such as spina bifida, can be screened for with blood tests and ultrasound, others are undetectable. Weighing against this increased risk is the fact that not all infants will be adversely affected by MTX exposure. Although 5 of 10 pregnancies in women receiving low-dose MTX for rheumatoid arthritis resulted in abortion (2 elective, 3 spontaneous), the other 5 women delivered healthy, full-term infants.[88] In this difficult situation, it is probably best to carefully discuss the issue of pregnancy termination with each couple individually. It is certainly preferable, however, to avoid this situation through careful counseling and effective contraception prior to initiation of MTX therapy.

CYCLOSPORINE

Cyclosporine (CyA) is useful for the treatment of refractory ulcerative colitis unresponsive to high-dose intravenous corticosteroid therapy.[89,90] In this role, its safety is of particular interest given the occasional presentation of fulminant ulcerative colitis during pregnancy, where delaying surgery for even just a few weeks may profoundly affect fetal viability. At 10 mg/kg/day, CyA showed no fetal toxicity in rats; however, at higher doses, renal tubular damage was noted, as is seen in adult humans.[78] It is likely that this effect relates directly to the general nephrotoxicity of CyA, rather than any specific effects on the fetus. CyA crosses the placenta, but the concentration of the drug in the newborn falls rapidly within days.[78]

The National Transplant Registry was established to study outcomes in all solid organ transplant recipients. The majority of the experience has been derived from female renal transplant recipients. Outcomes have shown no specific congenital abnormalities or birth defects associated with CyA use. There is a fairly high incidence of prematurity (56%) and LBW (49.5%), however.

In IBD, the literature is sparse and relegated to several case reports and one small recently published study in *American Journal of Gastroenterology* looking at 18 women with IBD of whom 5 patients required IV cyclosporine after high-dose IV steroids failed to achieve symptom control.[91] This study and the other case reports have shown no increase in the risk of congenital anomalies. These patients received CyA in the second or third trimesters.

In 2008, the first established case report describing the use of CyA in the first trimester was reported.[92] The case involved a young female with ulcerative colitis who failed high-dose steroids and was given CyA at the end of her first trimester. The patient delivered a healthy baby who weighed 6 lbs 4 oz with normal Apgar scores. The baby was delivered at 37 weeks gestation via cesarean. In another case report, a pregnant patient was treated for steroid-resistant severe colitis in the 29th week. The disease flare was controlled with the addition of CyA, and a healthy baby was delivered at 36 weeks.[93] Marion and colleagues reported on 5 patients (4 ulcerative colitis and 1 Crohn's disease) with severe colitis treated initially with intravenous and then oral CyA.[94] Four of the 5 patients had live births; one patient whose colitis had responded to CyA had a spontaneous abortion at 8 weeks. No congenital abnormalities were observed and no renal toxicity was noted in the neonates. Two of 4 infants were premature (<37 weeks) and weighed less than 2500 g. Two mothers needed a colectomy after delivery. These results were deemed favorable when compared to the results of surgery in the pregnant patient with severe colitis. In pregnancy, properly used and monitored CyA is probably as safe as AZA/6-MP. Use of CyA should be considered in cases of severe colitis as a means of avoiding urgent surgery and reaching a gestational age when the fetus can be safely delivered.

INFLIXIMAB

Infliximab (IFX) has dramatically improved the lives of many patients with Crohn's disease.[95] Given the peak incidence of IBD, it is not surprising that some women with Crohn's disease will inadvertently be exposed to infliximab either before conception or during pregnancy. Infliximab is currently FDA category B for pregnancy, which is surprising as it is a biologic; however, the limited studies thus far have shown relative safety in neonatal outcomes. The chimeric portion of the infliximab molecule contains human immunoglobulin (Ig) G1 constant region, which limits placental transfer during the first trimester. Maternal IgG concentrations in fetal blood increase from early in the second trimester through term, however, with most antibodies being acquired during the third trimester via placental transfer. This anti-tumor necrosis factor alpha (TNFα) agent is the medication in this class with the most safety literature thus far for pregnant IBD patients.

A single case report exists describing multiple congenital abnormalities and fetal death in a fetus exposed to infliximab; however, this mother had active luminal and fistulizing Crohn's disease and was also taking metronidazole, AZA, and 5-ASA.[96] Other case reports document the successful treatment of active Crohn's disease during pregnancy with infliximab.[97,98] A recent large study of postmarketing safety data by Katz et al suggested that inadvertent infliximab exposure either before conception or during pregnancy is safe and does not require termination of the pregnancy.[99] Among 82 pregnant Crohn's disease patients directly exposed to infliximab, live births occurred in 67%, miscarriages in 13%, and therapeutic termination in 20%, results not different from those expected for the general pregnant United States population or a population of pregnant women with CD not exposed to infliximab.[99] These findings were corroborated by data from the TREAT registry, a prospective registry of patients with Crohn's disease. The registry showed no fetal malformations, and the rates of miscarriage and neonatal complications were not statistically significant between IFX-treated and IFX-naïve patients.[99] In addition, a small number of pregnant patients with active Crohn's disease have been intentionally treated with infliximab with good outcome.[100] Interestingly, increased tumor necrosis factor has been associated with infertility, and TNFα blockade is being investigated as a potential therapy this condition.[101,102]

In 2005, Mahadevan et al performed a retrospective report on 10 women who had intentional infliximab use during pregnancy for induction or maintenance of remission in Crohn's disease.[103] All pregnancies resulted in healthy live births. Eight women had prior infliximab use and were maintained throughout pregnancy (mean of 5 weeks from last infliximab to start of pregnancy, mean dose 5 mg/kg, mean interval between doses 6.4 weeks). Two patients began infliximab in the first and third trimester, respectively.

Thus far, infliximab appears relatively safe to use during pregnancy with no obvious neonatal adverse events or congenital anomalies. What we do not yet know is the effect of infliximab on in utero and perinatal immune development of the infant.

A prospective study by Mahadevan et al in 2008 investigated 8 infants born to women with IBD (7 with CD and 1 with UC).[104] Seven of the patients were on maintenance infliximab, and 1 was on induction therapy. All women received infliximab in the third trimester. All infants received standard 6-month cycle of vaccines; their blood was collected up to 6 months postdelivery. Quantitative immunoglobulins A, G, and M; tetanus antibody titers; *Haemophilus influenzae* titers; and infliximab levels were drawn. The infants exposed to infliximab in utero generally mounted an appropriate response to routine childhood vaccinations. No child showed any immune deficits. Although 4 infants had decreased levels of IgM, the significance of this finding remains of unclear significance.

Two other anti-TNFα compounds are now approved for use in patients with Crohn's disease: adalimumab and etanercept. These formulations are administered subcutaneously and are in class B for pregnancy. At best in the literature, there have been case reports on adalimumab use during pregnancy in IBD patients.[105,106] In all cases, no increased incidence of congenital anomalies has been found.[105,106] A recently published abstract looking at pregnancy outcomes in women with autoimmune disease (mainly rheumatoid arthritis) exposed to adalimumab (OTIS project) found that pregnancy outcomes in the adalimumab-exposed group are comparable to disease-matched women with rheumatoid arthritis not treated with adalimumab (ADA) during pregnancy and women without rheumatoid arthritis with no exposure to ADA. Based on preliminary data from this ongoing study, there is no increased rate of congenital defects.[107]

Symptomatic Therapy

There exist little evidence-based data on the use of antidiarrheal and antispasmodic agents during pregnancy. Bulking agents are safe during pregnancy, as kaolin is a category B medication. Codeine has been used for many years during pregnancy without report of associated fetal abnormalities but is a category C medication. Drug dependence and withdrawal in the newborn can occur but are rare.[40] A recent cohort controlled study in 108 women taking loperamide during the first trimester found no association with fetal malformation, abortion, premature delivery, or birth weight.[108] In contrast, diphenoxylate with atropine, a category C medication in pregnancy, is teratogenic in animals, and fetal malformations have been observed in infants exposed to diphenoxylate during the first trimester.[108] Both loperamide and diphenoxylate are excreted in breast milk. Bismuth subsalicylate should also not be used during pregnancy because salicylate absorption can occur. Salicylates, in general, have been associated with prolonged labor, decreased birthweight, and increased perinatal mortality.[109] Anticholinergics and antispasmodics have been associated with non-life-threatening fetal malformations and are best avoided during pregnancy.[110]

SURGICAL THERAPY

Elective nonobstetric surgery in the pregnant patient without IBD performed in the second trimester does not increase perinatal mortality.[111] In the pregnant IBD patient, however, elective surgical intervention is uncommon. When the need for surgery is obvious, as in the patient with fulminant colitis, toxic megacolon, or perforation, decision-making is relatively easy. The more typical and difficult scenario is a patient with a flare of ulcerative colitis or Crohn's disease incompletely responsive to medical therapy. In this situation, the natural tendency is too push on with medical therapy in the hope that the patient may eventually respond. Unfortunately, this approach may only further increase the risk to both mother and fetus,[112] and little information exists to help guide the physician and patient in making the difficult decision to proceed to surgery. In the ill and pregnant IBD patient not responding to medical therapy, the greater risk to the fetus is continued maternal illness rather than surgical intervention.[113] Doing what is best for the mother generally ends up being what is best for the fetus.

Numerous case reports can be found documenting successful surgical intervention for treatment of severe colitis in the pregnant patient[113-116]; however, it is difficult to find even small case series.[117] Anderson and colleagues reported the outcomes in 4 pregnant women whose IBD flared between the 28th and 37th weeks of gestation. Three patients were treated medically and allowed to progress to labor. Two babies were stillborn and one child was normal. All 3 mothers required colectomy in the weeks after delivery. The fourth patient relapsed at 28 weeks gestation, had surgery for toxic megacolon at 31 weeks, and delivered at 34 weeks.[117] In patients with Crohn's disease, Hill and coworkers described 3 pregnant patients with intraperitoneal sepsis requiring surgery. All women recovered and delivered healthy infants.[118] As in these small case series, most isolated case reports also suggest proceeding to surgery when indicated.[112,114,115,117]

What operation to perform in the pregnant IBD patient depends on the disease and the specific indication for surgery. A variety of procedures have been performed, including panproctocolectomy, subtotal colectomy with ileostomy, hemicolectomy or segmental colectomy with primary anastomosis or ileostomy, and combined subtotal colectomy and cesarean section.[113] Two general points bear noting: First, primary anastomosis carries a greater risk of postoperative complications, and a temporary ileostomy is generally preferred. Second, if the fetus is sufficiently mature, cesarean section along with bowel resection is indicated.

Total proctocolectomy followed by IPAA is the preferred surgical procedure for ulcerative colitis. Ulcerative colitis patients who have had an IPAA and subsequently become pregnant typically do well, with little pouch dysfunction, either during the pregnancy or after delivery.[119,120] There is debate about whether women who have had IPAA should be allowed to deliver vaginally or whether cesarean section should be planned. In a study of 43 pregnancies in women who have had an IPAA, pregnancy was well-tolerated, with a complication rate lower than in women who had an ileostomy.[121] Although more cesarean sections were performed in women with IPAA, the authors felt that this was likely due to uncertainty about pouch function in this setting. An extended follow-up of women with an IPAA who delivered vaginally showed no adverse long-term effect on pouch function.[121] During pregnancy, however, women with IPAA may note increases in stool frequency, incontinence, and pad usage; these symptoms improved to baseline after delivery. Similarly, directly comparing pregnancy and delivery before and after IPAA in the same women (n = 37) has shown no differences in birth weight, duration of labor, pregnancy or delivery complications, vaginal delivery rates, or unplanned cesarean section.[122] Successful pregnancy and vaginal delivery do occur commonly after IPAA, despite the decrease in overall fertility. The mode of delivery in patients with an IPAA should be dictated by obstetric considerations.[121,122]

CONCLUSION

The past few years have seen significant additions to our knowledge of IBD and its relation to conception and pregnancy. Women with Crohn's disease appear to be at risk for early delivery and LBW infants, a significant finding given the association between LBW and the subsequent development of other illnesses later in life. Women with ulcerative colitis may be at increased risk for delivering children with congenital abnormalities, although this could be due to an unmeasured bias, such as disease activity or drug treatment. Despite lingering concerns, the preponderance of data supports the overall safety of the 5-ASA drugs, corticosteroids, and AZA/6-MP during pregnancy, and preliminary data suggest that inadvertent infliximab exposure may also be safe. Active disease, not drug treatment, remains the greatest risk to the pregnant mother and fetus. Despite recent advances, much of the available data remain tainted by small numbers and the inability to carefully assess the impact of disease activity on pregnancy course and fetal outcome. Until prospective, unbiased information arrives, the best advice is to recognize the limitations of our knowledge and carefully counsel each individual couple about the potential risks of IBD and its therapies during pregnancy. Although these risks are low, both potential parents and physicians are best served when such discussion takes place in advance of attempts at conception. To paraphrase an earlier author in this field,[123] the secret of the care of the pregnant IBD patient lies in caring for the patient before she becomes pregnant.

REFERENCES

1. Trachter AB, Rogers AI, Leiblum SR. Inflammatory bowel disease in women: impact on relationship and sexual health. *Inflamm Bowel Dis.* 2002;8:413-421.
2. Mayberry JF, Weterman IT. European survey of fertility and pregnancy in women with Crohn's disease: a case control study by European collaborative group. *Gut.* 1986;27:821-825.

3. Baird DD, Narendranathan M, Sandler RS. Increased risk of preterm birth for women with inflammatory bowel disease. *Gastroenterology.* 1990;99:987-994.
4. Ording KO, Juul S, Berndtsson I, Oresland T, Laurberg S. Ulcerative colitis: female fecundity before diagnosis, during disease, and after surgery compared with a population sample. *Gastroenterology.* 2002;122:15-19.
5. Khosla R, Willoughby CP, Jewell DP. Crohn's disease and pregnancy. *Gut.* 1984;25:52-56.
6. Hudson M, Flett G, Sinclair TS, Brunt PW, Templeton A, Mowat NA. Fertility and pregnancy in inflammatory bowel disease. *Int J Gynaecol Obstet.* 1997;58:229-237.
7. Fielding JF, Cooke WT. Pregnancy and Crohn's disease. *Br Med J.* 1970;2:76-77.
8. Baiocco PJ, Korelitz BI. The influence of inflammatory bowel disease and its treatment on pregnancy and fetal outcome. *J Clin Gastroenterol.* 1984;6:211-216.
9. Nielsen OH, Andreasson B, Bondesen S, Jarnum S. Pregnancy in ulcerative colitis. *Scand J Gastroenterol.* 1983;18:735-742.
10. Johnson P, Richard C, Ravid A, et al. Female infertility after ileal pouch-anal anastomosis for ulcerative colitis. *Dis Colon Rectum.* 2004;47:1119-1126.
11. Levi AJ, Fisher AM, Hughes L, Hendry WF. Male infertility due to sulphasalazine. *Lancet.* 1979;2:276-278.
12. Birnie GG, McLeod TI, Watkinson G. Incidence of sulphasalazine-induced male infertility. *Gut.* 1981;22:452-455.
13. O'Morain C, Smethurst P, Dore CJ, Levi AJ. Reversible male infertility due to sulphasalazine: studies in man and rat. *Gut.* 1984; 25:1078-1084.
14. Toth A. Reversible effect of salicylazosulfapyridine on semen quality. *Fertil Steril.* 1979;1:538-540.
15. Toovey S, Hudson E, Hendry WF, Levi AJ. Sulphasalazine and male infertility: reversibility and possible mechanism. *Gut.* 1981;22:445-451.
16. Narendranathan M, Sandler RS, Suchindran CM, Savitz DA. Male infertility in inflammatory bowel disease. *J Clin Gastroenterol.* 1989;11:403-406.
17. Burnell D, Mayberry J, Calcraft BJ, Morris JS, Rhodes J. Male fertility in Crohn's disease. *Postgrad Med J.* 1986;62:269-272.
18. Miller JP. Inflammatory bowel disease in pregnancy: a review. *J R Soc Med.* 1986;79:221-225.
19. Willoughby CP, Truelove SC. Ulcerative colitis and pregnancy. *Gut.* 1980;21:469-474.
20. Mogadam M, Korelitz BI, Ahmed SW, Dobbins WOD, Baiocco PJ. The course of inflammatory bowel disease during pregnancy and postpartum. *Am J Gastroenterol.* 1981;75:265-269.
21. Wolfson K, Cohen Z, McLeod RS. Crohn's disease and pregnancy. *Dis Colon Rectum.* 1990;33:869-873.
22. Bush M, Patel S, Lapinski R, Stone J. Perinatal outcomes in inflammatory bowel disease. *J Matern Fetal Med.* 2004;15:237-241.
23. Beaulieau DB, Otterson MF, Newcomer J, et al. Pregnancy complications and outcomes in the era of immunomodulator and biologic therapy: a tertiary referral center experience. *Gastroenterology.* 2005;128:A316.
24. Nwokolo CU, Tan WC, Andrews HA, Allan RN. Surgical resection in parous patients with distal ileal and colonic Crohn's disease. *Gut.* 1994;35:220-223.
25. Hanan IM, Kirsner JB. Inflammatory bowel disease in the pregnant woman. *Clin Perinatol.* 1985;12:669-682.
26. Fonager K, Sorensen HT, Olsen J, Dahlerup JF, Rasmussen SN. Pregnancy outcome for women with Crohn's disease: a follow-up study based on linkage between national registries. *Am J Gastroenterol.* 1998;93:2426-2430.
27. Kornfeld D, Cnattingius S, Ekbom A. Pregnancy outcomes in women with inflammatory bowel disease—a population-based cohort study. *Am J Obstet Gynecol.* 1997;177:942-946.
28. Nørgård B, Fonager K, Sorensen HT, Olsen J. Birth outcomes of women with ulcerative colitis: a nationwide Danish cohort study. *Am J Gastroenterol.* 2000;95:3165-3170.
29. Ludvigsson JF, Ludvigsson J. Inflammatory bowel disease in mother or father and neonatal outcome. *Acta Pediatr.* 2002;9:145-151.
30. Dominitz JA, Young JCC, Boyko EJ. Outcomes of infants born to mothers with inflammatory bowel disease: a population-based cohort study. *Am J Gastroenterol.* 2002;97:641-648.
31. Moser MA, Okun NB, Mayes DC, Bailey RJ. Crohn's disease, pregnancy, and birth weight. *Am J Gastroenterol.* 2000;95:1021-1026.
32. Nielsen OH, Andreasson B, Bondesen S, Jacobsen O, Jarnum S. Pregnancy in Crohn's disease. *Scand J Gastroenterol.* 1984;19:724-732.
33. Nørgård B, Puho E, Pedersen L, Czeizel AE, Sorensen HT. Risk of congenital abnormalities in children born to women with ulcerative colitis: a population-based, case-control study. *Am J Gastroenterology.* 2003;98:2006-2010.
34. Mahadevan U, Sandborn WJ, Li DK, Hakimian S, Kane S, Corley DA. Pregnancy outcomes in women with inflammatory bowel disease: a large community-based study from Northern California. *Gastroenterology.* 2007;133(4):1106-1112.
35. Nørgård B, Hundborg HH, Jacobsen BA, Nielsen GL, Fonager K. Disease activity in pregnant women with Crohn's disease and birth outcomes: a regional Danish cohort study. *Am J Gastroenterol.* 2007;102:1947-1954.
36. Porter RJ, Stirrat GM. The effects of inflammatory bowel disease on pregnancy: A case-controlled retrospective analysis. *Br J Obstet Gynecol.* 1986;93:1124-1131.
37. Cornish J, Tan E, Teare J, et al. A meta-analysis on the influence of inflammatory bowel disease on pregnancy. *Gut.* 2007;56:830-837.
38. Brandt LJ, Estabrook SG, Reinus JF. Results of a survey to evaluate whether vaginal delivery and episiotomy lead to perineal involvement in women with Crohn's disease. *Am J Gastroenterol.* 1995; 90:1918-1922.
39. Ilnyckyji A, Blanchard JF, Rawsthorne P, Bernstein CN. Perianal Crohn's disease and pregnancy: role of the mode of delivery. *Am J Gastroenterol.* 1999;94:3274-3278.
40. Present DH. Pregnancy and inflammatory bowel disease. In: Bayless TM, Hanauer SB, eds. *Advanced Therapy of Inflammatory Bowel Disease.* Hamilton, British Columbia: Decker Inc; 2001:613-618.
41. Cappell MS, Sidhom O. Multicenter, multiyear study of safety and efficacy of flexible sigmoidoscopy during pregnancy in 24 females with follow-up of fetal outcome. *Dig Dis Sci.* 1995;40:472-479.
42. Cappell MS, Colon VJ, Sidhom OA. A study at 10 medical centers of the safety and efficacy of 48 flexible sigmoidoscopies and 8 colonoscopies during pregnancy with follow-up of fetal outcome and with comparison to control groups. *Dig Dis Sci.* 1996;41:2353-2361.
43. Shoenut JP, Smelka RC, Silverman R, Yaffe CS, Micflikier AB. MRI in the diagnosis of Crohn's disease in two pregnant women. *J Clin Gastroenterol.* 1993;17:244-247.
44. Brent RL. The effects of embryonic and fetal exposure to x-ray, microwave, and ultrasound: counseling the pregnant and nonpregnant patient about the risks. *Semin Oncol.* 1989;16:347-368.
45. Warrell DW, Taylor R. Outcome for the foetus of mothers receiving prednisolone during pregnancy. *Lancet.* 1968;1:117-118.
46. Schade RR, Thiel DHV, Gavaler JS. Chronic idiopathic ulcerative colitis. Pregnancy and fetal outcome. *Dig Dis Sci.* 1984;29:614-619.
47. Fedorkow DM, Persaud D, Nimrod CA. Inflammatory bowel disease: a controlled study of late pregnancy outcome. *Am J Obstet Gynecol.* 1989;160:998-1001.

48. Moskovitz DN, Bodian C, Chapman ML, et al. The effect on the fetus of medications used to treat pregnant inflammatory bowel disease patients. *Am J Gastroenterol.* 2004;99:656-661.
49. Esbjörner E, Järnerot G, Wranne L. Sulphasalazine and sulphapyridine levels in children to mothers treated with sulphasalazine during pregnancy and lactation. *Acta Paediatr Scand.* 1987;76:137-142.
50. Mogadam M, Dobbins WO, Korelitz BI, Ahmed SW. Pregnancy in inflammatory bowel disease: effect of sulfasalazine and corticosteroids on fetal outcome. *Gastroenterology.* 1981;80:72-76.
51. Newman NM, Correy JF. Possible teratogenicity of sulphasalazine. *Med J Aust.* 1983;1:528-529.
52. Hoo JJ, Hadro TA. Possible teratogenicity of sulfasalazine [letter]. *N Engl J Med.* 1988;318:1128.
53. Nørgård B, Czeizel AE, Rockenbauer M, Olsen J, Sorensen HT. Population-based case control study of the safety of sulfasalazine use during pregnancy. *Aliment Pharmacol Ther.* 2001;15:483-486.
54. Moody GA, Probert C, Jayanthi V, Mayberry JF. The effects of chronic ill health and treatment with sulphasalazine on fertility amongst men and women with inflammatory bowel disease in Leicestershire. *Int J Colorectal Dis.* 1997;12:220-224.
55. Christensen LA, Rasmussen SN, Hansen SH. Disposition of 5-aminosalicylic acid an N-acetyl-5-aminosalicylic acid in fetal and maternal body fluids during treatment with different 5-aminosalicylic acid preparations. *Acta Obstet Gynecol Scand.* 1994;74:399-402.
56. Marteau P, Crand J, Devaux CB. Mesalazine in pregnancy: fetal outcome in 76 IBD patients treated with Pentasa. *Gastroenterology.* 1995;108:A871.
57. Habal FM, Hui G, Greenberg GR. Oral 5-aminosalicylic acid for inflammatory bowel disease in pregnancy: safety and clinical course. *Gastroenterology.* 1993;105:1057-1060.
58. Bell CM, Habal FM. Safety of topical 5-aminosalicylic acid in pregnancy. *Am J Gastroenterol.* 1997;92:2201-2202.
59. Diav-Citrin O, Park YH, Veerasuntharam G, et al. The safety of mesalamine in human pregnancy: a prospective controlled cohort study. *Gastroenterology.* 1998;114:23-28.
60. Nørgård B, Fonager K, Pedersen L, Jacobsen BA, Sprensen HT. Birth outcome in women exposed to 5-aminosalicylic acid during pregnancy: a Danish cohort study. *Gut.* 2003;52:243-247.
61. Roe FJ. Toxicologic evaluation of metronidazole with particular reference to carcinogenic, mutagenic, and teratogenic potential. *Surgery.* 1983;93:158-164.
62. Czeizel AE, Rockenbauer M. A population based case-control teratologic study of oral metronidazole treatment during pregnancy. *Br J Obstet Gynaecol.* 1998;105:322-327.
63. Greenberg F. Possible metronidazole teratogenicity and clefting [letter]. *Am J Med Genet.* 1985;22:825.
64. Burtin P, Taddio A, Ariburnu O, Einarson TR, Koren G. Safety of metronidazole in pregnancy: a meta-analysis. *Am J Obstet Gynecol.* 1995;172:525-529.
65. Caro-Paton T, Carvajal A, Diego IM, Martin-Arias LH, Requejo AA, Pinilla ER. Is metronidazole teratogenic? A meta-analysis. *Br J Clin Pharmacol.* 1997;44:179-183.
66. Linseman DA, Hampton LA, Branstetter DG. Quinolone-induced arthropathy in the neonatal mouse. Morphological analysis of articular lesions produced by pipemidic acid and ciprofloxacin. *Fundam Appl Toxicol.* 1995;28:59-64.
67. Berkovitch M, Pastuszak A, Garzarian M, Lewis M, Koren G. Safety of the new quinolones in pregnancy. *Obstet Gynecol.* 1994;84:535-538.
68. Loebstein R, Addis A, Ho E, et al. Pregnancy outcome following gestational exposure to fluoroquinolones: a multicenter prospective controlled study. *Antimicrob Agents Chemother.* 1998;42:1336-1339.
69. Fitzsimons R, Greenberger PA, Patterson R. Outcome of pregnancy in women requiring corticosteroids for severe asthma. *J Allergy Clin Immunol.* 1986;78:349-353.
70. Bulmash JM. Systemic lupus erythematosus and pregnancy. *Obstet Gynecol Annu.* 1978;7:153-194.
71. Bulmash JM. Rheumatoid arthritis and pregnancy. *Obstet Gynecol Annu.* 1979;8:223-276.
72. Pinsky L, DiGeorge AM. Cleft palate in the mouse: a teratogenic index of glucocorticoid potency. *Science.* 1965;147:402-403.
73. Rodriguez-Pinella E, Martinez-Frias ML. Corticosteroids during pregnancy and oral clefts: acase control study. *Teratology.* 1998;58:2-5.
74. Fraser FC, Sajoo A. Teratogenic potential of corticosteroids in humans. *Teratology.* 1995;51:45-46.
75. Beitens IZ, Bayarrd F, Ances IG, Kowarski A, Migeon CJ. The transplacental passage of prednisone and prenisolone in pregnancy near term. *J Pediatr.* 1972;81:936-945.
76. Alstead EM, Ritchie JK, Lennard-Jones JE, Farthing MJ, Clark ML. Safety of azathioprine in pregnancy in inflammatory bowel disease. *Gastroenterology.* 1990;99:443-446.
77. Sandborn WJ. A review of immune modifier therapy for inflammatory bowel disease: azathioprine, 6-mercaptopurine, cyclosporine, and methotrexate. *Am J Gastroenterology.* 1996;91:423-433.
78. Ramsey-Goldman R, Schilling E. Immunosuppressive drug use during pregnancy. *Rheum Clin NA.* 1997;23:149-167.
79. Zlatanic J, Korelitz BI, Rajapakse R, et al. Complications of pregnancy and child development after cessation of treatment with 6-mercaptopurine for inflammatory bowel disease. *J Clin Gastroenterol.* 2003;36:303-309.
80. Rajapaske RO, Korelitz BI, Zlatanic J, Baiocco PJ, Gleim GW. Outcome of pregnancies when fathers are treated with 6-mercaptopurine for inflammatory bowel disease. *Am J Gastroenterol.* 2000; 95:684-688.
81. Francella A, Dayan A, Bodian C, Rubin P, Chapman M, Present D. The safety of 6-mercaptopurine for childbearing patients with inflammatory bowel disease: a retrospective cohort study. *Gastroenterology.* 2003;124:9-17.
82. Nørgård B, Pedersen L, Fonager K, Rasmussen SN, Sorensen HT. Azathioprine, mercaptopurine and birth outcome: a population-based cohort study. *Aliment Pharmacol Ther.* 2003;17:827-834.
83. Jharap B, de Boer N, van der Woude CJ, et al. Thiopurine metabolite measurements during pregnancy in mother and child. *Gastroenterology.* 2008;134:A-69.
84. Feagan BG, Fedorak RN, Irvine EJ, et al. A comparison of methotrexate with placebo for the maintenance of remission in Crohn's disease. *N Engl J Med.* 2000;342:1627-1632.
85. Goldenberg M, Bider D, Admon D, Mashiach S, Oelsner G. Methotrexate therapy of tubal pregnancy. *Human Reprod.* 1993; 8:660-666.
86. Donnenfield AE, Pastuszak A, Noah JS, Schick B, Rose NC, Koren G. Methotrexate exposure prior to and during pregnancy. *Teratology.* 1994;49:79-81.
87. Briggs GG, Freeman RK, Yaffe SJ. *Drugs in pregnancy and lactation: A Reference Guide to Fetal and Neonatal Risk.* Baltimore, MD: Williams & Wilkins; 1998:702-705.
88. Kozlowski RD, Steinbrunner JV, MacKenzie AH, Clough JD, Wilke WS, Segal AM. Outcome of first-trimester exposure to low-dose methotrexate in eight patients with rheumatic disease. *Am J Med.* 1990;88:589-592.
89. Lichtiger A, Present D, Kornbluth A, et al. Cyclosporine in severe ulcerative colitis refractory to steroid therapy. *N Engl J Med.* 1994;330:1841-1845.
90. Cohen RD, Stein R, Hanauer SB. Intravenous cyclosporin in ulcerative colitis: a five year experience. *Am J Gastrorenterol.* 1999; 94:1587-1592.

91. Reddy D, Murphy SJ, Kane SV, Present DH, Kornbluth AA. Relapses of inflammatory bowel disease during pregnancy: in-hospital management and birth outcomes. *Am J Gastroenterol.* 2008;103:1203-1209.
92. Bertschinger P, Himmelmann A, Risti B, Follath F. Cyclosporine treatment of severe ulcerative colitis during pregnancy. *Am J Gastroenterol.* 1995;90:330.
93. Balzora S, Jacob V, Scherl E, Bosworth B. Cyclosporine in steroid refractory ulcerative colitis in the first trimester of pregnancy. *Am J Gastroenterol.* 2008;103:A663.
94. Marion JF, Rubin PH, Lichtiger S, Chapman M, Hanauer S, Present DH. Cyclosporine is safe for severe colitis complicating pregnancy [abstract]. *Am J Gastroenterol.* 1996;91:1975.
95. Feagan BG, Yan S, Bao W, Lichtenstein GR. The effects of infliximab maintenance therapy on health-related quality of life. *Am J Gastroenterol.* 2003;98:2232-2238.
96. Srinivasan R. Infliximab treatment and pregnancy outcome in active Crohn's disease. *Am J Gastroenterol.* 2001;96:2274-2275.
97. Burt MJ, Frizelle FA, Barbezat GO. Pregnancy and exposure to infliximab (anti-tumor necrosis factor-alpha monoclonal antibody). *J Gastroenterol Hepatol.* 2003;18:465-466.
98. James RL, Pearson LL. Successful treatment of pregnancy-triggered Crohn's disease complicated by severe recurrent life-threatening gastrointestinal bleeding [abstract]. *Am J Gastroenterol.* 2001;296:S295.
99. Katz JA, Antoni C, Keenan GF, Smith DE, Jacobs SJ, Lichtenstein GR. Outcome of pregnancy in women receiving infliximab for the treatment of Crohn's disease and rheumatoid arthritis. *Am J Gastroenterol.* 2004;99:2385-2392.
100. Mahadevan U, Kane S, Sandborn WJ, et al. Intentional infliximab use for maintenance or acute Crohn's disease (CD) flare in pregnancy. *Gastroenterology.* 2004;126:A629.
101. Sills ES, Perloe M, Tucker MJ, Kaplan CR, Palermo GD. Successful ovulation induction, conception, and normal delivery after chronic therapy with etanercept: a recombinant fusion anti-cytokine treatment for rheumatoid arthritis. *Am J Reprod Immunol.* 2001; 46:366-368.
102. Wallace DJ. The use of etanercept and other tumor necrosis factor-alpha blockers in infertility: it's time to get serious. *J Rheumatol.* 2003;30:1897-1899.
103. Mahadevan U, Kane S, Sandborn WJ, et al. Intentional infliximab use during pregnancy for induction or maintenance of remission in Crohn's disease. *Aliment Pharmacol Ther.* 2005;21:733-738.
104. Mahadevan U, Kane SV, Church JA, et al. The effect of maternal peripartum infliximab use on neonatal immune response. *Gastroenterology.* 2008;134:A499.
105. Mishkin DS, Van Deinse W, Becker JM, Farraye FA. Successful use of adalimumab (Humira) for Crohn's disease in pregnancy. *Inflamm Bowel Dis.* 2006;12:827-828.
106. Coburn LA, Wise PE, Schwartz DA. The successful use of adalimumab to treat active Crohn's disease of an ileoanal pouch during pregnancy. *Dig Dis Sci.* 2006;51:2045-2047.
107. Johnson D, Lyons Jones K, Chambers C. Pregnancy outcomes in women exposed to adalimumab: the OTIS autoimmune diseases in pregnancy project. *Am J Gastroenterol.* 2008;103(Suppl 1):958.
108. Einarson A, Mastroiacovo P, Arnon J, et al. Prospective, controlled, multicentre study of loperamide in pregnancy. *Can J Gastroenterol.* 2000;14:185-187.
109. Collins E. Maternal and fetal effects of acetominophen and salicylates in pregnancy. *Obstet Gynecol.* 1981;58:57S.
110. Bonapace ES, Fisher RS. Constipation and diarrhea in pregnancy. *Gastroenterol Clin NA.* 1998;27:197-211.
111. Levine W, Diamond B. Surgical procedures during pregnancy. *Am J Obstet Gynecol.* 1961;81:1046-1052.
112. Kelly MJ, Hunt TM, Wicks ACB, Mayne CJ. Fulminant ulcerative colitis and parturition: A need to alter current management? *Br J Obstet Gynecol.* 1994;101:166-167.
113. Subhani JM, Hamiliton MI. Review article: the management of inflammatory bowel disease during pregnancy. *Aliment Pharmacol Ther.* 1998;12:1039-1053.
114. Bohe MG, Ekelund GR, Genell SN, et al. Surgery for fulminating colitis during pregnancy. *Dis Colon Rectum.* 1983;26:119-122.
115. Boulton R, Hamilton M, Lewis A, Walker P, Pounder R. Fulminant ulcerative colitis in pregnancy. *Am J Gastroenterol.* 1994;89:931-933.
116. Greenfield C, Craft IL, Pounder RE, Lewis AAM. Severe ulcerative colitis during successful pregnancy. *Postgrad Med J.* 1983;59:459-461.
117. Anderson JB, Turner GM, Williamson RC. Fulminant ulcerative colitis in late pregnancy and the puerperium. *J R Soc Med.* 1987;80:492-494.
118. Hill J, Clark A, Scott NA. Surgical treatment of acute manifestations of Crohn's disease during pregnancy. *J R Soc Med.* 1997; 90:64-66.
119. Wax JR, Pinette MG, Cartin A, Blackstone J. Female reproductive health after ileal pouch anal anastomosis for ulcerative colitis. *Obstet Gynecol Surv.* 2003;58:270-274.
120. Ravid A, Richard CS, Spencer LM, et al. Pregnancy, delivery, and pouch function after ileal pouch-anal anastomosis for ulcerative colitis. *Dis Colon Rectum.* 2002;45:1283-1288.
121. Juhasz ES, Fozard B, Dozois RR, Ilstrup DM, Nelson H. Ileal pouch-anal anastomosis function following childbirth. An extended evaluation. *Dis Colon Rectum.* 1995;38:159-165.
122. Hahnloser D, Pemberton JH, Larson BGW, Harrington J, Farouk R, Dozois RR. Pregnancy and delivery before and after ileal pouch-anal anastomosis for inflammatory bowel disease: immediate and long-term consequences and outcomes. *Dis Colon Rectum.* 2004; 47:1127-1135.
123. Donaldson RM Jr. Management of medical problems in pregnancy—inflammatory bowel disease. *N Engl J Med.* 1985;312:1616-1619.

9 DIVERSION COLITIS

Eugeni Domènech, MD, PhD and Miquel A. Gassull, MD, PhD

Proximal diversion of the fecal stream remains an accepted and common surgical technique for the management of a wide range of conditions, such as benign or malignant colonic obstruction, colonic perforation (ie, trauma, diverticulosis), inflammatory processes (ie, diverticulitis), or perianal fistulas. Although, in the early 1970s, Morson and Dawson described the occurrence of inflammation in the bowel segments excluded from fecal stream,[1] this entity received little attention until 1981, when Glotzer et al reported the first 10 cases of what they called "*diversion-related colitis.*"[2] Since then, scarce data have been published in relation to its clinical presentation, epidemiology, pathogenesis, or medical treatment (Table 9-1).

DEFINITION

Diversion colitis (DC) has been defined as an inflammatory process that develops in the bypassed colorectal segment after surgical diversion of the fecal stream and that resolves when continuity is restored. This condition may occur as soon as 3 months after surgical diversion, and most patients will develop DC changes in the first 3 years.[3] Only a few studies have evaluated the real incidence of DC after surgical diversion. Ferguson and Siegel[4] reported the first endoscopic study evaluating the frequency of DC in 20 consecutive patients (those with inflammatory bowel disease [IBD] were excluded) scheduled for colostomy closure. Endoscopic findings were classified grossly as normal or "colitis" (including easy friability, edema, erythema, or ulceration). Although all the included patients were asymptomatic, 70% had endoscopic features of DC. There was no difference in terms of age, interval from colostomy to endoscopic examination, type (loop or end colostomy), or reason for colostomy between those patients with DC and those with normal endoscopy. Orsay et al,[5] in a similar study, evaluated 34 patients scheduled for colostomy closure who underwent endoscopic examination of the excluded segment prior to reanastomosis. As in the previously mentioned study, and after a mean interval between colostomy and endoscopy of 26 weeks, 74% of patients presented endoscopic features of mild to severe colitis. Despite this, none of them had symptoms. Whelan et al[6] found a higher incidence in a prospective study that included 53 patients, finding endoscopic evidences of colitis in 91% of the cases.

DC is clinically apparent only in a minority of patients; in these cases, clinical manifestations may develop from 1 month to decades after the diversion. Mucus discharge, rectal bleeding, and anal or abdominal pain are the most frequent symptoms, but this occurs in only 5% to 30% of patients with endoscopic or histologic evidence of DC.[6,7]

DIAGNOSIS

Diagnosis of DC relies on endoscopic and/or histologic findings. At endoscopy, diffuse granularity or nodularity (with or without erythema) is the most common finding. In severe cases, aphthous ulcers, or even large ulcerations with exudates and bleeding mucosal surface can be found. These features may be indistinguishable from those found in UC or Crohn's colitis.

Lichtenstein GR, ed.
Ulcerative Colitis: The Complete Guide to Medical Management (pp. 109-112).

TABLE 9-1

CHARACTERISTICS OF HISTOLOGIC AND ENDOSCOPIC STUDIES OF DIVERSION COLITIS

AUTHOR	N	STUDY DESIGN
Komorowski, 1990[11]	6	Patients with bypassed rectosigmoids and had biopsies of the bypassed segments. Biopsies were compared blindly with 6 cases of UC and 6 cases of CD.
Ma et al, 1990[7]	21	Patients diagnosed with DC by endoscopic or histologic features.
Yeong et al, 1991[20]	7	Histological features of 7 patients with underlying inflammatory diseases and defunctioned rectums.
Ferguson et al, 1991[4]	20	Patients scheduled for colostomy closure and underwent colonoscopy of the excluded segment.
Geraghty et al, 1991[9]	15	Specimens from surgical resection of defunctioned distal large bowel, 10 to 60 cm in length.
Haque et al, 1993[8]	37	Surgical specimens from patients with Hirschsprung's disease and had undergone colostomy and subsequent resection of the aganglionic segment with re-anastomosis.
Orsay et al, 1993[5]	34	Patients scheduled for colostomy closure and underwent colonoscopy of the excluded segment.
Whelan et al, 1994[6]	53	Endoscopic evaluation of the excluded segment in patients with fecal diversion. In 86% of the patients, colon proximal to the ostomy was also evaluated.

Histologic changes in DC have been described in detail in a few studies.[8,9] The primary microscopic characteristics of DC are increased chronic inflammatory infiltrates of the lamina propria and lymphoid hyperplasia with reactive germinal centers. These changes are usually limited to the upper part of the mucosa, and, when mild, they are often associated with a normal mucosal appearance at endoscopy. Some authors have defined these asymptomatic mild histological changes with normal endoscopy appearance as *"diversion reaction,"* which is thought to be an intermediate stage to DC.[8] Crypt structure is often altered, with branching, atrophy, and distortion of the crypts. In those cases with severe chronic inflammatory infiltrates, acute inflammation can also be seen with cryptitis, crypt abscesses, and mucosal erosions (more common over lymphoid nodules). Severe histologic lesions are usually seen in patients with more severe endoscopic lesions, but no correlation has been demonstrated with clinical manifestations. As seen with endoscopic findings, DC may histologically mimic idiopathic IBD. In fact, some authors have even reported the existence of granulomas in DC,[7] and others have proposed DC as a trigger for UC.[10] Komorowski[11] reported the results of a study in which biopsy specimens of 6 DC patients were blindly read, along with tissue taken from 6 UC patients and 6 patients with Crohn's colitis. Histologic features favoring DC included a variation in severity seen on multiple biopsy specimens taken from a single area, involvement limited to the distal bypassed segment, lack of mucin granulomas, or crypt atrophy.

Most cases of DC can be fairly readily distinguished from IBD on histologic examination. In DC, lymphoid hyperplasia is more prominent, and the proportion of lymphoid follicles with germinal centers is higher. The lymphoplasmacytosis is more concentrated in the superficial mucosa, and acute inflammation is localized predominantly to crypts. In contrast to Crohn's disease, DC is predominantly mucosal, diffuse, and usually more severe distally. In contrast to ulcerative colitis, architectural distortion is minimal, and the lymphoplasmacytic infiltrate is superficial rather than basal.[7,8]

PATHOGENESIS

The pathogenic mechanism by which DC develops in the majority of patients with diverted segments of the colon is still not known. Quantitative and qualitative changes in bacterial flora and nutritional deficiencies of the diverted segment are the main hypotheses that have been postulated. In normal conditions, short-chain fatty acids (SCFA) are the predominant solutes in the aqueous phase of colonic contents and stool, with n-butyric, propionic, and acetic acids accounting for 90% of them. These SCFA are produced by anaerobic bacterial fermentation of carbohydrate and are absorbed by colonocytes, in exchange for bicarbonate and simultaneous stimulation of sodium and water absorption. In fact, SCFA are the main energy source of human colonocytes, and this dependence is greater in the distal segments of the colon-rectum than in proximal segments of the colon[12,13]; colonocytes must assimilate these substrate from the lumen because plasma concentrations of SCFA are negligible.

Several studies have demonstrated that DC is not related to any specific infection nor is it related to colonization by a particular pathogen; and stool, lumen contents, or biopsy cultures from the excluded colonic segment have always been negative for any pathogens. Neut et al,[14] in the best microbiological study of DC, reported a mildly decreased total bacterial count in the excluded colorectum due to a significant reduction in the anaerobic bacterial count. These microbiological changes may lead to a decrease in SCFA production and, subsequently, a nutritional deficiency of the diverted colorectum. The treatment of diversion colitis has been studied in several small investigator-initiated trials. Harig et al[15] studied 4 patients with DC of the bypassed rectosigmoid in order to evaluate the presence of specific infection, decrease in anaerobic bacteria, and changes in the concentration of SCFA in the lumen contents. A breath hydrogen test after instillation of a glucose solution into the diverted colon and colostomy demonstrated that, whereas carbohydrate fermentation was present in the proximal colon (when carbohydrates were instilled in to the colostomy), there was an absence of carbohydrate-fermenting anaerobic bacterial flora in the diverted colon. As expected, cultures of luminal contents obtained from the bypassed segments revealed no enteric pathogenic bacteria. Finally, total SCFA concentration in these aspirates was very low, confirming the absence of bacterial fermentation. In the same study, patients were treated with irrigation of a solution of SCFA twice daily for 2 to 3 weeks; endoscopic and histologic evaluation was performed at baseline and after treatment protocol. A dramatic endoscopic improvement was noticed, especially when treatment was continued for a longer period. Histologically, acute changes (ie, acute inflammatory infiltrates, cryptitis, crypt abscesses) rapidly disappeared with SCFA treatment; however, chronic lesions (ie, increase in the number of plasma cells, lymphocytes, and prominence of lymphoid follicles) persisted despite endoscopic disappearance of the lesions. The authors concluded that, given the obtained results, a local nutritional deficiency leads to an inflammatory state in DC. In fact, in UC (in which endoscopic lesions may be identical to those seen in DC), it has been observed that there is a decrease in SCFA utilization by colonocytes with a consequent cellular energy deficiency.[16]

Unfortunately, these preliminary results were not confirmed by a posterior prospective, randomized, double-blind study that included 13 DC patients who were randomized to receive SCFA or isotonic saline rectal solutions for 14 days.[17] Although the period of treatment was shorter and the severity of lesions was lower than in the previous study by Harig et al,[15] endoscopic and histologic evaluations at baseline and after treatment protocol did not differ, calling into question this attractive hypothesis.

Recently, de Oliveira-Neto and de Aguilar-Nascimento[18] obtained successful results in a similar study conducted on 11 DC patients who were treated with irrigation of the diverted colorectal segment with a solution containing 5% soybean fibers (10% soluble and 90% insoluble). In turn, it seems that, although nutrient deficiency seems to play a pivotal role in the pathogenesis of DC, this is not only due to the decrease in anaerobe fermenting bacteria because a minimum amount must be present to produce SCFA from fiber irrigation.

Finally, Neut et al[19] reported a significant increase in the proportion of nitrate-reducing bacteria in DC patients compared to healthy controls. In addition, qualitative differences among this kind of bacteria were also demonstrated, with a higher proportion of aerobe nitrate-reducing strains (as *Pseudomonas species* was only encountered in DC patients). Hence, changes in bacterial flora of diverted segments may lead to an increased production of nitric oxide, playing an additional role in chronic inflammation.

The role of the bacteria-luminal content interaction in the colon should be more extensively investigated because bacterial changes induced by diversion may be similar to those in UC. We should also study why a certain type of bacteria is necessary to maintain a non-inflamed colon, whereas in the small intestine diversion leads to improvement of inflammation.

CONCLUSION

DC is an early and very common inflammatory disorder that involves the mucosa of the derived segments of the colon. DC is rarely symptomatic, but its major concern is to be distinguished from idiopathic IBD. Also, whereas DC is easily reversed by restoration of intestinal continuity, the diagnosis of IBD might prompt resection. The pathogenic mechanism by which DC develops is still unknown, but changes in bacterial flora (leading to a decrease in carbohydrate fermentation and an increase in nitric oxide production) and nutrient deficiencies may be involved.

REFERENCES

1. Morson BC, Dawson IMP. *Gastrointestinal Pathology*, 1st ed. London: Blackwell Scientific Publications; 1972:485.
2. Glotzer DJ, Glick ME, Goldman H. Proctitis and colitis following diversion of the fecal stream. *Gastroenterology*. 1981;80:438-441.
3. Korelitz BI, Cheskin LJ, Sohn N, Somers SC. The fate of the rectal segment after diversion of the fecal stream in Crohn's disease: its implications for surgical management. *J Clin Gastroenterol*. 1985;7:37-43.
4. Ferguson CM, Siegel RJ. A prospective evaluation of diversion colitis. *Am Surg*. 1991;57:46-49.

5. Orsay Ch P, Kim DO, Pearl RK, Abcarian H. Diversion colitis in patients scheduled for colostomy closure. *Dis Colon Rectum.* 1993;36:366-367.
6. Whelan RL, Abrason D, Kim DS, Hashmi HF. Diversion colitis: a prospective study. *Surg Endosc.* 1994;8:19-24.
7. Ma CK, Gottlieb C, Haas PA. Diversion colitis: a clinicopathologic study of 21 cases. *Hum Pathol.* 1990;21:429-436.
8. Haque S, Eisen RN, West AB. The morphologic features of diversion colitis: studies of a pediatric population with no other disease of the intestinal mucosa. *Hum Pathol.* 1993;24:211-219.
9. Geraghty JM, Talbot IC. Diversion colitis: histological features in the colon and rectum after defunctioning colostomy. *Gut.* 1991;32:1020-1023.
10. Lim AG, Langmead FL, Feakins RM, Rampton DS. Diversion colitis: a trigger for ulcerative colitis in the in-stream colon? *Gut.* 1999;44:279-282.
11. Komorowski RA. Histologic spectrum of diversion colitis. *Am J Surg Pathol.* 1990;14:548-554.
12. Roediger WE. Role of anaerobic bacteria in the metabolic welfare of the colonic mucosa in man. *Gut.* 1980;21:793-798.
13. Ruppin H, Bar-Meir S, Soergel KH, Wood CM, Schmitt MG Jr. Absorption of short-chain fatty acids by the colon. *Gastroenterology.* 1980;78:1500-1507.
14. Neut C, Colombel JF, Guillemot F, et al. Impaired bacterial flora in human excluded colon. *Gut.* 1989;30:1094-1098.
15. Harig JM, Soergel KH, Komorowski RA, Wood CM. Treatment of diversion colitis with short-chain-fatty acid irrigation. *N Engl J Med.* 1989;320:23-28.
16. Roediger WE. The colonic epithelium in ulcerative colitis: An energy-deficiency disease? *Lancet.* 1980;2:712-715.
17. Guillemot F, Colombel JF, Net Ch, et al. Treatment of diversion colitis by short-chain fatty acids: prospective and double-blind study. *Dis Colon Rectum.* 1991;34:861-864.
18. De Oliveira-Neto JP, De Aguilar-Nascimento JE. Intraluminal irrigation with fibers improves mucosal inflammation and atrophy in diversion colitis. *Nutrition.* 2004;20:197-199.
19. Neut C, Guillemot F, Colombel JF. Nitrate-reducing bacteria in diversion colitis: a clue to inflammation? *Dig Dis Sci.* 1997;42:2577-2580.
20. Yeong ML, Bethwaite PB, Prasad J, Isbister WH. Lymphoid follicular hyperplasia: a distinctive feature of diversion colitis. *Histopathology.* 1991;19:55-61.

10 Medication Adherence in Inflammatory Bowel Disease

Sunanda V. Kane, MD, MSPH, FACG, FACP, AGAF

Though literature on other chronic diseases, such as coronary artery disease, congestive heart failure, and diabetes, has tried to address the issue of medication nonadherence and its effect on disease outcomes, the impact of medication adherence on specific inflammatory bowel disease (IBD) outcomes has not been fully explored. The published literature on the efficacy of IBD maintenance medications underestimates the extent of the problem, as patients often conceal their failure to take medications as directed once outside of controlled clinical trial environments. The remainder of this chapter will discuss the state of knowledge regarding the issues surrounding nonadherence in the management of IBD, with special attention to ulcerative colitis, as the literature in this area is more substantial than that for Crohn's disease.

Current Data on Nonadherence

Nonadherence to Medications

Multiple studies have demonstrated the efficacy of aminosalicylates as first-line therapy to induce and maintain remission in ulcerative colitis.[1-5] These well-designed multicenter trials have used pill count and patient inquiry to assess adherence, with rates ranging from 70% to >95%. Based upon community-based follow-up studies in other chronic illnesses, the percentage of long-term adherence tends to be much lower, about 40% to 50%.[6] This wide variance across studies can be explained by 1) a study's definition of adherence, 2) the degree to which the investigators were proactive in adherence measures, and 3) patient population. Particularly after remission has been established, patients may not believe (or understand) the importance of continuing on maintenance therapy. Many patients openly admit they do not take their medications as prescribed; medication-taking probably makes patients more uncomfortably aware of their chronic illness status, they have a fear of long-term side effects from medications, and they question the need for medication in the setting of quiescent disease.

Patient adherence is defined as the extent to which an individual's behavior coincides with medical or health advice.[7] The term *adherence* replaces *compliance*, the latter a term that conveys a paternalistic concept of medical care and patient obedience to the physician's authority. Despite research attempting to profile nonadherent patients, there are no characteristics consistently linked to nonadherence. This is not surprising, given that patient nonadherence varies between and within individuals as well as across time, recommended behaviors, and diseases.

The issue of adherence was first introduced several decades ago, in several published studies addressing long-term sulfasalazine use in UC. Das and colleagues defined its metabolism in patients with ulcerative colitis, during both the active and quiescent phases of the disease. They subsequently studied the relationship between clinical status and serum concentrations of sulfasalazine and its metabolites.[8] Levels of total sulphapyridine (SP) were demonstrated to be different in slow versus rapid acetylators, and a serum concentration of 20 to 50 μg/mL appeared to coincide with clinical improvement in the absence of side effects.

Lichtenstein GR, ed.
Ulcerative Colitis: The Complete Guide to Medical Management (pp. 113-118)

One-year follow-up on 64 outpatients revealed that, of the 43 patients with quiescent disease, 32 with total SP levels above 20 μg/mL remained in remission.[9] Ten of 21 with active disease had levels below 20 μg/mL and remained symptomatic. The correlation between "therapeutic" levels and disease activity suggested that adherence was associated with an improved outcome and that following metabolite levels may be a method to monitor patient adherence.

In a second study, Van Hees and Van Tongeren measured urine levels of acetylated sulfasalazine as a marker for adherence in 51 patients 1 to 6 months after hospital discharge and in 171 outpatients over several years.[10] The authors found that nonadherence, as defined by undetectable urine levels, in the months after hospital discharge approximated 40%. In the cohort of outpatients followed on maintenance doses of sulfasalazine, 12% had undetectable urine levels at 6-month follow-up.

In a study by a group of Italian psychiatrists treating IBD patients, Nigro et al examined the effect of psychiatric disorders on adherence with medications.[11] They found a correlation between duration of disease and adherence but an inverse relationship between disease severity and the presence of significant psychiatric disorders with regular medication consumption. Their recommendation was preventive liaison interventions for these patients to improve disease outcomes.

In an attempt to understand the possible effect of adherence on disease outcome, Riley and colleagues included adherence as a potential factor leading to disease relapse in patients with quiescent UC.[12] Medication adherence was determined by pill count and direct patient inquiry. After 48 weeks, there was no difference in adherence rates between the patients who relapsed versus those who remained in remission. However, the total adherence for both groups was >95% throughout the study, making the interpretation of these findings difficult.

Farup et al, in their trial of mesalazine (European term for mesalamine) versus hydrocortisone foam enemas, incorporated the issue of tolerability, ease, and adherence into the data collection.[13] In this 4-week trial, patients were asked to mark on a 100-mm visual analog scale an assessment of their medication regimen with regard to ease of administration and practicality. Adherence, as measured by the return of unused bottles, was >80% at 2 weeks in both groups, then dropped to 73% for the foam patients but remained >90% for the mesalazine group. The authors suggested that the better outcome in the mesalazine group was in part due to convenience and simplicity and thus better adherence to that treatment regimen.

Shale and Riley, in another more recent prospective study, studied 98 outpatients with IBD who were prescribed maintenance delayed-release mesalazine.[14] Adherence was studied by both direct inquiry and by analysis of urine samples for the presence of 5-aminosalicylic acid (5-ASA) and N-acetyl 5-ASA. Demographic variables, disease- and treatment-related factors, quality of life, psychiatric morbidity, and aspects of the doctor-patient relationship were all assessed as possible determinants of adherence. Self-reporting revealed nonadherence (ie, taking less than 80% of the prescribed dose) in 42 patients (43%). Logistic regression revealed 3 times daily dosing (odds ratio [OR] 3.1, 95% confidence interval [CI] 1.8 to 8.4), full-time employment (OR 2.7, 95% CI 1.8 to 8.9), and depression (Hospital Anxiety and Depression rating scale >7) (OR 10.5, 95% CI (1.8 to 79) were the only independent predictors of nonadherence. Urinary drug measurements revealed 12 patients with no detectable 5-ASA or N-acetyl 5-ASA. Of interest, self-reporting correctly identified 66% of patients judged to be nonadherent on the basis of urinary drug measurements, but only 2 of the 12 patients with undetectable drug levels admitted to complete nonadherence.

In a recently published prevalence survey, Kane and colleagues found the overall adherence rate with a maintenance dose of Asacol to be only 40%.[15] Adherence was measured by pharmacy refill data rather than patient inquiry or pill count. The median amount of medication dispensed per patient was 71% (range, 8% to 130%) of the prescribed regimen over a 6-month period. Noncompliant patients were more likely to be male (67% versus 52%, $P<0.05$), single (68% versus 53%, $P=0.04$), and to have disease limited to the left side of the colon versus pancolitis (83% versus 51%, $P<0.01$). Sixty-eight percent of patients who took more than 4 prescription medications were found to be noncompliant versus only 40% of those patients taking fewer medications ($P = 0.05$). Age, occupation, a family history of IBD, length of remission, or quality-of-life score was not associated with nonadherence. Logistic regression identified that a history of more than 4 prescriptions (OR 2.5, 95% CI 1.4 to 5.7) and male gender (OR 2.06, 95% CI 1.17 to 4.88) increased the risk of nonadherence. Two statistically significant variables that were protective against nonadherence were endoscopy within the past 24 months (OR 0.96, 95% CI 0.93 to 0.99) and being married (OR 0.46, 95% CI 0.39 to 0.57).

The advent of biologic therapy and its intravenous administration potentially eases the burden of daily oral therapies. Regular infusions to some patients seem more attractive than pills or tablets frequently throughout the day. A study examining the adherence rate for scheduled infliximab appointments in a large tertiary IBD center found the no-show rate to be only 4%.[16]

Nonadherence With Non-Medication-Related Treatment and Therapies

Patient adherence rates with surveillance colonoscopy are not well-documented. In the only study that directly addressed this issue, Woolrich et al reported on 7 patients of their cohort of 121 who were found to have cancer.[17] In

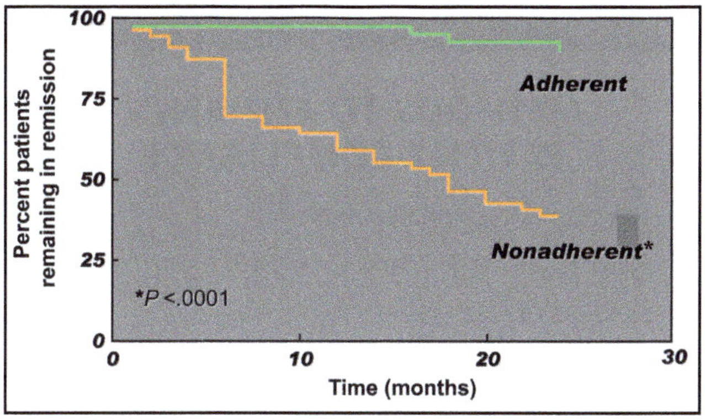

FIGURE 10-1. Nonadherence with medications is associated with disease recurrence.

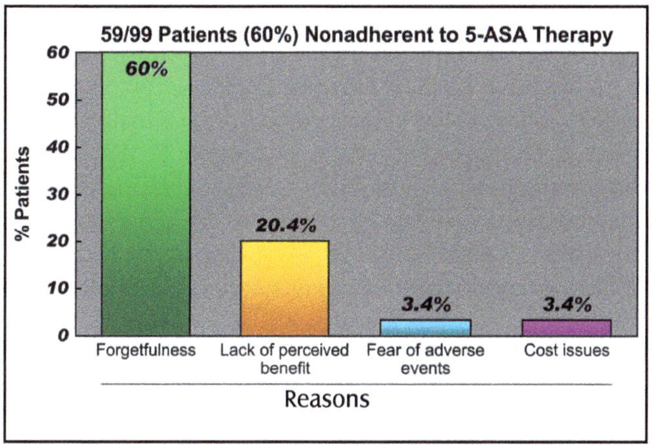

FIGURE 10-2. Reasons cited for patient nonadherence with maintenance medications.

2 of these patients, previous colonoscopy had found dysplasia in the setting of quiescent disease, and neither of these patients was adherent with recommendations for close follow-up colonoscopy or colectomy. It was the conclusion of the authors that quiescent disease was a risk factor for nonadherence with physician recommendations.

Long-term adherence rates with enteral feeding are dismal. In a dietary intervention trial by Levenstein et al, 24% (17/70) randomized to either a low residue or Mediterranean diet had dropped out prior to the end of the 24-month trial.[18] In another dietary intervention trial, adherence at 3 months for Ensure supplementation was only 39%.[19] In a postoperative recurrence study, patients were randomized to placebo, omega-3 fatty acid supplementation, or a low-carbohydrate diet. At the end of 12 months, only 16% of patients were adherent to the diet.[20]

ADHERENCE AND OUTCOMES

What data do we have that would compel a patient to continue taking medication in the setting of well-being? A prospective 2-year follow-up on a cohort of patients with quiescent UC was done to help answer this question.[21] Patients in remission were enrolled and then stratified by adherence based on the previous 6-month pharmacy refill data. At 6 months, 12 patients (12%) had clinical recurrence of disease symptoms, all of whom were noncompliant with medication. At 12 months, 19 of 86 patients had recurrent disease, 13 (68%) of whom were noncompliant. A multiple Cox proportional hazards model revealed that patients not compliant with medication had more than fivefold greater risk of recurrence than the compliant patients (hazard ratio 5.47, 95% CI 2.26 to 13.22, $P<0.001$; Figure 10-1). As part of the study, nonadherent patients were asked why they were not taking their medications.[22] The majority stated that they simply forgot one of their doses. Fewer than 10% of patients complained of side effects and cost (Figure 10-2).

The detrimental effects of tobacco smoking on Crohn's disease are well-known. Cosnes et al prospectively followed 59 patients who quit smoking and were able to remain adherent to the smoking cessation program.[23] During a median follow-up of 29 months, the risk for need for steroids or immunosuppressive medications was similar to that in nonsmokers and lower than in current smokers.

There are now several studies that suggest that documented medication consumption is protective for colon cancer, which is an important concern for the long-term natural history of UC. Moody et al studied 168 patients with UC diagnosed between 1972 and 1981 and correlated sulfasalazine nonadherence with risk of colorectal cancer.[24] A patient was classified as noncompliant if there was clear evidence in the medical record of medications not taken or if upon the advice of a physician medication was discontinued. Their crude colectomy rate was 23% in 10 years, with a 3% rate in those patients on maintenance sulfasalazine and 31% in patients either noncompliant or off all medications. Because the authors found colectomy rate and cancer incidence similar to previously published series, they concluded that medications were beneficial in reducing cancer risk. In a second retrospective case-control study, Pinczowski et al found that a record of at least a 3-month history of therapy with sulfasalazine had a protective effect for colon cancer.[25] There was a 62% reduction in risk with any history of therapy in the 102 patients studied. It is difficult to interpret this finding, however, as documentation of dose and duration of therapy for each patient was not known. However, a recent meta-analysis by Velayos et al demonstrated a 50% reduction in development of either dysplasia or colorectal cancer with continued use of 5-ASAs.[26]

Eaden and colleagues found in a case-control study that mesalamine at a dose of 1.2 g/day or greater reduced colorectal cancer risk by 91% in patients with UC compared to no treatment.[27] There was also a protective effect of more than 2 visits to the physician per year, but the same was not found for the number of surveillance colonoscopies. More data on mesalamine comes from investigators at Mount Sinai Medical Center in New York who followed patients whose colon biopsies were indeterminate for dysplasia.[28] Those patients on 2 g or more of 5-ASA per day did not progress to definite dysplasia, suggesting that any chemoprotective effect occurs early in the cancer progression pathway. Rubin and colleagues studied the University of Chicago experience with all forms of 5-ASA in ulcerative colitis patients.[29] The use of at least 1.2 g daily of a 5-ASA carried a 72% relative risk reduction for the development of colorectal cancer, when controlled for disease extent, duration, and folic acid use. In contrast, IBD patients on 5-ASA agents followed in Canada did not appear to have the same protective effect.[30]

METHODS TO OPTIMIZE ADHERENCE

Optimizing adherence is most effective when open lines of communication characterize the relationship between physician and patient (Table 10-1). Allowing the patient the time to voice his or her concerns and questions is the first step in effective education. Open-ended questions during a patient visit can be time-consuming, but setting an appropriate tone so as not to overestimate the patient's level of education is paramount in establishing a good relationship. One study from the psychology literature featuring IBD patients revealed that, when asked, their greatest concern was the uncertain nature of their disease.[31] In addition, patients expressed a significant concern about the effect of medications on their disease.

It has been suggested that physicians may overestimate patient comprehension in regard to instructions and education. Martin and colleagues showed that of IBD patients polled, 62% of ulcerative colitis patients felt ill-informed about their disease.[32] Though 86% of patients responding knew of the increased risk of cancer, only 44% knew that it was possible to screen for dysplasia and possible prevention of invasive cancer. Other literature also suggests that nonadherence is linked to patient noncomprehension.[33] A recent study (yet to be published in full form) reported that, in a GI outpatient clinic, 15% of patients did not know how their medication worked; 22% felt dissatisfied with their medications, primarily from unexpected side effects; and 12% admitted that they do not tell their physician all the medications that they take.[34]

A new model of patient adherence has been proposed in which effective patient-physician dialog is central to promoting patient adherence.[35] This theoretical framework is in part supported by findings that higher patient/physician discordance has been associated with unfavorable health outcomes as well as with decreased patient satisfaction, a

TABLE 10-1

METHODS TO ENHANCE PATIENT COMPLIANCE

- Communication regarding medication concerns
- Education about necessity of medications long-term
- Simplification of patient regimens as much as possible
- Provision of patient autonomy and self-management

variable that is related to poorer adherence. In a study of 153 patients, the nonadherence rate for IBD medications within 2 weeks of a clinic visit was 41%.[36] Eighty-one percent of these patients were found to have "nonintentional" nonadherent behavior (ie, forgetfulness or carelessness in taking medication). Intentional nonadherence was found to be associated with patients who were considered "nondistressed" by psychosocial measurements but showed high discordance with their physician in terms of disease activity. The clinical implications of these findings suggest that the therapeutic relationship can influence adherence just as much as individual clinical and psychosocial characteristics.

Simplifying patient regimens is an effective way to increase adherence. A recent pilot feasibility trial assessed short-term outcomes in patients on once-daily mesalamine compared to a conventional (twice or three times daily) regimen for maintenance of ulcerative colitis.[37] Secondary aims included overall medication consumption rates and patient satisfaction. Twenty-two patients were randomized and followed for 6 months. The number of clinical relapses after 6 months was similar in the once-daily and conventional dosing groups. Though there was no statistically significant difference in 6-month adherence rates between the 2 groups, there was a numerical advantage for overall consumption with a once-daily regimen. Patients in the once-daily group were generally more satisfied with their regimen as compared to the conventional dosing patients. There is an emerging trend toward once- and twice-daily dosing.[38,39] A recent study confirms maintenance of remission with once-a-day 1.5-g granulated mesalamine.[40,41]

Patient autonomy is also a means to enhance adherence with medications. Realizing the potential difficulties for long-term adherence with sulfasalazine, Dickinson et al studied continuous versus "on demand" sulfasalazine in 28 patients with quiescent ulcerative colitis.[42] Of the 18 patients in the "on demand" group directed to take 3 g of sulfasalazine per day starting within 24 hours of symptom recurrence, 7 relapsed within the study period and 4 within the first 2 months of the trial. Three of the 10 patients randomized to the continuous group relapsed. Adherence was measured by serum sulfapyridine levels every 4 months

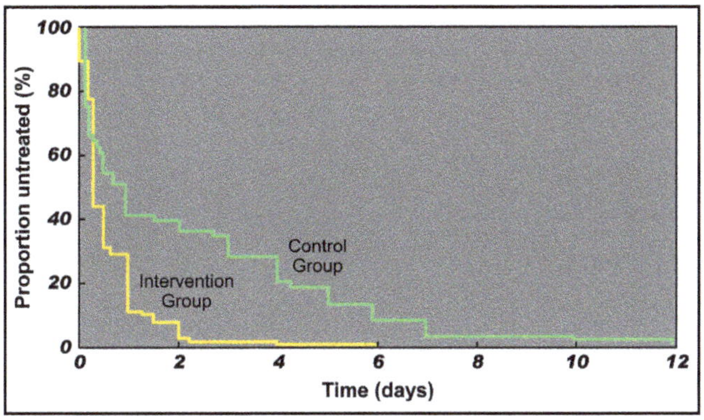

FIGURE 10-3. Self-management leads to improved disease outcomes.

for 1 year or until relapse and was reported as adequate for patients in either group. The authors concluded that because there was no difference in relapse rates between the 2 groups, and because by serologic testing sulfapyridine levels were therapeutic, an "on demand" regimen may be as efficacious as continuous therapy. These results were published as preliminary, and unfortunately no larger studies have been published to date that corroborate these results.

This patient-centered, self-management approach offers the opportunity to improve outcomes through patient education and empowerment. In a British study, 203 patients with UC were randomized to either routine treatment by a specialist or patient-centered self-management in the primary care setting.[43] Patient training included a written algorithm for treatment and a 15- to 30-minute training session. In the self-management group, relapses were treated significantly more rapidly than in the conventional group (14.8 versus 49.6 hours, $P<0.01$), had fewer office visits (0.9 versus 2.9/year, $P<0.01$), and the length of the flares that did occur was shorter (Figure 10-3).

CONCLUSION

Medication nonadherence is prevalent in chronic illnesses, and ulcerative colitis is no exception. The problem is still not well-understood because it is difficult to predict in whom and when nonadherence becomes a clinically important issue. As discussed previously, there are emerging data to show the long-term benefits of adherence, and the risks of nonadherence, with medications or other physician recommendations. Through physician and patient education, the clinical relevance of adherence can be emphasized, and outcomes will be improved in the long-term disease.

REFERENCES

1. An oral preparation of mesalamine as long-term maintenance therapy for ulcerative colitis: a randomized, placebo-controlled trial. The Mesalamine Study Group. *Ann Intern Med.* 1996;124:204-211.
2. Ardizzone S, Petrillo M, Molteni P, et al. Coated oral 5-aminosalicylic acid (Claversal) is equivalent to sulfasalazine for remission maintenance in ulcerative colitis: a double-blind study. *J Clin Gastroenterol.* 1995;21:287-289.
3. Fockens P, Mulder CJ, Tytgat GN, et al. Comparison of the efficacy and safety of 1.5 compared with 3.0 g oral slow-release mesalazine (Pentasa) in the maintenance treatment of ulcerative colitis. Dutch Pentasa Study Group. *Eur J Gastroenterol Hepatol.* 1995;7:1025-1030.
4. Green JR, Gibson JA, Kerr GD, et al. Maintenance of remission of ulcerative colitis: a comparison between balsalazide 3 g daily and mesalazine 1.2 g daily over 12 months. ABACUS Investigator group. *Aliment Pharmacol Ther.* 1998;12:1207-1216.
5. Miner P, Hanauer S, Robinson M, et al. Safety and efficacy of controlled-release mesalamine for maintenance of remission in ulcerative colitis. Pentasa UC Maintenance Study Group. *Dig Dis Sci.* 1995;40:296-304.
6. Miller NH. Compliance with treatment regimens in chronic asymptomatic diseases. *Am J Med.* 1997;102:43-49.
7. Haynes RB. Determinants of compliance: The disease and the mechanisms of treatment. In: Haynes RB, Taynor, DW, Sackett DL, eds. *Compliance in Health Care.* Baltimore, MD: Johns Hopkins University Press; 1979:1-21.
8. Das K, Estwood MA, McManus JPA, et al. The metabolisim of salicylazaosulphapyridine in ulcerative colitis. *Gut.* 1973;14:631-641.
9. Cowan GO, Das KM, Eastwood MA. Further studies of sulphasalazine metabolism in the treatment of ulcerative colitis. *Br Med J.* 1977;2:1057-1059.
10. van Hees PA, van Tongeren JH. Compliance to therapy in patients on a maintenance dose of sulfasalazine. *J Clin Gastroenterol.* 1982;4:333-336.
11. Nigro G, Angelini G, Grosso SB, et al. Psychiatric predictors of noncompliance in inflammatory bowel disease. Psychiatry and compliance. *J Clin Gastroenterol.* 2001;32:66-68.
12. Riley S, Mani V, Goddman MJ, et al. Why do patients with ulcerative colitis relapse? *Gut.* 1990;31:179-183.
13. Farup PG, Hovde O, Halvorsen FA, et al. Mesalazine suppositories versus hydrocortisone foam in patients with distal ulcerative colitis. A comparison of the efficacy and practicality of two topical treatment regimens. *Scand J Gastroenterol.* 1995;30:164-170.
14. Shale MJ, Riley SA. Studies of compliance with delayed-release mesalazine therapy in patients with inflammatory bowel disease. *Aliment Pharmacol Ther.* 2003;18:191-198.
15. Kane SV, Aikens J, Hanauer SB. Medication regimens are associated with nonadherence in quiescent ulcerative colitis. *Am J Gastroenterol.* 2002;97:S770.
16. Kane SV, Crivens L. Infliximab infusions are associated with high adherence rate. *Gastroenterol.* 2004;126:A476.
17. Woolrich AJ, DeSilva MD, Korelitz BI. Surveillance in the routine management of ulcerative colitis: the predictive value of low-grade dysplasia. *Gastroenterology.* 1992;103:431-438.
18. Levenstein L, Prantera C, Luzi C, D'Ubali A. Low residue or normal diet in Crohn's disease: a prospective controlled study in Italian patients. *Gut.* 1985;26:989-993.
19. Imes A, Pinchbeck B, Dinwoodie A, et al. Effect on Ensure, a defined formula diet, in patients with Crohn's disease. *Digestion.* 1986;35:158-169.
20. Lorenz-Mayer H, Bauer P, Nicolay C, et al. Omega-3 fatty acids and low carbohydrate diet for maintenance of remission in Crohn's disease: a randomized controlled multicenter trial. *Scan J Gastroenterol.* 1996;31:778-785.
21. Kane SV, Aikens J, Huo D, et al. Medication adherence is associated with improved outcomes in patients with quiescent ulcerative colitis. *Am J Med.* 2003;113:39-42.

22. Kane SV. Medication adherence and the physician-patient relationship. *Am J Gastroenterol.* 2002;97:1853.
23. Cosnes J, Beaugerie L, Carbonnel F, et al. Smoking cessation and the course of Crohn's disease: an intervention study. *Gastroenterology.* 2001;120:1093-1099.
24. Moody GA, Jayanthi V, Probert CS, et al. Long-term therapy with sulphasalazine protects against colorectal cancer in ulcerative colitis: a retrospective study of colorectal cancer risk and compliance with treatment in Leicestershire. *Eur J Gastroenterol Hepatol.* 1996;8:1179-1183.
25. Pinczowski D, Ekbom A, Baron J, et al. Risk factors for colorectal cancer in patients with ulcerative colitis: a case-control study. *Gastroenterology.* 1994;107:117-120.
26. Velayos FS, Terdiman JP, Walsh JM. Effect of 5-aminosalicylate use on colorectal cancer and dysplasia risk: a systematic review and metaanalysis of observational studies. *Am J Gastroenterol.* 2005;100:1345-1353.
27. Eaden J, Abrams K, Ekbom A, et al. Colorectal cancer prevention in ulcerative colitis: a case-control study. *Aliment Pharmacol Ther.* 2000;14:145-153.
28. Matula S, Croog V, Itzkowitz S, et al. Chemoprevention of colorectal neoplasia in ulcerative colitis: the effect of 6-mercaptopurine. *Clin Gastroenterol Hepatol.* 2005;3:1015-1021.
29. Rubin DT, LoSavio A, Yadron N, Huo D, Hanauer SB. Aminosalicylate therapy in the prevention of dysplasia and colorectal cancer in ulcerative colitis. *Clin Gastroenterol Hepatol.* 2006;4:1346-1350.
30. Bernstein CN, Blanchard JF, Metge C, et al. Does the use of 5-aminosalicylates in inflammatory bowel disease prevent the development of colorectal cancer? *Am J Gastroenterol.* 2003;98:2784-2788.
31. Drossman DA, Leserman K, Li Z, et al. The rating form of IBD patient concerns: a new measure of health status. *Psychosom Med.* 1991;53:701-712.
32. Martin A, Leone L, Fries W, et al. What do patients want to know about their inflammatory bowel disease. *Ital J Gastroenterol.* 1992;24:477-480.
33. Levy R, Feld AD. Increasing patient adherence to gastroenterology treatment and prevention regimens. *Am J Gastroenterol.* 1999;94:1733-1742.
34. Kane SV, Dang J. Medication taking behavior in a gastroenterology clinic: a disconnect between patient behavior and physician knowledge. *Gastroenterology.* 2004;126:A605.
35. Nobel LM. Doctor-patient communication and adherence to treatment. In: Myers LB, Midence K, eds. *Adherence to Treatment in Medical Conditions.* New York, NY: Harwood Academic Publishers; 1998:51-82.
36. Sewitch MJ, Abrahamowicz M, Barkun A, et al. Patient nonadherence to medication in inflammatory bowel disease. *Am J Gastroenterol.* 2003;98:1535-1544.
37. Kane SV, Huo D, Magnanti K. A pilot feasibility trial of once daily versus conventional dosing of mesalamine for treatment of ulcerative colitis. *Clin Gastroenterol Hepatol.* 2003;1:170-173.
38. Rubin DT, Rosen AA, Sedghi S, et al. Twice-daily balsalazide tablets improve patient quality of life after 2 and 8 weeks of treatment: results of a phase 3, randomized, double-blind, placebo-controlled, multicenter study [Abstract T1147]. *Gastroenterology.* 2008;134(Suppl 1):A494.
39. Bosworth BP, Pruitt RE, Gordon GL, et al. Balsalazide tablets 3.3 g twice daily improves signs and symptoms of mild-to moderate ulcerative colitis [abstract T1152]. *Gastroenterology.* 2008;134(Suppl 1):A495.
40. Lichtenstein G, Merchant K, Shaw A, Yuan J, Bortey E, Forbes W. Once-daily 1.5-g granulated mesalamine effectively maintains remission in patients with ulcerative colitis who switch from different 5-ASA formulations [abstract 1100]. *Am J Gastroenterol.* 2008;13(Suppl 1):s429-s430.
41. Kruis W, Kiudelis G, Racz I, et al. Once-daily versus three-times-daily mesalazine granules in active ulcerative colitis: a double-blind, double-dummy, randomised non-inferiority trial. *Gut.* 2009;58(2):233-240.
42. Dickinson RJ, King A, Wight DG, et al. Is continuous sulfasalazine necessary in the management of patients with ulcerative colitis? Results of a preliminary study. *Dis Colon Rectum.* 1985;28:929-930.
43. Robinson A, Thompson DG, Wilkin D, et al. Guided self-management and patient-directed follow-up of ulcerative colitis: a randomized trial. *Lancet.* 2001;358:976-981.

SECTION II

MEDICATIONS

General Principles of Medical Therapy of Ulcerative Colitis

Sonia Friedman, MD, FACP

Introduction

Ulcerative colitis (UC) is a chronic gastrointestinal disease that affects patients in the prime of their lives. In the United States alone, UC affects approximately 250,000 to 500,000 people with an incidence of 2 to 7 per 100,000 population per year. Most patients need to take chronic medications from diagnosis until death. Because UC almost always begins in the rectum, many patients need to take topical therapy in addition to multiple pills a day, which can have a significant impact on quality of life in addition to the disease process itself. Most patients with UC will have a normal lifespan and thus the medicine they take must be safe, have few side effects, and have simple dosing routines to which they adhere. Different factors such as stress, stopping smoking, NSAID use, and nonadherence to medical therapy can have a significant impact on disease activity, and physicians should take these factors into account when treating UC patients. In addition, different types of patients require different types of medical therapy, and the treatment goals of physicians should reflect those of their patients. Rather than relying solely on the physician's impression of disease activity, simple scales of clinical activity and quality of life can be used in the office to assess a patient's clinical status. This chapter discusses the impact of UC on quality of life and stresses the importance of appropriate and individualized medical therapy. To help physicians determine the efficacy of certain UC medications and reach treatment goals, this chapter offers a practical interpretation of clinical, endoscopic, and quality-of-life endpoints used in clinical trials. Most importantly, it provides a summary of the currently accepted medical therapies and recommendations for using these therapies in clinical practice.

Impact of Ulcerative Colitis on Quality of Life

Given its young age of onset, morbidity, and side effects of medical therapy, UC has a significant impact on quality of life. The McMaster Inflammatory Bowel Disease Questionnaire (long-form IBDQ) has been used to assess quality of life in both UC and Crohn's disease (CD) patients.[1] It is an inflammatory bowel disease (IBD)-specific instrument used in many clinical trials. Although it is a 32-item questionnaire, there is also a short form (short-form IBDQ) with 10 questions that has also been validated (Figure 11-1). The short-form IBDQ measures systemic and bowel symptoms, social impairment, and emotional health.[2] It is ideal for office use, and a patient's quality of life can be tracked from visit to visit. When compared to the general population, UC patients have an impaired quality of life in all 4 categories. The most frequent concerns of a UC patient are having an ostomy bag, developing cancer, the uncertain nature of the disease, and the need for surgery. In a recent quality of life study using the long-form IBDQ, symptom severity, rheumatic symptoms, and female gender were the strongest predictors of decreased quality of life.[3] All were statistically significant. In addition, active IBD (either UC or CD) has a negative impact on labor force participation,[4] personal relationships, and sexual health.[5]

Lichtenstein GR, ed.
Ulcerative Colitis: The Complete Guide to Medical Management (pp. 121-134).

This questionnaire is designed to find out how you have been feeling during the last 2 weeks. You will be asked about symptoms you have been having as a result of your inflammatory bowel disease, the way you have been feeling in general, and how your mood has been.

1. How often has the feeling of fatigue or of being tired and worn out been a problem for you during the last 2 weeks? Please indicate how often the feeling of fatigue or tiredness has been a problem for you during the last 2 weeks by picking one option: *(social)*
   1. All the time
   2. Most of the time
   3. A good bit of the time
   4. Some of the time
   5. A little of the time
   6. Hardly any of the time
   7. None of the time
2. How often during the last 2 weeks have you had to delay or cancel a social engagement because of your bowel problem? Please choose an option: *(social)*
   1. All the time
   2. Most of the time
   3. A good bit of the time
   4. Some of the time
   5. A little of the time
   6. Hardly any of the time
   7. None of the time
3. How much difficulty have you had, as a result of your bowel problems, doing leisure or sports activities you would have liked to have done during the last 2 weeks? Please choose an option: *(social)*
   1. A great deal of difficulty, activities made impossible
   2. A lot of difficulty
   3. A fair bit of difficulty
   4. Some difficulty
   5. A little difficulty
   6. Hardly any difficulty
   7. No difficulty; the bowel problems did not limit sports or leisure activities
4. How often during the last 2 weeks have you been troubled by pain in the abdomen? Please choose an option: *(bowel)*
   1. All of the time
   2. Most of the time
   3. A good bit of the time
   4. Some of the time
   5. A little of the time
   6. Hardly any of the time
   7. None of the time
5. How often during the last 2 weeks have you felt depressed or discouraged? Please choose an option: *(emotional)*
   1. All of the time
   2. Most of the time
   3. A good bit of the time
   4. Some of the time
   5. A little of the time
   6. Hardly any of the time
   7. None of the time
6. Overall, in the last 2 weeks, how much of a problem have you had with passing large amounts of gas? Please choose an option: *(bowel)*
   1. A major problem
   2. A big problem
   3. A significant problem
   4. Some trouble
   5. A little trouble
   6. Hardly any trouble
   7. No trouble
7. Overall, in the last 2 weeks, how much of a problem have you had maintaining or getting to the weight you would like to be? Please choose an option: *(systemic)*
   1. A major problem
   2. A big problem
   3. A significant problem
   4. Some trouble
   5. A little trouble
   6. Hardly any trouble
   7. No trouble
8. How often during the last 2 weeks have you felt relaxed and free of tension? Please choose an option: *(emotional)*
   1. None of the time
   2. A little of the time
   3. Some of the time
   4. A good bit of the time
   5. Most of the time
   6. Almost all of the time
   7. All of the time
9. How much of the time during the last 2 weeks have you been troubled by a feeling of having to go to the bathroom even though your bowels were empty? Please choose an option: *(bowel)*
   1. All of the time
   2. Most of the time
   3. A good bit of the time
   4. Some of the time
   5. A little of the time
   6. Hardly any of the time
   7. None of the time
10. How much of the time during the last 2 weeks have you felt angry as a result of your bowel problem? Please choose an option: *(emotional)*
    1. All of the time
    2. Most of the time
    3. A good bit of the time
    4. Some of the time
    5. A little of the time
    6. Hardly any of the time
    7. None of the time

FIGURE 11-1. Short quality of life in inflammatory bowel disease questionnaire (SIBDQ).

Stool frequency
0 = Normal number of stools for this patient
1 = 1-2 more stools than normal
2 = 3-4 more stools than normal
3 = 5 or more stools than normal

Findings of endoscopy
0 = Normal or inactive disease
1 = Mild disease (erythema, decreased vascular pattern, mild friability)
2 = Moderate disease (marked erythema, absent vascular pattern, friability, erosions)
3 = Severe disease (spontaneous bleeding, ulceration)

Rectal bleeding
0 = No blood seen
1 = Streaks of blood with stool less than half the time
2 = Obvious blood with stool most of the time
3 = Blood alone passed

Physician's global assessment
0 = Normal
1 = Mild disease
2 = Moderate disease
3 = Severe disease

FIGURE 11-2. The Mayo scoring system for assessment of ulcerative colitis activity.

MEASURES OF DISEASE ACTIVITY IN ULCERATIVE COLITIS

There have been many measures of disease activity that have been used in clinical UC trials. Truelove and Witts developed the first clinical activity index with disease classified as mild, moderate, or severe based on a variety of clinical, physical, and laboratory parameters.[6] Powell-Tuck et al incorporated additional variables, but their index has not been used extensively.[7] One of the most useful validated indices is the Mayo scoring system for assessment of UC activity (Figure 11-2).[8] It is quick and easy to use in the office to track a patient's symptoms. The Mayo index is realistic as it relies heavily on the patient's rather than the physician's assessment of disease. It takes into account stool frequency, rectal bleeding, endoscopic findings, and the physician's global assessment. The physician's global assessment acknowledges the 3 other criteria: the patient's recall of abdominal pain, general sense of well-being, and the patient's performance status. Patients in remission score less than or equal to 2 points and generally have solid bowel movements, no blood, and normal mucosa on endoscopy. Those with severe activity score 11 or 12 points and generally have multiple bloody bowel movements a day, spontaneous bleeding, and frank ulcerations on endoscopy. A partial Mayo score without endoscopy can be used to quickly assess disease activity.

THE PLACEBO EFFECT

In any discussion of medical therapy for UC, the placebo effect should be considered. Simply put, some patients get better without medical therapy. The disease course itself waxes and wanes, and patients may improve for reasons other than an added medication. There have been no observational studies of untreated UC patients, so all of the literature on the placebo effect comes from the placebo arm of randomized, controlled trials. In the largest systemic review and meta-analysis of the placebo response in 40 studies of UC, the clinical remission rate with placebo alone was 13% (95% confidence interval [CI] 9% to 18%) and the response rate was 28% (95% CI 23% to 33%).[9] The placebo remission rate was greater in trials with more frequent study visits, longer duration of follow-up, and longer duration of disease.

GENERAL PRINCIPLES OF MEDICAL THERAPY OF ULCERATIVE COLITIS

In choosing the correct medicine to treat UC, disease extent and activity should first be taken into account. UC involves the rectum in 95% of cases and may extend proximally in a symmetrical, circumferential, and continuous pattern to affect part or all of the large intestine. The major symptoms of UC are diarrhea, rectal bleeding, tenesmus, passage of mucous, and crampy abdominal pain. The severity of symptoms correlates with the extent of disease. Approximately 40% to 50% of patients have disease limited to the rectum and rectosigmoid, 30% to 40% have disease extending beyond the sigmoid but not involving the whole colon, and 20% have the presence of pancolitis. Patients with proctitis usually pass fresh blood or blood-stained mucous, either mixed with stool or streaked onto the surface of a normal or hard stool. They also have tenesmus, or urgency with a feeling of incomplete evacuation. They rarely have abdominal pain. With proctitis or proctosigmoiditis, proximal transit slows, which may account for the constipation that is commonly seen in patients with distal disease.

TABLE 11-1

ULCERATIVE COLITIS: DISEASE PRESENTATION

	MILD	MODERATE	SEVERE
Bowel movements	<4/day	4 to 6/day	>6/day
Blood in stool	Small	Moderate	Severe
Fever	None	<37.5°C mean	>37.5°C mean
Tachycardia	None	<90 mean pulse	>90 mean pulse
Anemia	Mild	>75%	≤75%
Sedimentation rate	<30 mm	>30 mm	

When disease extends beyond the rectum, blood is usually mixed with stool, or patients may have grossly bloody diarrhea. When the disease is severe, patients pass a liquid stool containing blood, pus, and fecal matter. Diarrhea is often nocturnal or postprandial. Severe cramping and abdominal pain can occur in association with severe attacks of the disease. Other symptoms in mild to moderate disease include anorexia, nausea, vomiting, fever, and weight loss. Other distinguishing features of mild, moderate, and severe disease are found in Table 11-1.

MEDICAL MANAGEMENT OF MILD TO MODERATE DISTAL COLITIS

5-ASA Agents: Topical Preparations

Patients with left-sided colitis have disease that is amenable to treatment with topical agents. These agents are extremely useful, yet often forgotten, first-line agents in treating distal disease. Suppositories can deliver mesalamine up to 20 cm from the anal verge, and enemas can deliver mesalamine up to the splenic flexure. Mesalamine foam has been tested in European studies. It is well-tolerated and just as effective as mesalamine enema preparations.[10,11] Remission rates for mesalamine suppositories, foam, and enemas vary between 50% and 75%. A recent meta-analysis confirmed that topical mesalamine is superior to placebo, oral mesalamine, and topical corticosteroids in inducing remission in left-sided UC.[12] Increased doses of topical mesalamine are not associated with increased remission rates over time. In fact, a trial assessing the efficacy of mesalamine enemas in nonrefractory patients with UC demonstrated that doses of 1, 2, and 4 g were equally efficacious for the induction of remission.[13] A combination of topical mesalamine and topical corticosteroids is superior to either therapy alone and is helpful in patients refractory to one or the other formulation.[14] Combination topical and oral mesalamine is superior to either therapy alone. A combination of oral mesalamine 2.4 g/d and 4 g/d of mesalamine enema was more effective in achieving clinical improvement than either agent alone.[15] A more recent study showed combination oral mesalamine 4 g/d and 1 g/d mesalamine enema more effective than oral therapy alone.[16]

For the maintenance of remission in left-sided UC, topical mesalamine is just as effective as oral preparations. Mesalamine suppositories in doses of 500 mg daily or twice a day are effective in maintaining remission with twice-a-day dosing being more effective. Ten percent of patients treated twice a day relapsed at 1 year, compared to 36% who did once-daily dosing.[17,18] The 500-mg suppository is now discontinued and has been replaced by 1000-mg once-daily suppositories. Mesalamine enemas in doses of 2 to 4 g maintained remission when dosed daily (78% effective), every other day (72% effective), or even every third day (65% effective).[12] The combination of oral mesalamine 1.6 g/d and mesalamine enema 2 g twice a week was more effective than the oral mesalamine alone.[19]

5-ASA Agents: Oral Preparations

Although topical therapy is the most effective treatment for distal UC, some patients complain of leakage, problems with retention, cramps, and bloating. Oral 5-ASA therapy is a viable alternative and can at least help decrease the frequency of topical preparations. The oral aminosalicylates include azo-bond conjugates (sulfasalazine, olsalazine, balsalazide), pH-dependent mesalamine with varied Eudragit (USP) coatings (Asacol, Apriso, Salofalk, Claversal; the last two are not available in the United States), and time-pH release formulations of mesalamine encapsulated into ethocellulose beads (Pentasa). Side effects of mesalamine agents and balsalazide are similar. Sulfasalazine is associated with well-recognized sulfapyride-induced toxicities; these include nausea, vomiting, dyspepsia, anorexia, and headache. More severe but less common side effects include allergic reactions, pancreatitis, hepatotoxicity, drug-induced connective tissue disease, bone marrow suppression, interstitial nephritis, hemolytic anemia, or megaloblastic anemia. Abnormal sperm counts, motility, and morphology are related to the sulfapyridine moiety and are not seen with the other mesalamine preparations. All patients taking sulfasalazine should be supplemented with folic acid 1 mg/d. Olsalazine is associated with a dose-dependent diarrhea in 18% of patients. All agents can cause an interstitial nephritis that is not dose-related. The rare risks of nephropathy, hepatotoxicity, pancreatitis, pulmonitis, and pericarditis require semiannual or annual therapeutic monitoring. Lialda (Multi Matrix [MMX] mesalamine) is a novel, once-daily high-strength (1.2-g tablet) formulation of mesalamine, utilizing MMX Multi Matrix System technology designed to deliver the active drug throughout the colon. Two studies have shown MMX mesalamine, given either once or twice a day in 2.4 g/d or 4.8 g/d doses, to be more effective than placebo.[20,21] This formulation is currently approved by the US Food and Drug Administration (FDA) for treatment of active ulcerative colitis with a dose of 2.4 to 4.8 g daily. A granulated formulation of mesalamine called Apriso (that releases mesalamine at a pH $\geq$6) that is administered once daily has recently been approved by the FDA at a dose of 1.5 g daily (4 375-mg capsules).[22,23] There is also a twice-daily 1.1-g formulation of balsalazide (GIAZO) under development.[24,25]

There are currently no data to support the superiority of one formulation over another in treating left-sided UC. There has been no study designed to assess the efficacy of one mesalamine derivative over another in the setting of left-sided UC. The recently updated Cochrane analysis found no difference in efficacy between oral 5-ASA drugs compared with sulfasalazine for the induction of remission.[26] There has been recent controversy, however, regarding the superiority of balsalazide in treating left-sided UC. In a trial by Green et al comparing mesalamine 2.4 g/d and balsalazide 6.75 g/d, balsalazide was superior in the induction of complete remission with a significantly shorter time to complete relief of symptoms.[27] This trial also suggested that left-sided UC patients responded better to balsalazide than mesalamine. Two later trials, however, showed similar efficacy of balsalazide 6.75 g/d and mesalamine 2.4 g/d in inducing remission in mild to moderate UC.[28,29] Patients with left-sided colitis have slow transit of stool in the right colon. One mechanism that might account for a postulated increased efficacy of azo-bond prodrugs in left-sided UC is the increased small intestinal secretion (shown with olsalazine and recently with sulfasalazine and balsalazide) and subsequent loosening of stools. This would allow more medication to be delivered to the inflamed left colon. The 5-ASA preparations are summarized in Table 11-2.

Corticosteroids: Topical Agents

Topical corticosteroids, available in the United States as a 100-mg hydrocortisone enema and a 10% hydrocortisone foam, are effective in acute therapy of distal UC but have not been effective in maintaining remission.[12] Budesonide, a corticosteroid that undergoes first-pass hepatic metabolism, has also been evaluated.[30] However, the optimal 2-g enema dose is not yet available in the United States. European studies have compared budesonide enemas and foam to the equivalent hydrocortisone or prednisolone formulations.[31] Each preparation is equally efficacious in inducing remission in distal UC. No steroid preparations have shown efficacy in maintaining remission.

Novel Agents for Left-Sided Disease

The most novel topical agent is epidermal growth factor (EGF) used as an enema in mild to moderate left-sided UC. EGF is a potent mitogenic peptide produced by salivary and duodenal Brunner's glands, which stimulates several components of the healing response. It enhances healing of skin wounds and, when given systemically, has shown to be beneficial for necrotizing enterocolitis in neonates. In the only human trial in UC, Sinha et al show a statistically significant remission rate at 2, 4, and 12 weeks.[32] In the future, this may be an option in patients with refractory disease. Because EGF influences the growth and repair of tissue, the long-term risk of colonic dysplasia and neoplasia with this drug still must be assessed.

Oral Steroids for Treating Left-Sided Colitis

Left-sided colitis may be more refractory in certain patients to treatment than extensive or pancolitis, and some patients will require oral prednisone to induce a remission. The usual starting dose is 40 mg of prednisone a day, usually in 1 or 2 divided doses.[33] There have been no randomized, placebo-controlled trials performed assessing the dose-response of various doses of oral corticosteroids in patients with IBD. An occasional patient may be refractory to 40 mg/d; in this case, the dose should be increased to 60 mg/d. Prednisone should be given at 40 mg/d or 60 mg/d until remission is achieved (usually 1 to 2 weeks) and tapered by 5 mg/week. There is no standard tapering schedule; many physicians will taper initially by 5 to 10 mg/week and then by 5 mg/week once a dose of 30 mg/d is reached. Steroids should be used in the acute setting only; they play no role in remission maintenance. Limited disease extent

TABLE 11-2

5-ASA PREPARATIONS

PREPARATION	FORMULATION	DELIVERY	DOSING (PER DAY)
Oral 5-ASA Preparations			
Azo-bond			
Sulfasalazine (500 mg) (Azulfidine)	Sulfapyridine-5-ASA	Colon	3 to 6 g (acute) 2 to 4 g (maintenance)
Olsalazine (250 mg) (Dipentum)	5-ASA-5-ASA	Colon	1 to 3 g
Balsalazide (750 mg) (Colazal)	Aminobenzoyl-alanine-5-ASA	Colon	6.75 to 9 g
Delayed-release			
Mesalamine (400, 800 mg) (Asacol)	Eudragit S (pH 7)	Distal ileum-colon	2.4 to 4.8 g (acute) 1.6 to 4.8 g (maintenance)
Claversal/Mesasal/Salofalk (250, 500 mg)	Eudragit L (pH 6)	Ileum-colon	1.5 to 3 g (acute) 1.5 to 3 g (maintenance)
Lialda (1.2 g)	(MMX mesalamine) (SPD476)	Ileum-colon	2.4 to 4.8 g
Sustained-release			
Mesalamine (375 mg) (Apriso)	Intellicor extended release	Ileum-colon	1.5 g (maintenance)
Rectal 5-ASA Preparations			
Mesalamine suppository (400, 500, 1000 mg) (Canasa)		Rectum	1 to 1.5 g (acute) 500 mg to 1 g (maintenance)
Mesalamine enema (1, 4 g) (Rowasa)	60 mL, 100 mL suspension	Rectum-splenic flexure	1 to 4 g (acute) 1 g/d to 3 g/week (maintenance)

should not deter the physician from using the full armamentarium of drugs to induce a remission. Intravenous (IV) corticosteroids or, even rarely, IV cyclosporine or IV infliximab can be used in patients with severe, refractory, left-sided colitis. The side effects of steroids can affect every organ system of the body, and patients should be cautioned about the risks including infection, hypertension, weight gain, fluid retention, acne, cataracts, emotional lability, myopathy, and osteonecrosis in 4% of patients.[34] The most significant long-term risk is loss of bone density. Bone loss occurs in 31% to 59% of patients with IBD, and steroid therapy compounds this risk.[35] The risk of steroid-induced bone loss is often greatest in the first few weeks of therapy when the highest doses are given, and patients should be started on calcium (1000 to 1500 mg/d) and vitamin D (800 U/d) when steroid therapy is initiated.

The American College of Gastroenterology has recently published guidelines for the diagnosis and management of osteoporosis in IBD.[36] A dual-energy x-ray absorptiometry (DEXA) scan should be considered in IBD patients with risk factors for osteoporosis, such as smoking, low body mass index, sedentary lifestyle, hypogonadism, family history of osteoporosis, and in the presence of nutritional deficiencies. IBD patients over the age of 60 are at greatest risk for fracture, and all of these patients should have DEXA scans done. Patients using corticosteroids beyond 3 months consecutively or who are recurrent users should also have bone density testing done. For patients with a T score of -2.5 or less, an oral bisphosphonate should be considered. A 12-month, randomized, double-blind, placebo-controlled trial with a 10-mg daily dose of alendronate significantly increased bone mineral density in patients with CD.[37] Most IBD patients with osteoporosis should see an endocrinologist to rule out secondary causes of bone loss.

Another often-neglected side effect of steroid therapy is suppression of the hypothalamic-pituitary axis. In a recent paper, 65% of patients had an abnormal cosyntropin test after only 2 to 3 months of a prednisone taper.[38] Hypothalamic-pituitary-adrenal axis suppression was noted in 30% to 100% of patients after receiving 2 to 8 weeks of topical steroid enemas (hydrocortisone, betamethasone phosphate, or prednisolone).[39-42] Physicians should be aware of this side effect, and some physicians actually suggest checking a cosyntropin test before discontinuing steroids.

MEDICAL MANAGEMENT OF MILD TO MODERATE EXTENSIVE COLITIS

5-ASA Agents: Oral Preparations

5-ASA agents are the first-line therapy for inducing remission in extensive mild to moderate UC. They may work by inhibiting activation of the transcription factor NF-κB, resulting in the suppression of proinflammatory gene expression in the inflamed mucosa.[43] The efficacy of sulfasalazine was demonstrated more than 40 years ago, and at daily doses of 2 to 6 g, it induces remission or clinical improvement in 64% to 80% of patients. The greater the dose, the greater the efficacy, and some patients require 6 to 8 g/d to induce a remission.[44-47] As detailed above, sulfasalazine has dose-limiting side effects, and 25% to 30% of patients will need to be switched to sulfa-free 5-ASA medications.

With the newer mesalamine derivatives, more 5-ASA can safely be delivered to the colon without dose-dependent side effects. These compounds are effective in inducing remission in 40% to 74% of UC patients in daily doses of 1.5 to 4.8 g. No study has determined the optimal mesalamine dosage, but in general, there is a dose-response curve with higher doses inducing higher rates of remission.[47-49] Balsalazide, olsalazine, and mesalamine are all equivalent to sulfasalazine when used at equal dosages.[28,50] In clinical practice, patients with more severe disease will require higher doses of 5-ASA agents than those with milder disease. Because the sulfa-free 5-ASA preparations are so safe and have so few side effects, physicians are free to increase the dosage as needed. Once-daily formulations of mesalamine have been effective in inducing remission in patients with mild to moderate UC.[21-23] Topical, in addition to oral, treatment still plays a role in extensive colitis by reducing symptoms of urgency, tenesmus, and distal inflammation.[15,16]

A maintenance regimen is almost always required when the initial attack is controlled. Clinical trials have tested various dosages for remission maintenance, and a recent meta-analysis showed that mesalamine at dosages from 0.8 to 4 g/d was superior in preventing relapse of disease, with a pooled OR of 0.47 (95% CI 0.36 to 0.62) and a number needed to treat of 6.[51] In this trial, a dose-dependent trend was not observed. Conversely, another trial showed the superiority of 3 g/d versus 1.5 g/d of mesalazine for maintaining remission.[52] The first once-daily formulation for maintenance of remission in patients with moderate to severe UC has been approved for use in patients in remission by using a granulated mesalamine formulation.[22,23] No trial published thus far has taken into account the severity and extent of inflammation nor the agent used to induce remission. In general, induction trials have not been connected to maintenance trials; each has been done independently. Many experts advocate that the doses of aminosalicylates used to induce remission should be used to maintain remission. There have been no blinded trials performed assessing this concept.

One of the problems with using 5-ASA agents is adherence to medications. Patients need to take large numbers of pills and often forget their midday dose. In one study, only about 40% of UC patients were adherent with mesalamine maintenance therapy.[53] Patients who were nonadherent had a higher risk of relapse than those who consumed more than 80% of their prescribed regimen.[54] Once-daily dosing of mesalamine was shown in a pilot study to improve adherence,[55] and studies are ongoing as to whether once-daily dosing also improves disease outcome.[20,21]

Oral/Topical Steroids

Prednisone at a starting dose of 40 mg/d should be used when a patient is flaring despite maximal 5-ASA therapy. The dose should be increased to 60 mg/d if 40 mg/d fails and continued until remission is achieved, usually for 1 or 2 weeks. The taper schedule is the same as in left-sided UC. Topical steroids are also helpful for symptoms of urgency and tenesmus, especially in patients who fail topical 5-ASA agents. Because mesalamine foam is not available in the United States, cortifoam is sometimes very helpful in controlling rectal symptoms. As opposed to enema therapy, patients do not often complain of leakage or incontinence with foam preparations. Given the severe side effects of oral steroids as detailed previously, it is comforting to know that, in population-based studies, only about a third of patients have required systemic steroid therapy. In a large population-based study, 63 of 185 UC patients (34%) required steroid therapy. Thirty-four of 63 (54%) UC patients went into complete remission, and 19 of 63 (30%) achieved partial remission after treatment with oral prednisone.[56] One-year outcomes for UC were prolonged response in 31 of 63 (49%), corticosteroid dependence in 14 of 63 (22%), and operation in 18 of 63 (29%). There is no role for steroids in maintaining remission in UC.

6-Mercaptopurine and Azathioprine

For steroid-dependent or refractory UC patients, 6-MP and AZA are attractive therapeutic options. Clinical experience and a handful of clinical trials demonstrate their usefulness as steroid-sparing agents and as maintenance therapy after induction of remission with IV cyclosporine. In a retrospective study from Mount Sinai Hospital of 105 refractory chronic UC patients, complete clinical remission was maintained with 6-MP in 68 patients (65%) and partial remission in 25 (24%).[57] Twelve patients (11%) failed to achieve remission. Patients in complete remission tapered off steroids completely, and those in partial remission tapered off 50% of their steroid dose. Of the complete responders who discontinued 6-MP, 87% relapsed. The use of AZA in corticosteroid-resistant and corticosteroid-dependent UC was demonstrated in a retrospective analysis of 56 patients, all of whom were taking steroids when AZA was initiated. Remission with complete elimination of corticosteroids was achieved in more than 60% of patients with continued AZA treatment.[58] The optimal duration of treatment with 6-MP/AZA is unknown, but 1 study suggests that patients should be treated indefinitely.[59] 6-MP/AZA are also useful in left-sided UC patients who cannot be weaned off steroids.

Common mistakes made by physicians when using these immunomodulators include underdosing them or stopping them after a period of time. Often, patients are started too late in the course of disease, after multiple courses of steroids, or are not started at all—even when unable to taper steroids after many months.[60] Current practice is to continue 6-MP/AZA long-term to maintain remission. Patients will often express concern about continuing to take these medications, but, thus far, there is no conclusive evidence that the drugs themselves are carcinogenic.[61] In a meta-analysis of 6 studies, Kandiel et al found a pooled relative risk of lymphoma of 4.18 in patients with CD on AZA or 6-MP. However, it is unknown whether this increased risk is due to the medications or the underlying CD.[62-64] Connell et al did not observe an increased risk of cancer over that expected in a population of 755 patients treated over a 30-year period of time.[65] Present et al reported a 3% rate of malignant lymphoma, with the incidence and type of tumors similar to those expected in the general population.[66] One study by Lewis et al showed that the benefits of AZA outweigh the risks even if there is assumed to be a 3-fold risk of lymphoma, and all patients who get lymphoma die[67]; and another found no increased risk of lymphoma with 6-MP use among IBD patients.[68] In population-based studies, there is a small increased risk of lymphoma, but this is associated with CD itself and not use of 6-MP/AZA.[69] A Mayo Clinic study found a slightly increased risk of Epstein-Barr virus-positive lymphoma in IBD patients treated with 6-MP/AZA.[70] However, there have been no specific studies examining the risk of lymphoma with different doses or duration of 6-MP/AZA. In addition, there are no data that examine the risk of a 6-MP/AZA-induced malignancy in patients with a personal or family history of cancer, and, in this case, 6-MP/AZA should be given only after consultation with the patient's oncologist.

Dosing of 6-MP/AZA is fairly straightforward after checking thiopurine methyltransferase (TPMT) genotype and phenotype. Checking TPMT genetics will not only help patients reach therapeutic levels more quickly than the usual 6 to 12 weeks, but will also help avoid severe toxicity in a handful of patients. TPMT is responsible for drug metabolism, and 1 in 300 individuals lack activity of this enzyme. An additional 11% of the population is heterozygote with intermediate enzyme activity. Both types are at increased risk of toxicity because of increased accumulation of thioguanine metabolites. There are physicians who advocate that patients who are homozygous (ie, wild type) for TPMT or who have normal TPMT enzyme activity should be dosed initially (after a small test dose for 2 weeks) at 1 to 1.5 mg/kg for 6-MP and 2 to 2.5 mg/kg for AZA.[71] 6-thioguanine (6-TG) and 6-methylmercaptopurine (6-MMP) levels can be checked to assess adherence and adequate dosage.

Although AZA and 6-MP are usually well-tolerated, pancreatitis occurs in 1% to 2% of patients, typically presents within the first few weeks of therapy, and is always completely reversible when the drug is stopped. Other side effects include nausea, fever, rash, and hepatitis. Some patients can be switched from 6-MP to AZA and vice versa if the side effect is nausea and vomiting and not fever or pancreatitis. Bone marrow suppression (particularly leukopenia) is dose related and often delayed, necessitating regular monitoring of the patient's complete blood count. In a recent analysis of patients who developed leukopenia,[72] it was found that those who are homozygous-deficient will have leukopenia develop within 6 weeks. It should be noted, however, that leukopenia in those individuals who do not lack the enzyme may develop months to several years later without any specific identifiable pattern. Thus, complete blood counts should be performed at approximately 2, 4, and 8 weeks after initiating therapy, regardless of TPMT status, and continued at least every 3 months thereafter. Liver enzymes should be tested concurrently. The complete blood count should be repeated every several months thereafter or every 2 weeks after a dose adjustment. 6-MP metabolite levels can be determined after 2 to 4 weeks of therapy or after a dose change, when a steady state is reached.

There may be a role for combination therapy with 5-ASA agents and 6-MP/AZA especially in patients who have high TPMT activity and thus overproduction of 6-MMP. Mesalamine theoretically inhibits TPMT, shunting more drug to 6-TG while reducing 6-MMP production. Because 6-TG had been shown to be the most important factor associated with treatment efficacy, adding mesalamine may allow more patients to achieve a therapeutic benefit with 6-MP/AZA.[73,74]

Nicotine

Current smokers are not as likely to develop UC as nonsmokers in the general population. Former smokers are more likely to develop the disease when compared with nonsmoker controls.[75] Former smokers, when compared with nonsmokers, are diagnosed at a younger age and have a greater degree of active disease at the time of diagnosis. Controlled trials have demonstrated that transdermal nicotine patches are effective in achieving clinical improvement[76] and remission[77] in mild to moderate UC with a dose-response effect between 15 and 25 mg of nicotine daily. Former smokers achieved greater benefit from the nicotine patch and tolerated it better. Transdermal nicotine in a daily dose of 15 mg/d was not effective in maintaining remission.[78] Side effects can be dose limiting and include contact dermatitis, lightheadedness, dizziness, nausea, and vomiting. Efficacy is generally less than that of 5-ASA agents (39% clinical improvement vs 9% placebo in one randomized, placebo-controlled trial).[76]

MEDICAL MANAGEMENT OF SEVERE TO FULMINANT COLITIS

Corticosteroids

The mainstays of treatment for severe UC are bowel rest, nutrition, and IV steroids. Typical starting regimens include hydrocortisone 100 mg IV q8h, prednisolone 30 mg IV q12h, and methylprednisolone 16 to 20 mg IV q8h. Although not proven to be superior to bolus infusions,[79] all 3 regimens may be given by continuous 24-hour infusion. IV steroids should be continued for 7 to 10 days until the patient is having solid bowel movements without blood and is taking adequate oral nutrition. A common mistake is to switch to oral prednisone too soon when the patient is not fully in remission. In this scenario, the patient will flare shortly after receiving oral steroids and will have to be rehospitalized. Both oral and IV steroids increase the risk of postoperative infectious complications.[80]

For patients who have not been on any corticosteroids within the previous 30 days, IV adrenocorticotropic hormone (ACTH) 120 units per 24 hours as a continuous infusion may be superior to IV hydrocortisone. One report randomized 66 patients to receive ACTH versus IV hydrocortisone. The remission rate was higher in those treated with ACTH only if they had not been previously treated with steroids (63% versus 27%).[81] In the group who had previously been treated with steroids, hydrocortisone was more effective than ACTH (25% versus 53%). ACTH is now not widely used because of the life-threatening side effect of bilateral adrenal hemorrhage.

Antibiotics

There is no proven role for antibiotics in the management of severe colitis. Controlled trials of intravenous metronidazole[82] and tobramycin[83] have demonstrated no therapeutic benefit when added to IV steroids. Most practice guidelines recommend adding antibiotics only if there are signs of toxicity or worsening symptoms despite maximal medical therapy. Occasionally, patients who are not responding to maximal medical therapy will have a superinfection with cytomegalovirus (CMV). It is important to do a sigmoidoscopy with biopsies and, if positive for CMV, start IV ganciclovir.

Total Parenteral Nutrition

Many physicians will add total parenteral nutrition (TPN) routinely in patients with severe colitis. Controlled trials on this subject, however, show no benefit as a primary therapy for UC.[84,85] In patients who cannot eat or who have significant nutritional deficiencies, TPN may play an adjunctive role.

Cyclosporine

IV cyclosporine CyA is a viable alternative for patients who fail IV corticosteroids.[86] The usual dose is 2 to 4 mg/kg/d given as a continuous IV infusion. High-dose IV cyclosporine (4 mg/kg) had no benefit over low-dose (2 mg/kg) in one large, double-blind, randomized, controlled trial.[87] Because the toxicity of cyclosporine is dose-dependent, and both doses are equally effective, the 2 mg/kg starting dose is recommended. For the 2 mg/kg dose, levels as measured by monoclonal radioimmunoassay or by the high-performance liquid chromatography assay should be maintained between 150 and 350 ng/mL. Levels as measured by the polyclonal radioimmunoassay should be maintained between 300 and 700 ng/mL. Side effects can be serious and include renal insufficiency, hypertension, infection, paresthesias, hypertrichosis, tremor, nausea, gingival hyperplasia, and seizures, especially with low magnesium levels and cholesterol levels less than 120 mg/dL.[88] Ciprofloxacin and metronidazole will increase cyclosporine levels and subsequent toxicity. Because of the risk for opportunistic infections with *Pneumocystis carinii*, one double-strength tablet 3 times a week of trimethoprim sulfamethoxazole should be given.

In one placebo-controlled, double-blind trial, 82% of patients with severe, steroid-refractory UC treated with IV CyA 4 mg/kg/d improved and were able to avoid colectomy in the short term.[86] Lower doses of cyclosporine (2 mg/kg/d) were equally effective with response rates of 87.5% and 85.7%, respectively.[87,89] Oral microemulsion cyclosporine[90,91] can also be successful in treating severe UC with response rates of 85% to 100% in 2 studies. As a single therapy, IV cyclosporine alone can be more successful than IV corticosteroids. In a Belgian study, 8 (53%) of 15 patients on IV methylprednisolone versus 9 (64%) of 14 patients on IV cyclosporine responded after 8 days.[90] At 12 months, 3 (37%) of 8 patients who initially received methylprednisolone maintained their remission on AZA versus 7 (78%) of 9 patients who initially received cyclosporine.[92] These data also highlight that 5-ASA should never be used as monotherapy after induction of remission with IV steroids or IV CyA. 6-MP/AZA should be used, often in addition to 5-ASA agents, in this setting. There is no prospective trial that evaluates the addition of 6-MP/AZA to CyA therapy, but retrospective series with follow-up from 3.5 to 5.5 years indicate a significantly higher long-term success rate when 6-MP/AZA is initiated during the oral CyA phase.[93] There are several reports that indicate that cyclosporine and 6-MP/AZA do not increase the risk of perioperative complications should these agents fail and a colectomy is needed.[94-96]

Given its toxicity, cyclosporine has limited indications in UC. If a patient fails to improve on IV corticosteroids after several days to at most a week, CyA should be initiated quickly before the patient gets too sick for any kind of medical therapy. Cyclosporine should not be used when severe colitis is fulminating or exsanguinating, or complicated by perforation, sepsis, or toxic dilatation. Here, the only therapy indicated is immediate colectomy. As determined by multivariable logistic regression analysis, factors on admission that are predictive of a colectomy (either immediate or by 9 months) are high white blood cell count, high percentage of band neutrophils, and a low albumin (<3 mg/dL).[97] Colectomy is sometimes a better option than cyclosporine. In a young person with a first attack of severe colitis, it is reasonable to give cyclosporine a try; but in a patient with decades of steroid dependency and an increasing risk of colon cancer, surgery is the better option. In addition, because of its toxicity, cyclosporine cannot be used as maintenance therapy. In patients who cannot tolerate immunomodulators, cyclosporine may not be worth considering.

Infliximab

Multiple studies show that infliximab can be effective in treating UC. However, no study has addressed whether specific subsets of patients are more likely to respond. Even in the large phase III studies that have been completed, IBD serologic markers have not been measured. The first randomized, placebo-controlled trial of infliximab in UC was in 11 severe steroid-refractory patients.[98] At 2 weeks, 0 of 3 patients (0%) receiving placebo responded and 4 of 8 patients (50%) receiving infliximab at various doses (5 mg/kg, 10 mg/kg, 20 mg/kg) responded. Open-label trials have had mixed results. Kaser et al reported initial clinical improvement in all 6 severe, steroid-refractory patients treated with 4 long-term remissions (mean 5.5 months) after a single dose of 5 mg/kg infliximab.[99] A study by Chey et al also had promising results; 14 of 16 severe refractory patients had initial responses to infliximab.[100] The patient population in this study, however, included patients with prior colon resections, a sigmoid stricture, and possible Crohn's disease. Recently, Su et al published their open-label experience in 27 patients, 33% with steroid-refractory and 37% with steroid-dependent UC. Eighty-nine percent received up to 3 infusions of infliximab, 5 mg/kg.[101] Response rates were significantly worse in the steroid-refractory group (33%) versus the steroid-responsive group (83%).

Since the data from the two large phase III studies (ACT 1 and ACT 2) have been published, it has been demonstrated that there is clearly a role for infliximab in the treatment of UC.[102] The potential risks of using infliximab are present; however, the benefit outweighs these risks in patients with active UC and hence the use of infliximab has been FDA-approved for treatment of these patients. ACT 1 and ACT 2 are randomized, double-blind trials of infliximab (5 mg/kg and 10 mg/kg) versus placebo in 724 patients with moderate to severe UC. In ACT 1, 69% of patients who received 5 mg/kg of infliximab and 61% of those who received 10 mg/kg responded at week 8, versus 37% of those who received placebo ($P<0.001$ for both infliximab arms versus placebo). In ACT 2, 64% (5 mg/kg) and 69% (10 mg/kg) responded at week 8, versus 29% placebo ($P<0.001$ for both comparisons). In both studies, all patients who received infliximab were more likely to have a clinical response at week 30 ($P \leq 0.002$ for both comparisons). In ACT 1, more patients who received infliximab had a clinical response at week 54 (5 mg/kg: 55%, 10 mg/kg: 54%) than those who received placebo (24%) ($P<0.001$). Infliximab also induced statistically significant remissions at weeks 8 and 30 in both ACT 1 (5 mg/kg: 47%, 41%; 10 mg/kg: 39%, 45%; placebo: 18%, 19%) and ACT 2 (5 mg/kg: 41%, 31%; 10 mg/kg: 33%, 43%; placebo: 7%, 13%), and at week 54 in ACT 1 (5 mg/kg: 42%; 10 mg/kg: 42%; placebo: 20%). Mucosal healing at weeks 8 and 30 in each study and at week 54 in ACT 1 occurred in significantly more patients in the infliximab

TABLE 11-3

ULCERATIVE COLITIS: MEDICAL MANAGEMENT

Active Disease: Extensive or Pancolitis

Mild	Moderate	Severe	Fulminant
5-ASA oral +/- 5-ASA enema/suppository or steroid enema/foam/suppository	5-ASA +/- 5-ASA enema/suppository or steroid enema/foam/suppository Prednisone	IV hydrocortisone IV cyclosporine	IV cyclosporine surgery IV infliximab

Maintenance

5-ASA oral +/- 5-ASA enema/suppository 6-MP/azathioprine

Active Disease: Proctitis or Proctosigmoiditis

Mild	Moderate	Severe
5-ASA enema/suppository or steroid enema/foam/suppository	5-ASA enema/suppository or steroid enema/foam/suppository	IV hydrocortisone, IV cyclosporine, IV infliximab
+/-	+	
5-ASA oral	5-ASA oral prednisone	

Maintenance

5-ASA enema/suppository +/- 5-ASA oral 6-MP/azathioprine

groups than in the placebo groups ($P \leq 0.009$) In addition, infliximab was steroid-sparing in both studies with mean dosages of corticosteroids decreased from 20 mg/d to between 5 and 10 mg/d depending on the study week and treatment arm. Depending on the study week and treatment arm, 18% to 27% of patients achieved clinical remission and were able to discontinue steroids.[102]

Common (>10%) side effects of infliximab include nausea, headache, upper respiratory infections, fatigue, and fever. More serious side effects include fungal and other invasive opportunistic infections. In a study looking at the safety profile of infliximab in 500 patients from the Mayo Clinic, 43 patients (8.6%) experienced a serious adverse event, of which 30 (6%) were related to infliximab.[103] Serious events attributed to infliximab included acute infusion reactions (3.8%) and serum sickness-like disease (2.8%). Three patients developed drug-induced lupus, and 1 patient developed a new demyelinating disorder. Forty-one (8.2%) patients had an infectious event attributed to infliximab, and 20 patients had a serious infection (2, fatal sepsis; 8, pneumonia; 6, viral infections; 2, abdominal abscesses; 1, cellulitis; 1, histoplasmosis). Nine patients had a malignant disorder, 3 of which were possibly related to infliximab. A total of 10 deaths were observed. For 5 of these patients (1%), the events leading to death were possibly related to infliximab. The mortality rate in this study is generally comparable with the expected excess of mortality reported in patients with Crohn's, particularly when considering that infliximab is indicated only for patients with moderate to severe disease refractory to conventional medical therapy.[104,105]

There have been 117 reported cases of disseminated tuberculosis related to infliximab. For this reason, patients should be evaluated for tuberculosis (TB) prior to infliximab therapy. Because the majority of IBD patients are anergic, a thorough evaluation for TB should also include a travel history and a chest x-ray.[106] Medical management of UC is summarized in Table 11-3.

CONCLUSION

The most important aspect of medical therapy of UC is individualizing each regimen to the needs of each patient.

Patients often see the severity of their disease differently than their physicians, and quality-of-life scales are helpful in determining the needs of the patient. Common mistakes in treating UC include failing to add topical therapy, especially in distal disease, underdosing with 5-ASA agents, and not starting or underdosing 6-MP/AZA. Steroids should be used to induce remission if needed and are ineffective in maintaining remission. IV cyclosporine should be used as a bridge to either immunomodulator therapy or sometimes surgery. Like steroids, cyclosporine cannot be continued long term. Finally, infliximab is no longer experimental in UC. It is a part of the standard armamentarium and should be used accordingly. The placebo response is real in UC and is increased with more physician visits.[9] Thus, in addition to medical therapy, physicians should keep in mind that sick UC patients need to be seen and assessed at regular intervals.

REFERENCES

1. Irvine EJ. Quality of life issues in patients with inflammatory bowel disease. *Am J Gastroenterol.* 1997;92:18S-24S.
2. Jowett SL, Seal CJ, Barton JR, Welfare MR. The short inflammatory bowel disease questionnaire is reliable and responsive to clinically important change in ulcerative colitis. *Am J Gastroenterol.* 2001;96(10):2921-2928.
3. Bernklev T, Jahnsen J, Aadland E, et al. Health-related quality of life in patients with inflammatory bowel disease five years after the initial diagnosis. *Scand J Gastroenterol.* 2004;39(4):365-373.
4. Boonen A, Dagnelie PC, Feleus A, et al. The impact of inflammatory bowel disease on labor force participation: results of a population sampled case-control study. *Inflamm Bowel Dis.* 2002;8(6):382-389.
5. Trachter AB, Rogers AI, Leiblum SR. Inflammatory bowel disease in women: impact on relationship and sexual health. *Inflamm Bowel Dis.* 2002;8(6):413-421.
6. Truelove SC, Witts LJ. Cortisone in ulcerative colitis: final report on a therapeutic trial. *BMJ.* 1955;4947:1041.
7. Powell-Tuck J, Bown RL, Lennard-Jones JE. A comparison of oral prednisolone given as single or multiple daily doses for active proctocolitis. *Scand J Gastroenterol.* 1978;13:833.
8. Schroeder KW, Tremaine WJ, Ilstrup DM. Coated oral 5-aminosalicylic acid therapy for mildly to moderately active ulcerative colitis. *N Engl J Med.* 1987;317(26):1625-1629.
9. Su C, Lewis JD, Goldberg B, Brensinger C, Lichtenstein GR. A meta-analysis of the placebo rates of remission and response in clinical trials of active ulcerative colitis. *Gastroenterology.* 2007;132(2):516-526.
10. Pokrotnieks J, Marlicz K, Paradowski L, et al. Efficacy and tolerability of mesalazine foam enema (Salofalk foam) for distal ulcerative colitis: a double-blind, randomized, placebo-controlled study. *Aliment Pharmacol Ther.* 2000;14(9):1191-1198.
11. Malchow H, Gertz B, CLAFOAM Study Group. A mesalazine foam enema (Claversal Foam) compared with standard liquid enema in patients with active distal ulcerative colitis. *Aliment Pharmacol Ther.* 2002;16(3):415-423.
12. Cohen RD, Woseth DM, Thisted RA, et al. A meta-analysis and overview of the literature on treatment options for left-sided ulcerative colitis and ulcerative proctitis. *Am J Gastroenterol.* 2000;95:1263-1276.
13. Hanauer SB. Dose-ranging study of mesalamine (PENTASA) enemas in the treatment of acute ulcerative proctosigmoiditis: results of a multicentered placebo-controlled trial. The U.S. PENTASA Enema Study Group. *Inflamm Bowel Dis.* 1998;4(2):79-83.
14. Mulder CJ, Fockens P, Meijer DW, et al. Beclomethasone diprionate (3 mg) versus 5-aminosalicylic acid (2 g) versus the combination of both (3 mg/2 g) as retention enemas in active ulcerative proctitis. *Eur J Gastroenterol Hepatol.* 1996;8:549-554.
15. Safdi M, DeMicco M, Sninsky C, et al. A double-blind comparison of oral versus rectal mesalamine versus combination therapy in the treatment of distal ulcerative colitis. *Am J Gastroenterol.* 1997;92:1867-1871.
16. Marteau P, Probert CS, Lindgren S, et al. Combined oral and enema treatment with Pentasa (mesalazine) is superior to oral therapy alone in patients with extensive mild/moderate active ulcerative colitis: a randomized, double blind, placebo controlled study. *Gut.* 2005;54:960-965.
17. Hanauer S, Good LI, Goodman MW, et al. Long term use of mesalazine (Rowasa) suppositories in remission maintenance of ulcerative proctitis. *Am J Gastroenterol.* 2000;95:1749-1954.
18. D'Albasio G, Paolizi P, Campieri M, et al. Maintenance treatment of ulcerative proctitis with mesalazine suppositories: a double-blind placebo-controlled trial. *Am J Gastroenterol.* 1998;93:799-803.
19. D'Albasio G, Pacini F, Camarri E, et al. Combination therapy with 5-aminosalicylic acid tablets and enemas for maintaining remission in ulcerative colitis: a randomized double-blind study. *Am J Gastroenterol.* 1997:1143-1147.
20. Lichtenstein GR, Kamm MA, Boddu P, et al. Effect of once or twice-daily MMX mesalamine (SPD476) for the induction of remission of mild to moderately active ulcerative colitis. *Clin Gastroenterol Hepatol.* 2007;5(1):95-102.
21. Kamm MA, Sandborn WJ, Gassull M, et al. Once-daily, high concentration MMX mesalamine in active ulcerative colitis. *Gastroenterology.* 2007;132:66-73.
22. Lichtenstein G, Merchant K, Shaw A, Yuan J, Bortey E, Forbes W. Once-daily 1.5-g granulated mesalamine effectively maintains remission in patients with ulcerative colitis who switch from different 5-ASA formulations [abstract 1100]. *Am J Gastroenterol.* 2008;13(suppl 1):s429-430.
23. Kruis W, Kiudelis G, Racz I, et al. Once-daily versus three-times-daily mesalazine granules in active ulcerative colitis: a double-blind, double-dummy, randomised non-inferiority trial. *Gut.* 2008;doi:10.1136.
24. Rubin DT, Rosen AA, Sedghi S, et al. Twice-daily balsalazide tablets improve patient quality of life after 2 and 8 weeks of treatment: results of a phase 3, randomized, double-blind, placebo-controlled, multicenter study [abstract T1147]. *Gastroenterology.* 2008;134(4 suppl 1):A494.
25. Bosworth BP, Pruitt RE, Gordon GL, et al. Balsalazide tablets 3.3 g twice daily improves signs and symptoms of mild-to-moderate ulcerative colitis [abstract T1152]. *Gastroenterology.* 2008;134(4 suppl 1):A495.
26. Sutherland L, MacDonald JK. Oral 5-aminosalicylic acid for the induction of remission in ulcerative colitis. *Cochrane Database Syst Rev.* 2003;(3):CD000543.
27. Green JR, Lobo AJ, Holdsworth CD, et al. Balsalazide is more effective and better tolerated than mesalamine in the treatment of acute ulcerative colitis. The Abacus Investigator Group. *Gastroenterology.* 1998;114:15-22.
28. Levine DS, Riff DS, Pruitt R, et al. A randomized, double-blind, dose-response comparison of balsalazide (6.75 g), balsalazide (2.25 g) and mesalamine (2.4 g) in the treatment of active, mild-to-moderate ulcerative colitis. *Am J Gastroenterol.* 2002;97:1398-1407.

29. Pruitt R, Hanson J, Safdi M, et al. Balsalazide is superior to mesalamine in the time to improvement of signs and symptoms of acute mild-to-moderate ulcerative colitis. *Am J Gastroenterol.* 2002;97:1283-1285.
30. Lindgren S, Lofberg R, Bergholm M, et al. Effect of budesonide enema on remission and relapse rate in distal ulcerative colitis and proctitis. *Scand J Gastroenterol.* 2002;37(6):705-710.
31. Bar-Meir S, Fidder HH, Faszczyk M, et al. Budesonide foam versus hydrocortisone acetate foam in the treatment of active ulcerative proctosigmoiditis. *Dis Colon Rectum.* 2003;46:929-936.
32. Sinha A, Nightingale J, West KP, et al. Epidermal growth factor enemas with oral mesalamine for mild-to-moderate left-sided ulcerative colitis or proctitis. *New Engl J Med.* 2003;349:350-357.
33. Baron JH, Connell AM, Kanaglunis TG, Lennard-Jones JE, Jones FA. Outpatient treatment of ulcerative colitis: comparison between three doses of oral prednisone. *BMJ.* 1962;2:441-443.
34. Vakil N, Sparberg M. Steroid-related osteonecrosis in inflammatory bowel disease. *Gastroenterology.* 1989;96:62-67.
35. Plevy SE. Corticosteroid-sparing treatments in patients with Crohn's disease. *Am J Gastroenterol.* 2002;97(7):1607-1617.
36. Bernstein C, Katz S. Guidelines for osteoporosis and inflammatory bowel disease: a guide to diagnosis and management for the gastroenterologist (monograph). *The American College of Gastroenterology*; 2003.
37. Haderslev KV, Tjellesen L, Sorensen HA, et al. Alendronate increases lumbar spine bone mineral density in patients with Crohn's disease. *Gastroenterology.* 2000;119(3):639-646.
38. Desramé J, Sabaté JM, Agher R, et al. Assessment of hypothalamic-pituitary-adrenal axis function after corticosteroid therapy in inflammatory bowel disease. *Am J Gastroenterol.* 2002;97(7):1785-1791.
39. Danielsson A, Hellers G, Lyrenas E, et al. A controlled randomized trial of budesonide versus prednisolone retention enemas in active distal ulcerative colitis. *Scand J Gastroenterol.* 1987;22:987-992.
40. Lofberg R, Ostergaard Thomsen O, et al. Budesonide versus prednisolone retention enemas in active distal ulcerative colitis. *Aliment Pharmacol Ther.* 1994;8(6):623-629.
41. Luman W, Gray RS, Pendek R, Palmer KR. Prednisolone metasulphobenzoate form retention enemas suppress the hypothalamo-pituitary-adrenal axis. *Aliment Pharmacol Ther.* 1994;8:255-258.
42. Lee DA, Taylor GM, James VH, Walker G. Plasma prednisolone levels and adrenocortical responsiveness after administration of prednisolone-21-phosphate as a retention enema. *Gut.* 1979;20:349-355.
43. Bantel H, Berg C, Vieth M, et al. Mesalazine inhibits activation of transcription factor NF-κB in inflamed mucosa of patients with ulcerative colitis. *Am J Gastroenterol.* 2000;95:3452-3457.
44. Baron JH, Connell AM, Lennard-Jones JE, et al. Sulphasalazine and salicylazosulphadimidine in ulcerative colitis. *Lancet.* 1962;1:1094-1096.
45. Dick AP, Grayson MJ, Carpenter RG, et al. Controlled trial of sulphasalazine in the treatment of ulcerative colitis. *Gut.* 1964;50:437-442.
46. Margolin ML, Krumholz MP, Fochios SE, et al. Clinical trials in ulcerative colitis: II. historical review. *Am J Gastroenterol.* 1988;83:227-243.
47. Kornbluth A, Sachar DB. Ulcerative guidelines in adults: American College of Gastroenterology practice parameters committee. *Am J Gastroenterol.* In press.
48. Stein RB, Hanauer SB. Medical therapy for inflammatory bowel disease. *Gastroenterol Clin N Amer.* 1999;28:297-321.
49. Lim WC, Hanauer SB. Controversies with aminosalicylates in inflammatory bowel disease. *Rev Gastroenterol Disord.* 2004;4(3):104-117.
50. Meyers S, Sachar DB, Present DH, et al. Olsalazine sodium in the treatment of ulcerative colitis among patients intolerant of sulphasalzine: a prospective, randomized, double-blind, dose-ranging clinical trial. *Gastroenterology.* 1987;93:1255-1262.
51. Sutherland L, Roth D, Beck P, et al. Oral 5-aminosalicylic acid for maintenance of remission in ulcerative colitis. *Cochrane Database Syst Rev.* 2002;4:CD000544.
52. Fockens P, Mulder CJ, Tygat GN, et al. Comparison of the efficacy and safety of 1.5 g compared with 3.0 g oral slow-release mesalazine (Pentasa) in the maintenance treatment of ulcerative colitis. Dutch Pentasa Study Group. *Eur J Gastroenterol Hepatol.* 1995;7:1025-1030.
53. Kane S, Cohen RD, Aikens JE, et al. Predictors of non-compliance with mesalamine in quiescent ulcerative colitis. *Am J Gastroenterol.* 2001;96:2929-2932.
54. Kane S, Huo D, Aikens J, Hanauer S. Medication nonadherence and the outcomes of patients with quiescent ulcerative colitis. *Am J Med.* 2003;114(1):39-43.
55. Kane S, Huo D, Kalyani M. A pilot feasibility study of once daily versus conventional dosing mesalamine for maintenance of ulcerative colitis. *Clin Gastroenterol Hepatol.* 2003;1:170-173.
56. Faubion WA, Loftus EV, Harmsen WS, Zinsmeister AR, Sandborn WJ. The natural history of corticosteroid therapy for inflammatory bowel disease: a population-based study. *Gastroenterology.* 2001;121:255-260.
57. George J, Present DH, Pou R, Bodian C, Rubin PH. The long-term outcome of ulcerative colitis treated with 6-mercaptopurine. *Am J Gastroenterol.* 1996;91(9):1711-1714.
58. Ardizzone S, Molteni P, Imbesi V, Bollani S, Bianchi Porro G, Molteni F. Azathioprine in steroid-resistant and steroid-dependent ulcerative colitis. *J Clin Gastroenterol.* 1997;25:330-333.
59. Lobel EZ, Korelitz BI, Xuereb MA, et al. A search for the optimal duration of treatment with 6-mercaptopurine for ulcerative colitis. *Am J Gastroenterol.* 2004;99(3):462-465.
60. Sachar DB. Ten common errors in the management of inflammatory bowel disease. *Inflamm Bowel Dis.* 2003;9(3):205-209.
61. Dubinsky M. Azathioprine, 6-mercaptopurine in inflammatory bowel disease: pharmacology, efficacy, and safety. *Clin Gastroenterol Hepatol.* 2004;2:731-743.
62. Kandiel A, Fraser AG, Korelitz Bi, et al. Increased risk of lymphoma among inflammatory bowel disease patients treated with azathioprine and 6-mercaptopurine. *Gut.* 2005;54:1121-1125.
63. Beaugerie L, Carrat F, Bouvier AM, et al, for the CESAME Study group. Excess risk of lymphoproliferative disorders (LPD) in inflammatory bowel diseases (IBD): interim results of the CESAME cohort [abstract 818]. *Gastroenterology.* 2008;134(4 suppl 1):A116.
64. Lewis JD, Gelfand JM, Troxel AB, et al. Immunosuppressant medications and mortality in inflammatory bowel disease. *Am J Gastroenterol.* 2008;103(6):1428-1435.
65. Connell WR, Kamm MA, Dickson, et al. Long-term neoplasia risk after azathioprine treatment in inflammatory bowel disease. *Lancet.* 1994;343:1249-1952.
66. Present DH, Meltzer SJ, Krumholz MP, et al. 6-mercaptopurine in the management of inflammatory bowel disease: short and long-term toxicity. *Ann Intern Med.* 1989;111:641-649.
67. Lewis JD, Schwartz JS, Lichtenstein GR. Azathioprine for maintenance of remission in Crohn's disease: benefits outweigh the risk of lymphoma. *Gastroenterology.* 2000;118:1018-1024.
68. Lewis JD, Bilker WB, Brensinger C, et al. Inflammatory bowel disease is not associated with and increased risk of lymphoma. *Gastroenterology.* 2001;121:1080-1087.
69. Bernstein CH, Blanchard JF, Kliewer E, et al. Cancer risk in patients with inflammatory bowel disease: a population-based study. *Cancer.* 2001;91:854-862.

70. Loftus EV, Tremaine WJ, Habermann TM, et al. Risk of lymphoma in inflammatory bowel disease. *Am J Gastroenterol.* 2000;95:2308-2312.
71. Seidman EG. Clinical use and practical application of TPMT enzyme and 6-mercaptopurine metabolite monitoring in IBD. *Rev Gastroenterol Disord.* 2003;3(Suppl 1):S30-S38.
72. Colombel JF, Ferrari N, Debuysere H, et al. Genotypic analysis of thiopurine S-methyltransferase in patients with Crohn's disease and severe myelosuppression during azathioprine therapy. *Gastroenterology.* 118(6):1025-1030.
73. Dewit O, Vanheurverzwyn R, Desager JP, et al. Interaction between azathioprine and aminosalicylates: an in vivo study in patients with Crohn's disease. *Aliment Pharmacol Ther.* 2002;16(1):79-85.
74. Hande S, Wilson-Rich N, Bousvaros A, et al. 5-aminosalicyclare therapy is associated with higher 6-thioguanine levels in adults and children with inflammatory bowel disease in remission on 6-mercaptopurine or azathioprine. *Inflamm Bowel Dis.* 2006;12(4):251-257.
75. Beaugerie L, Massot N, Carbonnel F, et al. Impact of cessation of smoking on the course of ulcerative colitis. *Am J Gastroenterol.* 2001;96:2113-2116.
76. Sandborn WJ, Tremaine WJ, Offord KP, et al. Transdermal nicotine for mildly to moderately active ulcerative colitis: a randomized, double-blind, placebo-controlled trial. *Ann Intern Med.* 1997;126:364-371.
77. Pullan RD, Rhodes J, Ganesh S. Transdermal nicotine for active ulcerative colitis. *N Engl J Med.* 1994;330:811-815.
78. Thomas GA, Rhodes J, Mani V, et al. Transdermal nicotine as maintenance therapy for ulcerative colitis. *N Engl J Med.* 1995;332:988-992.
79. Bossa F, Fiorella S, Caruso N, et al. Continuous infusion versus bolus administration of steroids in severe attacks of ulcerative colitis: a randomized, double-blind trial. *Am J Gastroenterol.* 2006;101:1-8.
80. Aberra FN, Lewis JD, Hass D, et al. Corticosteroids and immunomodulators: postoperative infectious complication risk in inflammatory bowel disease patients. *Gastroenterology.* 2003;125(2):320-327.
81. Meyers S, Sachar DB, Goldberg JD, et al. Corticotrophin versus hydrocortisone in the intravenous treatment of ulcerative colitis. *Gastroenterology.* 1983;85(2):351-357.
82. Chapman RW, Selby WS, Jewell DP. Controlled trial of intravenous metronidazole as an adjunct to corticosteroids in severe ulcerative colitis. *Gut.* 1986;27(10):1210-1212.
83. Mantzaris GJ, Hatzis A, Kontogiannis P, et al. Intravenous tobramycin and metronidazole as an adjunct to corticosteroids in acute, severe ulcerative colitis. *Am J Gastroenterol.* 1994;89(1):43-46.
84. Dickinson RJ, Ashton MG, Axon AT, et al. Controlled trial of intravenous hyperalimentation and total bowel rest as an adjunct to the routine therapy of acute colitis. *Gastroenterology.* 1980;79(6):1199-1204.
85. McIntyre PB, Powell-Tuck J, Wood SR, et al. Controlled trial of bowel rest in the treatment of severe acute colitis. *Gut.* 1986;27(5):481-485.
86. Lichtiger S, Present DH, Kornbluth A, et al. Cyclosporine in severe ulcerative colitis refractory to steroid therapy. *N Engl J Med.* 1994;330:1841-1845.
87. Van Assche G, D'haens G, Noman M, et al. Randomized, double-blind comparison of 4 mg/kg versus 2 mg/kg intravenous cyclosporine in severe ulcerative colitis. *Gastroenterology.* 2003;125(4):1025-1031.
88. Jani N, Regueiro MD. Medical therapy for ulcerative colitis. *Gastroenterol Clin N Am.* 2002;31:147-166.
89. Actis GC, Ottobrelli A, Pera A, et al. Continuously infused cyclosporin at low dose is sufficient to avoid emergency colectomy in acute attacks of ulcerative colitis without the need for high dose steroids. *J Clin Gastroenterol.* 1993;17:10-13.
90. Actis GC, Aimo G, Priolo G, Moscato D, Rizzetto M, Pagni R. Efficacy and efficiency of oral microemulsion cyclosporin versus intravenous and soft gelatin capsule cyclosporin in the treatment of severe, steroid-refractory ulcerative colitis: an open-label retrospective trial. *Inflamm Bowel Dis.* 1998;4:276-279.
91. Weber A, Fein F, Koch S, et al. Treatment of ulcerative colitis refractory to steroids therapy by oral emulsion cyclosporine (Neoral). *Inflamm Bowel Dis.* 2006;12(12):1131-1135.
92. D'Haens G, Lemmens L, Geboes K, et al. Intravenous cyclosporine versus intravenous corticosteroids as single therapy for severe attacks of ulcerative colitis. *Gastroenterology.* 2001;120:1323-1329.
93. Cohen RD, Stein R, Hanauer SB. Intravenous cyclosporin in ulcerative colitis: a five-year experience. *Am J Gastroenterol.* 1999;94(6):1587-1592.
94. Aberra FN, Lewis JD, Hass D, et al. Corticosteroids and immunomodulators: Postoperative infectious complication risk in inflammatory bowel disease patients. *Gastroenterology.* 2003;125(2):320-327.
95. Hyde GM, Jewell DP, Kettlewell MGW, et al. Cyclosporin for severe ulcerative colitis does not increase the rate of perioperative complications. *Dis Colon Rectum.* 2001;44:1436-1440.
96. Mahadevan U, Loftus E, Tremaine W, et al. Azathioprine or 6-mercaptopurine before colectomy for ulcerative colitis is not associated with increased postoperative complications. *Inflamm Bowel Dis.* 2002;8(5):311-316.
97. Rowe FA, Walker JH, Karp LC, Vasiliauskas EA, Plevy S, Targan SR. Factors predictive of response to cyclosporin treatment for severe steroid-resistant ulcerative colitis. *Am J Gastroenterol.* 2000;95:2000-2008.
98. Sands B, Tremaine WJ, Sandborn WJ, et al. Infliximab in the treatment of severe, steroid-refractory ulcerative colitis: a pilot study. *Inflamm Bowel Dis.* 2001;7(2):83-88.
99. Kaser A, Mairinger T, Vogel W, et al. Infliximab in severe steroid refractory ulcerative colitis: a pilot study. *Wien Klin Wochenshr.* 2001;113(23-24):930-933.
100. Chey WY, Hussain A, Ryan C, et al. Infliximab for refractory ulcerative colitis. *Am J Gastroenterol.* 2001;96:2373-2381.
101. Su C, Salzberg BA, Lewis JD, et al. Efficacy of anti-tumor necrosis factor therapy in patients with ulcerative colitis. *Am J Gastroenterol.* 2002;97(10):2577-2584.
102. Rutgeerts P, Sandborn WJ, Feagan BG, et al. Infliximab for induction and maintenance therapy for ulcerative colitis. *N Engl J Med.* 2005;353:2462-2476.
103. Colombel J, Loftus EV, Tremaine WJ. The safety profile of infliximab in patients with Crohn's disease: the Mayo Clinic experience in 500 patients. *Gastroenterology.* 2004;126:19-31.
104. Loftus EV Jr, Silverstein MD, Sandborn WJ, et al. Crohn's disease in Olmstead County, Minnesota 1940-1993: incidence, prevalence, and survival. *Gastroenterology.* 1998;114:1161-1168.
105. Jess T, Winther KV, Munkolm P, et al. Mortality and causes of death in Crohn's disease: follow-up of a population-based cohort in Copenhagen County, Denmark. *Gastroenterology.* 2002;122:1808-1814.
106. Mow WS, Abreau-Martin MT, Papadakis KA, et al. High incidence of anergy in inflammatory bowel disease patients limits the usefulness of PPD screening. *Clin Gastroenterol Hepatol.* 2004;2(4):309-313.

12

Assessment of Disease Activity in Ulcerative Colitis

Anthony L. Rosa, MD and Thomas A. Judge, MD

An objective evaluation of disease activity is essential for treating patients with inflammatory bowel disease (IBD). Throughout the years, many indices of disease activity have been proposed for both Crohn's disease (CD) and ulcerative colitis (UC). Perhaps the most recognized and widely used is the Crohn's disease activity index (CDAI) introduced by Best et al in 1976[1] and modified by Harvey and Bradshaw in 1980.[2] The most widely recognized disease activity index for patients with UC was introduced by Truelove and Witts in 1955.[3] These indices help the clinician assess severity of disease, make treatment decisions, and measure response to therapy when treating individual patients.

To date, there is no clear consensus among clinicians on specific parameters for monitoring disease activity in either ulcerative colitis or Crohn's disease. The development of an ideal disease activity index has been controversial with many classifications having been introduced, amended, defended, and discounted with great fervor. Some classification indices place emphasis on subjective complaints,[4] while others favor objective or endoscopic findings. Some require the use of elaborate equations and statistical calculations,[5] while others are quite simple to use in a clinical setting.[6]

Ideally, a perfect index of disease activity should consist of a simple, accurate, and reproducible method that integrates basic clinical, laboratory, and endoscopic data to guide when surgical intervention is appropriate and to predict when and in whom a poor outcome can be expected. Such an index should also serve as an effective means for clinicians to communicate the results of research trials. An ideal system must also strike a balance accounting for a patient's subjective feelings, without sacrificing objective descriptions of inflammation. This chapter will briefly trace the evolution of disease activity indices and review how the literature has shaped our current understanding of how to monitor activity in patients with severe, moderate, and mild UC.

Disease Activity Indices

Cameron and Rippman were the first to investigate predictive factors in ulcerative colitis in 1910. They demonstrated that a temperature of 101°F was associated with a high mortality rate in patients with colitis.[7] However, it was not until 1955 that Truelove and Witts developed the first index of disease activity.[3] Truelove, while pioneering his work on the effects of cortisone and sulfasalazine in UC, recognized that patients with varying degrees of illness could be described in terms of several symptoms and signs.[8] This observation resulted in a classification system of 5 variables that allows differentiation between mild, moderate, and severe colitis. A patient with severe UC is defined by Truelove and Witts' criteria as having more than 6 bloody bowel movements daily and at least 1 of the following: temperature greater than 37°C, pulse greater than 90 beats per minute, hemoglobin less than 10.0 g, or erythrocyte sedimentation rate (ESR) greater than 30 mm/h (Table 12-1).

In the final report on a therapeutic trial of cortisone in UC, the authors reported that the severity of disease at the beginning of treatment has a significant impact on outcome at 3 months. Severely ill patients had less of a response to steroid treatment than patients with moderate or mild degrees of illness. However, at each level of severity and for first attacks and relapses, patients treated with

Lichtenstein GR, ed.
Ulcerative Colitis: The Complete Guide to Medical Management (pp. 135-144)

TABLE 12-1

TRUELOVE AND WITTS' CLASSIFICATION OF DISEASE ACTIVITY IN ULCERATIVE COLITIS

Severe	Diarrhea >6 motions per day with blood
	Temperature >37°C
	Tachycardia >90 beats per minute
	Anemia with hemoglobin ≤10 g%
	ESR >30 mm/h
Mild	Diarrhea <4 motions per day without blood
	No fever
	No tachycardia
	Anemia with hemoglobin ≥10 g%
	ESR ≤30 mm/h
Moderately severe:	Between severe and mild

TABLE 12-2

BARON'S SIGMOIDOSCOPIC APPEARANCE SCALE

Sigmoidoscopic Appearance	
Nonhemorrhagic	No bleeding spontaneously
	No bleeding upon light touch
Moderately hemorrhagic	Bleeding upon light touch
	No bleeding spontaneously ahead of scope
Severely hemorrhagic	Spontaneous bleeding seen ahead of scope

steroids had a more favorable outcome than untreated controls.[3]

Truelove and Witts' classification scale has remained the most recognized and widely used tool for assessing disease activity in patients with UC to date. It is valuable to the general physician in the clinical setting where a quick, accurate, and reproducible measurement of disease severity is often needed. This is due, in part, to its intuitive design and ease of use in gathering required information.

Unfortunately, Truelove and Witts' criteria do not stand up as well in clinical trials where more stringent classification criteria are required to ensure accurate communication among physicians. Truelove and Witts' criteria has several limitations, such as strict definition of only 2 categories of severity of illness, an inability to account for either minor improvements or deteriorations in disease severity, the inability to accurately predict which patients will respond to medical treatment, and the lack of endoscopic data as an index parameter.

Clinicians often encounter patients who only meet some of the criteria for each degree of illness, making placement into one distinct category difficult and rather arbitrary. Powell-Tuck and colleagues addressed this issue by broadening the severity parameters of Truelove and Witts' criteria in 1978.[10] Additional clinical criteria included stool consistency, abdominal pain, anorexia, nausea/vomiting, general health, extracolonic manifestations, and abdominal tenderness. The authors also included sigmoidoscopic criteria based on a scoring system developed by Baron and colleagues in 1964 wherein it was established that interobserver variability of mucosal appearance was minimized when the observer rated the presence or absence of a clearly defined feature.[9] The features with greatest observer agreement pertained to bleeding and are summarized in Table 12-2. The end result is the St. Mark's Clinical Activity Score, a system of 10 clinical parameters wherein each parameter receives a graded numerical score based on severity (Table 12-3).[10] Two additional disease activity indices have been derived from the combination of Truelove and Witts clinical criteria and Baron's endoscopic assessment. In 1987, Sutherland et al presented a 12-point scoring system that was used to assess the clinical efficacy of mesalamine enema in the treatment of distal ulcerative colitis (Table 12-4).[11] Criteria were scored at 2 time-points based on diary assessments over the preceding 3-week interval. That year, a similar system was utilized by Schroeder and colleagues from the Mayo Clinic to assess the efficacy of oral mesalamine in the treatment of UC.[12] In contrast to the Sutherland index, the Mayo Score assesses clinical criteria over a 72-hour period. The primary difference between the Sutherland index and the Mayo Score is the calculation of the global physician rating of disease activity. Also in contrast to the Sutherland index, which scores the physician's qualitative assessment of disease activity to determine the physician global rating, the Mayo Score requires that the global physician rating include a consideration of the scores for each of the subunits (stool frequency, bleeding, mucosal appearance), a patient functional assessment (scored 0 to 3), in addition to the physician's clinical assessment of disease activity. Each of these 3 refined indices have continued to be used in clinical trials.

A simple clinical colitis index was introduced by Walmsley and colleagues in 1998 in an attempt to create a simple and reliable index of activity using a small number of clinical criteria.[6] The authors sought an index that could be calculated in the outpatient setting by a general practitioner without requiring a physical examination, sigmoidoscopic evaluation, or laboratory indices.[6] The index was established by recording the St. Mark's score in 57 patients with UC together with additional parameters, such as frequency of nocturnal bowel movements, urgency of defecation, subjective assessment of general well-being, and presence of extracolonic manifestations. The scores from 5 clinical parameters that best correlated with the St. Mark's score were used to devise the simple colitis index (Table 12-5). The index was subsequently validated by showing close correlation with the complex integrated disease activity index in 113 assessments of a different patient population.

Many indices of disease activity are limited by an inability to account for minor improvements or deteriorations in disease activity. The Truelove and Witts' index strictly defines criteria for mild and severe disease, but fails to clearly establish a definition of moderate disease. By default, patients who fail to meet criteria for severe or mild disease are grouped into the moderate disease category and represent a broad spectrum of disease activity ranging from

TABLE 12-3

ST. MARK'S CLINICAL ACTIVITY SCORE

Symptoms and Signs	Points
General Health	
Normal	0
Slightly impaired	1
Limited activities	2
Unable to work	3
Abdominal Pain	
None	0
Before or during motions	1
Prolonged	2
Bowel Frequency	
0 to 2	0
3 to 6	1
>6	2
Stool Consistency	
Formed	0
Semi-formed	1
Liquid	2
Anorexia	1
Nausea/vomiting	1
Extracolonic Manifestations	
None	0
One or mild	1
>One or severe	2
Abdominal Tenderness	
Mild	1
Marked	2
Rebound	3
Body Temperature (°C)	
<37.1	0
37.1 to 38	1
>38	2
Blood in stool	
None	0
Trace	1
More than trace	2
Sigmoidoscopy	
Nonhemorrhagic	0
Friable	1
Spontaneous bleeding	2

TABLE 12-4

SUTHERLAND INDEX/ MAYO SCORE

SYMPTOMS AND SIGNS	POINTS
Stool Frequency	
Normal	0
1 to 2 stools/day above normal	1
3 to 4 stools/day above normal	2
5 to 6 stools/day above normal	3
Rectal Bleeding	
None	0
Streaks of blood	1
Obvious blood	2
Mostly blood	3
Mucosal Appearance	
Normal	0
Mild friability	1
Moderate friability	2
Exudate with spontaneous bleeding	3
*Physician Rating of Disease Activity**	
Normal	0
Mild	1
Moderate	2
Severe	3

*Calculation of physician rating distinguishes these two indices.

TABLE 12-5

SIMPLE CLINICAL COLITIS ACTIVITY INDEX

SYMPTOM	SCORE
Bowel Frequency Per Day	
1 to 3	0
4 to 6	1
7 to 9	2
>9	3
Bowel Frequency Per Night	
1 to 3	1
4 to 6	2
Urgency of Defecation	
Hurry	1
Immediately	2
Incontinence	3
Blood in Stool	
Trace	1
Occasionally frank	2
Usually frank	3
General Well-Being	
Very well	0
Slightly unwell	1
Poor	2
Very poor	3
Terrible	4
Extracolonic features	1 per

less-moderate to severe-moderate disease. These patients may improve clinically but fail to demonstrate a change in clinical or endoscopic classification. This is commonly observed in tertiary-care centers where patients are seen in referral and often after extended courses of steroid therapy.

A solution to this problem is the activity index (AI), a regression analysis where an outcome variable is analyzed as a function of clinical and laboratory findings.[13,14] In 1992, Seo and colleagues[5] developed the complex integrated disease AI, an objective quantitative evaluation of disease severity in UC. By performing multiple stepwise regression analysis in 72 patients with UC evaluating 18 clinical, laboratory, and endoscopic parameters, they demonstrated that disease severity is significantly influenced by 5 factors: bloody stool, bowel movements, ESR, hemoglobin, and serum albumin (Table 12-6).[5] The AI values correlated with Truelove and Witts' criteria, but overlap existed, resulting in a misclassification rate of approximately 15%.[13] The calculations required to generate the AI are quite complex, such that the model may be best utilized in therapeutic trials rather than the clinical setting.

The quality of life in patients with IBD is significantly impaired, and many clinical indices are not capable of accounting for these impairments. The first assessment scale for health-related quality of life in patients with IBD (IBDQ-32) was established by Guyatt et al in 1989 as a tool to be used in clinical trials.[15] The original scale consisted of a 32-item questionnaire that measured the physical, social, and emotional impact on patients with IBD. The scale was later

TABLE 12-6

THE COMPLEX INTEGRATED DISEASE ACTIVITY INDEX

VARIABLE	SCORE	WEIGHT
Bloody stool		X 60
Little or none	0	
Present	1	
Bowel movements per day		X 13
≤4	1	
5 to 7	2	
≥8	3	
ESR (mm/h)		X 0.5
Hemoglobin (g/dL)		X -4
Albumin (g/dL)		X -15
Constant		200

expanded to include 36 items in 1992.[16] The reliability and responsiveness of the IBDQ-32 was validated by correlating it with a set of predicted criteria in patients with CD. The time required to completely fill out the questionnaire significantly limited its usefulness and prompted the development of a 9-question scale, the short inflammatory bowel disease questionnaire (SIBDQ) as a desirable alternative (Table 12-7).

The SIBDQ was validated in UC by Jowett and colleagues in 2001. They compared the results of the SIBDQ with the simple colitis activity index proposed by Walmsley et al and the complex integrated disease activity index proposed by Seo et al. Among 61 patients with varying degrees of UC, a strong correlation existed between the SIBDQ and the 2 UC indices. Furthermore, the SIBDQ was reliable and accurate in detecting changes in disease activity among these patients.[17] Similar findings were reported by Casellas et al.[18] These findings highlight that health-related quality of life may serve as another useful tool to assess severity in ulcerative colitis.

The physician global assessment (PGA) is a classification system that has been used in therapeutic trials assessing efficacy of mesalamine in acute UC.[19,20] Similar to the SIBDQ, it provides a means to document changes in a patient's status in response to specific therapeutic interventions. However, in contrast to the SIBDQ, the PGA is based entirely on the physician's assessment of improvement or worsening clinical status compared to baseline (Table 12-8).

The greatest challenge for any clinical activity index for UC has been its ability to accurately identify which patients will respond to medical treatment and enter clinical remission and which of those patients will require urgent surgical intervention. As highlighted by Goligher and colleagues, early colectomy in patients who fail medical treatment avoids significant morbidity and mortality.[21]

Treatment with IV glucocorticoids drastically reduced mortality in patients with ulcerative colitis in referral centers from 31% to 61% in the 1950s[22,23] to 5% to 9% in 1962.[24] However, mortality rates for patients with ulcerative colitis in nonreferral centers remained at 37% by 1974.[25] Lennard-Jones et al[26] attempted to define specific clinical parameters that could predict which group of patients would respond to IV glucocorticoids or fail medical treatment altogether, resulting in either colectomy or death. In a large retrospective trial examining 100 patients with UC admitted to the hospital between 1968 and 1972, the authors found that patients who had fewer than 8 daily bowel movements and a maximum temperature of 38°C after 24 hours of treatment were more likely to respond to medical treatment. Patients with more than 8 daily bowel movements and higher temperatures after 24 hours of treatment had an 80% chance of failing medical treatment and went on to require colectomy. Other features with high predictive values for early treatment failure were tachycardia, hypoalbuminemia, and the appearance of colonic dilatation, mucosal islands, or both on plain abdominal radiographs.[26]

Since Lennard-Jones and colleagues published their results in 1975, many others have attempted to find a simple clinical or laboratory parameter that could accurately predict treatment response. Buckell and colleagues reported that an elevated or rising C-reactive protein level was associated with urgent colectomy in 6 of 8 patients.[27] Others have tried to correlate first attack, extent of disease,[28] and the presence of 3 or more dilated loops of bowel on first abdominal radiograph[29] with a higher likelihood of failing IV medical treatment. None of these studies have yielded a particularly convincing or reproducible predictive parameter.

The need for a simple, early predictor of treatment outcome was reintroduced in 1994 when IV cyclosporine therapy was shown to be effective for patients with severe corticosteroid-resistant UC.[30] The addition of cyclosporine to the medical regimen for UC may inappropriately delay colectomy, making early recognition of treatment failure even more valuable. In 1996, Travis and colleagues[31] investigated 36 clinical, laboratory, and radiographic variables prospectively in an attempt to identify whether any markers could predict the need for surgery in patients not responding to IV corticosteroids and requiring cyclosporine. The authors found that after 3 days of intensive treatment with steroids and cyclosporine, those patients with greater than 8 daily stools and C-reactive protein of greater than 45 underwent urgent colectomy during that admission.[31] Patients on cyclosporine for greater than

TABLE 12-7

THE SHORT INFLAMMATORY BOWEL DISEASE QUESTIONNAIRE

1. How frequent have your bowel movements been during the past 2 weeks?
2. How often has the feeling of fatigue or being tired and worn out been a problem for you during the past 2 weeks?
3. How much energy have you had during the past 2 weeks?
4. How often during the past 2 weeks have you had to delay or cancel a social engagement because of your bowel problem?
5. How often during the past 2 weeks have you been troubled by cramps in your abdomen?
6. How often during the past 2 weeks have you felt generally unwell?
7. Overall, in the past 2 weeks, how much of a problem have you had with passing a large amount of gas?
8. How much of the time during the past 2 weeks have you been troubled by feeling nauseated or sick to your stomach?
9. How satisfied, happy, or pleased have you been with your personal life during the past 2 weeks?

TABLE 12-8

THE PHYSICIAN GLOBAL ASSESSMENT SCALE

1 = Complete symptom relief

2 = Marked symptom improvement

3 = Moderate symptom improvement

4 = Slight symptom improvement

5 = No changes in symptoms

6 = Worsened symptoms

7 days with more than 3 stools per day or visible blood have a 60% chance of continued symptoms and a 40% chance of requiring colectomy in the following months.

These results suggest that patients failing conventional medical therapy can be selected early for escalation of treatment with cyclosporine. Furthermore, the data provide clinically useful parameters for identifying patients who are likely to fail cyclosporine therapy and require colectomy.

In 1995, Seo and colleagues evaluated the prognostic potential of their activity index that was originally reported in 1992. Of 35 patients hospitalized with Truelove and Witts' moderate UC, 100% with AI <180 achieved complete medical remission. On the contrary, only 35% of patients with AI >180 achieved remission.[32] Significant overlap existed, making misclassification in approximately 14% and thus highlighting some inherent limitations in using activity indices as an alternative to solid clinical judgment.

ENDOSCOPIC DATA

Endoscopic evaluation has become a routine part of the clinical evaluation, because mucosal appearance has proven useful in assessing disease severity in patients with IBD. Endoscopy may be more valuable in assessing disease activity in UC than in CD, because the rectosigmoid mucosa is easily accessible via endoscopy, the endoscopic appearance of the mucosa has been described with minimal interobserver variation,[9] and severe symptoms tend to correlate with severe inflammation. However, many discrepancies remain.

To date, there is no direct correlation between histological findings and endoscopic appearance of colonic mucosa in ulcerative colitis. In 1956, Truelove and Richards were among the first to examine rectosigmoid biopsy specimens in 42 patients with UC and 24 controls. The authors categorized the clinical state of each subject into 1 of 3 groups: remission, mild/moderate, and severe. Sigmoidoscopic and histologic appearances were also categorized as normal, mild/moderate, and severe. Neither the sigmoidoscopic nor histologic findings correlated with the clinical state. More than half of the 40 specimens taken from patients in clinical remission showed evidence of inflammation.[33] Although it is commonly accepted that the histologic state may lag behind clinical improvement, the duration of this delay is uncertain.

Powell-Tuck and colleagues[34] compared 10 symptoms and clinical signs from the St. Mark's Clinical Activity Index (see Table 12-3) with the appearance of the rectal mucosa. Rectal mucosa was categorized into 1 of 3 groups: nonbleeding (grade 0) no bleeding spontaneously or on light touch; hemorrhagic (grade 1) bleeding upon light touch but no spontaneous bleeding; and hemorrhagic (grade 2) spontaneous bleeding seen ahead of the instrument. Most patients with nonhemorrhagic mucosa at sigmoidoscopy had no acute inflammation, and most with a hemorrhagic mucosa had moderate to severe inflammation; however, significant overlap occurred.[34] In a quantitative analysis of density of inflammation of cells in the lamina propria, there was a trend in increasing thickness among those with a hemorrhagic mucosa; however, this finding was not statistically significant. No histologic difference was observed between friable (grade 1) and hemorrhagic (grade 2) mucosa. Although no clinical variable was significantly associated with activity of disease well-being, increased stool consistency, diminished rectal bleeding, and decline in ESR were associated with improvement when hemorrhagic and nonhemorrhagic sigmoidoscopic appearance were compared.

Carbonnel and colleagues examined the endoscopic and clinical findings of 85 consecutive patients with attacks of ulcerative colitis in an attempt to evaluate the value and safety of colonoscopy in this setting.[38] They failed to demonstrate a strong correlation between endoscopic and clinical findings. Only 17% of patients with severe endoscopic disease met clinical criteria of severe disease based on Truelove and Witts' criteria. Unfortunately, baseline clinical severity was unknown as the patients studied were selected from a tertiary center population and had already received steroid treatment.

Nevertheless, the study demonstrated that severe endoscopic disease is a strong predictor of medical treatment failure and eventual colectomy. Of 46 patients with endoscopic signs of severe disease, 43 required colectomy. Conversely, 30 of 38 patients with endoscopic signs suggesting moderate disease went into clinical remission with continued medical treatment. It was concluded that colonoscopy accurately serves to identify patients at high risk for surgical intervention.

Several authors have considered a severe attack of UC a contraindication to colonoscopic surveillance because of the potential for colonic perforation, traumatic dilatation, and toxic megacolon.[35,36] Carbonnel and colleagues presented data to the contrary. They observed no perforations after performing colonoscopy in 85 patients with acute attacks of UC. Furthermore, as 92% of all colonic lesions were found distal to the splenic flexure, complete colonoscopic evaluation may be unnecessary in the acute setting. An unprepped, flexible sigmoidoscopy with minimal air insufflation may be all that is necessary to evaluate colonic mucosa and reduce risks associated with colonoscopic evaluation.[37] This may be especially true among patients in whom the diagnosis of UC is already firmly established.[38]

Endoscopic evaluation remains the most important modality for assessing disease activity in patients with mild to moderate disease. In a study reported by Wright and Truelove[39] utilizing a controlled diet, nearly 40% of patients remained symptom-free when a follow-up endoscopy at 1 year detected resolution of endoscopic lesions. However, only 18% of patients remained symptom-free when follow-up endoscopy at 1 year revealed persistent endoscopic lesions. Similar results were observed when histologic activity was evaluated.

Endoscopic evaluation of patients with UC is a critical component of cancer surveillance. Patients with UC have a 2.6- to 5.4-fold increased risk for developing colorectal cancer as compared to the general population.[40] Neoplasia in UC develops from flat mucosa, rather than the adenoma to cancer progression observed in the general population. The increased risk is proportional to duration of disease greater than 8 years and extent of colon involvement.[41,42] Chronic inflammation has been accepted as the inciting factor. A recent case-control study by Rutter and colleagues demonstrated that severity of colonoscopic and histologic inflammation correlates strongly with mucosal dysplasia in patients with long-standing UC.[43] This finding highlights the importance of endoscopic assessment of UC and may improve risk stratification for cancer screening in this population.

Current ACG recommendations support annual or biannual surveillance colonoscopy with multiple biopsies at regular intervals in patients with colitis for 8 to 10 years.[44] However, uniform guidelines for frequency of surveillance, number of biopsies, or number of sites do not exist.[45]

RADIOLOGIC DATA

Radiographic imaging studies have played an important role in the assessment of disease activity in UC. Typically, the inflammation in UC is superficial and progresses proximally from the anus in a confluent pattern.[46] In fulminant colitis, inflammation may extend deeper into the colonic wall, thus allowing correlation between severity and radiographic studies. Plain abdominal radiography alone is capable of detecting deep ulcerations in colonic mucosa and mucosal islands, seen as air-filled crevices and nodular intraluminal projections, respectively.[37] Additionally, abdominal x-rays are able to detect complications such as toxic megacolon and free air from colonic perforation.

The findings of double-contrast barium enema correlate with extent of disease and may be useful in patients with an established diagnosis with mild to moderate symptoms. Findings range from a fine, granular appearance of the rectosigmoid mucosa in early disease to the characteristic "collar-button ulcers" caused by ulceration into the submucosa of advanced disease. The findings of diffuse ulceration, absent haustral folds, narrowing, shortening, backwash

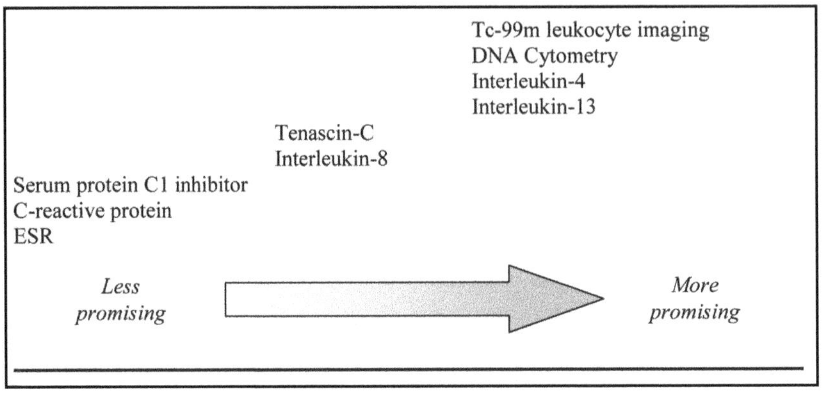

FIGURE 12-1. Potential of biological markers as indicators of severity in UC.

ileitis, and shortening of the colon have all been reported in chronic or "burnt-out" ulcerative colitis. The need for air insufflation and the risk of perforation have limited its use in severe ulcerative colitis. Early carcinomas may be erroneously interpreted as narrowing or stricture related to ulcerative colitis.

Computed tomography (CT) of the abdomen is not useful in assessing activity in mild disease. Patients with advanced disease may have varying degrees of mural thickening. Chronic disease often includes rectal narrowing and widening of the presacral space. These findings are nonspecific, and CT scanning does not play a major role in routine surveillance of disease activity.

High-resolution ultrasonography may be valuable in evaluating the extent of bowel wall involvement. Unfortunately, this modality is highly operator-dependent. Arienti and colleagues have reported good correlation with scintigraphy.[47]

NONINVASIVE STUDIES

Recent research has focused on objective, noninvasive laboratory surrogates for assessing disease severity in UC. During a flare of UC, neutrophils are attracted to areas of inflammation and are activated by numerous cytokines including interleukin-8 (IL-8). Activated neutrophils in the colonic mucosa release inflammatory mediators that may be responsible for local tissue damage. Radiolabeled human leukocytes with technetium Tc-99m hexamethyl propylene amine oxine (^{99m}Tc-HMPAO) migrate to areas of inflammation when reinjected. By using fecal collection or total body counts of radioactivity, ^{99m}Tc-HMPAO leukocyte imaging has shown promise as an accurate, quantitative, and noninvasive method for assessing degree of inflammation in UC.[48] Guimbaud and colleagues compared the results of ^{99m}Tc-HMPAO leukocyte imaging with colonoscopy and biopsy in 50 acute episodes of UC. They demonstrated that ^{99m}Tc-HMPAO leukocyte imaging correlated well with endoscopic and histologic assessment of inflammation.[49] There was also a correlation between the scintigraphic index, Truelove and Witts criteria, and biological markers such as IL-8.

^{99m}Tc-HMPAO leukocyte imaging has potential to serve as a noninvasive alternative to colonoscopy for assessing disease severity and monitoring treatment response; however, it may lack the sensitivity to detect disease where only mild macroscopic changes exist. Aburano and colleagues compared ^{99m}Tc-HMPAO leukocyte imaging with colonoscopy in 28 patients with UC. A close correlation with scintigraphy existed when there was colonoscopic appearance of marked granularity, edema, or severe ulceration of the mucosa. However, 82% of patients with slight macroscopic changes had normal ^{99m}Tc-HMPAO leukocyte imaging.[50]

Activation of Th2 lymphocytes with subsequent secretion of myriad proinflammatory cytokines has been implicated as a defining event in the inflammatory response in UC. Inoue et al examined RNA of rectal biopsy specimens from patients in an attempt to characterize local expression of cytokines such as IL-2, IL-4, IL-10, IL-13, IL-15, and interferon (IFN)-γ. These authors reported that the cytokines IL-4 and IL-13 were increased in mucosa of patients with active UC. They also reported a significant difference in IL-4 and IL-13 levels between active and inactive disease, suggesting that the degree of expression may correlate with disease activity.[51]

Many other biological markers have been investigated for their role in assessing disease severity. Determination of the synthetic phase of the cell cycle has been offered as an accurate assessment of disease activity in ulcerative colitis. In 1995, Bortoluzzi and colleagues reported that DNA cytometry of the rectal mucosa correlated with endoscopic, clinical, and histological indices of severity.[52] Mahmud et al reported that patients with active IBD have a higher concentration of microalbuminuria than patients in remission.[53] More recently, Riedl et al examined the value of tenascin-C in UC. Tenascin-C is a matrix protein that is elevated in states of tissue repair. The authors reported that serum tenascin-C levels were significantly higher in 47 patients than in controls and were significantly correlated with clinical and histologic indices of activity.[54]

Despite the potential promise of each of these biochemical markers in supplementing the assessment of disease activity, a consensus for appropriate use has not been established. None of these modalities should substitute for a complete assessment involving symptom evaluation, physical examination, basic laboratory testing, and endoscopic evaluation (Figure 12-1).

CONCLUSION

The assessment of disease activity in patients with ulcerative colitis requires frequent monitoring of clinical, laboratory, and endoscopic parameters. Hospitalized patients with acute attacks of UC require a daily physical examination with particular attention to the abdomen and monitoring of vital signs for temperature and heart rate. Stool should be assessed for frequency, consistency, and presence of blood. Laboratory evaluation in hospitalized patients should include complete blood count, ESR, C-reactive protein, electrolytes, and albumin. Abdominal imaging is useful to assess potential complications such as toxic megacolon and bowel wall perforation. Flexible sigmoidoscopy with minimal air insufflation to evaluate the degree of mucosal inflammation may be useful at the time of admission. If biopsies are obtained, an attempt to biopsy below the peritoneal reflection is usually performed. Repeat flexible sigmoidoscopy in 1 week is valuable to assess endoscopic response to treatment. In addition, the prudent use of activity indices may be valuable for the clinician to document response to treatment.

Delineation of the severity of mucosal inflammation in UC patients with mild to moderate disease are best assessed with endoscopic evaluation, which allows histologic and gross endoscopic appearance of colonic mucosa. Clinical indicators alone are less effective in providing accurate predicative information as compared with the combination of clinical and endoscopic data in this patient population. The role of radiographic studies in the routine assessment of UC patients has declined with the advent of improved endoscopic technologies, but may still provide important information in certain clinical settings. The utility of other noninvasive imaging studies and assessment of biological markers of inflammation remains to be defined. Ultimately, the inclusion of these various indicators in the evaluation of individual patients will be dictated by further validation in clinical trials, demonstration of their value in affecting therapeutic decisions, and their cost-effectiveness in clinical practice.

REFERENCES

1. Best WR, Becktel JM, Singleton JW, Kern F. Development of a Crohn's disease activity index: National Cooperative Crohn's disease study. *Gastroenterology.* 1976;70:339-444.
2. Harvey RF, Bradshaw JM. A simple index of Crohn's disease activity. *Lancet.* 1980;1:514.
3. Truelove SC, Witts LJ. Cortisone in ulcerative colitis: final report on a therapeutic trial. *Br Med J.* 1955;2:1041-1048.
4. Rutegard JN. Assessment profiles of disease severity in ulcerative colitis. *Dig Dis.* 1993;11(1):32-35.
5. Seo M, Okada M, Yao T, Ueki M, Arima S, Okumura M. An index of disease activity in patients with ulcerative colitis. *Am J Gastroenterol.* 1992;87(8):971-976.
6. Walmsley RS, Ayers RCS, Pounder RE, Allan RN. A simple clinical colitis activity index. *Gut.* 1998;43:29-32.
7. Cameron HC, Rippman CH. The post-mortem statistics of ulcerative colitis at Guy's Hospital from 1888 to 1907. *Guy's Hosp Rep.* 1910;64:353-371.
8. Singleton J. Clinical activity assessment in inflammatory bowel disease. *Dig Dis Sci.* 1987;32(12):42S-45S.
9. Baron JH, Connell AM, Lennard-Jones JE. Variation between observers in describing mucosal appearances in proctocolitis. *Br Med J.* 1964;1:89.
10. Powell-Tuck J, Brown RL, Lennard-Jones JE. A comparison of oral prednisone given as single or multiple daily doses for active proctocolitis. *Scand J Gastroenterol.* 1978;13:833-837.
11. Sutherland LR, Martin F, Greer S, et al. 5-aminosalicylic acid enema in the treatment of distal ulcerative colitis, proctosigmoiditis, and proctitis. *Gastroenterology.* 1987;92(6):1894-1898.
12. Schroeder KW, Tremaine WJ, Ilstrup DM. Coated oral 5-aminosalicylic acid therapy for mildly to moderately active ulcerative colitis: a randomized study. *N Engl J Med.* 1987;317(26):1625-1629.
13. Lashner BA. Prediction rules for ulcerative colitis. *Am J Gastroenterol.* 1995;90(10):1737-1738.
14. Wasson JH, Sox HC, Neff RK. Clinical prediction rules: application and methodological standards. *N Engl J Med.* 1985;313:793-799.
15. Guyatt G, Mitchell A, Irvine EJ. A new measure of health status for clinical trials in inflammatory bowel disease. *Gastroenterology.* 1989;96:804-810.
16. Love JR, Irvine EJ, Fedorak RN. Quality of life in inflammatory bowel disease. *J Clin Invest.* 1992;14:15-19.
17. Jowett SL, Seal CJ, Barton R, Welfare M. The short inflammatory bowel disease questionnaire is reliable and responsive to clinically important change in ulcerative colitis. *Am J Gastroenterol.* 2001;96(10):2921-2928.
18. Casellas F, Alcala M, Prieto L, Miro JA, Malagelada J. Assessment of the influence of disease activity on the quality of life of patients with inflammatory bowel disease using a short questionnaire. *Am J Gastroenterol.* 2004;99(3):457-461.
19. Hanauer S, Schwartz J, Robinson M, et al. Mesalamine capsules for treatment of active ulcerative colitis: results of a controlled trial. *Am J Gastroenterol.* 1993;88(8):1188-1197.
20. Levine D, Riff D, Pruitt R, et al. A randomized, double blind, dose-response comparison of balsalazide (6.75 g), balsalazide (2.25 g), and mesalamine (2.4 g) in the treatment of active, mild-to-moderate ulcerative colitis. *Am J Gastroenterol.* 2002;97(6):1398-1405.
21. Goligher JC, Hoffman DC, deDombal FT. Surgical treatment of severe attacks of ulcerative colitis, with special reference to the advantage of early operation. *Br Med J.* 1970;4:703-706.
22. Edwards FC, Truelove SC. The course and prognosis of ulcerative colitis. *Gut.* 1963;4:299-308.
23. Gallagher ND, Goulston SSM, Wyndham N, Morrow W. The management of fulminant ulcerative colitis. *Gut.* 1962;3:306-311.
24. Truelove SC, Jewell DP. Intensive intravenous regimen for severe attacks of ulcerative colitis. *Lancet.* 1974:1067-1070.
25. Ritchie JK. Results of surgery for inflammatory bowel disease: a further survey of one hospital region. *Br Med J.* 1974;1:264-268.
26. Lennard-Jones JE, Ritchie JK, Hilder W, Spicer CC. Assessment of severity in colitis: a preliminary study. *Gut.* 1975;16:579-584.

27. Buckell NA, Lennard-Jones JE, Hernandez MA, Kohn J, Riches PG, Wadsworth J. Measurement of serum proteins during attacks of ultraviolet as a guide to patient management. *Gut.* 1979;20:22-27.
28. Jarnerot G, Rolny P, Sandberg-Gertzen H. Intensive intravenous treatment of ulcerative colitis. *Gastroenterology.* 1985;89:1005-1013.
29. Chew CN, Nolan DJ, Jewell DP. Small bowel gas in severe ulcerative colitis. *Gut.* 1991;32:1535-1539.
30. Lichtiger S, Present D, Kornbluth A, et al. Cyclosporine in severe ulcerative colitis refractory to steroid therapy. *N Engl J Med.* 1994;330(26):1841-1845.
31. Travis SPL, Farrant JM, Ricketts C, Nolan DJ, Mortensen NM, Kettlewell MGW. Predicting outcome in severe ulcerative colitis. *Gut.* 1996;38:905-910.
32. Seo M, Okada M, Yao T, Okabe N, Maeda K, Oh K. Evaluation of disease activity in patients with moderately active ulcerative colitis: Comparisons between a new activity index and Truelove and Witts' classification. *Am J Gastroenterol.* 1995;90(10):1759-1763.
33. Truelove SC, Richards WCD. Biopsy studies in ulcerative colitis. *Br Med J.* 1956;1:1315-1318.
34. Powell-Tuck J, Day DW, Buckell NA, Wadsworth J, Lennard-Jones JE. Correlations between defined sigmoidoscopic appearances and other measures of disease activity in ulcerative colitis. *Dig Dis Sci.* 1982;27(6):533-537.
35. Harber GB. Role of endoscopy in inflammatory bowel disease. *Dig Dis Sci.* 1987;32 (Suppl):165-175.
36. Williams CB, Waye JD. Colonoscopy in inflammatory bowel disease. *Clin Gastroenterol.* 1978;7:701-717.
37. Rizzello F, Gionchetti P, Venturi A, Amadini C, Romagnoli R, Campieri M. Review article: monitoring activity in ulcerative colitis. *Aliment Pharmacol Ther.* 2002;16 (Suppl 4):3-6.
38. Carbonnel F, Lavergne A, Lemann M, et al. Colonoscopy of acute colitis: A safe and reliable tool for assessment of severity. *Dig Dis Sci.* 1994;39(7):1550-1557.
39. Wright R, Truelove SC. Serial biopsy in ulcerative colitis during the course of a controlled therapeutic trial of various diets. *Am J Dig Dis.* 1966;11:1854-1858.
40. Bernstein CN, Kliewer E, Wajda A, Blanchard JF. The incidence of cancer among patients with IBD: a population based study. *Cancer.* 2001;91:854-862.
41. Greenstein AJ, Sachar DB, Smith H. Cancer in ulcerative and left sided colitis: Factors determining risk. *Gastroenterology.* 1979;77:290-294.
42. Sugita A, Sachar DB, Bodian C. Colorectal cancer in ulcerative colitis: influence of anatomical extent and age at onset on colitis-cancer interval. *Gut.* 1991;32:167-169.
43. Rutter M, Saunders B, Wilkinson K. Severity of inflammation is a risk factor for colorectal neoplasia in ulcerative colitis. *Gastroenterology.* 2004;126:451-459.
44. Kornbluth A, Sachar DB. Ulcerative colitis practice guidelines in adults (update): American College of Gastroenterology, Practice Parameters Committee. *Am J Gastroenterol.* 2004;49:1371-1385.
45. Bernstein CN. Ulcerative colitis with low grade dysplasia. *Gastroenterology.* 2004;127:950-956.
46. Carucci L, Levine M. Radiographic imaging of inflammatory bowel disease. *Gastroenterol Clin N Am.* 2002;31:93-117.
47. Arienti V, Campieri M, Boriani L. Management of severe ulcerative colitis with the help of high resolution ultrasonography. *Am J Gastroenterol.* 1996;91:2163-2169.
48. Weldon MJ, Lowe C, Joseph AE, Maxwell JD. Review article: quantitative leucocyte scanning in the assessment of inflammatory bowel disease activity and its response to therapy. *Aliment Pharmacol Ther.* 1996;10(2):123-132.
49. Guimbaud R, Beades E, Chauvelot-Moachon L, et al. Technetium Tc 99m hexamethyl propylene amine oxine leukocyte scintigraphy in patients with ulcerative colitis: correlation with clinical, biologic, endoscopic, and pathologic intensity and local release of interleukin-8. *Gastrointest Endosc.* 1998;48(5):491-496.
50. Aburano T, Saito Y, Shuke N, et al. Tc-99m leukocyte imaging for evaluating disease severity and monitoring treatment response in ulcerative colitis: comparison with colonoscopy. *Clinical Nuclear Medicine.* 1998;23(8):509-513.
51. Inoue S, Matsumoto T, Iida M, et al. Characterization of cytokine expression in the rectal mucosa of ulcerative colitis: correlation with disease activity. *Am J Gastroenterol.* 1999;94(9):2441-2446.
52. Bortoluzzi F, Valentini M, Cernigoi C, et al. DNA flow cytometric evaluation of cell cycle distribution in ulcerative colitis: a proposed method for assessing severity of disease. *Gut.* 1995;36(1):50-54.
53. Mahmud N, McDonald G, Kelleher D, et al. Microalbuminuria correlates with intestinal histopathological grading in patients with inflammatory bowel disease. *Gut.* 1996;38(1):99-103.
54. Riedl S, Tandara A, Reinshagen M, et al. Serum tenascin-C is an indicator of inflammatory bowel disease activity. *Int J Colorect Dis.* 2001;16(5):285-291.

13

Current and Future Oral Mesalamine Derivative Use in Ulcerative Colitis

Lloyd Sutherland, MDCM, MSc, FRCP(C), FACP

The modern era for the therapy of inflammatory bowel disease (IBD) began with the work of Nana Svartz, a Swedish physician with an interest in rheumatoid arthritis and ulcerative colitis. She invited her local pharmaceutical company to produce a compound with both anti-inflammatory and antibiotic properties (based on the understanding at that time). Her observations of the effect of the new compound, sulfasalazine (SASP), on disease activity in patients with UC were published in 1942.[1] They provided the first effective pharmacologic therapy not only in the IBD field, but also in the entire field of gastroenterology.

The implications of Svartz's work, however, were not seriously addressed until the early 1960s, when the first trials in both the induction and maintenance of remission were performed. Investigators, mainly in the United Kingdom, undertook several randomized, controlled trials confirming that SASP, at a dosage of 4 g/d, was effective for both indications.[2-4] It is of interest that, by current standards, many of the early trials were poorly designed and were likely susceptible to type II error. Nevertheless, SASP was accepted as the drug of choice for patients with mild to moderate disease activity.

During the 1970s, the focus shifted to examination of the dose and duration of therapy required for patients who had entered remission after a course of corticosteroids. In addition, Azad Khan and colleagues showed that the effectiveness of SASP was related to its 5-ASA moiety.[5] This was demonstrated in a nonplacebo-controlled trial that compared efficacy of topical sulfasalazine to topical mesalamine and topical sulfapyridine. On the other hand, the toxicity of sulfasalazine was thought to be due primarily to the sulfapyridine component.[6] The two components are attached by an azo-bond, which is cleaved by bacterial action mainly in the colon and terminal ileum.

Several 5-ASA preparations have been formulated that contain active ingredients, without sulfapyridine. The most widely used is mesalamine, in which 5-ASA is either coated by an acrylic capsule that dissolves at pH >7 (Eudragit S: Asacol, Lialda) or pH >6 (Eudragit L: APRISO, Salofalk, Claversal, Mesasal, or Rowasa), or is contained within ethylcellulose-coated microspheres (Pentasa). Other 5-ASA preparations release 5-ASA after bacterial cleavage of an azo-bond: olsalazine is a dimer of two 5-ASA molecules, while balsalazide is composed of 5-ASA and 4-aminobenzoyl-β-alanine (ABA). Table 13-1 lists the available 5-ASA preparations and the amount of 5-ASA that is delivered with the usual daily dosages.

In this chapter, the efficacy and safety of this class of drugs, given either orally or topically, for induction and maintenance therapy are reviewed. Five key questions will be addressed:

1. Are 5-ASA preparations effective for the treatment of active UC?
2. Are 5-ASA preparations effective for maintenance of remission from UC?
3. Are the newer preparations more effective than SASP?
4. Are the newer preparations better tolerated than SASP?
5. Is combination therapy more effective than either oral or rectal treatment alone?

Lichtenstein GR, ed.
Ulcerative Colitis: The Complete Guide to Medical Management (pp. 145-156)

TABLE 13-1

5-ASA CONTENT OF 5-AMINOSALICYLATE PREPARATIONS

Preparation	5-ASA Content (%)	Usual Dosage (g/d)	5-ASA Delivered (g/d)
Sulfasalazine	38	4	1.6
Mesalamine	100	2.4 to 4.8	2.4 to 4.8
Olsalazine	100	2 to 3	2 to 3
Balsalazide	35	6.75	2.4

EFFECTIVENESS OF 5-AMINOSALICYLATES FOR INDUCTION OF REMISSION

Because the course of UC is characterized by unpredictable relapses and remissions, a placebo group is necessary to demonstrate efficacy. Systemic therapy is generally offered to patients with extensive disease, while topical preparations are most suitable for patients with distal colitis.

SYSTEMIC THERAPY

As pointed out already, oral SASP is effective for active disease at a dosage of 4 g/d, and many patients respond to lower dosages. A meta-analysis demonstrated that the newer 5-ASA formulations, including mesalamine and olsalazine, are superior to placebo for inducing remission.[7] Individual dose-ranging studies have shown that, in the case of mesalamine, 4 or 4.8 g/d doses are more effective than 1.6 or 2 g/d. Response rates of 60% to 80% have been achieved in some of these trials, with clinical remission in 25% to 40%. The various mesalamine preparations have not been directly compared to each other, but there is no evidence to suggest that one agent is superior to another in terms of efficacy or adverse effects.

The optimum dosage of olsalazine appears to be 3 g/d.[7,8] Even though it is more effective than 1.5 to 2 g/d, the use of higher doses of olsalazine is limited by the occurrence of watery diarrhea, especially in patients with pancolitis. In some cases, this complication might be confused with active colitis, leading to an underestimation of the efficacy of this agent. Olsalazine appears to be as effective as mesalamine at the same dosage.[9]

A dose effect has been demonstrated for balsalazide, with the optimum dosage for induction of remission appearing to be 6.75 g/d.[10] Balsalazide at this dosage appeared to be superior to mesalamine 2.4 g/d in one trial,[11] but its advantages were less clear in two larger studies.[10,12] Balsalazide appeared to work more quickly than mesalamine, with better results at 2 weeks.

TOPICAL THERAPY

Topical therapy allows the opportunity to deliver high concentrations of 5-ASA directly to the distal colon, while minimizing systemic absorption of medication and resultant adverse effects. The 5-ASA preparations are available as suppositories, enemas, foam preparations, and gels. In the United States, topical/rectal preparations of mesalamine include 1-g mesalamine suppositories (Canasa) and 4-g mesalamine enemas (Rowasa). The extent of spread of the drug depends on the form and characteristics of the preparation. Suppositories reliably deliver medication to the rectum.[13-15] Liquid enemas spread consistently within the sigmoid colon and often to the splenic flexure, depending on their volume.[13,15] Enemas of high viscosity facilitate retention of the contents in more proximal parts of the colon.[16] Foam preparations deliver medication uniformly to the inflamed sigmoid and descending colon,[17,18] and their contents persist at these sites for longer periods of time than do liquid enemas.[15] A 60-mL gel preparation has been shown to cover the sigmoid colon and, in one-half of cases, up to the descending colon.[19] Most of the studies have employed somewhat artificial conditions, however, including prolonged fasting or adopting a supine posture without allowing the patient to move for long periods of time. Therefore, the results might not be easily replicated in actual clinical practice.

SASP enemas and suppositories have been shown to be effective for induction of remission from UC.[20-22]

Systemic reviews have likewise shown that mesalamine enemas and suppositories are superior to placebo and achieve response rates of up to 80%.[13,23] No difference in efficacy has been demonstrated in the dosage range of 1 to 4 g/d in nonrefractory patients,[23] nor is there a consistent difference in efficacy among various types of formulations, although some may be more easily tolerated. Topical mesalamine is more effective than topical corticosteroids.[13] Hydrocortisone or prednisolone enemas have been available for treatment of distal colitis.[24] Table 13-2 provides a list of rectal steroid formulations; topical steroids are less effective than topical aminosalicylates.[13,25]

TABLE 13-2

RECTAL CORTICOSTEROID PREPARATIONS

MEDICATION	DOSE (MG)	FORMULATION
Hydrocortisone	80 to 100	Suppository, foam, or enema
Prednisolone-21-phosphate	20 to 40	Suppositories or enemas
Prednisolone metasulphobenzoate	20	Enema
Betamethasone	5 to 20	Enema
Tixocortol pivalate	250	Enema
Beclomethasone dipropionate	0.5 to 3	Enema
Budesonide	2	Enema

Why do oral, but not topical, 5-ASAs exhibit a dose effect in patients with active UC? Because the latter agents deliver 5-ASA directly and efficiently to the site of active inflammation, perhaps only small amounts (eg, 1 g/d) are required to induce remission. A dose response curve may exist at even smaller dosages, but this possibility has not been investigated. On the other hand, oral preparations release the active ingredient over a larger area of the colon and/or small bowel. It may be particularly difficult for an oral agent to deliver 5-ASA to the site of active disease when it is confined to the rectosigmoid colon. This is because of the occurrence of decreased colonic motility, which could result in release and absorption of the medication too proximally. Large doses of medication might therefore be required in such cases. It has recently been discerned that there is not a clear dose-response curve as was initially perceived to be present with use of oral mesalamine in patients with UC. In the ASCEND III trial, which assessed 2.4 vs 4.8 g of mesalamine, noninferiority was demonstrated.[26] In post-hoc subset analysis, it was demonstrated that those patients who had more difficult to treat disease had more benefit from higher-dose mesalamine (4.8 g/d).[27]

CONCLUSION

Oral agents are convenient to use and are suitable for extensive, as well as left-sided colitis. SASP and the newer 5-ASAs are all effective in the treatment of active UC. A dose effect has been shown in most individual trials and confirmed by meta-analysis. There is little conclusive evidence of the superiority of one agent over another, although balsalazide may be more effective than mesalamine in equimolar amounts and may work more rapidly. The various forms of mesalamine do not seem to differ in efficacy. The following dosage regimens appear to be roughly equivalent:

- Sulfasalazine 4 g/d
- Mesalamine 2.4 to 4.8 g/d
- Olsalazine 2 to 3 g/d
- Balsalazide 6.75 g/d
- MMX mesalamine 2.4 to 4.8 g/d[28,29]
- Mesalamine 1.5 g granulated[30,31]

Topical therapy provides rapid and effective relief of symptoms at low dosages and with little systemic effect. Various formulations are available, ie, suppositories for proctitis and liquid, foam, or gel enemas for disease in the sigmoid and descending colon. In general, larger enema volumes and viscous agents facilitate delivery of medication to the descending colon and even the splenic flexure.

EFFECTIVENESS OF 5-AMINOSALICYLATES FOR MAINTENANCE OF REMISSION

Strategies that prolong or maintain remission offer the greatest opportunity to provide long-term improvement in the patient's quality of life. Because maintenance therapy generally involves some inconvenience, expense, and possibly adverse effects, it is important to refine treatment so that the minimum amount of medication can be used.

A recent population-based study of the clinical course of UC found that 83% of patients relapsed in the first 10 years of diagnosis, but half (48%) were relapse-free during the last 5 years of the 10-year study period.[32] Another population-based study found that 50% of patients relapse in the first year after diagnosis.[33] Therefore, the need for effective maintenance therapy would seem to be clear. Dissanayake and Truelove reported that the risk of relapse did not decrease with increasing duration of disease,[34] which would suggest that maintenance therapy should be continued indefinitely. On the other hand, Ardizzone et al could not demonstrate a benefit from maintenance therapy after at least 2 years of remission,[35] but this study involved only a small number of patients and might have been subject to type II error. Incomplete healing of the mucosa despite clinical remission is also associated with early relapse, and certain endoscopic and histologic parameters are said to have predictive value.[36-38]

Maintenance therapy is given in one of 3 ways: 1) at the same dosage as effective therapy for active disease, 2) at half the effective induction dosage (as is done with H_2 antagonists), or 3) "on demand." A novel once-daily 1.5-g granulated mesalamine (taken as four 375-mg capsules) providing delayed and extended release of mesalamine to terminal ileum and colon provides effective maintenance of UC remission.[39] At present, this represents the only once-daily oral mesalamine preparation approved for maintenance of remission in the United States.

Systemic Therapy

SASP is effective for maintenance therapy at a dosage of 2 g/d,[34,40,41] which is half of the optimum induction dosage. Khan et al found that 2 g/d was superior to 1 g/d, whereas the advantage in efficacy of the 4 g/d dosage was offset by an increased risk of hematologic toxicity.[42] One small study found that on-demand therapy with SASP was shown to be as effective as continuous therapy.[43] More evaluation of this strategy is required.

The newer 5-ASAs have been shown to be effective for maintenance of remission in a number of clinical trials.[44] The minimum effective dosage of mesalamine may be 0.8 g/d, but most studies have used at least 1.2 g/d. Dosages greater than 1.5 g/d have not been proven to provide greater benefits[45] and are more expensive. Olsalazine has been shown to be effective for maintenance at dosages between 0.5 and 2 g/d, with no clear dose effect.[46,47] Diarrhea is a concern during long-term treatment. A dosage effect has been demonstrated for balsalazide, with 4 to 6 g/d being superior to 2 to 3 g/d.[48,49]

Balsalazide appears to be more effective than mesalamine in induction of remission, but does not differ from mesalamine in preventing relapse, according to a meta-analysis of 6 randomized, placebo-controlled trials.[50] One study comparing olsalazine to mesalamine found that the former was better at maintaining remission,[51] while another study showed no difference in effectiveness between the 2 agents in inducing endoscopic remission in patients with mild to moderate active UC within 12 weeks of treatment.[52] The ASCEND I and II trials suggested a dose-response curve for mesalamine.[53,54] In ASCEND II, response rates were 72% with 4.8 g of delayed-release mesalamine and 59% with 2.4 g delayed-release mesalamine in patients with mild to moderate UC; remission rates were similar at 24%.[54]

In the ASCEND III trial, however, there was no dose response demonstrated.[26] It is thus perceived that there is not a dose response for oral mesalamine. A post-hoc analysis demonstrated that there was a subset of patients who achieved benefit with higher dose of oral delayed-release mesalamine.[29]

Topical Therapy

Mesalamine enemas and suppositories are superior to placebo at maintaining remission from UC.[13,23,24] High-dose (4 g) enemas can be effective when used intermittently: 7 days per month, every third night, or twice per week. Such regimens should be associated with improved patient acceptance. Mesalamine suppositories are also effective at a dosage as small as 1 g three times per week.

A prospective blinded trial demonstrated that 1, 2, and 4 g were equally effective for induction of remission.[23] In practice, however, it seems reasonable to attempt to gradually reduce the number of enemas given per week, so as to forestall relapse and find the minimum effective maintenance dosage regimen. Because it is difficult to determine an individual patient's risk of relapse at a specific point in the course of his or her disease, treatment should be individualized.

Conclusion

Controlled clinical trials have demonstrated that 5-ASAs are more effective than placebo at maintaining remission from UC (Figure 13-1). The optimum dosage of oral SASP is probably 2 g/d, because higher dosages are associated with unacceptable levels of toxicity. A dose effect has been documented for balsalazide but not for mesalamine or olsalazine. Oral mesalamine, olsalazine, and balsalazide are superior to placebo and are probably roughly equivalent; however, isolated studies suggest that balsalazide and olsalazine may be better than mesalamine. Topical preparations are more effective than placebo at maintaining remission, but there is little conclusive evidence for the existence of a dose effect. Intermittent and on-demand therapy are options that have not been extensively tested, and the minimum effective regimen for an individual patient must be determined empirically.

It is worth noting that the 5-ASAs and infliximab have proven to be of benefit for the maintenance of remission from UC (Figure 13-2).[55] In contrast, corticosteroids and immunosuppressive agents are ineffective for this indication.[56,57] On the other hand, there is preliminary evidence that probiotics may be effective,[58,59] although more controlled studies are required.

Review: Oral 5-aminosalicylic acid for induction of remission in ulcerative colitis
Comparison: 01 5-ASA versus placebo
Outcome: 02 Failure to Induce Global/Clinical Remission or Improvement

Study	Treatment n/N	Control n/N	Peto Odds Ratio 95% Cl	Weight (%)	Peto Odds Ratio 95% Cl
01 Dose of 5-ASA: < 2 g					
Hanauer 1993	27/92	14/30		11.0	0.46 [0.19, 1.10]
Schroeder 1987	8/11	15/19		2.8	0.71 [0.13, 4.02]
Sninsky 1991	34/53	21/26		8.1	0.46 [0.17, 1.27]
Subtotal (95% Cl)	69/156	50/75		21.9	0.49 [0.26, 0.90]
Test for heterogeneity chi-square=0.21 df=2 P=0.8985					
Test for overall effect=–2.28 P=0.02					
02 Dose of 5-ASA: 2-2.9 g					
Feurle 1989	25/52	29/53		14.3	0.77 [0.36, 1.65]
Hanauer 1993	20/97	14/30		9.8	0.27 [0.11, 0.67]
Hetzel 1986	9/15	13/15		3.3	0.27 [0.05, 1.31]
Robinson 1988	29/50	34/48		12.3	0.58 [0.25, 1.31]
Sninsky 1991	32/53	21/26		8.4	0.40 [0.15, 1.08]
Sutherland 1990	37/45	18/22		4.8	1.03 [0.27, 3.85]
Subtotal (95% Cl)	152/312	129/194		52.9	0.51 [0.34, 0.76]
Test for heterogeneity chi-square=5.01 df=5 P=0.4144					
Test for overall effect=–3.31 P=0.0009					
03 Dose of 5-ASA: ≥3 g					
Hanauer 1993	15/95	13/30		8.6	0.21 [0.08, 0.55]
Schroeder 1987	10/38	16/19		6.9	0.10 [0.03, 0.30]
Sutherland 1990	26/47	18/22		7.6	0.32 [0.11, 0.92]
Zinberg 1990	3/7	6/8		2.1	0.29 [0.04, 2.12]
Subtotal (95% Cl)	54/187	53/79		25.2	0.20 [0.11, 0.35]
Test for heterogeneity chi-square=2.43 df=3 P=0.4881					
Test for overall effect=–5.50 P<0.00001					
Total (95% Cl)	275/655	232/348		100.0	0.40 [0.30, 0.53]
Test for heterogeneity chi-square=15.17 df=12 P=0.2321					
Test for overall effect=–6.23 P<0.0001					
			–1 –2 1 5 10		

FIGURE 13-1. Failure to induce global/clinical remission or improvement. (Reprinted from Sutherland LR, MacDonald JK. Oral 5-aminosalicylic acid for induction of remission in ulcerative colitis. *Cochrane Databaseof Systematic Reviews.* 2006;2[Art. No. CD000543].)

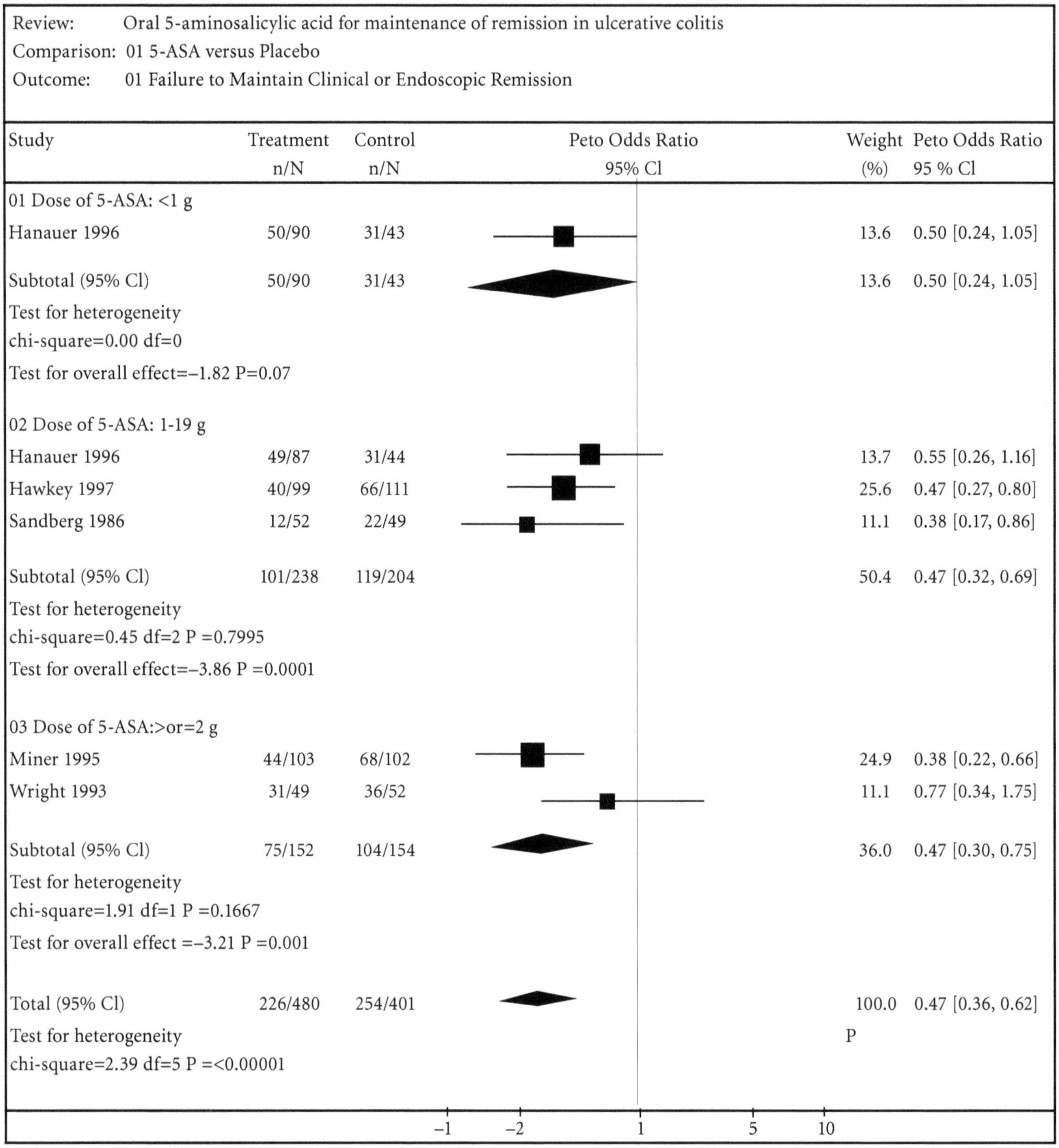

FIGURE 13-2. Failure to maintain clinical or endoscopic remission. (Reprinted from Sutherland: The Cochrane Library. 2004;4.)

EFFECTIVENESS OF SULFASALAZINE VERSUS NEWER AGENTS

Randomized controlled trials comparing SASP with the newer agents fail to demonstrate superior efficacy for the latter.[7,60] Moreover, many of the trials have utilized dosages of SASP with less 5-ASA content than the comparator drug. Perhaps SASP has therapeutic effects that are unrelated to the 5-ASA moiety. Alternatively, the newer agents may not reliably release as much 5-ASA as does SASP at the site of active disease.

Several studies have shown that SASP at a dosage of usually 1.5 to 2 g/d appears to be therapeutically equivalent to the mesalamine, olsalazine, or balsalazide at equimolar dosages for maintenance of remission.[60-62]

TABLE 13-3

ADVERSE EFFECTS FROM SULFASALAZINE

DOSE-RELATED	
Nausea	Fever
Abdominal pain	Folate deficiency
Diarrhea	Hemolytic anemia
Fatigue	Cytopenias
Malaise	Arthralgias and myalgias
Headache	Male infertility
IDIOSYNCRATIC	
Exacerbation of colitis	Pancreatitis
Hepatitis	Polyarteritis
Pneumonitis and pulmonary fibrosis	Interstitial nephritis
Pericarditis or myocarditis	Agranulocytosis
Lupus-like syndrome	Neuropathy
Skin rash or photosensitivity	Stevens-Johnson syndrome

TOLERABILITY OF SULFASALAZINE VERSUS NEWER AGENTS

SYSTEMIC THERAPY

One of the purported advantages of the newer 5-ASAa is that they would allow an increase in 5-ASA dosage without encountering sulfapyridine-related toxicity. In fact, mesalamine is tolerated well even at a dosage as high as 4.8 g/d, which is equivalent in 5-ASA content to 12 g/d of SASP. Meta-analyses have shown that the newer 5-aminosalicylates are better tolerated than SASP for induction of remission,[7] but not for maintenance therapy.[44]

It should also be noted that most comparative studies selected patients who had already been shown to be tolerant of SASP, which means that the SASP toxicity might have been underestimated. In trials involving patients with no previous exposure to SASP, however, the superior tolerability the mesalamine and balsalazide can be readily demonstrated.

On the other hand, olsalazine is associated with dose-related diarrhea and is the only new agent that is not more easily tolerated than SASP. It may be misleading, therefore, to include comparative trials of olsalazine with those involving other 5-ASAs. Although it may not be analogous to comparing apples with oranges, it may be like comparing oranges with tangerines.

TOPICAL THERAPY

Patients seem to tolerate suppositories well, even for long-term use, and prefer them to liquid enemas[63] or even foam preparations.[64] Gel preparations are better accepted than foams,[65] which are preferred over liquid enemas.[66] Most of the problems that patients experience with topical medications are more frequently encountered with liquid enemas: difficulty retaining or inserting the medication, leakage, interference with daily activities, and perianal or anal irritation or burning.

ADVERSE EFFECTS OF SULFASALAZINE

SASP has been associated with adverse effects in up to 45% of patients, which necessitates discontinuation of medication in approximately 20% of cases.[67,68] Adverse effects with this drug are divided into 2 groups: dose-related, presumably due to sulfapyridine and occurring more frequently in slow acetylators[69]; and idiosyncratic, which are more rare and serious. Some of the latter type of adverse effects have also been seen with mesalamine and other 5-ASAs and may constitute allergy or intolerance to 5-ASA itself. Examples of the most important adverse effects related to SASP are listed in Table 13-3.

Adverse Effects of Mesalamine

Although mesalamine is better tolerated than SASP, adverse effects still occur in up to 20% of patients taking the medication, although most clinical trials report that withdrawal due to adverse effects occurs in fewer than 10%.[70] Most investigators who have compared SASP with the newer agents reported fewer withdrawals with the latter.[7] Nevertheless, each of the idiosyncratic complications listed in Table 13-3 have also been associated with the newer 5-ASAs. Pancreatitis seems to be especially frequent, but this may be due to reporting bias due to increased awareness of this complication among physicians.

The toxicity of 5-ASA may be related to its systemic absorption, which is significantly lower with topical than with oral administration of the drug.[71] Because it appears to be affected by the pH of the intestinal lumen, absorption of 5-ASA is reduced more during active colitis than when the disease is quiescent,[72] despite the presence of inflamed mucosa.

Olsalazine-Induced Diarrhea

Diarrhea is the only dose-related symptom that is reported more frequently with any of the newer 5-ASAs (specifically olsalazine) than with SASP. Up to 36% of patients taking olsalazine in clinical trials experience this symptom, and approximately 10% to 20% have needed to withdraw from treatment because of it.[7,73] The incidence of diarrhea may be ameliorated by taking the medication with or immediately after meals or by slowly increasing the dosage.[73]

Diarrhea seems to be more frequent in patients with pancolitis than in those with proctosigmoiditis or distal colitis. Olsalazine has been shown, in a dose-dependent manner, to stimulate fluid secretion and inhibit salt and water absorption in the small intestine and colon in both normal human volunteers and experimental animals.[74,75] It appears that the increased fluid load that is delivered to the colon can readily be absorbed by normal subjects,[76,77] but not by patients with extensive colitis.[75] There is experimental[78] and clinical[79] evidence that tolerance to the diarrhea effect of olsalazine occurs.

Most patients and physicians are able to distinguish between drug-induced diarrhea and an exacerbation of colitis, which has also been reported with both SASP[80,81] and mesalamine.[82-84] The latter is characterized by increased diarrhea (often bloody), nocturnal diarrhea, urgency, abdominal cramps, fevers, myalgias, and arthralgias, often beginning within 24 to 48 hours of starting the medication and resolving within a similar period of time after discontinuing it. Olsalazine-induced diarrhea, on the other hand, is watery, non-bloody, and not associated with other features of active inflammation. Sigmoidoscopy may be helpful in equivocal cases.

Nephrotoxicity

There is some controversy about the association between interstitial nephritis and mesalamine. This complication has rarely been reported with the use of SASP, but there are many case reports linking it to mesalamine.[85-88] Fever, rash, arthralgias, and eosinophilia can accompany this condition, but most cases are asymptomatic. Interstitial nephritis might be due to decreased renal blood flow or to direct tubular toxicity.

Evaluation of sensitive markers of tubular dysfunction have not clearly implicated 5-ASA in causing either tubular damage or renal failure.[89-91] In fact, tubular dysfunction is more closely correlated with the activity or severity of IBD. Overt renal disease, including glomerular and tubular defects, has been reported as a complication of IBD itself.[89,90] Moreover, microalbuminuria can occur in patients with untreated IBD.[92,93]

Renal compromise is a very infrequent occurrence in patients taking 5-ASA, according to large surveys.[94,95] In fact, it appears that interstitial nephritis is likely to be a poorly recognized extraintestinal manifestation of IBD. The most recent study, conducted in the United Kingdom, found an association between 5-ASAs (both mesalamine and SASP) and nephrotoxicity, which could be partly explained by the underlying bowel disease.[95] The risk of renal disease was low, however, and in only a few cases could interstitial nephritis and the link to 5-ASA be established with certainty.

Pregnancy

The 5-ASAs are generally accepted for use in pregnancy,[96,97] despite the fact that SASP and sulfapyridine can readily cross the blood-brain barrier.[98] There may be a concern about its use while nursing, however, because both sulfapyridine and mesalamine can be excreted in breast milk.[99,100] This may result in diarrhea in infants who are breastfed.[101,102]

Conclusion

Sulfasalazine is associated with a variety of adverse effects that limit the ability to use this drug in high doses. Although most of the dose-related toxicity has been attributed to the sulfapyridine moiety, several of the potentially serious reactions (notably pancreatitis) have also been reported with the newer 5-ASAs. Secretory diarrhea is a specific complication of olsalazine and appears to be dose-related. Strategies to reduce its occurrence include taking the medication with meals or slowly increasing the dosage, and it might subside with time. Although there are many case reports of nephrotoxicity with the use of mesalamine, especially interstitial nephritis, it appears that this might be an extraintestinal manifestation of IBD per se. The 5-ASAs are generally thought to be safe for use during pregnancy (category B), but are excreted in breast milk. The ability to demonstrate superior tolerability of the newer agents, compared with SASP, in clinical trials is impaired by the inclusion criteria, which often specify previous tolerance to the latter agent.

EFFECTIVENESS OF COMBINATION THERAPY

Randomized controlled trials have shown that mesalamine enemas are at least as effective as oral SASP or mesalamine, provide more rapid relief of symptoms, and are associated with fewer adverse effects.[103,104] The combination of topical and oral 5-ASA also appears to be superior to either modality alone.[105] Most of the latter studies could be criticized because the total amount of the 5-ASA administered in the combination therapy arm was greater than that given in the other arms. In a study that overcame this problem, no difference in either the efficacy or the speed of action of combination could be demonstrated.[106] Nevertheless, clinical experience verifies the concept that topical therapy provides rapid relief of symptoms of UC. This is probably due to the fact that many symptoms of UC, such as rectal urgency and bleeding, are due in large part to inflammation in the rectum, even in patients with more extensive disease.

Combination therapy with mesalamine enemas and tablets maintain remission more effectively than oral 5-ASA alone and is associated with reduced overall health-care utilization.[107,108] This strategy might be too cumbersome for the typical patient in remission and should be reserved for patients who have demonstrated a propensity to rapid or frequent relapse. A recent study has shown that adding topical mesalamine improves two-thirds of patients with universal colitis.[109]

THE FUTURE ROLE OF 5-AMINOSALICYLATES

So what is the future of 5-ASA? It is clearly effective in the induction and maintenance of remission from UC and should continue to be the agent of first choice for both indications. It is not likely that increasing the dosage of these agents would improve their effectiveness. Adherence to treatment could be enhanced, however, by simplifying the dosage regimen. A once-daily formulation for induction therapy would be especially welcome. Further research on the minimum effective dosage for maintenance therapy is also required. We now have once-daily dosing for the induction of remission in UC,[28,29,31] and a once-daily granulated mesalamine is approved for maintenance of remission.[30] This work would allow the potential of the discovery made by Dr. Svartz to be fully realized.[110]

REFERENCES

1. Svartz N. Salazopyrin, a new sulfanilamide preparation. *Acta Med Scand.* 1942;110:577-598.
2. Baron JH, Connell AM, Lennard-Jones JE, Jones FA. Sulphasalazine and salicylazosulphadimidine in ulcerative colitis. *Lancet.* 1962;1:1094.
3. Dick AP, Grayson MJ, Carpenter RG, Petrie A. Controlled trial of sulphasalazine in the treatment of ulcerative colitis. *Gut.* 1964;50:437.
4. Lennard-Jones JE, Longmore AJ, Newell AC, Wilson CW, Jones FA. An assessment of prednisone, salazopyrin, and topical hydrocortisone hemisuccinate used as out-patient treatment for ulcerative colitis. *Gut.* 1960;1:217-222.
5. Khan AK, Piris J, Truelove SC. An experiment to determine the active therapeutic moiety of sulphasalazine. *Lancet.* 1977;2(8044):892-895.
6. Myers B, Evans DNW, Rhodes J, et al. Metabolism and urinary excretion of 5-aminosalicylic acid in healthy volunteers when given intravenously or released for absorption at different sites in the gastrointestinal tract. *Gut.* 1987;28:196-200.
7. Sutherland LR, MacDonald JK. Oral 5-aminosalicylic acid for induction of remission in ulcerative colitis. *Cochrane Database Syst Rev.* 2006;(2):CD000543.
8. Zinberg J, Molinas S, Das KM. Double-blind placebo-controlled study of olsalazine in the treatment of ulcerative colitis. *Am J Gastroenterol.* 1990;85(5):562-566.
9. Kruis W, Brandes JW, Schreiber S, et al. Olsalazine versus mesalazine in the treatment of mild to moderate ulcerative colitis. *Aliment Pharmacol Ther.* 1998;12(8):707-715.
10. Levine DS, Riff DS, Pruitt R, et al. A randomized, double blind, dose-response comparison of balsalazide (6.75 g), balsalazide (2.25 g), and mesalamine (2.4 g) in the treatment of active, mild-to-moderate ulcerative colitis. *Am J Gastroenterol.* 2002;97(6):1398-1407.
11. Green JR, Lobo AJ, Holdsworth CD, et al. Balsalazide is more effective and better tolerated than mesalamine in the treatment of acute ulcerative colitis. The Abacus Investigator Group. *Gastroenterology.* 1998;114(1):15-22.
12. Pruitt R, Hanson J, Safdi M, et al. Balsalazide is superior to mesalamine in the time to improvement of signs and symptoms of acute mild-to-moderate ulcerative colitis. *Am J Gastroenterol.* 2002;97(12):3078-3086.
13. Marshall JK, Irvine EJ. Putting rectal 5-aminosalicylic acid in its place: the role in distal ulcerative colitis. *Am J Gastroenterol.* 2000;95(7):1628-1636.
14. Marshall JK, Irvine EJ. Rectal aminosalicylate therapy for distal ulcerative colitis: a meta-analysis. *Aliment Pharmacol Ther.* 1995;9(3):293-300.
15. Campieri M, Corbelli C, Gionchetti P, et al. Spread and distribution of 5-ASA colonic foam and 5-ASA enema in patients with ulcerative colitis. *Dig Dis Sci.* 1992;37(12):1890-1897.
16. Otten MH, De Haas G, Van den Ende R. Colonic spread of 5-ASA enemas in healthy individuals, with a comparison of their physical and chemical characteristics. *Aliment Pharmacol Ther.* 1997;11(4):693-697.
17. Wilding IR, Kenyon CJ, Chauhan S, et al. Colonic spreading of a non-chlorofluorocarbon mesalazine rectal foam enema in patients with quiescent ulcerative colitis. *Aliment Pharmacol Ther.* 1995;9(2):161-166.

18. Farthing MJ, Rutland MD, Clark ML. Retrograde spread of hydrocortisone containing foam given intrarectally in ulcerative colitis. *Br Med J.* 1979;2(6194):822-824.
19. Gionchetti P, Venturi A, Rizzello F, et al. Retrograde colonic spread of a new mesalazine rectal enema in patients with distal ulcerative colitis. *Aliment Pharmacol Ther.* 1997;11(4):679-684.
20. Palmer KR, Goepel JR, Holdsworth CD. Sulphasalazine retention enemas in ulcerative colitis: a double-blind trial. *Br Med J (Clin Res Ed).* 1981;282(6276):1571-1573.
21. Frühmorgen P, Demling L. On the efficacy of ready-made-up commercially available salicylazosulphapyridine enemas in the treatment of proctitis, proctosigmoiditis and ulcerative colitis involving rectum, sigmoid and descending colon. *Hepatogastroenterology.* 1980;27(6):473-476.
22. Serebro H, Kay S, Javett S, Abrahams C. Sulphasalazine rectal enemas: Topical method of inducing remission of active ulcerative colitis affecting rectum and descending colon. *Br Med J.* 1977;2(6097):1264.
23. Hanauer SB. Dose-ranging study of mesalamine (PENTASA) enemas in the treatment of acute ulcerative proctosigmoiditis: results of a multicentered placebo-controlled trial. The U.S. PENTASA Enema Study Group. *Inflamm Bowel Dis.* 1998;4(2):79-83.
24. Marshall JK, Irvine EJ. Rectal corticosteroids versus alternative treatments in ulcerative colitis: A meta-analysis. *Gut.* 1997;40(6):775-781.
25. Hanauer S. Medical therapy for ulcerative colitis. In: Sartor RB, Sandborn WJ, eds. *Kirsner's Inflammatory Bowel Diseases.* 6th ed. Philadelphia, PA: WB Saunders; 2004:510-511.
26. Sandborn WJ, Regula J, Feagan B, et al. Efficacy and safety of delayed-release oral mesalamine at 4.8 g/d (800 mg tablet) in the treatment of moderately active ulcerative colitis: results of the ASCEND III study [abstract 702]. *Gastroenterology.* 2008;134(4 suppl 1):A99.
27. Hanauer SB, Ramsey D, Sandborn W. Increased efficacy of delayed-release mesalamine 4.8 g/d (800 mg tablet) compared to 2.4 g/d (400 mg tablet) for treatment of moderately active ulcerative colitis in patients with a history of more difficult to treat disease: combined analysis from three randomized, double-blind, active-controlled trials [abstract 1085]. *Am J Gastroenterol.* 2008;103:S424.
28. Lichtenstein GR, Kamm MA, Boddu P, et al. Effect of once or twice-daily MMX mesalamine (SPD476) for the induction of remission of mild to moderately active ulcerative colitis. *Clin Gastroenterol Hepatol.* 2007;5(1):95-102.
29. Kamm MA, Sandborn WJ, Gassull M, et al. Once-daily, high concentration MMX mesalamine in active ulcerative colitis. *Gastroenterology.* 2007;132:66-73.
30. Lichtenstein G, Merchant K, Shaw A, Yuan J, Bortey E, Forbes W. Once-daily 1.5-g granulated mesalamine effectively maintains remission in patients with ulcerative colitis who switch from different 5-ASA formulations [abstract 1100]. *Am J Gastroenterol.* 2008;13(suppl 1):429-430.
31. Kruis W, Kiudelis G, Racz I, et al. Once-daily versus three-times-daily mesalazine granules in active ulcerative colitis: a double-blind, double-dummy, randomised non-inferiority trial. *Gut.* 2008;doi:10.1136.
32. Solberg IC, Lygren I, Jahnsen J, et al. Clinical course during the first 10 years of ulcerative colitis: results from a population-based inception cohort (IBSEN Study). *Scand J Gastroenterol.* 2009;44(4):431-440.
33. Moum B, Ekbom A, Vatn MH, et al. Clinical course during the 1st year after diagnosis in ulcerative colitis and Crohn's disease. results of a large, prospective population-based study in southeastern Norway, 1990-93. *Scand J Gastroenterol.* 1997;32(10):1005-1012.
34. Dissanayake AS, Truelove SC. Proceedings: a controlled therapeutic trial of long-term maintenance treatment of ulcerative colitis with sulphasalazine (salazopyrin). *Gut.* 1973;14(10):818.
35. Ardizzone S, Petrillo M, Imbesi V, et al. Is maintenance therapy always necessary for patients with ulcerative colitis in remission? *Aliment Pharmacol Ther.* 1999;13(3):373-379.
36. Nishio Y, Ando T, Maeda O, et al. Pit patterns in rectal mucosa assessed by magnifying colonoscope are predictive of relapse in patients with quiescent ulcerative colitis. *Gut.* 2006;55(12):1768-1773.
37. Higaki S, Nohara H, Saitoh Y, et al. Increased rectal wall thickness may predict relapse in ulcerative colitis: a pilot follow-up study by ultrasonographic colonoscopy. *Endoscopy.* 2002;34(3):212-219.
38. Bitton A, Peppercorn MA, Antonioli DA, et al. Clinical, biological, and histologic parameters as predictors of relapse in ulcerative colitis. *Gastroenterology.* 2001;120(1):13-20.
39. Lichtenstein G, Merchant K, Shaw A, Yuan J, Bortey E, Forbes W. Once-daily 1.5-g granulated mesalamine effectively maintains remission in patients with ulcerative colitis who switch from different 5-ASA formulations. *Am J Gastroenterol.* 2008;13(suppl 1): s429-430(abstract 1100).
40. Khan AK, Howes DT, Piris J, Truelove SC. Optimum dose of sulphasalazine for maintenance treatment in ulcerative colitis. *Gut.* 1980;21(3):232-240.
41. Dronfield MW, Langman MJ. Comparative trial of sulphasalazine and oral sodium cromoglycate in the maintenance of remission in ulcerative colitis. *Gut.* 1978;19(12):1136-1139.
42. Khan AZ, Nurazzaman, Truelove. The effect of the acetylator phenotype on the metabolism of sulphasalazine in man. *J Med Genet.* 1983;20(1):30-36.
43. Dickinson RJ, King A, Wight DG, Hunter JO, Neale G. Is continuous sulfasalazine necessary in the management of patients with ulcerative colitis? Results of a preliminary study. *Dis Colon Rectum.* 1985;28(12):929-930.
44. Sutherland L, Macdonald JK. Oral 5-aminosalicylic acid for maintenance of remission in ulcerative colitis. *Cochrane Database Syst Rev.* 2006;(2):CD000544.
45. The Mesalamine Study Group. An oral preparation of mesalamine as long-term maintenance therapy for ulcerative colitis. a randomized, placebo-controlled trial. *Ann Intern Med.* 1996;124(2):204-211.
46. Zinberg J, Molinas S, Das KM. Double-blind dose-finding study of olsalazine versus sulphasalazine as maintenance therapy for ulcerative colitis. *Eur J Gastroenterol Hepatol.* 1995;7(5):391-396.
47. Kruis W, Judmaier G, Kayasseh L, et al. Double-blind dose-finding study of olsalazine versus sulphasalazine as maintenance therapy for ulcerative colitis. *Eur J Gastroenterol Hepatol.* 1995;7(5):391-396.
48. Kruis W, Schreiber S, Theuer D, et al. Low dose balsalazide (1.5 g twice daily) and mesalazine (0.5 g three times daily) maintained remission of ulcerative colitis but high dose balsalazide (3.0 g twice daily) was superior in preventing relapses. *Gut.* 2001;49(6):783-789.
49. Levine DS, Riff DS, Pruitt R, et al. A randomized, double blind, dose-response comparison of balsalazide (6.75 g), balsalazide (2.25 g), and mesalamine (2.4 g) in the treatment of active, mild-to-moderate ulcerative colitis. *Am J Gastroenterol.* 2002;97(6):1398-1407.
50. Rahimi R, Nikfar S, Rezaie A, Abdollahi M. Comparison of mesalazine and balsalazide in induction and maintenance of remission in patients with ulcerative colitis: a meta-analysis. *Dig Dis Sci.* 2009;54:712-721.
51. Courtney MG, Nunes DP, Bergin CF, et al. Randomised comparison of olsalazine and mesalazine in prevention of relapses in ulcerative colitis. *Lancet.* 1992;339(8804):1279-1281.
52. Kruis W, Brandes JW, Schreiber S, et al. Olsalazine versus mesalazine in the treatment of mild to moderate ulcerative colitis. *Aliment Pharmacol Ther.* 1998;12(8):707-715.

53. Hanauer SB, Sandborn WJ, Dallaire C, et al. Delayed-release oral mesalamine 4.8 g/day (800 mg tablets) compared to 2.4 g/day (400 mg tablets) for the treatment of mildly to moderately active ulcerative colitis: The ASCEND I trial. *Can J Gastroenterol.* 2007;21(12):827-834.
54. Hanauer SB, Sandborn WJ, Kornbluth A, et al. Delayed-release oral mesalamine at 4.8 g/day (800 mg tablet) for the treatment of moderately active ulcerative colitis: The ASCEND II trial. *Am J Gastroenterol.* 2005;100(11):2478-2485.
55. Rutgeerts P, Sandborn WJ, Feagan BG, et al. Infliximab for induction and maintenance therapy for ulcerative colitis. *N Engl J Med.* 2005;353(23):2462-2476.
56. Bianchi Porro G, Cassinotti A, Ferrara E, Maconi G, Ardizzone S. Review article: the management of steroid dependency in ulcerative colitis. *Aliment Pharmacol Ther.* 2007;26(6):779-794.
57. Lennard-Jones JE, Misiewicz JJ, Connell AM, Baron JH, Jones FA. Prednisone as maintenance treatment for ulcerative colitis in remission. *Lancet.* 1965;1(7378):188-189.
58. Heilpern D, Szilagyi A. Manipulation of intestinal microbial flora for therapeutic benefit in inflammatory bowel diseases: review of clinical trials of probiotics, pre-biotics and synbiotics. *Rev Recent Clin Trials.* 2008;3(3):167-184.
59. Fedorak RN, Dieleman LA. Probiotics in the treatment of human inflammatory bowel diseases: update 2008. *J Clin Gastroenterol.* 2008;42 Suppl 2:S97-S103.
60. Nikfar S, Rahimi R, Rezaie A, Abdollahi M. A meta-analysis of the efficacy of sulfasalazine in comparison with 5-aminosalicylates in the induction of improvement and maintenance of remission in patients with ulcerative colitis. *Dig Dis Sci.* 10.1007/s10620-008-0481-x.
61. McIntyre PB, Rodrigues CA, Lennard-Jones JE, et al. Balsalazide in the maintenance treatment of patients with ulcerative colitis, a double-blind comparison with sulphasalazine. *Aliment Pharmacol Ther.* 1988;2(3):237-243.
62. Kane SV, Bjorkman DJ. The efficacy of oral 5-ASAs in the treatment of active ulcerative colitis: a systematic review. *Rev Gastroenterol Disord.* 2003;3(4):210-218.
63. Campieri M, Gionchetti P, Belluzzi A, et al. 5-Aminosalicylic acid as enemas or suppositories in distal ulcerative colitis? *J Clin Gastroenterol.* 1988;10(4):406-409.
64. Farup PG, Hovde O, Halvorsen FA, Raknerud N, Brodin U. Mesalazine suppositories versus hydrocortisone foam in patients with distal ulcerative colitis: a comparison of the efficacy and practicality of two topical treatment regimens. *Scand J Gastroenterol.* 1995;30(2):164-170.
65. Gionchetti P, Ardizzone S, Benvenuti ME, et al. A new mesalazine gel enema in the treatment of left-sided ulcerative colitis: a randomized controlled multicentre trial. *Aliment Pharmacol Ther.* 1999;13:381-388.
66. Malchow H, Gertz B. A new mesalazine foam enema (Claversal Foam) compared with a standard liquid enema in patients with active distal ulcerative colitis. *Aliment Pharmacol Ther.* 2002;16:415-423.
67. Nielsen OH. Sulfasalazine intolerance: a retrospective study of the reasons for discontinuing treatment with sulfasalazine in patients with chronic inflammatory bowel disease. *Scand J Gastroenterol.* 1982;17:389-393.
68. Scott DL, Dacre JE. Adverse reactions to sulfasalazine: the British experience. *J Rheumatol Suppl.* 1988;16:17-21.
69. Chen M, Xia B, Chen B, et al. N-acetyltransferase 2 slow acetylator genotype associated with adverse effects of sulphasalazine in the treatment of inflammatory bowel disease. *Can J Gastroenterol.* 2007;21(3):155-158.
70. Rachmilewitz D. Coated mesalazine (5-aminosalicylic acid) versus sulphasalazine in the treatment of active ulcerative colitis: a randomised trial. *Br Med J.* 1989;298(6666):82-86.
71. Dilger K, Trenk D, Rössle M, et al. A clinical trial on absorption and N-acetylation of oral and rectal mesalazine. *Eur J Clin Invest.* 2007;37(7):558-565.
72. Nugent SG, Kumar D, Rampton DS, Evans DF. Intestinal luminal pH in inflammatory bowel disease: possible determinants and implications for therapy with aminosalicylates and other drugs. *Gut.* 2001;48(4):571-577.
73. Travis SP, Tysk C, de Silva HJ, et al. Optimum dose of olsalazine for maintaining remission in ulcerative colitis. *Gut.* 1994;35(9):1282-1286.
74. Raimundo AH, Patil DH, Frost PG, Silk DB. Effects of olsalazine and sulphasalazine on jejunal and ileal water and electrolyte absorption in normal human subjects. *Gut.* 1991;32(9):1087.
75. Wadworth AN, Fitton A. Olsalazine. A review of its pharmacodynamic and pharmacokinetic properties, and therapeutic potential in inflammatory bowel disease. *Drugs.* 1991;41(4):647-664.
76. Fallingborg J, Christensen LA, Jacobsen BA, et al. Effect of olsalazine and mesalazine on intraluminal pH of the duodenum and proximal jejunum in healthy humans. *Scand J Gastroenterol.* 1994;29(6):498-500.
77. Raimundo AH, Patil DH, Frost PG, Silk DB. Effects of olsalazine and sulphasalazine on jejunal and ileal water and electrolyte absorption in normal human subjects. *Gut.* 1991;32(3):270-274.
78. Berglindh T, Landström E, Bergqvist E. Induction of and adaptation to olsalazine induced intestinal volume load. *Scand J Gastroenterol Suppl.* 1988;148:24-28.
79. Nilsson A, Danielsson A, Löfberg R, et al. Olsalazine versus sulphasalazine for relapse prevention in ulcerative colitis: A multicenter study. *Am J Gastroenterol.* 1995;90(3):381-387.
80. Shanahan F, Targan S. Sulfasalazine and salicylate-induced exacerbation of ulcerative colitis. *N Engl J Med.* 1987;317(7):455.
81. Chakraborty TK, Bhatia D, Heading RC, Ford MJ. Salicylate induced exacerbation of ulcerative colitis. *Gut.* 1987;28(5):613-615.
82. Kapur KC, Williams GT, Allison MC. Mesalazine induced exacerbation of ulcerative colitis. *Gut.* 1995;37(6):838-839.
83. Rutgeerts P. Comparative efficacy of coated, oral 5-aminosalicylic acid (Claversal) and sulphasalazine for maintaining remission of ulcerative colitis. International Study Group. *Aliment Pharmacol Ther.* 1989;3(2):183-191.
84. Goldstein F, DiMarino AJ Jr. Diarrhea as a side effect of mesalamine treatment for inflammatory bowel disease. *J Clin Gastroenterol.* 2000;31(1):60-62.
85. Patel H, Barr A, Jeejeebhoy KN. Renal effects of long-term treatment with 5-aminosalicylic acid. *Can J Gastroenterol.* 2009;23(3):170-176.
86. de Jong DJ, Tielen J, Habraken CM, Wetzels JF, Naber AH. 5-Aminosalicylates and effects on renal function in patients with Crohn's disease. *Inflamm Bowel Dis.* 2005;11(11):972-976.
87. Van Biervliet S, Raes A, Vande Walle J, et al. Mesalazine interstitial nephritis presenting as colitis ulcerosa exacerbation. *Acta Gastroenterol Belg.* 2006;69(3):321-322.
88. Tadic M, Grgurevic I, Scukanec-Spoljar M, et al. Acute interstitial nephritis due to mesalazine. *Nephrology (Carlton).* 2005;10(2):103-105.
89. Herrlinger KR, Noftz MK, Fellermann K, Schmidt K, Steinhoff J, Stange EF. Minimal renal dysfunction in inflammatory bowel disease is related to disease activity but not to 5-ASA use. *Aliment Pharmacol Ther.* 2001;15(3):363-369.
90. Fraser JS, Muller AF, Smith DJ, Newman DJ, Lamb EJ. Renal tubular injury is present in acute inflammatory bowel disease prior to the introduction of drug therapy. *Aliment Pharmacol Ther.* 2001;15(8):1131-1137.
91. Schreiber S, Hämling J, Zehnter E, et al. Renal tubular dysfunction in patients with inflammatory bowel disease treated with aminosalicylate. *Gut.* 1997;40(6):761-766.

92. Poulou AC, Goumas KE, Dandakis DC, et al. Microproteinuria in patients with inflammatory bowel disease: is it associated with the disease activity or the treatment with 5-aminosalicylic acid? *World J Gastroenterol.* 2006;12(5):739-746.
93. Mahmud N, McDonald GS, Kelleher D, Weir DG. Microalbuminuria correlates with intestinal histopathological grading in patients with inflammatory bowel disease. *Gut.* 1996;38(1):99-103.
94. Gisbert JP, Luna M, González-Lama Y, et al. Effect of 5-aminosalicylates on renal function in patients with inflammatory bowel disease: 4-year follow-up study. *Gastroenterol Hepatol.* 2008;31(8):477-484.
95. Van Staa TP, Travis S, Leufkens HG, Logan RF. 5-aminosalicylic acids and the risk of renal disease: a large British epidemiologic study. *Gastroenterology.* 2004;126(7):1733-1739.
96. Rahimi R, Nikfar S, Rezaie A, Abdollahi M. Pregnancy outcome in women with inflammatory bowel disease following exposure to 5-aminosalicylic acid drugs: a meta-analysis. *Reprod Toxicol.* 2008;25(2):271-275.
97. Diav-Citrin O, Park YH, Veerasuntharam G, et al. The safety of mesalamine in human pregnancy: a prospective controlled cohort study. *Gastroenterology.* 1998;114:23-28.
98. Datta RK, Antopol W. Influence of methadone and sulfapyridine on mouse liver and brain ribonuclease and deoxyribonuclease. *Pharmacology.* 1973;9(2):97-106.
99. Christensen LA. 5-Aminosalicylic acid containing drugs: delivery, fate, and possible clinical implications in man. *Dan Med Bull.* 2000;47(1):20-41.
100. Ambrosius Christensen L, Rasmussen SN, Hansen SH, Bondesen S, Hvidberg EF. Salazosulfapyridine and metabolites in fetal and maternal body fluids with special reference to 5-aminosalicylic acid. *Acta Obstet Gynecol Scand.* 1987;66(5):433-435.
101. Mottet C, Juillerat P, Pittet V, et al. Pregnancy and breastfeeding in patients with Crohn's disease. *Digestion.* 2007;76(2):149-160.
102. Silverman DA, Ford J, Shaw I, Probert CS. Is mesalazine really safe for use in breastfeeding mothers? *Gut.* 2005;54(1):170-171.
103. Gionchetti P, Rizzello F, Venturi A, et al. Comparison of oral with rectal mesalazine in the treatment of ulcerative proctitis. *Dis Colon Rectum.* 1998;41(1):93-97.
104. Kam L, Cohen H, Dooley C, Rubin P, Orchard J. A comparison of mesalamine suspension enema and oral sulfasalazine for treatment of active distal ulcerative colitis in adults. *Am J Gastroenterol.* 1996;91(7):1338-1342.
105. d'Albasio G, Pacini F, Camarri E, et al. Combined therapy with 5-aminosalicylic acid tablets and enemas for maintaining remission in ulcerative colitis: a randomized double-blind study. *Am J Gastroenterol.* 1997;92(7):1143-1147.
106. Vecchi M, Meucci G, Gionchetti P, et al. Oral versus combination mesalazine therapy in active ulcerative colitis: a double-blind, double-dummy, randomized multicentre study. *Aliment Pharmacol Ther.* 2001;15(2):251-256.
107. Safdi M, DeMicco M, Sninsky C, et al. A double-blind comparison of oral versus rectal mesalamine versus combination therapy in the treatment of distal ulcerative colitis. *Am J Gastroenterol.* 1997;92(10):1867-1871.
108. Frieri G, Pimpo M, Galletti B, et al. Long-term oral plus topical mesalazine in frequently relapsing ulcerative colitis. *Dig Liver Dis.* 2005;37(2):92-69.
109. Marteau P, Probert CS, Lindgren S, et al. Combined oral and enema treatment with Pentasa (mesalazine) is superior to oral therapy alone in patients with extensive mild/moderate active ulcerative colitis: a randomized, double blind, placebo controlled study. *Gut.* 2005;54:960-965.
110. Svartz N. Sulfasalazine: II. Some notes on the discovery and development of salazopyrin. *Am J Gastroenterol.* 1988;83(5):497-503.

14

Current and Future Topical Mesalamine Derivatives in Ulcerative Colitis

Jeffrey W. Nathanson, MD and Russell D. Cohen, MD

Sulfasalazine has been used in the treatment of ulcerative colitis (UC) for more than 50 years. In 1977, Khan et al demonstrated that mesalamine (also referred to as mesalazine or 5-ASA) was the therapeutically active component of sulfasalazine.[1] Since then, a number of different mesalamine derivatives have been developed, each with its own specific delivery system.

Topical formulations of mesalamine offer several unique advantages as a means of drug delivery. More than two-thirds of all patients with UC have endoscopic involvement distal to the splenic flexure.[2] The great majority of these cases are mild to moderate in severity.[2] For these patients, administering mesalamine rectally delivers treatment directly to the site of maximal inflammation while potentially minimizing the frequency of systemic adverse effects. Topical mesalamine is the most effective mesalamine therapy for the treatment of active distal UC and has an important role in the maintenance of disease remission.

The delivery formulations of topical mesalamine that currently exist include liquid enemas, suppositories, foams, and gels (Table 14-1). This chapter summarizes the pharmacokinetics, safety, and efficacy of each of these formulations in the management of distal UC. In addition, 2 agents closely related to mesalamine, 4-ASA and N-acetyl-5-ASA, will be reviewed.

MESALAMINE (5-ASA)

Liquid Enemas

Background

Mesalamine liquid rectal suspension enemas have been a mainstay of topical therapy for distal UC for 2 decades. They consist of micronized 5-ASA particles suspended in an aqueous solution. Several formulations are commercially available in Canada and Europe (Salofalk, Asacol, Pentasa), but only Rowasa is currently available in the United States. Each Rowasa enema contains 4 g of 5-ASA in a 60-mL aqueous suspension. Inactive ingredients include carbomer 934P, edentate disodium, potassium acetate, potassium metabisulfite, purified water, and a sodium benzoate preservative.[3] Multiple scintigraphic studies have labeled mesalamine liquid enemas with radioisotopes and shown consistent proximal spread of the enema to at least the splenic flexure (Figure 14-1).[4-8] Van Bodegraven et al studied the retrograde spread of 3 ^{99m}Tc labeled mesalamine enemas (2 g/30 mL, 4 g/60 mL, and 1 g/100 mL) in 31 UC patients. Scintigraphic images demonstrated that the enema with the largest volume (1 g/100 mL) was associated with more consistent proximal coating of the colon, independent of disease activity.[9] Otten et al compared the physical and chemical

Lichtenstein GR, ed.
Ulcerative Colitis: The Complete Guide to Medical Management (pp. 157-172)

TABLE 14-1

SOME OF THE MESALAMINE FORMULATIONS CURRENTLY AVAILABLE WORLDWIDE

Formulation	Common Brand Names	Available Dosages
Liquid enema	*United States:* Rowasa	4 g/60 mL
	Other countries: Asacol, Asamax, Pentasa, Quintasa, Salofalk	1 g, 2 g, or 4 g/60 mL 1 g, 2 g, or 4 g/100 mL
Suppository	*United States:* Canasa	1000 mg
	Other countries: Asacol, Asalex, Asalit, Asamax, Asazine, Bufexan, Claversal, Colitofalk, Lextrasa, Pentasa, Quintasa, Salofalk	250 mg, 400 mg, 500 mg, 1000 mg
Foam	*United States:* None	–
	Other countries: Asacol, Claversal, Salofalk	1 g/30 mL, 1g or 2 g/60 mL 2 g/120 mL
Gel	*United States:* None	–
	Other countries: Enterasin	2 g/60 mL

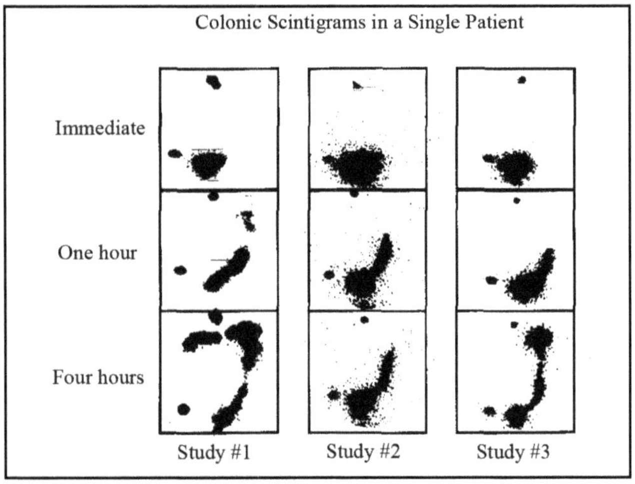

FIGURE 14-1. Serial colonic scintigrams over time in a single patient administered mesalamine liquid enemas during 3 studies separated by at least 24 hours. (Reprinted with permission from Vitti RA, Meyers F, Knight LC, Siegel JA, Malmud LS, Fisher RS. Quantitative distribution of radiolabeled 5-aminosalicylic acid enemas in patients with left-sided ulcerative colitis. *Dig Dis Sci.* 1989;34(11):1792-1797.)

characteristics of Salofalk and Asacol 2 g enemas administered to 12 healthy volunteers and found the higher viscosity preparation (Asacol) reached a substantially larger portion of the colon, demonstrated better bowel wall adherence and retention time, and reached a higher specific surface area per gram active compound.[10]

PHARMACOKINETICS

Several studies have demonstrated that mesalamine liquid enemas are poorly absorbed from the colon.[11,12] Almer et al reported a median peak plasma value of total 5-ASA of 0.92 at a median of 11 hours after administration of a 4-g/60-mL mesalamine enema to 10 UC patients.[8,13] Campieri et al administered a single dose of 3 different mesalamine liquid enemas (2 g/100 mL, 4 g/100 mL, and 4 g/200 mL) to 7 patients with UC in remission and 5 with active disease. Peak plasma values of total 5-ASA were achieved after 3 to 6 hours and never exceeded 7 µg/mL.[14] In neither study did 5-ASA or its metabolite, acetyl 5-ASA (Ac-5-ASA), accumulate in plasma with repeated daily administration, and, in several patients, both were undetectable at 24 hours. Although aminosalicylates are largely eliminated by the kidneys, urinary 5-ASA and Ac-5-ASA values were low in both studies, indicating poor absorption at steady-state conditions. Campieri noted 24-hour urinary recovery of Ac-5-ASA was lower among patients with active disease than among those in remission (10% versus 19%; $P < 0.01$), suggesting that 5-ASA exerts its therapeutic benefit primarily through local action. Bondesen et al reported that mesalamine administered in a slightly acidic, buffered enema suspension resulted in significantly lower plasma concentrations than the same dose of mesalamine administered in a neutral suspension.[15]

Mesalamine liquid enemas appear to act directly on the colonic mucosa, concentrating at the site of inflammation. Schoonjans et al used fluorescence to demonstrate characteristic 5-ASA uptake within the epithelial cells and the lamina propria of rectal mucosa that correlated strongly with 5-serum concentrations of 5-ASA (r=0.84; *P*<0.005) and acetyl-5-ASA (r=0.80; *P*<0.005).[16] Moreover, mesalamine liquid enemas appear to achieve a higher mucosal concentration in the distal colon than oral mesalamine. Frieri et al randomized 22 patients to either 2.4 g oral mesalamine (Asacol) or 2.4 g oral mesalamine (Asacol) plus 4 g/100 mL mesalamine liquid enema. After 2 weeks, rectal mucosal biopsies revealed mesalamine levels approximately 20 times greater in patients in the combination therapy group than with oral mesalamine (52.1 ng/mg, range: 13.6 to 122.1 versus 0.2 ng/mg, range: 0.2 to 9.7; *P*<0.0001). The effect was evident up to the splenic flexure where mucosal mesalamine concentrations were twice as much on combination therapy versus oral therapy alone (46.6 ng/mg, range: 6 to 112.6 versus 15.9 ng/mg, range 2.3 to 42.4; *P*=0.01).[17] Not only does the clinical activity in UC correlate better with tissue than with plasma concentrations,[18,19] but higher rectal mucosal concentrations appear to translate into better clinical efficacy.[18,20]

ADVERSE EFFECTS

Due to poor colonic absorption, the incidence of adverse effects with mesalamine enemas is very low and significantly less than with the oral formulations. The most frequently cited adverse effects with Rowasa enemas were abdominal pain (8.1%), headache (6.5%), flatulence (6.1%), nausea (5.8%), and flu-like symptoms (5.3%), all similar to placebo. Less commonly, fever, rash, joint pain, headaches, dizziness, peripheral edema, and hair loss have been reported. Patients may complain of local symptoms related to the difficulty and inconvenience of drug instillation, including pain on insertion of the enema tip, hemorrhoids, perianal itching or burning, constipation, and diarrhea.[3] Rowasa contains potassium metabisulfite, a sulfite that may cause allergic-type reactions in certain susceptible individuals. Although there are no adequate and well-controlled studies of mesalamine enemas in pregnant women, teratologic studies in rats and rabbits using oral doses up to 5 and 8 times, respectively, the maximum recommended human dose have revealed no evidence of harm to the embryo or the fetus.[21,22] Bell et al reported normal full-term deliveries and no fetal abnormalities in 16 women with ulcerative proctosigmoiditis or proctitis prospectively followed through 19 pregnancies while being maintained on either mesalamine enemas or suppositories.[23] Rowasa is classified by the FDA as a pregnancy category B drug.

CLINICAL TRIALS

Treatment of Active Disease

Uncontrolled Studies

In the mid-1980s, a number of uncontrolled studies described success with mesalamine enemas in UC patients with mild to moderately active distal disease who had already failed therapy with oral sulfasalazine,[24,25] steroid enemas,[24,25] and oral steroids.[26,27]

Placebo-Controlled Trials

Several randomized, controlled trials have shown mesalamine liquid enemas to be superior to placebo in the treatment of mild to moderately active distal UC. Vantrappen et al[28] randomized 20 patients with mild to moderately active distal UC refractory to sulfasalazine and steroid enemas to the addition of a 1.5 g/100 mL mesalamine liquid enema once daily or placebo. Eight-week clinical, endoscopic, and histologic improvement was significantly greater with mesalamine (11 versus 3, *P*<0.05; 10 versus 2, *P*<0.05; and 10 versus 2, *P*<0.05, respectively).[28] Sutherland et al[29] blindly randomized 153 patients with mild to moderately active distal UC to either a 4 g/60 mL mesalamine enema once daily or placebo. Six-week improvement rates were higher for the mesalamine-treated patients (63% versus 29%; *P*<0.001).[29] Campieri et al blindly randomized 113 patients with mild to moderately active distal UC to either a 1 g/100 mL, a 2 g/100 mL, or a 4 g/100 mL mesalamine enema once daily or placebo. After 30 days, all patients who were taking mesalamine enemas (regardless of dose) showed significantly better clinical, endoscopic, and histologic improvement than those who received placebo (*P*<0.01).[30] In a separate study, Campieri et al blindly randomly allocated 50 patients with mild to moderately active distal UC to receive either a daily 2 g/100 mL mesalamine enema, a 10 g/100 mL sucralfate enema, or placebo enema for 1 month. Clinical, endoscopic, and histologic improvement was observed in a significantly greater number of patients in the mesalamine enema group (94%, 88%, and 83%, respectively) than seen with either sucralfate (22%, 22%, and 17%, respectively) or placebo (14%, 14%, and 7%, respectively; *P*<0.01).[30] Hanauer et al randomly allocated 287 patients with mild to moderately active distal UC to treatment with either a 1 g/100 mL, a 2 g/100 mL, or a 4 g/100 mL mesalamine enema once daily or placebo for 8 weeks. A significantly greater percentage of patients receiving mesalamine enemas (regardless of dose) than placebo demonstrated clinical, endoscopic, and histologic improvement.[31]

Comparison to Topical Steroids

A number of studies have also compared the efficacy of mesalamine enemas to several different topical steroids in the treatment of mild to moderately active distal UC. Some,[32,33] but not all,[34] trials have shown mesalamine enemas to be superior to hydrocortisone enemas. Campieri et al blindly randomized 86 patients with mild to moderately active distal UC to receive either a daily 4 g/100 mL mesalamine enema or a 100 g/100 mL hydrocortisone enema for 15 days. Clinical, endoscopic, and histologic remission rates were higher with mesalamine (93% versus 57%, 93% versus 54%, and 77% versus 33%, respectively; *P*<0.0005).[32] Friedman et al blindly randomized 18 patients with mild to moderately active distal UC refractory to 100 mg hydrocortisone enemas to treatment with either a daily 4 g/100 mL mesalamine enema or continued therapy with hydrocortisone enemas. After 3 weeks, clinical improvement was superior with mesalamine (7 of 9 versus 1 of 9 patients; $P<0.05$).[33] However, Porro et al blindly randomized 52 patients with mild to moderately active distal UC to receive either a daily 1 g/100 mL mesalamine enema or a 100 mg/60 mL hydrocortisone enema for 3 weeks. They found no significant difference in clinical, endoscopic, and histologic improvement, although a trend toward benefit in clinical activity was seen with mesalamine ($P=0.07$).[34]

Similar results have been shown with mesalamine and prednisolone enemas in the treatment of mild to moderately active distal UC. The Danish 5-ASA Group reported similar 4-week improvement or remission rates in 123 patients blindly randomized to either a daily 1 g/100 mL mesalamine enema or a 25 mg/100 mL prednisolone enema (77% versus 72%; P=NS).[35] Another study by Mulder et al reported no significant difference in 28-day clinical, endoscopic, or histologic improvement rates in 29 patients randomly assigned treatment with either a daily 3 g/40 mL mesalamine liquid enema or a 30 mg/40 mL prednisolone enema (74% versus 79%, 73% versus 86%, and 73% versus 57%, respectively; P=NS).[36]

Three therapeutic trials have compared mesalamine enemas to rectal formulations of budesonide, a locally acting steroid with a high first-pass metabolism in the liver and low systemic effects, in patients with mild to moderately active distal UC. Mulder et al randomized 62 patients to either a daily 4 g/60 mL mesalamine enema or a 2 mg/100 mL budesonide enema. They failed to show a significant difference in endoscopic grading, disease extent, histology, or in clinical improvement, although the mesalamine-treated patients had significantly more formed stools ($P<0.05$).[37] In a single-blind study, Lemann et al randomized 97 patients to treatment with either a daily 1 g/100 mL mesalamine enema or a 2 mg/100 mL budesonide enema. Clinical remission rates were higher with mesalamine (60% versus 38%; $P=0.03$), with no difference in endoscopic and histologic scores.[38] In an open pilot study, Rufle et al reported similar improvement rates between 33 patients randomized to either a 4 g/60 mL mesalamine enema daily or a 1 mg/50 mL budesonide rectal foam twice daily (67% versus 71%; P=NS).[39]

The incremental benefit of combining rectal corticosteroids with mesalamine liquid enemas was studied by Mulder et al, who blindly randomized 60 patients to either 4 weeks of a nightly 1 g/100 mL mesalamine enema, a 3 mg/100 mL beclomethasone dipropionate enema, or an enema containing both drugs. Clinical, endoscopic, and histologic improvement was comparable between those patients who received the mesalamine enema and the beclomethasone dipropionate enema-treated patients (76% versus 70%, 71% versus 75%, 48% versus 50%, respectively; P=NS), but was significantly greater in those given the combination enema (100%, 95%, and 95%, respectively; $P<0.05$), without a higher incidence of adverse effects.[40]

Comparison to Oral Mesalamine

Four randomized, double-blind, double-dummy trials have compared the efficacy of mesalamine liquid enemas in the treatment of mild to moderately active distal UC to any one of several oral mesalamine formulations currently available. Kam et al[41] blindly randomized 37 patients to either a 4 g/60 mL mesalamine liquid enema once daily or 4 g of oral sulfasalazine daily in divided doses (500 mg tablets). While both treatments produced a similar improvement in the disease activity index, patients treated with mesalamine enemas showed an earlier response in patient global improvement scores (61% versus 12% at week 2; $P= 0.02$, 88% versus 43% at week 4; $P=0.04$), and fewer adverse events (42% versus 83%; $P=0.02$).[41] Safdi et al[42] randomized 60 patients to either a 4 g/60 mL mesalamine enema once daily, 2.4 g oral mesalamine daily in divided doses (Asacol 400 mg tablets), or a combination of the 2 treatments. Most outcomes were similar between the groups, although more patients experienced cessation of rectal bleeding with combination therapy than with either enemas or tablets alone (89% versus 69% versus 46%; $P=0.013$), and bleeding cessation was achieved in fewer days with combination therapy (11.9 days) than with either the mesalamine enema (24.8 days; $P=0.04$) or tablet (25.5 days; $P=0.002$).[42] Of note in the Safdi study, the total dose of mesalamine administered to patients in the combination therapy arm (6.4 g/d) was greater than that given to the mesalamine enema-treated patients (4 g/d) or those who received oral therapy alone (2.4 g/d). However, similar total doses were studied by Vecchi et al,[43] who randomized 130 patients to either 4 g oral mesalamine daily in divided doses (Salofalk, 500 mg tablets) or a 2 g/60 mL mesalamine enema daily plus 2 g oral mesalamine daily in divided doses (Salofalk, 500 mg tablets). After 6 weeks, both the oral therapy and the combination therapy achieved unusually high rates of clinical remission (82% versus 87%), but neither the rate of clinical remission nor the time to achieve remission (22.2 days versus 20.2 days) was significantly different between groups.[43] Marteau et al[44] randomized 127 patients to treatment with 4 g oral mesalamine (Pentasa, 500 mg tablets) daily in divided doses and either a 1 g mesalamine enema (Pentasa) or placebo nightly for the first 4 weeks of therapy.[44] Improvement was significantly greater with combination therapy than oral therapy alone at 4 weeks (89% versus 62%; $P=0.0008$) and at 8 weeks (86% versus 68%; $P=0.03$). Remission, however, was only significantly greater with combination therapy at 8 weeks (64% versus 43%; $P=0.03$).

Dosing Studies

Dose-ranging studies have been performed in an effort to determine the optimal dose of mesalamine enema to induce improvement or remission in patients with mild to moderately active distal UC. Powell-Tuck and colleagues found no significant differences in clinical, endoscopic, or histologic improvement rates in 25 patients randomized to a 28-day course of daily 1 g or 2 g mesalamine enemas.[45] Campieri et al randomized 113 patients to 30-day treatment with either a nightly placebo or a 1 g/100 mL, 2 g/100 mL, or 4 g/100 mL mesalamine enema. Clinical, endoscopic, and histologic improvement rates were higher with mesalamine than placebo, but no significant differences were found between the different concentrations of mesalamine.[30] Hanauer et al conducted a similar double-blind trial randomizing 287 patients to either a daily 1 g/100 mL, 2 g/100 mL, or 4 g/100 mL mesalamine enema or placebo enema for 8 weeks. Improvement rates by physician global assessment were similar among mesalamine doses (67%, 65%, and 75%, respectively; P=NS) and superior to placebo (27%; $P<0.05$).[31]

Meta-Analysis

Our group conducted a meta-analysis on the various treatment options reported in the literature for mild to moderately active distal UC and calculated the pooled advantage of mesalamine enemas over placebo in inducing clinical improvement was 52.3% (95% confidence interval [CI] 19.8 to 84.7) at 2 weeks and 56% (95% CI 8.3 to 103.7) at 4 weeks. For clinical remission, the week 2 and week 4 data were 35.4% (95% CI 21.0 to 49.7) and 57.1% (95% CI 41.1 to 73.2), respectively.[46] Reviewing a broader range of studies that fell within acceptable guidelines, we concluded that mesalamine liquid enemas were more efficacious than either topical steroids or oral mesalamine and that efficacy was independent of dose. In a separate meta-analysis, Marshall et al pooled data from the 5 randomized, controlled studies that compared mesalamine enemas to either hydrocortisone or prednisolone enemas and concluded that the pooled odds ratio (OR) for inducing disease remission significantly favored the mesalamine enemas.[47]

Maintenance of Remission

Uncontrolled Studies

By the late 1980s, uncontrolled studies of the use of mesalamine enemas in the maintenance of remission in patients with distal UC were published. McPhee et al reported on 39 patients followed for as long as 3 years while taking mesalamine enemas for maintenance of remission: 19 patients experienced a total of 25 episodes of relapse, although 92% of these episodes responded successfully to enema retreatment.[48] Biddle et al retrospectively reviewed the clinical outcomes of 90 patients with colitis refractory to sulfasalazine and/or corticosteroids who were subsequently treated with mesalamine enemas. Remission rates were 54% and 80% at 12 and 34 weeks, respectively, with subsequent intermittent enema dosing for at least 1 year (Figure 14-2). Relapses were seen in 41 patients (84 relapses), which responded as well to enema retreatment as they did to the first course of therapy, regardless of whether the relapse occurred after discontinuation of mesalamine enemas or during a tapering of the dose.[49]

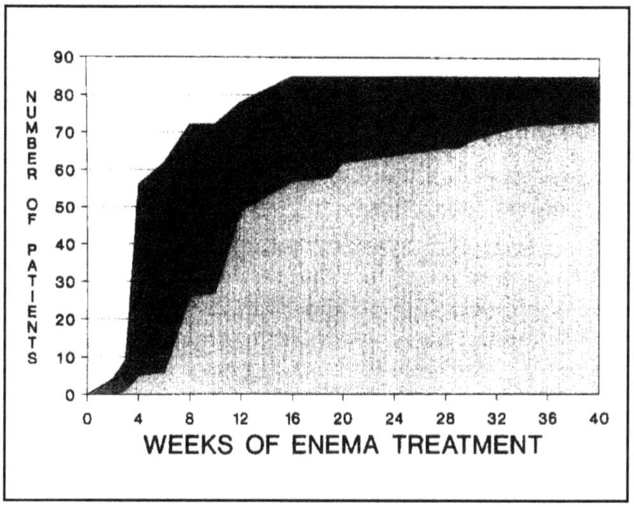

FIGURE 14-2. Rates of improvement and remission in patients with distal UC for first course of treatment with mesalamine liquid enemas. (Reprinted with permission from Biddle WL, Miner PB Jr. Long-term use of mesalamine enemas to induce remission in ulcerative colitis. *Gastroenterology.* 1990;99(1):113-118.)

Placebo-Controlled Trials

Biddle et al blindly randomized 25 patients with distal UC in remission to receive a daily enema containing either 1 g/60 mL mesalamine or placebo. Remission was maintained in 9 of 12 patients receiving mesalamine enemas at 1 year, while 11 of 13 patients receiving placebo relapsed after a mean of 16 weeks ($P<0.005$).[50]

Comparison to Oral Mesalamine

Three randomized studies have compared mesalamine enemas to oral mesalamine in the maintenance of remission in distal UC. Andreoli et al reported no difference in clinical or endoscopic remission rates at 6 months between 31 patients randomized to either a 4 g/100 mL mesalamine enema every third night or 2 g oral sulfasalazine daily.[51] Similar relapse rates were reported by d'Albasio et al among 60 patients randomized to either a 4 g mesalamine enema daily for the first 7 days of each month or 2 g oral sulfasalazine daily in divided doses (1 year relapse rates: 20% versus 24%; P=NS; 2 year relapse rates: 37% versus 43%; P=NS), with similar mean time to relapse and relapse severity.[52] However, Mantzaris et al found that patients treated with a 4 g mesalamine enema every third night were significantly less likely to relapse than those receiving 1.5 g oral mesalamine daily in divided doses (Salofalk, 500 mg tablets; 26% versus 68%; $P<0.001$).[53]

D'Albasio et al randomized 72 patients to receive either combination therapy with 1.6 g oral mesalamine daily in divided doses (Asacol, 400 mg tablets) plus a 4 g/100 mL mesalamine liquid enema twice weekly or 1.6 g oral mesalamine in divided doses (Asacol, 400 mg tablets) plus a placebo enema. After 1 year, the rate of relapse in the combination therapy group was significantly less than the rate in the oral therapy alone group (39% versus 69%; $P=0.04$).[54]

Dosing Studies

Sutherland et al randomized 29 patients with distal UC in remission to receive either a 2 g/60 mL or a 4 g/60 mL mesalamine liquid enema once daily and found no significant difference in the rate of relapse.[55] The optimal frequency of maintenance therapy with mesalamine enemas was studied by Guarino et al,[56] who examined 14 patients with distal UC who had achieved remission with nightly 4 g mesalamine liquid enemas and systematically tapered the frequency of enema administration. Although relapse was common, complete remission was again induced in all but 1 patient with reinitiation of nightly mesalamine enemas. At follow-up of between 5 and 16 months, 1 patient was on no therapy, 8 were maintained on enemas every third night, 3 on enemas every second night, and 3 on a nightly schedule. Miner et al[57] randomized 157 patients with distal UC in remission to a 4 g mesalamine liquid enema to be administered every night, every other night, or every third night, or a placebo enema as sole therapy. At 24 weeks, the relapse rates were similar between the mesalamine groups, but were significantly less in the nightly and every other night treatment groups as compared to placebo.[57]

Meta-Analysis

Marshall et al combined data from the 3 randomized studies cited that compared mesalamine liquid enemas to oral mesalamine in the maintenance of remission in patients with distal UC, with a pooled OR favoring the enemas (2.3; 95% CI 1.1 to 4.8).[58] In a separate review, our group calculated that varying the mesalamine enema dosing intervals only minimally decreased efficacy from 78% (nightly) to 72% (every second night) to 65% (every third night).[46]

Suppositories

Background

Mesalamine suppositories are commonly used in the treatment of distal UC and are considered the treatment of choice when disease is confined to the distal sigmoid colon (proctosigmoiditis) or rectum (proctitis). Several formulations are commercially available in Canada and Europe (ie, Salofalk, Asacol, Pentasa, Claversal), but only Canasa is currently sold in the United States. Each Canasa suppository contains 1000 mg of mesalamine in a hard fat base (saturated vegetable fatty acid esters). The suppository is manually inserted completely into the rectum with gentle pressure, pointed end first, and should be retained for at least 1 to 3 hours to achieve the maximum benefit.[59]

Williams et al used ^{99m}Tc-labeled mesalamine suppositories and showed that in healthy volunteers and patients with IBD, the ^{99m}Tc-labeled mesalamine remained localized to the rectum and sigmoid colon.[60]

Pharmacokinetics

Jacobsen et al compared local and systemic bioavailability of a 1 g mesalamine suppository to a 1 g mesalamine enema dosed twice daily for 1 week. Plasma concentrations of 5-ASA and acetylated-5-ASA did not exceed 6 μmol/L and 8 μmol/L, respectively, nor did either accumulate during a 12-hour dose interval. At the end of treatment, feces and urine were collected for 48 hours and 5-ASA and Ac-5-ASA concentrations measured. The fecal water concentration was significantly higher following suppository treatment (55.7 mmol/L) than after enema treatment (31.7 mmol/L) ($P<0.01$). In addition, total urinary recovery was less following suppository treatment (median 10%; range 2% to 24%) than with enema treatment (median 14%; range 7% to 35%). These findings suggest the more limited spread of mesalamine suppositories results in less systemic absorption than with mesalamine enemas.[61]

Aumais et al[62] administered a single 500-mg mesalamine suppository followed by 500 mg every 8 hours for 5 days to 16 healthy volunteers and 9 patients with ulcerative proctitis. After a single dose in patients, mean 5-ASA half-life was 5.0 hours. At steady state, means were 89.1 ng/mL for C_{min}, 361.1 ng/mL for C_{min}, and 7.1 hours for half-life. The mean amount of 5-ASA and Ac-5-ASA recovered in the urine after a single dose in patients was 9.5 mg and 186.8, respectively, over 30 hours. The mean amount of 5-ASA and Ac-5-ASA recovered in urine after the last dose at steady state was 11.7 mg and 142.9 mg, respectively, over 30 hours. Patients were noted to have significantly greater mean systemic bioavailability of mesalamine after a single dose than healthy volunteers (35% versus 14%; $P=0.0145$). Importantly, rectal biopsies were performed and tissue concentrations of 5-ASA and Ac-5-ASA measured. 5-ASA was the main moiety found in biopsy specimens, and mean rectal 5-ASA concentrations were significantly greater in patients (167.8 ng/mg tissue [range: 1.4 to 541.6]) than in healthy volunteers (22.3 ng/mg tissue [range 0.02 to 139.31]) ($P=0.016$). Mesalamine delivered by suppository appears to concentrate in inflamed rectal mucosa, and clinical studies suggest higher rectal mucosal concentrations translate into better clinical efficacy.[18,20] The efficacy of mesalamine suppositories appears to be independent of dose and administration schedule.[46,63]

Adverse Effects

There is little systemic absorption of mesalamine from suppositories, so the incidence of adverse effects is very low and, of note, significantly less than with oral formulations of mesalamine. The most frequently cited adverse effects in patients treated with Canasa were dizziness (3.0%), fever (1.2%), rash (1.2%), acne (1.2%), and colitis (1.2%), all similar to placebo. Patients may experience difficulty with drug instillation and rectal pain (1.8%).[59] Although there are no adequate and well-controlled studies of mesalamine suppositories in pregnant women, teratologic studies in rats and rabbits using oral doses up to 5 and 8 times, respectively, the maximum recommended human dose have revealed no evidence of harm to the embryo or the fetus.[21,22]

CLINICAL TRIALS

Treatment of Active Disease

Uncontrolled Studies

Several early reports touted the use of mesalamine suppositories in the treatment of active ulcerative proctosigmoiditis and proctitis refractory to conventional therapies. Small uncontrolled studies noted clinical as well as endoscopic improvement following mesalamine suppository therapy in patients with active ulcerative proctosigmoiditis and proctitis. In addition, these early studies suggested patients might prefer the relative ease of suppository administration compared to the inconvenience and potential discomfort of various enema formulations.[64,65]

Placebo-Controlled Trials

Several randomized, controlled trials have demonstrated the superiority of a variety of doses of mesalamine suppositories to placebo in the treatment of active distal proctosigmoiditis and proctitis. Williams et al[66] blindly randomized 79 patients with active ulcerative proctitis to suppositories containing either 1.5 g of mesalamine (500 mg each, divided doses) or placebo. Reduction in the disease activity index (DAI) was superior after 6 weeks with mesalamine (80.4% versus 36.8%; $P<0.05$). Mean reduction in DAI was also superior among 94 patients randomized to suppositories containing 1.0 g of mesalamine (500 mg each, divided doses) than with placebo (74.7% versus 34.2%; $P<0.001$), as was the physician's final global assessment (79.2% versus 26.2%; $P<0.001$).[66]

Campieri et al showed superior clinical, endoscopic, and histologic improvement or remission in 62 patients with active ulcerative proctosigmoiditis blindly randomized to either 1.5 g mesalamine suppositories daily in divided doses (500-mg suppository) or placebo (28 versus 10, 25 versus 7, and 21 versus 4, respectively; $P<0.01$).[67] Remission rates were also superior to placebo (but not different among doses of mesalamine) in a blinded trial of 94 patients with active ulcerative proctosigmoiditis randomized to receive 4 weeks of therapy with either 1.5 g or 1 g of mesalamine suppositories (500-mg suppository) or placebo (74%, 69%, versus 39%, respectively; $P<0.01$).[68]

Kohn et al reported superior 6-week clinical and endoscopic remission rates with two 500-mg mesalamine suppositories (78.2%) versus placebo (31.8%; $P<0.02$) in 48 patients with active ulcerative proctitis,[69] while Ngo et al found superior week 2 endoscopic and clinical remission rates with 1-g mesalamine suppositories (69% and 65%, respectively) than with placebo (33% and 25%, respectively; $P<0.01$).[70]

Comparison to Topical Steroids

One randomized, controlled study has compared mesalamine suppositories to topical steroids in the treatment of active ulcerative proctosigmoiditis and proctitis. Farup et al[71] randomized 79 patients to treatment with either 1-g mesalamine suppositories daily in divided doses (500-mg suppository) or 178-mg hydrocortisone foam enemas twice daily. The overall difference in DAI scores favored mesalamine ($P=0.02$), but only for proctitis, while the therapies were comparable in the proctosigmoiditis patients. However, a greater percentage of patients rated suppositories as more practical, more tolerable, and easier to use than foam ($P<0.05$), and greater patient preference was mirrored in a significantly higher compliance at 4 weeks among patients treated with suppositories (100% versus 73%; $P=0.03$).[70]

Comparison to Oral Mesalamine

Gionchetti et al[72] randomized 58 patients with active ulcerative proctitis to either 1.2-g mesalamine suppositories daily in divided doses (400-mg suppository) or 2.4 g oral mesalamine daily in divided doses (Asacol, 400-mg tablets). Improvement in mean DAI was significantly greater with suppositories than with oral mesalamine at 2 weeks (2.59 versus 5.72; $P<0.001$) and at 4 weeks (1.48 versus 3.48; $P<0.001$). The physician's global assessment rated a significantly greater percentage of patients receiving suppositories as "much improved" compared to those taking oral mesalamine at 2 weeks (65.5 versus 17.2; $P<0.01$) and at 4 weeks (82.7 versus 34.5; $P<0.01$). Clinical, endoscopic, and histologic rates of remission were also significantly greater in the mesalamine suppository group than in the oral mesalamine group at 2 weeks (62% versus 20.9%, 51.7% versus 13.8%, and 37.9% versus 6.8%, respectively; $P<0.01$) and at 4 weeks (89.6% versus 41.4%, 72.4% versus 34.5%, and 62% versus 17.2%, respectively; $P<0.01$). In addition, while no patients in the mesalamine suppository group experienced adverse effects, 6 patients treated with oral mesalamine did, although all were of mild intensity and no patient had to withdraw from the study.[72]

Comparison to Other Topical Mesalamines

Campieri et al did not show a difference in clinical, endoscopic, or histologic improvement rates between 39 patients with active ulcerative proctosigmoiditis randomized to receive either a 1-g mesalamine suppository twice daily or a 2-g/100 mL mesalamine liquid enema once daily for 1 month.[73] However, patients in the suppository group were significantly more likely to report no problems, while the enema-treated patients described minor problems or complaints ($P<0.01$).[73]

Dosing Studies

Several studies have attempted to define the optimal dose of mesalamine suppository to achieve maximal benefit while minimizing potential toxicity and inconvenience. Campieri et al noted no significant difference in clinical or endoscopic improvement between patients treated for 1 month with 400 mg 3 times a day, 250 mg 5 times a day, or 1 g twice a day.[74] Massa et al also found no difference in clinical, endoscopic, or histologic response in patients given 500-mg mesalamine suppositories 2 times a day versus 3 times a day.[75] Campieri et al reported similar remission rates among patients with active ulcerative proctosigmoiditis randomized to either 500 mg mesalamine suppositories dosed 3 times a day or 2 times a day (74% versus 69%; *P*=NS), although both were significantly more effective than placebo (39%; *P*<0.01).[68]

Gionchetti et al performed a randomized, single-blind study in 50 patients with active ulcerative proctosigmoiditis comparing 2 different suppository formulations of mesalamine. Half of the patients were administered a 1-g slow-release mesalamine suppository (Pentasa) once daily; the other half received a standard 500-mg glycerin-based mesalamine suppository (Claversal). After 2 weeks, clinical and endoscopic remission were significantly higher in the Pentasa group than in the Claversal group (64% versus 28% and 52% versus 24%, respectively; *P*<0.01). By 4 weeks, however, clinical and endoscopic remission were no longer significantly different (84% versus 80%, 76% versus 72%, respectively; *P*=NS), suggesting a possible quicker response to Pentasa. Also of note, the patient's evaluation for tolerability and practicality showed that the Pentasa suppository was significantly superior to the Claversal suppository.[76] Lamet et al randomized 99 patients with mild-to-moderate proctitis to either a 500-mg mesalamine suppository (Canasa) twice daily or a 1-g suppository nightly.[63] After 6 weeks, mean DAI fell in both groups: 6.6 ± 1.5 (SD) to 1.6 ± 2.3 (SD) in the 500-mg twice daily group versus 6.1 ± 1.5 (SD) to 1.3 ± 2.2 in the 1-g nightly group, with no significant difference in efficacy, adverse events, or adherence.

Meta-Analysis

Our group's meta-analysis and overview of the literature of the management of active ulcerative proctitis[46] confirmed that, after 4 weeks of therapy, the pooled advantage of 1.5-g mesalamine suppositories daily over placebo in achieving clinical improvement was 52% (95% CI 37.8 to 66.3), in inducing clinical remission was 44.3% (95% CI 29.4 to 59.1), and in inducing endoscopic remission was 33.3% (95% CI 18.5 to 48.0). Pooled data for other doses of mesalamine, as well as different durations of treatment, was more limited due to the paucity of studies suitable for combination in a meta-analysis, but suggested that mesalamine suppositories showed a duration, but not a dose, response in inducing clinical remission.

Maintenance of Remission

Uncontrolled Studies

A number of uncontrolled studies reported success in using mesalamine suppositories as a means of maintaining remission in patients with ulcerative proctosigmoiditis and proctitis. Campieri et al reported superior 6- to 12-month maintenance of remission with mesalamine suppositories containing 800 mg in divided doses (400-mg suppository) than with 1000 mg delivered in a single dose (83% versus 53%) in 37 patients with ulcerative proctosigmoiditis.[74] Casellas et al reported 1-year relapse in 5 of 32 patients (16%) with distal UC treated with a single 500-mg suppository once daily.[77]

Placebo-Controlled Trials

D'Arienzo et al[78] blindly randomized 30 patients with proctosigmoiditis or proctitis in remission to receive either 800-mg mesalamine suppositories daily in divided doses (400 mg suppository) or placebo suppositories. At 1 year, 92% of the mesalamine group and 21% of the placebo group remained in remission by clinical, endoscopic, and histologic criteria (*P*<0.001). D'Albasio et al[79] reported lower rates of relapse at 1 year with 1-g mesalamine suppositories daily in divided doses (500 mg suppository) (10%) compared to one 500-mg mesalamine suppository daily (32%; *P*=0.03), or placebo (47%; *P*=0.007) in 111 blindly randomized proctitis patients. Hanauer et al[80] found a 500-mg mesalamine suppository once-a-day was significantly more effective than placebo in preventing relapse at 12 and 24 months (61% versus 12% and 45% versus 9%, respectively; *P*<0.001) in 65 patients with ulcerative proctitis blindly randomized to either therapy (Figure 14-3). Marteau et al[81] compared the efficacy of a 1-g slow release mesalamine suppository (Pentasa) 3 times a week to placebo in 95 proctitis patients. They found a lower risk of relapse with mesalamine at 3, 6, and 9 months (19% versus 38%; *P*=0.035, 29% versus 54%; *P*=0.017, and 38% versus 60%; *P*=0.031), but only a trend by 12 months (48% versus 62%; *P*=0.18). In addition, 61% of the mesalamine patients who relapsed subsequently achieved remission again by using the mesalamine suppositories on a daily basis.

Dosing Studies

In the study previously mentioned, D'Albasio et al[79] reported 1-year relapse rates of 10% for 1-g mesalamine suppositories in divided doses, versus 32% (*P*=0.03) for a single daily 500-mg suppository, and 47% for placebo (*P*=0.007).

Foam

BACKGROUND

Rectal foam represents an alternative means of delivering mesalamine to the inflamed mucosa of patients with

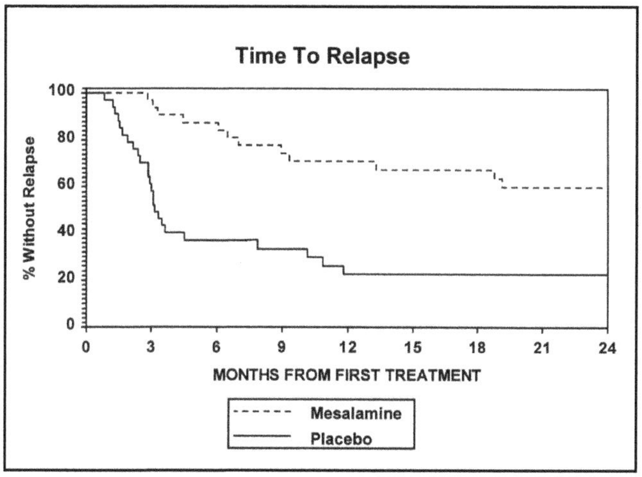

FIGURE 14-3. Kaplan-Meier survival curve. Relapse rates for patients with distal UC on maintenance therapy with mesalamine suppositories versus placebo. (Reprinted with permission from Hanauer S, Good LI, Goodman MW, et al. Long-term use of mesalamine (Rowasa) suppositories in remission maintenance of ulcerative proctitis. *Am J Gastroenterol.* 2000;95(7):1749-1754.)

distal UC. Foam, as opposed to liquid enemas, offers the advantage of expanded volume, prolonged retention, and more uniform coating of the colonic mucosa. Currently, there are no mesalamine foam formulations available in the United States, but several brands (Salofalk, Asacol, Claversal) are commercially available in Canada and Europe. The mesalamine is typically formulated in an aqueous solution and stored in a spray canister that is fit with a dispensing valve. Actuation of the valve initiates a rapid expansion of an inert gas propellant and activation of a surfactant that, together, generates foam that is administered intrarectally.

Campieri et al[82] described the retrograde spread of mesalamine foam generated in a chlorofluorocarbon based aerosol. In a pilot study, 2 different strengths of mesalamine foam were compared in 4 patients with distal UC. Methylene blue (2%) was added to the foam, and at 3 hours, colonoscopy demonstrated more consistent spread to the splenic flexure of a 4 g/20 mL mesalamine foam compared to that of a 2 g/10 mL mesalamine foam.[82] More recently, Wilding evaluated the degree of dispersion of a 2 g/120 mL non-chlorofluorocarbon mesalamine foam in 10 patients with UC. Using gamma scintigraphy, the foam was observed to spread as far as the descending colon in 9 out of 10 patients. All patients retained the foam for the full 4-hour imaging period, and, on average, 23% of the dose was still present in the descending colon 4 hours later.[83]

Compared to mesalamine liquid enemas, mesalamine foam appears to achieve equal or greater retrograde spread. In a small, randomized, crossover study, Campieri et al used scintigraphy to compare the colonic distribution of a 4 g/20 mL mesalamine foam to a 4 g/100 mL mesalamine liquid enema in 10 patients with distal UC. In 6 patients, the same segment was reached with both formulations, but in another 3 patients, a greater spread was observed with the foam. In only 1 patient did the enema result in more proximal spread. The foam reached the upper limit of disease in all cases, while the enema failed in 2 cases. In addition, the study suggested more uniform spread and greater persistence of the mesalamine foam compared to liquid enemas. At 2 hours, the foam had significantly better homogeneity scores than the enema in the descending colon ($P<0.02$) and in the sigmoid colon ($P<0.02$). At 4 hours, persistence scores were also higher for the foam than the enema in the descending colon ($P<0.03$) and in the sigmoid colon ($P<0.05$). The authors suggested these findings might be attributable to the physical properties of the foam, such as greater surface coating, mucosal adhesion, and volumetric expansion.[82]

PHARMACOKINETICS

Although there are to date no published pharmacokinetic studies of mesalamine foam, an unpublished report noted that the administration of a 2-g 5-ASA rectal foam led to the same plasma 5-ASA level as a 4-g 5-ASA liquid enema (Salofalk).[84]

ADVERSE EFFECTS

There are no published studies that have been designed specifically to assess the adverse effects of mesalamine foam. However, it is believed that, like other topical formulations of mesalamine, there is likely little systemic absorption of mesalamine foam, and, as a result, the incidence of adverse effects is presumed to be quite low. In addition, clinical trials that have reported on the efficacy of mesalamine foam have also noted relatively few adverse events. Adverse events reported have included abdominal pain, bloating, flatulence, tenesmus, nausea, and headache.[84-86] In a double-blind, placebo-controlled study of mesalamine foam, Pokrotnieks et al reported the incidence of treatment-adverse events to be no greater than placebo (11% versus 19%; P=NS).[87] With rare exception, adverse events have been mild to moderate in nature; in only one study was a severe adverse event attributed to mesalamine foam (severe abdominal pain with rectal discharge).[85]

CLINICAL TRIALS

Treatment of Active Disease

Placebo-Controlled Studies

Pokrotnieks et al[87] blindly randomized 111 patients with mild to moderately active distal UC to either a 2 g/60 mL mesalamine foam once daily or placebo for 6 weeks. Clinical and endoscopic remission were significantly more likely among those patients treated with mesalamine foam than placebo (65% versus 40% $P=0.008$; and 57% versus 37%, $P=0.047$, respectively; Figure 14-4), and there was a trend toward histologic improvement in the mesalamine

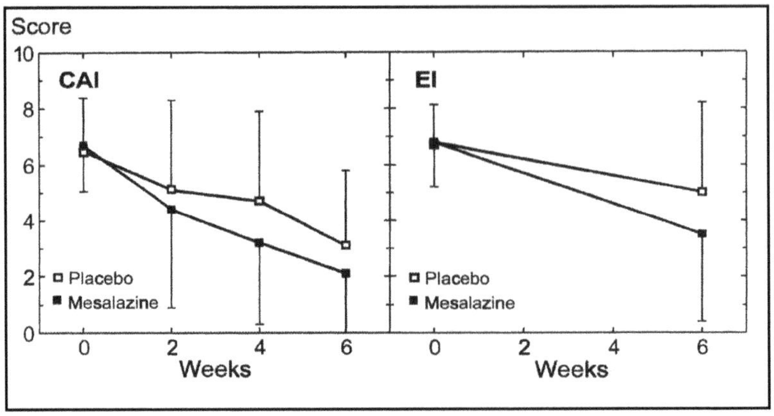

FIGURE 14-4. Mean Clinical Disease Activity Index (CAI) and Endoscopic Index (EI) scores (± standard deviation) in patients with distal UC treated with mesalamine foam enemas versus placebo. (Reprinted with permission from Pokrotnieks J, Marlicz K, Paradowski L, Margus B, Zaborowski P, Greinwald R. Efficacy and tolerability of mesalazine foam enema (Salofalk foam) for distal ulcerative colitis: A double-blind, randomized, placebo-controlled study. *Aliment Pharmacol Ther.* 2000;14(9):1191-1198.)

group (59% versus 41%; P=0.068). A statistically significantly higher percentage of patients reported a therapeutic benefit as early as 2 weeks (75% versus 55%; P = 0.028).[87]

Comparison to Topical Steroids

Lee et al blindly randomized 295 patients with mild to moderately active distal UC to treatment with either a 2 g/120 mL mesalamine foam or a 20 mg/30 mL prednisolone foam once daily for 4 weeks. Clinical remission was achieved in a significantly greater number of patients in the mesalamine group than in the prednisolone group (52% versus 31%; P<0.001). After 4 weeks, mesalamine-treated patients were noted to be significantly less likely to have blood in their stools (67% versus 40%; P<0.001) or have tenesmus 2 or more days per week (15% versus 29%; P=0.038), but more likely to have 3 or more days with abnormal stool consistency (39% versus 23%; P=0.001). There was a trend toward higher endoscopic remission rates with the mesalamine foam (40% versus 31%; P=0.10), but no difference in histologic remission was noted (27% versus 21%; P=NS).[85] In a separate analysis of the same clinical trial, Lee et al noted significantly fewer patients with blood in the stool as early as 2 weeks (P=0.014), suggesting a quicker onset of clinical effect with mesalamine foam.[85]

Comparison to Oral Mesalamine

Hinojosa et al randomized 111 patients with mild to moderately active distal UC to 6 weeks of therapy with either a 1-g mesalamine foam once daily, 3-g oral mesalamine daily in divided doses (1-g tablets), or combined treatment. There was a trend toward higher remission rates with mesalamine foam alone (74%) or combination therapy (66%) compared to those who received only oral mesalamine (50%) (P=0.142).[88]

Comparison to Other Topical Mesalamines

Three randomized, controlled trials have demonstrated mesalamine rectal foam to be at least as effective in treating mild to moderately active distal UC as mesalamine liquid enemas. Campieri et al performed a multicenter, single-blinded study in which 1 arm randomized 117 patients to either a 2 g/10 mL mesalamine foam or a 2 g/50 mL mesalamine liquid enema daily while the second arm randomized 116 patients to either a 4 g/20 mL mesalamine foam or a 4 g/100 mL mesalamine liquid enema daily. The remission rates were higher with the foam at 10 days (54% versus 31%; P<0.05) but not after 3 weeks (83% versus 74%; P=NS) in the first arm, with only a trend toward higher remission rates with the foam in the second arm. Combining the results of both arms, the difference between clinical remission rates favoring foam over enemas was 16% (OR 2.38, 95% CI 1.27 to 4.46; P<0.01) at 10 days, but not at 3 weeks (OR 1.62, 95% CI 0.92 to 2.86; P=NS). Endoscopic and histologic improvement and remission rates were similar between products.[86] Ardizzone et al reported no difference in either clinical or endoscopic remission in 195 patients randomized to either a 2-g mesalamine foam or a 2-g mesalamine liquid enema,[89] while Malchow et al reported similar rates of clinical and endoscopic remission (65% versus 70, P=NS and 38% versus 38%, P=NS) among 266 patients randomized to either a 2-g mesalamine foam or a 4 g/60 mL mesalamine liquid enema once daily for 4 weeks, despite the double-dose of mesalamine in the enema formulation.[84]

There is also evidence to suggest that mesalamine foam may better tolerated and, overall, more acceptable to patients than mesalamine liquid enemas. For many, liquid enemas can be uncomfortable, inconvenient, require prolonged retention, and be complicated by leakage and staining of

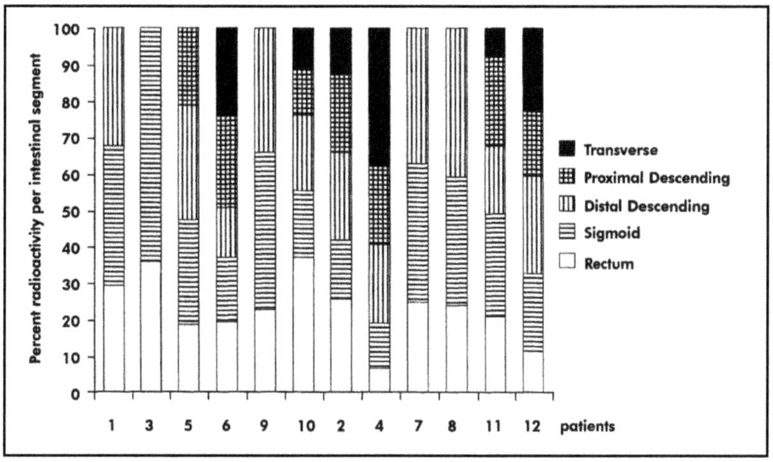

FIGURE 14-5. Intestinal segment of maximum spread and regional distribution of radioactivity (% dose) of the radiolabeled mesalamine gel administered to 12 patients. (Reprinted with permission from Gionchetti P, Venturi A, Rizzello F, et al. Retrograde colonic spread of a new mesalazine rectal enema in patients with distal ulcerative colitis. *Aliment Pharmacol Ther.* 1997;11(4):679-684.)

clothing. Because of its smaller volume and better adhesive properties, mesalamine foam appears to be more easily retained and less likely to trigger urgency or incontinence. It does not require administration at bedtime and, because of its convenient small size dosage unit, can be easily carried and managed. Campieri et al found that a higher proportion of patients receiving mesalamine foam reported good acceptance than those who were taking mesalamine enemas (81% versus 49%; $P<0.01$). Among patients treated with foam, 81% preferred foam to their previous use of enema, reporting that foam was more comfortable, more practical, easier to retain, and interfered less with their evening routine.[86] In the study by Malchow et al, however, there was no significant difference in quality of life scores between mesalamine foam and enemas.[84] Similarly, Ardizzone et al noted patient acceptance of mesalamine foam to be similar to that for liquid enemas.[89]

Gel

Background

Mesalamine rectal gel represents the newest addition to the armamentarium of mesalamine topical formulations. It consists of a high-viscosity thixotropic mesalamine suspension that, in theory, offers better adhesion and, hence, better distribution to the colonic mucosa. Although there are at present no mesalamine gel formulations commercially sold in the United States, Enterasin gel is available in Europe. Enterasin gel is stored in a spray canister fitted with a dispensing valve. The spray system consists of a two-chamber device: an inner chamber (a flexible polyethylene-coated aluminum bag) containing the mesalamine suspension and an outer chamber (an airtight can) filled with pressurized nitrogen acting as a propellant. Upon activation of the valve, the pressurized nitrogen squeezes the inner bag containing the gel suspension, which is released into the colon via a disposable rectal applicator.[90]

Gionchetti et al labeled a 4 g/60 mL mesalamine rectal gel with 100 MBq ^{99m}technetium sulphur colloid and measured proximal spread in 12 patients with active distal UC. The gel reached beyond the sigmoid colon in 11 out of 12 patients, to the transverse colon in 6 out of 12 patients, and effectively coated the upper limit of disease in all cases (Figure 14-5). Maximal retrograde progression was achieved within 3 to 4 hours, suggesting that the delivery of gel was gradual. Semiquantitative analysis demonstrated a fairly uniform distribution of gel, and in none of the patients was there any significant backflow of gel after maximum retrograde progression.[90]

Pharmacokinetics

Gionchetti et al measured plasma levels of 5-ASA and Ac-5-ASA in 12 patients with active distal UC administered a 4 g/60 mL mesalamine gel. Systemic absorption of mesalamine gel was low, as evidenced by mean 5-ASA values of 0.9, 1.2, and 1.1 µg/mL, respectively, at 2, 4, and 6 hours after dosing, and Ac-5-ASA values of 2.0, 2.6, and 2.8 µg/mL, respectively, at the same time points.[90]

Adverse Events

There have been only 2 published reports to date of the use of mesalamine rectal gel, and neither has reported serious adverse events. In the first study by Gionchetti et al, designed to assess retrograde spread of the new gel formulation, none of the 12 patients reported adverse reactions attributable to the gel.[90] In the second, larger study, one patient developed renal colic and another insomnia, but neither was thought to be related to the gel.[91] Because of the low systemic absorption of the gel, it is presumed that the incidence of adverse events will be low.

CLINICAL TRIALS

Comparison to Other Topical Mesalamines

Gionchetti et al randomized 103 patients with mild to moderately active distal UC to either a 2 g/60 mL mesalamine gel or a 2 g/120 mL mesalamine foam once daily. After 4 weeks, both gel and foam significantly reduced the mean total DAI scores from baseline, but there was no significant difference in the number of patients who achieved clinical, endoscopic, or histologic remission between groups (76% versus 69%, 51% versus 52%, and 30% versus 30%, respectively; *P*=NS). However, the mesalamine gel was significantly better tolerated than the foam, as patients taking the foam had significantly more difficulty in retention, abdominal bloating, and discomfort during administration (25% versus 6%, 50% versus 26%, and 48% versus 26%, respectively; *P*<0.05). It is unclear whether this was attributable to the increased viscosity of the gel, or simply its smaller volume.[91]

PARA-AMINOSALICYLIC ACID (4-AMINOSALICYLIC ACID)

BACKGROUND

Para-aminosalicylic acid, commonly referred to as 4-aminosalicylic acid (4-ASA), has been evaluated as a topical agent in the management of distal UC. 4-ASA is structurally similar to 5-ASA, differing only in the position of the amine group. The sodium salt of 4-ASA is more stable than 5-ASA, and animal studies have suggested that it might have greater anti-inflammatory activity.[92]

PHARMACOKINETICS

There are no published studies that have described the pharmacokinetics of rectally administered 4-ASA. However, oral ingestion of 4-ASA at therapeutic doses has been reported to result in intraluminal concentrations of 4-ASA similar to those of 5-ASA following oral administration of mesalamine.[93] It is very possible that, as is the case with topical mesalamine, topical 4-ASA is poorly absorbed from the colon, although data are lacking.

ADVERSE EVENTS

For many years, oral 4-ASA had been used extensively in the treatment of tuberculosis, and its relative safety as an oral agent has been well-established. Data regarding its use as a topical agent are much more limited, but in the few studies describing its use in the treatment of distal UC, no significant adverse events have been reported. In one study, a single patient developed malaise, nausea, and fever within 2 days of starting 4-ASA enema that was thought to be most consistent with an idiosyncratic reaction.[94]

CLINICAL TRIALS

TREATMENT OF ACTIVE DISEASE

Placebo-Controlled Trials

Three small, randomized, placebo-controlled trials have shown 4-ASA liquid enemas to be an effective therapy in the treatment of mild to moderately active distal UC. Selby et al conducted a 2-week, double-blind study randomizing 52 patients to daily enemas containing 1 g/100 ml, 2g/100 mL 4-ASA, or placebo. Pooling the data between the 4-ASA groups showed greater clinical and endoscopic improvement than with placebo (80% versus 41% and 72% versus 32%, respectively; *P*<0.005).[95] Gandolfo et al conducted a similar study in 45 patients with mild to moderately active distal UC, and showed greater improvement in symptoms with the 1 g (but not 2 g) 4-ASA enema than placebo (*P*<0.05). Thirty-five of the patients continued on open-label 4-ASA experienced 1 year of clinical remission and improvement rates of 46% and 31%, respectively.[96] Ginsberg et al randomized 25 patients to either a 2 g/60 mL 4-ASA liquid enema once daily or placebo. Improvement in clinical, endoscopic, and histologic parameters were noted in 83% of patients who received 4-ASA enemas versus 15% for placebo (p <0.005), with successful salvage of 9 of the 11 failed placebo patients who were treated subsequently with open-label 4-ASA.[97]

Comparison to Topical Steroids

O'Donnell et al reported no clinical or histological differences in 53 patients randomized to receive either a 2 g/50 mL 4-ASA liquid enema or a 20 mg/50 mL prednisolone enema once daily for 6 weeks.[94] A second, double-blind study by Sharma et al randomized 40 patients to either a 2 g/50 mL 4-ASA liquid enema or 20 mg/50 mL prednisolone enema for 4 weeks. Although there was no significant difference in clinical improvement between the 2 groups, the patients treated with 4-ASA showed significantly greater endoscopic and histologic improvement (*P*<0.001).[98] Marshall et al analyzed both studies and calculated the pooled OR for symptomatic improvement to be 3.88 (95% CI 1.29 to 11.64) favoring 4-ASA.[47]

Comparison to Topical Mesalamine

Two studies have directly compared 4-ASA and 5-ASA liquid enemas. In a double-blind study conducted by Campieri et al, 63 patients with mild to moderately active distal UC were treated with either a 2-g 4-ASA liquid enema or a 2-g 5-ASA liquid enema once daily. After 15 days, clinical, endoscopic, and histologic improvement was similar, whether the patient was treated with 4-ASA or 5-ASA (77% versus 81%, 77% versus 78%, and 41% versus 46%, respectively; *P*=NS).[99] In a multicenter, open-label trial, Marteau et al randomized 50 patients with mild to moderately active distal UC to receive either a 2-g 4-ASA liquid enema or a 1-g 5-ASA liquid enema once daily for 4 weeks. Although there was no significant difference between groups in clinical and endoscopic improvement, tolerance scores were significantly better with 4-ASA (0.46 ± 0.77 versus 1.00 ± 0.73; $P=0.03$).[100]

N-ACETYL-5-AMINOSALICYLIC ACID

N-acetyl-5-aminosalicylic acid (Ac-5-ASA), a metabolite of 5-ASA, has been studied as a liquid enema in the treatment of distal UC. In a double-blind, controlled trial, Willoughby et al randomized 43 patients with either clinical or endoscopic evidence of mild to moderately active UC to either a 2 g/100 mL Ac-5-ASA liquid enema twice a day or placebo. After 2 weeks, endoscopic and histologic improvement was significantly greater in patients treated with Ac-5-ASA (10 versus 2, $P<0.02$; and 13 versus 5, $P<0.05$).[101] However, a second controlled study of Ac-5-ASA failed to show efficacy.[102]

FUTURE DIRECTIONS

Topical mesalamine therapy is an essential part of the medical management of distal UC. There is strong evidence from randomized, controlled trials to support rectal mesalamine as first-line treatment for patients with mild to moderately active distal UC. Mesalamine liquid enemas have been the formulation most well-studied, although their mode of delivery can at times be uncomfortable and inconvenient for patients, which may limit compliance. Mesalamine foam and gel may offer a more acceptable alternative for patients, but more studies are needed comparing the efficacy, tolerability, and practicality of these formulations to liquid enemas. Until more studies become available, the choice of formulation should depend on the extent of disease and on the patient's preference. For active ulcerative proctitis, however, mesalamine suppositories are generally considered the treatment of choice.

Future directions include the development of new formulations of mesalamine gels and foams and low-dose mesalamine enemas. Combination topical therapies with mesalamine and corticosteroids, including budesonide or one of the other potent novel corticosteroid formulations that undergo first-pass metabolism in the liver and thus have lower systemic side effects, are also under development. Finally, the development of rectally absorbed biological therapies such as the anti-ICAM-1 anti-sense oligonucleotide[103] raise the potential for combination therapies of these exciting agents and the "tried and true" mesalamine products.

REFERENCES

1. Khan AK, Piris J, Truelove SC. An experiment to determine the active therapeutic moiety of sulphasalazine. *Lancet.* 1977;2(8044):892-895.
2. Farmer RG, Easley KA, Rankin GB. Clinical patterns, natural history, and progression of ulcerative colitis: a long-term follow-up of 1116 patients. *Dig Dis Sci.* 1993;38(6):1137-1146.
3. *Rowasa.* Montvale, NJ: Thompson PDR; 2004;58.
4. Campieri M, Lanfranchi GA, Brignola C, et al. Retrograde spread of 5-aminosalicylic acid enemas in patients with active ulcerative colitis. *Dis Colon Rectum.* 1986;29(2):108-110.
5. Vitti RA, Meyers F, Knight LC, Siegel JA, Malmud LS, Fisher RS. Quantitative distribution of radiolabeled 5-aminosalicylic acid enemas in patients with left-sided ulcerative colitis. *Dig Dis Sci.* 1989;34(11):1792-1797.
6. Tiel-van Buul MM, Mulder CJ, van Royen EA, Wiltink EH, Tytgat GN. Retrograde spread of mesalazine (5-aminosalicylic acid)-containing enema in patients with ulcerative colitis. *Clin Pharmacokinet.* 1991;20(3):247-251.
7. Chapman NJ, Brown ML, Phillips SF, et al. Distribution of mesalamine enemas in patients with active distal ulcerative colitis. *Mayo Clinic Proceedings.* 1992;67(3):245-248.
8. Almer S, Ekberg S, Strom M. Retrograde distribution of a new 5-aminosalicylic acid enema in patients with ulcerative colitis. *Gastroenterol Clin Biol.* 1992;16(6-7):564-568.
9. van Bodegraven AA, Boer RO, Lourens J, Tuynman HA, Sindram JW. Distribution of mesalazine enemas in active and quiescent ulcerative colitis. *Aliment Pharmacol Ther.* 1996;10(3):327-332.
10. Otten MH, De Haas G, Van den Ende R. Colonic spread of 5-ASA enemas in healthy individuals, with a comparison of their physical and chemical characteristics. *Aliment Pharmacol Ther.* 1997;11(4):693-697.
11. Gionchetti P, Belluzzi A, Campieri M, et al. 5-Aminosalicylic acid in patients with ulcerative colitis in remission: plasma levels after administration of a new rectal enema. *Methods Find Exp Clin Pharmacol.* 1988;10(10):667-669.
12. Dew MJ, Cardwell M, Kidwai NS, Evans BK, Rhodes J. 5-amino-salicylic acid in serum and urine after administration by enema to patients with colitis. *J Pharm Pharmacol.* 1983;35(5):323-324.
13. Rosenberg L, Palmer JR, Zauber AG, Warshauer ME, Stolley PD, Shapiro S. A hypothesis: Nonsteroidal anti-inflammatory drugs reduce the incidence of large-bowel cancer. *J Natl Cancer Inst.* 1991;83(5):355-358.
14. Campieri M, Lanfranchi GA, Boschi S, et al. Topical administration of 5-aminosalicylic acid enemas in patients with ulcerative colitis: studies on rectal absorption and excretion. *Gut.* 1985;26(4):400-405.
15. Bondesen S, Nielsen OH, Jacobsen O, et al. 5-Aminosalicylic acid enemas in patients with active ulcerative colitis: influence of acidity on the kinetic pattern. *Scand J Gastroenterol.* 1984;19(5):677-682.
16. Schoonjans R, De Vos M, Schelfhout AM, Praet M, Elewaut A. Distribution and concentrations of 5-aminosalicylic acid in rectosigmoid biopsy specimens after rectal administration. *Dis Colon Rectum.* 1996;39(7):788-793.
17. Frieri G, Pimpo MT, Andreoli A, et al. Prevention of post-operative recurrence of Crohn's disease requires adequate mucosal concentration of mesalazine. Gruppo Italiano per lo Studio del Colon e del Retto. *Aliment Pharmacol Ther.* 1999;13(5):577-582.
18. Frieri G, Giacomelli R, Pimpo M, et al. Mucosal 5-amino-salicylic acid concentration inversely correlates with severity of colonic inflammation in patients with ulcerative colitis. *Gut.* 2000;47(3):410-414.

19. Hussain F, Ajjan R, Grundman M, Bolton R, Riley S. Mucosal aminosalicylate levels correlate with clinical activity in patients with ulcerative colitis. *Gut.* 1997;40(Suppl 1):A23.
20. Naganuma M, Iwao Y, Ogata H, et al. Measurement of colonic mucosal concentrations of 5-aminosalicylic acid is useful for estimating its therapeutic efficacy in distal ulcerative colitis: comparison of orally administered mesalamine and sulfasalazine. *Inflamm Bowel Dis.* 2001;7(3):221-225.
21. Marteau P, Devaux CB. Mesalazine during pregnancy. *Lancet.* 1994;344(8938):1708-1709.
22. Ota T, Fujimura T, Hongyo T, Kawase S. Prenatal and postnatal study of mesalazine in rats. *Oyo Yakuri.* 1994;47(6):513-522.
23. Bell CM, Habal FM. Safety of topical 5-aminosalicylic acid in pregnancy. *Am J Gastroenterol.* 1997;92(12):2201-2202.
24. Barber GB, Lee DE, Antonioli DA, Peppercorn MA. Refractory distal ulcerative colitis responsive to 5-aminosalicylate enemas. *Am J Gastroenterol.* 1985;80(8):612-614.
25. Kandel G, Prokipchuk EJ. 5-ASA enemas for refractory distal ulcerative colitis. An open trial. *J Clin Gastroenterol.* 1987;9(5):536-540.
26. Hanauer S, Schultz P. Efficacy of 5-ASA for steroid dependent ulcerative colitis. *Gastroenterology.* 1986;90(5):1449.
27. Fedotin MS. Five-aminosalicylic acid enemas in treatment of ulcerative colitis. *Mo Med.* 1985;82(6):301-303.
28. Vantrappen G, Coremans G, Janssens J, Rutgeerts P. Does intercurrent hepatitis have a beneficial effect on the course of Crohn's disease? *Gastroenterology.* 1983;84(4):843-845.
29. Sutherland LR, Martin F, Greer S, et al. 5-Aminosalicylic acid enema in the treatment of distal ulcerative colitis, proctosigmoiditis, and proctitis. *Gastroenterology.* 1987;92(6):1894-1898.
30. Campieri M, Gionchetti P, Belluzzi A, et al. Optimum dosage of 5-aminosalicylic acid as rectal enemas in patients with active ulcerative colitis. *Gut.* 1991;32(8):929-931.
31. Hanauer SB. Dose-ranging study of mesalamine (PENTASA) enemas in the treatment of acute ulcerative proctosigmoiditis: results of a multicentered placebo-controlled trial. The U.S. PENTASA Enema Study Group. *Inflamm Bowel Dis.* 1998;4(2):79-83.
32. Campieri M, Lanfranchi GA, Bazzocchi G, et al. Treatment of ulcerative colitis with high-dose 5-aminosalicylic acid enemas. *Lancet.* 1981;2(8241):270-271.
33. Friedman LS, Richter JM, Kirkham SE, DeMonaco HJ, May RJ. 5-Aminosalicylic acid enemas in refractory distal ulcerative colitis: a randomized, controlled trial. *Am J Gastroenterol.* 1986;81(6):412-418.
34. Porro GB, Ardizzone S, Petrillo M, Fasoli A, Molteni P, Imbesi V. Low Pentasa dosage versus hydrocortisone in the topical treatment of active ulcerative colitis: a randomized, double-blind study. *Am J Gastroenterol.* 1995;90(5):736-739.
35. Topical 5-aminosalicylic acid versus prednisolone in ulcerative proctosigmoiditis: a randomized, double-blind multicenter trial. Danish 5-ASA Group. *Dig Dis Sci.* 1987;32(6):598-602.
36. Mulder CJ, Tytgat GN, Wiltink EH, Houthoff HJ. Comparison of 5-aminosalicylic acid (3 g) and prednisolone phosphate sodium enemas (30 mg) in the treatment of distal ulcerative colitis: a prospective, randomized, double-blind trial. *Scand J Gastroenterol.* 1988;23(8):1005-1008.
37. Mulder TP, Verspaget HW, Janssens AR, de Bruin PA, Pena AS, Lamers CB. Decrease in two intestinal copper/zinc containing proteins with antioxidant function in inflammatory bowel disease. *Gut.* 1991;32(10):1146-1150.
38. Lemann M, Galian A, Rutgeerts P, et al. Comparison of budesonide and 5-aminosalicylic acid enemas in active distal ulcerative colitis. *Aliment Pharmacol Ther.* 1995;9(5):557-562.
39. Rufle W, Fruhmorgen P, Huber W, Kimmig JM. Budesonide foam as a new therapeutic principle in distal ulcerative colitis in comparison with mesalazine enema: an open, controlled, randomized and prospective multicenter pilot study. *Z Gastroenterol.* 2000;38(4):287-293.
40. Mulder CJ, Fockens P, Meijer JW, van der Heide H, Wiltink EH, Tytgat GN. Beclomethasone dipropionate (3 mg) versus 5-aminosalicylic acid (2 g) versus the combination of both (3 mg/2 g) as retention enemas in active ulcerative proctitis. *Eur J Gastroenterol Hepatol.* 1996;8(6):549-553.
41. Kam L, Cohen H, Dooley C, Rubin P, Orchard J. A comparison of mesalamine suspension enema and oral sulfasalazine for treatment of active distal ulcerative colitis in adults. *Am J Gastroenterol.* 1996;91(7):1338-1342.
42. Safdi M, DeMicco M, Sninsky C, et al. A double-blind comparison of oral versus rectal mesalamine versus combination therapy in the treatment of distal ulcerative colitis. *Am J Gastroenterol.* 1997;92(10):1867-1871.
43. Vecchi M, Meucci G, Gionchetti P, et al. Oral versus combination mesalazine therapy in active ulcerative colitis: a double-blind, double-dummy, randomized multicentre study. *Aliment Pharmacol Ther.* 2001;15(2):251-256.
44. Marteau P, Probert CS, Lindgren S, et al. Combined oral and enema treatment with Pentasa (mesalazine) is superior to oral therapy alone in patients with extensive mild/moderate active ulcerative colitis: a randomised, double blind, placebo controlled study. *Gut.* 2005;54(7):960-965.
45. Powell-Tuck J, Parkins R. Controlled comparison of enemas containing 1g and 2g 5 aminosalicylic acid in patients with ulcerative proctosigmoiditis. *Gut.* 1984;25:A1143.
46. Cohen RD, Woseth DM, Thisted RA, Hanauer SB. A meta-analysis and overview of the literature on treatment options for left-sided ulcerative colitis and ulcerative proctitis. *Am J Gastroenterol.* 2000;95(5):1263-1276.
47. Marshall JK, Irvine EJ. Rectal corticosteroids versus alternative treatments in ulcerative colitis: a meta-analysis. *Gut.* 1997;40(6):775-781.
48. McPhee MS, Swan JT, Biddle WL, Greenberger NJ. Proctocolitis unresponsive to conventional therapy: response to 5- aminosalicylic acid enemas. *Dig Dis Sci.* 1987;32(12 Suppl):76S-81S.
49. Biddle WL, Miner PB Jr. Long-term use of mesalamine enemas to induce remission in ulcerative colitis. *Gastroenterology.* 1990;99(1):113-118.
50. Biddle WL, Greenberger NJ, Swan JT, McPhee MS, Miner PB Jr. 5-Aminosalicylic acid enemas: effective agent in maintaining remission in left-sided ulcerative colitis. *Gastroenterology.* 1988;94(4):1075-1079.
51. Andreoli A, Spinella S, Levenstein S, Prantera C. 5-ASA enema versus oral sulphasalazine in maintaining remission in ulcerative colitis. *Ital J Gastroenterol.* 1994;26(3):121-125.
52. d'Albasio G, Trallori G, Ghetti A, et al. Intermittent therapy with high-dose 5-aminosalicylic acid enemas for maintaining remission in ulcerative proctosigmoiditis. *Dis Colon Rectum.* 1990;33(5):394-397.
53. Mantzaris GJ, Hatzis A, Petraki K, Spiliadi C, Triantaphyllou G. Intermittent therapy with high-dose 5-aminosalicylic acid enemas maintains remission in ulcerative proctitis and proctosigmoiditis. *Dis Colon Rectum.* 1994;37(1):58-62.
54. d'Albasio G, Pacini F, Camarri E, et al. Combined therapy with 5-aminosalicylic acid tablets and enemas for maintaining remission in ulcerative colitis: A randomized double-blind study. *Am J Gastroenterol.* 1997;92(7):1143-1147.
55. Sutherland LR, Martin F. 5-aminosalicylic acid enemas in the maintenance of remission in distal ulcerative colitis and proctitis. *Can J Gastroenterol.* 1987;1(1):3-6.

56. Guarino J, Chatzinoff M, Berk T, Friedman LS. 5-Aminosalicylic acid enemas in refractory distal ulcerative colitis: Long-term results. *Am J Gastroenterol.* 1987;82(8):732-737.
57. Miner PB Jr, Daly R, Nester T. The effect of varying dose intervals of mesalamine enemas for the prevention of relapse in distal ulcerative colitis. *Gastroenterology.* 1994;106(4):A736.
58. Marshall JK, Irvine EJ. Putting rectal 5-aminosalicylic acid in its place: the role in distal ulcerative colitis. *Am J Gastroenterol.* 2000;95(7):1628-1636.
59. Canasa. Montvale, NJ: Thompson PDR; 2004;58.
60. Williams CN, Haber G, Aquino JA. Double-blind, placebo-controlled evaluation of 5-ASA suppositories in active distal proctitis and measurement of extent of spread using 99mTc- labeled 5-ASA suppositories. *Dig Dis Sci.* 1987;32(12 Suppl):71S-75S.
61. Jacobsen BA, Abildgaard K, Rasmussen HH, et al. Availability of mesalazine (5-aminosalicylic acid) from enemas and suppositories during steady-state conditions. *Scand J Gastroenterol.* 1991;26(4):374-378.
62. Aumais G, Lefebvre M, Tremblay C, et al. Rectal tissue, plasma and urine concentrations of mesalazine after single and multiple administrations of 500 mg suppositories to healthy volunteers and ulcerative proctitis patients. *Aliment Pharmacol Ther.* 2003;17(1):93-97.
63. Lamet M, Ptak T, Dallaire C, et al. Efficacy and safety of mesalamine 1 g HS versus 500 mg BID suppositories in mild to moderate ulcerative proctitis: a multicenter randomized study. *Inflamm Bowel Dis.* 2005;11(7):625-630.
64. Kornbluth AA, Salomon P, Sachar DB, et al. ACTH-induced adrenal hemorrhage: a complication of therapy masquerading as an acute abdomen [see comments]. *J Clin Gastroenterol.* 1990;12(4):371-377.
65. Borkje B, Riedel B, Berstad A, Maartmann-Moe H. Effect of mesalazine (mesasal®) suppositories in patients with ulcerative proctitis or proctosigmoiditis. *Scand J Gastroenterol.* 1993;28:A49.
66. Williams CN. Role of rectal formulations: Suppositories. *Scand J Gastroenterol Suppl.* 1990;172:60-62.
67. Campieri M, Gionchetti P, Belluzzi A, et al. Topical treatment with 5-aminosalicylic in distal ulcerative colitis by using a new suppository preparation: a double-blind placebo controlled trial. *Int J Colorectal Dis.* 1990;5(2):79-81.
68. Campieri M, De Franchis R, Bianchi Porro G, Ranzi T, Brunetti G, Barbara L. Mesalazine (5-aminosalicylic acid) suppositories in the treatment of ulcerative proctitis or distal proctosigmoiditis: a randomized controlled trial. *Scand J Gastroenterol.* 1990;25(7):663-668.
69. Kohn A, Luzi C, Iurato S, et al. 5-ASA suppositories: a double blind trial in ulcerative proctitis. *Lit Rev Ther IBD.* 1992;32:A173.
70. Ngo Y, Gelinet JM, Ivanovic A, et al. Efficacy of a daily application of mesalazine (Pentasa) suppository with progressive release, in the treatment of ulcerative proctitis: a double-blind versus placebo randomized trial. *Gastroenterol Clin Biol.* 1992;16(10):782-786.
71. Farup PG, Hovde O, Halvorsen FA, Raknerud N, Brodin U. Mesalazine suppositories versus hydrocortisone foam in patients with distal ulcerative colitis: a comparison of the efficacy and practicality of two topical treatment regimens. *Scand J Gastroenterol.* 1995;30(2):164-170.
72. Gionchetti P, Rizzello F, Venturi A, et al. Comparison of oral with rectal mesalazine in the treatment of ulcerative proctitis. *Dis Colon Rectum.* 1998;41(1):93-97.
73. Campieri M, Gionchetti P, Belluzzi A, et al. 5-Aminosalicylic acid as enemas or suppositories in distal ulcerative colitis? *J Clin Gastroenterol.* 1988;10(4):406-409.
74. Campieri M, Gionchetti P, Belluzzi A, et al. 5-Aminosalicylic acid suppositories in the management of ulcerative colitis. *Dis Colon Rectum.* 1989;32(5):398-399.
75. Massa P, Michetti P, Dodero M. 5-ASA suppositories in topical treatment of ulcerative colitis (UC). *Gastroenterology.* 1990;98(5):A189.
76. Gionchetti P, Rizzello F, Venturi A, et al. Comparison of mesalazine suppositories in proctitis and distal proctosigmoiditis. *Aliment Pharmacol Ther.* 1997;11(6):1053-1057.
77. Casellas F, Vaquero E, Armengol JR, Malagelada JR. Practicality of 5-aminosalicylic suppositories for long-term treatment of inactive distal ulcerative colitis. *Hepatogastroenterology.* 1999;46(28):2343-2346.
78. D'Arienzo A, Panarese A, D'Armiento FP, et al. 5-Aminosalicylic acid suppositories in the maintenance of remission in idiopathic proctitis or proctosigmoiditis: a double-blind placebo-controlled clinical trial. *Am J Gastroenterol.* 1990;85(9):1079-1082.
79. d'Albasio G, Paoluzi P, Campieri M, et al. Maintenance treatment of ulcerative proctitis with mesalazine suppositories: a double-blind placebo-controlled trial. The Italian IBD Study Group. *Am J Gastroenterol.* 1998;93(5):799-803.
80. Hanauer S, Good LI, Goodman MW, et al. Long-term use of mesalamine (Rowasa) suppositories in remission maintenance of ulcerative proctitis. *Am J Gastroenterol.* 2000;95(7):1749-1754.
81. Marteau P, Crand J, Foucault M, Rambaud JC. Use of mesalazine slow release suppositories 1 g three times per week to maintain remission of ulcerative proctitis: a randomised double blind placebo controlled multicentre study. *Gut.* 1998;42(2):195-199.
82. Campieri M, Corbelli C, Gionchetti P, et al. Spread and distribution of 5-ASA colonic foam and 5-ASA enema in patients with ulcerative colitis. *Dig Dis Sci.* 1992;37(12):1890-1897.
83. Wilding IR, Kenyon CJ, Chauhan S, et al. Colonic spreading of a non-chlorofluorocarbon mesalazine rectal foam enema in patients with quiescent ulcerative colitis. *Aliment Pharmacol Ther.* 1995;9(2):161-166.
84. Malchow H, Gertz B. A new mesalazine foam enema (Claversal Foam) compared with a standard liquid enema in patients with active distal ulcerative colitis. *Aliment Pharmacol Ther.* 2002;16(3):415-423.
85. Lee FI, Jewell DP, Mani V, et al. A randomised trial comparing mesalazine and prednisolone foam enemas in patients with acute distal ulcerative colitis. *Gut.* 1996;38(2):229-233.
86. Campieri M, Paoluzi P, D'Albasio G, Brunetti G, Pera A, Barbara L. Better quality of therapy with 5-ASA colonic foam in active ulcerative colitis: a multicenter comparative trial with 5-ASA enema. *Dig Dis Sci.* 1993;38(10):1843-1850.
87. Pokrotnieks J, Marlicz K, Paradowski L, Margus B, Zaborowski P, Greinwald R. Efficacy and tolerability of mesalazine foam enema (Salofalk foam) for distal ulcerative colitis: a double-blind, randomized, placebo-controlled study. *Aliment Pharmacol Ther.* 2000;14(9):1191-1198.
88. Hinojosa J, Agueda A, Panes J, de Sola CM, Fernandez-Blanco I, Gassull MA. Multicenter, randomized trial comparing oral, topic, and oral plus topic mesalazine treatment in active distal ulcerative colitis. *Gastroenterology.* 2000;118(4):A4168.
89. Ardizzone S, Doldo P, Ranzi T, et al. Mesalazine foam (Salofalk foam) in the treatment of active distal ulcerative colitis: a comparative trial vs Salofalk enema. The SAF-3 study group. *Ital J Gastroenterol Hepatol.* 1999;31(8):677-684.
90. Gionchetti P, Venturi A, Rizzello F, et al. Retrograde colonic spread of a new mesalazine rectal enema in patients with distal ulcerative colitis. *Aliment Pharmacol Ther.* 1997;11(4):679-684.
91. Gionchetti P, Ardizzone S, Benvenuti ME, et al. A new mesalazine gel enema in the treatment of left-sided ulcerative colitis: a randomized controlled multicentre trial. *Aliment Pharmacol Ther.* 1999;13(3):381-388.
92. Lover MJ. Use of 4-aminosalicylic acid as an anti-inflammatory agent. US patent 4 440 763. April 3, 1984.

93. John A, Dickey K, Fenwick J, Sussman B, Beeken W. Pneumatosis intestinalis in patients with Crohn's disease. *Dig Dis Sci.* 1992;37(6):813-817.

94. O'Donnell LJ, Arvind AS, Hoang P, et al. Double blind, controlled trial of 4-aminosalicylic acid and prednisolone enemas in distal ulcerative colitis. *Gut.* 1992;33(7):947-949.

95. Selby WS, Bennett MK, Jewell DP. Topical treatment of distal ulcerative colitis with 4-amino-salicylic acid enemas. *Digestion.* 1984;29(4):231-234.

96. Gandolfo J, Farthing M, Powers G, et al. 4-Aminosalicylic acid retention enemas in treatment of distal colitis. *Dig Dis Sci.* 1987;32(7):700-704.

97. Ginsberg AL, Beck LS, McIntosh TM, Nochomovitz LE. Treatment of left-sided ulcerative colitis with 4-aminosalicylic acid enemas: a double-blind, placebo-controlled trial. *Ann Intern Med.* 1988;108(2):195-199.

98. Sharma MP, Duphare HV, Dasarathy S. A prospective randomized double blind trial comparing prednisolone and 4-aminosalicylic acid enemas in acute distal ulcerative colitis. *J Gastroenterol Hepatol.* 1992;7(2):173-177.

99. Campieri M, Lanfranchi GA, Bertoni F, et al. A double-blind clinical trial to compare the effects of 4- aminosalicylic acid to 5-aminosalicylic acid in topical treatment of ulcerative colitis. *Digestion.* 1984;29(4):204-208.

100. Marteau P, Halphen M. Comparative randomized open study of the efficacy and tolerance of enemas with 2 g of 4-amino-salicylic acid (4-ASA) and 1 gr of 5-amino-salicylic acid (5-ASA) in distal forms of hemorrhagic rectocolitis. *Gastroenterol Clin Biol.* 1995;19(1):31-35.

101. Willoughby CP, Truelove SC. Ulcerative colitis and pregnancy. *Gut.* 1980;21(6):469-474.

102. Binder V, Halskov S, Hvidberg EF, et al. A controlled study of 5-acetyl-aminosalicylic acid (5-Ac-ASA) as enema in ulcerative colitis. *Scand J Gastroenterol.* 1981;16:1122.

103. Miner P, Wedel M, Bane B, Bradley J. An enema formulation of alicaforsen, an antisense inhibitor of intercellular adhesion molecule-1, in the treatment of chronic, unremitting pouchitis. *Aliment Pharmacol Ther.* 2004;19(3):281-286.

15

Antibiotics in Ulcerative Colitis

Kim L. Isaacs, MD, PhD

BACKGROUND

The inflammatory process in ulcerative colitis (UC) is thought, at least in part, to be due to an aggressive host immune response to normal luminal bacteria.[1] This concept is supported by work performed in animal models of chronic intestinal inflammation. The development of spontaneous colitis in mice and rats requires the presence of luminal bacteria.[2] Colitis is not expressed in susceptible animals raised in a germ-free environment. Specific subsets of enteric bacteria appear to lead to a more aggressive colitis in rats and mice. Pretreatment of these animals with antibiotics attenuates the inflammatory response in the colon.[3] Table 15-1 reviews some of the representative animal models of colitis and the impact of bacteria/antibiotics on disease expression.

One of the first drugs that was used for treatment of UC was sulfasalazine, which consists of an antibacterial agent (sulfapyridine) and an anti-inflammatory agent (5-ASA).[4] Based on the antibacterial activity of this agent and efficacy of sulfasalazine in UC, it has been proposed that bacteria may play a role in the initiation and perpetuation of UC in humans. However, subsequent studies have indicated that 5-ASA is the active moiety and sulfapyridine is primarily a carrier. There have been multiple reports of both the first episode and exacerbations of UC being precipitated by or associated with a co-existing bacterial infection, such as *Clostridium difficile* and *Salmonella*.[5]

If bacteria play a role in initiating and perpetuating the inflammatory response, then manipulation of the host bacteria with antibiotics and probiotics is a sensible approach to the treatment of UC.[6,7] There is a clear role of antibiotics in the treatment of complications of UC, for example, bacterial superinfection with *Clostridium difficile* or toxic megacolon where there is a concern for bacterial translocation across the diseased colonic mucosa. Less clear is the clinical evidence of the role of antibiotics in the primary treatment of UC. In this chapter, we will review the clinical trial data for the use of antibiotics in UC.

CLINICAL TRIALS

Antibiotics

Truelove and Jewell proposed use of an intensive IV regimen for the treatment of severe attacks of UC that included both IV steroids and tetracycline.[8] The rationale for antibiotics in this regimen was to prevent infectious complications related to the severity of the illness. There was a 60% improvement in patients treated aggressively with this regimen. The impact of antibiotics cannot be separated from the effects of the IV steroids in this trial[9]; those data were re-evaluated retrospectively, and there was no difference in outcome between patients who had received antibiotics and those who had not.[10] Subsequently, there have been several controlled trials evaluating the role of antibiotics in the treatment of UC (Table 15-2).

Intravenous Antibiotics

Chapman et al reported the experience of a double-blind, placebo-controlled trial of IV metronidazole as adjunctive therapy in patients hospitalized with severe UC.[11]

Lichtenstein GR, ed.
Ulcerative Colitis: The Complete Guide to Medical Management (pp. 173-178)

TABLE 15-1

THE EFFECT OF A GERM-FREE ENVIRONMENT OR ANTIBIOTICS ON REPRESENTATIVE ANIMAL MODELS OF COLITIS[23]

Animal Model	Germ-Free Environment	Antibiotic Effect
Guinea pig Carrageenan-induced colitis[23,24]	No colitis	Colitis is decreased by metronidazole and clindamycin
Mouse DSS-induced colitis[25]	Both decreased and increased colitis	Colitis is decreased by ciprofloxacin, imipenem/vancomycin
Rat TNBS colitis[26]	No data	Colitis is decreased by amoxicillin/clavulanic acid
HLA B27 rat colitis[25]	No colitis	Colitis is decreased by metronidazole, vancomycin/imipenem
IL-10 knockout mouse colitis[27]	No colitis	Decreased colitis by metronidazole, ciprofloxacin, vancomycin, imipenem

Thirty-nine patients were randomized upon admission to 500 mg of metronidazole or placebo IV every 8 hours. The patients also received IV corticosteroids, total parenteral nutrition, and hydrocortisone enemas twice a day. They were assessed for response to therapy at 5 days. Seventy-four percent (14/19) of patients treated with IV metronidazole and 70% (14/20) of patients who received placebo showed significant improvement. The remainder of the patients were nonresponders and went on to surgical therapy. These data suggest that the routine use of IV metronidazole in this patient population likely does not improve the odds of responding to standard aggressive IV steroid therapy.[11] The antimicrobial spectrum of activity of metronidazole includes anaerobic bacteria and protozoa.[12]

Mantzaris and colleagues combined IV metronidazole with IV tobramycin for treatment of UC in a similar group of patients. Thirty-nine patients who were hospitalized for severe UC were randomized to 500 mg of metronidazole every 8 hours plus tobramycin (4 mg/kg tid) or placebo.[13] As in the Chapman study, the patients received IV corticosteroids, parenteral nutrition, and hydrocortisone enemas. The patients were evaluated after 10 days of therapy for clinical efficacy; 63.15% (12/19) of those treated with the antibiotic combination and 65% (12/20) treated with placebo had a clinical improvement. The remainder of patients underwent colectomy due to lack of improvement. There was no clear difference between the groups. It appears that, in this patient population, expanding the gram-negative coverage of the antibiotic therapy did not lead to an improved clinical response.[13]

It is possible that the broad-spectrum antibiotics that were used in these trials targeted the wrong populations of luminal bacteria. Mantzaris et al elected to study the same population of severely ill UC patients with adjunctive antibiotic treatment with intravenous ciprofloxacin.[14] Ciprofloxacin is a fluoroquinolone with a wide antibacterial spectrum, of which the main activity is against aerobic gram-negative bacilli. This group studied 55 consecutive patients admitted to the hospital with a diagnosis of severe UC. The standard treatment protocol was the same as used in the metronidazole/tobramycin trial. Added to this therapy was 400 mg bid of IV ciprofloxacin or placebo. As a result, 79.3% (23/29) of patients treated with ciprofloxacin and 77% (20/26) of patients treated with placebo improved. The remainder of the patients underwent colectomy.[14]

In summary, 3 placebo-controlled trials in patients with severe UC requiring hospitalization for intensification of therapy did not show any added advantage of IV antibiotics as adjunctive therapy.[11,13,14] In this situation, antibiotics should be used for infectious complications, such as bacteremia or toxic megacolon with a high risk of bacterial translocation. Response to intensive IV therapy with IV steroids in this population is affected by duration of the current exacerbation, severity of endoscopic lesions, and the presence of Truelove and Witts severity criteria.[15] It is important to conjecture that the disease itself may be too severe and too far advanced for antibiotic therapy to make a meaningful impact in this population of patients.

Oral Antibiotics

The placebo-controlled trials of oral antibiotics in patients with ulcerative colitis show more promise as potential adjunctive therapy in the treatment of acute ulcerative colitis. These trials show that the patient population tends to be less ill than those who received the IV therapies,

TABLE 15-2

CLINICAL TRIALS OF ANTIBIOTICS IN ULCERATIVE COLITIS

PI	Drug	N	Days	Outcome
Chapman[11]	Metronidazole 500 mg IV q 8 hours versus placebo	39 hospitalized patients with severe UC	5 days	No difference between metronidazole and placebo groups
Mantzaris[13]	Metronidazole (500 mg q 8 hours) and tobramycin (4 mg/kd tid) IV versus placebo	39 hospitalized patients with severe UC	10 days	No difference between metronidazole/ tobramycin group and placebo
Mantzaris[14]	Ciprofloxacin 400 mg IV bid versus placebo	55 hospitalized patients with severe UC	10 days	No difference between ciprofloxacin group and placebo
Dickinson[16]	Vancomycin 500 mg oral q 6 hours versus placebo	40 patients: 33 UC, 7 CD	7 days	No clinical difference, trend to less need for surgery in vancomycin-treated UC group
Burke[17]	Tobramycin 120 mg oral tid	84 patients with acute relapse of UC	1 week	Short-term benefit with higher clinical remission and improved histology scores in antibiotic-treated group. No difference in rate of relapse after 2 years
Mantzaris[18]	Ciprofloxacin 250 mg bid oral vs placebo	70 patients mild to moderate UC, also treated with steroids, 5-ASAs	14 days	No difference between the groups based on clinical parameters, endoscopy, and histology
Turunen[19]	Ciprofloxacin 500 to 750 mg oral bid versus placebo	83 patients poorly responding to IV steroids and 5-ASA	6 months	Treatment failure of 23% in antibiotic-treated group versus 44% in placebo group
Gionchetti[20]	Rifaximin 400 mg bid oral versus placebo	24 patients who had failed 7 to 10 days of IV steroids	10 days	NS trend towards clinical improvement in antibiotic group (64% versus 42%) Significant decrease in bleeding and stool frequency. Significant improvement in endoscopy

and the antibiotics are given orally. Oral administration of antibiotics potentially gives the greatest exposure of the drug to the luminal bacteria that may be driving the inflammatory response in UC.

Dickinson and his co-workers took 40 consecutive patients with IBD (33 UC and 7 CD) and randomized them to 500 mg of vancomycin orally every 6 hours or placebo.[16] This was given for 7 days in addition to "standard" medical therapy. There was no significant difference in clinical outcome between the 2 groups, although there was an apparent decrease in the need for surgery in patients who received the active drug.[16] The potential bacterial targets of this regimen include gram-positive bacteria and *Clostridium difficile. Clostridium difficile* was not isolated from any of the stool cultures from these patients.

Burke et al studied 84 patients with an acute relapse of UC. These patients were randomized to receive oral tobramycin or placebo for 1 week in addition to standard oral prednisone therapy.[17] At the end of the acute therapy, 74% (31 of 42) who had received tobramycin had attained a symptomatic remission while only 43% (18 of 42) in the placebo group were in a symptomatic remission. Histology scores in the tobramycin-treated group were also significantly better ($P<0.05$) than in the placebo group.[18] The patients were then followed to the point of relapse. Relapse consisted of rectal bleeding and an increase in stool frequency to 3 times per day. Relapse rate was examined at 1 and 2 years. There was no statistically significant difference in the rate of relapse at 2 years in those who had received short-term tobramycin (20% with SE 6.3%) as compared to those who had received placebo (12% with SE 5.1%). The investigators suggest that the lack of a durable benefit over the study period points towards a short-term change or effect on the luminal flora.[17]

Oral ciprofloxacin has been studied in 2 placebo-controlled trials in UC. Mantzaris and colleagues randomized 70 patients with mild to moderate UC to oral ciprofloxacin at 250 mg bid or placebo for 14 days.[18] The patients were also treated with oral prednisolone, hydrocortisone enemas, and olsalazine for 7 to 9 weeks. The patients were assessed at the end of the study drug period (day 14) and at the end of the steroid therapy. There were no differences between the 2 groups with respect to clinical status, endoscopic evaluation, and histology at the end of the study period (7 to 9 weeks). Response rate in both groups was greater than 70%.[18] This trial is plagued by one of the same issues that is seen in the IV trials in the more severely ill patients. The duration of antibiotic therapy was short, and a highly effective therapy (IV or oral steroids) was being initiated at the same time as the antibiotic. With this combination of therapies, the effect of the antibiotic therapy may be diluted by the positive effect of the steroid therapy.

Turunen and co-workers avoided this potential difficulty by looking at oral ciprofloxacin in a 6-month treatment trial in patients who were poorly responding to therapy with steroids and mesalamine.[19] The only intervention at trial initiation was the addition of oral ciprofloxacin (500 to 750 mg bid) or placebo to the patient's active medical regimen. Steroids were tapered during the trial. Clinical and endoscopic evaluations were carried out at 0, 3, 6, and 12 months. A total of 83 patients were enrolled into the trial. Treatment failure was defined as both a lack of endoscopic and clinical response to the drug therapy. During the active treatment phase of the study, the treatment failure rate was 21% versus 44% in the treated group as compared to the placebo group (*P*=0.2). Endoscopic evaluation was significantly better at the 3-month but not the 6-month evaluation in the ciprofloxacin-treated group.[19]

In a small, placebo-controlled trial, Gionchetti and colleagues administered Rifaximin, a UC.[20] The patients studied were hospitalized patients who had failed 7 to 10 days of IV methylprednisolone. Patients received 400 mg po bid of rifaximin or placebo orally for 10 days as a supplement to the standard steroid therapy. A total of 24 patients were studied; 64.3% (9/14) of rifaximin-treated and 41.7% (5/12) of placebo-treated patients showed clinical improvement (NS). As compared to the placebo, there was a significant decrease in stool frequency and rectal bleeding and a significant improvement in the sigmoidoscopy score. The drug was safe and well-tolerated.[20] This pilot study in a very ill population suggests that oral administration of an antibiotic may be a useful adjunctive therapy for ulcerative colitis.

Casellas and co-workers provided further evidence that antibiotic therapy in patients with UC may help attenuate the mucosal inflammatory response. This group looked at the effect of the addition of enterically coated amoxicillin-clavulanic acid on the intestinal inflammation in patients with active UC.[21] Three groups of patients were compared. One group received methylprednisolone, one group received amoxicillin-clavulanic acid, and the final group received methylprednisolone plus amoxicillin-clavulanic acid. The patients were treated for 5 days. Pre- and post-treatment assessment of mucosal release of eicosanoids and IL-8 were done using rectal dialysis. The metabolic activity of the gut flora was assessed using a lactulose breath test. A total of 30 patients were studied. Both the amoxicillin-clavulanic acid and the methylprednisolone significantly decreased the mucosal release of the inflammatory mediators. As expected, only the antibiotic therapy inhibited the excretion of hydrogen on the lactulose breath test. This study suggests that the resident gut bacteria play an important role in the release of gut inflammatory mediators in active UC. [21]

FUTURE DIRECTIONS

Currently, there are no clinical trial data that support the routine use of antibiotics as primary therapy for active UC. The IV antibiotic trials as adjunctive agents to steroids in severe UC have uniformly shown no benefit. The trials that show the most promise are those that use oral broad-spectrum agents in patients with milder disease. The science behind the attempts at impacting on colitis disease activity by manipulating the native luminal flora remains appealing. Our focus at this point should be to study larger groups of patients with milder disease activity using oral antibiotics. Nonabsorbable broad-spectrum antibiotics that have their main activity in the lumen of the gut are likely candidates for success that should be studied. Rifaximin would fit this category well. Oral ciprofloxacin may have some role in the therapy of UC and can be used as an adjunct to standard therapy. Antibiotics should continue to be used for complications of UC, such as toxic megacolon with bacterial translocation.

REFERENCES

1. Podolsky DK. *Inflammatory bowel disease.* 2002;347:417-429.
2. Sellon RK, Tonkonogy S, Schultz M, et al. Resident enteric bacteria are necessary for development of spontaneous colitis and immune system activation in interleukin-10-deficient mice. *Infect Immunol.* 1998;66:5224-5231.

3. Rath HC, Schultz M, Freitag R, et al. Different subsets of enteric bacteria induce and perpetuate experimental colitis in rats and mice. *Infect Immun.* 2001;69:2277-2285.
4. Swartz N. Salazopyridin, a new sulfanilaminde preparation. *Acta Med Scand.* 1942;118:540-549.
5. Kochhar R, Ayyagari A, Goenka M, Dhali G, Aggarwal R, Mehta S. Role of infectious agents in exacerbations of ulcerative colitis in India: a study of Clostridium difficile. *J Clin Gastroenterol.* 1993;16:26-30.
6. Sartor RB, Borody TJ, Warren EF, et al. Therapeutic manipulation of the enteric microflora in inflammatory bowel diseases: antibiotics, probiotics, and prebiotics. *Gastroenterology.* 2004;126:1620-1633.
7. Campieri M, Gionchetti P, Rizzello F, et al. Bacteria as the cause of ulcerative colitis. *Gut.* 2001;48:132-135.
8. Truelove S, Jewell D. Intensive intravenous regimen for severe attacks of ulcerative colitis. *Lancet.* 1974;1:1067-1070.
9. Truelove S, Willoughby C, Lee E, Kettlewell M. Further experience in the treatment of severe attacks of ulcerative colitis. *Lancet.* 1978;2:1086-1088.
10. Jarnerot G, Rolny P, Sandberg-Gertzen H. Intensive intravenous treatment of ulcerative colitis. *Gastroenterology.* 1985;89:1005-1013.
11. Chapman R, Selby W, Jewell D. Controlled trial of intravenous metronidazole as an adjunct to corticosteroids in severe ulcerative colitis. *Gut.* 1986;27:1210-1212.
12. Edwards D. Nitroimidazole drugs: action and resistance mechanisms. I. Mechanisms of action. *J Antimicrob Chemother.* 1993;31:9-20.
13. Mantzaris GJ, Hatzis A, Kontogiannis P, et al. Intravenous tobramycin and metronidazole as an adjunct to corticosteroids in acute, severe ulcerative colitis. *Am J Gastroenterol.* 1994;89:43-46.
14. Mantzaris GJ, Petraki K, Archavlis E, et al. A prospective randomized controlled trial of intravenous ciprofloxacin as an adjunct to corticosteroids in acute, severe ulcerative colitis. *Scand J Gastroenterol.* 2001;36:971-974.
15. Carbonnel, Gargouri, Lemann, et al. Predictive factors of outcome of intensive intravenous treatment for attacks of ulcerative colitis. *Aliment Pharmacol Ther.* 2000;14:273-279.
16. Dickinson RJ, O'Connor HJ, Pinder I, Hamilton I, Johnston D, Axon AT. Double blind controlled trial of oral vancomycin as adjunctive treatment in acute exacerbations of idiopathic colitis. *Gut.* 1985;26:1380-1384.
17. Burke DA, Axon AT, Clayden SA, et al. The efficacy of tobramycin in the treatment of ulcerative colitis. *Aliment Pharmacol Ther.* 1990;4:123-129.
18. Mantzaris GJ, Archavlis E, Christoforidis P, et al. A prospective randomized controlled trial of oral ciprofloxacin in acute ulcerative colitis. *Am J Gastroenterol.* 1997;92:454-456.
19. Turunen U, Farkkila M, Hakala K, et al. Long-term treatment of ulcerative colitis with ciprofloxacin: a prospective, double-blind, placebo-controlled study. *Gastroenterology.* 1998;115:1072-1078.
20. Gionchetti P, Rizzello F, Ferrieri A, et al. Rifaximin in patients with moderate or severe ulcerative colitis refractory to steroid-treatment: A double-blind, placebo-controlled trial. *Dig Dis Sci.* 1999;44:1220-1221.
21. Casellas F, Borruel N, Papo M, et al. Anti-inflammatory effects of enterically coated amoxicillin-clavulanic acid in active ulcerative colitis. *Inflamm Bowel Dis.* 1998;4:1-5.
22. Sartor RB, Sandborn W. *Kirsner's Inflammatory Bowel Diseases.* 6th ed. Philadelphia, PA: Saunders; 2004.
23. Onderdonk A, Hermos J, Dzink J, Bartlett J. Protective effect of metronidazole in experimental ulcerative colitis. *Gastroenterology.* 1978;74:521-526.
24. Onderdonk A, Hermos J, Bartlett J. The role of the intestinal microflora in experimental colitis. *Am J Clin Nutr.* 1977;30:1819-1825.
25. Rath H, Schultz M, Freitag R, et al. Different subsets of enteric bacteria induce and perpetuate experimental colitis in rats and mice. *Infect Immunol.* 2001;69:2277-2285.
26. Videla S, Vilaseca J, Guarner F, et al. Role of intestinal microflora in chronic inflammation and ulceration of the rat colon. *Gut.* 1994;35:1090-1097.
27. Madsen K, Doyle J, Tavernini M, Jewell L, Rennie R, Fedorak R. Antibiotic therapy attenuates colitis in interleukin 10 gene-deficient mice. *Gastroenterology.* 2000;118:1094-1105.

16

Oral and Parenteral Corticosteroids in Ulcerative Colitis

Leonard Baidoo, MD and Gary R. Lichtenstein, MD, FACP, FACG, AGAF

The etiology of ulcerative colitis remains elusive; however, it is perceived that the complex interaction of environmental, genetic, and immunologic factors play a role in its pathogenesis.[1] Medications that target immuno-inflammatory pathways are effective in the treatment of patients with UC. Since 1955, corticosteroids have been demonstrated to be effective for the treatment and rapid relief of symptoms in patients with UC,[2] subsequent to its mechanism of action on the immunoinflammatory pathways. Corticosteroids produce consistent and rapid clinical benefit, but also have potential to cause significant therapy-related side effects—some of which may be quite debilitating and substantially impair a patient's quality of life. In spite of its recognized potential adverse effects (particularly when used at high doses and over prolonged periods of time), corticosteroids remain one of the main treatments of ulcerative colitis.[3,4]

Mechanism of Action

The effects of corticosteroids are mediated by specific intracytoplasmic glucocorticoid receptors. Because most cells can express glucocorticoid receptors, corticosteroids can affect the functioning of a large variety of cells. The beneficial as well as deleterious effects of corticosteroids are a result of these multifactorial and widespread effects and are not explained by any particular action. Activated glucocorticoid receptors regulate the expression of certain target genes.[5,6] The end result is either the induction or suppression of the transcription of various steroid-responsive target genes, many of which are obviously involved in the inflammatory process. Corticosteroids inhibit early events such as increased vascular permeability, vasodilatation, leukocyte infiltration, and the release of inflammatory cytokines such as IL-1, IL-2, IL-8, IL-6, α-interferon, TNF adhesion molecule (intercellular AM-1), vascular cell AM-1, endothelial lymphocyte AM, E-selectin (CD62), lymphocyte adhesion molecule, colony stimulating factor, cytologic phospholipase A2, inducible nitric oxide synthase, prostaglandins, and leukotrienes.[7-9]

Corticosteroids also act to suppress later processes, including neovascular proliferation and fibroblast activation. The direct and indirect inhibition of the production of various proinflammatory cytokines, adhesion molecules, and inflammatory enzymes at the molecular level is responsible for the potent anti-inflammatory effects of corticosteroids. The cellular effects of such regulation include impaired intercellular reactions that are essential to antigen presentation, inflammatory cell activation, impaired migration of immune cells to sites of inflammation and increasing the number of circulatory polymorphonuclear leukocytes, and impaired phagocytic and degenerative functions.[6,10,11]

In vitro evidence suggests that corticosteroids can suppress intestinal mucosal natural killer cell activity.[12] Furthermore, corticosteroids have been shown to reduce plasma exudation from postcapillary vessels at inflammatory sites.[13] Finally, corticosteroids stimulate water and sodium absorption in the gastrointestinal tract and thus reduce diarrhea (Table 16-1).[14]

Efficacy and Use of Corticosteroids

Approximately one-third of patients with UC will require corticosteroid therapy during the course of their

Lichtenstein GR, ed.
Ulcerative Colitis: The Complete Guide to Medical Management (pp. 179-190)

TABLE 16-1

CORTICOSTEROID FORMULATIONS: COMMONLY AVAILABLE GLUCOCORTICOID PREPARATIONS

Drug	Route of Administration	Relative Potency
Hydrocortisone	IV, po, suppository, enema	1x
Prednisone	IV, po	4x
	IV, po	5x
Dexamethasone	IV, po	10x
Budesonide	po	15x

IV indicates intravenous; po, by mouth

disease (based on population-based cohort studies), and approximately 1 in 6 of these patients will experience a clinical response to these agents within a month. Once corticosteroids are initiated, a 1-year prolonged response is seen in 49%, corticosteroid dependence in 22%, and 29% required a colectomy.[15] It should be stressed that this is representative of what transpired prior to the era of biologic use. Corticosteroids are efficacious for induction of remission in patients with mild, moderate, or severe colitis, regardless of disease distribution.[16] The original study by Truelove and Witts[2] in 1955 reported a remission rate of 40% for patients treated with oral cortisone (100 mg per day for 6 weeks of therapy). In that study, 75% of patients with mild disease achieved remission compared with 31% of patients with severe colitis. Subsequent studies have evaluated the optimal dose, duration of therapy, and route of administration for corticosteroids. One study demonstrated that treatment with 40 to 80 mg per day of oral prednisone achieved remission rates of 84% in mild disease, 80% in moderate disease, and 47% in severe disease.[17] A dose response has been documented for prednisone 20 to 60 mg daily; however, the modest benefits of higher doses are offset by increased steroid-related side effects. The use of higher doses of corticosteroids is associated with a substantial increase in the risk for side effects without appreciable clinical benefits.[16,18]

Corticosteroids are used to induce remission in patients with moderate to severe ulcerative colitis initially or in those patients who are intolerant of or fail mesalamine. A dose of prednisone 40 to 60 mg per day should be maintained until symptoms resolve (this historically requires 1 to 3 weeks). Most clinicians use once-a-day dosing; however, some physicians advocate "split dosing" 3 to 4 times a day. Note that this approach may be helpful in patients who remain symptomatic after a trial of once-daily dosing, especially if they are bothered by nocturnal bowel movements. This suggestion has yet to be validated or studied in a randomized, controlled study. This level of therapy may take up to 2 weeks or more for symptoms to resolve. At this time, when remission has been achieved, corticosteroids should be gradually tapered. Once the decision is made to start oral corticosteroid therapy for the treatment of UC, no appropriate rationale exists for starting corticosteroids at a lower dose to prevent steroid side effects. This approach to treatment leads to inadequate clinical response and overall longer duration of steroid therapy. Likewise, premature tapering of steroids before complete response is achieved will most likely lead to rapid relapse of symptoms.[19] In general, the rate of corticosteroid tapering is the equivalent of 5 mg of prednisone weekly until cessation of corticosteroids, although some advocate a slower rate of taper at 2.5 mg weekly at lower doses such as 20 mg of prednisone.

Patients who fail to respond adequately to oral prednisone (or other oral formulations at equivalent doses) should be hospitalized and given IV corticosteroids in the form of methylprednisolone (48 to 60 mg prednisolone daily) or hydrocortisone (300 to 400 mg of hydrocortisone daily) as a continuous infusion for 7 to 10 days. A response should be observed within 3 days. Otherwise, alternate therapies should be considered for this patient cohort. When using doses of 300 to 400 mg of hydrocortisone daily, most patients respond within 5 days. A recent study suggested that after 3 days of such intensive IV treatment, 85% of patients with persistent frequent stools (>8 per day) or raised CRP (>40 mg/d) will eventually need a colectomy.[16] Another option for consideration is the use of infliximab. Recent data presented in the ACT 1 and 2 trials demonstrated the efficacy of infliximab for patients with moderate to severe ulcerative colitis.[20,21] This was confirmed by Jarnerot et al, who showed that infliximab is an effective and safe rescue therapy in patients experiencing an acute severe or moderately severe attack of ulcerative colitis not responding to conventional treatment, including corticosteroids.[22] As of this point in time, there have been no comparative trials (either noninferiority or superiority in design) performed that were adequately powered and randomized and that compared infliximab and corticosteroids for treatment of UC. IV adrenocorticotropic hormone (ACTH) may be more effective than methylprednisolone for UC patients who have not received prior corticosteroid treatment.[25]

Forty-eight to 80% of patients will respond to this IV regimen. Most practitioners will treat severe UC for 7 to 10 days with IV corticosteroids before moving on to other medical therapy (infliximab or cyclosporine A usually in combination with 6-MP or AZA) or surgery.

Corticosteroids have not been demonstrated to be effective agents for maintenance of remission in UC.[23,24] Once remission is achieved with corticosteroids, maintenance must be continued with immunomodulators (such as AZA or 6-MP) or infliximab. Mesalamine derivatives have been demonstrated to be effective for induction and maintenance of remission of patients with UC who have not been recently treated with corticosteroids. There have not yet been trials performed that evaluated the efficacy of mesalamine derivatives in patients who have been recently treated with corticosteroids. (In other words, a patient is more likely to stay in remission once tapered off steroids when using mesalamine compared to a patient not receiving mesalamine.) Recently, it has been demonstrated that infliximab is effective to induce and maintain remission in patients with UC.[20,21] It is important to make a distinction between steroid dependence and the concept of maintenance benefit. Maintenance therapies illustrate a dose response in a population of patients, as compared to steroid dependence, which focuses on an individual patient who is unable to wean below a specific dose prior to flaring (Table 16-2).

TABLE 16-2

INDICATIONS FOR CORTICOSTEROID USE IN ULCERATIVE COLITIS

- Acute treatment of moderate disease (oral corticosteroids)
- Acute treatment of severe disease (IV corticosteroids)
- Acute treatment of proctitis and proctosigmoiditis (topical corticosteroids)
- No role for maintenance of remission with corticosteroid therapy

NONSYSTEMIC CORTICOSTEROIDS

Because conventional systemic corticosteroids have the potential to cause serious side effects, a formulation of corticosteroid that preserves the benefits of steroids and yet minimizes their adverse effects is desirable.

Budesonide is a topically active glucocorticoid that is structurally related to 16-hydroxy-prednisolone.[25] Budesonide has a very high affinity for corticosteroid receptors (15 times that of prednisolone and 195 times that of hydrocortisone).[26] The majority of the drug is converted by the cytochrome P450 system in the liver to inactive metabolites, and only 10% to 15% of the drug reaches the systemic circulation.[27] This results in similar therapeutic efficacy as systemic corticosteroids, but only about 30% of adverse effects are noted. Budesonide was initially used for the treatment of asthma and allergic rhinitis,[28] but in the last few years has been available for the treatment of IBD in the United States. The current preparation of budesonide (Entocort) is formulated to allow the slow release of the drug, mainly in the ileum, cecum, and ascending colon. The capsule of budesonide consists of 1-mm acid-stable microcapsules. The microcapsules are composed of an inner sugar core surrounded by budesonide in ethyl cellulose and an outer acrylic-based resin coating (Eudragit-L) that dissolves at a pH of 5.5 or higher. Fifty to 70% of the controlled ileal release (CIR) budesonide formulation is absorbed in the ileocolonic region with a mean absorption time of 6.4 hours and a systemic bioavailability of 9% in healthy volunteers.[27] A single placebo-controlled trial has evaluated the efficacy of enteric-coated budesonide in UC. This trial has demonstrated that budesonide was no more effective than placebo when assessing patients with distal UC.[29] In another trial, budesonide enemas were compared to prednisolone enemas. Budesonide enema (2 mg administered for 8 weeks) controlled active distal UC in a similar percentage of patients as the prednisolone enema (36% versus 47%) with fewer corticosteroid side effects (Table 16-3).[30]

Budesonide does not have a role in maintenance of remission in UC. The role of budesonide in the treatment of UC is still uncertain.

Topical administration of corticosteroids is an effective modality of treatment for distal ulcerative colitis.[31,32] Although it has been perceived to be an effective therapy as an adjuvant treatment for pancolitis, its role as such has never been formally tested in a controlled fashion. Preparations are available in the form of suppositories, foams, or enemas. Suppositories are useful for the treatment of proctitis, while enemas and foams are useful for more extensive left-sided disease. Radionucleotide scintigraphy studies have demonstrated enema tracer spread to the splenic flexure. Foams are very useful in patients with severe urgency and tenesmus, and many patients prefer foam preparations to enemas due to the ease of administration and ability for retention. In several studies evaluating the efficacy of corticosteroid enemas, 60% of patients with distal colitis treated with topical hydrocortisone (80 to 100 mg), prednisolone (20 to 49 mg), or betamethasone (5 to 20 mg) showed an improvement.[33,34] Although topically applied corticosteroids have less systemic absorption, and therefore, fewer side effects than oral steroids, plasma concentrations can be such that suppression of the pituitary-adrenal-hypothalamic pathway does occur.

TABLE 16-3

STUDIES EVALUATING EFFICACY OF BUDESONIDE FOR TREATMENT OF ULCERATIVE COLITIS

Reference	Title	No. of Patients	Type of Study	Results
Hanauer et al[30]	Budesonide enema for the treatment of active, distal UC and proctitis: dose ranging study	233	Randomized, double-blind, multicenter	Budesonide enema is both effective and safe for the treatment of active distal UC 2 mg/100 mL is the lowest effective dose
Lofberg et al[31]	Oral budesonide versus prednisolone in patients with active extensive and left-sided UC	72	Randomized, double-blind, controlled	Oral budesonide seems to give an overall treatment result in active UC approaching that of prednisolone without suppression of plasma cortisol levels
Lindgren et al	Effect of budesonide enema on remission and relapse rate in distal UC and proctitis	149	Dose ranging, controlled, double-blind, multicenter with 2 parallel groups	Budesonide enema 2 mg once daily appears to be the optimal dosage in active distal UC Twice-weekly dosing did not maintain remission

CORTICOSTEROID DEPENDENCE AND RESISTANCE

Although corticosteroids can lead to dramatic success in achieving clinical remission, a large proportion of patients experience recurrent symptoms while the corticosteroid dose is being reduced or shortly after corticosteroids are withdrawn. In a population-based study of 109 patients, corticosteroid dependence (ie, relapse within 30 days after prednisolone treatment had finished or relapse at reduction impeding the discontinuation of prednisolone therapy at 1 year) was seen in 36% of patients at 1 year.[35] There seems to be a clinical pattern associated with corticosteroid dependence. Corticosteroid-dependent patients tend to be younger and more frequently smokers.[36]

Patients vary widely with respect to their response to corticosteroid therapy and the development of side effects. Some patients are hypersensitive to corticosteroids, such that a low dose of corticosteroids can lead to severe side effects, while others do not experience any clinical response or side effects to high doses during long-term therapy. In severe UC, 44% of patients do not respond to 5 to 7 days of hydrocortisone (100 mg IV every 6 hours) plus rectal hydrocortisone (100 mg bid). Similar findings have been reported in other inflammatory diseases, such as rheumatoid arthritis and systemic lupus erythematosus. This will suggest a common underlying mechanism. Generalized resistance and tissue-specific corticosteroid resistance are increasingly recognized to be responsible for these variable corticosteroid responses.[36,37] The mechanism of corticosteroid resistance is not yet entirely clear, but the 2 possibilities commonly described are either true resistance to corticosteroids or decreased bioavailability (Table 16-4).

ADVERSE EFFECTS OF CORTICOSTEROIDS

The widespread use of corticosteroids in UC is associated with an increased incidence of adverse effects that may involve the gastrointestinal system, the metabolic system, neuropsychiatric well-being, musculoskeletal system, endocrine system, the skin, eyes, cardiovascular system, and increased infection (Table 16-5).

The adverse effects of corticosteroids vary depending on many factors including route of administration, duration and dosage of therapy, gender, and individual sensitivity to corticosteroids. Short-term therapy may result in

TABLE 16-4

PROPOSED BIOLOGICAL MECHANISMS OF CORTICOSTEROID RESISTANCE

	Mechanisms	Effect
Receptor or postreceptor pathways	Cytokine-mediated inhibition of corticosteroid receptor (CR) ligand binding or the subsequent transcriptional regulation	Decreased T cell response to corticosteroids (eg, IL-2, IL-4)
	Cytokine-mediated inhibition or activation of NF-κB activity	Increased T cell response to corticosteroids (eg, IL-10)
		Decreased T cell response to corticosteroids (eg, TNFα)
	Polymorphisms in the CR gene	Impaired binding of corticosteroids to CRs
Prereceptor pathways	Increased binding capacity of serum albumin to corticosteroids	Decreased availability of corticosteroids to CRs
	Constitutive high multi-drug resistance gene expression in the peripheral lymphocytes and intestinal mucosal cells, resulting in efflux of intracellular corticosteroids	Decreased intracellular availability of corticosteroids to CRs

TABLE 16-5

POTENTIAL ADVERSE EFFECTS ASSOCIATED WITH SYSTEMIC CORTICOSTEROID THERAPY

Cutaneous

Atrophy

Striae

Vascular effects, purpura

Hair changes

Pigmentary changes

Acne, acneiform eruptions

Infections

Easy bruising

Cardiovascular

Hypertension

Edema

Atherosclerosis

Gastrointestinal

Nausea, vomiting

Peptic ulcer disease (with NSAIDs)

Intestinal perforation

Pancreatitis

Esophagitis

Gynecological/Obstetrical

Amenorrhea

Fetal effects

Neuropsychiatric

Psychosis

Peripheral neuropathy

Pseudo tumor cerebri

Depression/mood disorders

Impaired cognitive functions

Seizures

Metabolic

Hyperglycemia

Hyperlipidemia

continued

TABLE 16-5 (CONTINUED)

POTENTIAL ADVERSE EFFECTS ASSOCIATED WITH SYSTEMIC CORTICOSTEROID THERAPY

Obesity	Impaired fibroplasia
Hypocalcemia	Decreased mitotic rate
Hypokalemic alkalosis	**OPHTHALMOLOGIC**
Buffalo hump	Cataracts
MUSCULOSKELETAL	Glaucoma
Osteoporosis	Infection
Aseptic osteonecrosis	Exophthalmos
Growth retardation	Hemorrhage
Muscle atrophy	**ENDOCRINE**
Myopathy	Hypothalamic-pituitary-adrenal axis suppression
HEMATOLOGIC	**PEDIATRIC**
Leukocytosis	Growth retardation
Lymphopenia	
Eosinopenia	
Immunosuppression	

Adapted from Nesbitt LT. Minimizing complications from systemic corticosteroid use. *Dermatol Clin.* 1995;13:925-939.

NSAID = Nonsteroidal anti-inflammatory drug

the following adverse effects: mood changes, insomnia, gastrointestinal intolerance, weakness, increased appetite, fluid retention and weight gain, increased susceptibility to infections, amenorrhea, elevated blood sugar, slow wound healing, acne, and striae.

Long-term supraphysiological doses (ie, the equivalence of 7.5 mg of prednisone daily) of corticosteroid usually lead to more serious consequences such as osteoporosis, osteonecrosis, cataracts, and hypothalamic-pituitary-adrenal axis suppression.[40] Osteoporosis is a primary musculoskeletal complication of chronic corticosteroid therapy. Patients with IBD have an increased prevalence of reduced bone mineral density (BMD) relative to healthy controls.[41] Osteoporosis is present in 30% to 45% of patients in some series of patients with Crohn's disease, and its rate is somewhat lower in patients with ulcerative colitis.[42] The pathophysiology of osteopenia in UC is unclear, but is likely multifactorial. The inflammatory process itself in IBD, through the release of cytokines such as IL-1, TNFα, IL-6, and colony-stimulating factors, can lead to low BMD.[43] Clinical studies have demonstrated that UC patients who have never received corticosteroids are also at increased risk of developing reduced BMD. IL-6 has been found to enhance the differentiation of osteocytes to osteoclasts. IL-1 and TNFα stimulate the osteoclasts in the bone, resulting in excessive resorption.[44] Other proposed etiologies of osteopenia in IBD include relative immobility due to disease flare and impaired absorption of vitamin D, calcium, and other nutrients in the small bowel. Furthermore, in contrast to patients with osteoporosis resulting from the postmenopausal state, corticosteroid use affects trabecular bone to a greater extent than cortical bone. It has been well-demonstrated that patients with IBD have a significantly higher prevalence of reduced bone density in the hips (cortical bones) than in vertebrae (trabecular bones). These observations support the notion that factors other than corticosteroid use are important in the pathogenesis of osteoporosis in IBD.

Osteoporosis occurs more commonly in patients with IBD than the general population, but the relative importance of corticosteroid use versus underlying chronic inflammation as risk factors remains controversial. In a population-based study of 273 UC patients, Loftus et al[47] showed that the use of corticosteroids did not appear to significantly influence the risk of osteoporotic fractures. Despite the uncertainty as to how much corticosteroids contribute to the development of osteoporosis in IBD, we know that long-term supraphysiological corticosteroid therapy use alone is one of the most common causes of osteoporosis. In addition, van Staa et al[48] showed that average daily doses of 2.5 to 7.5 mg and more than 7.5 mg of prednisone daily result in relative fracture risks of 1.77 and 2.27, respectively, compared to controls. This deleterious effect is not reduced by alternate-day doses.[49] It has been demonstrated by Bernstein et al[50] that individuals with IBD have a 40% increase in fracture risk compared to individuals in the general population (incidence rate ratio = 1.41, confidence interval [CI] 1.27 to 1.56, $P<0.001$). Corticosteroid-associated bone loss is both dose and duration dependent. The greatest damage usually occurs during the first few weeks to months of therapy, underscoring the importance of prompt preventive measures.[50,51] The pathogenesis of osteoporosis secondary to corticosteroids has been studied extensively. Corticosteroids inhibit absorption of calcium in the intestine and promote excretion of calcium in the kidneys, which may result in secondary hyperparathyroidism.[51] This stimulates bone resorption by osteoclasts. In women, corticosteroids suppress circulating estrogen (by reducing follicle-stimulating hormone-induced estrogen production), thus reducing its role in inhibiting IL-6, a stimulator of osteoclastic activity. In men, corticosteroid use reduces blood testosterone concentrations. Furthermore, recent evidence in human and animal models suggests that corticosteroids lead to defective osteoblastogenesis, osteoblast apoptosis, and osteocyte apoptosis. The defective osteoblast production and premature death of the osteoblasts contribute to the incomplete repair and resorption of cavities and loss of bone. The enhanced apoptosis of osteocytes and possibly corticosteroid-induced inhibition of angiogenesis could contribute to osteonecrosis.[52] Corticosteroids tend to cause more demineralization in trabecular bones than cortical bones because of a higher turnover rate. Symptoms of osteoporosis include bone pain, spontaneous fracture, and vertebral collapse. Many patients will experience no symptoms early on, despite progressive damage to the bone.

Corticosteroid-induced myopathy is an uncommon complication. The pathogenesis of this condition is not known. Corticosteroid-induced myopathy can occur with any corticosteroid preparation. Patients with corticosteroid-induced myopathy present with insidious onset of proximal muscle weakness and muscle wasting. Myalgia or muscle tenderness is absent. Lower extremity weakness usually occurs first and is most severe.[53,54] There are no consistent relations with age and gender. However, corticosteroid-induced myopathy is rare with use of corticosteroid doses of less than 10 mg/d of prednisone or its equivalent, and higher doses of corticosteroid tend to cause more rapid onset of weakness.[53] Establishing the diagnosis of corticosteroid-induced myopathy is difficult. Creatine phosphokinase and electromyography are usually normal, but they are useful in excluding other causes of myopathy. In animal and human studies, muscle biopsy may show nonspecific atrophy in type IIb-fast twitch fiber without signs of necrosis or inflammation.[55] Certain clinical features can help to make the diagnosis. The onset of weakness follows initiation of or increase in corticosteroid therapy. Other features of Cushing's syndrome may be present. Furthermore, a useful test is to observe the muscle strength after decreasing or stopping the corticosteroid therapy. Weakness due to steroid myopathy will begin to improve 3 to 4 weeks after a sufficient dose alteration.[56]

Growth retardation is a major concern in children on long-term corticosteroid therapy. The mechanism is thought to be impaired collagen synthesis, compromised growth hormone effect, inhibited epiphyseal maturation, and retarded long bone growth. Adolescents receiving chronic corticosteroid therapy may not achieve expected height. Alternate-day or low-dose daily therapy may minimize the growth retardation.[57]

The risk of infection is increased among patients on chronic corticosteroids. In a study pooling data from 71 controlled clinical trials, Stuck et al[58] showed that the risk of infection is not increased with a daily dose of less than 10 mg. However, for doses greater than 10 mg daily, the overall rate of lethal and nonlethal infectious complications was 12.7% in the corticosteroid-treated patients and 8% in the controls ($P<0.001$). A study of 159 patients by Aberra et al showed that preoperative use of corticosteroids in patients with IBD who are undergoing elective bowel surgery is associated with an increase risk of postoperative infectious complications. Patients receiving corticosteroids had an adjusted OR for any major infectious complications of 3.69 (95% CI 1.24 to 10.97) and 5.54 (95% CI 1.12 to 27.26), respectively.[59]

Hypothalamic-pituitary-adrenal axis suppression is related to both dose and duration of therapy.[59] Suppression usually occurs at doses above physiological levels for 4 weeks or longer.[59,60] Schlaghecke et al[61] evaluated 279 patients on chronic corticosteroid therapy and 50 normal subjects using a corticotropin-releasing hormone stimulation test. Among corticosteroid-treated patients, 15% had no response, 48% had blunted responses, and 37% had normal responses. After long-term supraphysiological corticosteroid therapy, ACTH levels may not normalize for several months, and cortisol levels may not return to normal after 6 to 12 months.[62] Risk of Addisonian crises during surgery or infection may last for even 1 year after the discontinuation of long-term corticosteroid therapy.[62] Uncontrolled studies suggest that hypothalamic-pituitary-adrenal axis suppression may be minimized by single morning doses and by alternate-day dosing.[40,60]

A number of cutaneous side effects can occur in patients on corticosteroids. Telangiectasia, striae, and purpura are common.[38] Hirsutism and increased vellus hair may occur. Corticosteroid-associated acneiform eruptions are common and usually present on the back and chest. In addition, patients on chronic corticosteroids are more susceptible to bacterial and fungal infection of the skin.[38]

A host of metabolic derangements can occur with corticosteroids. Hyperglycemia occurs 4 times more often in patients on corticosteroids than controls.[62] Weight gain is a common result of therapy with corticosteroids and is related to both increased appetite and fluid retention. After 2 months of corticosteroid therapy, 10% to 15% of patients developed edema and increased facial fat. Other metabolic changes associated with corticosteroid therapy include hyperlipidemia, hypokalemia, and hypocalcemia.[62,63]

Corticosteroid use has been associated with an increase in blood pressure through their effect on sodium retention and by vasoconstriction. In a meta-analysis pooling data from 93 double-blind, randomized control trials,[64] Conn and Poynard studied more than 8700 patients who had been randomized to receive mean daily doses of 35 mg of prednisone or its equivalent for a mean duration of 64 days. Corticosteroid-treated patients were 4 to 5 times more likely than controls to develop hypertension. In a study on elderly Crohn's patients,[65] the relative risk for hypertension in corticosteroid-treated patients was 1.46. However, with lower doses, the relationship between hypertension and corticosteroid therapy is not as clear. Jackson et al evaluated the changes in blood pressure in 129 patients with asthma and in 66 patients with rheumatoid arthritis.[66] When adjusted for age, the mean daily prednisone doses of 6.7 and 8.4 mg in asthma and rheumatoid arthritis groups, respectively, were not associated with the development of hypertension. The blood pressure effect from corticosteroids usually occurs after the first 2 weeks of therapy.[59]

A variety of neuropsychiatric disorders are associated with corticosteroid therapy, including hypomania; irritability; insomnia; restlessness; fatigue; impaired memory, concentration, and attention; depression; and overt psychosis.[67] Corticosteroid-associated psychosis appears to occur more often with higher corticosteroid doses, and with some variation, its onset is usually early in the therapy. Mood and personality changes, headache, and insomnia are common dose-related side effects. Depression can be seen during the tapering phase of the corticosteroid therapy. Cognitive disorders can occur in association with corticosteroid-related psychosis. Impaired concentration and attention is seen in 79% of patients with corticosteroid-related neuropsychiatric changes, and intermittent memory impairment in 71%.[68] Lewis and Smith reviewed 93 cases of corticosteroid-induced syndrome and 29 corticosteroid efficacy studies in various medical illnesses and reported a 7.1% incidence of persistent memory impairment in corticosteroid treatment.[69] Possible mechanisms of corticosteroid effect on cognition may include direct binding of postsynaptic receptors, indirect genomically mediated alterations in the levels of biogenic amines and neuropeptides via the corticosteroid receptor, alterations in memory-related electrophysiological responses, and direct neurotoxicity leading to hippocampal cell loss.[67] Elderly patients are more susceptible to the development of corticosteroid-related neuropsychiatric changes.[65]

Cataracts are the most common ocular side effects of chronic corticosteroid therapy. Children are most at risk for this complication.[57] The pathogenesis of cataract formation in patients on corticosteroids is not clear. Black et al[68] demonstrated that the dosage and duration of corticosteroid therapy were directly proportional to the development of cataracts.

USE OF CORTICOSTEROIDS IN SPECIAL ULCERATIVE COLITIS SITUATIONS

Corticosteroid Use in Pregnancy

Corticosteroids may cross the placenta and can be transferred into breast milk, but the ratio of fetal to maternal serum concentrations depend on which type of corticosteroids used. Prednisolone is better metabolized compared to dexamethasone, and even then fecal serum levels are approximately 10% of maternal levels.[70] In spite of the theoretical possibility of adrenal suppression in babies born to UC patients on corticosteroids, in practice, it rarely happens.[71] If steroids must be used during pregnancy, use a formulation that is well-metabolized like prednisone or prednisolone. The same principles of use (ie, doses and duration used in non-pregnant patients) must apply in pregnant patients. Avoid using steroids in the first trimester of pregnancy if possible due to the possible side effect of cleft palate. Among patients with IBD, corticosteroid therapy has not been found to be harmful to the fetus.[72-76] In one study of 531 pregnant women,[72] 168 received corticosteroids for an extended period of time, mostly during the second and third trimesters. There was no increased incidence of spontaneous abortions, prematurity, stillbirth, or developmental defects. When necessary, corticosteroids can be used safely during pregnancy to control active UC.

Corticosteroids and Lactation

Corticosteroids are transferred to breast milk usually at concentrations of 5% to 25% of maternal serum concentrations. Such concentrations are not thought to be clinically significant, and no adverse effects have been noted. Corticosteroids are safe for breastfeeding, and mothers on steroids should be encouraged to continue breastfeeding if they so desire.[74]

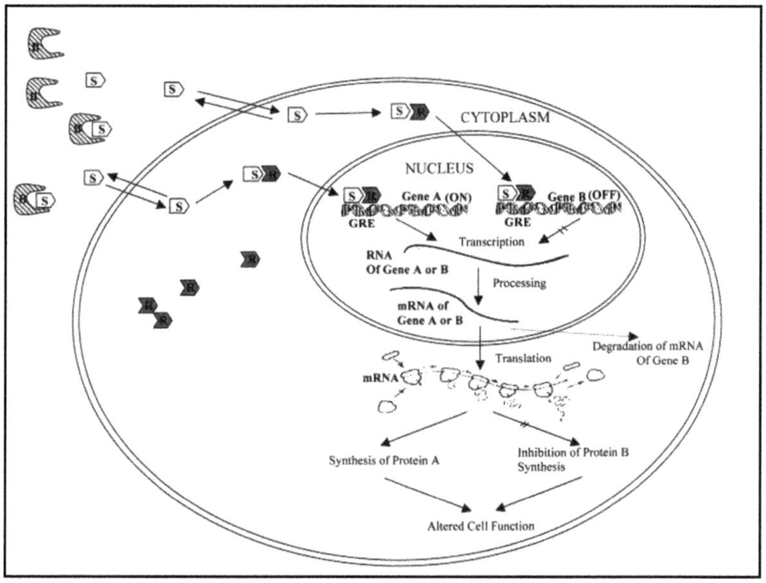

FIGURE 16-1. Schematic representation of corticosteroid action on cells of the immune system. Corticosteroid molecules (Ss) are transported to steroid binding proteins (Bs). Dissociated corticosteroid molecules cross the cell membrane freely. Once inside the cytoplasm, they bind to their receptors (Rs). The corticosteroid/receptor complexes translocate to the nucleus, where they bind to the glucocorticoid response elements (GREs) in the promoter region of steroid-responsive target genes, either promoting (ON) or suppressing (OFF) the transcription of a particular gene. Altered cellular function results from the combination of increased production of certain proteins and decreased production of others. (Adapted from Boumpas DT, Paliogianni F, Anastassiou ED. Glucocorticoids action on the immune system: Molecular and cellular aspects. *Clin Ex Rheum.* 1991;9:414-423.)

CONCLUSION

Oral and parenteral corticosteroids are effective for the treatment of moderate to severe active ulcerative colitis regardless of disease distribution to induce remission. Once the decision is made to use corticosteroids, high doses (the equivalent of 40 to 60 mg of prednisone daily) should be used, and the dose must be maintained at this high level until the patient's symptoms resolve. The corticosteroid dose is then tapered gradually. Corticosteroids have no role in the maintenance of remission. Topical corticosteroids in liquid and foam formulation are effective as short-term therapy for active distal UC when assessed in a controlled fashion. Not all patients respond to corticosteroid therapy (ie, steroid resistance), and some patients who respond are either unable to taper off medication or relapse shortly after the discontinuation of corticosteroids (ie, steroid dependence). Population studies suggest that about 50% of UC patients will never require corticosteroid therapy. Of UC patients treated with corticosteroids, 54% achieve remission, 30% obtain partial response, and 16% do not respond. After 1 year of treatment with corticosteroids, prolonged response can be expected in 44% of patients, corticosteroid dependence in 22%, and colectomy in 29%.[15]

For UC patients, no other class of drug acts as rapidly and consistently as corticosteroids do to control disease activity and alleviate symptoms and promote endoscopic and histologic improvement. Unfortunately, no other group of medicines produces such varied and difficult-to-manage adverse effects as corticosteroids.

Attention to appropriate patient selection, timing and duration of treatment, as well as dose and formulation will maximize the benefit of corticosteroids and minimize adverse effects in patients with ulcerative colitis. Corticosteroids have an important role in the treatment of ulcerative colitis if appropriate use and limitations are recognized.

REFERENCES

1. Fiocchi C. Inflammatory bowel disease: Etiology and pathogenesis. *Gastroenterology.* 1998;115:182-205.
2. Truelove SC, Witts LF. Cortisone in ulcerative colitis: final report on a therapeutic trial. *BMJ.* 1955;2:1041-1048.
3. Kornbluth A, Sachar DB. Ulcerative colitis: practice guidelines in adults. *Am J Gastroenterol.* 1997;92:204-211.
4. Sands BE. Therapy of inflammatory bowel disease. *Gastroenterology.* 2000;118:568-582.
5. Boumpas DT, Paliogianni F, Anastassiou ED. Glucocorticoids action on the immune system: molecular and cellular aspects. *Clin Ex Rheum.* 1991;9:414-423.
6. Barnes PT, Adcock I. Anti-inflammatory action of steroids: molecular mechanism. *Trends Pharmacol Sci.* 1993;14:436-441.

7. Schneiber S, Nikolaus S, Hampe J. Activation of nuclear factor kappa B in inflammatory bowel disease. *Gut.* 1998;42:477-487.
8. Van der Burg B, Liden J, Okert A, et al. Nuclear factor kb repression in anti-inflammatory and immune suppression by glucocorticoids. *Trends Endocrinol Metab.* 1997;8:152-157.
9. Van der Stolpe A, Caldenhoun E, et al. Glucocorticoid-mediated repression of intercellular adhesion molecule-1 expression in human monocytic and bronchial epithelial cell lines. *Amer J Resp Cell Mol Biol.* 1993;8:340-347.
10. Schreiber AD, Parsons J, McDermott P, et al. Effect of corticosteroids on the human monocyte, IgG and complement receptors. *J Clin Invest.* 1975;56:1184-1197.
11. Pitzalis C, Kingsley G, Panayi G. Adhesion molecules in rheumatoid arthritis: Role in the pathogenesis and prospects for therapy. *Ann Rheum Dis.* 1994;53:287-288.
12. Van Ierssel AJ, Mieremet-Ooms, Van der Zon JM, et al. Suppression of intestinal natural killer cell by corticosteroids. *Aliment Pharm Ther.* 1997;11;347-353.
13. Carnuccio R, Di Rosa M, Guerrasteo B, et al. Vasocortin: a novel glucocorticoid-induced anti-inflammatory protein. *Br J Pharmacol.* 1987;90:443-445.
14. Hanauer SB. Inflammatory bowel disease. *N Engl J Med.* 1996;334:841-848.
15. Faubion WA, Loftus EV, Harmsen WS, Zinmeister AR, Sandborn WJ. The natural history of corticosteroid therapy for inflammatory bowel disease: a population-based study. *Gastroenterology.* 2001;121:255-260.
16. Travis SPL, Farrant JM, Ricketts C, et al. Predicting outcome in severe ulcerative colitis. *Gut.* 1996;38:905-910.
17. Kjeidsen J. Treatment of ulcerative colitis with high doses of oral prednisone: the rate of remission, the need for surgery and the effect of prolonged treatment. *Scand J Gastroenterol.* 1993;28:821-826.
18. Baron T, Connell A, Kanagham T, et al. Outpatient treatment of ulcerative colitis. Comparison between three doses of oral prednisone. *BMJ.* 1962;2:441-443.
19. Hanauer SB. Medical therapy for ulcerative colitis. In: Kirsner JB, et al. *Inflammatory Bowel Disease.* 5th ed. Philadelphia, PA: WB Saunders Co; 2000:529-556.
20. Rutgeerts P, Feagan BG, Olson A, et al. A randomized placebo-controlled trial of infliximab therapy for active ulcerative colitis: Act I trial. *Gastroenterology.* 2005;128:A105.
21. Sandborn WJ, Rahmilewitz D, Hanauer SB, et al. Infliximab induction and maintenance therapy for ulcerative colitis: act II trial. *Gastroenterology.* 2005;128:A104.
22. Jarnerot G, Hertervig E, Friis-Liby I, Blomquist L, et al. Infliximab as rescue therapy in severe to moderately severe ulcerative colitis: a randomized, placebo-controlled study. *Gastroenterology.* 2005;128:1805-1811.
23. Hawthorne AB, Travis SPL, and the BSG Inflammatory Bowel Disease Clinical Trial Network. Outcomes of important management of severe ulcerative colitis. *Gut.* 2002;50:A16.
24. Lennard-Jones JE, Shivananda S, the EC-IBD Study Group. Clinical uniformity of inflammatory bowel disease at presentation and during the first year of disease in north and south Europe. *Eur J Gastroenterol Hepatol.* 1997;9:353-359.
25. Lichtiger S, Present DH, Kornbluth A, et al. Cyclosporine in severe ulcerative colitis refractory to steroid therapy. *N Engl J Med.* 1994;330:1841-1845.
26. Brattsand R. Overview of newer glucocorticosteroid preparation for inflammatory bowel disease. *Can J Gastroenterol.* 1990;4:407-414.
27. Dahlberg E, Thalen A, Brattsand R, et al. Correlation between chemical structure, receptor binding and biological activity of some novel, highly active 16∞ 17∞ acetal-substituted glucocorticoid. *Mol Pharmacol.* 1984;25:70-78.
28. Edsbacker S, Wollmer P, Nilsson A, et al. Pharmacokinetics and gastrointestinal transit of budesonide controlled ileal release (CIR) capsule. *Gastroenterology.* 1993;104(Suppl):A695.
29. Brogden RN, McTavish D. Budesonide. An updated review of its pharmacological properties and therapeutic efficacy in asthma and rhinitis. *Drugs.* 1992;44:373-407.
30. Hanuaer SB, Robinson M, Pruitt R, et al. Budesonide enema for the treatment of active, distal ulcerative colitis and proctitis: a dose ranging study. US Budesonide Enema Study Group. *Gastroenterology.* 1998;115(3):58-64.
31. Lofberg R, Danielsson A, Schr O, et al. Oral budesonide versus prednisolone in patients with active extensive and left sided ulcerative colitis. *Gastroenterology.* 1996;110:1713-1718.
32. Lofberg R, Ostergaard Thomson O, Langholz E, et al. Budesonide versus prednisolone enemas in active distal ulcerative colitis. *Aliment Pharmacol Ther.* 1994;8:623-629.
33. Marshal J, Irvine E. Rectal corticosteroid versus alternative treatment for ulcerative colitis—A meta analysis. *Gut.* 1997;40:775-781.
34. Marshall JK, Irvine EJ, Steinhart AH, Thabane M. Rectal corticosteroids for induction in ulcerative colitis. *Cochrane Database. Proctocols.* 2003;Issue 1.
35. Marshall JK, Irvine EJ, Steinhart AH, Thabane M. Rectal corticosteroids for maintenance of remission in ulcerative colitis. *Cochrane Data Review. Protocols.* 2003;Issue 1.
36. Mulder CT, Tytgat GN. Review article. Topical corticosteroids in inflammatory bowel disease. *Aliment Pharmacol Ther.* 1993;7:125-130.
37. Munkholm P, Langholz E, Davidson M. Frequency of glucocorticoid resistance and dependency in CD. *Gut.* 1994;35:360-362.
38. Franchimort DP, Louis E, et al. Clinical pattern of corticosteroid dependent CD. *Eur J Gastroenterol Hepatol.* 1998;10:821-825.
39. Barnes PT, Greening AP, Crompton GK. Glucocorticoid resistance in asthma. *Am J Respir Crit Care Med.* 1995;152:S124-S140.
40. Leung DY, Hamid Q, Vottero A, et al. Association of glucocorticoid insensitivity with increased expression of glucocorticoid receptor beta. *J Exp Med.* 1997;186:1567-1574.
41. Farrell RJ, Murphy A, Long A, et al. High multidrug resistance (P-glycoprotein 170) expression in inflammatory bowel disease patients who fail medical therapy. *Gastroenterology.* 2000;118:279-288.
42. Nesbitt LT. Minimizing complications from systemic corticosteroid use. *Dermatol Clin.* 1995;13:925-939.
43. Compston JE, Judd D, Crawley EO, et al. Osteoporosis in patients with inflammatory bowel disease. *Gut.* 1987;28:410-415.
44. Fromm H. Consequences of reduced absorption. In: Scholmeric J, Krius W, Goebell H, et al. *Inflammatory Bowel Disease, Pathophysiology as the Basis of Treatment. Falk Symposium 67.* Dordrecht, The Netherlands: Kluver; 1993:231-239.
45. Fries W, Giacomin D, Plebani M, Martin A. Effect of experimental colitis on bone metabolism in the rat. *Digestion.* 1994;55:229-233.
46. Manoglas SC, Jilka RL. Bone marrow, cytokines, and bone remodeling: emerging insight into the pathophysiology of osteoporosis. *N Engl J Med.* 1995;332:305-311.
47. Loftus EV Jr, Achenbach SJ, Sandborn WJ, Tremaine WJ, Oberg AL, Melton LJ. Risk of fracture in ulcerative colitis: a population based study from Olmsted County, Minnesota. *Clin Gastroenterol Hepatol.* 2000;1(6):465-473.
48. van Staa TP, Leufkens HG, Abenhaim L, et al. Use of corticosteroids in the United Kingdom. *QJM.* 2000;93:105-111.
49. Gluck OS, Murphy WA, Hahm TJ, Hahm B. Bone loss in adults receiving alternate day glucocorticoid therapy: a comparison with daily therapy. *Arthritis Rheum.* 1981;24:892-898.

50. Bernstein CN, Blanchard JF, Leslie W, et al. The incidence of fractures among patients with inflammatory bowel disease: a population-based cohort study. *Ann Intern Med.* 2000;133:795-799.
51. LoCascio V, Bonucci E, Imbimbo B, et al. Bone loss in response to long term glucocorticoid therapy. *Bone Miner.* 1990;8:39-51.
52. Valentine JF, Sninsky CA. Prevention and treatment of osteoporosis in patients with inflammatory bowel disease. *Am J Gastroenterol.* 1999;94:878-883.
53. Weinstein RS, Jilka RL, Parfitt AM, Manoglagas SC. Inhibition of osteoblastogenesis and promotion of apoptosis of osteoblasts and osteocytes by glucocorticoids: potential mechanisms of their deleterious effects on bone. *J Clin Invest.* 1998;102:274-282.
54. Bowyer SL, LaMothe MP, Hollister JR. Steroid myopathy: Incidence and detection in a population with asthma. *J Allergy Clin Immunol.* 1985;76:234-242.
55. Decramer M, Stas KJ. Corticosteroid-induced myopathy involving respiratory muscles in patients with chronic obstructive pulmonary disease or asthma. *Am Rev Respir Dis.* 1992;146:800-802.
56. Wilcox PG, Hards JM, Bockhold K, et al. Pathologic changes and contractile properties of the diaphragm in corticosteroid myopathy in hamsters. *Am J Respir Cell Mol Biol.* 1989;1:191-199.
57. Askari A, Vignos PJ, Moskowitz RW. Steroid myopathy in connective tissue disease. *Am J Med.* 1976;61:485-492.
58. Stuck AE, Minder CE, Frey FJ. Risk of infectious complication in patients taking corticosteroids. *Rev Infect Dis.* 1989;11(6):954-963.
59. Lucky AW. Principles of the use of glucocorticoids in the growing child. *Pediatr Dermatol.* 1984;1:226-235.
60. Aberra FN, Lewis JD, Hass D, Rombeau JL, Osborne B, Lichtenstein GR. Corticosteroids and immunomodulators: postoperative infectious complication risk in inflammatory bowel disease patients. *Gastroenterology.* 2003;125:610-612.
61. Schurmeyer TH, Tsokos GC, Avgerinos PC, et al. Pituitary adrenal responsiveness to corticotrophin releasing hormone in patients receiving chronic, alternate day clucocorticoid therapy. *J Clin Endocrinol Metab.* 1985;61:22-27.
62. Schlaghecke K, Kornely E, Santen RT, Ridderskamp P. The effect of long term glucocorticoid therapy on pituitary adrenal responses to exogenous corticotrophin releasing hormone. *N Engl J Med.* 1992;326:226-230.
63. Axelod L. Side effects of glucocorticoid therapy. In: Schleimer RP, Claman HN, Oronsky A, eds. *Anti-inflammatory Steroid Action: Basic and Clinical Aspects.* New York, NY: Academic Press; 1989:377-408.
64. Wolverton SE. Glucocorticoids. In: Wolverton SE, Wilkins JK, eds. *Systemic Drugs for Skin Diseases.* Philadelphia, PA: WB Saunders; 1991:87-124.
65. Conn HO, Poynard T. Corticosteroids and peptic ulcers; meta-analysis of adverse events during steroid therapy. *Intern Med.* 1994;236:619-632.
66. Jackson SH, Beeves DG, Myers K. Does long-term low dose corticosteroid therapy cause hypertension? *Clin Sci (Lond).* 1981;61 (Suppl 7);381s-383s.
67. Akerkar GA, Peppercorn MA, Hamel MB. Corticosteroid-associated complications in elderly patients. *Am J Gastroenterol.* 1997;92:461-464.
68. Wolkowitz OM, Reus VI, Canick J, et al. Glucocorticoid medication, memory and steroid psychosis in medical illness. *Ann N Y Acad Sci.* 1997;823:81-96.
69. Hall RC, Popkin MK, Stickney SK, Gardner ER. Presentation of the steroid psychosis. *Nerv Mental Dis.* 1979;167:229-236.
70. Lewis DA, Smith RE. Steroid-induced psychiatric syndromes. *Affect Disord.* 1983;5:319-332.
71. Black RL, Oglesby RB, von Sallmann L, et al. Posterior subcapsular cataracts induced by corticosteroids in patients with rheumatoid arthritis. *JAMA.* 1960;174:166-171.
72. Beitens IZ, Bayarrd F, Ances IG, Kowarski A, Migeon CJ. The transplacental passage of prednisone and prednisolone in pregnancy near term. *J Pediatr.* 1972;81:936-945.
73. Frazer FC, Sajoo A. Teratogenic potential of corticosteroids in humans. *Teratology.* 1995;51:45-46.
74. Mogadam M, Dobbins WO, Korelitz BI, Ahmed SW. Pregnancy in inflammatory bowel disease: effect of sulfasalazine and corticosteroids on fetal outcome. *Gastroenterology.* 1981;80:72-79 Abstract.
75. Willoughby CP, Truelove SC. Ulcerative colitis and pregnancy. *Gut.* 1980;21:467-474.
76. Connell W, Miller A. Treating inflammatory bowel disease during pregnancy: risks and safety of drug therapy [abstract]. [published erratum appears in *Drug Saf.* 1999;21:456] *Drug Saf.* 1999;21:311-323.

17

Topical Corticosteroid Use in Ulcerative Colitis

Seymour Katz, MD, FACP, MACG

Rectal therapy has been accepted as co-partnering with oral therapy in the management of mild to moderate ulcerative colitis. Rectal corticosteroid enemas have been used for more than 50 years, yet experience favors topical 5-ASA as the more effective therapy. Safety issues include additional risk factors with prolonged topical corticosteroid use. Newer formulations using a first-pass metabolism feature (budesonide or beclomethasone dipropionate [BDP]) are worthwhile for short-term use only. Corticosteroid foams or suppositories have a similar but lesser role than 5-ASA products. Pouchitis offers a new challenge and is responsive to (topical) rectal budesonide in a limited experience. Although not well-studied, one approach to therapy is alternating daily doses of rectal 5-ASA with a topical corticosteroid. The safety and efficacy of this approach has not yet been established.

Rectal therapy for IBD can be traced to Osler's therapy in the 19th century of a small enema of 2 oz starch with 20 drops of Laudanum (opium); if unsuccessful, then astringents such as silver nitrate in 2 to 4 pints of warm water were applied rectally in the dorsal position with hips elevated.[1] Glucocorticoid enemas were first shown to be effective 51 years ago in the United Kingdom by Truelove[2] and by Bargen[3] at the Mayo Clinic and have become a standard component of UC therapy.[4]

Rectal delivery of glucocorticoids by liquid enemas can extend to the splenic flexure[5] and occasionally more proximally.[6] Rectal foam dispenses medication to the rectum and distal descending colon,[7] whereas suppositories release their drug only locally in the rectum.[8]

This review will detail the experience with such agents, including the pharmacology of glucocorticoids given rectally as well as the topically active first-pass metabolism corticosteroids (budesonide, BDP, and prednisolone metasulphabenzoate).

The efficacy of topical delivery of therapeutic agents (5-ASA, glucocorticoids) is influenced by multiple factors including colonic motility, intraluminal pH, extent and characteristics of IBD, and the vagaries of drug dispersion. Clinical response rates can vary from 35% to 75%. Ideally, topical first-pass metabolism corticosteroids would seem the best option to avoid extensive bioavailability with resultant systemic side effects.[4,9]

Of all of the drugs listed in Table 17-1, budesonide is the most extensively studied (in enema, foam, and suppository) and serves as the paradigm of topical nonsystemic glucorticoid therapy.

Glucocorticoids

Mechanisms of Action

Glucocorticoid activity is dependent on specific glucocorticoid receptors (GR) found on chromosome 5. The GR-α isoform is the physiologically important form. GR-β does not bind glucocorticoids,[10,11] and GR-γ is a variant that may alter GR-α activity. Glucocorticoids bind to GR-α as a homodimer to specific glucocorticoid response elements (GREs), which activate gene expression. DNA

Lichtenstein GR, ed.
Ulcerative Colitis: The Complete Guide to Medical Management (pp. 191-202)

TABLE 17-1

TOPICAL SYSTEMIC CORTICOSTEROIDS

Hydrocortisone (in alcohol or as hemisuccinate sodium)
Prednisolone-21-phosphate
Betamethasone

NONSYSTEMIC STEROIDS

Prednisolone metasulfobenzoate
Tixocortol pivalate
Fluticasone propionate
Beclomethasone dipropionate
Budesonide

binding of the GR, which activates gene expression, may be repressed by monomer protein-protein interactions that are also capable of DNA binding. This GRE pathway is crucial to survival.[12] Many glucorticoid effects (eg, anti-inflammatory and immunosuppressive) require the interaction of the GR with activating protein 1 (AP-1) and NF-κB transcription factors. These transcription factors are also capable of repressing GR-dependent transcription. The overall expected effect is GR-dependent transcription and activation of lymphocytes to result in apoptosis and anti-inflammatory effects.[13]

RESISTANCE: WHY DOESN'T IT WORK

Thirty percent of patients given glucocorticoids will not enter remission and are considered steroid-resistant. If such resistance can be clearly related to IL-2 delivery, conceivably Basiliximab (which interrupts IL-2 signaling) may offer a benefit. Lymphocyte steroid resistance may be the key for glucorticoid failure in UC,[14] but this conclusion is hampered by varied lymphocyte sensitivity in normal subjects as well.[15]

The impact of steroid resistance has been detailed in studies from the Mayo Clinic and Scandinavia. Faubion et al[16] recorded a complete 30-day steroid-induced remission in 58%, partial in 26% (84% total), and a failure in 16%. One-year follow-up revealed 38% of CD patients so treated required surgery as did 24% of UC patients. Munkholm et al[17] had reported a similar steroid-induced remission at 30 days (48% complete, 38% partial, total 80%) and no response in 20%. Interestingly, the failure of steroid responsiveness was not related to the severity of disease (ie, remission rates of 48% in severe versus 35% in moderate disease) in the initial oral cortisone study.[18]

There may be a rare familial disorder of altered glucorticoid receptors resulting in mutations that encode GR.[19-21] These patients lack functional glucorticoid receptors in target organs, yet counterintuitively these patients with poor glucorticoid responses still suffer the ravages of glucorticoid adverse events. Such glucorticoid resistance appears unrelated to abnormalities in steroid absorption,[22-24] metabolism, or number of glucorticoid receptors. GR isoform variations may play a role, ie, a greater preponderance of GR-β isoforms that do not bind glucocorticoids have been found in steroid-resistant UC patients.[25] The actual concentration of GR-β is small compared to GR-α.[26] GR-γ may affect glucorticoid binding as an alternative theory of glucorticoid resistance.[27,28] Other thoughts on glucorticoid resistance include impaired binding or a reduced number of receptors available for binding of DNA, resulting in a GR-ligand complex failure to activate the appropriate genes.[29]

Glucocorticoids modulate transcription factors and cytokines. IL-4/IL-2 promote steroid resistance *in vitro*[30] and murine cell lines.[31] IL-2 reduces nuclear translocation of GR by adding a Janus Kinase (JAK) inhibitor. JAK inhibitors block IL-2 receptor signaling and restores responsiveness to glucocorticoids. STAT5 is associated with nuclear GR and, when phosphorylated by IL-2 binding, will inhibit nuclear translocations of GR. In a STAT5 knockout mouse model, IL-2 fails to induce steroid resistance.[30] IL-2 and IL-4 cytokines increase p38 mitogen-activated protein (MAP) kinase, which phosphorylates GRs associated with steroid resistance[32] and reduces antiproliferative glucorticoid activity.[30] Steroid-resistant patients usually produce more IL-2 than steroid-sensitive patients.

NF-κB regulates cytokine synthesis with a peculiar epithelial cell distribution in steroid-resistant patients, yet this is also found in lamina propria macrophages in steroid-sensitive patients.[33] The conclusion seems inescapable that lymphocyte resistance to glucocorticoids results from signaling pathways activated by IL-2. Conceivably, inhibiting IL-2 overcomes this resistance. Unfortunately, *in vitro* activated lymphocyte studies show a surprisingly low IL-2 production, which was not correlated with steroid sensitivity.

Membrane cytokine binding activates transcription factor in the receptor complex and produces inflammation. Glucocorticoids oppose this process by promoting apoptosis to lessen inflammation.[34]

Genetic factors in addition to the glucorticoid receptor disorders, at work in steroid resistance, include the multidrug resistance 1 (MDR1) gene. The MDR1 gene product, a P-glycoprotein 170 found in colonic and jejunal tissue,[35] transports glucocorticoids and reduces intracellular fluid drug and glucorticoid concentrations. High levels of P-glycoprotein 170 are protective in UC but may be down-regulated by inflammation.[36] It is uncertain if MDR1 polymorphisms relate to steroid resistance.

TABLE 17-2

MECHANISMS OF STEROID RESISTANCE

GENETIC

- GR mutations
- MDR1 gene
- HLA Class II DRB1*0103

ACQUIRED

- Abnormal steroid absorption or metabolism—*not proven*
- Altered glucocorticoid receptor concentrations—*not proven*
- Greater presence of GR-β and GR-γ isoforms—*possible*
- Lessened affinity of ligand for glucocorticoid receptors—*not proven*
- Reduced glucocorticoid receptor affinity to bind DNA—*possible*
- Altered expressions of transcription factors/cytokines —possible

Reprinted with permission from Creed TJ, Probert CSJ. Steroid resistance in inflammatory bowel disease—Mechanisms and therapeutic strategies. *Aliment Pharmacol Ther.* 2007;25:111-122.

TABLE 17-3

RECTAL HYDROCORTISONE—PHARMACOLOGY

	ULCERATIVE COLITIS	CONTROLS
Bioavailability (%)	16.4 ± 14.8	30.0 ± 15.1
C_{max}(nM)	277 ± 215	610 ± 334

With foam: bioavailability, 2%; C_{max}, 35 ng/mL

Reprinted with permission from Petitjean O, Wendling JL, Tod M, et al. Pharmacokinetics and absolute rectal bioavailability of hydrocortisone acetate in distal colitis. *Aliment Pharmacol Ther.* 1992;6:351-357.

HLA Class II allele DRB1*0103 may be a "surrogate" marker for steroid resistance because it is associated with severe disease and high risk for colectomy (Table 17-2).[37]

OTHER MECHANISMS OF ACTION

The actual benefit of glucocorticoids in controlling diarrhea in IBD may also include the significant stimulation of ATPase activity, the number of ATPase molecules, and apical 5'-nucleotidase, all of which precede the observable morphologic effect on inflammation as detected by endoscopy or histology.[38]

Rectal potential differences (PDs) as a measure of ion transport across the rectal mucosa improved after glucocorticoids (both topical and systemic therapy) as well as with 5-ASA enemas. The clinical utility and significance of this observation remains unexplored.[39]

GLUCOCORTICOID ABSORPTION FROM RECTOCOLON

Glucocorticoid receptors are present in most human cells. This widespread receptor presence may well explain the systemic glucocorticoids' adverse event history.[40] Rectal glucocorticoids are presumed to provide lesser systemic bioavailability and plasma concentration than oral glucocorticoids. Nevertheless, plasma concentrations of prednisolone given rectally have been reported as equivalent to orally administered glucocorticoids.[41,42]

The bioavailability is further reduced with foam preparations (2%) with even lower plasma peak levels (Table 17-3).[43]

Although decreased glucocorticoid receptor sites are reported in PMN leukocytes of prior steroid-treated patients, similar reduced receptor sites have been reported in glucorticoid naïve and normal control patients.[44] Topical glucocorticoids are effective, but systemic absorption does occur.[45] Rapidly metabolized budesonide was effective with maintenance of normal ACTH levels in 90% of patients at 6 weeks.[46]

NONSYSTEMIC FIRST-PASS METABOLISM GLUCOCORTICOIDS

BUDESONIDE

PHARMACOKINETICS

Budesonide is a nonhalogenated corticosteroid that has the highest known affinity for the glucocorticoid receptor, yet with a remarkably low rate of corticosteroid systemic side effects. It is a 1:1 mixture of epimers (22R)- and (22S)-, which are quickly metabolized with a half-life of 2.7 ± 0.6 hours. Budesonide's metabolism requires hydroxylation mainly by cytochrome *P*450 isoenzyme CYP3A4 found in highest concentration in the hepatocytes and intestinal epithelium[48] and is 88% protein bound. Because oral budesonide is cleared significantly in the intestinal mucosa and first pass through the liver (at a rate approaching hepatic blood flow), the resultant bioavailability borders on 10%.[49,50] When given rectally, budesonide may reach the splenic flexure[51] with a reported bioavailability up to 15%

TABLE 17-4

BUDESONIDE ENEMAS FOR ACTIVE DISTAL ULCERATIVE COLITIS[59,60,65]

	Budesonide, 2 mg (n = 20)	Placebo (n = 20)	Budesonide, 2 mg (n = 28)	Prednisolone, 31 mg (n =28)
Failure (%)	35	80*		
Plasma cortisol				
After 4 weeks (mmol/L)	446 ± 91	447 ± 89		
Complete remission (%)			52	24*
Objective improvement (%)			93	75*
ΔPlasma cortisol (mmol/L)			+11	-127

*P<0.05 versus budesonide

Reprinted with permission from Schölmerich J. Review article: systemic and topical steroids in inflammatory bowel disease. *Aliment Pharmacol Ther.* 2004;20(Suppl 4):66-74.

in proctitis or left-sided UC patients.[52] Elimination is correlated with drug exposure concentration and duration of surface contact, which will vary with inducers of CYP3A4 (eg, rifampicin, dilantin) and inhibitors (grapefruit juice, ketoconazole, etc).[53]

Topical budesonide enemas can reach the splenic flexure within 15 minutes of administration. Maximal plasma levels from absorption of this route occurred within 1 to 3 hours (1.5 ± 0.9 hours).[54] Eight-week use of European pH-released budesonide formulation (Budenofalk) resulted in identifiable drug levels in the descending colon, sigmoid, and rectal mucosa (15 to 60 ng/g) in biopsies from UC patients.[55]

Budesonide has demonstrated efficacy both orally and rectally with fewer corticosteroid side effects due to its low (systemic) bioavailability. Budesonide enema therapy at 6 weeks was significantly more effective than placebo with maintenance of normal ACTH levels.[46]

There is a predominant impression that rectal steroid use is diminishing based on the reports of successful 5-ASA therapy in 80% of UC patients.[56] The Mayo Clinic's analysis recorded only 34% of UC requiring steroids.[16] Rectal therapy fares better than oral therapy in most cases of distal colitis,[57] although considerable improvement in bleeding, bowel motion frequency, and mucosal healing in left-sided disease and proctitis has been noted with high-dose oral 5-ASA alone (ASCEND data). 5-ASA preparations appear more effective than topical corticosteroids.[58] Budesonide enemas are as effective as prednisone enemas and significantly better than placebo (Table 17-4).[46,59-64]

Budesonide foam is equivalent in efficacy to hydrocortisone foam[66] but 5-ASA enemas may have better efficacy than budesonide or standard glucocorticoid enemas.[67,68] Budesonide foam is comparable in efficacy to 5-ASA enemas[69] and no different than betamethasone enema therapy.[70]

Further Experience With Budesonide as the Paradigm of Rapidly Acting First-Pass Metabolism Glucocorticoids

In one study, 23/44 (52%) budesonide foam (2 mg) patients entered remission versus 14/38 (37%) receiving hydrocortisone foam (hydrocortisone acetate 100 mg). Although numerically greater, the budesonide foam group's results did not achieve statistical significance. Three percent of the budesonide foam group had low plasma cortisol levels. There were no significant adverse events. Remission criteria were strict, corresponding to a DAI of 0 in this 8-week study.[66]

Budesonide Foam Versus Enema in Active Ulcerative Proctitis and PS

A large 449-patient randomized, controlled trail revealed a 60% remission rate with budesonide foam versus 66% rate with budesonide enema on a per protocol basis (*P*=0.02) for non-inferiority of foam. Eighty-four percent of patients preferred the easier application and tolerability of foam. Given a 15% noninferiority margin, 541 patients had to be enrolled, making this the largest rectal therapy trial for distal UC. Still, 49% of those patients previously treated with oral 5-ASA and 41% of those treated with rectal 5-ASA

TABLE 17-5

BDP VERSUS 5-ASA ENEMAS VERSUS COMBINATION IN DISTAL ULCERATIVE COLITIS[71]

4 WEEKS	BDP, 3 MG (N = 20)	5-ASA, 1 G (N = 21)	COMBINATION (N = 20)
Endoscopic Remission (%)	30	10	37
Clinical Improvement (%)	70	76	100
Endoscopic Improvement (%)	75	71	100

Reprinted with permission from Mulder CJ, Fockens P, Meijer JW, et al. Beclomethasone dipropionate (3 mg) versus 5-aminosalicylic acid (2 g) versus the combination of both (3 mg/2 g) as retention enemas in active ulcerative proctitis. *Eur J Gastroenterol Hepatol.* 1996;8:549-553.

previously who received budesonide foam achieved remission. Similarly, 50% of those patients previously treated with oral 5-ASA and 60% of those treated with rectal 5-ASA previously who received budesonide enemas achieved remission. There were high rates of endoscopic (50% foam, 54% budesonide) and histologic (51% foam, 57% enema) remission.[72]

A rectal budesonide foam remission rate of 60% is comparable to rectal 5-ASA remission (53%) and considerably higher than placebo in published studies.[73] Greater acceptance of the foam (84%) over enema (6%) was impressive but predictable. Although increased flatulence with foam preparations has been reported,[74] this may be related to incorrect usage or product variation regarding volume and pressure effects.

The role of oral budesonide in the therapy of pouchitis was revisited in an Italian study of 20 patients given budesonide C.I.R. 9 mg daily for 8 weeks.[75] Fifteen of 20 patients entered remission with a median drop in their Pouchitis Disease Activity Index (PDAI) from 14 to 3 (remission defined as ≤4 in this chapter, elsewhere combined PDAI ≤7)[76] and improved IBDQ score (102 to 182). These patients were unresponsive to a prior 4-week course of antibiotics.

Prior experience with budesonide enemas showed efficacy comparable to metronidazole in a double-blind randomized controlled trial (RCT). Whether this response is sustained or maintenance therapy is required in that 10% to 15% of patients developing chronic pouchitis will await further long-term trials.

OTHER RAPIDLY METABOLIZABLE GLUCOCORTICOIDS

BECLOMETHASONE DIPROPIONATE

The risks of corticosteroid systemic effects are considerably reduced when using first-pass metabolism agents such as budesonide or beclomethasone dipropionate (BDP). The anti-inflammatory activity is retained.[77-80] BDP has been useful when combined with oral 5-ASA as well.[81]

Two hundred seventeen UC patients entered a single-blind, randomized, controlled trial of either BDP 3 mg enema or 5-ASA 1 g enema daily for 6 weeks. A significant DAI decrease ($P<0.05$) occurred in 36.7% BDP and 29.2% 5-ASA treated patients. An initial problem in interpretation (other than lacking a placebo arm) was a 15.7% (34 patients) dropout rate: 18 in the BDP group (16.2%) and 16 (15.1%) in the 5-ASA group. A total of 203 patients were eventually included in the ITT analysis. Both agents were equivalent in efficacy (ie, DAI score) and sigmoidoscopic appearance, with BDP better for the moderate UC patients (DAI 7 to 10; ie, 28.8% remission versus 5.9% 5-ASA), especially in left-sided disease. There was no adrenal suppression, and morning plasma cortisol levels were unchanged. Both budesonide and BDP appear effective and safe with their first-pass metabolism feature.[82] BDP enemas were as effective as conventional glucocorticoids, with a diminished effect on plasma cortisol.[83]

BDP enema in combination with oral 5-ASA was better than either drug alone (Table 17-5).[71]

In general, distal versus left-sided UC when refractory to 5-ASA can be treated with glucocorticoid enemas. Topical budesonide (enemas or foam) is a reasonable alternative to standard steroid enema therapy.

CLINICAL EXPERIENCE WITH TOPICAL GLUCOCORTICOIDS

In 1997, Marshall and Irvine reported a meta-analysis of 33 reviewed rectal corticosteroid studies that met their "strict" inclusion criteria of 83 published reports.[72]

Inclusion criteria required randomization, disease distal to splenic flexure, a predefined symptom score, and no inclusion of Crohn's patients or duplicate reporting of trial data. The response rates based on symptomatic, endoscopic, and histologic criteria for conventional oral glucocorticoids (hydrocortisone, prednisolone, or betamethasone) were

TABLE 17-6

POOLED RESPONSE RATES FOR RECTAL PREPARATIONS (ALL TRIALS)

Remission (%)

	Symptomatic	Endoscopic	Histologic
Glucocorticoids (conventional)	45	34	30
Topical glucorticoids	46	31	23
5-ASA	52	39	32
Placebo	9	17	

Response (%)

	Symptomatic	Endoscopic	Histologic
Glucocorticoids (conventional)	77	66	52
Topical glucocorticoids	73	69	55
5-ASA	81	75	65
Placebo	34	38	

Adapted from Marshall JK, Irvine EJ. Rectal corticosteroids versus alternative treatments in ulcerative colitis: A meta-analysis. *Gut.* 1997;40:775-781.

77%, 66%, and 58% with remission rates of 45%, 34%, and 29%. The response to topical corticosteroids (budesonide, BDP, prednisolone, or metasulphobenzoate) was 73%, 69%, and 55% with remission rates of 46%, 31%, and 23%.

5-ASA preparations resulted in improvement in 81%, 75%, and 65% with remission recorded as 58%, 41%, and 38%. Placebo response rates were 34% symptom and 38% endoscopic improvement, and remission rates of symptomatic and endoscopic criteria were 9% and 17%.

They concluded that although topical corticosteroids were 32% superior to placebo, 7 trials proved 5-ASA to be superior to corticosteroids when considering clinical, endoscopic, and histologic standard of remission, and this occurred even with discrepant volumes of instilled medication (eg, 30 cc prednisolone foam versus 120 cc 5-ASA foam).[84]

Throughout all these analyses, a placebo benefit of 30% and a remission placebo rate of 10% must be kept in mind when evaluating efficacy.[85] Foam and suppositories will provide a higher response rate in distal UC[86] and better patient compliance.[87] As anticipated, higher endoscopic and histologic remission rates accrued with longer treatment duration[59-61,67,68,84,86,88-95] and with lower relapse rates.[96,97]

Their meta-analysis concluded that rectal 5-ASA is comparable to rectal glucocorticoids for improvement, but is better for inducing remission. This was consistent across symptomatic, endoscopic, and histologic outcomes. 5-ASA was as effective as budesonide in 2 trials regarding improvement and remission but failed to meet all endpoints. Adverse events were comparable for all rectal preparations of budesonide, albeit with less endogenous cortisol suppression than conventional glucocorticoids based on serum cortisol determinations.

They concluded that the role of rectal corticosteroids was an alternative distal colitis treatment in patients failing or intolerant to 5-ASA preparations, and 5-ASA preparations were superior to glucocorticoids in active disease as well as maintenance of remission (Table 17-6).

In 2000, Cohen et al[98] revisited therapy for left-sided UC and proctitis via a meta-analysis of the accumulated literature through 1997 and concluded that topical 5-ASA was superior to oral therapies or topical glucocorticoids. In left-sided disease, 5-ASA's higher remission rate over glucocorticoid enemas was not dose-dependent. Similarly 5-ASA suppositories were superior to glucocorticoid topical therapy in ulcerative proctitis but no dose-response could be established. Overall, the authors concluded remission and improvement rates of 10% to 80% of 5-ASA enemas over oral 5-ASA and glucocorticoid enemas.

Confounding features of meta-analyses open to criticism include different study populations, methodologies, and variation in study design. Odds ratios can be exaggerated by 17% if studies are not double-blinded,[99] 30% if lacking randomization,[100] 41% if inadequate concealment of treatment allocation, or 30% if unclear concealment.[99]

In a detailed analytic review of therapeutic trials for left-sided ulcerative proctitis, Regueiro et al in 2006 evaluated the literature from 1995 through September 2005.[101] Their assessment required multiple high-quality, randomized, controlled trials with consistent results to merit "A+" grade down to "D" for expert opinion only. Trials of therapeutic efficacy were excellent only if specifically designed for left-sided disease, with positive results compared to placebo or a comparative drug.

Rectally administered corticosteroids rated A+ on evidence and excellent efficacy with a clear advantage of 4 to 5 times more likely to have symptomatic and endoscopic improvement than placebo. Pooled OR was 0.21 (95% CI 0.07 to 0.71) for symptom and 0.27 (95% CI 0.10 to 0.77) for endoscopic improvement.[73]

Rapidly (first-pass) metabolized, rectally administered corticosteroids (budesonide, BDP) were effective in inducing and maintaining remission.[66,70,102,103]

Comparison studies of rectal 5-ASA versus rapidly metabolized glucocorticoids were of comparable efficacy (Table 17-7).[67,71,82]

Rapidly metabolized glucocorticoids are as effective as conventional glucocorticoids or 5-ASA enemas and are safe for induction of remission. As part of an analysis of efficacy of combined oral and topical therapy as superior to monotherapy, combined rectal therapy of both 5-ASA enema (2 g/100 cc) and BDP enemas (3 mg/100 cc) revealed significant clinical, endoscopic, and histologic improvements referable to monotherapy; 100% of patients were clinically improved at 4 weeks.[71]

Rectal glucocorticoids for maintenance of remission fare poorly and should be considered ineffective for this indication; in addition, there are the added adverse effects that it carries (osteoporosis, cataracts, avascular necrosis, etc). Indeed, there was no value or gain of oral glucocorticoids over placebo after 6 months (as noted in the earliest study in 1965).[104] The oral steroid therapy data from the Mayo Clinic are clearly unfavorable for any sustained benefit, ie, the 1-month combined partial and complete remission note of 84% diminished to 49% without glucocorticoids at 1 year, 22% of patients became dependent on glucocorticoids, and 29% required colectomy.[16]

No benefit was noted with a maintenance dose of rectal hydrocortisone 100 mg biweekly for 6 months.[105] No rectal budesonide (2 mg biweekly) maintenance benefit versus placebo could be established.[106]

Proctitis may become a vexing problem when active. 5-ASA or glucocorticoid suppositories given 2 to 3 times daily may be helpful even with the expected difficulty of retaining them with refractory disease.[101]

5-ASA or glucocorticoid enemas and glucocorticoid foam have been the mainstays of topical therapy for rectosigmoid UC. Occasionally, enema preparations may skip (or bypass) the inflamed irritable rectal sigmoid due to instillation with the patient on his or her left side. Suppositories are recommended 2 to 3 times daily as supplemental rectal medication until relief is achieved.[107]

CONCLUSION

Rectal therapy with glucocorticoids and 5-ASA are effective in inducing remission in ulcerative proctitis and left-sided ulcerative colitis (Table 17-8). 5-ASAs orally and rectally are preferred. Glucocorticoid enemas are effective, but there are concerns regarding systemic absorption unless first-pass metabolism corticosteroids are used (budesonide or BDP). There is little to no support for rectal glucocorticoids for maintenance of remission, as does exist for rectal 5-ASA. Rectal glucocorticoids or rectal 5-ASA in combination with oral 5-ASA is more effective than monotherapy.[108] Rectal corticosteroids and 5-ASA suppositories are effective treatment for ulcerative proctitis.

REFERENCES

1. Osler W. *The Principles & Practice of Medicine,* 1st ed. New York, NY: D. Appleton & Co; 1892.
2. Truelove SC. Treatment of ulcerative colitis with local hydrocortisone. *BMJ.* 1956;2:1267-1272.
3. Bargen JA. *Chronic Ulcerative Colitis: A Lifelong Study.* Springfield, IL: Charles C. Thomas; 1969.
4. Mulder CJJ, Tygat GNJ. Topical corticosteroids in inflammatory bowel disease. *Aliment Pharmacol Ther.* 1993;7:125-130.
5. Jay M, Digenis GA, Foster TS, et al. Retrograde spreading of hydrocortisone enema in inflammatory bowel disease. *Dig Dis Sci.* 1986;31:139-144.
6. Swarbrick ET, Loose H, Lennard-Jones JE. Enema volume as an important factor in successful topical corticosteroid treatment of colitis. *Proc Royal Soc Med.* 1974;67:753-754.
7. Farthing MJG, Rutland MD, Clark ML. Retrograde spread of hydrocortisone containing foam given intrarectally in ulcerative colitis. *BMJ.* 1979;2:822-824.
8. Jay M, Beihn RM, Digenis GA, et al. Disposition of radiolabelled suppositories in humans. *J Pharm Pharmacol.* 1985;37:266-268.
9. Friend DR. Review article: issues in oral administration of locally acting glucocorticosteroids for treatment of inflammatory bowel disease. *Aliment Pharmacol Ther.* 1998;12:591-603.
10. Hollenberg SM, Weinberger C, Ong ES, et al. Primary structure and expression of a functional human glucocorticoid receptor cDNA. *Nature.* 1985;318:635-641.
11. Encio IJ, Detera-Wadleigh SD. The genomic structure of the human glucocorticoid receptor. *J Biol Chem.* 1991;266:7182-7188.
12. Reichardt HM, Kaestner KH, Tuckermann J, et al. DNA binding of the glucocorticoid receptor is not essential for survival. *Cell.* 1998;93:531-541.
13. Stocklin E, Wissler M, Goiulleux M, et al. Functional interactions between Stat5 and the glucocorticoid receptor. *Nature.* 1996;383:726-728.
14. Hearing SD, Norman M, Probert CSJ, et al. Predicting therapeutic outcome in severe ulcerative colitis by measuring in vitro steroid sensitivity of proliferating peripheral blood lymphocytes. *Gut.* 1999;45:382-388.
15. Hearing SD, Norman M, Smyth C, et al. Wide variation in lymphocyte steroid sensitivity among healthy human volunteers. *J Clin Endocrinol Metab.* 1999;84:4149-4154.

TABLE 17-7

RANDOMIZED CONTROLLED TRIALS OF TREATMENT FOR ACTIVE L-UC: TOPICALLY ACTIVE CORTICOSTEROIDS[101]

Authors, Year	Study Design	Treatment 1 Compared to	Treatment 2	Results
Lofberg et al,[102] 1996	RCT, double blind, (n = 72)	Oral budesonide 10 mg	Prednisolone 40 mg	Endoscopic scores: budesonide comparable efficacy to prednisolone after 9 weeks
Campieri et al,[82] 1998	RCT, double blind, (n = 157)	BDP enema (3 mg/60 mL)	PSP enema (30 mg/60 mL)	Clinical and endoscopic remission with BDP 29% and PSP 25% at 4 weeks (P=NS)
Hanauer et al,[110] 1998	RCT, double blind, (n = 233)	Budesonide enema, varying strengths: 0.5, 2.0, 8.0 mg/100 mL	Placebo	Remission at 6 weeks: budesonide 0.5 mg/100 mL, 7% (P=NS) budesonide 2.0 mg/100 mL, 19% ($P \leq 0.05$) budesonide 8.0 mg/100 mL, 27% ($P<0.001$)
Lindgren et al,[103] 2002	RCT, double blind, (n = 149)	Budesonide enema, varying strengths: Induction, 2.0, 4.0 mg/100 mL; remission, 2.0 mg/100 mL	Placebo	2-mg dose induces remission; no effect on maintenance of remission
Bar-meir et al,[66] 2003	RCT, open label, (n = 251)	Budesonide foam 2 mg (Budenofalk)	Hydrocortisone acetate foam 100 mg (Colifoam)	Remission rates: BDP 55% and hydrocortisone acetate 51% at 8 weeks
Hammond et al,[70] 2004	RCT, open label (n = 38)	Budesonide 2 mg/50 mL foam	Betamethasone 5 mg/100 mL	Mean Life Quality Index score at 4 weeks: budesonide foam 2.9 and betamethasone enema 2.1 ($P<0.09$)

*BDP = Beclomethasone dipropionate; PSP = Prednisolone sodium phosphate; RCT = randomized controlled trial

Reprinted with permission from publisher, adapted from Regueiro M, Loftus Jr EV, Steinhart AH, et al. Medical management of left-sided ulcerative colitis and ulcerative proctitis: critical evaluation of therapeutic trials. *Inflamm Bowel Dis.* 2006;12:979-994.

16. Faubion W, Loftus E, Harmsen W, et al. The natural history of corticosteroid therapy for inflammatory bowel disease: a population-based study. *Gastroenterology.* 2001;121:255-260.
17. Munkholm P, Langholz E, Davidsen M, et al. Frequency of glucocorticoid resistance and dependency in Crohn's disease. *Gut.* 1994;35:360-362.
18. Truelove S, Witts L. Cortisone in ulcerative colitis. *BMJ.* 1995;ii:1041-1048.
19. Hurley D, Accili D, Stratakis C, et al. Point mutation causing a single amino acid substitution in the hormone binding domain of the glucocorticoid receptor in familial glucocorticoid resistance. *J Clin Invest.* 1991;87:680-686.
20. Karl M, Lamberts S, Detera-Wadleigh S, et al. Familial glucocorticoid resistance caused by a splice site deletion in the human glucocorticoid receptor gene. *J Clin Endocrinol Metab.* 1993;73:683-689.
21. Malchoff D, Brufsky A, Reardon G, et al. A mutation of the glucocorticoid receptor in primary cortisol resistance. *J Clin Invest.* 1993;91:1918-1925.
22. Lane S, Lee S. Glucocorticoid receptor characteristics in monocytes of patients with corticosteroid resistant bronchial asthma. *Am Rev Respir Dis.* 1991;143:1020-1024.
23. Lane SJ, Atkinson AB, Swaminathan R, et al. Hypothalamic-pituitary-adrenal axis in corticosteroid-resistant bronchial asthma. *Am J Respir Crit Care Med.* 1996;153:557-560.
24. Flood L, Lofberg R, Syierna P, et al. Glucocorticoid receptor mRNA in patients with ulcerative colitis: a study of responders and nonresponders to glucocorticosteroid therapy. *Inflamm Bowel Dis.* 2001;7:202-209.
25. Bantel H, Domschke W, Schulze-Osthoff K. Molecular mechanisms of glucocorticoid resistance. *Gastroenterology.* 2000;119:1178-1179.
26. Matthews JG, Ito K, Barnes PJ, et al. Defective glucocorticoid receptor nuclear translocation and altered histone acetylation patterns in glucocorticoid-resistant patients. *J Allergy Clin Immunol.* 2004;113:1100-1108.
27. Ray DW, Davis JR, White A, et al. Glucocorticoid receptor structure and function in glucocorticoid-resistant small cell lung carcinoma cells. *Cancer Res.* 1996;56:3276-3280.
28. Rivers C, Levy A, Hancock J, et al. Insertion of an amino acid in the DNA-binding domain of the glucocorticoid receptor as a result of alternative splicing. *J Clin Endocrinol Metab.* 1999;84:4283-4286.
29. Kam JC, Szefler SJ, Surs W, et al. Combination IL-2 and IL-4 reduces glucocorticoid receptor-binding affinity and T cell response to glucocorticoids. *J Immunol.* 1993;151:3460-3466.
30. Goleva E, Kisich KO, Leung DYM. A role for STAT5 in the pathogenesis of IL-2 induced glucocorticoid resistance. *J Immunol.* 2002;169:5934-5940.
31. Bantel H, Domschke W, Schulze-Ostohoff K, et al. Abnormal activation of transcription factor NF-B involved in steroid resistance in chronic inflammatory bowel disease. *Am J Gastroenterol.* 2000;95:1845-1846.
32. Walker K, Potter J, House A. Variable inhibition of mitogen-induced blastogenesis in human lymphocytes by prednisolone in vitro. *Transplant Proc.* 1985;17:1676-1678.
33. Irusen E, Matthews JG, Takahashi A, et al. p 38 Mitogen-activated protein kinase-induced glucocorticoid receptor phosphorylation reduces its activity: role in steroid-insensitive asthma. *J Allergy Clin Immunol.* 2002;109:649-657.
34. Creed TJ, Probert CSJ. Steroid resistance in inflammatory bowel disease—mechanisms and therapeutic strategies. *Aliment Pharmacol Ther.* 2007;25:111-122.
35. Ho G, Nimmo E, Tenesa A, et al. Allelic variations of the multidrug resistance gene determine susceptibility and disease behavior in ulcerative colitis. *Gastroenterology.* 2005;128:288-296.
36. Bouma G, Crusius J, Garcia-Gonzalez M. Genetic markers in clinically well defined patients with ulcerative colitis. *Clin Exp Immunol.* 1995;115:294-300.
37. Hanauer SB, Sandborn WJ, Kornbluth A, et al. Delayed-release oral mesalamine at 4.8 g/day (800 mg tablet) for the treatment of moderately active ulcerative colitis: The ASCEND II Trial. *Am J Gastroenterol.* 2005;100:2478-2485.
38. Scheurlen C, Allgayer H, Hardt M, et al. Effect of short-term topical corticosteroid treatment on mucosal enzyme systems in patients with distal inflammatory bowel disease. *Hepatogastroenterol.* 1998;45:1539-1545.
39. Pienkowski P, Fioramonti J, Skalli F, et al. Effects of corticoids, 5-aminosalycilic acid and sucralfate on the potential difference of the rectum in inflammatory colitis in man. *Gastroenterol Clin Biol.* 1989;13:202-207.
40. Andus T, Targan SR. Corticosteroids. In: Targan S, Shanahan F, eds. *Inflammatory Bowel Disease: From Bench to Bedside.* Baltimore, MD: Williams & Wilkins; 1993:487-502.
41. Powell Tuck J, Lennard-Jones JE, May CS, et al. Plasma prednisolone levels after administration of prednisolone-21 phosphate as a tetnetion enema in colitis. *BMJ.* 1976;1:193-195.
42. Lee DAH, Taylor GM, James VHT, et al. Plasma prednisolone levels and adrenocortical responsiveness after administration of prednisolone-21 phosphate as a retention enema. *Gut.* 1979;20:349-355.
43. Petitjean O, Wendling JL, Tod M, et al. Pharmacokinetics and absolute rectal bioavailability of hydrocortisone acetate in distal colitis. *Aliment Pharmacol Ther.* 1992;6:351-357.
44. Campieri M, Gionchetti P, Belluzzi A, et al. 5-Aminosalicylic acid as enemas or suppositories in distal ulcerative colitis? *J Clin Gastroenterol.* 1988;10:406-409.
45. Hanauer SB, Kane S. The pharmacology of anti-inflammatory drugs in inflammatory bowel disease. In: Kirsner JB, ed. *Inflammatory Bowel Disease.* 5th ed. Philadelphia, PA: WB Saunders; 2000.
46. Hanauer SB, Robinson M, Pruitt R, et al. Budesonide enema for the treatment of active, distal ulcerative colitis and proctitis: a dose-ranging study. U.S. Budesonide Enema Study Group. *Gastroenterology.* 1998;115:525-532.
47. Klotz U, Schwab M. Topical delivery of the therapeutic agents in the treatment of inflammatory bowel disease. *Adv Drug Deliv Rev.* 2005;57:267-279.
48. Jönsson G, Åström A, Andersson P. Budesonide is metabolized by cytochrome P4503A (CYP3A4) enzymes in human liver. *Drug Metab Dispos.* 1995;23:137-142.
49. Spencer CM, McTavish D. Budesonide: a review of its pharmacological properties and therapeutic efficacy in inflammatory bowel disease. *Drugs.* 1995;50:854-872.
50. McKeage K, Goa KL. Budesonide (Entocort® EC Capsules): a review of its therapeutic use in the management of active Crohn's disease in adults. *Drugs.* 2002;62:2263-2282.
51. Nilsson M, Edsbäcker S, Larsson P, et al. *Dose-proportional kinetics of budesonide controlled ileal release (CIR) capsules*, Poster Abstract. No. 1783P, 10th World Congr Gastroenterol, Los Angeles, Oct 2-1, 1994.
52. Danielsson Å, Edsbäcker S, Löfberg R, et al. Pharmacokinetics of budesonide enema in patients with distal ulcerative colitis or proctitis. *Aliment Pharmacol Ther.* 1993;7:401-407.
53. Seidegård J. Reduction of the inhibitory effect of ketoconazole on budesonide pharmacokinetics by separation of their time of administration. *Clin Pharmacol Ther.* 2000;67:13-17.
54. Nyman-Pantelidis M, Nilsson Å, Wagner ZG, et al. Pharmacokinetics and retrograde colonic spread of budesonide enemas in patients with distal ulcerative colitis. *Aliment Pharmacol Ther.* 1994;8:617-622.

55. Peña AS, Kolkman JJ, Greinwald R, et al. Pharmacokinetics after single and multiple oral dosing of budesonide pH-modified-release capsules in patients with distal ulcerative colitis. In: Dignass A, Gross V, Buhr HJ, et al, eds. *Topical Steroids in Gastroenterology and Hepatology.* Dordrecht: Kluwer Academic Publisher; 2004:30-35.
56. Sutherland LR, May GR, Shaffer EA. Sulfasalazine revisited: ameta-analysis of 5-aminosalicylic acid in the treatment of ulcerative colitis. *Ann Intern Med.* 1993;118:540-549.
57. Hamilton I, Pinder IF, Dickinson RJ, et al. A comparison of prednisolone enemas with low-dose oral prednisolone in the treatment of acute distal ulcerative colitis. *Dis Colon Rectum.* 1984;27: 701-702.
58. Kornbluth AA, Salomon P, Sacks HS, et al. Meta-analysis of the effectiveness of current drug therapy of ulcerative colitis. *J Clin Gastroenterol.* 1993;16:215-218.
59. Danielsson A, Hellers G, Lyrenäs E, et al. A controlled randomized trial of budesonide versus prednisolone retention enemas in active distal ulcerative colitis. *Scand J Gastroenterol.* 1987;22:987-992.
60. Danielsson A, Löfberg R, Persson T, et al. A steroid enema, budesonide, lacking systemic effects for the treatment of distal ulcerative colitis or proctitis. *Scand J Gastroenterol.* 1992;27:9-12.
61. Löfberg R, Ostergaard-Thomsen O, Langholz E, et al. Budesonide versus prednisolone retention enemas in active distal ulcerative colitis. *Aliment Pharmacol Ther.* 1994;8:623-629.
62. Matzen P. Budesonide enema in distal ulcerative colitis. A randomized dose-response trial with prednisolone enema as positive control. *Scand J Gastroenterol.* 1991;26:1225-1230.
63. Bianchi-Porro G, Prantera C, Campieri M, et al. Comparative trial of methylprednisolone and budesonide enemas in active distal ulcerative colitis. *Eur J Gastroenterol Hepatol.* 1994;6:125-130.
64. Bayless T, Sninsky C, for the U.S. Budesonide Enema Study Group. Budesonide enema is effective alternative to hydrocortisone enema in active distal ulcerative colitis [abstract]. *Gastroenterology.* 1995;108:A778.
65. Schölmerich J. Review article: Systemic and topical steroids in inflammatory bowel disease. *Aliment Pharmacol Ther.* 2004;20(Suppl 4):66-74.
66. Bar-Meir S, Fidder HH, Faszczyk M, et al. International Budesonide Study Group. Budesonide foam versus hydrocortisone acetate foam in the treatment of active ulcerative proctosigmoiditis. *Dis Colon Rectum.* 2003;46:929-936.
67. Lėmann M, Galian A, Rutgeerts P, et al. Comparison of budesonide and 5-aminosalicylic acid enemas in active distal ulcerative colitis. *Aliment Pharmacol Ther.* 1995;9:557-562.
68. Lamers C, Meijer J, Engels L, et al. Comparative study of the topically acting glucocorticosteroid budesonide and 5-aminosalicylic acid enema therapy of proctitis and proctosigmoiditis [abstract]. *Gastroenterology.* 1991;100:A223.
69. Rufle W, Fr'ühmorgen P, Huber W, et al. Budesonide foam as a new therapeutic principle in distal ulcerative colitis in comparison with mesalazine enema: an open, controlled, randomized and prospective multicenter pilot study. *Z Gastroenterol.* 2000;38:287-293.
70. Hammond A, Andus T, Gierend M, et al. Open, randomized multicentre trial comparing safety and efficacy of budesonide foam with betamethasone enema in patients with active distal ulcerative colitis. *Hepatogastroenterol.* 2004;51:1345-1349.
71. Gross V, Bar-Meir S, Lavy A, et al. Budesonide foam versus budesonide enema in active ulcerative proctitis and proctosigmoiditis. *Aliment Pharmacol Ther.* 2006;23:303-312.
72. Marshall JK, Irvine EJ. Rectal corticosteroids versus alternative treatments in ulcerative colitis: a meta-analysis. *Gut.* 1997;40:775-781.
73. Malchow H, Gertz B, the Clafoam Study Group. A new mesalazine foam enema (Claversal Foam) compared with a standard liquid enema in patients with active distal ulcerative colitis. *Aliment Pharmacol Ther.* 2002;16:415-423.
74. Gionchetti P, Rizzello F, Poggioli G, et al. Oral budesonide in the treatment of chronic refractory pouchitis. *Aliment Pharmacol Ther.* 2007;25(10):1231-1236.
75. Sandborn WJ, Tremaine WJ, Batts KP, et al. Pouchitis after ileal pouch-anal anastomosis: a pouchitis disease activity index. *Mayo Clin Proc.* 1994;69:409-415.
76. Mulder CJ, Endert E, Van der Heide H, et al. Comparison of beclomethasone dipropionate (2 and 3 mg) and prednisolone sodium phosphate enemas (30 mg) in the treatment of ulcerative proctitis: an adrenocortical approach. *Neth J Med.* 1989;35:18-24.
77. Kumana CR, Seaton T, Meghji M, et al. Beclomethasone dipropionate enemas for treating inflammatory bowel disease without producing Cushing's syndrome or hypothalamic pituitary adrenal suppression. *Lancet.* 1982;1:579-583.
78. Bansky G, Buhler H, Stamm B, et al. Treatment of distal ulcerative colitis with beclomethasone enemas: high therapeutic efficacy without endocrine side effects: a prospective, randomised, double blind trial. *Dis Colon Rectum.* 1987;30:288-292.
79. Harris DM. Some properties of beclomethasone dipropionate and related steroids in man. *Postgrad Med J.* 1975;51(Suppl 4):20-25.
80. D'Arienzo A, Manguso F, Bennato R, et al. Beclomethasone dipropionate (3 mg) enemas combined with oral 5-ASA (2.4 g) in the treatment of ulcerative colitis not responsive to oral 5-ASA alone. *Ital J Gastroeneterol Hepatol.* 1998;30:254-257.
81. Gionchetti P, D'Arienzo A, Rizzello F, et al. Topical treatment of distal active ulcerative colitis with beclomethasone dipropionate or mesalamine—A single-blind randomized controlled trial. *J Clin Gastroenterol.* 2005;30:291-297.
82. Campieri M, Cottone M, Miglio F, et al. Beclomethasone dipropionate enemas versus prednisolone sodium phosphate enemas in the treatment of distal ulcerative colitis. *Aliment Pharmacol Ther.* 1998;12:361-366.
83. Mulder CJ, Fockens P, Meijer JW, et al. Beclomethasone dipropionate (3 mg) versus 5-aminosalicylic acid (2 g) versus the combination of both (3 mg/2 g) as retention enemas in active ulcerative proctitis. *Eur J Gastroenterol Hepatol.* 1996;8:549-553.
84. Lee FI, Jewell DP, Mani V, et al. A randomised trial comparing mesalazine and prednisolone foam enemas in patients with acute distal ulcerative colitis. *Gut.* 1996;38:229-233.
85. Ilnycki A, Shanahan F, Anton PA, et al. The placebo response in ulcerative colitis [abstract]. *Gastroenterology.* 1996;110:A929.
86. Farup PG, Hovde O, Halvorsen FA, et al. Mesalazine suppositories versus hydrocortisone foam in patients with distal ulcerative colitis. *Scand J Gastroenterol.* 1995;30:164-170.
87. Ruddell WSJ, Dickinson RJ, Dixon MF, et al. Treatment of distal ulcerative colitis (proctosigmoiditis) in relapse: comparison of hydrocortisone enemas and rectal hydrocortisone foam. *Gut.* 1980;21:885-889.
88. Sharma MP, Duphare HV, Dasarathy S. A prospective randomized double blind trial comparing prednisolone and 4-aminosalicylic acid enemas in acute distal ulcerative colitis. *J Gastroenterol Hepatol.* 1992;7:173-177.
89. Friedman LS, Richter JM, Kirkham SE, et al. 5-Aminosalicylic acid enemas in refractory distal ulcerative colitis; a randomized controlled trial. *Am J Gastroenterol.* 1986;81:412-418.
90. Mulder CJJ, Endert E, Van der Heide H, et al. Comparison of 5-aminosalicylic acid (3 g) and prednisolone phosphate sodium enemas (30 mg) in the treatment of distal ulcerative colitis; A prospective, randomized, double-blind trial. *Scand J Gastroenterol.* 1988;23:1005-1008.

91. O'Donnell LFK, Arvind AS, Cameron D, et al. Double blind, controlled trials of 4-aminosalicylic acid and prednisolone enemas in distal ulcerative colitis. *Gut.* 1992;33:947-949.
92. Tarpila S, Turunen U, Seppala K, et al. Budesonide enema in active haemorrhagic proctitis: a controlled trial against hydrocortisone foam enema. *Aliment Pharmacol Ther.* 1994;8:591-595.
93. Cobden I, Al-Mardini H, Zaitoun A, et al. Is topical therapy necessary in acute distal ulcerative colitis? Double-blind comparison of high-dose oral mesalazine versus steroid enemas in the treatment of active distal ulcerative colitis. *Aliment Pharmacol Ther.* 1991;5:513-522.
94. Grace RH, Gent AI, Hellier MD. Comparative trial of sodium cromoglycate enemas with prednisolone enemas in the treatment of ulcerative colitis. *Gut.* 1987;28:88-92.
95. Halpern Z, Sold O, Baratz M, et al. A controlled trial of beclomethasone versus betamethasone enemas in distal ulcerative colitis. *J Clin Gastroenterol.* 1991;13:38-41.
96. Meyers S, Janowitz HD. The natural history of ulcerative colitis: an analysis of the placebo response. *J Clin Gastroenterol.* 1989;11:33-37.
97. Riley SA, Mani V, Goodman MJ, et al. Microscopic activity in ulcerative colitis: what does it mean? *Gut.* 1991;32:174-178.
98. Cohen RD, Woseth DM, Thisted RA, et al. A meta-analysis and overview of the literature on treatment options for left-sided ulcerative colitis and ulcerative proctitis. *Am J Gastroenterol.* 2000;95:1263-1276.
99. Schulz KF, Chalmers I, Hayes RJ, et al. Empirical evidence of bias. Dimensions of methodological quality associated with estimates of treatment effects in controlled trials. *JAMA.* 1995;273:408-412.
100. Peto R. Why do we need systematic overviews of randomized trials? *Stat Med.* 1987;6:233-244.
101. Regueiro M, Loftus EV Jr, Steinhart AH, et al. Medical management of left-sided ulcerative colitis and ulcerative proctitis: critical evaluation of therapeutic trials. *Inflamm Bowel Dis.* 2006;12:979-994.
102. Lofberg R, Danielsson J, Suhr O, et al. Oral budesonide versus prednisolone in patients with active extensive and left-sided ulcerative colitis. *Gastroenterology.* 1996;10:1713-1718.
103. Lindgren S, Lofberg R, Bergholm L, et al. Effect of budesonide enema on remission and relapse rate in distal ulcerative colitis and proctitis. *Scand J Gastroenterol.* 2002;37:705-710.
104. Rizzello F, Gionchetti P, D'Arienzo A, et al. Oral beclomethasone dipropionate in the treatment of active ulcerative colitis: A double-blind placebo-controlled study. *Aliment Pharmacol Ther.* 2002;16:1109-1116.
105. Lennard-Jones JE, Misiewicz J, Connell AM, et al. Prednisone as maintenance treatment for ulcerative colitis in remission. *Lancet.* 1965;191:188-189.
106. Truelove SC. Treatment of ulcerative colitis with local hydrocortisone hemisuccinate sodium: a report on a controlled therapeutic trial. *Br Med J.* 1958;1072-1077.
107. Lindgren S, Suhr O, Persson T, et al. Treatment of active distal ulcerative colitis (UC) and maintenance of remission with Entocort enema: a randomized controlled dosage study. *Gut.* 1997;41:A223(Abstr.).
108. MacDermott RP, Green JA. Refractory ulcerative colitis treatment. *Gastroenterol Hepatol.* 2007;3:64-69.
109. Regueiro M, Loftus EV Jr, Steinhart H, et al. Clinical guidelines for the medical management of left-sided ulcerative colitis and ulcerative proctitis: summary statement. *Inflamm Bowel Dis.* 2006;12:972-978.
110. Hanauer SB. Dose-ranging study of mesalamine (PENTASA) enemas in the treatment of acute ulcerative proctosigmoiditis: results of a multicentered placebo-controlled trial. The U.S. PENTASA Enema Study Group. *Inflam Bowel Dis.* 1998;4:79-83.
111. Sutherland LR, Martin F. 5-Aminosalicylic acid enemas in treatment of distal ulcerative colitis and proctitis in Canada. *Dig Dis Sci.* 1987;32:64S-66S.
112. Danish 5-ASA Group. Topical 5-aminosalicylic acid versus prednisolone in ulcerative proctosigmoiditis. A randomized, double-blind multicenter trial. *Dig Dis Sci.* 1987;32:598-602.
113. Farmer RG, Schumacher OP. Treatment of ulcerative colitis with hydrocortisone enemas: relationship of hydrocortisone absorption, adrenal suppression, and clinical response. *Dis Colon Rectum.* 1970;13:355-361.
114. Luman W, Gray RS, Pendek R, et al. Prednisolone metasulphobenzoate foam retention enemas suppress the hypothalamo-pituitary-adrenal axis. *Aliment Pharmacol Ther.* 1994;8:255-258.
115. Lennard-Jones JE, Baron JH, Connell AM, et al. A double blind controlled trial of prednisolone-21-phosphate suppositories in the treatment of idiopathic proctitis. *Gut.* 1962;3:207-210.
116. Watkinson G. Treatment of ulcerative colitis with topical hydrocortisone hemisuccinate sodium: a controlled trial employing restricted sequential analysis. *Br Med J.* 1958;2:1077-1082.
117. Campieri M, Lanfranchi GA, Bazzocchi GG, et al. Treatment of ulcerative colitis with high-dose 5-aminosalicylic acid enemas. *Lancet.* 1981;2:270-271.
118. Porro GB, Ardizzone S, Petrillo M, et al. Low Pentasa dosage versus hydrocortisone in the topical treatment of active ulcerative colitis: a randomized, double-blind study. *Am J Gastroenterol.* 1995;90:736-739.
119. Campieri M, Gionchetti P, Belluzzi A, et al. Efficacy of 5-aminosalicylic acid enemas versus hydrocortisone enemas in ulcerative colitis. *Dig Dis Sci.* 1987;32:67S-70S.
120. Lucidarme D, Marteau P, Foucault M, et al. Efficacy and tolerance of mesalazine suppositories versus hydrocortisone foam in proctitis. *Aliment Pharmacol Ther.* 1997;11:335-340.
121. Lennard-Jones JE, Longmore AJ, Newell AC, et al. An assessment of prednisone, salazopyrine and topical hydrocortisone hemisuccinate used as outpatient treatment for ulcerative colitis. *Gut.* 1960;1:217-222.
122. Gionchetti P, Rizzello F, Venture A, et al. Comparison of mesalazine suppositories in proctitis and distal proctosigmoiditis. *Aliment Pharmacol Ther.* 1997;11:1053-1057.
123. Danish Budesonide Study Group. Budesonide enema in distal ulcerative colitis. A randomized dose-response trial with prednisolone enema as positive control. *Scand J Gastroenterol.* 1991;26:1225-1230.

18

6-Mercaptopurine and Azathioprine Use in Ulcerative Colitis

Marla C. Dubinsky, MD

BACKGROUND

Immunomodulator therapy has become an integral part of the management of inflammatory bowel disease (IBD) patients. The most commonly used immunomodulators, 6-MP and AZA, belong to the family of drugs known as the thiopurines. 6-MP was first synthesized in 1951 by Gertrude Elion and was widely used for children with acute lymphoblastoid leukemia (ALL). Subsequently, AZA was synthesized as a pro-drug for 6-MP; it was found to be superior to 6-MP for kidney rejection and rheumatoid arthritis and was approved for these indications. To date, there is no evidence to suggest that either drug is superior to the other in IBD, and thus both thiopurines are used for Crohn's disease (CD) and ulcerative colitis (UC). Although the use of these drugs in IBD has significantly increased over the past 5 to 10 years, there still remains a discrepancy between need and use among IBD patients. Safety concerns, bone marrow suppression in particular, and delayed onset of action most likely drive this incongruity. The advent of pharmacogenetics and therapeutic drug monitoring in IBD has addressed some of these concerns; however, an understanding of the pharmacology and metabolism of thiopurines is critical to optimizing the effects of thiopurines in our IBD patients. The available clinical trial data on the use of thiopurines in UC are considerably less than that reported for CD; and unlike CD, the efficacy of these drugs based on the evidence for both induction and maintenance of a steroid-free remission remains under question. These therapies, however, remain widely used in UC based on clinical experience and the therapeutic benefits observed among our patients.

PHARMACOKINETICS

Although 6-MP and its prodrug AZA are often used interchangeably there are pharmacological differences between the 2 compounds. Studies have shown that the bioavailability of AZA may be superior to that of 6-MP with a range of 27% to 83%.[1,2] Once absorbed, AZA is rapidly converted via a nonenzymatic process to 6-MP and S-methyl-4-nitro-5-thioimidazole. AZA is 55% of 6-MP by molecular weight, and 88% of AZA is converted to 6-MP such that a conversion factor of 2.08 must be taken into account when calculating equivalent doses of 6-MP and AZA. 6-MP (or AZA converted to 6-MP) undergoes a complex biotransformation to its inactive and active metabolites via competing catabolic and anabolic metabolic pathways (Figure 18-1). 6-MP undergoes extensive first-pass catabolism by xanthine oxidase (XO), which is present in both the intestinal mucosa and liver, limiting the systemic bioavailability of thiopurines. 6-MP also serves as a substrate for the thiopurine methyltransferase (TPMT) enzyme, which methylates 6-MP to the inactive methylated-mercaptopurine metabolite (6-MeMP). Like XO, TPMT may be present in the intestinal mucosa and may also contribute to the pre-systemic catabolism of 6-MP. The hypoxanthine phosphoribosyltransferase (HPRT) enzyme is paramount to the initiation of the anabolic transformation of 6-MP to its active metabolites. The intracellular activation of 6-MP yields the first active intermediate metabolite, thioinosine monophosphate (TiMP), which is then rapidly converted to thioguanine nucleotides (6-TGN). The cytotoxic and immunosuppressive effects of thiopurines were, until recently, presumed to be primarily mediated via the

Lichtenstein GR, ed.
Ulcerative Colitis: The Complete Guide to Medical Management (pp. 203-214)

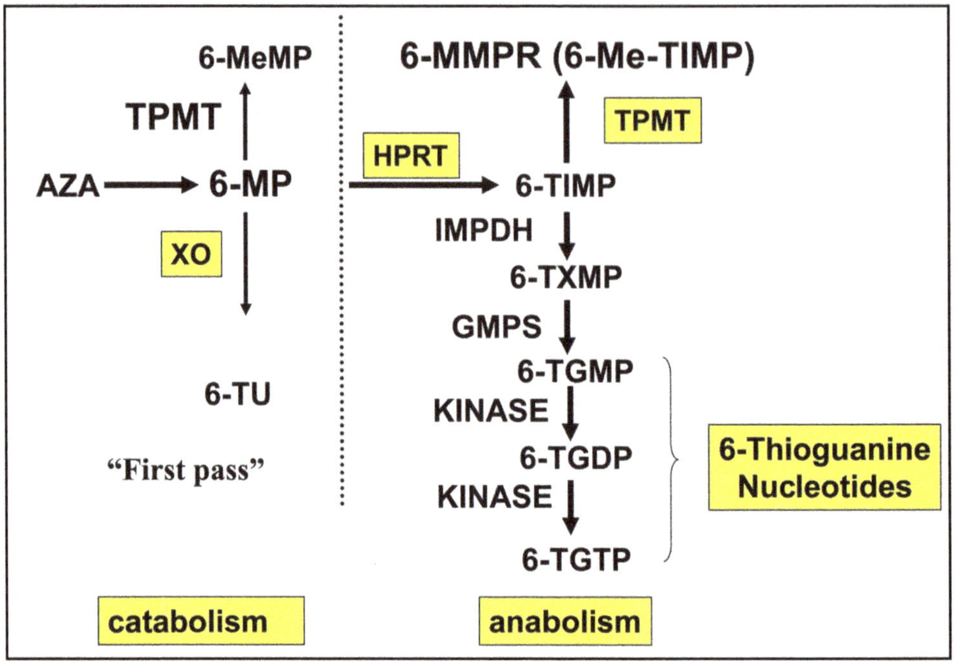

FIGURE 18-1. The metabolism of thiopurines.

incorporation of 6-TGN into cellular nucleic acids—ultimately resulting in inhibition of lymphocyte proliferation. Recent advances in the understanding of the mechanism of action of thiopurines, however, suggests that the 6-thioguanine triphosphate (6-thio-GTP) nucleotide may play an important role in the process of signaling lymphocyte apoptosis by inhibiting Rac1 activation in T cells.[3] As illustrated in Figure 18-1, 6-thio-GTP is likely the final nucleotide in the activation pathway of thiopurines. Further research is needed to examine the potential therapeutic role of 6-thio-GTP in patients with IBD and perhaps other autoimmune disorders.

The major enzymatic process that competes with the intracellular activation pathway is the thiol methylation of TiMP by TPMT. Although these methylated metabolites (Me-TiMP or 6-MMPR) have been shown in vitro to inhibit denovo purine synthesis, in vivo evidence is lacking as to their role in the mechanism of action of thiopurines.[4] It has been demonstrated that not all individuals tolerate methylate thiopurines equally and that the genetic variability in TPMT enzyme activity is responsible for the majority of the individual differences observed in both the efficacy and toxicity of thiopurines. Population-based studies have demonstrated that TPMT activity is inherited as an autosomal co-dominant trait.[5] The frequency distribution of the TPMT polymorphisms reveals that 1 in 300 (0.3%) individuals have low to absent enzyme activity (homozygous $TPMT^L$), 11% have intermediate (heterozygous $TPMT^H$/$TPMT^L$), and 89% have normal to high levels of activity (homozygous/wild type $TPMT^H$). Although a number of variant TPMT alleles have been described, TPMT*3A, a double mutant (A719G and G460A), is the most frequently occurring mutant allele and predominates in Caucasians (Figure 18-2). Each mutant, however, TPMT*3B (G460A) and TPMT*3C (A710G), can occur independently. Although mutant allele frequencies may be similar among different ethnicities, the prevalent mutant alleles do differ such that TPMT*3C is most common among African Americans.[6] TPMT*3C is also the prevalent mutant allele among the Chinese population; however, the frequency of mutant alleles appears lower than among Caucasians.[7] The degree of reduction in TPMT activity and immunoreactive protein varies based on the mutant allele present in an individual.[8] TPMT*3B mutation alone is associated with a 9-fold reduction in catalytic activity, whereas the TPMT*3C leads to a 1.4-fold reduction. The presence of both mutations (TPMT*3A), however, is associated with a complete loss of enzyme activity. Similarly, the less common mutant TPMT*2 leads to complete loss of activity. Four other rare TPMT alleles have since been described.[9]

TPMT methylation competes with the activation pathway and influences the relative proportion of intracellular active 6-TGN produced by a given individual. This inverse relationship between TPMT and 6-TGN has important implications in both the efficacy and toxicity of thiopurines. Patients with intermediate or absent TPMT activity can produce significantly higher concentrations of 6-TGN. The negative correlation between TPMT and 6-TGN was first reported in the treatment of childhood leukemia[10] and has since been confirmed among pediatric IBD patients.[11] The most noteworthy of the safety implications is that TPMT deficiency is associated with major elevations in 6-TGN levels, and patients experience profound, potentially life-threatening, myelo-

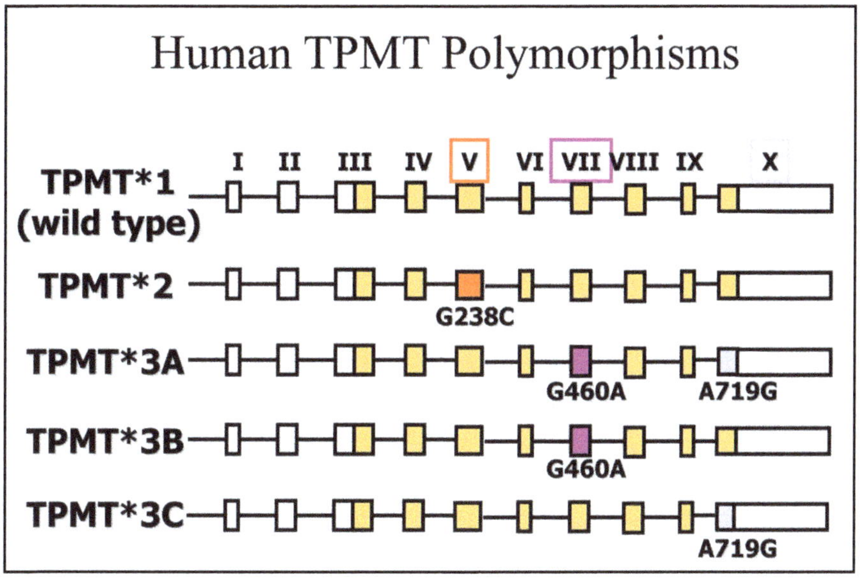

FIGURE 18-2. Genetic TPMT polymorphisms.

suppression when treated with standard or even low-dose therapy.[12,13]

Concomitant medications may also influence TPMT enzyme activity and can affect the safety and efficacy of thiopurines. It has been demonstrated among IBD patients that 5-ASA-containing compounds cause in vitro inhibition of recombinant human TPMT.[14] The clinical correlate of this interaction has been reported with both 6-MP and olsalazine.[15] Caution should be taken when coadministering 5-ASAs and thiopurines, as TPMT inhibition may increase the risk of developing myelosuppression. This effect may also vary depending on the 5-ASA an individual is receiving, such that mesalamine may have the greatest effect on the metabolism of thiopurines.[16] A recent study suggested that, although an interaction between AZA and 5-ASAs does exist, an alternate mechanism to TPMT inhibition might be responsible for the change in thiopurine pharmacokinetics.[17] After 5-ASA withdrawal, the mean 6-TGN levels significantly decreased without significant changes in TPMT activity or blood counts. This effect may be additive in patients already genetically determined to produce lower levels of the TPMT enzyme, such that diligent blood count monitoring is necessary. Patients receiving concomitant allopurinol must be carefully monitored as they are at risk of marked myelosuppression given its blockade of xanthine oxidase, an important enzyme for the catabolism of thiopurines. A recent study suggests that certain IBD patients may benefit from adding allopurinol to 6-MP/AZA as an iatrogenic mechanism of altering the metabolite profile in favor of 6-TGN production.[18]

ADVERSE EVENTS

The adverse events associated with thiopurines may be categorized as either non dose-dependent (allergic/idiosyncratic) or dose-dependent. Both the Pearson and Cochrane analyses[19,20] have reported that adverse events severe enough to cause withdrawal from the controlled trials occurred more frequently among 6-MP/AZA treated patients as compared to placebo (9% versus 2%). However, the number needed to treat (NNT) to observe an adverse event in 1 patient was approximately 15.

Hypersensitivity Reactions

Approximately 5% to 10% of patients are unable to tolerate thiopurines regardless of what dose is administered and irrespective of their underlying drug metabolism (non dose-dependent). These allergic reactions typically occur within 2 to 4 weeks of initiating therapy and are characterized by a "flu-like" illness, malaise, fevers, nausea, rash, abdominal pain, pancreatitis, and rarely a drug hepatitis. A certain proportion of patients who experienced an allergic reaction initially to AZA may be successfully rechallenged with 6-MP.[21] The theory is that the patient is reacting to the imidazole ring found on AZA but not 6-MP. This type of "thiopurine switch," however, is not recommended for patients who experienced pancreatitis. In general, the majority of patients who experienced idiosyncratic reactions require alternate immunomodulators such as methotrexate. Although once a promising alternative for patients allergic to 6-MP/AZA, thioguanine (6-TG), a sister compound to 6-MP, has been shown to cause significant liver toxicity and is not safe in IBD patients.[22]

Myelosuppression

The most commonly observed dose-dependent adverse event is myelosuppression, most commonly manifested as leukopenia. The frequency of leukopenia reported in the literature varies from 2.2% to 15% of patients.[23,24] This wide range is due to the different cut points chosen to define leukopenia (<2000 versus <4000) in the literature. The majority of leukopenic events respond to dose reduction or discontinuation; however, infectious complications do increase when the white blood cell count (WBC) is less than 2000, and these patients must be carefully monitored. Connell et al[23] observed that leukopenia (WBC <3000) was observed in 28 of 739 (3.8%) patients and 9 of 28 patients had a WBC less than 2000. Two of these 9 patients died of sepsis. Present et al[24] reported that 7.4% of patients experienced an infectious complication, which does not appear to be significantly increased over that expected in a control population. Moreover, it is believed that the risk of infection, including those attributed to opportunistic organisms, is highest in patients on multiple immunosuppressants, with steroids significantly contributing to that risk. Now that infliximab has been added to the therapeutic pyramid, caution should be taken and patients closely monitored for infectious complications. Thrombocytopenia can occur in conjunction with leukopenia or can be an isolated incident. If the drop in platelet count does not improve with dose reduction and/or cessation of therapy, then patients should undergo further evaluation, focusing on the potential hepatotoxic effect of thiopurines. Pharmacogenetic testing with TPMT may reduce the number of leukopenic events occurring in thiopurine-treated patients

Hepatotoxicity

Although the exact mechanisms remain unclear, thiopurines appear to affect the liver in a variety of ways. A certain proportion of patients may experience mild elevations in transaminases.[25] Recent evidence suggests that this form of mild toxicity is dose-dependent and that there may be a biochemical explanation for this form of liver toxicity, which will be described further.[11,26] The majority of such patients respond to dose reduction such that cessation of therapy is rarely necessary. Moreover, the liver enzymes may normalize on their own without any dose changes. For those patients who do not normalize their enzymes over time, the long-term consequences remain unknown and merit further exploration. The potentially serious hepatic effects of thiopurines were brought to the forefront when nodular regenerative hyperplasia (NRH) was observed in both leukemia and IBD patients treated with 6-TG, the sister compound to 6-MP.[22,27] NRH has also recently been described in IBD patients treated with AZA,[28] and thus raises the level of concern for the potential hepatotoxic effects of all thiopurines. Although the exact mechanism of thiopurine-related NRH remains unknown, it has been proposed that it is more idiosyncratic in nature than dose- or metabolite-dependent.

Malignancy

The relationship of malignancy and thiopurines remains a controversial topic. Connell et al did not observe an increased risk of cancer over that expected in a population of 755 patients treated over a 30-year period.[29] Present et al reported a 3% rate of malignant lymphoma, with the incidence and type of tumors similar to that expected in a background population.[24] Lewis et al first reported, using a hypothetical Markov model, that the benefits of thiopurines outweigh the risks, including malignancy.[30] Subsequently, the same group performed a retrospective cohort study using the General Practice Research Database UK database and concluded that there did not appear to be an increase risk of lymphoma associated with 6-MP use among IBD patients.[31] Population-based studies suggest the possibility of a small increased risk for the development of cancer in CD patients; however, the use of immunomodulators do not significantly increase that risk.[32,33] Results from the Mayo Clinic have suggested that the treatment of IBD patients with thiopurines appears to be associated with a small increased risk of Epstein-Barr virus-positive lymphoma.[34] A more recent meta-analysis suggested a 4-fold increased risk of lymphoma in IBD patients treated with AZA/6-MP. The study reported that the increased risk of lymphoma could be a result of the medications, the severity of the underlying disease, or a combination of the two.[35] It is unclear if this is a dose-dependent phenomenon, and further studies are needed to examine the potential implications of the inherited variations in 6-MP/AZA metabolism on the possible carcinogenic effect of thiopurines.

PREGNANCY

The safety of thiopurines in pregnancy also remains a controversial topic given the conflicting data as well as the lack of prospective data reported among IBD patients. 6-MP is rated as a category D medication, or positive evidence of risk to the fetus, according to the FDA (based on animal studies). A Danish cohort study based on data from a population-based prescription registry, the Danish Birth Registry and the Hospital Discharge Registry, examined the risk of congenital malformations and perinatal mortality among IBD patients treated with 6-MP.[36] In order to examine the risk of congenital malformations, 9 pregnancies exposed 30 days before conception or during the first trimester were included; and to examine preterm birth and low birthweight, 10 pregnancies exposed during the entire pregnancy were included. Outcomes were compared with those of 19,418 pregnancies in which no drugs were prescribed to the mothers. Fifty-five percent of the exposed women had IBD, and 45% had other diseases. Adjusted OR for congenital malformations, perinatal mortality, pre-term birth, and low birthweight were 6.7 (95% confidence interval [CI] 1.4 to 32.4), 20.0 (2.5 to 161.4), 6.6 (1.7 to 25.9), and 3.8 (0.4 to 33.3), respectively. The results of this small study suggest that there is an increased risk of congenital malformations, perinatal mortality, and pre-term birth in children born to women treated with AZA or mercaptopurine during pregnancy. The results were no longer significant when a woman with autoimmune hepatitis was removed from the analysis. Another study reported the outcome of 72 pregnancies in patients with IBD who were previously treated with 6-MP with 3 different doses of 50, 75, and 100 mg/d, for a median duration of 18 months, along with long-term follow-up of the children.[37] Group 1 (patients with IBD who conceived 6 months to 22 years after stopping 6-MP [median 72 months]) included 72 pregnancies carried by 29 women. There were 51 live births (4 premature), 16 spontaneous abortions, 1 stillbirth, 2 therapeutic abortions due to abnormal amniocentesis, and 2 ectopic pregnancies. The total incidence of fetal loss was 29.2%. In group 2 (patients with IBD who never received 6-MP prior to conception), 75 women had 140 pregnancies resulting in 120 live births (8 premature), 18 spontaneous abortions, and 2 stillbirths. There were no cases of ectopic pregnancies or abnormal amniocentesis. The total incidence of fetal loss was 14.3%. The incidence of fetal loss was higher in women with IBD who had been previously treated with 6-MP compared with those who had not. As per the authors' conclusions, it is unclear if the increased fetal loss was related to the older age at conception in the 6-MP group, longer duration of disease, initially more severe disease, or use of 6-MP. There was no increase in the incidence of developmental defects when the mothers had been treated with 6-MP prior to pregnancy. Francella et al evaluated the potential toxicity of 6-MP, based on a retrospective review of the records of 485 patients who had received the drug.[38] Of the 462 patients who were contacted, 155 conceived at least one pregnancy after developing IBD. Pregnancies were analyzed as to whether the patient had taken 6-MP before or at the time of conception, as compared to those IBD patients who had their pregnancies before taking 6-MP. Based on their findings, there was no statistical difference in spontaneous abortion rate, abortion secondary to a birth defect, major congenital malformations, neoplasia, or increased infections among male or female patients taking 6-MP compared with controls (RR = 0.85 [0.47 to 1.55], P=0.59). The authors concluded that 6-MP use before or at the time of conception or during pregnancy appears to be safe. It should be noted that further studies are clearly needed and therapeutic decisions during pregnancy must be a collaborative effort between the patient and the treating physician based on best available evidence. The risk of both the patient and the fetus must be appreciated in the face of active disease as well as a thiopurine-induced remission. With regard to breastfeeding, low concentrations of AZA are found in breast milk, and in most cases nursing is not recommended because of unknown risk of long-term immunosuppression and carcinogenesis to the child. That being said, it has been suggested that postpartum is a high-risk state for women, and it may be deleterious to stop 6-MP during this time. The data in such cases are lacking, rendering recommendations difficult.

CLINICAL TRIALS

The efficacy of AZA and 6-MP for both the induction and maintenance of a disease-free remission in CD has been evaluated in a number of controlled, clinical trials. There are, however, limited data for such indication in UC. AZA and 6-MP were first introduced into the treatment of UC in the 1960s by both Bean and Bowen.[39,40] Encouraging results prompted controlled trials in UC. Jewell and Truelove reported on the value of AZA in acute relapse of UC as well as maintenance of remission.[41] All patients with active disease were randomized to steroids plus AZA (2.5 mg/kg/d) or steroids plus placebo. As expected, there was no difference in efficacy between the 2 groups when assessed at 4 weeks (Table 18-1). There was, however, a trend toward endoscopic and histologic improvement in the AZA-treated group. After 12 months, there were more treatment failures in the placebo-treated group than the AZA group. However, when arbitrarily grouping patients based on number of flares during the first year of therapy, there did not appear to be a significant difference between the 2 groups (P=0.18; Table 18-2). The numbers were very small as well, due to the fact that some patients were reduced from 2.5 mg/kg/d to 1.5 mg/kg/d, making interpretation of these data and extrapolation to clinical practice very difficult. A small study examined the efficacy of AZA as compared to sulfasalazine after just 3 months of therapy. Caprilli found no difference in efficacy among the 2 drugs, such that both were efficacious in reducing clinical symptoms and improving endoscopic and histologic lesions.[42] Kirk and Lennard-Jones reported that, although disease activity did decrease as compared to baseline in the AZA-treated group, it did not differ from the placebo-treated group. The dose of steroids, however, was significantly lower among the AZA-treated patients at 6 months (see Table 18-1).[43]

Population-based natural history studies have shown that, in the absence of immunomodulators, 29% of patients necessitating steroid therapy will undergo colectomy 12 months after initiating steroids.[44] To date, thiopurines remain the therapy of choice for the successful

TABLE 18-1

INDUCTION OF REMISSION IN ULCERATIVE COLITIS: PLACEBO-CONTROLLED TRIALS

Study	Total No. of Patients	Efficacy Measure	Efficacy (Drug)	Efficacy (Placebo)	P Value	Thiopurine Starting Dose (mg/kg/d)	Treatment Duration (Months)
Part 1: Jewell[41]	80	Remission %	78	68	NS	AZA 2.5	1
Kirk[43]	44	Disease activity score and prednisone dose	2.3 mg/d	13.6 mg/d	<0.001	AZA 2.0 to 2.5	6

TABLE 18-2

MAINTENANCE OF REMISSION IN ULCERATIVE COLITIS: PLACEBO-CONTROLLED TRIALS

Study	Total No. of Patients	Efficacy Measure	Efficacy (Drug)	Efficacy (Placebo)	P Value	AZA Starting Dose	Treatment Duration (Months)
Part 2: Jewell[41]	80	Remission %	40	23	NS	1.5 to 2.5 (mg/kg/d)	12
Hawthorne[46]	67	Relapse %	59	36	0.04	100 mg/d	12
Rosenberg[45]	30	Mean prednisone dose (mg/d)	7.9 mg	15.8 mg	<0.05	1.5 (mg/kg/d)	6

maintenance of a steroid-free quiescent disease state. The timing of the introduction of thiopurines in patients dependent on corticosteroids for disease remission may vary among clinicians. In general, it is recommended that thiopurines be added to the therapeutic regimen in patients failing to wean off corticosteroids during their first attempt at tapering the dose, or alternatively after a second attempt. The steroid withdrawal studies conducted in UC have supported the addition of AZA to steroid-treated patients (see Table 18-2).

Rosenberg et al conducted a steroid withdrawal study and found that AZA permits reduction of steroid dose without worsening of disease as measured at 6 months.[45] A total of 7 of 16 patients were able to discontinue steroids without worsening of symptoms, compared to only 1 of 14 treated with placebo. Moreover, the average steroid reduction in the AZA group at the end of the trial was -11.5 mg/d compared to -6.1 mg/d in the placebo group. To date, the most referenced study highlighting the benefits of long-term AZA in UC is the study reported by Hawthorne et al.[46] The objective of this study was to determine whether AZA can prevent relapse in UC employing a 1-year placebo-controlled, double-blind trial of withdrawal or continuation of AZA. The 1-year relapse rate was 36% for patients continuing AZA and 59% for those withdrawn and placed on placebo. The authors concluded that AZA maintenance treatment was beneficial for a minimum of 2 years if patients were already in remission on AZA.

Based on these reports, AZA appears to be most effective as a steroid-sparing agent and in maintaining a steroid-free remission, thus limiting its use as monotherapy for induction. In UC patients resistant to corticosteroids, cyclosporine (CyA) may serve as an effective medical alternative to surgery in the face of moderate to severe disease activity. The safety concerns surrounding long-term CyA generally renders this drug an unacceptable maintenance therapy. If CyA is indeed being used to decrease the rate of colectomy, patients need to be able to respond to a safer long-term maintenance therapy. The experience from the University of Chicago demonstrates that the rate of colectomy is decreased in patients receiving 6-MP/AZA and CyA, as compared to CyA alone.[47] If patients have already failed what is considered appropriate dosing and duration of thiopurines, clinicians may want to rethink the use of CyA given its toxicity profile; surgery may be a more appropriate alternative. This highlights again the concept of optimizing thiopurine therapy to maximize the therapeutic benefit of thiopurines in the role in which they have been implicated.

The use of infliximab in combination with thiopurines in general has a different therapeutic implication than what was just described for combination steroids and thiopurines. A large majority of patients receiving infliximab for UC manifest disease activity despite corticosteroids and/or thiopurines.[48] These patients require infliximab for the control of symptoms. If patients remain on suboptimal doses of thiopurines, there is a greater probability that they will require both induction and maintenance infliximab for control of disease activity and for steroid-sparing. There are, however, a subgroup of patients who remain refractory to thiopurines despite appropriate dosing and who rely on infliximab for maintenance of a steroid-free remission. In such cases, despite the lack of efficacy of thiopurine monotherapy, the combination of thiopurines and infliximab may offer a therapeutic advantage over infliximab alone. Roblin et al recently demonstrated evidence of a drug interaction between infliximab and AZA.[49] They found the level of active 6-TGN metabolites measured post-infusion was highly predictive of clinical response to infliximab, such that higher 6-TGN levels were measured in responders (478) as compared to nonresponders (257). An additional benefit of combination therapy is the immunomodulatory properties of thiopurines that may confer protection against the development of antibodies to infliximab (ATI). It has been shown that the formation of ATIs is lower in CD patients receiving concomitant thiopurine therapy.[50] This phenomenon has both efficacy and safety implications. It has been suggested that ATI formation contributes to attenuation of response to infliximab over time, which can significantly impact patient outcomes. Theoretically, by reducing the titer of anti-infliximab antibodies, more of the active drug would be available to exert its biologic properties. From a safety perspective, the frequency of infusion reactions may be reduced by decreasing the formation of ATIs, which in turn will have a direct effect on the proportion of patients who can tolerate infliximab, thus maximizing the therapeutic benefits.[51] The majority of evidence to date comes from the CD literature, and, as the new data are revealed from the UC infliximab trials, more information will be available for combination therapy.

Once initiated, the question then remains as to how long thiopurine therapy should be continued and whether or not there is any benefit to this form of therapy after a certain period of time. The initial results from a retrospective analysis based on a small number of CD patients suggested that there may no longer be a benefit to therapy after 4 to 5 years of continued treatment.[52] However, this study did show that there is a higher relapse rate in patients who discontinued therapy early at the 5-year mark as compared to those remaining on therapy (75% versus 32%). In a follow-up study, Lemann et al tested patients in remission after 42 months of AZA therapy to see whether stopping AZA was less effective than its continuation.[53] Based on their results, they could not conclude that continuation was superior to stopping therapy because the relapse rate was relatively low in the placebo group (21%). Further withdrawal studies are warranted. However, until then, patients should be informed about the possibility of "indefinite" therapy, and clinicians may want to consider the indication for initiating therapy when deciding which patients will have a lower relapse rate after withdrawal. Rosenberg showed that patients can receive long-term benefit from at least 2 years of AZA and demonstrated that a substantial proportion of patients flared after therapy was discontinued.[45]

The notion of disease-modifying therapies has recently been brought to the forefront with the introduction of biological therapies to our therapeutic armamentarium; more specifically, the concept that mucosal healing may be an outcome that serves as a potential marker or perhaps even a predictor of altering the natural history of disease. In an unblinded and uncontrolled study published by D'Haens et al,[54] the majority of patients on AZA were able to achieve near to complete healing of the colonic and ileal mucosa.

PHARMACOGENETICS AND THERAPEUTIC DRUG MONITORING

Pharmacogenetics

TPMT methylates thiopurine metabolites at the expense of the formation of 6-TGN. However, patients with less than normal TPMT expression and activity can produce significantly higher concentrations of 6-TGN. This inverse relationship between TPMT and 6-TGN has important implications in both the efficacy and toxicity of thiopurines. The most significant safety implication is the association between TPMT deficiency and the development of potentially fatal myelosuppression when treated with standard or even low-dose therapy secondary to major elevations in 6-TGN as reported in the oncology literature.[55,56] The association between TPMT and myelosuppression in IBD patients was published by Colombel et al, who reported that 27% of

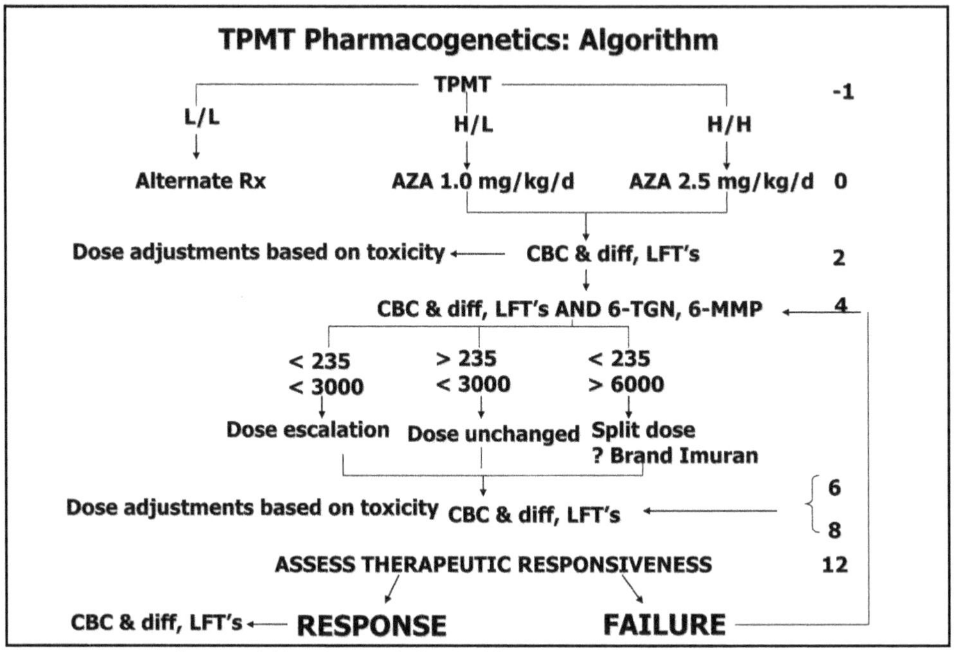

FIGURE 18-3. Proposed TPMT and thiopurine metabolite algorithm.

IBD patients experienced leukopenia and/or thrombocytopenia attributable to abnormal TPMT activity.[57] Moreover, TPMT deficiency (homozygote mutant) accounted for 10% of the cases, and the median time to onset of bone marrow suppression was 1 month, while 17% of cases were TPMT heterozygotes. This study also brought attention to the fact that not all myelosuppression—in fact a minority of cases in this study—is secondary to low TPMT activity. Also, patients should be regularly monitored with complete blood counts, and secondary causes such as concomitant medications or concurrent viral illness should be considered. Other reports outside of the IBD literature also support the positive association between TPMT and leukopenia and have proposed screening patients for low TPMT activity prior to initiating thiopurine therapy to identify at-risk individuals and to modify dosing.[58,59] The a priori knowledge of an individual's TPMT activity can identify those patients prone to early leukopenic events when treated with standard doses of thiopurines as a result of intermediate TPMT levels. Moreover, the 1 in 300 individuals at risk for potentially life-threatening complications can be rapidly identified, and alternate immunomodulators can be administered. Intermediate TPMT activity is certainly not a contraindication for thiopurine use. Typically, these patients can safely receive thiopurines at lower doses (30% to 50% of standard dose), and dose escalation can be successful while patients are monitored closely with regular blood counts and possibly 6-TGN concentrations.[60,61] For the majority of thiopurine recipients (≅ 90%), clinicians can safely administer an optimal starting dose of 6-MP (1 to 1.5 mg/kg/d) and AZA (2.0 to 2.5 mg/kg/d) as a result of normal to high TPMT activity. Despite the apparent safety advantage to employing pharmacogenetic TPMT-based dosing over empiric or weight-based strategies, controversy still remains as to whether TPMT-based dosing really does maximize patient safety. Both a prospective[62] and retrospective[63] study, presented in abstract form only, have attempted to answer this question in IBD; however, too few patients and the inability to capture those patients who would have either discontinued therapy due to early leukopenia or already had a dose reduction prior to evaluation makes these studies difficult to interpret. Until definitive information is available, clinicians will continue to individualize dosing based on their own practice experience and preference. Whether it is empiric or TPMT-based dosing, patients require regular blood count and liver chemistry monitoring throughout the duration of thiopurine therapy. At minimum, blood counts should be monitored every 2 weeks for the first month, and clinicians may consider monthly monitoring thereafter for 2 months, followed by every 2 months for 4 months and every 3 months thereafter. In patients who do not get TPMT prior to dose initiation, clinicians may consider weekly monitoring for the first 6 weeks of therapy, as early leukopenia can occur in TPMT-deficient patients treated with standard doses. Additionally blood counts should be monitored 2 to 3 weeks after any dose escalation and then resume their individualized monitoring schedule. Figure 18-3 illustrates an algorithmic approach to pharmacogenetic testing and therapeutic drug monitoring.

In contrast to what we know about the influence of TPMT deficiency on myelosuppression, the safety implications of having high TPMT activity remains unclear. As mentioned earlier, hepatotoxicity is, in part, a dose-dependent safety concern in patients receiving thiopurines. Elevated levels of 6-MMP have been shown to be associated with an increased frequency of hepatotoxicity as defined by elevations in transaminases more than 2 times over normal.[11,26] These findings suggest that the accumulation of 6-MMP could play an important role in the pathogenesis of 6-MP-induced hepatic toxicity. Given that TPMT results in the formation of 6-MMP, it would be a rational assumption that patients with high TPMT produce potentially hepatotoxic levels of 6-MMP. Erythrocyte TPMT activity levels parallel the enzyme activity in other tissues, particularly the liver, and thus it could be hypothesized that the first-pass catabolism of the drug in the liver by higher than normal TPMT activity may lead to the accumulation of higher levels of 6-MMP. Liver-associated biochemical laboratory abnormalities typically normalize in a timely manner in response to dose reduction as a result of a decrease in 6-MMP levels. Not all patients experience an elevation in transaminases in association with high 6-MMP levels, and few merit a significant dose reduction; however these patients should be closely monitored. There is often a debate as to whether the addition of these tests to the management of thiopurine-treated IBD patients is cost-effective. A decision analysis performed by Winter et al reported that TPMT screening was cost-effective, taking into account direct costs associated with leukopenia and infectious complications and costs per life years saved.[64] Another decision analysis was performed to estimate the potential costs and effectiveness of TPMT screening and metabolite monitoring as disease management strategies for CD. This study demonstrated that the utilization of TPMT screening and metabolite monitoring strategies within a community-care setting improves therapeutic outcomes and reduces costs for steroid-treated chronically active CD patients.[65]

Although TPMT plays an important role in the safe administration of thiopurines, further studies are needed to determine whether TPMT activity is an independent predictor of efficacy or whether 6-TGN level remains a more significant factor in determining thiopurine response. Cuffari et al reported that patients with a TPMT level less than 15.3 U/mL have a 6.2-fold increased likelihood of response to AZA and found the TPMT levels to be an independent predictor.[66] Further studies are needed to further separate the role of TPMT as a predictor as compared to the 6-TGN level.

Therapeutic Drug Monitoring

The importance of metabolite monitoring and TPMT activity was first brought to our attention through the research initiated in childhood ALL.[12,13] Initial studies in IBD were conducted in the pediatric age group and reported that 6-TGN was shown to be significantly and independently associated with therapeutic response.[11,67] This study demonstrated that significantly higher median 6-TGN levels were observed at points of clinical response (312) versus nonresponse (199). Further analysis revealed that the best probability of treatment response was not significantly increased until 6-TGN levels were greater than 235. Also, the OR of a therapeutic response for a 6-TG level higher than a cutoff of 235 was 5.0 as compared to when the levels were below this cut-point. A certain percentage of patients did achieve a therapeutic response with levels less than 235; however, this response rate was almost less than half the proportion of patients (78%) achieving therapeutic response when levels were more than 235. Subtherapeutic dosing, or (based on these studies) perhaps more appropriately subtherapeutic 6-TGN levels, is the most common reason why patients are not responding to thiopurines. Cuffari et al demonstrated that most patients who did not initially respond to low-dose thiopurine therapy who underwent dose escalation responded well once they achieved 6-TGN levels higher than 250.[68] Gupta et al similarly showed that the likelihood of response did not increase significantly at 6-TGN levels higher than 235; however, serial metabolite measurements in children with active disease showed that increasing 6-TGN levels correlated with disease remission.[69] Mardini et al evaluated the role of metabolite monitoring in clinical practice and found that metabolite levels may be helpful to adjust dosing in order to achieve clinical remission and avoid unnecessary dose adjustments.[70] Despite these initial positive studies, there remains conflicting data on the clinical utility of monitoring in IBD. Lowry et al observed that 6-TGN levels did not correlate with disease activity as measured by the IBDQ for quality of life outcome.[71] Belaiche et al similarly did not find a correlation between 6-TGN levels and clinical response; however, they did find metabolite monitoring useful to confirm compliance and supported its role in nonresponders to safely allow for dose escalation.[72] Table 18-3 lists the various studies published to date on the utility of 6-MP metabolite levels in IBD patients.[11,67-72] These discrepancies may be attributed to the variability in the outcome measure of response and the patient population studied. A recent meta-analysis pooled available data to provide a more precise estimate of the association between 6-TGN levels and IBD activity. This study reported that patients with 6-TGN levels above a level of 235 were more likely to be in remission (62%) than those below the threshold value (36%) (pooled OR 3.3; 95% CI 1.7 to 6.3; $P<0.001$).[73] Prospective randomized, dose-optimization studies are currently underway to determine if individualized (pharmacogenetics/TPMT- and pharmacokinetic/6-TGN-based) dosing is superior, both in safety and efficacy, to weight-based dosing.

Perhaps the most significant role of metabolite monitoring is in defining therapeutic failures. Noncompliance and under-dosing remain the most common reasons for therapeutic failure. Both of these can be uncovered by measuring 6-MP metabolite levels. When both 6-TGN and 6-MMP levels are undetectable, there is a high likelihood

TABLE 18-3

REPORTS OF 6-MP METABOLITE MONITORING IN IBD

Study	Total No. of Patients	Patient Population	Outcome Measure	Correlation Between 6-TGN and Disease Activity
Cuffari[66]	25	Children	HBI	Yes
Dubinsky[11]	93	Children	HBI	Yes
Lowry[71]	170	Adults	IBDQ	No
Belaiche[72]	28	Adults	CDAI	No
Cuffari[67]	82	Adults	HBI	Yes
Gupta[69]	101	Children	PCDAI/TLW	No
Dubinsky[26]	51	Adults	HBI	Yes

that the patient is not adhering to therapy. However, a subgroup of patients continues to fail therapy despite dose escalation and receiving standard or even higher than standard doses of thiopurines. These patients can be divided into 2 distinct subgroups and are defined biochemically by their metabolite profiles. The most common subgroup is composed of patients *resistant* to thiopurines and biochemically characterized by the persistence of subtherapeutic 6-TGN (<235) and the preferential shunting toward excessive potentially hepatotoxic 6-MMP levels upon 6-MP/AZA dose escalation.[26] Individuals unmask this metabolic profile when they are challenged with higher doses of the drug. There is a small group of *refractory* patients who, despite therapeutic (>235) and often potentially toxic 6-TGN (>450) levels, are unable to benefit from the immunosuppressive properties of these therapies. The identification of these 2 subgroups early on the course of therapy can significantly improve patient outcomes by moving patients quickly to alternate immunomodulator therapy.

FUTURE DIRECTIVES

6-MP and AZA remain an important part of UC management. The role of these therapies continues to evolve in the management of IBD patients with a focus on disease modification and altering the natural history of disease. The introduction of pharmacogenetic testing and drug monitoring has significantly improved the management of patients receiving thiopurine therapy. The safety advantage of TPMT screening prior to drug initiation has become an important part of clinical practice and can have a significant impact on patient outcome from both a safety and efficacy perspective. The knowledge of an individual's metabolic preference for 6-TGN or 6-MMP production and, hence, propensity to respond or to be resistant to 6-MP/AZA is also very important for the optimization of the most commonly used immunomodulator for the long-term treatment of IBD. These alternate management strategies still require further evaluation, and prospective studies are currently underway to validate the therapeutic benefits of metabolite monitoring in management of IBD patients.

REFERENCES

1. Van Os EC, Zins BJ, Sandborn WJ, et al. Azathioprine pharmacokinetics after intravenous, oral, delayed release oral and rectal foam administration. *Gut.* 1996;39:63-68.
2. Ding TL, Benet LZ. Comparative bioavailability and pharmacokinetic study of azathioprine and 6-mercaptopurine in the rhesus monkey. *Drug Metab Dispos.* 1979;7:373-377.
3. Tiede I, Fritz G, Strand S, et al. CD28-dependent Rac1 activation is the molecular target of azathioprine in primary human CD4+ T lymphocytes. *J Clin Invest.* 2003;111:1133-1145.
4. Lennard L. The clinical pharmacology of 6-mercaptopurine. *Eur J Clin Pharmacol.* 1992;43:329-339.
5. Weinshilboum RM, Sladek SL. Mercaptopurine pharmacogenetics: Monogenic inheritance of erythrocyte thiopurine methyltransferase activity. *Am J Hum Genet.* 1980;32:651-662.
6. Hon YY, Fessing MY, Pui CH, Relling MV, Krynetski EY, Evans WE. Polymorphism of the thiopurine S-methyltransferase gene in African-Americans. *Human Molecular Genetics.* 1999;8:371-376.

7. Lee FJ, Kalow W. Thiopurine S methyltransferase activity in a Chinese population. *Clin Pharm Ther.* 1993;54:28-33.

8. Tai HL, Krynetski EY, Yates CR, et al. Thiopurine S methyltransferase deficiency: two nucleotide transitions define the most prevalent mutant allele associated with loss of catalytic activity in Caucasians. *Am J Hum Genet.* 1996;58:694-702.

9. Otterness DM, Szumlanski CL, Wood TC, Weinshilboum RM. Human thiopurine methyltransferase pharmacogenetics: kindred with a terminal exon splice junction mutation that results in loss of activity. *J Clin Invest.* 1998;101:1036-1044.

10. Lennard L, Van Loon JA, Weinshilboum RM. Pharmacogenetics of acute azathioprine toxicity: relationship to thiopurine methyltransferase genetic polymorphism. *Clin Pharmacol Ther.* 1989;46:149-154.

11. Dubinsky MC, Lamothe S, Yang HY, et al. Pharmacogenomics and metabolite measurement for 6-mercaptopurine therapy in inflammatory bowel disease. *Gastroenterology.* 2000;118:705-713.

12. Lennard L, Lilleyman JS. Variable 6-mercaptopurine metabolism and treatment outcome in childhood lymphoblastic leukemia. *J Clin Oncol.* 1989;7:1816-1823.

13. Lennard L, Van Loon JA, Weinshilboum RM. Pharmacogenetics of acute azathioprine toxicity: relationship to thiopurine methyltransferase genetic polymorphism. *Clin Pharmacol Ther.* 1989;46:149-154.

14. Szumlanski CL, Weinshilboum RM. Sulphasalazine inhibition of thiopurine methyltransferase: possible mechanism for interaction with 6-mercaptopurine and azathioprine. *Br J Clin Pharm.* 1995;39:456-459.

15. Lewis LD, Benin A, Szumlanski CL, et al. Olsalazine and 6-mercaptopurine-related bone marrow suppression: a possible drug-drug interaction. *Clin Pharm Ther.* 1997;62:464-475.

16. Lowry PW, Franklin CL, Weaver AL, et al. Leukopenia resulting from a drug interaction between azathioprine or 6-mercaptopurine and mesalamine, sulphasalazine, or balsalazide. *Gut.* 2001;49:656-664.

17. Dewitt O , Vanheuverzwyn R, Desager JP, Horsmans Y. Interaction between azathioprine and aminosalicylates: an in vivo study in patients with Crohn's disease. *Aliment Pharmacol Ther.* 2002;16:79-85.

18. Sparrow MP, Hande SA, Friedman S, et al. Allopurinol safely and effectively optimizes thioguanine metabolites in inflammatory bowel disease patients not responding to azathioprine and mercaptopurine. *Aliment Pharmacol Ther.* 2005;22:441-446.

19. Pearson DC, May GR, Fick GH, Sutherland LR. Azathioprine and 6-Mercaptopurine in Crohn's disease: a meta-analysis. *Ann Intern Med.* 1995;123:132-142.

20. Sandborn W, Sutherland L, Pearson D, May G, Modigliani R, Prantera C. Azathioprine or 6-mercaptopurine or inducing remission of Crohn's disease. *Cochrane Database of Systematic Reviews.* 2000;3.

21. McGovern DP, Shobowale-Bakre E, Duley J, et al. Early azathioprine intolerance in IBD patients is imidazole-related and independent of thiopurine methyl transferase (TPMT) activity. *Gastroenterology.* 2000;118:A890.

22. Dubinsky MC, Vasiliauskas EA, Singh H, et al. 6-thioguanine (6-TG) can cause serious liver injury in inflammatory bowel disease (IBD) patients. *Gastroenterology* 2003;125:298-303.

23. Connell WR, Kamm MA, Ritchie JK, Lennard-Jones JE. Bone marrow toxicity caused by azathioprine in inflammatory bowel disease: 27 years of experience. *Gut.* 1993;34:1081-1085.

24. Present DH, Meltzer SJ, Krumholz MP, Wolke A, Korelitz BI. 6-Mercaptopurine in the management of inflammatory bowel disease: short- and long-term toxicity. *Ann Intern Med.* 1989;111:641-649.

25. Kirschner BS. Safety of azathioprine and 6-mercaptopurine in pediatric patients with inflammatory bowel disease. *Gastroenterology.* 1998;115:813-821.

26. Dubinsky MC, Hassard PV, Seidman EG, et al. Preliminary evidence suggests that 6-MP metabolite profiles provide a biochemical explanation for 6-MP resistance in patients with inflammatory bowel disease. *Gastroenterology.* 2002;122:904-915.

27. Stork LC, Broxson EH, Sather H, et al. Oral 6-thioguanine causes late onset splenomegaly and portal hypertension in a subset of children with acute lymphoblastic leukemia. *Gastroenterology.* 2002;122A:T833.

28. Daniel F, Cadranel JF, Seksik P, et al. Azathioprine induced nodular regenerative hyperplasia in IBD patients. *Gastroenterologie Clinique et Biologique.* 2005;29:600-603.

29. Connell WR, Kamm MA, Dickson M, Balkwill AM, Ritchie JK, Lennard-Jones JE. Long-term neoplasia risk after azathioprine treatment in inflammatory bowel disease. *Lancet.* 1994;343(8908):1249-1952.

30. Lewis JD, Schwartz JS, Lichtenstein GR. Azathioprine for maintenance of remission in Crohn's disease: benefits outweigh the risk of lymphoma. *Gastroenterology.* 2000;118:1018-1024.

31. Lewis JD, Bilker WB, Brensinger C, Deren JJ, Vaughn DJ, Strom BL. Inflammatory bowel disease is not associated with an increased risk of lymphoma. *Gastroenterology.* 2001;121:1080-1087.

32. Bernstein CH, Blanchard JF, Kliewer E, Wajda A. Cancer risk in patients with inflammatory bowel disease: a population based study. *Cancer.* 2001;91:854-862.

33. Loftus EV, Tremaine WJ, Habermann TM, Harmsen WS, Zinsmeitser AR, Sandborn WJ. Risk of lymphoma in inflammatory bowel disease. *Am J Gastroenterol.* 2000;95:2308-2312.

34. Dayharsh GA, Loftus EV Jr, Sandborn WJ, et al. Epstein-Barr virus-positive lymphoma in patients with inflammatory bowel disease treated with azathioprine or 6-mercaptopurine. *Gastroenterology.* 2002;122:72-77.

35. Kandiel A, Fraser AG, Korelitz BI, Brensinger C, Lewis JD. Increased risk of lymphoma among inflammatory bowel disease patients treated with azathioprine and 6-mercaptopurine. *Gut.* 2005;54:1121-1125.

36. Norgard B, Pedersen L, Fonager K, Rasmussen SN, Sorensen HT. Azathioprine, mercaptopurine and birth outcome: a population-based cohort study. *Aliment Pharmacol Ther.* 2003;17:827-834.

37. Zlatanic J, Korelitz BI, Rajapakse RM, et al. Complications of pregnancy and child development after cessation of treatment with 6-mercaptopurine for inflammatory bowel disease. *J Clin Gastroenterol.* 2003;36(4):303-309.

38. Francella A, Dyan A, Bodian C, Rubin P, Chapman M, Present DH. The safety of 6-mercaptopurine for childbearing patients with inflammatory bowel disease: a retrospective cohort study. *Gastroenterology.* 2003;124:9-17.

39. Bean RH. The treatment of chronic ulcerative colitis with 6-mercaptopurine. *Medical Journal of Australia.* 1962;49:592-593.

40. Bowen GE, Irons GV, Rhodes JB. Early experience with azathioprine in ulcerative colitis. *JAMA.* 1966;195:460-464.

41. Jewell DP, Truelove SC. Azathioprine in ulcerative colitis: final report on controlled therapeutic trial. *Br Med J.* 1974;4:627-630.

42. Caprilli R, Carratu R, Babbini M. A double blind comparison of the effectiveness of azathioprine and sulfasalazine in idiopathic proctocolitis. *Dig Dis.* 1975;20:115-120.

43. Kirk AP, Lennard-Jones JE. Controlled trial of azathioprine in chronic ulcerative colitis. *Br Med J.* 1982;284:1291-1292.

44. Faubion WA Jr, Loftus EV Jr, Harmsen WS, Zinsmeister AR, Sandborn WJ. The natural history of corticosteroid therapy for inflammatory bowel disease: a population-based study.[see comment]. *Gastroenterology.* 2001;121:255-260.

45. Rosenberg JL, Levin B, Wall AJ, et al. A controlled trial of azathioprine in the management of Crohn's disease. *Dig Dis.* 1975;20:721-726.
46. Hawthorne AB, Logan RF, Hawkey CJ, et al. Randomized controlled trial of azathioprine withdrawal in ulcerative colitis. *Br Med J.* 1992;305:20-22.
47. Cohen RD, Stein R, Hanauer SB. Intravenous cyclosporine in ulcerative colitis: a five-year experience. *Am J Gastroenterol.* 1999;94:1587-1592.
48. Sandborn W, Rachmilewitz D, Hanauer SB, et al. Infiximab induction and maintenance therapy for ulcerative colitis: The ACT 2 trial. *Gastroenterology.* 2005;128:A-104.
49. Roblin X, Serre-Debeauvais F, Phelip JM, Besssard G, Bonaz B. Drug interaction between infliximab and azathioprine in patients with Crohn's disease. *Aliment Pharmacol Ther.* 2003;18:917-925.
50. Baert F, Noman M, Vermeire S, et al. Influence of immunogenicity on the long-term efficacy of infliximab in Crohn's disease. *New Engl J Med.* 2003;348:601-608.
51. Farrell RJ, Alsahli M, Jeen YT, Falchuk KR, Peppercorn MA, Michetti P. Intravenous hydrocortisone premedication reduces antibodies to infliximab in Crohn's disease: a randomized controlled trial. *Gastroenterology.* 2003;124(4):917-924.
52. Bouhnik Y, Lemann M, Mary JY, et al. Long-term follow-up of patients with Crohn's disease treated with azathioprine or 6-mercaptopurine. *Lancet.* 1996;347:215-219.
53. Lemann M, Bouhnik Y, Colombel JF, et al. Randomized, double blind placebo controlled multicenter, azathioprine withdrawal trail in Crohn's disease. *Gastroenterology.* 2002;122:A23.
54. D'Haens G, Geboes K, Rutgeerts P. Endoscopic and histologic healing of Crohn's (ileo-) colitis with azathioprine. *Gastrointest Endosc.* 1999;50:667-671.
55. Lennard L, Rees CA, Lilleyman JS, Maddocks JL. Childhood leukemia: A relationship between intracellular 6-MP metabolites and neutropenia. *Br J Clin Pharmacol.* 1983;16:358-363.
56. Lennard L, Gibson BES, Nicole T, Lilleyman JS. Congenital thiopurine methyltransferase deficiency and 6-mercaptopurine toxicity during treatment for acute lymphoblastic leukemia. *Arch Dis Child.* 1993;69:577-579.
57. Colombel JF, Ferrari N, Debuysere H, et al. Genotypic analysis of thiopurine S-methyltransferase in patients with Crohn's disease and severe myelosuppression during azathioprine therapy. *Gastroenterology.* 2000;118:1025-1030.
58. Black AJ, McLeod HL, Capell HA, et al. Thiopurine methyltransferase genotype predicts therapy-limiting severe toxicity from azathioprine. *Ann Intern Med.* 1998;129:716-718.
59. Sebbag L, Boucher P, Davelu P, et al. Thiopurine S methyltransferase gene polymorphism ispredictive of azathioprine-induced myelosuppression in heart transplant recipients. *Transplantation.* 2000;69:1524-1527.
60. Regueiro M, Mardini H. Determination of thiopurine methyltransferase genotype or phenotype optimizes initial dosing of azathioprine for the treatment of Crohn's disease. *J Clin Gastroenterol.* 2002;35:240-244.
61. Campbell S, Kingstone K, Ghosh S. Relevance of thiopurine methyltransferase activity in inflammatory bowel disease patients maintained on low dose azathioprine. *Aliment Pharmacol Ther.* 2002;16:389-398.
62. Seddik M, Texier F, Ferrari N, et al. Hiopurine methyl transferase genotyping does not predict azathioprine induced myelosuppression in Crohn's disease. *Gastroenterology.* 2003;124:A192.
63. Curvers W, Derijks L, Stokkers P, et al. No predictive value of TPMT genotyping for leukopenia or hepatotoxicity during azathioprine therapy in inflammatory bowel disease. *Gastroenterology.* 2003:124:A49.
64. Winter J, Walker A, Shapiro D, Gaffney D, Spooner RJ, Mills PR. *Aliment Pharmacol Therapeut.* 2004;20:593-599.
65. Dubinsky MC, Reyes E, Ofman J, Chiou CF, Wade S, Sandborn WJ. A cost-effectiveness analysis of alternative disease management strategies in patients with Crohn's disease treated with azathioprine or 6-mercaptopurine. *Am J Gastroenterol.* 2005;100:2239-2247.
66. Cuffari C, Dassopoulos T, Turnbough L, Thompson RE, Bayless TM. Thiopurine methyltransferase activity influences clinical response to azathioprine in inflammatory bowel disease. *Clin Gastroenterol Hepatol.* 2004;5:410-417.
67. Cuffari C, Théorêt Y, Latour S, Seidman EG. 6-mercaptopurine metabolism in Crohn's disease: correlation with efficacy and toxicity. *Gut.* 1996;39:401-406.
68. Cuffari C, Hunt S, Bayless T. Utilization of erythrocyte 6-thioguanine metabolite levels to optimise azathioprine therapy in patients with inflammatory bowel disease. *Gut.* 2001;48:642-646.
69. Gupta P, Gokhale R, Kirschner B. 6-Mercaptopurine levels in children with inflammatory bowel disease. *J Pediatr Gastroenterol Nutr.* 2001;33:450-454.
70. Mardini HE, Arnold GL. Utility of measuring 6-methylmercaptopurine and 6-thioguanine nucleotide levels in managing inflammatory bowel disease patients treated with 6-mercaptopurine in a clinical practice setting. *J Clin Gastroenterol.* 2003;36:390-395.

Azathioprine Metabolism in Inflammatory Bowel Disease

A Physician's Guide to Metabolite Testing

19

Carmen Cuffari, MD

Critical-dose drugs are therapeutic agents that demonstrate a wide inter-patient variability in drug metabolism.[1] These inherent differences in pharmacokinetics are perceived to influence patient responsiveness to therapy and patient susceptibility to drug-induced cytotoxicity.[2,3] 6-MP and its prodrug AZA are 2 examples of critical-dose drugs that are well-known for their immunosuppressive and lymphocytotic effects in the management of patients with lymphoma and leukemia. Their immunosuppressive properties are mediated through their interference with protein synthesis and nucleic acid metabolism in the sequence that follows antigen stimulation, as well as by their cytotoxic effects on lymphoid cells.[4,5]

The metabolism of 6-MP and AZA occurs intracellularly along the competing routes catalyzed by hypoxanthine phosphoribosyltransferase and TPMT, giving rise to 6-TG and 6-MMP, respectively (Figure 19-1).[4] 6-TG is the active ribonucleotide of 6-MP that functions as a purine antagonist. The incorporation of these antimetabolites into lymphocyte DNA and RNA interferes with nucleic acid metabolism, thereby inducing lymphocytotoxicity and immunosuppression.[6,7]

An apparent genetic polymorphism has been observed in TPMT activity in both the Caucasian and African American populations. Negligible activity was noted in 0.3%, and low levels (<5U/mL of blood) in 11% of individuals.[1] TPMT enzyme deficiency is inherited as an autosomal recessive trait, and, to date, 10 mutant alleles and several silent and intronic mutations have been described.[8] In patients with the heterozygous TPMT genotype, 6-MP metabolism is shunted preferentially into the production of 6-TG nucleotides. Although 6-TG nucleotides are thought to be lymphocytotic and beneficial in the treatment of patients with leukemia and lymphoma, patients with low (<5) TPMT activity are at risk for bone marrow suppression by achieving potentially toxic erythrocyte 6-TG levels on standard doses of 6-MP.[4,9,10] Despite low TPMT enzyme activity levels, therapeutic erythrocyte 6-TG metabolite levels can still be achieved without untoward cytotoxicity by lowering the dose of 6-MP 10-fold to 15-fold.[11]

These pharmacogenetic differences in 6-MP and AZA metabolism are also known to influence clinical responsiveness to therapy in patients with leukemia. Patients with high TPMT activity shunt 6-MP metabolism away from the production of 6-TG nucleotides and into the preferential formation of 6-MMP metabolites. Despite the use of conventional therapeutic 6-MP dosing practices, these patients with leukemia remain either refractory to maintenance 6-MP therapy or at an increased risk for a disease relapse. This inherent variability in 6-MP metabolism has led many pediatric oncologists to implement pharmacogenomic screening prior to instituting maintenance therapy in patients with critical disease states, including lymphoma and leukemia.[11]

Ulcerative colitis (UC) and Crohn's disease (CD) are also regarded as critical disease states that are often difficult to manage clinically. Although 6-MP and AZA have proven clinical efficacy in the induction and maintenance of remission in patients with steroid-dependent disease, therapeutic responsiveness to therapy ranges from 20% to 70% and is independent of drug dose.[13-18] Indeed, the wide therapeutic dosing range used in clinical practice today, as well as the variation in clinical response time, would

Lichtenstein GR, ed.
Ulcerative Colitis: The Complete Guide to Medical Management (pp. 215-220)

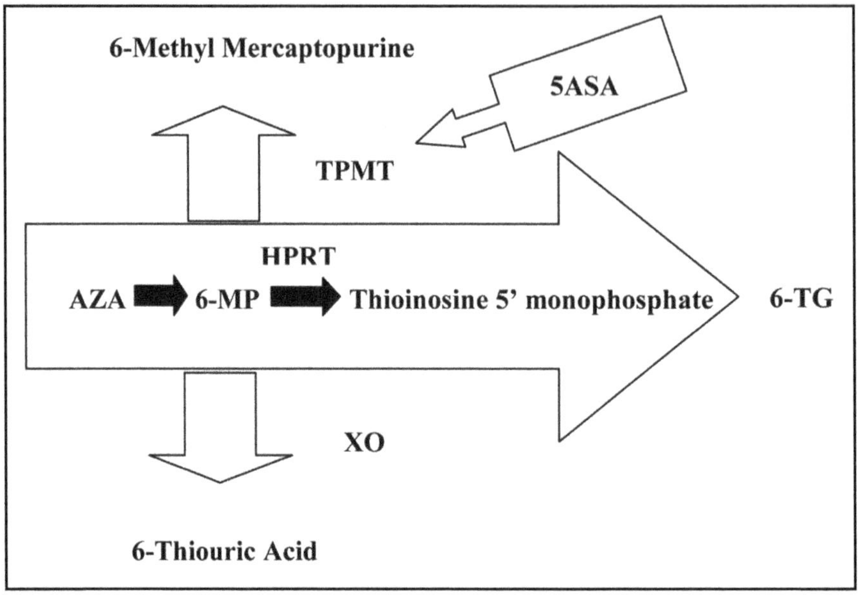

FIGURE 19-1. The metabolism of AZA (AZA, azathioprine; 6-MP, 6-mercaptopurine; TPMT, thiopurine methyl transferase; XO, xanthine oxidase; HPRT, hypoxanthine phosphoribosyltransferase; 5-ASA, mesalamine).

suggest that pharmacokinetic differences in drug metabolism may also influence clinical responsiveness to therapy.

Herein, we will review the metabolism of 6-MP and its prodrug AZA as it applies to the management of patients with IBD. Moreover, the role of metabolite testing will be discussed based on our literature review, and several recommendations will be made on applying this technology in clinical practice.

AZATHIOPRINE METABOLISM IN INFLAMMATORY BOWEL DISEASE

6-MP and its parent compound AZA are well-known for their immunosuppressive properties in the treatment of IBD.[19] In active CD, when combined with corticosteroids, AZA induces remission faster and more frequently with a median response time of 12 to 16 weeks.[14] Furthermore, AZA has proven efficacy in maintaining long-term remission and eliminating the need for corticosteroids in improving quality of life in about 75% of patients.[13]

Pearson's meta-analysis of several well-controlled clinical trials in patients with CD has affirmed that the clinical response to AZA therapy is largely dependent on duration of therapy. Indeed, patients who are weaned from prednisone before AZA can achieve its effect do not have a favorable clinical response to therapy.[13] Interestingly, a therapeutic response would seem to require a delay in clinical response time of at least 4 months of continuous AZA therapy in most patients.[17] However, not all patients respond favorably. As a consequence, many clinicians are either reluctant to prescribe these slow-acting agents subsequent to the delayed clinical response times, or they will prematurely discontinue drug therapy in patients with a less than favorable clinical response.

Most often, physicians will measure drug efficacy based on either an improvement in their patients' clinical symptoms and quality of life or their ability to maintain remission while weaning off of corticosteroid therapy. In general, physicians will tend to rely on their clinical judgment and experience in determining the dose of AZA to be used in treating patients with IBD.[13] Colonna and co-workers have proposed that clinical responsiveness to therapy can best be achieved by tailoring the dose of 6-MP to induce leukopenia in patients with CD. In 51 patients with moderate to severe CD on long-term 6-MP therapy, clinical responsiveness correlated well with drug-induced leukopenia. None of their patients developed clinical signs of bone marrow suppression, required hospitalization for concurrent infection, or required transfusions despite total leukocyte counts less than 5000.[18] A true separation between immunosuppression and cytotoxicity has yet to be defined because the dosing of 6-MP and AZA has been based largely on clinical outcome. Indeed, the wide range in AZA dose used in clinical practice would suggest that a safe and established therapeutic dose has yet to be determined. As a consequence, the clinician must always remain aware of potential adverse effects, including allergic reactions, hepatitis, pancreatitis, bone marrow suppression, and lymphoma while attempting to achieve an optimal therapeutic response.[20] In comparison, the pediatric oncologist will effectively tailor the dose of either 6-MP or AZA based on the measure of erythrocyte 6-TG metabolite levels. Indeed, the notion of a therapeutic window of clinical efficacy and toxicity based on the measurement of AZA therapy has

TABLE 19-1

6-TG METABOLITE LEVELS: CORRELATION WITH CLINICAL EFFICACY

STUDY	N	SETTING	CLINICAL CORRELATION
Cuffari[21]	25	Adolescent CD	6-TG α clinical response
Dubinsky[22]	95	Ped. IBD >4 mo	6-TG >235*
Gupta[23]	54	Ped. IBD	NS
Belaiche[24]	24	Adult IBD	NS
Cuffari[25]	82	Adult IBD	6-TG >250* colitis/fistula
Achar[26]	60	Adult IBD	6-TG >260
Lowry[27]	170	Adult IBD	NS
Cuffari[3]	101	Adult IBD	6-TG >234 (PPV 86%)

*pmol/8 x 10^8 RBCs

now become the standard of care in post-pediatric practices in the treatment of patients with leukemia.

The measurement of erythrocyte 6-TG and 6-MMP metabolite levels by means of high-pressure liquid chromatography (HPLC) has now become a useful clinical tool for documenting patients' compliance to therapy.[21] In our preliminary study, erythrocyte 6-TG metabolite levels showed a strong inverse correlation with disease activity in adolescent patients with CD.[21] Although a wide range of erythrocyte 6-TG levels was associated with clinical responsiveness to therapy, patients with 6-TG levels more than 250 pmol/8 x 10^8 RBCs were uniformly asymptomatic. Moreover, the lack of clinical response was clearly associated with low erythrocyte 6-TG metabolite level. In 1 patient, noncompliance was easily suspected in view of very low erythrocyte 6-TG levels, and was subsequently confirmed by the patient involved. To date, a number of studies in both the pediatric and adult literature have supported the notion of therapeutic drug monitoring in patients with IBD. However, a uniform consensus has not yet been reached because of the absence of well-controlled clinical trials (Table 19-1). Prospective clinical trials are needed in order to develop a therapeutic window of efficacy and toxicity based on the measure of erythrocyte AZA metabolite levels, as is done when prescribing critical dosed drugs, including anticonvulsant, antimicrobial, and allograft rejection therapies.

In comparison, erythrocyte 6-MMP levels have not been shown to correlate with clinical responsiveness to therapy. Furthermore, the wide inter-patient variability in erythrocyte 6-MMP levels may be secondary to inherent differences in TPMT activity present within the population, as discussed previously. However, a recent study by Dubinsky and co-workers would suggest that very high erythrocyte 6-MMP levels may also reflect a patient's refractoriness to therapy and susceptibility to drug-induced hepatotoxicity.[28]

THIOPURINE METHYL-TRANSFERASE PHARMACOGENOMICS

Genetic polymorphism in TPMT enzyme activity can be qualitatively measured by genotype testing. It has been proposed that genotype testing alone is useful in identifying patients at risk for 6-MP and AZA-induced toxicity. Eleven percent of the population is considered heterozygous carriers of the TPMT deficient allele and is potentially at risk for drug-induced leukopenia. Furthermore, in homozygous recessive patients with absent TPMT enzyme activity, there is the added risk of severe, irreversible bone marrow suppression. Since then, there have been a number of similar cases of irreversible bone marrow suppression both in patients with IBD on maintenance AZA therapy and in patients with leukemia on standard doses of 6-MP.[29,30] Interestingly, a number of secondary malignancies, including acute myelogenous leukemia and brain tumors, have been insinuated as related to the use of maintenance 6-MP therapy in patients with leukemia and the heterozygous TPMT genotype.[31,32] Although 6-TG and 6-MMP metabolites were not measured in those patients, it may be assumed that these patients were potentially exposed to high-maintenance 6-TG metabolite levels despite presumed therapeutic 6-MP dosing.

In comparison, Black and co-workers[33] showed that patients with Crohn's disease and a "mutant" TPMT allele also incurred significant drug-induced leukopenia on standard doses of AZA therapy and were compelled to discontinue treatment. In contrast, patients with the wild-type allele achieved a good clinical response while on AZA therapy without untoward cytotoxicity. This study and others would suggest that all patients with the heterozygote allele are at an increased risk for drug toxicity and should not be prescribed AZA or 6-MP therapy. However, this would exclude 11% of the population who could potentially benefit from 6-MP therapy.[33]

The influence of pharmacogenomics on AZA metabolism is compounded by the putative inhibitory effect that sulfasalazine and related salicylate compounds have on TPMT activity.[34] As with AZA and 6-MP, mesalamine must be metabolized by n-acetyl transferase (NAT-1) into its active n-acetyl 5-ASA metabolite. Interestingly, there are variant NAT-1 alleles present within the population that may potentially affect 5-ASA metabolism. Patients with the variant NAT-1 allele do not convert 5-ASA effectively into its active n-acetyl 5-ASA metabolite. Because 5-ASA has been shown to interfere with TPMT activity in vitro, patients with the variant NAT-1 allele may be predisposed to AZA and 6-MP induced cytotoxicity. Recently, Proujansky and colleagues have shown that inherent differences in 5-ASA metabolism may predict complications to 6-MP therapy.[35] This study showed that patients with the NAT-1 variant allele were at a significantly increased risk for 6-MP related cytotoxicity, including pancreatitis. Although sulfasalazine and related mesalamine compounds may have a direct inhibitory effect on TPMT activity, a recent study showed TPMT activity may increase after 4 months of continuous AZA therapy.[3]

The genetic polymorphism in TPMT activity observed in the general population may also have far-reaching implications regarding patient responsiveness to therapy and clinical response time, as previously discussed. Ten percent of the population is considered to be rapid metabolizers of 6-MP and AZA and in theory would require larger than standard doses of the drugs in order to achieve any therapeutic drug benefit. In these patients, 6-MP metabolism is shunted away from 6-TG production and into the formation of 6-MMP. Patients with leukemia and high TPMT activity are considered to be at an increased risk for disease recurrence. Furthermore, a recent study in children with IBD also suggests that these patients remain refractory to therapy despite a presumed therapeutic drug-dosing regimen. Moreover, despite an aggressive escalation in AZA dosage, these patients remained refractory to AZA therapy.[36]

AZA metabolism is influenced by inherent differences in TPMT activity present within the population. Instead of using a fixed dosage of either AZA or 6-MP for induction therapy, the knowledge of TPMT activity levels may allow physicians to predict clinical response and effectively dose AZA in order to maximize efficacy while minimizing the risk of toxicity. In a recently published prospective open-label study, the response rate to induction AZA therapy was highest in patients with less than average (<12 U/mL blood) TPMT activity and was correlated with achieving high erythrocyte (>250) 6-TG metabolite levels. Indeed, the knowing of the low (<5) TPMT activity before initiating AZA therapy in 2 patients led to a low dosing strategy (1 mg/kg/d) with a favorable clinical response without untoward side effects.[3] A study by Kaskas and co-workers[37] would also suggest that an effective low (0.25 mg/kg/d) treatment approach can be safely and effectively adopted in patients with the homozygous recessive genotype. Both of these studies would support the contention that a low-dose treatment strategy may be used to treat those patients with low TPMT activity.

Another study also showed that patients with above-average TPMT activity levels were less likely to respond to AZA therapy and more likely to require higher dosages (2 mg/kg/d) of AZA from the outset in order to optimize erythrocyte 6-TGn metabolite levels.[3] Patients with above-average (>12) TPMT activity had a mean erythrocyte 6-TGn level that leveled off below a presumed therapeutic (<250) treatment level after 8 weeks of continuous AZA therapy. Patients with TPMT activity levels ≤12 U/mL blood achieved high (>250) mean erythrocyte 6-TG levels after 16 weeks of induction AZA. This occurred even though both groups received a similar dosage of AZA. Clinically, 69% of patients with TPMT activity levels ≤12 U/mL blood achieved a clinical response with therapeutic erythrocyte 6-TGn metabolite levels after 4 months of continuous therapy, while only 30% patients with above-average (>12) TPMT activity achieved a clinical response.

High hepatic TPMT activity may draw most of the 6-MP from the plasma, thereby limiting the amount of substrate available for the bone marrow and peripheral leukocytes.[38] This concept of rapid AZA metabolism interfering with therapeutic response could explain the low response rate in a controlled trial in Crohn's disease that compared high dose oral (2 mg/kg/d) AZA therapy with and without initiating a short course of high-dose IV (40 mg/kg) AZA therapy. That study was confined to individuals with upper normal or high levels of TPMT enzyme activity so that the intravenous azathioprine treatment group could be studied safely. Even at 2 mg/kg/d of oral AZA therapy, only 20% of these rapid metabolizers in both groups achieved clinical remission,[39] a clinical response that is lower than that reported in most consecutive patient publications.[13-18]

CLINICAL APPLICATION

The careful monitoring of a complete blood count (CBC) and erythrocyte 6-TGn metabolite levels are appropriate in patients with either low or above-average (>12) TPMT levels in order to avoid either excessive 6-TGn or the unpredictable shunting of 6-MP metabolism into the

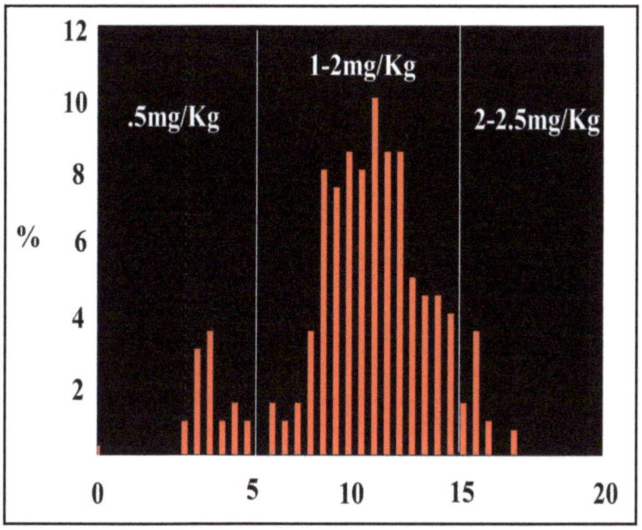

FIGURE 19-2. Azathioprine dosage recommendations based on TPMT phenotype.

production of 6-MMP metabolites,[3] respectively. It remains the authors' opinion that relying on either the WBC or mean corpuscular volume as the only measure of dosing adequacy should be used with caution.[18,40] The putative cytotoxicity of methylated metabolites in developing 6-MP-induced leukopenia would suggest that leukopenia may not be an appropriate endpoint for all patients on antimetabolite therapy, especially in those patients with high TPMT activity. Previously, several studies have entertained a therapeutic index of clinical responsiveness to AZA therapy in different groups of patients on maintenance antimetabolite therapy based on achieving therapeutic erythrocyte 6-TGn levels between 235 and 260 picomol/8 x 10^8 RBCs.[21,24,26] Recent studies would also support the same notion.[3] However, the therapeutic index for clinical responsiveness to induction therapy may be higher.[3] In a recent study, high (>290) erythrocyte 6-TGn level showed a positive predictive value of 86% for obtaining a favorable clinical response to induction AZA therapy.

Knowing the TPMT status in a patient may aid the physician in utilizing a variable AZA dosing strategy in patients with IBD. Patients with absent TPMT should not receive AZA therapy. Those with very low (<5) TPMT activity can be effectively treated with 1 mg/kg/d while monitoring CBC and erythrocyte 6-TG levels. Patients with TPMT activity between 5 and 12 U/mL blood have an increased likelihood of responding to a more moderate dosing strategy, such as 1.5 mg/kg/d. In patients with above-average (>12) TPMT activity, AZA therapy may have to be started at 2.0 mg/kg/d in order to achieve a favorable clinical response. However, higher dosages, such as 2.5 mg/kg/d may be needed for those with very high (>20) TPMT enzyme activity (Figure 19-2).[3] We also recommend that if a patient has not responded clinically despite presumed therapeutic 6-TGn levels, another treatment approach needs to be considered. Prospective controlled trials are needed to determine whether individualized AZA dosing strategies that are based on the inherent differences in TPMT activity can be utilized in order to improve therapeutic effectiveness and clinical response time, and lessen adverse side effects.

REFERENCES

1. Weinshilboum RN, Sladek Sl. Mercaptopurine pharmacogenetics: Monogenic inheritance of erythrocyte thiopurine methyl transferase activity. *Am J Hum Genet.* 1980;32:651-662.
2. Evans WE, Horner M, Chu YQ, et al. Altered mercaptopurine metabolism, toxic effects, and dosage requirements in a thiopurine methyltransferase deficient child with acute lymphoblastic leukemia. *J Pediatr.* 1991;119:985-989.
3. Cuffari C, Dassoupolus T, Bayless TM. Thiopurine methyl-transferase activity influences clinical response to azathioprine therapy in patients with IBD. *Clin Gastroenterol Hepatol.* 2004;2:410-417.
4. Lennard L. The clinical pharmacology of 6-mercaptopurine in acute lymphoblastic leukemia. *Eur J Clin Pharmacol.* 1992;43:329-339.
5. Bostrom B, Erdman G. Cellular pharmacology of 6-mercaptopurine in acute lymphoblastic leukemia. *Am J Pediatr Hematol Oncol.* 1993;15:80-86.
6. Christie NT, Drake S, Meyn RE. 6-thioguanine induced DNA damage as a determinant of cytotoxicity in cultured hamster ovary cells. *Cancer Res.* 1986;44:3665-3671.
7. Fairchild CR, Maybaum J, Kennedy KA. Concurrent unilateral chromatid damage and DNA strand breaks in response to 6-thioguanine treatment. *Biochem Pharmacol.* 1986;35:3533-3541.
8. Alves S, Prata MJ, Ferreira F, Amorim A. Screening of thiopurine methyl s-transferase mutations by horizontal conformation-sensitive gel electrophoresis. *Human Mutation.* 2000;15:246-253.
9. Lennard L, Rees CA, Lilleyman JS, et al. Childhood leukemia: a relationship between intracellular 6-mercaptopurine metabolites and neutropenia. *Br J Clin Pharmacol.* 1993;16:359-363.
10. Zimm S, Collins JM, Riccardi R, et al. Variable bioavailability of oral mercaptopurine: is maintenance chemotherapy in acute lymphoblastic leukemia being optimally delivered. *N Engl J Med.* 1983;308:1005-1009.
11. McLeod HL, Relling MV, Liu Q, Pui CH, Evans WE. Polymorphic thiopurine methyl transferase in erythrocytes is indicative of activity in leukemic blasts from children with acute lymphoblastic leukemia. *Blood.* 1995;85:1897-1902.
12. Kombluth A, Sachar DB, Salomon P. Crohn's disease. In: Sleisenger MH, Fordtran JS, eds. *Gastrointestinal Diseases.* Philadelphia, PA: WB Saunders; 1998:1708-1734.
13. Pearson DC, May GR, Fick GH, et al. Azathioprine and 6-mercaptopurine in Crohn's disease: a meta-analysis. *Ann Intern Med.* 1995;122:132-142.
14. Ewe K, Press AG, Singe CC, et al. Azathioprine combined with prednisolone or monotherapy with prednisolone in active Crohn's disease. *Gastroenterology.* 1993;105:367-372.
15. Korelitz BI, Adler DJ, Mendelsohn RA, et al. Long-term experience with 6-mercaptopurine in the treatment of Crohn's disease. *Am J Gastroenterol.* 1993;88:1198-1205.
16. Present DH, Korelitz BI, Wisch N, et al. Treatment of Crohn's disease with 6-mercaptopurine: along-term, randomized, double-blind study. *N Engl J Med.* 1980;302:981-987.
17. O'Brien JJ, Bayless TM, Bayless JA. Use of azathioprine or 6-mercaptopurine in the treatment of Crohn's disease. *Gastroenterology.* 1991;101:39-46.

18. Colonna T, Korelitz BI. The role of leukopenia in 6-mercaptopurine-induced remission of refractory Crohn's disease. *Am J Gastroenterol.* 1993;89:362-366.
19. Brogan M, Hiserot J, Olicer M. The effects of 6-mercaptopurine on natural killer cell activities in Crohn's disease. *J Clin Immunol.* 1985;5:204-211.
20. Present DH, Meltzer SJ, Krumholz MP, et al. 6-mercaptopurine in the management of inflammatory bowel disease: short and long-term toxicity. *Ann Intern Med.* 1995;111:641-649.
21. Cuffari C, Theoret Y, Latour S, et al. 6-mercaptopurine metabolism in Crohn's disease: correlation with efficacy and toxicity. *Gut.* 1996;39:401-406.
22. Dubinsky MC, Lamothe S, Yang HY, et al. Pharmacogenomics and metabolite measurement for 6-mercaptopurine therapy in inflammatory bowel disease. *Gastroenterology.* 2000;118;705-713.
23. Gupta P, Gokhlae R, Kirschner BS. 6-mercaptopurine metabolite levels in children with inflammatory bowel disease. *J Pediatr Gastroenterol Nutr.* 2001;33:450-454.
24. Belaiche J, Desager JP, Horsman Y, Louis E. Therapeutic drug monitoring of azathioprine and 6-mercaptopurine metabolites in Crohn's disease. *Scand J Gastroenterol.* 2001;36:71-76.
25. Cuffari C, Hunt S, Bayless TM. Utilization of erythrocyte 6-thioguanine metabolite levels to optimize therapy in IBD. *Gut.* 2001;48:642-646.
26. Achar JP, Stevens T, Brzezinski A, Seidner D, Lashner B. 6-thioguanine levels versus white blood cell counts in guiding 6-mercaptopruine and azathioprine therapy. *Am J Gastroenterol.* 2000;95:A272.
27. Lowry PW, Franklin CL, Weaver AL, et al. Leukopenia resulting from a drug interaction between azathioprine or 6-mercaptopurine and mesalamine, sulphasalazine or balsalazide. *Gut.* 2001;49:656-664.
28. Dubinsky MC, Yang H, Hassard PV, et al. 6-MP metabolite profiles provide a biochemical explanation for 6-MP resistance in patients with inflammatory bowel disease. *Gastroenterology.* 2002;122:904-915.
29. Gearry RB, Barclay ML, Burt MJ, Collett JA, Chapman BA. Thiopurine drug effects in a population of New Zealand patients with inflammatory bowel disease. *Pharmacoepidemiol Drug Saf.* 2004;13:563-567.
30. Evans WE, Homer M, Chu YQ. Altered mercaptopurine metabolism, toxic effects, and dosage requirements in a thiopurine methyl transferase deficient child with acute lymphoblastic leukemia. *J Pediatr.* 1991;119:985-989.
31. Thomsen JB, Schroder H, Kristinsson J, et al. Possible carcinogenic effect of 6-mercaptopurine on bone marrow stem cells. *Cancer.* 1999;86:1080-1086.
32. McLeod HL, Krynetski EY, Relling MV, Evans WE. Genetic polymorphism of thiopurine methyltransferase and its clinical relevance for childhood acute lymphoblastic leukemia. *Leukemia.* 2000;14(4):567-572.
33. Black AJ, McLeod HL, Capell HA. Thiopurine methyl transferase predicts therapy-limiting severe toxicity from azathioprine. *Ann Intern Med.* 1998;129:716-718.
34. Szumlanski C, Weinshilboum RN. Sulphasalazine inhibition of thio methyl transferase: possible mechanism of interaction with 6-mercaptopurine. *Br J Clin Pharmacol.* 1995;39:456-459.
35. Proujansky R, Maxwell M, Johnson J, et al. Molecular genotyping predicts complications of 6-mercaptopurine therapy in childhood IBD. *Gastroenterology.* 1999;116:A800.
36. Lennard L, Lilleyman JS. Variable mercaptopurine metabolism and treatment outcome in childhood lymphoblastic leukemia. *J Clin Oncol.* 1989;7:1816-1823.
37. Kaskas BA, Louis E, Hinderof U, et al. Safe treatment of thiopurine S-transferase deficient Crohn's disease patients with azathioprine. *Gut.* 2003;52:140-142.
38. Szumlanski C, Weinshilboum RM. Sulphasalazine inhibition of thiopurine methyltransferase: possible mechanism for interaction with 6-mercaptopurine and azathioprine. *Br J Pharmacol.* 1995;39:1505-1506.
39. Sandborn WJ, Tremaine WJ, Wolfe DC, et al. Lack of effect of intravenous administration on time to respond to azathioprine for steroid-treated Crohn's disease. *Gastroenterology.* 1999;117:527-535.
40. Garza A, Sninsky CA. Changes in red cell mean corpuscular volume (MCV) during azathioprine or 6-mercaptopurine therapy for Crohn's disease may indicate optimal dose titration. *Gastroenterology.* 2001;120:A3166.

20 METHOTREXATE IN THE TREATMENT OF ULCERATIVE COLITIS

Ellen J. Scherl, MD, FACP, AGAF; Vinita Elizabeth Jacob, MD; Brian P. Bosworth, MD; Ryan Urquhart Warren, MD; and Harrison Lakehomer, BA

Methotrexate, a folate antagonist and potent anti-inflammatory agent, is an analog of dihydrofolic acid that inhibits dihydrofolate reductase and folate-dependent enzymes that are pivotal in the synthesis of purines and pyrimidines.[1-3] It is an effective therapy in rheumatoid arthritis, Crohn's disease, and psoriasis.[4-9] The efficacy of methotrexate in the treatment of ulcerative colitis (UC) is not yet established.

The majority of UC patients have moderate disease,[10] and two-thirds of UC patients requiring steroid induction therapy become either steroid-dependent or steroid-refractory.[11,12] Furthermore, one-third of UC patients will require colectomy over time.[13]

Unlike total proctocolectomy and ileostomy, the current surgery—ileal pouch-anal anastomosis—is not curative for UC. Postoperative complications of pouchitis, decreased fecundity, and fistulizing Crohn's disease are now recognized and raise the question of the role of immunomodulators in UC similar to the established role in Crohn's disease.[14-17] Furthermore, 15% of UC patients have indeterminate colitis or unrecognized Crohn's disease. Serologic markers may identify a subgroup of immunologically vulnerable UC patients more likely to develop postoperative Crohn's disease and more likely to respond to Crohn's disease therapeutic strategies including limited use of steroids and aggressive early immunomodulator and biologic therapy.[18-20] These factors raise the question of limited steroid therapy and more aggressive immunomodulators including methotrexate in moderate-to-severe UC.

The current indications for immunomodulator therapy in UC are steroid-dependent and steroid-refractory UC.[21-25] Azathioprine and 6-mercaptopurine (6-MP) are purine analogs that modulate immune responses by inhibiting the synthesis of nucleic acid, resulting in anti-proliferative effects on activated lymphocytes.[26-28]

Both azathioprine and 6-MP are widely used as maintenance in Crohn's disease but are less well established in steroid-dependent UC.[21-23] Cyclosporine is effective in steroid-refractory UC.[24,25,29] Infliximab is indicated for steroid-dependent UC.[30] While methotrexate is established for both induction and maintenance of remission for Crohn's disease prior to use of infliximab or in combination with infliximab,[7-9] its role has been less well-studied in either induction or maintenance of remission in UC. Approximately one-third of patients with Crohn's disease or UC are intolerant or unresponsive to optimized dosing of 6-MP or azathioprine.[31-33]

MECHANISM OF ACTION

Methotrexate is an analog of dihydrofolic acid with a substitution of a hydroxyl group by an amino acid and an insertion of a methyl group allowing methotrexate to enter the cell by active transport or facilitated diffusion. It inhibits dihydrofolate reductase and inhibits the synthesis of purines and pyrimidines. These molecular mechanisms explain its antiproliferative effect although the anti-inflammatory effects remain to be elucidated. It is felt that, in part, the anti-inflammatory effects of methotrexate are related to binding adenosine on target cells, which may lead to inhibition of TNFα and other proinflammatory cytokines.[34-36]

Lichtenstein GR, ed.
Ulcerative Colitis: The Complete Guide to Medical Management (pp. 221-226)

TOXICITY

The most common adverse events associated with low-dose methotrexate use in UC are nausea, vomiting, occasional diarrhea, abdominal pain, and increased liver transaminase levels. Rare central nervous system effects such as insomnia and paresthesias have been described, and infectious events have also been noted along with bone marrow suppression, but these effects are transient. Methotrexate-induced pneumonitis may be severe or life-threatening. Hepatic fibrosis and cirrhosis are concerns with long-term maintenance therapy, but data suggest that even with cumulative doses of greater than 1.5 g there is no significant toxicity.[3,36,37]

Neurotoxicity is rare with low-dose methotrexate and is mostly related to higher doses.[38,39] While the mechanism is not clear, high-dose methotrexate has been shown to decrease 5-methyltetrahydrofolate in the cerebrospinal fluid of some patients not given folate rescue, which underscores the importance of folate supplementation in methotrexate low- or high-dose treatment.[39]

Methotrexate is contraindicated in pregnancy because of its teratogenicity and must be discontinued 6 months prior to conception. Folic acid plays a significant role in hematopoiesis and the growth and development of the central nervous system.[40] During pregnancy, methotrexate may pose a risk to normal fetal development, as folic acid deficiency can lead to fetal abnormalities.[40] Neural tube defects leading to conditions such as spina bifida and anencephaly in the fetus can result from administration of methotrexate during pregnancy.[41] High-dose methotrexate has been shown to induce spontaneous abortion in the third trimester.[41] Whether low-dose methotrexate with folic acid supplementation will have the same effect is not clear. Pending further trials, the authors speculate that perhaps the category X should be re-evaluated in low-dose methotrexate with folate replacement. Nonetheless, methotrexate is also contraindicated in breastfeeding. Folic acid supplementation at a dose of 1 to 5 mg per day is common when prescribing methotrexate.[42] In addition, the risk of lymphoproliferative disorders observed in thiopurines is not associated with methotrexate in the treatment of rheumatoid arthritis, psoriasis, and Crohn's disease.[43-45]

Hypersensitivity pneumonitis, although rare, is a recognized complication of methotrexate use. A baseline chest x-ray as well as follow-up monitoring of complete blood counts and liver chemistries is advocated.[46-48] The risk of methotrexate-associated hepatotoxicity is low in patients who do not have one of the following risk factors: obesity, diabetes mellitus, history of excessive or long-term ethanol use, elevated baseline hepatocellular laboratory chemistries, a cumulative dose of methotrexate exceeding 1.5 g total drug dose, and daily dosing of methotrexate.[3,46]

INDUCTION AND MAINTENANCE TRIALS

In patients with UC, there are an increasing number of studies evaluating the effectiveness of methotrexate on the induction of remission. However, there has only been one double-blind, placebo-controlled trial by Oren et al[49] in 1996 evaluating the effectiveness of oral methotrexate in chronic steroid-dependent UC patients. No benefit over placebo was found in this study, thus leading to current management guidelines that do not include methotrexate as evidence-based therapy for steroid-dependent UC.[46,50,51]

Oren's group included UC patients who were clearly defined as steroid-dependent if they had received steroids (at ≥7.5 mg/day) for at least 4 months during the preceding year and if they had a Mayo Clinic score of 7 or higher.[49] If patients were on immunosuppressives instead of or in addition to steroids, they had to be off the immunosuppressives for at least 3 months before entry into the study. Of the 67 patients in the study, 30 were assigned to receive methotrexate 12.5 mg orally once a week for 9 months, and 37 patients were assigned to receive placebo. The results showed that 14 out of the 30 patients receiving methotrexate (47%) and 18 of the 37 patients receiving placebo (49%) went into clinical remission with withdrawal of the steroids during the 9-month period. The methotrexate group reached remission within a mean time of 4.1 months while the placebo group's mean time to remission was 3.4 months. There clearly were no statistically significant differences between the 2 groups in the proportion of patients inducted into clinical remission or mean time to remission.

The conclusion from this study is that ultra-low-dose methotrexate (12.5 mg weekly via oral dosing) is not effective in inducing remission in the chronic steroid-dependent UC patient. However, no conclusion can be made in regard to whether higher oral doses or parenteral administration of methotrexate would have made a difference. Theoretically, there should be no problem with oral absorption in the UC patient as this drug is absorbed in the small bowel. The Crohn's trial showing the effectiveness of methotrexate in induction of remission by Feagan in 1995 used higher doses parenterally.[8]

Another randomized trial that evaluated methotrexate in UC was published by Maté-Jiménez in 2000.[52] This study did not have a placebo arm and involved 34 UC patients enrolled who were once again steroid-dependent. The patients were randomized to 6-mercaptopurine 1.5 mg/kg/day, methotrexate 15 mg weekly, or 5-aminosalicylic acid 3 g/day for 30 weeks. Seven of the 12 patients (58%) assigned to methotrexate—11/14 (79%) in the 6-MP group and 2/8 (25%) in the 5-ASA group—went into clinical remission with withdrawal of steroids by week 30. This study corroborated Oren's results that there was no significant benefit in using oral methotrexate at a dose of 15 mg/week over 30 weeks over 6-MP or 5-ASA. These results were also replicated in the maintenance phase of the study where 1/12 (8%) patients given methotrexate initially—7/14 (50%) given 6-MP and 0/8 (0%) given 5-ASA—maintained their clinical remission through week 76 of the trial.

On the other hand, some uncontrolled studies do suggest that methotrexate may be of benefit in UC.[53,54] Cummings et al[55] in 2005 published a chart review on patients treated with oral methotrexate at the inflammatory bowel disease clinics of Oxford and Wycombe General Hospital in the UK and concluded that oral methotrexate at 20 mg orally weekly was moderately effective in steroid-dependent or refractory UC patients. The study involved 42 patients with UC either steroid refractory or steroid dependent who were given azathioprine and developed intolerance to the medication (31/42) or remained medically refractory to it (11/42). The mean dose of methotrexate was approximately 20 mg orally per week for a period of 30 weeks. Remission was achieved in 42% of the patients, defined as complete withdrawal of steroids for more than 3 months and response (good, partial, or failure of response). There was a good response in 54% and partial response in 18%. Side effects occurred in 23% of patients with 10% stopping treatment.

Paoluzi's group[56] in 2002 performed an open-label clinical trial in which methotrexate was used as salvage therapy in steroid-dependent or steroid-refractory UC patients who were refractory or intolerant to azathioprine. Forty-two patients were treated with azathioprine at a dose of 2 mg/kg on a daily basis and then transitioned to methotrexate 12.5 mg weekly via intramuscular injection for 6 months if they did not respond or were intolerant to azathioprine. Ten patients showed lack of response (n=2) or intolerance (n=8), and all 10 responded to methotrexate with 60% induced into complete clinical remission and 40% with clinical improvement. Patients who are intolerant or refractory to 6-MP/azathioprine may be candidates for infliximab or may be considered for methotrexate.[55,57-59] A recent retrospective study evaluated 32 patients with UC of whom 72% were intolerant and 28% were unresponsive to 6-MP or thiopourine.[60] An induction dose of methotrexate 25 mg/week was given either orally (20 patients) or intramuscularly (12 patients), and a maintenance dose of 20 mg/week was given for an average of 1 year. Clinical response was achieved in 68% of UC patients comprising 7 out of 9 (78%) patients in the 6-MP/azathioprine refractory group and nearly two-thirds (15 out of 23) of patients in the intolerant group. Steroid withdrawal occurred in 7 out of 19 patients. Although the numbers are small, there was no difference in clinical response between the oral and intramuscular administration groups. Adverse events occurred in 17.4% of patients and required discontinuation in 8.3%. Generally, 25 mg/week oral or intramuscular methotrexate was effective and well-tolerated in UC.

Only one-third of steroid-exposed Crohn's disease patients achieve mucosal healing.[61] Steroid-sparing with thiopurine 6-MP/azathioprine or methotrexate achieves clinical efficacy but mucosal healing is generally achieved in only approximately one-third of patients.[53,62] However, 2 small series reported higher rates of mucosal healing associated with methotrexate.[63,64]

There appears to be an emerging role for methotrexate in UC, especially in the 6-MP/azathioprine refractory or intolerant population. Cases of UC and indeterminant colitis are not cured by ileal pouch-anal anastomosis and therefore may require maintenance immunomodulator therapy. A re-evaluation of the role of methotrexate in treating UC is needed. Larger randomized controlled trials evaluating both steroid-free remission and mucosal healing in both thiopurine-naïve and thiopurine-intolerant/refractory UC patients are warranted. While waiting for randomized controlled trials, we may consider the role of methotrexate 25 mg/week intramuscularly with replacement folic acid 1 to 5 mg per day in 6-MP naïve or experienced UC patients.

REFERENCES

1. Schröder O, Stein J. Low dose methotrexate in inflammatory bowel disease: current status and future directions. *Am J Gastroenterol.* 2003;98(3):530-537.
2. El-Matary W, Vandermeer B, Griffiths AM. Methotrexate for maintenance of remission in ulcerative colitis. *Cochrane Database Syst Rev.* 2009 Jul 8;(3):CD007560.
3. Te HS, Schiano TD, Kuan SF, Hanauer SB, Conjeevaram HS, Baker AL. Hepatic effects of long-term methotrexate use in the treatment of inflammatory bowel disease. *Am J Gastroenterol.* 2000;95(11):3150-3156.
4. Schnabel A, Gross WL. Low-dose methotrexate in rheumatic diseases—efficacy, side effects, and risk factors for side effects. *Semin Arthritis Rheum.* 1994;23(5):310-327.
5. Klippel JH, Decker JL. Methotrexate in rheumatoid arthritis. *N Engl J Med.* 1985;312(13):853-854.
6. Weinblatt ME, Coblyn JS, Fox DA, et al. Efficacy of low-dose methotrexate in rheumatoid arthritis. *N Engl J Med.* 1985;312(13):818-822.
7. Feagan BG, Fedorak RN, Irvine EJ, et al. A comparison of methotrexate with placebo for the maintenance of remission in Crohn's disease. North American Crohn's Study Group Investigators. *N Engl J Med.* 2000;342(22):1627-1632.
8. Feagan BG, Rochon J, Fedorak RN, et al. Methotrexate for the treatment of Crohn's disease. The North American Crohn's Study Group Investigators. *N Engl J Med.* 1995;332(5):292-297.
9. Feagan BG, McDonald JWD, Panaccione R, et al. A randomized trial of methotrexate (MTX) in combination with infliximab (IFX) for the treatment of Crohn's disease (CD). *Gastroenterology.* 2008;134(4 suppl 1):682c.
10. Langholz E, Munkholm P, Nielsen OH, Kreiner S, Binder V. Incidence and prevalence of ulcerative colitis in Copenhagen county from 1962 to 1987. *Scand J Gastroenterol.* 1991;26(12):1247-1256.
11. Munkholm P, Langholz E, Davidsen M, Binder V. Frequency of glucocorticoid resistance and dependency in Crohn's disease. *Gut.* 1994;35(3):360-362.

12. Faubion WA Jr, Loftus EV Jr, Harmsen WS, Zinsmeister AR, Sandborn WJ. The natural history of corticosteroid therapy for inflammatory bowel disease: a population-based study. *Gastroenterology.* 2001;121(2):255-260.
13. Langholz E, Munkholm P, Davidsen M, Binder V. Course of ulcerative colitis: analysis of changes in disease activity over years. *Gastroenterology.* 1994;107(1):3-11.
14. Olsen KO, Juul S, Berndtsson I, Öresland T, Laurberg S. *Gastroenterology.* 2002;122:15-19.
15. Koltun WA, Schoetz DJ, Roberts PL, Murray JJ, Coller JA, Veidenheimer MC. Indeterminate colitis predisposes to perineal complications after ileal pouch-anal anastomosis. *Dis Colon Rectum.* 1991;34(10):857-860.
16. Ståhlberg D, Gullberg K, Liljeqvist L, Hellers G, Löfberg R. Pouchitis following pelvic pouch operation for ulcerative colitis. Incidence, cumulative risk, and risk factors. *Dis Colon Rectum.* 1996;39(9):1012-1018.
17. Farouk R, Pemberton JH, Wolff BG, Dozois RR, Browning S, Larson D. Functional outcomes after ileal pouch-anal anastomosis for chronic ulcerative colitis. *Ann Surg.* 2000;231(6):919-926.
18. Vasiliauskas EA, Plevy SE, Landers CJ, et al. Perinuclear antineutrophil cytoplasmic antibodies in patients with Crohn's disease define a clinical subgroup. *Gastroenterology.* 1996;110(6):1810-1819.
19. Joossens S, Reinisch W, Vermeire S, et al. The value of serologic markers in indeterminate colitis: a prospective follow-up study. *Gastroenterology.* 2002;122(5):1242-1247.
20. Fleshner PR, Vasiliauskas EA, Kam LY, et al. High level perinuclear antineutrophil cytoplasmic antibody (pANCA) in ulcerative colitis patients before colectomy predicts the development of chronic pouchitis after ileal pouch–anal anastomosis. *Gut.* 2001;49(5):671-677.
21. Hawthorne AB, Logan RF, Hawkey CJ, et al. Randomised controlled trial of azathioprine withdrawal in ulcerative colitis. *BMJ.* 1992;305(6844):20-22.
22. Ardizzone S, Maconi G, Russo A, et al. Randomised controlled trial of azathioprine and 5-aminosalicylic acid for treatment of steroid dependent ulcerative colitis. *Gut.* 2006;55(1):47-53.
23. Timmer A, McDonald JW, Macdonald JK. Azathioprine and 6-mercaptopurine for maintenance of remission in ulcerative colitis. *Cochrane Database Syst Rev.* 2007;(1):CD000478.
24. Lichtiger S, Present DH, Kornbluth A, et al. Cyclosporine in severe ulcerative colitis refractory to steroid therapy. *N Engl J Med.* 1994; 330:1841-1845.
25. Shibolet O, Regushevskaya E, Brezis M, Soares-Weiser K. Cyclosporine A for induction of remission in severe ulcerative colitis. *Cochrane Database Syst Rev.* 2005;(1):CD004277.
26. Hitchings GH. Selective inhibitors of dihydrofolate reductase (Nobel Lecture). *Angewandte Chemie International Edition in English.* 2003;28(7):879-885.
27. Schroll S, Sarlette A, Ahrens K, Manns MP, Göke M. Effects of azathioprine and its metabolites on repair mechanisms of the intestinal epithelium in vitro. *Regul Pept.* 2005;131(1-3):1-11.
28. Tiede I, Fritz G, Strand S, et al. CD28-dependent Rac1 activation is the molecular target of azathioprine in primary human CD4+ T lymphocytes. *J Clin Invest.* 2003;111(8):1133-1145.
29. D'Haens G, Lemmens L, Geboes K, et al. Intravenous cyclosporine versus intravenous corticosteroids as single therapy for severe attacks of ulcerative colitis. *Gastroenterology.* 2001;120(6):1323-1329.
30. Rutgeerts P, Sandborn WJ, Feagan BG, et al. Infliximab for induction and maintenance therapy for ulcerative colitis. *N Engl J Med.* 2005;353(23):2462-2476.
31. Dubinsky MC, Lamothe S, Yang HY, et al. Pharmacogenomics and metabolite measurement for 6-mercaptopurine therapy in inflammatory bowel disease. *Gastroenterology.* 2000;118(4):705-713.
32. Ansari A, Arenas M, Greenfield SM, et al. Prospective evaluation of the pharmacogenetics of azathioprine in the treatment of inflammatory bowel disease. *Aliment Pharmacol Ther.* 2008;28(8):973-983.
33. Ansari A, Hassan C, Duley J, et al. Thiopurine methyltransferase activity and the use of azathioprine in inflammatory bowel disease. *Aliment Pharmacol Ther.* 2002;16(10):1743-1750.
34. Cronstein BN, Naime D, Ostad E. The antiinflammatory mechanism of methotrexate. Increased adenosine release at inflamed sites diminishes leukocyte accumulation in an in vivo model of inflammation. *J Clin Invest.* 1993;92(6):2675-2682.
35. Krump E, Lemay G, Borgeat P. Adenosine A2 receptor-induced inhibition of leukotriene B4 synthesis in whole blood ex vivo. *Br J Pharmacol.* 1996;117(8):1639-1644.
36. Schröder O, Stein J. Low dose methotrexate in inflammatory bowel disease: current status and future directions. *Am J Gastroenterol.* 2003;98(3):530-537.
37. Kozarek RA, Bredfeldt JE, Rosoff LE, et al. Does chronic methotrexate (MTX) cause liver toxicity when used for refractory inflammatory bowel disease *Gastroenterology.* 1991;100:A223.
38. Raghavendra S, Nair MD, Chemmanam T, Krishnamoorthy T, Radhakrishnan VV, Kuruvilla A. Disseminated necrotizing leukoencephalopathy following low-dose oral methotrexate. *Eur J Neurol.* 2007;14(3):309-314.
39. Vezmar S, Schüsseler P, Becker A, Bode U, Jaehde U. Methotrexate-associated alterations of the folate and methyl-transfer pathway in the CSF of ALL patients with and without symptoms of neurotoxicity. *Pediatr Blood Cancer.* 2009;52(1):26-32.
40. Lloyd ME, Carr M, McElhatton P, Hall GM, Hughes RA. The effects of methotrexate on pregnancy, fertility and lactation. *QJM.* 1999;92(10):551-563.
41. Hausknecht RU. Methotrexate and misoprostol to terminate early pregnancy. *N Engl J Med.* 1995;333(9):537-540.
42. van Ede AE, Laan RF, Blom HJ, De Abreu RA, van de Putte LB. Methotrexate in rheumatoid arthritis: an update with focus on mechanisms involved in toxicity. *Semin Arthritis Rheum.* 1998; 27(5):277-292.
43. Kandiel A, Fraser AG, Korelitz BI, Brensinger C, Lewis JD. Increased risk of lymphoma among inflammatory bowel disease patients treated with azathioprine and 6-mercaptopurine. *Gut.* 2005 Aug;54(8):1121-1125.
44. Rosh JR, Gross T, Mamula P, Griffiths A, Hyams J. Hepatosplenic T-cell lymphoma in adolescents and young adults with Crohn's disease: a cautionary tale? *Inflamm Bowel Dis.* 2007;13(8):1024-1030.
45. Beaugerie L, Seksik P, Carrat F. Thiopurine therapy is associated with a three-fold decrease in the incidence of advanced colorectal neoplasia in IBD patients with longstanding extensive colitis: results from the CESAME cohort. *Gastroenterology.* 2009;5(1): A-54.
46. Lichtenstein GR, Hanauer SB, Sandborn WJ. Practice Parameters Committee of American College of Gastroenterology. Management of Crohn's disease in adults. *Am J Gastroenterol.* 2009;104(2):465-483.
47. Travis SP, Stange EF, Lémann M, et al. European evidence based consensus on the diagnosis and management of Crohn's disease: current management. *Gut.* 2006;55 Suppl 1:i16-35.
48. Lichtenstein GR, Abreu MT, Cohen R, Tremaine W; American Gastroenterological Association. American Gastroenterological Association Institute medical position statement on corticosteroids, immunomodulators, and infliximab in inflammatory bowel disease. *Gastroenterology.* 2006;130(3):935-939.

49. Oren R, Arber N, Odes S, et al. Methotrexate in chronic active ulcerative colitis: a double-blind, randomized, Israeli multicenter trial. *Gastroenterology.* 1996;110(5):1416-1421.
50. Kornbluth A, Sachar DB. Ulcerative colitis practice guidelines in adults (update): American College of Gastroenterology, Practice Parameters Committee. *Am J Gastroenterol.* 2004;99:1371-1385.
51. Long MD, Plevy SE. Poorly responsive ulcerative colitis in the hospital. *Clin Gastroenterol Hepatol.* 2009;7(6):635-640.
52. Maté-Jiménez J, Hermida C, Cantero-Perona J, Moreno-Otero R. 6-mercaptopurine or methotrexate added to prednisone induces and maintains remission in steroid-dependent inflammatory bowel disease. *Eur J Gastroenterol Hepatol.* 2000;12(11):1227-1233.
53. Kozarek RA, Patterson DJ, Gelfand MD, et al. Methotrexate induces clinical and histologic remission in patients with refractory inflammatory bowel disease. *Ann Intern Med.* 1989;110(5):353-356.
54. Baron TH, Truss CD, Elson CO, et al. Low-dose oral methotrexate in refractory inflammatory bowel disease. *Dig Dis Sci.* 1993; 38(10):1851-1856.
55. Cummings JR, Herrlinger KR, Travis SP, Gorard DA, McIntyre AS, Jewell DP. Oral methotrexate in ulcerative colitis. *Aliment Pharmacol Ther.* 2005;21(4):385-389.
56. Paoluzi OA, Pica R, Marcheggiano A, et al. Azathioprine or methotrexate in the treatment of patients with steroid-dependent or steroid-resistant ulcerative colitis: results of an open-label study on efficacy and tolerability in inducing and maintaining remission. *Aliment Pharmacol Ther.* 2002;16(10):1751-1759.
57. Lémann M, Zenjari T, Bouhnik Y, et al. Methotrexate in Crohn's disease: long-term efficacy and toxicity. *Am J Gastroenterol.* 2000; 95(7):1730-1734.
58. Soon SY, Ansari A, Yaneza M, Raoof S, Hirst J, Sanderson JD. Experience with the use of low-dose methotrexate for inflammatory bowel disease. *Eur J Gastroenterol Hepatol.* 2004;16(9):921-926.
59. Mack DR, Young R, Kaufman SS, Ramey L, Vanderhoof JA. Methotrexate in patients with Crohn's disease after 6-mercaptopurine. *J Pediatr.* 1998;132(5):830-835.
60. Wahed M, Louis-Auguste JR, Baxter LM, et al. Efficacy of methotrexate in Crohn's disease and ulcerative colitis patients unresponsive or intolerant to azathioprine/mercaptopurine. *Aliment Pharmacol Ther.* 2009;30(6):614-620.
61. Olaison G, Sjödahl R, Tagesson C. Glucocorticoid treatment in ileal Crohn's disease: relief of symptoms but not of endoscopically viewed inflammation. *Gut.* 1990;31(3):325-328.
62. D'Haens G, Geboes K, Rutgeerts P. Endoscopic and histologic healing of Crohn's (ileo-) colitis with azathioprine. *Gastrointest Endosc.* 1999;50(5):667-671.
63. Panaccione R. The use of methotrexate is associated with mucosal healing in Crohn's disease. *Gastroenterology.* 2005;128(Suppl):A49.
64. Mañosa M, Naves JE, Leal C, et al. Does methotrexate induce mucosal healing in Crohn's disease? *Inflamm Bowel Dis.* 2009: DOI 10.1002/ibd.21015.

21

Calcineurin Inhibitors (Cyclosporine, Tacrolimus, Sirolimus) and Mycophenolate Mofetil Use in Ulcerative Colitis

Hans Herfarth, MD, PhD and Jürgen Schölmerich, MD, PhD

Immunomodulatory therapies with the calcineurin inhibitors cyclosporine and, more recently, tacrolimus play an important role in the management of patients with severe, steroid-refractory or steroid-dependent ulcerative colitis. Sirolimus, another inhibitor of calcineurin, and a potential alternative drug, mycophenolate mofetil, may be appropriate therapeutic options for the treatment of patients with severe ulcerative colitis. Currently, there is inadequate published controlled literature that allows us to establish firm guidelines regarding treatment of patients with these drugs.

BACKGROUND

Mechanisms of Action of Cyclosporine, Tacrolimus, Sirolimus, and Mycophenolate Mofetil

Cyclosporine and tacrolimus are both drugs that target intracellular signalling pathways, which are activated as a consequence of T cell receptor activation. Cyclosporine and tacrolimus do not act, per se, as immunosuppressive agents. They bind to the so-called immunophilins, which is cyclophilin in the case of cyclosporine and FK506-binding protein in the case of tacrolimus.[1] If such a binding between one of the drugs and the respective immunophilin occurs, a complex is formed that binds the phosphatase calcineurin and inhibits the calcineurin catalyzed dephosphorylation essential to permit movement of the nuclear factor of activated T cells (NFAT) into the nucleus. NFAT is required for transcription of IL-2 and other growth- and differentiation-associated cytokines. Sirolimus also binds to the FK506-binding protein, but in contrast to tacrolimus this complex does not affect calcineurin activity. Rather it binds to and inhibits the so-called mammalian kinase target of rapamycin (mTOR), which is a key enzyme in cell cycle progression. In contrast to cyclosporine, tacrolimus, and sirolimus, mycophenolate mofetil is a prodrug that is rapidly hydrolyzed to the active drug mycophenolic acid. Mycophenolic acid is a selective, noncompetitive, and reversible inhibitor of inosine monophosphate dehydrogenase. This is one of the key enzymes in the de novo pathway of guanine nucleotide synthesis, a pathway of cell proliferation in B and T lymphocytes. However, in contrast to B and T cells, other cell types can use salvage pathways. Thus, mycophenolate mofetil selectively inhibits B and T lymphocyte proliferation and other B and T cell functions such as antibody formation, cellular adhesion, and migration.

PHARMACOKINETICS

Cyclosporine (Sandimmune, Neoral)

Cyclosporine, which is a cyclic polypeptide consisting of 11 amino acids produced as a metabolite by the fungus species *Tolypocladium inflatum*,[2] is available in an IV and an oral formulation. Intravenously, the doses mostly investigated in clinical studies in UC are 2 to 4 mg/kg/d and orally 6 to 8 mg/kg/d. By oral application, cyclosporine

Lichtenstein GR, ed.
Ulcerative Colitis: The Complete Guide to Medical Management (pp. 227-236)

has a wide range of bioavailability (1% to 89%, mean 30%) that is influenced by age, ethnicity, variability of bile flow, nutrition, drug interactions, and co-morbidities.[3] A modified microemulsion (Neoral) possesses a more uniform and slightly increased bioavailability, which necessitates dosage adjustments in case of a switch between the original soft gelatin capsules and the microemulsion formulation. The published half-life of cyclosporine is dependent on the age and the specific patient population being evaluated and varies between 5 and 18 hours. Cyclosporine is metabolized in the liver by the CYP3A (cytochrome P3A) enzyme system. Its metabolites are excreted principally through the bile, and only 6% are excreted in the urine, requiring dosage adjustments in the case of hepatic dysfunction. No adjustments are necessary for dialysis or renal failure patients. Cyclosporine interacts with a wide variety of drugs that affect cyclosporine blood concentrations such as calcium channel blockers, antifungal agents, antibiotics, glucocorticoids, and HIV-protease inhibitors.[3] Of note, grapefruit juice is known to increase cyclosporine blood concentrations by inhibiting the CYP3A system.[3]

Monitoring of Blood Concentrations of Cyclosporine

Cyclosporine can be measured by a variety of methods; however, in the fully published controlled clinical trials investigating the continuous IV application of cyclosporine in patients with active UC (Table 21-1), a monoclonal radioimmunoassay or a monoclonal fluorescence polarization immunoassay was employed. The use of HPLC is currently believed to be the best assay available for measuring cyclosporine levels. In these trials, the clinical response did not correlate with the cyclosporine concentrations (see Table 21-1),[4,5] which were all above 200 ng/mL (trough levels), suggesting this level as the lowest possible blood concentration.

Tacrolimus (FK 506, Prograf)

Tacrolimus is a macrolide antibiotic produced by *Streptomyces tsukubaensis*[6] and is available in an IV and an oral formulation. It is usually dosed intravenously 0.01 to 0.02 mg/kg/d and orally 0.1 to 0.2 mg/kg/d. The absorption of tacrolimus in the gastrointestinal tract ranges from 5% to 67%.[3] Its half-life is approximately 12 hours. Like cyclosporine, tacrolimus is metabolized by the CYP3A4 enzyme system and is excreted as the parent drug or as its metabolites in the bile. Tacrolimus is not dependent on bile or mucosal integrity for absorption. Less than 1% is excreted unchanged in the urine. The drug interactions are similar to the interactions of cyclosporine as described previously.[7]

Monitoring of Blood Concentrations of Tacrolimus

No controlled trial demonstrated a correlation of clinical effectiveness with the whole blood concentration of tacrolimus. The target range for tacrolimus is initially 10 to 15 ng/mL; however, tacrolimus has to be adjusted often because of rising creatinine concentrations, indicating nephrotoxicity. In a study by Sandborn et al including patients with CD, the mean final oral tacrolimus dose at week 10 of the study was 0.16 mg/kg/d with mean final blood concentrations of 8.3 ng/mL.[8] Fellermann et al reported mean tacrolimus blood levels of 13.1 ng/mL (range 7.6 to 17) during IV administration and 9.2 ng/mL(range 0.7 to 14) if tacrolimus was administered orally.[9]

Sirolimus (Rapamycin, Rapamune)

Sirolimus is a macrocyclic lactone produced by *Streptomyces hygroscopicus*[10] and is available as an oral formulation. It has a bioavailability of 15%.[3] Similar to the other calcineurin inhibitors, sirolimus is also metabolized by the CYP3A4 enzyme system, and metabolites are found in feces and urine. The half-life is approximately 62 hours in renal transplant patients. In comparison to cyclosporine, it is less nephrotoxic.[11] The drug interactions are similar to cyclosporine or tacrolimus, due to the similar metabolic pathway.

Mycophenolate Mofetil (Cell-Cept)

Mycophenolate mofetil is the 2-morpholinoethyl ester of mycophenolic acid[12] and is available as an oral preparation (capsule, tablet, or suspension) and as an IV formulation. After administration by both routes, the parent drug is cleared and metabolized to mycophenolic acid, which has a half-life of about 16 hours. Mycophenolic acid is metabolized to the inactive mycophenolic acid glucuronide by the Uridine 5'-diphospho-glucuronosyltransferase (UDP)-glucuronosyltransferase in the gastrointestinal tract, the liver, and possibly the kidney. Mycophenolic acid glucuronide is nearly 90% excreted in the urine.[13] Plasma concentrations of mycophenolic acid and mycophenolic acid glucuronide are increased in patients with renal insufficiency. Co-administration of drugs, which affect the enterohepatic circulation such as cholestyramine, metronidazole, or norfloxacin, decrease the plasma concentrations of mycophenolic acid.[14]

ADVERSE EVENTS

If patients with severe UC are treated with immunosuppressive regimens such as cyclosporine or tacrolimus, one should be aware of opportunistic infections (eg, *pneumocystis carinii* pneumonia) because the patients receiving

TABLE 21-1

EFFICACY OF CYCLOSPORINE IN PATIENTS WITH SEVERE ULCERATIVE COLITIS: PROSPECTIVE CONTROLLED TRIALS

Study	Patients (N)	Cyclosporine (mg/kg/d)	Mean Cyclosporine Blood Level (ng/mL)	Mean Time to Response Days (Range)	Response After 8 Days	Colectomy	Remission at 6 Months	Remission at 12 Months
Lichtiger[20]	11	4	482 (339 to 653)#	7 (3 to 14)	9/11 (82%)**	3/11 (27%)	n.d	n.d.
D'Haens[22]	14	4	376 (212 to 488)#	5 (2 to 8)	9/14 (64%)	2/14 (10%)	8/9 (89%)*	7/9 (78%)*
Van Assche[29]	38	4	332 ± 43##	4 (1 to 7)	32/38 (84%)	5/38 (13%)	n.d.	n.d.
	35	2	237 ± 33##	4 (1 to 8)	32/35 (86%)	3/35 (9%)	n.d.	n.d.

* Long-term response of patients who initially responded to cyclosporine and were maintained on a therapy with azathioprine.

** No exact time point given in the study.

Immunoassay: mean (range)

Immunoassay: mean ± SD; At days 0 and 1, doses were calculated per kilogram body weight; from day 2 until day 8, blood levels were strictly controlled to vary between 150 and 250 ng/mL in the 2 mg/kg/d and 250 to 350 in the 4 mg/kg/d group.

TABLE 21-2

MOST COMMON ADVERSE REACTIONS TO CYCLOSPORINE

ADVERSE EFFECT	FREQUENCY
Paresthesias	26%
Hypertrichosis	13%
Hypertension	11%
Tremor	7%
Nausea and vomiting	6%
Renal insufficiency	6%
Headache	5%
Hepatotoxicity	3%
Infection	3%
Gingival hyperplasia	2%
Seizures	1%
Anaphylaxis	0.3%

Adverse events in 343 IBD patients treated with high-dose cyclosporine.[5,51] The frequency of adverse events in this patient population was 0.94 events per patient. By decreasing the dose, most of these events could be reversed—indicating the dose relationship of the observed adverse events.

TABLE 21-3

KNOWN SIDE EFFECTS OF TACROLIMUS

ADVERSE EFFECT	FREQUENCY
Tremor	50%
Hyperglycemia	34%
Hypertension	16%
Infection	13%
Rise of creatinine >25% from baseline	8%
Headache	8%
Alopecia	8%

Adverse events in 38 patients with steroid-refractory colitis (33 ulcerative colitis, 5 indeterminate colitis) receiving either intravenous 0.01 to 0.02 mg/kg/d or oral 0.1 to 0.2 mg/kg/d tacrolimus.[48]

these drugs often receive multimodal immunosuppressive regimens (eg, steroids + cyclosporine + AZA). In this case, a preventive antibiotic therapy with trimethoprim-sulfamethoxazole is recommended.[15] Additionally, when applying calcineurin inhibitors (cyclosporine, tacrolimus, sirolimus), there is a considerable risk for new-onset diabetes mellitus, which, in a meta-analysis of patients after solid organ transplantation, occurred in 10% of patients.[16]

CYCLOSPORINE

The most common adverse reactions of cyclosporine in all patient groups are nephrotoxicity, tremor, hirsutism, hypertension, hyperlipidemia, and gum hyperplasia (Table 21-2).[17] Predictors of cyclosporine nephropathy are older age, a dose exceeding 5 mg/kg/d orally, and a 30% rise in creatinine levels from baseline.[18]

TACROLIMUS

Known side effects of tacrolimus are nephrotoxicity, neurotoxicity, gastrointestinal-related complaints (nausea, vomiting), hypertension, and the development of diabetes, which has been demonstrated to occur in about 17% (Table 21-3).[16]

SIROLIMUS

The use of sirolimus is associated with an increase in serum cholesterol and triglycerides. Compared to cyclosporine and tacrolimus, sirolimus is not nephrotoxic. Adverse events include bone marrow toxicity (anemia, leukopenia, thrombocytopenia), fever, and gastrointestinal side effects (nausea, vomiting).

MYCOPHENOLATE MOFETIL

The most important adverse effects seen with the use of mycophenolate mofetil are gastrointestinal-related side effects such as vomiting, diarrhea, and bone marrow suppression (leukopenia).[13,19]

CLINICAL TRIALS

CYCLOSPORINE

Intravenous cyclosporine has been investigated in 3 prospective controlled trials in patients with severe UC, which were published as full articles (see Table 21-1). The first study published in 1994 by Lichtiger et al

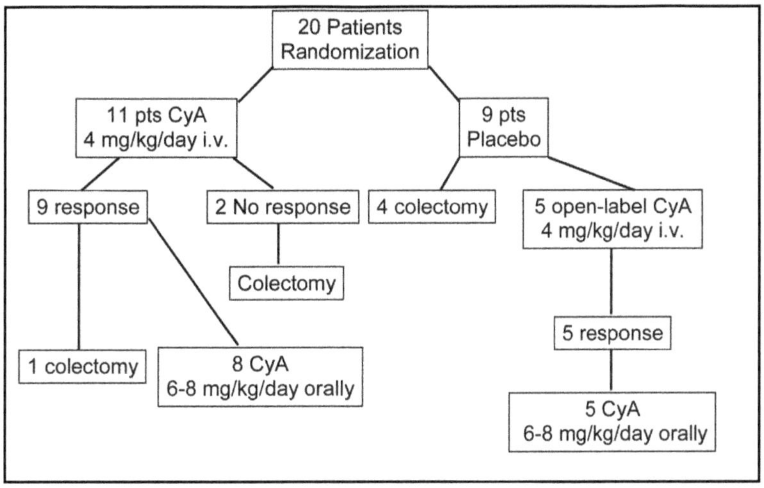

FIGURE 21-1. Results of the first prospective, placebo-controlled trial of cyclosporine in severe UC refractory to steroid therapy. (Adapted from Lichtiger S, Present DH, Kornbluth A, et al. Cyclosporine in severe ulcerative colitis refractory to steroid therapy. *N Engl J Med.* 1994;330:1841-1845.)

demonstrated the clinical efficacy of a continuous IV administration of cyclosporine in 20 patients in a placebo-controlled trial,[20] after the same group had already published their experience in a small open-label trial.[21] They reported a response in 9 of 11 patients receiving IV cyclosporine in a dose of 4 mg/kg/d after a mean of 7 days (Figure 21-1). D'Haens compared the efficacy of IV cyclosporine (4 mg/kg/d) with methylprednisolone 40 mg/d in a randomized, double-blind, controlled trial in 30 patients with a steroid-refractory attack of UC.[22] After 8 days, patients who had a response received the same medication orally in combination with AZA. Nine of 14 patients (64%) had a response to cyclosporine therapy, compared to 8 of 15 (53%) to methylprednisolone (one patient was withdrawn from the study due to the presence of *C. difficile* toxin in the stool). The mean time to response was 5.2 ± 0.9 days (range 2 to 8) in the cyclosporine group. All the responders to IV cyclosporine were discharged on oral cyclosporine (Neoral), and AZA was started. After 6 and 12 months, 89% and 78% of the patients, respectively, initially controlled with cyclosporine maintained their remission on AZA.

Actis was the first to report in an open-label trial that cyclosporine might also be effective in lower doses of 1 to 2 mg/kg/d,[23] which was also confirmed in another retrospective analysis by Rayner et al.[24] In a randomized, double-blind, controlled trial, the dose of 2 mg/kg/d cyclosporine was compared to 4 mg/kg/d cyclosporine (both administered by continuous infusion) by van Assche et al, who could demonstrate similar effectiveness (see Table 21-1) and a trend to a lower incidence of hypertension in the 2 mg/kg/d group. Therefore, it is likely that lower doses of cyclosporine (2 mg/kg/d) and lower cyclosporine blood levels could be applied by continuous infusion with probably fewer toxic side effects. Unfortunately, none of the previously named studies (as well as a large retrospective study including 86 patients) described a reliable predictor of treatment failure of cyclosporine that could separate these sick patients with severe UC for immediate surgery (Table 21-4).[25]

After responding to IV cyclosporine, it is generally recommended that the patient should be switched to oral cyclosporine (4 to 6 mg/kg/d; Figure 21-2). Additionally, the start of AZA (2 to 2.5 mg/kg/d) or 6-MP (1 to 1.5 mg/kg/d) should be initiated as a long-term maintenance treatment while the patient is still on cyclosporine. This is because the probability of preventing colectomy in the patients responding to IV cyclosporine in the next 5 years is 40% in patients treated with cyclosporine alone, compared to 66% in patients who are also treated with AZA or 6-MP (Table 21-5, also see Figure 21-2).[26,27] Therefore, most of the patients will be on 3 immunosuppressive drugs for a short-term period (steroids, cyclosporine, and AZA). In this case, for the prevention of *Pneumocystis carinii* infections, therapy with trimethoprim-sulfamethoxazole is recommended—similar to patients with AIDS with low CD4+ lymphocyte counts.[28-30]

Results of numerous, mostly retrospective, studies of oral as well as IV cyclosporine have been published so far. In a recently published analysis by Loftus et al,[5] the overall response rate (which is defined as the avoidance of colectomy) of 604 patients studied in 42 trials was 70% (422 of 604). The preferred route of administration was continuous IV application at a mean dose of 4 mg/kg/d (range 4 to 15 mg/kg/d) with an observed improvement of the patients within 1 to 2 weeks.

TABLE 21-4

CHARACTERISTICS OF PATIENTS TREATED WITH INTRAVENOUS CYCLOSPORINE DUE TO SEVERE ULCERATIVE COLITIS

	No Colectomy	Colectomy
N (female/male)	72 (46/26)	14 (8/6)
Age (mean ± SEM)	39.9 ± 12.7	46.0 ± 6.5
Disease duration (yrs)	6.2 ± 5.2	5.2 ± 4.1
Disease location		
Pancolitis	41.7%	64.3%
Left-sided colitis	58.3%	35.7%
Duration IV CyA (days)	8.9 ± 1.7	10.0 ± 3.2
CyA blood concentrations (ng/mL)	322 ± 66	339 ± 54

A total of 86 patients were treated.[25] No significant differences between the patients undergoing colectomy and the patients responding to the therapy could be demonstrated in this retrospective analysis.

TABLE 21-5

CUMULATIVE PROBABILITY OF CLINICAL RELAPSE OR COLECTOMY AFTER THE ADMINISTRATION OF INTRAVENOUS CYCLOSPORINE

Cumulative Probability of	1 Year	3 Years	5 Years
Clinical relapse	42%	72%	77%
Colectomy	29%	35%	42%

Cumulative probability of clinical relapse or colectomy after the administration of intravenous cyclosporine for severe, steroid-refractory UC (n = 27 patients, retrospective analysis).[52] Responders to IV cyclosporine were treated with AZA without oral cyclosporine as maintenance therapy.

ORAL CYCLOSPORINE MICROEMULSION FORMULATION (NEORAL)

Three small uncontrolled trials suggest that the microemulsion formulation of cyclosporine is as effective as the IV application. In the report by Actis et al, the short-term response rate was 100% in 14 patients being treated with oral microemulsion cyclosporine compared to a historical cohort of 40 patients receiving IV cyclosporine.[31] In both groups, the doses were titrated to ensure whole-blood drug concentrations of approximately 200 ng/mL. In another small trial, the same group reported a response rate of 89% in patients with chronic active steroid-dependent colitis.[32] A fast response to the therapy with Neoral in a mean time of 3.6 days was also reported by Navazo et al in 9 of 10 patients with acute steroid-resistant colitis.[33] The initial dose was 7 to 7.5 mg/kg/d adjusted to maintain whole-blood cyclosporine trough levels between 250 and 350 ng/mL. However, larger prospective studies (especially in patients with severe steroid-resistant UC) are missing to really compare the oral with the IV regimen.

OUTCOME IN CASE OF CYCLOSPORINE FAILURE

Similar to results of patients treated perioperatively with AZA,[34] there does not seem to be a higher complication rate in patients undergoing proctocolectomy after failing cyclosporine than in patients failing steroids only.[35-37]

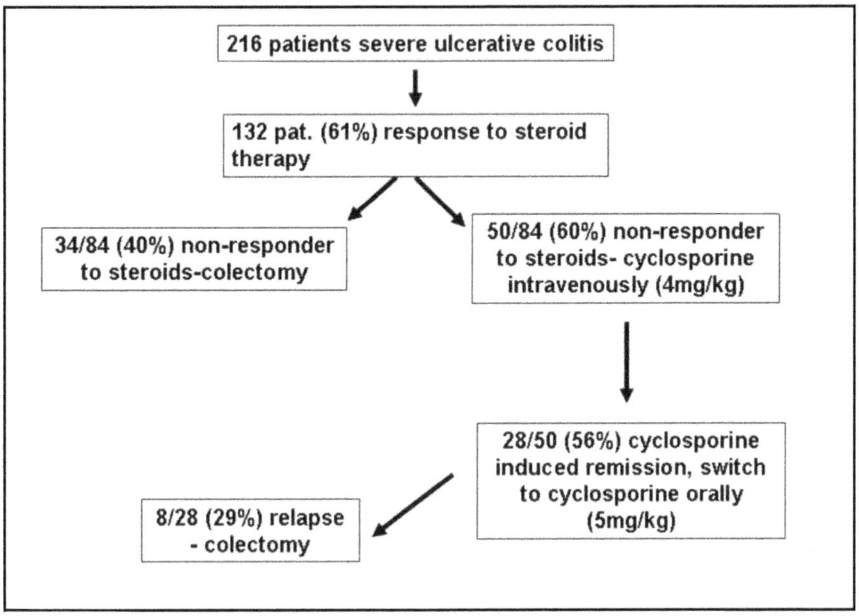

FIGURE 21-2. Short- and long-term efficacy of IV cyclosporine in patients admitted to a tertiary hospital with acute severe UC. The short-term efficacy was 56%; during a mean follow-up of 19 months, the long-term efficacy was only 40%, because 8 of the patients relapsed while being on oral cyclosporine. (Adapted from Hyde GM, Thillainayagam AV, Jewell DP. Intravenous cyclosporin as rescue therapy in severe ulcerative colitis: time for a reappraisal? *Eur J Gastroenterol Hepatol.* 1998;10:411-413.)

CYCLOSPORINE ENEMAS

Whereas 4 small, uncontrolled trials suggested a clinical efficacy of cyclosporine enemas in UC,[38-41] the only controlled trial that investigated the local application of cyclosporine as an enema in patients with left-sided colitis demonstrated no clinical benefit.[42] Forty patients were randomized to receive either nightly cyclosporine (350 mg) or placebo enemas. At 4 weeks, 8 of 20 patients (40%) who received cyclosporine showed clinical improvement compared with 9 of 20 patients (45%) who received placebo. One patient receiving cyclosporine had reversible neutropenia attributable to sulfasalazine, and another patient receiving cyclosporine was unable to tolerate the enema vehicle. No other toxicity was noted during the trial. Blood cyclosporine levels were detectable in only 2 patients.

TACROLIMUS

One placebo-controlled trial investigated the efficacy of 2 different trough levels of orally administered tacrolimus (high tacrolimus [HT] and low tacrolimus [LT] trough levels, 10 to 15 ng/l and 5 to 10 ng/mL, respectively) compared to placebo in 63 patients with refractory ulcerative colitis.[43] After 14 days, 68% in the HT, 38% in the LT, and 10% in the placebo group had a partial response, defined as a reduction of the DAI of more than 4 points with improvement of all categories. Clinical remission defined as a DAI ≤2 was observed in 20%, 10%, and 6% in the HT, LT, and placebo group, respectively. There are several small open-label trials published that investigate the clinical efficacy of tacrolimus in patients with UC.[9,44-48] Bousvaros et al demonstrated a response rate of 69% with 0.2 mg/kg/d tacrolimus administered orally in 14 pediatric patients with severe steroid-refractory colitis (10 UC, 2 Crohn's colitis, 2 indeterminate colitis).[45] Of the responders, 45% underwent colectomy at 6 months and 65% after 12 months despite concomitant immunosuppressive therapy with AZA or 6-MP in the majority of the patients. Fellermann et al published the results of 38 patients with refractory colitis (33 with UC and 5 with indeterminate colitis) in the largest retrospective study so far in 2002.[48] Two other publications of the same group reported the results of a smaller number of patients, which were most likely included in the analysis of 2002.[9,47] The patients were either treated with 0.01 to 0.02 mg/kg/d tacrolimus IV or 0.1 to 0.2 mg/kg/d orally. Forty-seven percent (18/38) of the patients responded to the treatment, 11 of 38 patients achieved remission (29%) by 14 days. After 3 months of treatment (the initial IV-treated patients were switched to orally administered tacrolimus after 14 days), 34% of the patients (13/38) were in remission, and another 26% (10/38) had improved. The colectomy rate was 34% in a mean observation period of 16.2 months. Baumgart et al reported on 23 patients with severe UC; they had a response in 96% and a remission in 74% of the patients. Three patients (13%), all having initially responded to tacrolimus, underwent colectomy either due to adverse effects that necessitated the discontinuation of the drug (n = 1) or due to unwillingness to undergo long-term immunosuppression (n = 2).[46] Hogenauer et al demonstrated similar results as Baumgart et al in a small retrospective analysis in 9 patients with UC.[44]

Sirolimus

There are currently no published clinical trials using sirolimus in patients with UC.

Mycophenolate Mofetil

There are only scarce reports of patients with UC treated with orally administered mycophenolate mofetil. In an analysis of all published data in 2004 by Loftus et al,[5] 19 patients with a response rate of 47% (9/19) were identified. The overall mean dose in these reports, which included mainly patients with CD, was 2 g/d with 20% adverse events reported in these series.

FUTURE DIRECTIVES

The IV application of cyclosporine can be regarded as an established therapeutic option in patients with severe, steroid-refractory UC. However, one should always be aware of the considerable toxicity of this therapy, and the treatment should be conducted in specialized centers. There is some evidence that tacrolimus is similarly effective as cyclosporine, but this therapeutic option has to be further investigated in prospective trials. The limited experience with mycophenolate mofetil makes it impossible to recommend this drug for usage outside of controlled trials, which is even more true for sirolimus, for which no clinical data in IBD are available thus far. The main clinical issue that needs to be tackled in the future is the maintenance of remission in those patients who respond to cyclosporine or tacrolimus, because both drugs are only "bridging therapies." Right now, AZA is used as a maintenance therapy, but the outcome is far from optimal (as shown previously). Therefore, future drug developments should focus on therapies that can be used not only for short term, but also as a reliable maintenance therapy. Despite this, clinicians treating patients with severe colitis should always keep in mind that restorative proctocolectomy represents a valuable alternative therapeutic possibility that should not always be used as the "last exit," especially because this procedure also protects from the well-known increased colorectal cancer risk in UC.[49,50]

REFERENCES

1. Martinez-Martinez S, Redondo JM. Inhibitors of the calcineurin/NFAT pathway. *Curr Med Chem.* 2004;11:997-1007.
2. Borel JF, Kis ZL. The discovery and development of cyclosporine (Sandimmune). *Transplant Proc.* 1991;23:1867-1874.
3. Kapturczak MH, Meier-Kriesche HU, Kaplan B. Pharmacology of calcineurin antagonists. *Transplant Proc.* 2004;36:25S-32S.
4. Sandborn WJ, Tremaine WJ, Lawson GM. Clinical response does not correlate with intestinal or blood cyclosporine concentrations in patients with Crohn's disease treated with high-dose oral cyclosporine. *Am J Gastroenterol.* 1996;91:37-43.
5. Loftus CG, Egan LJ, Sandborn WJ. Cyclosporine, tacrolimus, and mycophenolate mofetil in the treatment of inflammatory bowel disease. *Gastroenterol Clin North Am.* 2004;33:141-169.
6. Kino T, Goto T. Discovery of FK-506 and update. *Ann N Y Acad Sci.* 1993;685:13-21.
7. Moreno M, Latorre A, Manzanares C, et al. Clinical management of tacrolimus drug interactions in renal transplant patients. *Transplant Proc.* 1999;31:2252-2253.
8. Sandborn WJ, Present DH, Isaacs KL, et al. Tacrolimus for the treatment of fistulas in patients with Crohn's disease: a randomized, placebo-controlled trial. *Gastroenterology.* 2003;125:380-388.
9. Fellermann K, Ludwig D, Stahl M, David-Walek T, Stange EF. Steroid-unresponsive acute attacks of inflammatory bowel disease: immunomodulation by tacrolimus (FK506). *Am J Gastroenterol.* 1998;93:1860-1866.
10. Thomson AW, Starzl TE. New immunosuppressive drugs: Mechanistic insights and potential therapeutic advances. *Immunol Rev.* 1993;136:71-98.
11. Mota A, Arias M, Taskinen EI, et al. Sirolimus-based therapy following early cyclosporine withdrawal provides significantly improved renal histology and function at 3 years. *Am J Transplant.* 2004;4:953-961.
12. Allison AC, Eugui EM. Mycophenolate mofetil and its mechanisms of action. *Immunopharmacology.* 2000;47:85-118.
13. Shaw LM, Korecka M, DeNofrio D, Brayman KL. Pharmacokinetic, pharmacodynamic, and outcome investigations as the basis for mycophenolic acid therapeutic drug monitoring in renal and heart transplant patients. *Clin Biochem.* 2001;34:17-22.
14. Naderer OJ, Dupuis RE, Heinzen EL, Wiwattanawongsa K, Johnson MW, Smith PC. The influence of norfloxacin and metronidazole on the disposition of mycophenolate mofetil. *J Clin Pharmacol.* 2005;45:219-226.
15. Loftus CG, Loftus EV Jr, Sandborn WJ. Cyclosporin for refractory ulcerative colitis. *Gut.* 2003;52:172-173.
16. Heisel O, Heisel R, Balshaw R, Keown P. New onset diabetes mellitus in patients receiving calcineurin inhibitors: a systematic review and meta-analysis. *Am J Transplant.* 2004;4:583-595.
17. Burke JF Jr, Pirsch JD, Ramos EL, et al. Long-term efficacy and safety of cyclosporine in renal-transplant recipients. *N Engl J Med.* 1994;331:358-363.
18. Feutren G, Mihatsch MJ. Risk factors for cyclosporine-induced nephropathy in patients with autoimmune diseases. International Kidney Biopsy Registry of Cyclosporine in Autoimmune Diseases. *N Engl J Med.* 1992;326:1654-1660.
19. Fulton B, Markham A. Mycophenolate mofetil: a review of its pharmacodynamic and pharmacokinetic properties and clinical efficacy in renal transplantation. *Drugs.* 1996;51:278-298.
20. Lichtiger S, Present DH, Kornbluth A, et al. Cyclosporine in severe ulcerative colitis refractory to steroid therapy. *N Engl J Med.* 1994;330:1841-1845.
21. Lichtiger S. Cyclosporine therapy in inflammatory bowel disease: Open-label experience. *Mt Sinai J Med.* 1990;57:315-319.
22. D'Haens G, Lemmens L, Geboes K, et al. Intravenous cyclosporine versus intravenous corticosteroids as single therapy for severe attacks of ulcerative colitis. *Gastroenterology.* 2001;120:1323-1329.
23. Actis GC, Ottobrelli A, Pera A, et al. Continuously infused cyclosporine at low dose is sufficient to avoid emergency colectomy in acute attacks of ulcerative colitis without the need for high-dose steroids. *J Clin Gastroenterol.* 1993;17:10-13.
24. Rayner CK, McCormack G, Emmanuel AV, Kamm MA. Long-term results of low-dose intravenous ciclosporin for acute severe ulcerative colitis. *Aliment Pharmacol Ther.* 2003;18:303-308.
25. Arts J, D'Haens G, Zeegers M, et al. Long-term outcome of treatment with intravenous cyclosporin in patients with severe ulcerative colitis. *Inflamm Bowel Dis.* 2004;10:73-78.

26. Cohen RD, Stein R, Hanauer SB. Intravenous cyclosporin in ulcerative colitis: a five-year experience. *Am J Gastroenterol.* 1999;94:1587-1592.
27. Campbell S, Ghosh S. Combination immunomodulatory therapy with cyclosporine and azathioprine in corticosteroid-resistant severe ulcerative colitis: the Edinburgh experience of outcome. *Dig Liver Dis.* 2003;35:546-551.
28. Daperno M, Sostegni R, Rocca R, et al. Review article: medical treatment of severe ulcerative colitis. *Aliment Pharmacol Ther.* 2002;16 Suppl 4:7-12.
29. Van Assche G, D'Haens G, Noman M, et al. Randomized, double-blind comparison of 4 mg/kg versus 2 mg/kg intravenous cyclosporine in severe ulcerative colitis. *Gastroenterology.* 2003;125:1025-1031.
30. Glück T, Geerdes-Fenge HF, Straub RH, et al. Pneumocystis carinii pneumonia as a complication of immunosuppressive therapy. *Infection.* 2000;28:227-230.
31. Actis GC, Aimo G, Priolo G, Moscato D, Rizzetto M, Pagni R. Efficacy and efficiency of oral microemulsion cyclosporin versus intravenous and soft gelatin capsule cyclosporin in the treatment of severe steroid-refractory ulcerative colitis: an open-label retrospective trial. *Inflamm Bowel Dis.* 1998;4:276-279.
32. Actis GC, Volpes R, Rizzetto M. Oral microemulsion cyclosporin to reduce steroids rapidly in chronic active ulcerative colitis. *Eur J Gastroenterol Hepatol.* 1999;11:905-908.
33. Navazo L, Salata H, Morales S, et al. Oral microemulsion cyclosporine in the treatment of steroid-refractory attacks of ulcerative and indeterminate colitis. *Scand J Gastroenterol.* 2001;36:610-614.
34. Aberra FN, Lewis JD, Hass D, Rombeau JL, Osborne B, Lichtenstein GR. Corticosteroids and immunomodulators: Postoperative infectious complication risk in inflammatory bowel disease patients. *Gastroenterology.* 2003;125:320-327.
35. Pinna-Pintor M, Arese P, Bona R, et al. Severe steroid-unresponsive ulcerative colitis: outcomes of restorative proctocolectomy in patients undergoing cyclosporin treatment. *Dis Colon Rectum.* 2000;43:609-613.
36. Fleshner PR, Michelassi F, Rubin M, Hanauer SB, Plevy SE, Targan SR. Morbidity of subtotal colectomy in patients with severe ulcerative colitis unresponsive to cyclosporine. *Dis Colon Rectum.* 1995;38:1241-1245.
37. Hyde GM, Jewell DP, Kettlewell MG, Mortensen NJ. Cyclosporine for severe ulcerative colitis does not increase the rate of perioperative complications. *Dis Colon Rectum.* 2001;44:1436-1440.
38. Sandborn WJ, Tremaine WJ, Schroeder KW, Steiner BL, Batts KP, Lawson GM. Cyclosporine enemas for treatment-resistant, mildly to moderately active, left-sided ulcerative colitis. *Am J Gastroenterol.* 1993;88:640-645.
39. Winter TA, Dalton HR, Merrett MN, Campbell A, Jewell DP. Cyclosporine A retention enemas in refractory distal ulcerative colitis and pouchitis. *Scand J Gastroenterol.* 1993;28:701-704.
40. Ranzi T, Campanini MC, Velio P, Quarto di Palo F, Bianchi P. Treatment of chronic proctosigmoiditis with cyclosporine enemas. *Lancet.* 1989;2:97.
41. Brynskov J, Freund L, Thomsen OO, Andersen CB, Rasmussen SN, Binder V. Treatment of refractory ulcerative colitis with cyclosporine enemas. *Lancet.* 1989;1:721-722.
42. Sandborn WJ, Tremaine WJ, Schroeder KW, et al. A placebo-controlled trial of cyclosporine enemas for mildly to moderately active left-sided ulcerative colitis. *Gastroenterology.* 1994;106:1429-1435.
43. Ogata H, Matsui T, Nakamura M, et al. A randomised dose finding study of oral tacrolimus (FK506) therapy in refractory ulcerative colitis. *Gut.* 2006;55:1255-1262.
44. Hogenauer C, Wenzl HH, Hinterleitner TA, Petritsch W. Effect of oral tacrolimus (FK 506) on steroid-refractory moderate/severe ulcerative colitis. *Aliment Pharmacol Ther.* 2003;18:415-423.
45. Bousvaros A, Kirschner BS, Werlin SL, et al. Oral tacrolimus treatment of severe colitis in children. *J Pediatr.* 2000;137:794-799.
46. Baumgart DC, Wiedenmann B, Dignass AU. Rescue therapy with tacrolimus is effective in patients with severe and refractory inflammatory bowel disease. *Aliment Pharmacol Ther.* 2003;17:1273-1278.
47. Fellermann K, Herrlinger KR, Witthoeft T, Homann N, Ludwig D, Stange EF. Tacrolimus: a new immunosuppressant for steroid-refractory inflammatory bowel disease. *Transplant Proc.* 2001;33:2247-2248.
48. Fellermann K, Tanko Z, Herrlinger KR, et al Response of refractory colitis to intravenous or oral tacrolimus (FK506). *Inflamm Bowel Dis.* 2002;8:317-324.
49. Winther KV, Jess T, Langholz E, Munkholm P, Binder V. Long-term risk of cancer in ulcerative colitis: a population-based cohort study from Copenhagen County. *Clin Gastroenterol Hepatol.* 2004;2:1088-1095.
50. Itzkowitz SH, Harpaz N. Diagnosis and management of dysplasia in patients with inflammatory bowel diseases. *Gastroenterology.* 2004;126:1634-1648.
51. Sandborn WJ. A critical review of cyclosporine therapy in inflammatory bowel disease. *Inflamm Bowel Dis.* 1995;1:48-63.
52. Domenech E, Garcia-Planella E, Bernal I, et al. Azathioprine without oral ciclosporin in the long-term maintenance of remission induced by intravenous ciclosporin in severe, steroid-refractory ulcerative colitis. *Aliment Pharmacol Ther.* 2002;16:2061-2065.
53. Hyde GM, Thillainayagam AV, Jewell DP. Intravenous cyclosporin as rescue therapy in severe ulcerative colitis: time for a reappraisal? *Eur J Gastroenterol Hepatol.* 1998;10:411-413.

22

INFLIXIMAB USE IN ULCERATIVE COLITIS

Wojciech Blonski, MD, PhD; Antoni Stadnicki, MD, PhD;
Gary R. Lichtenstein, MD, FACP, FACG, AGAF; and Anne Burke, MD

Inflammatory bowel disease (IBD) encompasses Crohn's disease and ulcerative colitis, which are chronic, spontaneously relapsing disorders. The causes of these diseases are unknown, but genetic and environmental factors appear to interact via an immunologically mediated pathogenetic mechanism. There is convincing evidence that the pathogenesis of IBD involves immunological hyperresponsiveness within the gastrointestinal tract mucosa. The inciting stimulus is unknown but possibilities include luminal bacteria (normal or pathogenic flora), epithelial HLA haplotypes, and other environmental factors (eg, a transient nonspecific injury). Under normal circumstances, the inflammatory response is followed by a local suppression of inflammation to allow healing and a return to normal. In patients with IBD, individual genetic susceptibility may lead to amplification of the normal immune response.

The mainstays of medical therapy in UC have historically been the 5-ASA derivatives and corticosteroids during periods of flare. These agents are effective in the majority of patients. However, for those who are steroid-resistant, therapeutic options are limited. Cyclosporine A has recently been shown to be an agent capable of inducing remission in patients with severe disease; however, its adverse effect profile, including hypertension and renal impairment, makes it less than ideal as a long-term agent for the treatment of UC. Therefore, therapeutic options are limited for steroid-resistant or refractory patients.

INFLIXIMAB

Infliximab is a chimeric, monoclonal antibody (human-murine) directed against tumor necrosis factor alpha (TNFα) of approximate molecular weight of 149,000 Daltons. In infliximab, the entire variable domain is derived from a murine anti-TNFα hybridoma and is attached to a human IgG_1 constant region derived from plasmid expression vectors.[1-5] Chimeric antibodies, such as infliximab, are less immunogenic than murine antibodies and can persist for more than 2 weeks in human circulation compared to only 2 days for murine antibodies.[3]

PHARMACOKINETICS

There are limited pharmacokinetic data available on infliximab. Data from clinical studies using single IV infusions of infliximab (5, 10, 20 mg/kg) showed a linear and direct relationship between the dose administered, the maximum serum concentration, and the area under the concentration time curve.[6] Its route of metabolism and excretion is unknown,[7] and the rate of clearance is dose independent.[6] A single dose of infliximab 5 mg/kg had a serum half-life of 9.5 days, remaining primarily in the vascular compartment (volume of distribution at steady state = 3 liters).[6] Serum infliximab levels decline in an exponential fashion and are usually undetectable at week 12.[8] Repeat dosing, 10 mg/kg every 8 weeks for 4 doses, does not result in accumulation of infliximab.[8]

Lichtenstein GR, ed.
Ulcerative Colitis: The Complete Guide to Medical Management (pp. 237-254)

Mechanism of Action

The mechanism of action of infliximab is not clear but likely involves interference with the functions of TNFα. The variable region of this antibody binds to both soluble and transmembrane TNFα with high affinity and specificity while the constant region mediates its effector functions including antibody-dependent cellular toxicity, complement fixation, and antibody clearance and apoptosis of T lymphocytes.[2-4,9]

Therapeutic Use

The use of infliximab has been approved by the FDA, in combination with methotrexate, for reducing the signs and symptoms, inhibiting the progression of structural damage, and improving physical function in patients with moderately to severely active rheumatoid arthritis who have had an inadequate response to methotrexate.[2,10,11] Infliximab is also indicated for reducing the signs and symptoms and inducing and maintaining clinical remission in patients with moderately to severely active CD who have had an inadequate response to conventional therapy. In addition, infliximab is indicated for reducing the number of draining enterocutaneous and rectovaginal fistulas and maintaining fistula closure in patients with fistulizing CD.[2,10,11] Moreover, infliximab has been approved by the FDA for reducing signs and symptoms in patients with active ankylosing spondylitis or psoriatic arthritis.[2] Recently, infliximab has been approved by the FDA for reducing signs and symptoms, inducing and maintaining clinical remission and mucosal healing, and eliminating corticosteroid use in patients with moderately to severely active UC who have had an inadequate response to conventional therapy of UC.

TNFα in Inflammation and Inflammatory Bowel Disease

TNFα: Molecular Effects

TNFα is a 26-kd protein produced mainly by activated macrophages and also by other inflammatory cells.[12,13] Endotoxin lipopolysaccharide (LPS) is the major stimulator for TNFα, but other cytokines may play a role. TNFα is expressed on the cell membrane, cleaved into its active 17-kd form. It promotes the expression of a variety of downstream signaling molecules, including cytokines (IL-6, IL-8, and IL–1), adhesion molecules (ICAM and VCAM), and inducible nitric oxide synthase,[13,14] which in turn lead to activation of macrophages, priming of neutrophils, altered epithelial permeability, enhanced production of acute-phase reactants, and stimulation of protease synthesis and release, causing tissue injury resulting in recruitment of additional immune cells.[15] In addition, the gene products influence cell growth and differentiation; apoptosis and necrosis; immunomodulation and antiviral activity, and are mitogenic to lymphocytes, fibroblasts, and other cells.[16]

Effects of Infliximab on TNFα

Infliximab, in vitro and in vivo, inhibits TNFα-induced priming of neutrophils and their adherence to endothelial cells.[17] It induces apoptosis in peripheral monocytes,[18] and accelerates the apoptosis of subsets of T lymphocytes, which have TNFα expression on their cell surface.[19,20] Infliximab causes a rapid and specific increase in apoptosis of T lymphocytes in gut mucosa without affecting peripheral blood mononuclear cells,[20] decreases production of granulocyte-macrophage colony stimulating factor by intestinal T cells,[21,22] and inhibits the expression of ICAM-1.[23]

There is a clear increase in circulating lymphocytes and monocytes and a concomitant decrease in circulating neutrophils 2 to 4 weeks after infliximab infusion.[24]

In summary, infliximab reduces the production of proinflammatory and chemotactic cytokines, decreases the activity of neutrophils, and induces apoptosis in lymphocytes and mononuclear cells.

Role of TNFα in Inflammatory Bowel Disease

TNFα is a major inflammatory cytokine with properties relevant to intestinal inflammation.[25] It attracts circulating cells to the sites of inflammation, activates coagulation and induces edema, and takes part in granuloma formation.[26] In addition, it increases intestinal permeability and influences epithelial cell growth, induces epithelial cell apoptosis, and affects gastrointestinal integrity by stimulating mucosal mesenchymal cells to secrete matrix-degrading metalloproteinases.[27-30]

The current knowledge emphasizes the role of immunological factors in the development of IBD.[15] CD is characterized by domination of Th_1 lymphocytes in the intestinal mucosa, whereas UC is characterized by domination of Th_2 lymphocytes in colonic mucosa.[31] The immune response in UC is characterized by the production of TGF β and IL-5 and downregulation of IL-4 production.[31-33] The diminished IL-4 response is associated with activating natural killer (NK) cells and IL-13 secretion.[34] Studies have shown increased levels of TNFα in the colonic mucosa, serum, and stool of patients with UC, and the degree of elevation correlates with disease activity.[35-41] Another study has found elevated levels of IL-6, IL-8, TNFα, and TNFα receptor, p55 and p75, which correlated the degree of inflammation.[42,43] TNFα-secreting cells are increased in the mucosa and submucosa of inflamed intestine in both CD and UC, but TNFα levels are higher in CD patients.[44-46] Increased expression of IL-8, TNFα, and interferon-γ m-RNA has been detected even in inactive UC, suggesting that these cytokines play a pivotal role in the relapses of UC.[47] It was suggested that TNFα is one possible mediator of the increased IL-8 synthesis in active UC.[48,49] IL-8 is

TABLE 22-1

RANDOMIZED PLACEBO-CONTROLLED TRIALS OF INFLIXIMAB IN PATIENTS WITH ULCERATIVE COLITIS

Author	Number of Patients	Dose	Treatment	Response N (%) [*]	P-value
Sands et al[56]	11	Single	Infliximab patients: 8 Placebo patients: 3	4 (50) [14 days] 0 (0) [14 days]	P=0.124
Probert et al[57]	43	Multiple	Infliximab patients: 23 Placebo patients: 20	9 (39) [6 weeks] 6 (30) [6 weeks]	P=0.76
Ochsenkuhn et al[60]	13	Multiple	Infliximab patients: 6 Prednisolone patients: 7	5 (83.3) [3 weeks and 13 weeks] 6 (85.7) [3 weeks and 13 weeks]	P=0.7
Rutgeerts et al (ACT 1)[58]	364	Multiple	Infliximab patients: 243 Placebo patients: 121	159 (65.4) [8 weeks] 45 (37.2) [8 weeks]	P<0.001
Rutgeerts et al (ACT 2)[58]	364	Multiple	Infliximab patients: 241 Placebo patients: 123	161 (66.8) [8 weeks] 36 (29.3) [8 weeks]	P<0.001
Järnerot et al[59]	45	Single	Infliximab patients: 24 Placebo patients: 21	not reported	–

* Time from initial administration of the studied drug when the response was evaluated.

thought to mediate local mucosal recruitment and activation of neutrophils in UC.[49] It has also been suggested that TNFα is involved in cell injury in the colonic epithelium in UC by increasing antibody-dependent cellular cytotoxicity activity.[50] These findings prompted the evaluation of anti-TNFα treatment in UC.

ANIMAL DATA ON ANTI-TNFα USE IN ULCERATIVE COLITIS

Infusion of TNFα in rodent models results in acute and chronic inflammation of the intestine, with focal ulceration of the cecum, weight loss, hepatomegaly, bile duct proliferation, periportal inflammation, leukocytosis, and anemia.[51] Anti-TNFα antibodies reduced the severity of intestinal inflammation down-regulation of the production of inflammatory cytokines.[52] Unlike rodent models, the cotton-top tamarin (the *Saguinus Oedipus*) spontaneously develops a colitis that more closely resembles human UC. This colitis only develops when the animal is in captivity. It is responsive to 5-ASA and corticosteroids and is associated with the subsequent development of adenocarcinoma and primary sclerosing cholangitis.[53,54] Watkins et al have studied the effect of an engineered human monoclonal anti-TNFα antibody (CD571) in this model.[53] All 6 animals in this study received intramuscular injection of CDP571 antibody (20 mg/kg) in 6 doses every 6 days,[53] and all responded to the anti-TNFα treatment with increased body weight, improved stools consistency, and decreased mucosal inflammation on histologic scoring.[53] During 18 months of follow-up, 4 animals remained disease-free and required no further therapy. The 2 remaining animals relapsed between 8 months and 1 year after the last dose of CD571 and obtained additional therapy with olsalazine.[53] The results of this study suggested that treatment by anti-TNFα antibody in humans might also be effective.[53]

HUMAN DATA ON ANTI-TNFα USE IN ULCERATIVE COLITIS

The first studies of anti-TNFα antibody in humans followed from the work of Watkins et al and used the human monoclonal antibody CDP571.[53] Fifteen patients with mild to moderate UC received a single dose of 5 mg/kg. Nine patients did not receive steroids, and 6 were steroid-refractory.[55] In the first 2 weeks following administration of the drug, 10 patients (6 who did not receive steroids and 4 steroid-refractory) showed improvement in Powell-Tuck clinical symptom scores, sigmoidoscopy score, and decreased inflammatory markers—erythrocyte sedimentation rate

(ESR), serum C reactive protein (CRP), and IL-6 plasma concentration.[55] However, a statistically significant improvement was noted only for the clinical scores and ESR.[55]

There have been 5 randomized, double-blind, controlled trials (5 with placebo control[56-59] and 1 with prednisolone control[60]) of infliximab for UC. Enrollment criteria varied slightly, but included 840 patients with moderate to severe steroid-resistant UC (n = 827)[56-59] or nonsteroid-resistant UC (n = 13).[60] Data from these studies are summarized in Table 22-1.

In the study by Sands et al, 11 patients with severe UC (Truelove and Witts score >10) refractory to steroids received either a single infusion of 5 (n = 3), 10 (n = 3), or 20 (n = 2) mg/kg infliximab (8 patients) or placebo (3 patients).[56] Within 2 weeks of infusion, all placebo patients, but only 4 (50%) infliximab patients, required colectomy.[56] Clinical response was correlated with decreases in ESR, serum levels of CRP, and circulating IL-6.[56] The decrease in modified Truelove and Witts criteria was noted in all 5 of 8 infliximab patients, 4 of whom avoided colectomy.[56]

There is only one negative study of all the controlled studies to date assessing infliximab. Probert et al evaluated 43 patients with moderately severe UC.[57] Patients were assessed using the UC symptom score (UCSS) (stool frequency, rectal bleeding, sigmoidoscopic appearance, and the global assessment by physician). In addition, the endoscopic appearance was assessed using the Baron scale. Patients were randomized to receive infliximab (n = 23) 5 mg/kg or placebo (n = 20). There was no difference in clinical or endoscopic response rates between the 2 groups at 0 or 6 weeks post-infusion (see Table 22-1). A modest decrease in steroid dose was seen in the treated group between 0 and 6 weeks post-infusion. In follow-up, 20 patients received open-label infliximab 10 mg/kg; 11 had received infliximab 5 mg/kg and 9 had received placebo. Clinical remission was achieved in 27% and 11%, respectively, which was not statistically significantly different.[57]

Two recent multicenter, randomized, double-blind, placebo-controlled, parallel-treatment group trials (ACT 1, ACT 2) evaluated infliximab use in patients with moderate or severe active UC refractory to standard therapy including 5-ASA, corticosteroids, or immunosuppressants.[58] Active UC was defined as a Mayo score of ≥6 points (on a 12-point scale) and endoscopy subscore of ≥2 points. There were 364 patients randomized in each study. The data from these 2 trials are presented in Table 22-2.

In the ACT 1 study, enrollment criteria included patients who met at least one of the following criteria: current treatment with oral corticosteroids and 6-MP or AZA; failure to successfully taper, tolerate, or respond to corticosteroids within the past 18 months; and failure to tolerate or respond to 6-MP or AZA within the previous 5 years.

In the ACT 1 trial, patients received either infliximab 5 mg/kg (n = 121), infliximab 10 mg/kg (n = 121), or placebo (n = 122) at weeks 0, 2, and 6, then every 8 weeks through week 46.[58] Patients continued their corticosteroids and immunosuppressants as clinically indicated. The primary endpoint was clinical response at week 8, defined as a decrease in the Mayo score of ≥30% and ≥3 points accompanied by a decrease in the rectal bleeding score of ≥1 or a rectal bleeding score of 0 or 1 at week 8. The major secondary endpoints were clinical remission at week 8, mucosal healing at week 8, clinical response at week 30, and clinical remission at week 30. Clinical remission was defined as Mayo score ≤2 with no individual subscore >1, whereas mucosal healing was defined as endoscopy subscore of 0 or 1.[58]

Clinical response occurred in 69.4% and 61.5% of patients treated with infliximab 5 mg/kg and 10 mg/kg, respectively ($P<0.001$), and in 37.2% of placebo-treated patients at week 8. Clinical response was also found in 52.1% and 50.8% of patients treated with infliximab 5 mg/kg and 10 mg/kg, respectively ($P<0.001$ and $P=0.002$, respectively), and in 29.8% of patients receiving placebo at week 30.[58]

Clinical remission was achieved at week 8 in 38.8% and 32.0% of infliximab-treated patients 5 mg/kg and 10 mg/kg, respectively ($P<0.001$ and $P=0.002$, respectively), and in 14.9% of patients receiving placebo. At week 30, 33.9% of patients receiving infliximab 5 mg/kg ($P=0.001$), 36.9% of patients receiving infliximab 10 mg/kg ($P<0.001$), and 15.7% of placebo-treated patients maintained their clinical remission.[58] In addition, the proportion of patients who were able to discontinue corticosteroids while in clinical remission at week 30 was twofold greater in the combined infliximab treatment group than in the placebo (21.7% versus 10.1%; $P=0.039$) group.[58]

The ACT 2 trial included patients who either received concurrent treatment with corticosteroids, AZA, 6-MP, or aminosalicylates, or who failed to tolerate or respond to corticosteroids, AZA, 6-MP, or aminosalicylates.[58] In this study, patients received either infliximab 5 mg/kg (n = 121), infliximab 10 mg/kg (n = 120), or placebo (n = 123) at weeks 0, 2, 6, 14, and 22. Patients continued their corticosteroids and immunosuppressants as clinically indicated. The primary endpoints were the same as in the ACT 1 trial.[58,59] At week 8, clinical response occurred in 64.5% and 69.2% of patients treated with infliximab 5 mg/kg and 10 mg/kg, respectively ($P<0.001$), and in 29.3% of placebo-treated patients.[58]

At week 30, 47.1% and 60.0% of patients treated with infliximab 5 mg/kg and 10 mg/kg, respectively ($P<0.001$), and 26.0% of patients receiving placebo maintained their clinical response.[58] Clinical remission was achieved at week 8 in 33.9% and 27.5% of patients treated with infliximab 5 mg/kg and 10 mg/kg, respectively ($P<0.001$), and in 5.7 % of patients receiving placebo. At week 30, 25.6%

TABLE 22-2

THE ACT 1 AND ACT 2 TRIALS EVALUATING INFLIXIMAB IN PATIENTS WITH MODERATE TO SEVERE UC REFRACTORY TO STANDARD THERAPY, INCLUDING 5-ASA, CORTICOSTEROIDS, OR IMMUNOSUPPRESSANTS

Trial	Number of Patients	Treatment	Clinical Response [%]*		Mucosal Healing [%]**		Clinical Remission [%]***		Discontinuation of Corticosteroids at Week 30
			Week 8	Week 30	Week 8	Week 30	Week 8	Week 30	
ACT 1[58]	121	Infliximab (5 mg/kg)	69.4	52.1	62.0	50.4	38.8	33.9	Infliximab group: 21.7%
	121	Infliximab (10 mg/kg)	61.5	50.8	59.0	49.2	32.0	36.9	
	122	Placebo	37.2	29.8	33.9	24.8	14.9	15.7	Placebo group: 10.1%
		P-value (infliximab versus placebo)	$P<0.001$ $P<0.001$	$P<0.001$ $P=0.002$	$P<0.001$ $P<0.001$	$P<0.001$ $P<0.001$	$P<0.001$ $P=0.002$	$P=0.001$ $P<0.001$	$P=0.0039$
ACT 2[58]	121	Infliximab (5 mg/kg)	64.5	47.1	60.3	46.3	33.9	25.6	Infliximab 5 mg/kg 18.3%
	120	Infliximab (10 mg/kg)	69.2	60.0	61.7	56.7	27.5	35.8	Infliximab 10 mg/kg 27.3%
	123	Placebo	29.3	26.0	30.9	30.1	5.7	10.6	Placebo group: 3.3%
		P-value (infliximab versus placebo)	$P<0.001$ $P<0.001$	$P<0.001$ $P<0.001$	$P<0.001$ $P<0.001$	$P=0.009$ $P<0.001$	$P<0.001$ $P<0.001$	$P=0.003$ $P<0.001$	$P<0.001$ $P=0.010$

*Clinical response: decrease in the Mayo score of ≥30% and ≥3 points, accompanied by decrease in rectal bleeding score of ≥1 or a rectal bleeding score of 0 or 1 at week 8.

**Mucosal healing: endoscopy subscore of 0 or 1.

***Clinical remission: Mayo score ≤2 with no individual subscores >1.

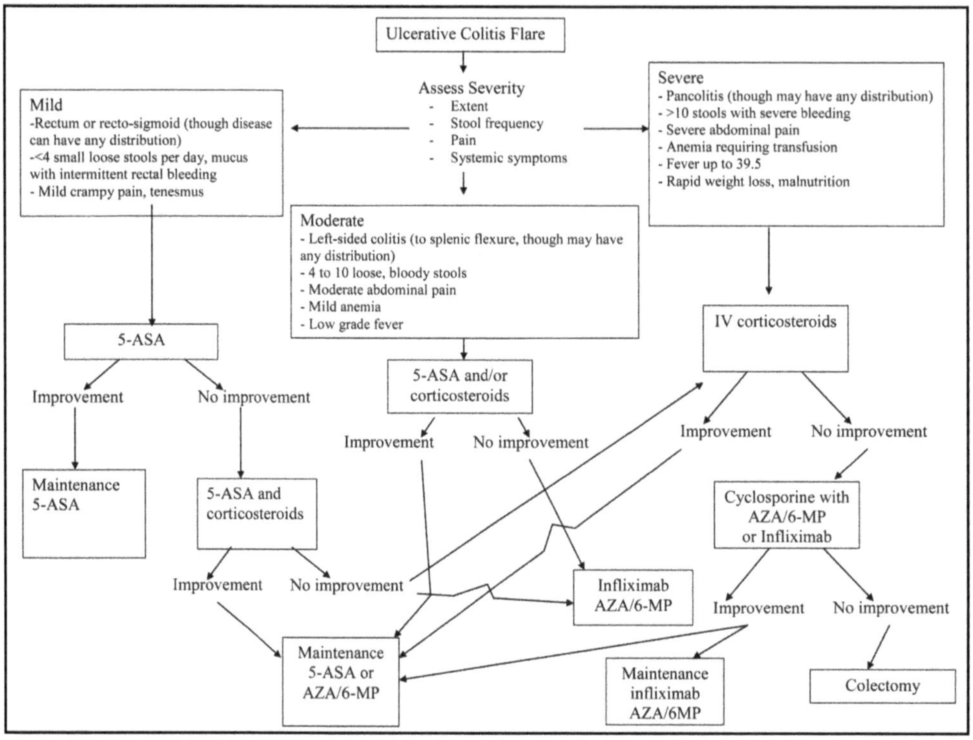

Figure 22-1. Management of ulcerative colitis.

of patients receiving infliximab 5 mg/kg (P=0.003), 35.8% of patients receiving infliximab 10 mg/kg (P<0.001), and 10.6% of placebo-treated patients maintained their clinical remission. In addition, the proportion of patients who were able to discontinue corticosteroids while in clinical remission at week 30 was sixfold greater in patients treated with infliximab 5 mg/kg (18.3%, P<0.001) and ninefold greater in patients treated with infliximab 10 mg/kg (27.3%, P=0.010) than in the placebo (3.3%) group.[58]

A landmark double-blind, placebo-controlled study by Järnerot et al evaluated the efficacy of infliximab in patients with severe or moderately-severe UC unresponsive to conventional therapy.[59] In order to be included in the study, the patients were required to have a "fulminant colitis index" ≥8 on the third day of the treatment with IV corticosteroids or a Seo-index >150 on the fifth, sixth, or seventh day of the treatment with IV corticosteroids. There were 45 patients included in this study who received either a single infusion of 4 to 5 mg infliximab (n = 24) or placebo (n = 21) and were followed for up to 90 days. Overall, 29% of patients treated with infliximab underwent colectomy, with the median time between infusion and surgical procedure of 8 days. This was in contrast to 66% of placebo-treated patients who were subject to colectomy in the median time of 4 days following the infusion (P=0.017).[59]

There has been one randomized prednisolone-controlled trial in which patients received infliximab 5 mg/kg for 3 doses (7 patients) versus prednisolone 1.5 mg/kg for 2 weeks (6 patients).[60] Treatment response, at 3 weeks and 3 months, was defined as a decrease in median activity score to less than 10 points. Five (83%) infliximab-treated patients and 6 (85%) prednisolone-treated patients achieved clinical response.[60]

The previous data, particularly the study by Sands et al[56] and the ACT 1 and ACT 2 trials,[58] suggest that infliximab may be of benefit in severe UC, and there is potential that in the future infliximab will become the standard therapy for these patient populations. Furthermore, recent data from Scandinavia have shown impressive efficacy in acute severe or moderately severe UC unresponsive to IV corticosteroids.[59]

One retrospective analysis from 4 medical centers evaluated the efficacy of infliximab in 27 patients with UC who received single or multiple infusions of infliximab.[61] Twelve patients (44%) achieved remission, 6 (22%) had a partial response, whereas 9 (33%) had no response (5 of whom required colectomy).[62] The median time to response was 4 days, and the median duration of response was 8 weeks.[61] A clinical response was more likely in those who were steroid-sensitive compared with steroid-refractory patients (83% versus 33%). Nine of the 18 responders experienced a total of 19 relapses, all but one of which were successfully treated with further infliximab.[61]

There have also been 11 other open-labeled, uncontrolled, retrospective studies assessing the use of infliximab in patients with UC.[62-72] Those studies included 6 to 20 patients who received single or multiple infusions of infliximab 5 mg/kg or 10 mg/kg.[62-72] In these studies, the initial response

TABLE 22-3

OPEN-LABEL STUDIES IN ADULT PATIENTS WITH ULCERATIVE COLITIS TREATED WITH INFLIXIMAB

Authors	Number of Patients	Design	Dose	Response	Sustained Remission	Steroid-Free Remission
Chey et al[62]	8	Retrospective	Single	100% (1 week)	Not reported	-
Chey et al[63]	16	Retrospective	Single or multiple	88% (>4 months)	25% (7 to 10 months)	-
Kaser et al[64]	6	Retrospective	Single	100% (7 days)	57% (5.5 months)	-
Fleisher et al[70]	17	Retrospective	Multiple	82% (4 weeks)	76% (12 weeks)	-
Kohn et al[65]	13	Retrospective	Single	77% (6 days)	69% (10.1 months)	69% (10.1 months)
Actis et al[66]	8	Retrospective	Single or multiple	50% (7 to 30 days)	25% (1 to 7 months)	25%
Kugathasan et al[68]	15	Retrospective	Not reported	73%: • 13% complete response • 60% partial response	Not reported	-
Su et al[61]	27	Retrospective	Single or multiple	66%: • 44% (remission) (1 to 21 days) • 22% (partial response) • Response in 33% steroid-refractory patients and 83% nonsteroid-refractory	33% (at least 1 month) infliximab reinfusion resulted in 97% response)	11%
Gornet et al[67]	18	Retrospective	Single or multiple	89% (7 days)	39% (1 month)	-
Cooper et al[69]	14	Retrospective	Single or multiple	36%	Not reported	-
Bermejo et al[71]	7	Retrospective	Single or multiple	86%	Not reported	83%
Shen et al[72]	8	Retrospective	Single or multiple	37.5%	12.5% (1.5 years)	-

rate to infliximab ranged from 37.5% to 100%, whereas the sustained response rate ranged from 25% to 76%.[62-72] In two studies, response was achieved in less than 50% patients.[69,72] All open-label studies are summarized in Table 22-3.[61-72] Based on the data derived from the clinical trials, we propose the medical approach to patients with UC, which is presented in Figure 22-1.

Adverse Events

Adverse Events in Patients With Ulcerative Colitis Treated With Infliximab

The data on safety and toxicity with the use of infliximab in UC are not as extensive as the data from patients who had CD and used infliximab. The 2 largest trials evaluating infliximab in patients with UC, ACT 1 and ACT 2, observed similar rates of adverse events in the placebo and infliximab recipients.[58] The reported adverse events occurred in 84% of patients treated with infliximab and 77% of those treated with placebo, and serious adverse events were reported in 13% of those receiving active drug and 20% of those receiving placebo. The incidence of infections (31% for infliximab and 30% for placebo) and infusion reactions (11% for infliximab and 9% for placebo) was similar between treatment groups. The most notable adverse events occurred in patients treated with infliximab and included pneumonia (n = 5), tuberculosis (n = 1), optic neuritis (n = 1), multifocal motor neuropathy (n = 1), and drug-induced lupus (n = 1). ATI developed in 6% and 3% of patients treated with infliximab 5 mg/kg and 10 mg/kg, respectively.[58]

Additional data regarding safety of infliximab evaluated in 4 trials in patients with UC, a total of 112 patients, (61 infliximab, 51 control) are summarized in Table 22-1.[56,57,59,60] The reported rates of serious adverse events are 0% to 36% across 3 studies, including a 10% rate of life-threatening adverse events in one group (this was seen in both the infliximab and placebo control arms).[56,57,60] This finding cannot be distinguished from the side effects observed from corticosteroids alone, as multivariable analysis was not performed. Sands et al noted 87.5% of infliximab-treated subjects had nonserious adverse events, which resolved with appropriate management.[56] Järnerot et al observed the similar prevalence of generalized side effects in both the infliximab and placebo groups.[59]

The role of infliximab in UC is not yet fully established, but its role is evolving, and thus far there has been toxicity in some patients; however, this toxicity cannot be dissociated from use of other concurrent medications such as corticosteroids.

Adverse Events in Patients With Crohn's Disease and Rheumatoid Arthritis Treated With Infliximab

Much of the information learned regarding the safety of infliximab stems from its use in CD or rheumatoid arthritis (RA). However, in determining acceptable risk of a therapy, the magnitude of benefit is also important, and efficacy in UC cannot be inferred from the CD data. Infliximab has been evaluated in several clinical trials. There is a wealth of data concerning the prevalence of adverse events in patients with CD or RA treated with infliximab. Clinical safety of infliximab has been well-evaluated in 3 randomized, placebo-controlled clinical trials on patients with luminal and fistulizing CD (ACCENT I: 573 CD patients, ACCENT II: 282 CD patients, and ATTRACT: 428 RA patients) and in one retrospective analysis of 500 patients with CD.[73-77] The data from these studies are presented in Table 22-4. Adverse event data from these trials are discussed later.

Infusion-Related Reactions

Infusion reactions to infliximab are divided into acute (<24 hours after the infusion) or delayed (1 to 14 days after the infusion) and as mild, moderate, and severe.[78]

Most acute reactions to infliximab are non-IgE-mediated acute hypersensitivity reactions and present as fever, chest pain, hypertension or hypotension, and dyspnea. The usual approach is to slow or stop the infusion and to treat symptomatically with diphenhydramine, acetaminophen, antihistamines, and corticosteroids.[11,78] The infusion can usually be completed at a slower rate. Future infusions should be preceded by acetaminophen and an antihistamine agent.

Antibodies to Infliximab

Delayed infusion reactions are divided into serum sickness-like reactions, characterized by the presence of antibodies to infliximab (ATI) (previously called human anti-chimeric antibodies, HACA) and into others, such as lupus-like reactions, viral-type syndrome, IBD flare, and nonspecific reactions. Delayed infusion reactions to infliximab are usually of mild to moderate severity, presenting with arthralgia, myalgias, fever, urticarial rash, and malaise and typically respond to acetaminophen, antihistamines, and steroids.[78]

Randomized controlled studies reported that 11% to 17% of patients developed ATI during treatment with infliximab.[73-76] The presence of ATI increases twofold the risk of infusion reaction, occurring in 16% to 30% of patients with ATI and 8% to 16% of those without ATI.[73-76]

It was shown that the presence of ATI, particularly at concentrations ≥8.0 μg/mL in plasma, predicts a higher risk of infusion reactions when given in an episodic fashion.[79] Delayed hypersensitivity reactions were observed in 10 of 40 patients re-exposed to infliximab after a 2- to 4-year hiatus.[80] Symptoms developed 3 to 12 days following the infusion and resolved 24 to 96 hours after treatment with corticosteroids.[80] In large series, the occurrence of this reaction is noted to occur in 17% of individuals.[73]

TABLE 22-4

CLINICAL SAFETY OF INFLIXIMAB IN CLINICAL, RANDOMIZED, PLACEBO-CONTROLLED TRIALS AND RETROSPECTIVE SAFETY ANALYSIS IN PATIENTS WITH CD AND RA

	ACCENT I[73,74]			ACCENT II[75]		ATTRACT[76]		COLOMBEL ET AL[77]
Disease	CD			CD		RA		CD
Number of patients	573			282*		428		500
Follow-up time	54 weeks			54 weeks		30 weeks		17 months
Design	RCT			RCT		RCT		Retrospective
Induction	Infliximab 5 mg/kg IV			Infliximab 5 mg/kg IV		Methotrexate po or IV		Infliximab IV
	A Placebo	B Infliximab 5 mg/kg	C Infliximab 10 mg/kg	A Placebo	B Infliximab 5 mg/kg	A Placebo	B Infliximab 3 to 10 mg/kg	
All AE [%]	Not reported	Not reported	Not reported	92	89	All patients: 80		Not reported
Serious AE [%]	29	28	22	23	14	16	9 to 13	8.6
Infusion reactions [%]	13	32	24	17	16	Not reported		3.8
Infusions reactions by ATI status [%]•	ATI positive: 36 ATI negative: 24			ATI positive: 30 ATI negative: 16		Not reported		Not reported
Serious infusion reactions [%]	0.5	2	0.5	All patients: 0.3		0	0	0.4
Serum-sickness like reactions [%]	2	3	3	Not reported	Not reported	Not reported	Not reported	
Serious infection [%]	4	4	3	6	3	6	1-6	3
Malignancy [%]	1.1	1.5	0.5	0		0	0.9	1.8
Mortality rate per patient year	0	0.01	0	0		0.06	0.01	0.01

*Number of patients included in safety analysis through week 54. Total of 306 patients were enrolled in this trial.

•Among patients with evaluable samples.

The presence of ATI is also associated with decreased infliximab concentrations at 4 weeks and a shorter duration of response.[79] The occurrence of a delayed hypersensitivity-like reaction is not an absolute contraindication to re-infusion of infliximab. Premedication with corticosteroids and histamine-1 receptor antagonists is an appropriate management scheme in this patient population.

Various strategies have been used to prevent the development of ATI and subsequent infusion reactions. Administration of corticosteroids or immunomodulators with infliximab decreases the likelihood of developing ATI from approximately 20% to approximately 5%[73,75,77]; however, infusion reactions were noted in 19% to 89% of patients who were already receiving concomitant corticosteroids or immunosuppressants.[73,77] A more effective strategy seems to be the use of maintenance infliximab. The use of maintenance infliximab decreased the formation of ATI from 30% to approximately 7%.[72,74] The presence of ATI was associated with a 12% absolute increase in infusion reactions.[74] However, ATIs were not associated with the increase in serious infusion reactions or serum sickness-like reactions.[74] Nevertheless, repeat exposure increases the risk of development of ATI, which was documented in 61% of patients after 5 infusions.[79]

DEVELOPMENT OF ANTI-DOUBLE-STRANDED DNA ANTIBODIES AND DRUG-INDUCED LUPUS-LIKE SYNDROME

Treatment with infliximab has been shown to cause the formation of autoantibodies to antinuclear antibodies (ANA), double-stranded DNA (anti-dsDNA), and drug-induced lupus-like syndrome in 46% to 56%, 16% to 34%, and 0.2% to 0.7% of infliximab-treated patients, respectively.[73,75,76,81] The equivalent rates in placebo-treated patients were 18% to 35%, 0% to 11%, and 0%, respectively. Typically, the drug-induced lupus-like syndrome is mild, without involvement of other major organs (specifically CNS or renal) and resolves on discontinuation of the therapy and treatment with corticosteroids.[82-87] The natural history of ANA has been documented in an observational study of 125 patients treated with infliximab. All patients were ANA negative (titers <1:40) before treatment. Seventy-one patients (57%) developed ANA, usually after 1 or 2 infusions. ANA titers had a female preponderance 3:1 and were associated with a papulosquamous or butterfly rash.[88] A high ANA titer (>1:80) occurred in 43 (60.5%) of 71 ANA-positive subjects and when present was associated with other autoantibodies (anti-dsDNA 32.5%, anti-ssDNA 39.5%, and antihistone 20.9%). Two of the 125 patients (1.6%), both with ANA >1:80, presented with a drug-induced lupus-like syndrome associated with a butterfly rash, myalgias, and polyarthralgias, but without major organ involvement. ANA remained positive in 56 of 71 ANA-positive patients (79%) after a median of 12 months follow-up.[88]

It should be stressed that anti-dsDNA antibodies are reversible, and there have been suggestions that patients can be retreated with infliximab once reversion to negative anti-ds-antibodies has occurred.

NEUROLOGIC EVENTS

A review of the FDA Adverse Events Reporting System revealed 20 case reports suggestive of demyelination associated with anti-TNFα antibodies.[89]

Paresthesias and visual disturbances were most common, but confusion, gait disturbance, apraxia, facial palsy, and Guillain-Barré syndrome also occurred.[89] All neurologic events were temporally associated with anti-TNFα therapy, with partial or complete resolution on discontinuation. One patient developed a positive rechallenge phenomenon (reappearance of symptoms upon re-exposure to the agent),[89] but another individual tolerated reinstitution of anti-TNFα therapy in lower dose without further neurologic sequelae.[90] A recent study has demonstrated that patients with IBD have a higher rate of demyelinating diseases, with significant incidence rate ratio of 2.63 for UC and 2.12 for CD when compared with matched controls.[91] Therefore, future studies are needed to assess the relationship between anti-TNFα therapy and the prevalence of demyelinating diseases in IBD patients.[91]

INFECTIONS

Infections requiring antimicrobial therapy are more common in patients with CD or RA who require immunosuppression or disease-modifying therapy compared to patients not on immunosuppression, but this rate is not increased further in those on infliximab. In randomized, controlled trials, bacterial infections occurred in 30% to 34% of patients on infliximab and in 21% to 37% of patients on placebo.[73-76] Likewise, serious infections occurred in 3% to 4% of patients on infliximab and in 4% to 6% on placebo.[73-76] The majority of infections involved the upper respiratory tract and urinary tract.[11] Data from the manufacturer, postmarketing surveillance, and case reports document the occurrence of opportunistic infections such as nocardiosis, cytomegalovirus, histoplasmosis, invasive pulmonary aspergillosis, and others.[10,92-95]

TUBERCULOSIS

Data from the FDA Adverse Event Reporting System[95] and from a review by Rutgeerts in 2003[24] report an incidence of tuberculosis in 70 of 147,000 patients (0.047%) and 350 of 400,000 patients (0.08%), respectively. This rate is higher than expected, even allowing for the increased incidence of other opportunistic infections seen with infliximab.[96] Therefore, anti-TNFα treatment should be considered a risk factor for the reactivation of tuberculosis, and patients under consideration of infliximab should be evaluated for latent tuberculosis. A suggested algorithm is outlined in Figure 22-2.[11,96-99]

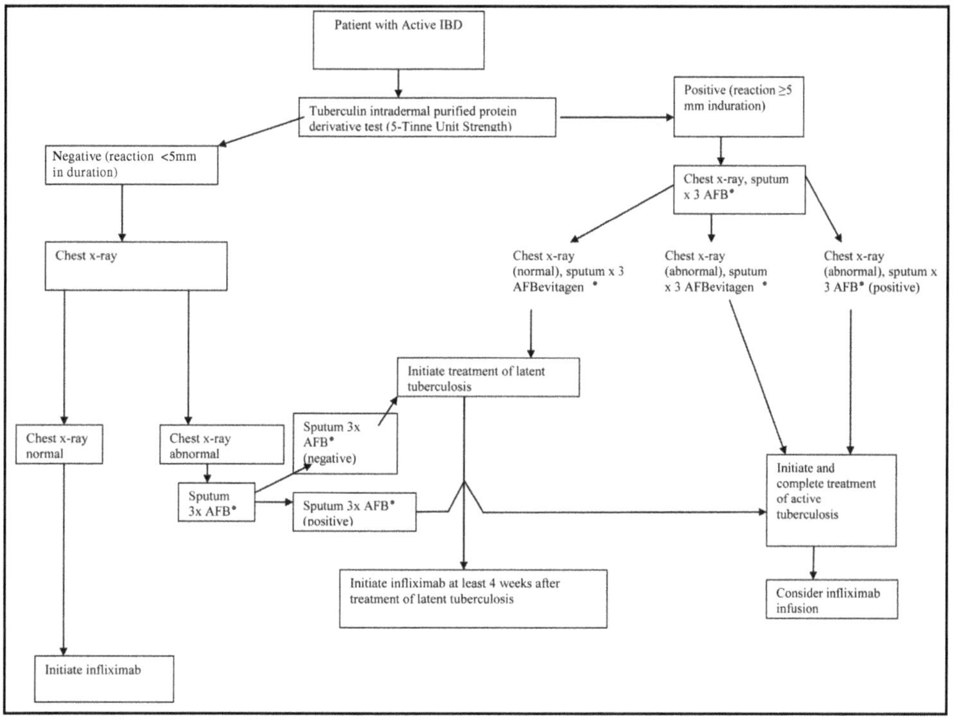

FIGURE 22-2. The approach to the patient with IBD who is under consideration for treatment with infliximab.

Before initiating infliximab therapy, a history of travel and immigration; previous tuberculosis exposure; symptoms such as chronic cough, weight loss, as well as previous antituberculous treatment; and previous tuberculosis immunization should be evaluated.[11,96-98] All patients should receive a tuberculin test and a chest x-ray, given the high prevalence of anergy in the IBD population. It has been suggested that those individuals with positive tuberculin test (≥5 mm of induration) should be tested for *Mycobacterium tuberculosis* in 3 consecutive sputum or gastric aspirates.[98,99] Those whose chest radiographs show images consistent with residual tuberculosis should proceed to computed tomography of the chest and referral to a pulmonary specialist.[98] Patients with a positive tuberculin test and abnormal chest x-ray should undergo treatment for active tuberculosis for 6 to 12 months.[11,98] Therapy with infliximab should be deferred until the end of treatment for active tuberculosis.[98] Patients with positive tuberculin test but with a normal chest x-ray should be treated for latent tuberculosis for 9 months.[11,98] Therapy with infliximab may be started after at least 4 weeks of antituberculous therapy to ensure they tolerate antituberculous medications well.[98] Patients with a negative tuberculin test and normal chest x-ray may proceed on to infliximab therapy without further intervention.[11,98] Regardless of the results of the tuberculin test, those with abnormal chest x-ray should have sputum or gastric aspirates evaluated for the *Mycobacterium tuberculosis* and, in case of positive outcome, should proceed on to treatment of active tuberculosis with the remainder being treated for latent tuberculosis.[11,98] Should active tuberculosis develop during treatment with infliximab, the infliximab should be stopped, and standard antituberculous treatment with 3 or 4 drugs should be initiated.[98]

REACTIVATION OF HEPATITIS B

There have been 2 case reports of fulminant and acute hepatitis B (HBV) related to treatment with infliximab in patients with RA.[100,101] In a series of patients with CD and chronic quiescent HBV, 2 patients developed a severe reactivation of HBV on discontinuation of infliximab.[102] Based on these observations, it has been proposed that patients under consideration for treatment with infliximab should be tested for hepatitis B markers, and those positive for surface antigen (HBsAg) should receive therapy with lamivudine or adefovir dipivoxil to prevent the reactivation of hepatitis B.[102] Furthermore, hepatitis B vaccination is also recommended in patients with IBD who lack immunity to HBV.[102]

LYMPHOMA AND TREATMENT OF IBD

There has been some controversy regarding the prevalence of lymphoma in patients with IBD. Two retrospective, hospital-based studies including 6752 patients with IBD found significantly increased risk of lymphoma in patients with IBD, with IBD acting as an independent risk factor for lymphoma.[103,104] More recently, a population-based study by Lewis et al including 16,996 patients with IBD established that the risk of lymphoma in patients with IBD is not significantly increased over that of the general population (relative risk 1.2).[105] The characteristics of IBD patients with and without lymphoma were generally similar. In this retrospective analysis, the authors did not demonstrate an increase of lymphoma in those using AZA or 6-MP, but could not preclude the possibility of increased risk of lymphoma in patients treated with immunomodulators.[105] However, Lewis et al have demonstrated in their meta-analysis of 6 previous studies a significant fourfold increase in the risk of lymphoma in patients with IBD treated with AZA/6-MP.[106] There were 5 hospital-based studies and 1 population-based study included in this meta-analysis, which may represent the potential source of bias.[106] It remains uncertain if this increased risk is a consequence of disease activity or a result of the immunosuppressants 6-MP and AZA.

LYMPHOMA AND INFLIXIMAB

At this time, the current experience does not suggest the presence of an increased risk for development of lymphoma in IBD patients treated with infliximab.[24] However, continued vigilance is appropriate because the duration of follow-up of patients with IBD treated with infliximab is short.[24] In addition, caution should be considered when recommending infliximab in patients with a history of prior malignancy (R. Diamond, written communication, October 2004). Their course remains uncertain because this cohort of patients are excluded from the clinical trials.

Data from the 3 randomized, controlled trials using infliximab in CD (n = 952) documented 2 cases of lymphoma (0.2%) in patients with infliximab exposure.[73,74,81] A retrospective analysis of safety data from 500 patients with CD who were receiving AZA and then received infliximab reported an additional 2 cases (0.4%).[77] In addition, the Crohn's Therapy, Resource, Evaluation, and Assessment Tool (TREAT) registry studying long-term safety of infliximab in CD, following prospectively more than 5000 patients with CD, reported a similar prevalence of lymphomas in patients treated with infliximab and those on other treatment (R. Diamond, written communication, October 2004).[107]

A trial of infliximab in 342 patients with RA reported one case of lymphoma (0.3%) in the infliximab arm and none in the placebo arm.[76] The authors also reported 3 additional cases of lymphoma among 555 infliximab-treated RA patients (0.55%) in another 6 clinical trials.[76] It should be noted that, unlike patients with IBD, those with RA have been found to have an increased risk of lymphoma.[108-110] In February 2003, postmarketing surveillance had documented 71 cases (45 in RA, 20 in CD) of lymphoma among 365,000 patients treated with infliximab.[24]

OTHER MALIGNANCIES AND INFLIXIMAB

Nine cases of nonlymphomatous malignancies have been reported in the 1283 patients from the 3 major clinical trials of infliximab, an incidence of 0.7%.[73-76] In addition, retrospective safety analysis in 500 patients with CD treated with infliximab found 7 cases of such malignancies (1.4%).[77] The most common malignancies included breast cancer, colorectal cancer, and malignant melanoma (R. Diamond, written communication, October 2004). There was no apparent association between dose of infliximab or time from treatment and development of malignancy (R. Diamond, written communication, October 2004). The TREAT registry reports a similar incidence of malignancies in CD patients treated and not treated with infliximab.[107]

In summary, the existing data do not indicate an increased incidence of lymphoma or nonlymphomatous malignancies in patients treated with infliximab. However, continued vigilance is recommended because the total experience of infliximab therapy and the duration of follow-up remains somewhat limited (R. Diamond, written communication, October 2004).[24]

HEMATOLOGIC ABNORMALITIES

Hematologic adverse events are uncommon in CD patients treated with infliximab. According to the manufacturer, the rates of anemia (4%), leukopenia (<1%), and thrombocytopenia (<1%) were similar in both patients treated with infliximab (n = 1678) and placebo (n = 192) in clinical trials (R. Diamond, written communication, October 2004). It is important to stress that many patients are often concurrently treated with infliximab and immunomodulators, thus making it hard to distinguish the responsible agent for hematologic abnormalities if they do develop.

OTHER ADVERSE EVENTS

Isolated cases of aseptic meningitis,[111,112] polymyositis,[113] anaphylaxis-like reactions,[114,115] acute idiopathic pancreatitis,[116] and reversible cholestatic liver disease[117] have been reported in patients receiving infliximab therapy.

INFLIXIMAB IN PREGNANCY

There are very limited data on the effects of infliximab in pregnancy. Infliximab reacts only with TNFα of human and chimpanzee origin, thus meaningful animal studies are nonexistent, and a positive pregnancy test excludes patients from infliximab clinical trials (R. Diamond, written communication, October 2004). Mouse studies using an analogous antibody that reacts with mouse TNFα showed no maternal toxicity, embryotoxicity, or teratogenicity (R. Diamond, written communication, October 2004).

Katz et al reported pregnancy outcomes in 96 women with CD or RA, 53 of whom (55%) were exposed to infliximab within 3 months of conception and 30 of whom first received infliximab during the first trimester.[118] Sixty-four pregnancies resulted in 32 live births (67%), 14 miscarriages (15%), and 18

TABLE 22-5

THE CHARACTERISTICS OF PATIENTS PARTICIPATING IN THE CLINICAL, RANDOMIZED, PLACEBO-CONTROLLED TRIAL EVALUATING THE EFFICACY OF INFLIXIMAB IN PATIENTS WITH MODERATE TO SEVERE HEART FAILURE (ATTACH)

ATTACH Study[127]	Placebo	Infliximab 5 mg/kg	Infliximab 10 mg/kg
Number of patients	49	50	51
Serious adverse events [%]	29.2	23.5	44.0
Frequency of heart failure [%]	8.3	2.0	22.0
14 weeks			
Worsening clinical status	8	10	22
Hospitalization	2	2	8
Deaths	0	0	1
28 weeks			
Worsening clinical status	14	16	31
Hospitalization	5	3	11
Deaths	1	2	5
Patients who discontinued treatment	1	2	5

therapeutic terminations (19%).[118] There was no significant difference in outcome between patients with CD or RA, and results were similar to historical controls (66% live birth, 17% miscarriages, and 20% therapeutic terminations).[118] Population-based case-control studies do not show an elevated risk of spontaneous abortion, stillbirth, or neonatal death in patients with IBD.[119-122] However, significant risk of preterm delivery (<37 weeks), low birthweight (<2500 g), and congenital malformations in women with IBD has been demonstrated.[119-122] Katz et al followed the women's partners of 14 men receiving infliximab who conceived within 3 months of infliximab exposure. Among these 14 pregnancies, there were 7 live births, 1 miscarriage, 3 ongoing pregnancies, and 3 unknown outcomes.[118] However, number of patients is too small to reach the conclusive results. The TREAT registry reported 66 pregnancies among more than 5000 patients either receiving or not receiving infliximab, with similar rates of miscarriage and neonatal complications among the infliximab-treated and untreated groups.[107] At present, infliximab is category B, meaning that animal studies have revealed no evidence of harm to the fetus. It should be cautioned that there are no adequate and well-controlled studies in pregnant women.[123] However, the limited data available do not suggest increased rates of adverse outcomes in pregnancy.

It is not known if infliximab is excreted with breast milk. The examination of human milk from one nursing female patient with CD who was treated with infliximab showed that either infliximab is not secreted to human milk or its concentration in milk is low and undetectable by standard assays.[124] A recent study has shown that high infliximab levels in the serum of the infant whose mother used infliximab during pregnancy continued to decrease despite the studies reporting that infliximab is not likely to be transmitted via breast milk.[125] Nevertheless, at this time it is recommended that either nursing or infliximab should be discontinued.[10]

INFLIXIMAB AND CONGESTIVE HEART FAILURE

TNFα has negative inotropic effects on the heart and in animal models, may promote fibrosis, hypertrophy, and cardiomyopathy.[126] Serum levels of TNFα are increased in patients with heart failure, and the extent of the elevation is directly related to the severity of the disease.[126] In a study to evaluate whether TNFα inhibition with infliximab could have favorable effects in patients with moderate to severe heart failure (New York Heart Association class III to IV), 150 patients were randomized to receive infliximab 10 mg/kg, infliximab 5 mg/kg, or placebo.[126] Outcomes were worse in the patients treated with infliximab at 10 mg/kg with a markedly increased number of hospitalizations and a trend toward increased symptoms and mortality in this group of patients (Table 22-5).[126]

In addition, new onset of heart failure has been reported to the manufacturer. Case reports have included patients younger than 50 years of age, without known pre-existing cardiovascular disease.[10] Thus, infliximab at doses greater than 5 mg/kg is contraindicated in patients with moderate to severe (New York Association class III or class IV) heart failure.[10,126] However, the safety of infliximab in asymptomatic left ventricular dysfunction or mild symptoms of heart failure has to be determined.[126]

It was recently suggested that induction therapy with infliximab and AZA (top-down therapy) is superior to sequential therapy (step-up) with aminosalicylates and glucocorticosteroids for reducing exposure to glucocorticosteroids in patients with Crohn's.[127] The top-down therapy resulted in attaining remission in 74.5% of patients, compared to step-up therapy attaining remission in 48.1% (P=0.006).[127] The longstanding remission was achieved in 77% of patients who were not treated with glucocorticosteroids.[127] Therefore, it was suggested that therapy with glucocorticosteroids is not necessary for inducing remission in moderate or severe Crohn's disease.[127]

CONCLUSION

Unlike the wealth of data available on infliximab use in CD, the data in UC are less extensive and evolving. The majority of the data (5 of 6 prospective studies) does support the use of infliximab in UC. The benefit for patients in these studies is quite significant. There is a single study by Probert et al[57] not suggesting efficacy in this patient population. The two most recent trials evaluating treatment with infliximab in 728 patients with moderate to severe UC demonstrated that infliximab induces and maintains clinical response, clinical remission, and mucosal healing and permits the tapering of corticosteroids while maintaining remission. The weight of evidence suggests that infliximab will have a significant role in the treatment of UC in patients who are refractory to steroids and immunosuppressive therapy (AZA or 6-MP) or who are steroid-dependent and desire to attempt steroid withdrawal while maintaining remission. This approach has been a step-up approach. In the future, it is uncertain whether a top-down approach will become the standard. The role of infliximab in UC will continue to evolve as more data continue to be collected and further trials define appropriate patient populations that may benefit from it.

REFERENCES

1. Valle E, Gross M, Bickston SJ. Infliximab. *Expert Opin Pharmacother.* 2001;2:1015-1025.
2. Remicade (Infliximab) for IV injections. Package insert, Centocor Inc, 2005.
3. Breedveld FC. Therapeutic monoclonal antibodies. *Lancet.* 2000;355:735-740.
4. Knight DM, Trinh H, Le J, et al. Construction and initial characterization of a mouse-human chimeric anti-TNF antibody. *Mol Immunol.* 1993;30:1443-1453.
5. Bell S, Kamm MA. Antibodies to tumour necrosis factor-α as treatment for Crohn's disease. *Lancet.* 2000;355:858-859.
6. Wagner C, Mace K, De Woody K, et al. Infliximab treatment benefits correlate with pharmacodynamic parameters in Crohn's disease patients. *Digestion.* 1998;59(Suppl 3):124-125.
7. Mouser JF, Hyams JS. Infliximab: A novel chimeric monoclonal antibody for the treatment of Crohn's disease. *Clin Ther.* 1999;21:932-942.
8. Sandborn WJ, Hanauer SB. Antitumor necrosis factor therapy for inflammatory bowel disease: a review of agents, pharmacology, clinical results and safety. *Inflamm Bowel Dis.* 1999;5:119-133.
9. Sandborn WJ, Targan SR. Biologic therapy of inflammatory bowel disease. *Gastroenterology.* 2002;122:1592-1608.
10. Remicade (infliximab) prescribing information. Centecor, 2004.
11. Sandborn WJ, Hanauer SB. Infliximab in the treatment of Crohn's disease: a user's guide for clinicians. *Am J Gastroenterol.* 2002;97:2962-2972.
12. Vassalli P. The pathophysiology of tumor necrosis factors. *Annu Rev Immunol.* 1992;10:411-452.
13. Lichtenstein GR. Chemokines and cytokines in inflammatory bowel disease and their application to disease treatment. *Current Opin Gastroenterol.* 2000;16:83-88.
14. Eigler A, Sinha B, Hartmann G, Endres S. Taming TNF: strategies to restrain this proinflammatory cytokine. *Immunol Today.* 1997;18:487-492.
15. Su CG, Judge TA, Lichtenstein GR. The role of biological therapy in inflammatory bowel disease. *Drugs Today.* 2001;37:121-133.
16. Luster MI, Simeonova PP, Gallucci R, Matheson J. Tumor necrosis factor α and toxicology. *Crit Rev Tox.* 1999;29:491-511.
17. Siegel SA, Shealy DJ, Nakada MT, et al. The mouse/human chimeric monoclonal antibody cA2 neutralizes TNF in vitro and protects transgenic mice from cachexia and TNF lethality in vivo. *Cytokine.* 1995;7:15-25.
18. Schmidt M, Luegering N, Luegering A, et al. Infliximab exerts anti-inflammatory capacity in IBD by induction of apoptosis in monocytes. *Gastroenterology.* 2001;118:A664.
19. van Deventer SJ. Review article: targeting TNF alpha as a key cytokine in the inflammatory processes of Crohn's disease—The mechanisms of action of infliximab. *Aliment Pharmacol Ther.* 1999;13(Suppl 4):3-8.
20. ten Hove T, van Montfrans C, Peppelenbosch MP, van Deventer SJ. Infliximab treatment induces apoptosis of lamina propria T lymphocytes in Crohn's disease. *Gut.* 2002;50:206-211.
21. Agnholt J, Kelsen J, Brandsborg B, Jakobsen NO, Dahlerup JF. Increased production of granulocyte-macrophage colony-stimulating factor in Crohn's disease: a possible target for infliximab treatment. *Eur J Gastroenterol Hepatol.* 2004;16:649-655.
22. Kirman I, Whelan RL, Nielsen OH. Infliximab: mechanism of action beyond TNF-alpha neutralization in inflammatory bowel disease. *Eur J Gastroenterol Hepatol.* 2004;16:639-641.
23. Lorenz HM, Antoni C, Valerius T, et al. In vivo blockade of TNF-alpha by intravenous infusion of a chimeric monoclonal TNF-alpha antibody in patients with rheumatoid arthritis: short term cellular and molecular effects. *J Immunol.* 1996;156:1646-1653.
24. Rutgeerts P, Van Assche G, Vermeire S. Optimizing anti-TNF treatment in inflammatory bowel disease. *Gastroenterology.* 2004;126:1593-1610.
25. Sands BE. Novel therapies for inflammatory bowel disease. *Gastroenterol Clin N Am.* 1999;28:323-351.
26. Van Deventer SJH. Tumor necrosis factor and Crohn's disease. *Gut.* 1997;40:443-448.

27. Kaiser GC, Polk DB. Tumor necrosis factor alpha regulates proliferation in a mouse intestinal cell line. *Gastroenterology.* 1997;112:1231-1240.
28. Heyman M, Darmon N, Dupont C, et al. Mononuclear cells from infants allergic to cow's milk secrete tumor necrosis factor alpha, altering intestinal function. *Gastroenterology.* 1994;106:1514-1523.
29. Pender SL, Fell JM, Chamow SM, Ashkenazi A, MacDonald TT. A p55 TNF receptor immunoadhesin prevents T cell-mediated intestinal injury by inhibiting matrix metalloproteinase production. *J Immunol.* 1998;160:4098-4103.
30. Piguet PF, Vesin C, Guo J, Donati Y, Barazzone C. TNF-induced enterocyte apoptosis in mice is mediated by the TNF receptor 1 and does not require p53. *Eur J Immunol.* 1998;28:3499-3505.
31. Podolsky DK. Inflammatory bowel disease. *N Engl J Med.* 2002;347:417-429.
32. Papadakis KA, Targan SR. Role of cytokines in the pathogenesis of inflammatory bowel disease. *Annu Rev Med.* 2000;51:289-298.
33. Fuss IJ, Neurath M, Boirivant M, et al. Disparate CD4+ lamina propria (LP) lymphokine secretion profiles in inflammatory bowel disease. Crohn's disease LP cells manifest increased secretion of IFN-gamma, whereas ulcerative colitis LP cells manifest increased secretion of IL-5. *Immunol.* 1996;157:1261-1270.
34. Fuss IJ. Cytokine network in inflammatory bowel disease. *Curr Drug Targets Inflamm Allergy.* 2003;2:101-112.
35. Guimbaud R, Bertrand V, Chauvelot-Moachon L, et al. Network of inflammatory cytokines and correlation with disease activity in ulcerative colitis. *Am J Gastroenterol.* 1998;93:2397-2404.
36. Nicholls S, Stephens S, Braegger CP, Walker-Smith JA, MacDonald TT. Cytokines in stools of children with inflammatory bowel disease or infective diarrhoea. *J Clin Pathol.* 1993;46:757-760.
37. Saiki T, Mitsuyama K, Toyonaga A, Ishida H, Tanikawa K. Detection of pro- and anti-inflammatory cytokines in stools of patients with inflammatory bowel disease. *Scand J Gastroenterol.* 1998;33:616-622.
38. Murch SH, Lamkin VA, Savage MO, Walker-Smith JA, MacDonald TT. Serum concentrations of tumour necrosis factor α in childhood chronic inflammatory bowel disease. *Gut.* 1991;32:913-917.
39. Nielsen OH, Gionchetti P, Ainsworth M, et al. Rectal dialysate and fecal concentrations of neutrophil gelatinase-associated lipocalin, interleukin-8, and tumor necrosis factor-alpha in ulcerative colitis. *Am J Gastroenterol.* 1999;94:2923-2928.
40. Tsukada Y, Nakamura T, Iimura M, Iizuka BE, Hayashi N. Cytokine profile in colonic mucosa of ulcerative colitis correlates with disease activity and response to granulocytapheresis. *Am J Gastroenterol.* 2002;97:2820-2828.
41. Maeda M, Watanabe N, Neda H, et al. Serum tumor necrosis factor activity in inflammatory bowel disease. *Immunopharmacol Immunotoxicol.* 1992;14:451-461.
42. Ishiguro Y. Mucosal proinflammatory cytokine production correlates with endoscopic activity of ulcerative colitis. *J Gastroenterol.* 1999;34:66-74.
43. Hadziselimovic F, Emmons LR, Gallati H. Soluble tumour necrosis factor receptors p55 and p75 in the urine monitor disease activity and the efficacy of treatment of inflammatory bowel disease. *Gut.* 1995;37:260-263.
44. Murch SH, Braegger CP, Walker-Smith JA, MacDonald TT. Location of tumour necrosis factor α by immunohistochemistry in chronic inflammatory bowel disease. *Gut.* 1993;34:1705-1709.
45. Cappello M, Keshav S, Prince C, Jewell DP, Gordon S. Detection of mRNAs for macrophage products in inflammatory bowel disease by in situ hybridisation. *Gut.* 1992;33:1214-1219.
46. Breese EJ, Michie CA, Nicholls SW, et al. Tumor necrosis factor alpha-producing cells in the intestinal mucosa of children with inflammatory bowel disease. *Gastroenterology.* 1994;106:1455-1466.
47. Masuda H, Iwai S, Tanaka T, Hayakawa S. Expression of IL-8, TNF-α and INF-γ m-RNA in ulcerative colitis, particularly in patients with inactive phase. *J Clin Lab Immunol.* 1995;46:111-123.
48. Patel RT, Bain I, Youngs D, Keighley MRB. Cytokine production in pouchitis is similar to that in ulcerative colitis. *Dis Colon Rectum.* 1995;38:831-837.
49. Raab Y, Gerdin B, Ahlstedt S, Hallgren R. Neutrophil mucosal involvement is accompanied by enhanced local production of interleukin-8 in ulcerative colitis. *Gut.* 1993;34:1203-1206.
50. Watanabe N, Maeda M, Okamoto T, et al. Tumor necrosis factor and interferon-gamma augment anticolon antibody-dependent cellular cytotoxicity in ulcerative colitis. *Immunopharmacol Immunotoxicol.* 1996;18:15-26.
51. Sartor RB. Cytokines in intestinal inflammation: Pathophysiological and clinical considerations. *Gastroenterology.* 1994;106:533-539.
52. Powrie F, Leach MW, Mauze S, Menon S, Caddle LB, Coffman RL. Inhibition of Th1 responses prevents inflammatory bowel disease in scid mice reconstituted with CD45RBhi CD4+ T cells. *Immunity.* 1994;1:553-562.
53. Watkins PE, Warren BF, Stephens S, Ward P, Foulkes R. Treatment of ulcerative colitis in the cottontop tamarin using antibody to tumour necrosis factor alpha. *Gut.* 1997;40:628-633.
54. Warren BF, Watkins PE. Animal models of inflammatory bowel disease. *J Pathol.* 1994;172:313-316.
55. Evans RC, Clarke L, Heath P, Stephens S, Morris AI, Rhodes JM. Treatment of ulcerative colitis with an engineered human anti-TNF alpha antibody CDP571. *Aliment Pharmacol Ther.* 1997;11:1031-1035.
56. Sands BE, Tremaine WJ, Sandborn WJ, et al. Infliximab in the treatment of severe, steroid-refractory ulcerative colitis: a pilot study. *Inflamm Bowel Dis.* 2001;7:83-88.
57. Probert CSJ, Hearing SD, Schreiber S, et al. Infliximab in moderately severe glucocorticoid resistant ulcerative colitis: a randomized controlled trial. *Gut.* 2003;52:998-1002.
58. Rutgeerts P, Sandborn WJ, Feagan BG, et al. Infliximab for induction and maintenance therapy for ulcerative colitis. *N Engl J Med.* 2005;353:2462-2476.
59. Järnerot G, Hertervig E, Friis-Liby I, et al. Infliximab as rescue therapy in severe to moderately severe ulcerative colitis: a randomized, placebo-controlled study. *Gastroenterology.* 2005;128:1805-1811.
60. Ochsenkuhn T, Sackmann M, Goeke B. Infliximab for acute, not steroid-refractory ulcerative colitis: a randomized pilot study. *Eur J Gastroenterol Hepatol.* 2004;16:1167-1171.
61. Su C, Salzberg BA, Lewis JD, et al. Efficacy of anti-tumor necrosis factor therapy in patients with ulcerative colitis. *Am J Gastroenterol.* 2002;97:2577-2584.
62. Chey WY, Hussain A, Ryan C, Potter GD, Shah A. Infliximab for refractory ulcerative colitis. *Am J Gastroenterol.* 2001;96:2373-2381.
63. Chey WY. Infliximab for patients with refractory ulcerative colitis. *Inflamm Bowel Dis.* 2001;7(Suppl. 1):S30-S33.
64. Kaser A, Mairinger T, Vogel W, Tilg H. Infliximab in severe steroid-refractory ulcerative colitis: a pilot study. *Wien Klin Wochenschr.* 2001;113:930-933.
65. Kohn A, Prantera C, Pera A, Cosintino R, Sostegni R, Daperno M. Anti-tumor necrosis factor alpha (infliximab) in the treatment of severe ulcerative colitis: result of an open study on 13 patients. *Dig Liver Dis.* 2002;34:626-630.
66. Actis GC, Bruno M, Pinna-Pintor M, Rossini FP, Rizzetto M. Infliximab for treatment of steroid-refractory ulcerative colitis. *Dig Liver Dis.* 2002;34:631-634.
67. Gornet JM, Couve S, Hassani Z, et al. Infliximab for refractory ulcerative colitis or indeterminate colitis: an open-label multicentre study. *Aliment Pharmacol Ther.* 2003;18:175-181.

68. Kugathasan S, Prajapati DN, Kim JP, et al. Infliximab outcome in children and adults with ulcerative colitis. *Gastroenterology.* 2002;122:A615.
69. Cooper JM, Patterson DJ, Thirlby RC. Infliximab for ulcerative colitis: Not a cure for severe disease. *Gastroenterology.* 2003;124: A818.
70. Fleisher MR, Rubin SD, Levine AE, et al. Infliximab in the treatment of steroid-naive ulcerative colitis. *Am J Gastroenterol.* 2001;96:S291-S292.
71. Bermejo F, Lopez-Sanroman A, Hinojosa J, Castro L, Jurado C, Gomez-Beldal AB. Infliximab induces clinical, endoscopic and histological responses in refractory ulcerative colitis. *Rev Esp Enferm Dig.* 2004;96:94-101.
72. Shen EH, Das KM. Current therapeutic recommendations. Infliximab for ulcerative colitis. *J Clin Gastroenterol.* 2004;38:741-745.
73. Hanauer SB, Feagan BG, Lichtenstein GR, et al; ACCENT I Study Group. Maintenance infliximab for Crohn's disease: The ACCENT I randomised trial. *Lancet.* 2002;359:1541-1549.
74. Hanauer SB, Wagner CL, Bala M, et al. Incidence and importance of antibody responses to infliximab after maintenance or episodic treatment in Crohn's disease. *Clin Gastroenterol Hepatol.* 2004;2:543-553.
75. Sands BE, Anderson FH, Bernstein CN, et al. Infliximab maintenance therapy for fistulizing Crohn's disease. *N Engl J Med.* 2004;350:876-885.
76. Maini R, St Clair EW, Breedveld F, et al. Infliximab (chimeric anti-tumour necrosis factor alpha monoclonal antibody) versus placebo in rheumatoid arthritis patients receiving concomitant methotrexate: a randomised phase III trial. ATTRACT Study Group. *Lancet.* 1999;354:1932-1939.
77. Colombel JF, Loftus EV Jr, Tremaine WJ, et al. The safety profile of infliximab in patients with Crohn's disease: the Mayo clinic experience in 500 patients. *Gastroenterology.* 2004;126:19-31.
78. Cheifetz A, Smedley M, Martin S, et al. The incidence and management of infusion reactions to infliximab: a large center experience. *Am J Gastroenterol.* 2003;98:1315-1324.
79. Baert F, Noman M, Vermiere S, et al. Influence of immunogenicity on the long-term efficacy of infliximab in Crohn's disease. *N Engl J Med.* 2003;348:601-608.
80. Hanauer SB, Rutgeerts PJ, D'Haens G, et al. Delayed hypersensitivity to infliximab (Remicade) re-infusion after a 2-4 year interval without treatment. *Gastroenterology.* 1999;116:A731.
81. Kavanaugh A, Keenan G, DeWoody K , et al. Long term follow up of patients treated with Remicade in clinical trials. *Arthritis Rheum.* 2001;44(suppl 9):S81.
82. Rutgeerts P, D'Haens G, Targan S, et al. Efficacy and safety of retreatment with anti-tumor necrosis factor antibody (infliximab) to maintain remission in Crohn's disease. *Gastroenterology.* 1999;117:761-769.
83. Charles PJ, Smeenk RJ, De Jong J, Feldmann M, Maini RN. Assessment of antibodies to double-stranded DNA induced in rheumatoid arthritis patients following treatment with infliximab, a monoclonal antibody to tumor necrosis factor alpha: findings in open-label and randomized placebo-controlled trials. *Arthritis Rheum.* 2000;43:2383-2390.
84. Favalli EG, Sinigaglia L, Varenna M, Arnoldi C. Drug-induced lupus following treatment with infliximab in rheumatoid arthritis. *Lupus.* 2002;11:753-755.
85. Debandt M, Vittecoq O, Descamps V, Le Loet X, Meyer O. Anti-TNF-alpha-induced systemic lupus syndrome. *Clin Rheumatol.* 2003;22:56-61.
86. Ali Y, Shah S. Infliximab-induced systemic lupus erythematosus. *Ann Intern Med.* 2002;137:625-626.
87. Klapman JB, Ene-Stroescu D, Becker MA, Hanauer SB. A lupus-like syndrome associated with infliximab therapy. *Inflamm Bowel Dis.* 2003;9:176-178.
88. Vermeire S, Noman M, Van Assche G, et al. Autoimmunity associated with anti-tumor necrosis factor alpha treatment in Crohn's disease: a prospective cohort study. *Gastroenterology.* 2003;125:32-39.
89. Mohan N, Edwards ET, Cupps TR, et al. Demyelination occurring during anti-tumor necrosis factor alpha therapy for inflammatory arthritides. *Arthritis Rheum.* 2001;44:2862-2869.
90. Cisternas M, Gutierrez M, Jacobelli S. Successful rechallenge with anti-tumor necrosis factor alpha for psoriatic arthritis after development of demyelinating nervous system disease during initial treatment: comment on the article by Mohan et al. *Arthritis Rheum.* 2002;46:3107-3108.
91. Gupta G, Gelfand JM, Lewis JD. Increased risk for demyelinating diseases in patients with inflammatory bowel disease. *Gastroenterology.* 2005;129:819-826.
92. Lee JH, Slifman NR, Gershon SK, et al. Life-threatening histoplasmosis complicating immunotherapy with tumor necrosis factor alpha antagonists infliximab and etanercept. *Arthritis Rheum.* 2002;46:2565-2570.
93. Kamath BM, Mamula P, Baldassano RN, Markowitz JE. Listeria meningitis after treatment with infliximab. *J Pediatr Gastroenterol Nutr.* 2002;34:410-412.
94. De Rosa FG, Shaz D, Campagna AC, Dellaripa PE, Khettry U, Craven DE. Invasive pulmonary aspergillosis soon after therapy with infliximab, a tumor necrosis factor-alpha-neutralizing antibody: a possible healthcare-associated case? *Infect Control Hosp Epidemiol.* 2003;24:477-482.
95. Warris A, Bjorneklett A, Gaustad P. Invasive pulmonary aspergillosis associated with infliximab therapy. *N Engl J Med.* 2001;344:1099-1100.
96. Keane J, Gershon S, Wise RP, et al. Tuberculosis associated with infliximab, a tumor necrosis factor alpha-neutralizing agent. *N Engl J Med.* 2001;345:1098-1104.
97. Mow WS, Abreu-Martin MT, Papadakis KA, Pitchon HE, Targan SR, Vasiliauskas EA. High incidence of anergy in inflammatory bowel disease patients limits the usefulness of PPD screening before infliximab therapy. *Clin Gastroenterol Hepatol.* 2004;2:309-313.
98. Salmon D, on behalf of the GTI and AFSSAPS. Recommendations about the prevention and management of tuberculosis in patients taking infliximab. *Joint Bone Spine.* 2002;69:170-172.
99. American Thoracic Society. Targeted tuberculin testing and treatment of latent tuberculosis infection. *Am J Respir Crit Care Med.* 2000;161:S221-S247.
100. Michel M, Duvoux C, Hezode C, Cherqui D. Fulminant hepatitis after infliximab in a patient with hepatitis B virus treated for an adult onset still's disease. *J Rheumatol.* 2003;30:1624-1625.
101. Ostuni P, Botsios C, Punzi L, Sfriso P, Todesco S. Hepatitis B reactivation in a chronic hepatitis B surface antigen carrier with rheumatoid arthritis treated with infliximab and low dose methotrexate. *Ann Rheum Dis.* 2003;62:686-687.
102. Esteve M, Saro C, Gonzalez-Huix F, Suarez F, Forne M, Viver JM. Chronic hepatitis B reactivation following infliximab therapy in Crohn's disease patients: need for primary prophylaxis. *Gut.* 2004;53:1363-1365.
103. Greenstein AJ, Gennuso R, Sachar DB, et al. Extraintestinal cancers in inflammatory bowel disease. *Cancer.* 1985;56:2914-2921.

104. Masel SL, Hanauer SB. Increased association of lymphoma and inflammatory bowel disease. *Gastroenterology.* 2000;118 (Suppl. 2):A119.
105. Lewis JD, Bilker WB, Brensinger C, Deren JJ, Vaughn DJ, Strom BL. Inflammatory bowel disease is not associated with an increased risk of lymphoma. *Gastroenterology.* 2001;121:1080-1087.
106. Kandiel AE, Fraser AJ, Korelitz BI, Brensinger CM, Lewis JD. Increased risk of lymphoma among inflammatory bowel disease patients treated with azathioprine and 6-mercaptopurine. *Gut.* 2005;54:1121-1125.
107. Lichtenstein GR, Cohen RD, Feagan BG, et al. Safety of infliximab in Crohn's disease: Data from the 5000-Patient TREAT registry. *Gastroenterology.* 2004;126:A54.
108. Tennis P, Bombardier C, Malcolm E, Downey W. Validity of rheumatoid arthritis diagnoses listed in the Saskatchewan Hospital Separations Database. *J Clin Epidemiol.* 1993;46:675-683.
109. Wolfe F, Mitchell DM, Sibley JT, et al. The mortality of rheumatoid arthritis. *Arthritis Rheum.* 1994;37:481-494.
110. Wolfe F, Michaud K. Lymphoma in rheumatoid arthritis: the effect of methotrexate and anti-tumor necrosis factor therapy in 18,572 patients. *Arthritis Rheum.* 2004;50:1740-1751.
111. Marotte H, Charrin JE, Miossec P. Infliximab-induced aseptic meningitis. *Lancet.* 2001;358:1784.
112. Kashyap AS, Kashyap S. Infliximab-induced aseptic meningitis. *Lancet.* 2002;359:1252.
113. Musial J, Undas A, Celinska-Lowenhoff M. Polymyositis associated with infliximab treatment for rheumatoid arthritis. *Rheumatology* (Oxford). 2003;42:1566-1568.
114. Farrell RJ, Shah SA, Lodhavia PJ, et al. Clinical experience with infliximab therapy in 100 patients with Crohn's disease. *Am J Gastroenterol.* 2000;95:3490-3497.
115. O'Connor M, Buchman A, Marshall G. Anaphylaxis-like reaction to infliximab in a patient with Crohn's disease. *Dig Dis Sci.* 2002;47:1323-1325.
116. Triantafillidis JK, Cheracakis P, Hereti IA, Argyros N, Karra E. Acute idiopathic pancreatitis complicating active Crohn's disease: favorable response to infliximab treatment. *Am J Gastroenterol.* 2000;95:3334-3336.
117. Menghini VV, Arora AS. Infliximab-associated reversible cholestatic liver disease. *Mayo Clin Proc.* 2001;76:84-86.
118. Katz JA, Antoni C, Keenan GF, Smith DE, Jacobs SJ, Lichtenstein GR. Outcome of pregnancy in women receiving infliximab for the treatment of Crohn's disease and rheumatoid arthritis. *Am J Gastroenterol.* 2004;99:2385-2392.
119. Alstead EM, Nelson-Piercy C. Inflammatory bowel disease in pregnancy. *Gut.* 2003;52:159-161.
120. Norgard B, Fonager K, Pedersen L, Jacobsen BA, Sorensen HT. Birth outcome in women exposed to 5-aminosalicylic acid during pregnancy: a Danish cohort study. *Gut.* 2003;52:243-247.
121. Dominitz JA, Young JC, Boyko EJ. Outcomes of infants born to mothers with inflammatory bowel disease: a population-based cohort study. *Am J Gastroenterol.* 2002;97:641-648.
122. Ludvigsson JF, Ludvigsson J. Inflammatory bowel disease in mother or father and neonatal outcome. *Acta Paediatr.* 2002;91(2):145-151.
123. Meadows M. *Pregnancy and the drug dilemma.* http://www.fda.gov/fdac/features/2001/301_preg.html (Accessed on November 18, 2004).
124. Peltier M, James D, Ford J, Wagner C, Davis H, Hanauer S. Infliximab levels in breast milk of a nursing Crohn's patient. *Am J Gastroenterol.* 2001;96(Suppl):S312.
125. Vasiliauskas E, Dubinsky M, Barry M, Targan S. High serum levels of infliximab detected in the newborn of a mother receiving infliximab during pregnancy. *Gastroenterology.* 2005;128:A-26.
126. Chung ES, Packer M, Lo KH, Fasanmade AA, Willerson JT, Anti-TNF Therapy Against Congestive Heart Failure Investigators. Randomized, double-blind, placebo-controlled, pilot trial of infliximab, a chimeric monoclonal antibody to tumor necrosis factor-alpha, in patients with moderate-to-severe heart failure: Results of the anti-TNF Therapy Against Congestive Heart Failure (ATTACH) trial. *Circulation.* 2003;107:3133-3140.
127. Hommes D, Baert F, Van Assche G, et al. Management of recent onset Crohn's disease: a controlled, randomized trial comparing step-up and top-down therapy. *Gastroenterology.* 2005;129:371.

23

Other Tumor Necrosis Factor-Alpha Antagonists in Ulcerative Colitis

Joshua R. Korzenik, MD

Until recently, ulcerative colitis (UC) was theorized to be unlikely to respond to anti-tumor necrosis factor-alpha (TNFα) agents. This preconception of the efficacy of anti-TNFα therapy in UC was not based on evidence from clinical studies but on hypotheses concerning the pathophysiology of UC. Crohn's disease (CD), which can respond dramatically to anti-TNFα therapy, is seen as a paradigm of a type 1 helper T cell (Th1) disease with TNFα as well as interferon-γ and IL-2 elevated. However, UC is suggested to be closer to a type 2 helper T cell (Th2) cytokine profile, in which TNFα is not significantly elevated, with increased levels of transforming growth factor β, IL-5, and IL-13 (though not IL-1 through IL-4). Small studies of infliximab in UC were equivocal, with results ranging from near universal improvement to responses comparable to placebo rates. The 2 large multicenter studies of infliximab, ACT 1 and ACT 2, confirmed a significant benefit in moderate to severe UC in an outpatient setting,[1] in addition to a placebo-controlled trial in hospitalized patients with UC, failing to improve on IV glucocorticoids.[2]

However, this chapter is not a review of infliximab in UC but rather a survey of anti-TNFα therapies other than infliximab. Its brevity is testimony to the limited research that has been conducted with anti-TNFα agents other than infliximab in UC. However, new studies evaluating golimumab, a humanized anti-TNFα for treatment of moderate-to-severe UC, are being conducted. In a few years, this area will expand, and the choice of potential TNFα agents is likely to parallel the growing options for CD. Ongoing investigations are exploring a variety of strategies for suppressing TNFα in UC, including golimumab and adalimumab (Humira; Abbott Laboratories, Abbott Park, Illinois), a fully human anti-TNFα antibody, which has demonstrated efficacy in Crohn's disease. At present, the available data are limited to a small open-label study of the anti-TNFα antibody CDP571, and four cases of UC treated with thalidomide.

Tumor Necrosis Factor and Ulcerative Colitis

TNFα is a proinflammatory cytokine central to mucosal protection. In the aberrant immune response seen in IBD, levels of TNFα have been demonstrated as increased in both patients with CD and UC in specimens isolated from colonic mucosa,[3] stool,[4] serum,[5] neutrophils,[6] and monocytes.[7,8] Soluble TNFα receptors are elevated in active UC, and levels correlate with clinical activity.[9] TNFα-converting enzyme (TACE), which serves to cleave TNFα from the cell surface, is raised in UC as well, though not in Crohn's disease.[10] Despite the identification of this elevation of TNFα in UC, the use of anti-TNFα agents has met with skepticism because of assumptions of the nature of the pathophysiology of UC as a Th2-driven disease, in which TNFα is not a dominant cytokine. The recent positive trials of infliximab in UC has challenged this wisdom, forcing a reconsideration of either the pathophysiology of UC, the mechanisms of action of infliximab, or both.

Golimumab

Like infliximab, golimumab binds with high affinity human TNFα and inhibits TNFα bioactivity. It contains

Lichtenstein GR, ed.
Ulcerative Colitis: The Complete Guide to Medical Management (pp. 255-258)

human variable regions, whereas infliximab contains mouse variable regions. Preclinical in vitro studies have shown that golimumab has high affinity for soluble TNFα and inhibits TNFα binding to the TNFα receptor. A phase III multicenter, randomized, placebo-controlled trial is currently evaluating the efficacy of golimumab induction and maintenance therapy in the treatment of patients with moderate to severe UC. This agent is being developed in both IV and subcutaneous forms.

CDP571

The only specific anti-TNFα agent, other than infliximab, about which a study has been completed and published is CDP571 (Celltech Therapeutics Ltd, Slough, UK), a humanized, though not fully human, anti-TNFα antibody. Unlike infliximab, an IgG1 antibody, CDP571 is an IgG4 subclass antibody that does not activate complement, differing from IgG1, which does activate complement. This antibody also differs from infliximab (which is 25% murine) in being only 10% murine. This reduced murine component offered the hope that it would be less immunogenic. Studies in CD suggested a steroid-sparing effect, as well as a decrease in disease activity judged by CDAI response, but the remission rates were poor.[11,12] Consequently, further development in Crohn's has been abandoned. Still, during the early days of investigation of this compound in CD, a single-dose, open-label study of CDP571 was conducted by Evans et al.[13] Fifteen patients were enrolled with mild to moderate UC and were treated with 1 IV dose of CDP571 at 5 mg/kg. Most patients had left-sided disease (11/15) with the remainder, pancolitis. Nine patients were not receiving steroids while 6 were considered steroid-refractory. Disease activity was assessed by the Powell-Tuck score, a visual analogue scale and a patient diary. Sigmoidoscopy was performed at weeks 0, 2, 4, and 8.

The therapy was generally well-tolerated with 9 of the 15 experiencing minor adverse events; 1 patient was hospitalized for worsening UC, and 3 patients had mild upper respiratory tract infection. No infusion reaction or other allergic reactions were noted.

The duration of the study was through week 8 after the infusion, and 5 of the 15 patients were withdrawn due to treatment failure prior to that time point, with the remaining 10 completing the study. A modest decrease in disease activity was seen at week 1, but it was not statistically significant at week 2. A mild decrease was also seen in C reactive protein (baseline: 6.0 mg/L to week 1: 5.0 mg/L), which was also statistically significant at week 1 but not week 2. A minor decrease in the visual analogue score did not reach statistical significance at any time point. The sigmoidoscopic score and histologic evaluation failed to demonstrate any significant change, though there was a trend toward an improvement (score at week 0: 2.3 to week 2: 1.2). Response was not influenced by use of steroids, with 6 of 9 having a response in the steroid-free group while 4 of 6 had a response in the steroid-resistant group. The pharmacokinetic studies identified a half-life of about 7 days of the antibody. Of note was a minor increase in low levels of anti-idiotype antibodies to CDP571 in 11 of 15, though that was not felt to be clinically significant and had no impact on response.

Given the short half-life and the modest clinical benefit, the investigators concluded that repeat dosing with a higher dose was necessary to demonstrate a more significant and durable response.

THALIDOMIDE

Thalidomide was initially abandoned as a therapeutic agent after it was associated with phocomelia. Its use has been relatively recently revived for a variety of diseases, in part after it was identified as having a primary effect in vivo of reducing TNFα levels by destabilizing its mRNA, suggesting a potential use in IBD.[14] However, thalidomide is a weak TNFα suppressant and also is nonspecific. Several other cytokines are diminished by thalidomide as well, in particular NFκB, a transcription factor that regulates the expression of a number of important proinflammatory cytokines, including IL-1α, IL-2, IL-6, and IL-12, among others. In decreasing IL-12 and augmenting IL-4, thalidomide may also act by shifting a Th1-type response toward a Th2-type response, which may be beneficial for CD, but in theory is less useful for UC.[15]

The efficacy of thalidomide in UC is minimally described in case reports, despite that the initial report recommending the use of thalidomide in IBD was in a UC patient in 1979.[16] Otherwise, a recent open-label series of 11 patients with IBD, including 4 patients with ulcerative colitis, examined the use of thalidomide in this patient population. Two UC patients withdrew early, but the other 2 demonstrated a marked improvement—as did the remaining Crohn's patients.[17]

Lazzerini et al examined the effects of thalidomide 1.5 to 2.5 mg/kg/d in 28 children and adolescents with refractory moderate-severe inflammatory bowel disease (IBD) (19 CD, 9 UC).[18] Overall, 21 of 28 (75%) patients (17 CD, 4 UC) achieved remission and 16 of 20 (80%) patients were able to suspend their use of steroids. The mean duration of remission was 34.5 months. Neuropathy occurred in 7 patients, but this adverse effect was reversible and was only with cumulative doses over 28 g. Other side effects requiring thalidomide suspension were vertigo/somnolence in one patient and agitation/hallucinations in another patient.

STA 5326 AND RDP-58

Novel therapeutic targets that have failed to show significant efficacy in IBD include STA5326 (apilimod) and RDP-58 (delmitide).[19] STA5326 is a small-molecule compound that selectively inhibits the IL-12 protein family, including the IL-12 and IL-23. A phase IIb clinical trial for Crohn's disease failed to show significant efficacy and was terminated.

RDP-58 (delmitide) is a minimally absorbed, D-amino acid decapeptide with established anti-inflammatory properties. In a randomized study by Travis et al involving 93 patients with ulcerative colitis, a significantly greater proportion of patients given RDP-58 200 mg or 300 mg showed treatment success (71% and 72%) compared with placebo 43% ($P = 0.016$).[20] However, further trials in IBD have not been conducted because of failed phase II trials (data unpublished).

CONCLUSION

Infliximab has provided a window by which to evaluate anti-TNFα therapy in UC. Its robust response raises questions of exploring novel, more effective anti-TNFα formulations with improved molecular construction and administration. Golimumab is a humanized anti-TNFα agent that is being developed for IV and subcutaneous administration. Studies are ongoing and show promise in the treatment of UC. Up until the present, other anti-TNFα agents for the treatment of CD may not necessarily translate into efficacy in the treatment of UC. The few patients treated with CDP571 and thalidomide represent a complete summary of the reported clinical experience with anti-TNFα agents, other than infliximab in UC. While these reports are not strongly supportive of a role for anti-TNFα agents in UC, the success of infliximab in UC, however surprising to some, has cleared the way for other agents that are likely to demonstrate efficacy. A more extensive set of studies of anti-TNFα alternatives for UC can be anticipated in the near future. Trials of adalimumab in UC are underway. These newer anti-TNFα medications could not be theorized to be less or more effective than infliximab in UC. In addition, most of the adverse events observed with infliximab are likely to be a class effect associated with all anti-TNFα medications, with the exception of infusion reactions that might be largely associated with the development of antibodies to the murine portion of infliximab. Still, any biologic is antigenic, however similar to human antibodies, and likely to induce antibody formation.

At present, even with infliximab, existing data provide little information with regard to predictors of response to anti-TNFα therapy: which subgroups or individual patient characteristics identify those with a better or worse response, which individuals are at higher risk of complications. These agents are appropriate for only a minority of patients with UC. Most importantly, physicians caring for these patients must have the necessary information and use judgment to determine who is appropriate for treatment with these therapies. The guidelines evolving for treatment of individuals with Crohn's with anti-TNFα antibodies should not be automatically applied to the parallel patient group with UC. However, golimumab holds promise for treatment of UC and will hopefully diminish the need for colectomy. While surgery is sometimes considered a therapy for UC rather than a failure of medical therapy, with the introduction of novel anti-TNFα agents such as golimumab, we may have more options for medical therapy in the treatment of UC. The existence of a surgical cure, however harsh, changes the equation in evaluating the relative risks and benefits of anti-TNFα agents and identifying appropriate candidates for these medications.

REFERENCES

1. Rutgeerts P, Sandborn WJ, Feagan BG, et al. Infliximab for induction and maintenance therapy for ulcerative colitis. *N Engl J Med.* 2005;353(23):2462-2476.
2. Jarnerot, G, Hertervig E, Friis-Liby I, et al. Infliximab as rescue therapy in severe to moderately severe ulcerative colitis: a randomized, placebo-controlled study. *Gastroenterology.* 2005;128:1805-1811.
3. Murch SH, Braegger CP, Walker-Smith JA, MacDonald TT. Location of tumour necrosis factor alpha by immunohistochemistry in chronic inflammatory bowel disease. *Gut.* 1993;34:1705-1709.
4. Braegger CP, Nicholls S, Murch SH, Stephens S, MacDonald TT. Tumour necrosis factor alpha in stool as a marker of intestinal inflammation. *Lancet.* 1992;339:89-91.
5. Murch SH, Lamkin VA, Savage MO, Walker-Smith JA, MacDonald TT. Serum concentrations of tumour necrosis factor alpha in childhood chronic inflammatory bowel disease. *Gut.* 1991;32:913-917.
6. Nikolaus S, Bauditz J, Gionchetti P, Witt C, Lochs H, Schreiber S. Increased secretion of pro-inflammatory cytokines by circulating polymorphonuclear neutrophils and regulation by interleukin 10 during intestinal inflammation. *Gut.* 1998;42:470-476.
7. Bouma G, Oudkerk Pool M, Scharenberg JG, et al. Differences in the intrinsic capacity of peripheral blood mononuclear cells to produce tumor necrosis factor alpha and beta in patients with inflammatory bowel disease and healthy controls. *Scand J Gastroenterol.* 1995;30:1095-1100.
8. Reinecker HC, Steffen M, Witthoeft T, et al. Enhanced secretion of tumour necrosis factor-alpha, IL-6, and IL-1 beta by isolated lamina propria mononuclear cells from patients with ulcerative colitis and Crohn's disease. *Clin Exp Immunol* 1993;94:174-181.
9. Hanai H, Watanabe F, Yamada M, et al. Correlation of serum soluble TNF-alpha receptors I and II levels with disease activity in patients with ulcerative colitis. *Am J Gastroenterol.* 2040;99:1532-1538.
10. Brynskov J, Foegh P, Pedersen G, et al. Tumour necrosis factor alpha converting enzyme (TACE) activity in the colonic mucosa of patients with inflammatory bowel disease. *Gut.* 2002;51:37-43.

11. Feagan BG, Sandborn WJ, Baker JP, et al. A randomized, double-blind, placebo-controlled trial of CDP571, a humanized monoclonal antibody to tumour necrosis factor-alpha, in patients with corticosteroid-dependent Crohn's disease. *Aliment Pharmacol Ther.* 2005;21:373-384.
12. Sandborn WJ, Feagan BG, Radford-Smith G, et al. CDP571, a humanised monoclonal antibody to tumour necrosis factor alpha, for moderate to severe Crohn's disease: a randomised, double blind, placebo controlled trial. *Gut.* 2004;53:1485-1493.
13. Evans RC, Clarke L, Heath P, Stephens S, Morris AI, Rhodes JM. Treatment of ulcerative colitis with an engineered human anti-TNFalpha antibody CDP571. *Aliment Pharmacol Ther.* 1997;11:1031-1035.
14. Moreira AL, Sampaio EP, Zmuidzinas A, Frindt P, Smith KA, Kaplan G. Thalidomide exerts its inhibitory action on tumor necrosis factor alpha by enhancing mRNA degradation. *J Exp Med.* 1993;177:1675-1680.
15. Ginsburg PM, Dassopoulos T, Ehrenpreis ED. Thalidomide treatment for refractory Crohn's disease: a review of the history, pharmacological mechanisms and clinical literature. *Ann Med.* 2001;33:516-525.
16. Waters MF, Laing AB, Ambikapathy A, Lennard-Jones JE. Treatment of ulcerative colitis with thalidomide. *BMJ.* 1979;1:792.
17. Bariol C, Meagher AP, Vickers CR, et al. Early studies on the safety and efficacy of thalidomide for symptomatic inflammatory bowel disease. *J Gastroenterol Hepatol.* 2002;17:135-139.
18. Lazzerini M, Martelossi S, Marchetti F, et al. Efficacy and safety of thalidomide in children and young adults with intractable inflammatory bowel disease: long-term results. *Aliment Pharmacol Ther.* 2007;25(4):419-427.
19. Peyrin-Biroulet L, Desreumaux P, Sandborn WJ, Colombel J-F. Crohn's disease: beyond antagonists of tumour necrosis factor. *Lancet.* 2008;372(9632):67-81.
20. Travis S, Yap LM, Hawkey C, et al. RDP58 is a novel and potentially effective oral therapy for ulcerative colitis. *Inflamm Bowel Dis.* 2005;11(8):713-719.

Novel Biological Agents for the Treatment of Ulcerative Colitis

24

Gert Van Assche, MD, PhD, FRCP and Paul Rutgeerts, MD, PhD, FRCP

Despite the therapeutic efficacy of the biological agent infliximab in Crohn's disease (CD), the development of agents specifically interacting with an immune pathway has not led to registered novel therapeutics in ulcerative colitis (UC). Recently, more biological agents have entered development programs in this indication (Table 24-1), but (contrary to the situation in CD) many of these programs have originally been driven by interest from investigators involved in patient care and not by the pharmaceutical industry. Several reasons may underlie this discrepancy in "market interest" between CD and UC. First, the immunopathogenesis of UC is not well-defined, and this hinders the selection of a clear target pathway. Even so, the lack of a paradigm about cytokines driving the inflammatory reaction in UC prevents extrapolation to other diseases, such as rheumatoid arthritis, spondyloarthropathy, or psoriasis, as is the case for CD. Finally, colectomy with ileal pouch anastomosis is viewed as a good solution for refractory UC, despite all the possible long-term inconveniences associated with this procedure. Nevertheless, in recent years, several novel biological agents have entered clinical trials in UC. Some of them have already been evaluated in randomized, controlled trials. Others still need to move from open-label pilot trials to placebo-controlled studies. Many of the therapeutic strategies, such as anti-TNFα agents or selective adhesion molecule blocking antibodies, have been tested in parallel with or following the trials in CD. Others, such as interferons, anti-CD25 antibodies, or anti-CD3 antibodies, have been initially or more extensively evaluated in UC.

Anti-Tumor Necrosis Factor Strategies

The development of anti-TNFα strategies in UC therapy is discussed in other chapters and will not be extensively dealt with here. The chimeric humanized anti-TNFα IgG1 antibody infliximab (Remicade) has been evaluated in several open-label trials for refractory moderate to severe UC. The early data on efficacy were not unequivocal, and only the recently published large, controlled trials ACT 1 and ACT 2 conclusively demonstrated the efficacy of infliximab in active UC.[1] A first placebo-controlled trial enrolled 43 patients with active UC resistant to glucocorticosteroids.[2] Patients were treated at weeks 0 and 2 with 5 mg/kg infliximab or placebo IV. At 6 weeks, no difference in clinical remission was observed between infliximab- and placebo-treated patients (39% infliximab versus 30% placebo). Also, the median improvement in Baron activity score was not different between groups. Patients were offered open-label 10 mg/kg infliximab IV if they did not respond after 6 weeks. Of the patients treated with open-label infliximab 10 mg/kg, remission was achieved in 27% (3/11) and 11% (1/9) in the original infliximab and the placebo group, respectively. A more recent Italian study included 20 patients with moderate to severe (Mayo score ≥6) disease to receive infliximab 5 mg/kg IV at 0, 2, and 6 weeks, and every 8 weeks thereafter, or glucocorticosteroids 0.7 to 1 mg/kg for 1 week with gradual tapering afterwards.[3] Preliminary results showed that all patients (10/10) in both groups achieved clinical remission. After a median of 10 months follow-up, 9/10 (infliximab) and 8/10 (corticosteroids) patients were still in clinical remission.

Lichtenstein GR, ed.
Ulcerative Colitis: The Complete Guide to Medical Management (pp. 259-272)

TABLE 24-1

NOVEL BIOLOGICAL AGENTS EVALUATED IN ACTIVE ULCERATIVE COLITIS

Compound Name	Molecular Structure	Efficacy in Ulcerative Colitis	Targeted Study Population	Development Phase*
Infliximab Remicade, Centocor	Chimeric, anti-TNFα, IgG1 monoclonal antibody	Efficacious in open-label trials, negative PCT	Moderate and severe disease medically refractory	Large phase III trials ongoing
CDP-571 UCB, Celltech	Humanized, anti-TNFα IgG4 monoclonal antibody	Efficacious in open-label trial	Moderate disease, medically refractory	Development halted (peg CDP-870, Fab fragment further developed)
RDP-58	Small molecule, topical, oral administration, cytokine inhibitor (TNFα, IL-1, IL-12)	Efficacious in PCT	Moderate disease, medically refractory	
Natalizumab Antegren, Elan, Biogen	Humanized mouse anti-human α4 integrin monoclonal antibody (IgG4)	Efficacious in open-label pilot study	Moderate disease, medically refractory	Phase II
LDP-02 (MLN-02) Millennium, Genentech	Humanized mouse anti-human α4β7 integrin monoclonal antibody	Efficacious in phase I and II trials	Mild to moderate disease, medically refractory	Development halted
ISIS 2303 Alicaforsen, ISIS Pharmaceuticals	Antisense oligonucleotide to ICAM-1 mRNA	Efficacious as topical agent in open-label trial for pouchitis	Active left-sided disease	Phase II and III trials in UC with enemas
Daclizumab Protein Design Labs, Zenapax (Roche)	Humanized anti-CD25 IgG1 monoclonal antibody	Efficacious in open-label trial, negative PCT	Mild to moderate disease, medically refractory	Development in UC stopped
Basiliximab Simulect, Novartis	Humanized anti-CD25 IgG1 monoclonal antibody	Efficacious in open-label trial	Steroid-refractory, moderate to severe disease	
IFN-β 1a (Rebif), Serono	Recombinant human interferon-β 1a	Efficacious in open-label trial, no clear activity in PCT	Mild to moderate disease, medically refractory	
Peg IFNα Schering-Plough	Pegylated human recombinant interferon-α	Negative PCT	Mild to moderate disease, medically refractory	
Visilizumab Nuvion, Protein design labs	Humanized anti-CD3 IgG2 monoclonal antibody	Efficacious in phase I open-label trial	Severe steroid-refractory disease	Phase I and II dose finding study ongoing

(continued)

TABLE 24-1 (CONTINUED)

NOVEL BIOLOGICAL AGENTS EVALUATED IN ACTIVE ULCERATIVE COLITIS

(CONTINUED)

Compound Name	Molecular Structure	Efficacy in Ulcerative Colitis	Targeted Study Population	Development Phase*
KGF-II Repifermin	Recombinant human keratinocyte growth factor II	Negative PCT	Mild to moderate disease, medically refractory	Development halted
EGF enema	Recombinant human epidermal growth factor	Efficacious in PCT as a topical agent	Moderate disease in combination with mesalamine	

PCT: placebo-controlled trial

*Information on development phase is subject to change; if blank no details were known to the authors.

Those patients relapsing were successfully treated either with infliximab at shorter intervals or with infliximab at 0, 2, and 6 weeks (placebo group). These data suggest but do not prove that infliximab may be as efficacious as glucocorticosteroids in patients with active UC not treated with steroids.

Two large multicenter trials sufficiently powered to assess the true therapeutic potential of infliximab in active moderate to severe UC have now been published.[1] The Active Colitis Trials, ACT 1 and ACT 2, enrolled 728 patients in 171 centers worldwide. Each of the trials recruited patients with clinically and endoscopically active disease. Patients were randomized to receive infliximab 5 mg/kg, infliximab 10 mg/kg, or placebo at weeks 0, 2, and 6, and then every 8 weeks thereafter for 22 weeks (ACT 1) or 46 weeks (ACT 2) in total. Apart from the duration of treatment, the main difference between the 2 trials was the fact that patients in ACT 2 were allowed to fail only mesalamine, whereas in ACT 1 only patients failing steroids and/or purine-analogues were eligible. In ACT 1, the clinical response at week 8 (following a 3-dose induction with infliximab) was 69% and 62% for patients receiving infliximab 5 and 10 mg/kg, respectively, compared with 37% of those who received placebo ($P<0.005$ for both comparisons). In ACT 2, very similar results were obtained in clinical response at week 8 with 65% and 69% of patients receiving infliximab 5 and 10 mg/kg, respectively, compared with 26% of those who received placebo ($P<0.001$ for both comparisons). In both studies, the proportions of patients who achieved clinical response at weeks 8, 30, or 54 (ACT 1) or clinical remission at weeks 30 or 54 (ACT 1) were several-fold higher among infliximab-treated patients than placebo-treated patients. At week 54, 16% of patients on placebo, 35% on 5 mg/kg and 34% on 10 mg/kg infliximab were in remission ($P=0.001$ for both comparisons). Sustained remission at weeks 8, 30, and 54 was observed in fewer patients, but again significant differences were observed between the placebo- and infliximab-treated groups (ACT 1 placebo 7%, infliximab 5 and 10 mg 20%). Endoscopic mucosal healing was also significantly more frequent in infliximab-treated patients. At week 8, approximately 30% of placebo-treated and 60% of infliximab-treated patients had complete mucosal healing or only mild lesions, and this difference remained significant at week 30 in both ACT 1 and ACT 2 and at 54 weeks in ACT 1. A recent Scandinavian trial also demonstrated that in severe colitis failing intravenous steroids, patients treated with infliximab 5 mg/kg IV single dose were more likely than those treated with placebo to improve and avoid colectomy.[4]

CDP-571, a humanized anti-TNFα IgG4 antibody, has been evaluated in a small, open-label trial that showed some improvement in clinical scores, although the effect was short-lived.[5] Recently RDP58, an interesting small molecule that inhibits the production of several cytokines (including TNFα) at a post-transcriptional level, has been studied in moderately active UC. In a randomized trial, patients received placebo or 100, 200, or 300 mg of RDP58 daily for 4 weeks.[6] Both high doses resulted in very high clinical remission rates (72% and 70% versus 40% in placebo-treated patients). Also, histological scores decreased more in RDP58-treated patients. In this trial, the placebo remission rate of 40% was exceptionally high. Nevertheless, the drug appeared to be safe and is appealing due to its oral route of administration and its very low absorption. This low systemic bioavailability could have favorable implications for the side effect profile.

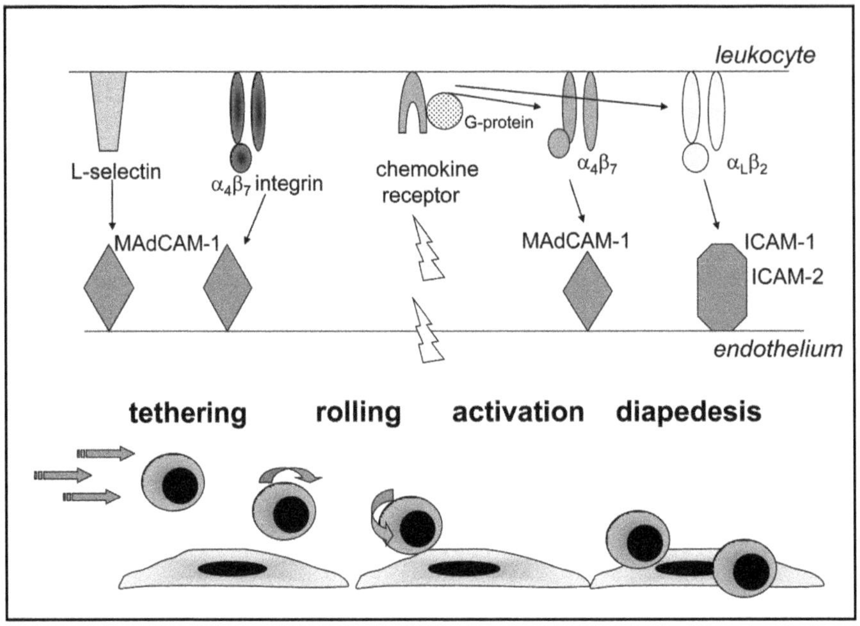

FIGURE 24-1. Schematic depiction of the different stages in leukocyte adhesion occurring in the intestinal wall. The principal interactions occurring in the HEV of Peyer's patches are represented. The leukocytes escape from the shear stresses in the blood flow to adhere and, after activation, to squeeze through the endothelial layer. Primary adhesion occurs through selectins and nonactivated integrins. Second-stage adhesion is mediated by integrins, activated through the chemokine receptors. $\alpha_4\beta_7$ integrins interacting with MadCAM-1 are gut selective adhesion molecules.

SELECTIVE ADHESION MOLECULE INHIBITION

Background and Rationale

Even if the pathogenesis of UC is still incompletely understood, the crucial role of T cells and other "blood-borne" leukocytes in the pathogenesis of IBD is beyond this discussion. The journey of leukocytes from the blood to antigen-rich organs, such as the gut or the lungs, is guided by an elaborate system of traffic signals or adhesion molecules.[7] Primary adhesion slowing down the fast-moving leukocytes occurs through engagement of the selectin class of molecules. Secondary adhesion molecules, all members of the integrin family, will definitively stop the lymphocytes to allow migration (Figure 24-1).

The integrins interact with specific ligands, the addressins, on the endothelium. Because there is some specificity to addressin distribution, adhesion molecules do not only serve to facilitate lymphocyte migration but also contribute to tissue-specific lymphocyte trafficking. T effector cells and T memory cells with a high density of membrane bound $\alpha_4\beta_7$ integrin, so-called gut-homing cells, directly engage with mucosal addressin cellular adhesion molecule-1 (MadCAM-1).[8-12] Naïve T cells and T effector cells also engage their $\alpha_L\beta_2$ integrin to connect with ICAM-1, but this interaction occurs in most organs. Because the interaction of $\alpha_4\beta_7$ integrin with MadCAM-1 is a gut-specific phenomenon, it has instigated the concept of "selective adhesion molecule inhibition" in gastrointestinal drug development.

The crucial role of adhesion molecules in inflammatory disorders makes them interesting targets for drug development.[13] Pioneering studies with anti-adhesion strategies have been undertaken in asthma where antagonists of T helper-2 specific chemokines and inhibitors of $\alpha_4\beta_1$ integrins have been shown to induce profound anti-inflammatory effects. In IBD, anti-adhesion therapy has focused on 2 pathways: the α_4 integrin/MadCAM-1 and the β_2 integrin/ICAM-1 interaction.

Anti-α_4 Integrin Antibodies

Animal Studies and Pharmacokinetics

Two monoclonal antibodies have been selected for drug development and subsequently studied in a primate model and in clinical trials. Millennium (formerly leukocyte) developed a specific humanized $\alpha_4\beta_7$ integrin monoclonal antibody, MLN-02. Elan Pharmaceuticals (now Elan-Biogen) developed a humanized α_4 integrin IgG4 antibody, natalizumab (Antegren). The only conceptual difference between the 2 compounds resides in the specificity of MLN-02 for blocking the $\alpha_4\beta_7$-MadCAM-1 interaction, whereas natalizumab also inhibits the $\alpha_4\beta_1$-VCAM-1 binding. Both compounds were first tested in the cotton-top tamarin.[14,15] This South American primate develops chronic colitis when kept in captivity. Both anti-α_4 integrin antibodies and anti-$\alpha_4\beta_7$ integrin antibodies proved to markedly ameliorate spontaneous colitis in cotton-top tamarin colitis. Administration of the antibody markedly improved the clinical and histological scores in the colitic animals. The clinical response was mirrored by improvement of histologic changes and by a reduction of mucosal T cells and neutrophils.

Phase I and II trials in humans have demonstrated that the anti-α_4 integrin antibody, natalizumab, is tolerated well at doses ranging from 1.0 to 3.0 mg/kg; administration of this dose results in sustained serum levels of natalizumab for 3 to 8 weeks.[16-18] In the pioneering trials with this antibody, dose ranges between 1 and 6 mg were used. Further pharmacokinetic modelling, however, demonstrated that over a wide range of body weights, the 300-mg dose induced sustained serum levels. Therefore, this dose is now used in most clinical trials with natalizumab. The compound has a serum half-life of 5 to 9 days.

The humanized anti-$\alpha_4\beta_7$-integrin antibody, MLN-02, only inhibits gut-specific MadCAM-1 mediated leukocyte adhesion. Therefore, this compound is only being developed for UC and CD and not for multiple sclerosis. The t1/2 of this antibody is comparable to that of natalizumab and doses from 0.15 to 2.0 mg/kg have been used in clinical trials.

Clinical Trials in Ulcerative Colitis

LDP-02 (MLN-02), the humanized anti-$\alpha_4\beta_7$ integrin antibody, has been most extensively studied in UC. A phase I/II, double-blind, placebo-controlled, ascending dose trial was initiated to evaluate the safety and pharmacokinetics of MLN-02 in 28 patients with moderate UC.[19] Patients were treated with a single dose of 0.15 mg/kg MLN-02 s.c., a single dose of 0.15, 0.5, or 2.0 mg/kg IV, or placebo. The trial was designed to evaluate tolerability and not efficacy. Nevertheless, it should be noted that a complete endoscopic and clinical remission at day 30 was observed in 3/5 patients receiving a dose of 0.5 mg/kg IV. This dose saturated $\alpha_4\beta_7$ binding for up to 30 days.

In a follow-up phase II trial, 181 patients were included and received either 0.5 or 2.0 mg/kg of MLN-02 or placebo twice with a 28-day interval.[20] Remission rates on day 43 were significantly higher in actively treated (33%: 0.5 mg/kg; 34%: 2.0 mg/kg) than in placebo-treated patients (15%, P=0.03). The LDP-02 drug was generally tolerated well, and infusion reaction with angioedema was seen in only 1 patient when the 2 trials were combined. Headache was the most commonly reported side effect. Although this adverse event occurred more often in LDP-02-treated than in placebo-treated patients, no clear dose-response relationship was observed.

Natalizumab (humanized monoclonal α_4 integrin IgG4 antibody) has been evaluated in 1 uncontrolled study including patients with moderately active UC.[21] Patients in this trial had a Powell-Tuck score of 4 or more and were allowed to take stable doses of aminosalicylates, AZA, or corticosteroids. A total of 10 patients were included and received a single dose of 3 mg/kg natalizumab IV. Patients were evaluated every 2 weeks through to week 8 and at week 12 post-infusion. Although uncontrolled, a significant improvement in the Powell-Tuck score was observed at week 2 with a median of 6 compared to 10 at baseline (P=0.004). Quality of life, assessed with the IBDQ, increased from a median of 101 at baseline to 161 at week 4 post-infusion. Tolerability of natalizumab was good. Serious adverse events, all hospitalizations, were observed in 3/10 patients, but these were not regarded as related to natalizumab administration by the investigators. Extensive clinical trial experience in Crohn's disease has shown that natalizumab has a good toxicity profile and that immunogenicity (anti-natalizumab antibodies) is low and probably does not affect the serum half-life of natalizumab.

Anti-ICAM-1 Antisense Oligonucleotides

The proof of concept for the use of anti-ICAM strategies in human IBD was found in animal models. Both blocking anti-ICAM-1 antibodies and ICAM-1 antisense oligonucleotides have been successfully used in animal models of IBD.[22,23] Clinical trials investigating the therapeutic potential of anti-ICAM agents have been exclusively conducted with antisense oligonucleotides to ICAM-1 (Table 24-1). Antisense oligonucleotides hybridize to a specific RNA molecule, most often messenger RNA (mRNA), and consecutively prevent the translation of the protein encoded by the RNA. Several placebo-controlled, randomized trials with an ICAM antisense oligonucleotide (ISIS-2302; Alicaforsen) have been performed in active steroid-treated CD.[24-26] Alicaforsen binds to the 3' untranslated region of the mRNA and prevents further translation. These trials have produced conflicting results.

In an open-label trial, 15 patients with active UC received Alicaforsen enemas 240 mg every night for 6 weeks.[27] The patients showed a 46% reduction in mean DAI and 33% rate of remission (ie, complete mucosal healing) at the end of treatment. However, results from controlled trials in active UC will provide more insight in the therapeutic potential of the Alicaforsen enemas.

Future Perspectives

At this moment, the precise role of selective adhesion molecule inhibiting agents in active UC is hard to define. Evidence from trials has been limited and ambiguous, although anti-α_4 integrin agents seem most promising. Although the safety profile of this class of biological drugs appears to be acceptable, more efficacy data are needed to decide on their therapeutic potential.

TABLE 24-2

SPECIFIC CHARACTERISTICS OF THE ANTI-CD25 ANTIBODIES DACLIZUMAB AND BASILIXIMAB

	Basiliximab	Daclizumab
Commercial name	Simulect (Novartis)	Zenapax (Roche)
Humanization	Chimeric	Humanized
Isotype	IgG1	IgG1
Serum half-life	7 days	20 days
UC trial design	Open-label	Open-label, PCT
Trial population	Steroid-refractory, moderate and severe disease	Medically refractory, mild to moderate disease
Doses used in UC	40 mg (fixed dose)	1.0 to 2.0 mg/kg
UC trial outcome	Efficacy in open-label trial	Efficacy in open-label trial, PCT negative

PCT: placebo-controlled trial

ANTI-INTERLEUKIN-2 RECEPTOR (CD25) ANTIBODIES

BACKGROUND AND RATIONALE

The efficacy of medical immunosuppression with cyclosporine in the treatment of severe UC has been clearly established.[28-30] The macrolide compounds cyclosporine and tacrolimus downregulate lymphocyte activation and proliferation by inhibiting IL-2 synthesis through the inhibition of the calcineurin pathway. IL-2 interacts with specific receptors on the T lymphocyte membrane to induce a clonal expansion of T effector cells.[31] The role of the activated IL-2 receptor (CD25) in UC is somewhat controversial because it has been shown that IL-2 cytokine or IL-2 receptor knockouts develop spontaneous colitis.[32-34] Indeed, regulatory T cells, a subclass of lymphocytes directed at controlling exaggerated immune responses, are CD25-CD4 positive. Therefore, inhibition of CD25 may theoretically downscale the inflammatory reaction, but may also unleash uncontrolled inflammation. Recently, humanized monoclonal antibodies that neutralize the binding capacity of the high affinity IL-2 receptor (CD25) on antigen-exposed T lymphocytes have been developed. These antibodies have been registered in the prevention of acute renal transplant rejection.[35-37] Ample clinical trial evidence has been gathered in various indications. Not only solid-organ transplantation, but also psoriasis, uveitis, and asthma. Protein Design Labs (Fremont, CA) developed daclizumab (Zenapax), a humanized monoclonal antibody of the human IgG1 isotype.[38] Novartis developed a chimeric anti-CD25, monoclonal IgG1 antibody, basiliximab.[36] Both antibodies have been evaluated in acute UC. Daclizumab is marketed worldwide by Roche as Zenapax for the prevention of renal transplants. Basiliximab is marketed by Novartis for the same indication (Table 24-2).

PHARMACOKINETICS

In daclizumab, the human IgG1 framework is derived from the Eumyeloma antibody and the murine hypervariable sequence from the MAT antibody. Daclizumab is administered as a 15-min IV infusion at a dose of 1.0 to 2.0 mg/kg. At this dose, the compound has a serum half-life ($t_{1/2}$) of 20 days, and it has a small distribution volume mostly confined to the vascular compartment.[38] Basiliximab on the other hand saturates IL-2R (CD25) for 36 ± 14 days when administered perioperatively in renal transplant patients. In adults, the antibody has a serum half-life of 7 days.[36]

CLINICAL TRIALS IN ULCERATIVE COLITIS

Daclizumab was first evaluated in an open-label pilot trial in 10 patients with chronically active UC at a dose of 1 mg/kg IV twice with a 4-week interval. Patients were allowed but not obliged to fail any standard UC treatment such as steroids, aminosalicylates, or immunosuppressives.[39] Clinical, endoscopic, and histologic evolution was scored at regular intervals. CD25 immunohistochemistry was followed in mucosal biopsies. The primary study endpoint was clinical improvement at week 8. One patient dropped out at week 4 due to persistent disease activity. The median clinical activity score decreased from a median

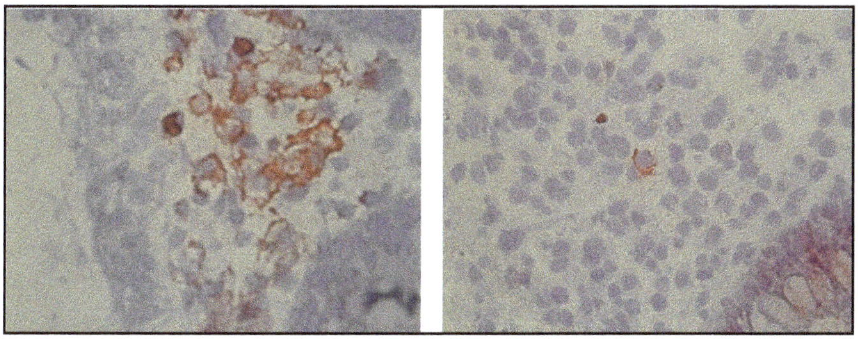

FIGURE 24-2. Decrease of CD25 positive staining in the colonic mucosa after treatment with daclizumab 1 mg/kg in a patient with moderate UC. Immunohistochemical stain of CD25+ cells in brown before (left) and 4 weeks after treatment (right).

of 8 (95% confidence interval [CI] 7.2 to 9.2) at baseline to 3.5 (95% CI 1.4 to 4.9) at week 8, $P<0.005$. Of the ten patients enrolled in the trial, 5 were considered to be in clinical remission at week 8. Endoscopic scores were significantly decreased at week 8 (week 0: 8, 95% CI 6.3 to 8.5; week 8: 5.0, 95% CI 2.6 to 6.3; $P<0.01$). However, not all patients considered to be in clinical remission achieved endoscopic remission. Mucosal biopsies showed a significant decrease in CD25+ cells, and there was a trend toward lower histology scores at week 8. CRP levels dropped substantially even 2 weeks after the first infusion of daclizumab. Nausea was most frequently reported as an adverse event, but always in patients who were concomitantly started on AZA (Figure 24-2).

This encouraging open-label trial triggered a large multicenter trial in North America and Belgium. Again, patients with moderately active colitis (Mayo score 6 to 10 inclusive) were included. A little more than the target population of 150 patients were enrolled to receive daclizumab 2 mg/kg every 2 weeks for 6 weeks, daclizumab 1 mg/kg every 4 weeks (weeks 0 and 4), and placebo every 4 weeks (weeks 2 and 6), or placebo every 2 weeks. The high dose of 2.0 mg/kg has been demonstrated to saturate all CD25 binding sites on peripheral lymphocytes. The primary endpoint was remission as defined by a score of 0 on the rectal bleeding and endoscopy scores and a score of 0 or 1 on the other components of the Mayo score. Complete data from this trial are not available, but an interim analysis announced in a press release by Protein Design Labs showed no significant difference in remission rates at week 8 between the 3 groups.[40]

Basiliximab was evaluated also in an open-label pilot trial in 10 patients with refractory moderate to severe UC.[41] However, only patients failing at least 14 days of prednisolone ≥30 mg or 7 days of IV hydrocortisone at adequate doses were eligible. Patients were assessed at regular intervals for 24 weeks with the UC severity score (UCSS) and a histological score for the endoscopic biopsies. All patients received a single infusion of basiliximab 40 mg over 5 minutes. Of the 10 patients included (7 moderate and 3 severe disease), as many as 9 were in clinical remission (UCSS <2) within 8 weeks. One patient was referred for colectomy at day 9. Parallel with clinical improvement, endoscopic and histologic scores decreased dramatically in basiliximab patients. The response to this antibody was not durable, because 8/9 patients who initially achieved remission relapsed anywhere between week 4 and week 20. As in the trial with daclizumab, a decrease in CRP levels was observed during the course of the study. Interestingly, the authors also studied the effects of basiliximab on the in vitro steroid sensitivity of peripheral blood lymphocytes. IL-2 and IL-2R are considered to have an important role in lymphocyte steroid resistance. In 7 UC patients with quiescent disease and in 32 healthy volunteers, 22% were found to have steroid-resistant lymphocytes. Lymphocytes from all these "resistant" patients became steroid responsive after incubation with basiliximab, and at low doses the antibody demonstrated synergistic effects with dexamethasone. Recently, preliminary data of an expanded study including 30 patients (20 moderate and 10 severe disease) were presented as an abstract. In the moderately active group, 70% of patients had achieved remission and 95% clinical improvement by week 8. In the severe group, 5/10 (50%) did well, and 50% needed a colectomy.

Safety

In the clinical trials for refractory UC, anti-IL2R agents were generally well-tolerated. Nausea was most often reported with daclizumab, and pyrexia was observed in 1 patient treated with basiliximab. All other adverse events were minor; in solid-organ transplantation, these antibodies have a good safety profile. Nonetheless, the risk of serious infections appears to be increased.[38] However, it should be noted that, in this indication, anti-IL2R antibodies have always been used in combination with triple immune suppressive regimens.

Future Perspectives

Although the pilot trials with daclizumab and basiliximab have produced very promising results, the negative outcome of the large, randomized, controlled daclizumab trial in refractory active UC has questioned somewhat the therapeutic potential of these agents. Of course, there are several differences between the 2 antibodies: basiliximab is a chimeric antibody (similar to infliximab), whereas daclizumab is humanized. The chimeric nature of basiliximab may preclude chronic retreatment, but may induce a higher intrinsic efficacy. Second, the binding affinity for CD25 is higher in the case of basiliximab. Finally, basiliximab has only been used in steroid-refractory patients, whereas daclizumab has been tested in patients failing any kind of standard therapy. However, the negative result of the placebo-controlled daclizumab trial urges a controlled trial with basiliximab in this indication before it will be accepted as a true candidate for further development.

ANTI-CD3 THERAPY

Background and Rationale

The interest in anti-CD3 antibodies as powerful immunosuppressive agents is not new. More than a decade ago, OKT3, a mouse monoclonal antibody specifically targeted at the human CD3 complex on T-cells, was introduced in the clinic as part of induction anti-rejection regimens for solid-organ transplantation. Like for every murine monoclonal, the clinical application of this antibody has been limited by the induction of neutralizing anti-murine antibodies. Moreover, OKT3 induces a severe cytokine release syndrome caused by T cell activation. This activation results from OKT3-mediated cross-linking of CD3-expressing T cells and FC receptor bearing cells. Even if the cytokines and immune pathways underlying UC are still incompletely characterized, there is a rationale for eliminating activated lymphocytes as a therapeutic strategy in this immune-mediated disease.

Protein Design Labs developed a mouse monoclonal antibody, M291, which competes with OKT3 for binding CD3 expressing cells. Based on this antibody, a humanized non-Fc-receptor binding antibody, huM291, was engineered, and this compound has been tested in UC.[42]

Pharmacokinetics

The pharmacodynamics and effects on the immune system of humanized M291, visilizumab, or Nuvion, have been studied in pioneering graft versus host disease (GVHD) studies. The human IgG2 isotype of huM291 has the longest serum half-life of all IgG2 antibodies. HuM291 has a serum half-life between 103 and 177 hours, depending on the dose used.[42] Early studies in GVHD demonstrated that administration of the antibody results in T cell depletion and that serum levels below 100 ng/mL are needed for peripheral T cells to start recovering.[43] The compound causes little or no activation of resting T cells but induces apoptosis of antigen-activated cycling T cells. When compared to OKT3, visilizumab is more potent in inducing T cell death. The antibody functions as a partial agonist of the T cell receptor and, as a consequence, visilizumab-treated T cells are anergic to antigen cells. Functional studies in GVHD indeed showed that the remaining circulating T cells had a decreased ability to proliferate when exposed to alloantigens, such as phytohemagglutinin. This anergy is reversed by the administration of IL-2.

Clinical Trials in Ulcerative Colitis

An open-label, phase I and II trial in severe steroid-refractory colitis was initiated in several US academic centers, and preliminary results of the first 10 patients have been reported.[44] Eight patients received a 15 μg/kg IV visilizumab bolus on 2 consecutive days, and 2 others 10 μg/kg. After a month, 7/8 patients from the 15 μg/kg group (and at 15 days 2/2 patients in the 10 μg/kg groups) had achieved remission (Modified Truelove and Witts Severity Index, MTWSI <4) and 8/8 had a clinic response (MTWSI <10). All 8 patients in the high-dose group showed also endoscopic improvement, and endoscopic lesions were absent or only mild in 6/8 patients. Most patients in remission managed to fully taper their concomitant steroid treatment.

An extension of this original trial included a total of 24 patients enrolled in the original 15 μg/kg cohort (n = 8) and 16 more in the 10 μg/kg group.[45] Clinical improvement (MTWSI <10) was observed in 84% (19/24) and remission in 66%. At baseline, 87% of patients had a maximal score of 3 on the endoscopy severity index compared to 8% at day 30. Sixteen patients had sustained remission beyond 30 days of treatment for up to 16 months. Colectomy had to be performed for recurrence of colitis in 1 patient at day 102 post-treatment. A phase I and II dose-finding, dose-escalating phase I trial is currently enrolling patients in North America and Europe.

Safety

Although the open-label nature of the phase I trial precludes a final statement on the clinical efficacy of Nuvion in severe UC, the preliminary data are impressive. However, some side effects appear to be consistently associated with anti-CD3 treatment. Cytokine release symptoms, characterized by chills, fever, malaise, and arthralgias, were present in 100% and 75% of patients in the 15 and 10 μg/kg group, respectively. A transient but marked decrease in T cells was observed in most patients, but by day 30 sustained severe suppression of CD3-CD4+ cells (total counts <200/μL) was only present in 1/12 (10 μg) and in 2/8 (15 μg) evaluable patients at day 30. By day 60, T cell counts had returned to normal in all patients. Also, patients experienced a transient increase in whole blood Epstein-Barr virus (EBV) DNA levels. This is of importance, taking into account that EBV reactivation is considered to be the cause of post-transplant lymphoproliferative disorder (PTLD). In trials with visilizumab for the treatment of GVHD, PTLD linked to increase in EBV DNA titers has been observed. Prophylactic treatment with rituximab, based on increased EBV viral load monitoring, appears to prevent PTLD in this indication. In the ongoing phase I and II trials, patients with significantly increased EBV viral loads at baseline enter the trial at the lowest dose reached in the gradual dose escalation (5, 7.5, 10, or 12.5 μg/kg) with permanent monitoring for dose-limiting toxicity.

Future Perspectives

Although the first open-label experience with the anti-CD3 antibody, visilizumab (Nuvion), are encouraging, more dose-finding data establishing the minimally effective dose and eventually placebo-controlled trials with effective medical immune suppressive therapy as a rescue are needed to correctly assess the therapeutic potential in severely active colitis. The side effect profile of the antibody precludes downstaging to more moderate disease at this moment.

INTERFERON THERAPY (IFNα AND IFNβ)

Background and Pharmacokinetics

Although the exact cytokine profiles involved in the pathogenesis are largely unknown, several proinflammatory cytokines, such as TNFα, IFNγ, and IL-1β, are increased in the serum and in the inflamed bowel wall of UC patients. However, IFNγ (and to a lesser extent TNFα) is typically secreted by lymphocytes with a T helper 1 phenotype, and several lines of evidence indicate that UC may be a T helper 2-driven disease. Interferon-α and -β have been widely used as immunomodulatory therapy in other indications, in which they have been shown to downregulate proinflammatory cytokines. In multiple sclerosis, IFNβ 1b has been shown to inhibit the production of several proinflammatory cytokines such as IFNγ and TNFα, and trigger lymphocytes to release anti-inflammatory IL-10.[46] T helper 2-predominant diseases appear to benefit from IFNα therapy,[47] whereas T helper 1-driven illnesses may be worsened by administration of this cytokine. Also, patients with quiescent UC treated for concomitant chronic active hepatitis showed no worsening of symptoms.[48] Both IFNα 2a and pegylated IFNα 2a have been used to treat active UC. Renal elimination is the main route of clearance for IFNα. Pegylation of the compound facilitates subcutaneous (SC) administration and prolongs the serum half-life from 5 to 80 hours. Also, the time to peak serum concentration increases from 6 to 72 hours. IFNβ 1b, on the other hand, has also been explored for efficacy and safety in UC. This cytokine administered subcutaneously has a short serum half-life of 5 hours with a time to peak serum concentration of 1 to 8 hours.

Clinical Trials in Ulcerative Colitis

IFNβ 1b has been first explored in an open-label pilot study including 25 steroid-refractory patients.[49] These patients were treated 3 times per week with 0.5 million units (MIU) of natural human IFNβ 1b IV or 1.0 MIU recombinant human IFNβ for a duration of 1 year. A very high remission rate of 88% (22/25) was observed in this trial. No differences were observed between the 2 types of IFNβ 1b. In a subsequent placebo-controlled trial, 97 steroid-refractory patients were included.[50] In the 3 treatment groups (placebo, IFNβ 1b 1 MIU, or IFNβ 1b 3 MIU SC 3 times per week for 8 weeks), remission rates were 38%, 30%, and 58%, respectively. The most recent placebo-controlled trial with IFNβ 1b included 18 patients (2:1 randomization) with moderately active UC failing mesalamine but not steroids or immunosuppressives.[51] The trial was designed as a double-blind, dose-escalating trial, and patients with no improvement at every 2-week interval were given increasing doses of IFNβ 1b (22, 44, 88 μg) or matching placebo. If improvement was observed at any of these time points, patients entered a maintenance phase at the same dose level. Patients reached a study endpoint when achieving remission or having completed the full dosing schedule. Eighteen patients were included, and 17 were analyzed (misallocation of treatment in 1 patient). Clinical response and endoscopically proven remission was achieved in 50% and 30% of IFN treated and in 14% and 0% of placebo-treated patients. No clear dose response was observed. Improvement was observed after a mean of 28 ± 11 days.

IFNα 2a was first evaluated in a 6-month open-label trial including 28 patients with moderately active colitis at a dose of 3 to 9 MIU 3 times per week.[52] Of these patients, 82% achieved clinical and endoscopic remission after 6 months of treatment. Subsequently, Madsen et al reported the efficacy of this cytokine given as an enema for left-sided disease.[53]

More recently, however, a randomized, controlled trial failed to show efficacy of peg IFNα 2a in moderately active UC.[54] In this trial, 60 patients received placebo, 0.5, or 1.0 μg/kg peg IFNα 2a once weekly for 12 weeks. The study was designed to assess safety, but efficacy endpoints were also assessed. Serious adverse events were reported more frequently in actively treated patients, and injection site reactions and flu-like symptoms were present in more than 50% of these patients. No differences in clinical, endoscopic, and histologic efficacy were observed. Study dropouts due to lack of efficacy were 55%, 32%, and 38% in the placebo, peg IFNα 2a 0.5, and 1.0 μg groups respectively.

Safety

Interferons have been widely used in immune therapy of viral disease and in cancer treatment. The overall safety profile of these cytokines administered subcutaneously appears to be good. In the placebo-controlled trial with peg IFNα, 4/6 of the excess serious adverse events included hospitalizations for worsening disease.[54] This may reflect a lack of efficacy, but is probably not an extra burden to the safety profile. More relevant are milder side effects such as injection site reactions, headache, and flu-like syndrome, which have been observed in other illnesses with peg IFNα. In the placebo-controlled trial with IFNβ 1b, injection site reactions and flu-like symptoms were the most commonly reported side effects considered to be possibly or probably related to the study drug. However, only 1 patient of 10 in the IFNβ 1b-treated group withdrew because of treatment-related side effects, and flu-like symptoms were also observed in 25% of placebo-treated patients (versus 30% in IFNβ 1b treated).

Future Perspectives

The data available at the moment from randomized, controlled trials do not support treatment of moderately active UC with IFNβ 1b or peg IFNα. There was a trend toward higher clinical and endoscopic remission rates in patients treated with peg IFNα as compared to placebo, but the low number of patients included limits the value of this observation. Further trials are warranted, but the commonly observed side effects, such as injection site reactions and flu-like symptoms, may shift the development to more severely ill patients as an alternative to oral corticosteroids.

GROWTH FACTORS

Background

The rationale to use growth factors to treat UC is the ability of these molecules to accelerate the regeneration of the colonic mucosa. Unlike CD, UC is primarily a mucosal disease, and the extension of mucosal ulcerations determines the severity of the disease. Several growth factors, such as trefoil factor, transforming growth factor-b, keratinocyte growth factor (KGF), and epidermal growth factor (EGF), have been implicated in the preservation of mucosal integrity and the regeneration of damaged mucosa.[55] KGF, for instance, stimulates the proliferation of enterocytes in vitro, and in animal models a combination of recombinant human KGF-1 (fibroblast growth factor-7) and KGF-2 (Repifermin; fibroblast growth factor-10) ameliorates the experimental colitis. EGF is a potent mitogenic peptide secreted from duodenal and salivary glands and has been used in uncontrolled trials to improve necrotizing enterocolitis in children and to heal skin wounds as a topical agent.

Clinical Trials in Ulcerative Colitis

Repifermin, KGF-2, has been studied in a placebo-controlled trial including 88 patients with moderately active UC. Patients were randomized to receive placebo or Repifermin 1 to 50 μg/kg IV for 5 days. Repifermin was not superior to placebo to induce clinical improvement at the doses used, but the safety analysis was beneficial.[56]

EGF formulated as an enema has been used in a smaller placebo-controlled trial to treat mild to moderate UC in combination with oral mesalamine.[57] Twenty-four patients were randomized (1:1) to receive placebo (100 mL inert enema) or EGF (5 μg in 100 mL enemas). After 2 weeks of treatment, as many as 83% (10/12) of actively treated patients achieved disease remission versus 8% (1/12) of placebo patients. This remission was sustained in all patients throughout week 4 and started to wean off after 8 to 12 weeks.

Safety and Future Perspectives

Safety concerns appear to represent the Achilles heal of growth factor treatment in UC. Most of these compounds, with EGF being a strong example, have mitogenic properties. Longstanding UC is characterized by an increase in colorectal carcinoma (as discussed in other chapters). Therefore, the seemingly impressive results obtained with EGF should be confirmed in future trials and confronted with careful analysis of the dysplastic and carcinogenic potential of these growth factors (Figure 24-3).

GENERAL CONCLUSION AND FUTURE PERSPECTIVES

Although the clinical development of biological agents in Crohn's disease has clearly outpaced the progress in UC, some progress has been achieved in recent years. After initial conflicting data with the use of infliximab in active UC, 2 large, controlled trials in moderate to severe and 1 controlled trial in severe disease have conclusively shown efficacy for this anti-TNFα antibody in patients with UC. In moderately active colitis, the role of anti-α_4 integrin antibodies and other selective adhesion molecule inhibitors should be further explored. The preliminary evaluation of anti-IL-2 receptor antibodies looked promising in this

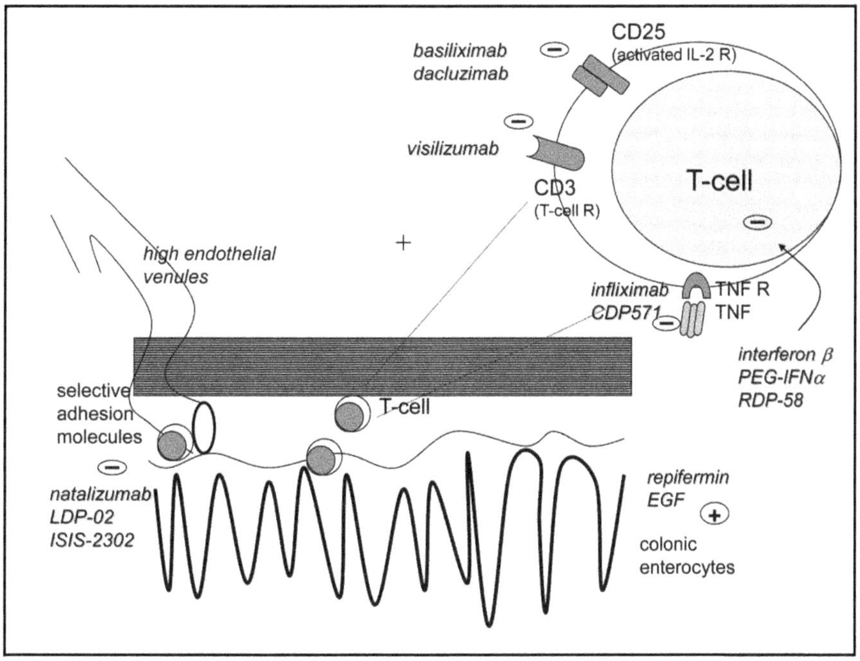

FIGURE 24-3. Immune pathways targeted with novel biological agents in ulcerative colitis.

indication, but the negative result of daclizumab in a randomized trial forces us to reconsider the potential of basiliximab until placebo-controlled data confirm the open-label experience. Clinical trial experience with growth factors has been ambiguous. EGF enemas appear to have the most potential of all agents, but uncertainty remains about its putative upregulation of proto-oncogene expression. This is extremely relevant in a population who is already at a higher risk for colorectal dysplasia and cancer than the general population. Inteferon-β 1a may be efficacious in moderately active colitis, but the data with pegylated IFNα 2a are less convincing. Both interferons carry a burden of subjective intolerance to injections of the drug.

The anti-CD3 antibody, visilizumab (Nuvion), has shown some very promising data in open-label experience and may be an alternative to colectomy for many patients and bridge them to the delayed effect of purine-analogues. However, the efficacy and safety of this antibody that temporarily depletes T cells from the circulation should be compared to those of cyclosporine. This nonbiological agent has been shown to dramatically improve severe colitis in 70% to 80% of patients and to prevent colectomy in the long term in 50%.

Despite the significant advantage achieved with the introduction of the anti-TNFα antibody infliximab in the treatment options of patients with refractory UC, more randomized, controlled data are needed for all new biological agents under development for active UC. Gradually, however, the biological endpoints of these studies, such as analysis of circulating and tissue leukocytes, histology, and functional T cell studies, provide new insights in the still enigmatic pathogenesis of UC. For instance, it is clear that the strict distinction between T helper 2-driven immune processes in UC and T helper 1-predominant inflammation in CD is challenged by results from the trials discussed in this chapter. A more accurate knowledge of cytokines and immune pathways that drive the inflammatory reaction in UC will facilitate a priori selection of novel biologicals for future development.

REFERENCES

1. Rutgeerts P, Sandborn WJ, Feagan BG, et al. Infliximab for induction and maintenance therapy for ulcerative colitis. *N Engl J Med.* 2005;353:2462-2476.
2. Probert CS, Hearing SD, Schreiber S, et al. Infliximab in moderately severe glucocorticoid resistant ulcerative colitis: a randomised controlled trial. *Gut.* 2003;52(7):998-1002.
3. Armuzzi A, Lupascu A, Fedeli P, De Pascalis B, Gasbarrini G, Gasbarrini A. Infliximab in the treatment of moderate to severe glucocorticoid dependent ulcerative colitis: a randomized methylprednisolone controlled trial [abstract]. *Gastroenterology.* 2004;126:A464.
4. Jarnerot G, Hertervig E, Friis-Liby I, et al. Infliximab as rescue therapy in severe to moderately severe ulcerative colitis: a randomized, placebo-controlled study. *Gastroenterology.* 2005;128:1805-1811.
5. Evans RC, Clarke L, Heath P, et al. Treatment of ulcerative colitis with an engineered human anti-TNFalpha antibody CDP571. *Aliment Pharmacol Ther.* 1997;11:1031-1035.
6. Travis S, Yap L, Hawkey CJ. Novel and effective therapy for ulcerative colitis: Results of parallel, prospective, placebo-controlled trials [abstract]. *Am J Gastroenterol.* 2003;98:S239.

7. Berlin C, Bargatze RF, von Adrian UH, et al. α_4 integrins mediate lymphocyte attachment and rolling under physiologic flow. *Cell.* 1995;80:413-422.
8. Briskin M, Winsor-Hines D, Shyjan A, et al. Human mucosal addressin cell adhesion molecule-1 is preferentially expressed in intestinal tract and associated lymphoid tissue. *Am J Pathol.* 1997;151:97-110.
9. Hamann JA, Andrew D, Jablonski-Westrich D, Holtzman B, Burtcher EC. Role of α_4 integrins in lymphocyte homing to muocsal tissues in vivo. *J Immunol.* 1994;152:3282-3293.
10. Wagner N, Lohler J, Kunkel EJ, et al. Critical role for β_7 integrins in formation of the gut-associated lymphoid tissue. *Nature.* 1996;382:366-370.
11. Kunkel EJ, Ramos CL, Steeber DA, et al. The roles of L-selectin, beta 7 integrins and P-selectin in leukocyte rolling and adhesion in high endothelial venules of Peyer's patches. *J Immunol.* 1998;161:2449-2456.
12. Kuhlman P, Moy VT, Lollo BA, Brain AA. The accessory function of murine intercellular adhesion molecule-1 in T lymphocyte activation. *J Immunol.* 1991;146:1773-1782.
13. Bernstein CN, Sargent M, Gallatin WM. β2 integrin/ICAM expression in Crohn's disease. *Clin Immunol Immunopathol.* 1998;86:147-160.
14. Hesterberg PE, Winsor-Hines D, Briskin MJ, et al. Rapid resolution of chronic colitis in the cotton-top tamarin with an antibody to a gut-homing integrin $\alpha_4\beta_7$. *Gastroenterology.* 1996;111:1373-1380.
15. Podolsky DK, Lobb R, King N, et al. Attenuation of colitis in the cotton-top tamarin by anti-alpha 4 integrin monoclonal antibody. *J Clin Invest.* 1993;82:372-380.
16. Rutgeerts P, Colombel J, Enns R, et al. Subanalyses of a phase III study on the evaluation of natalizumab in active Crohn's disease therapy-1 (ENACT 1). *Gut.* 2003;52:A329.
17. Ghosh S, Goldin E, Gordon FH, et al. Natalizumab for active Crohn's disease. *N Engl J Med.* 2003;348:24-32.
18. Gordon FH, Clament WY, Lai Y, et al. A randomized placebo controlled trial of a humanized monoclonal antibody to α4 integrin in active Crohn's disease. *Gastroenterology.* 2001;121:268-274.
19. Feagan BG, McDonald J, Greenberg G, et al. An ascending dose trial of a humanized $\alpha_4\beta_7$ antibody in ulcerative colitis (UC) [abstract]. *Gastroenterology.* 2000;118:A874.
20. Feagan BG, Greenberg G, Wild G, et al. A randomized placebo controlled trial of a humanized alpha4beta7 antibody in ulcerative colitis [abstract]. *Am J Gastroenterol.* 2003;98:S248.
21. Gordon FH, Hamilton MI, Donoghue S, et al. A pilot study of treatment of active ulcerative colitis with natalizumab, a humanized monoclonal antibody to alpha4 integrin. *Aliment Pharmacol Ther.* 2002;16:699-705.
22. Hamamoto N, Maemua K, Hirata I, Murano M, Sasaki S, Katsu K. Inhibition of dextran sulphate sodium (DSS)–induced colitis in mice by intracolonically administered antibodies against adhesion molecules ELAM-1 or ICAM-1. *Clin Exp Immunol.* 1999;117:462-468.
23. Burns RC, Rivera-Nieves J, Moskaluk CA, Matsumoto S, Cominelli F, Ley K. Antibody blockade of ICAM-1 and VCAM-1 ameliorates inflammation in the SAMP-1/Yit adoptive transfer model of Crohn's disease in mice. *Gastroenterology.* 2001;121:1428-1436.
24. Yacyshyn BR, Bowen-Yacyshyn MB, Jewell L, et al. A placebo-controlled trial of ICAM-1 antisense oligonucleotide in the treatment of Crohn's disease. *Gastroenterology.* 1998;114:1133-1142.
25. Yacyshyn BR, Cey WY, Goff J, et al. A randomised, placebo-controlled trial of an antisense ICAM-1 inhibitor (ISIS 2302) in steroid-dependent Crohn's disease showed clinical improvement at high serum levels [abstract]. *Gastroenterology.* 2001;120:A280.
26. Schreiber S, Nikolaus S, Malchow H, et al. Absence of efficacy of subcutaneous antisense ICAM-1 treatment of chronic active Crohn's disease. *Gastroenterology.* 2001;120:1339-1346.
27. Miner PB Jr, Geary RS, Matson J, et al. Bioavailability and therapeutic activity of alicaforsen (ISIS 2302) administered as a rectal retention enema to subjects with active ulcerative colitis. *Aliment Pharmacol Ther.* 2006;23(10):1427-1434.
28. Lichtiger S, Present DH, Kornbluth A, et al. Cyclosporine in severe ulcerative colitis refractory to steroid therapy. *N Engl J Med.* 1994;330:1841-1845.
29. Sandborn WJ. A critical review of cyclosporin therapy in inflammatory bowel disease. *Inflamm Bowel Dis.* 1995;1:48-63.
30. D'Haens G, Lemmens L, Geboes K, et al. Intravenous cyclosporine versus intravenous corticosteroids as single therapy for severe attacks of ulcerative colitis. *Gastroenterology.* 2001;120:1323-1329.
31. Willerford DM, Chen J, Ferry JA, Davdison L, Ma A, Alt FW. Interleukin-2 receptor alpha chain regulates the size and content of the peripheral lymphoid component. *Immunity.* 1995;3:521-530.
32. Poussier P, Ning T, Chen J, Benerjee D, Julius M. Intestinal inflammation in IL-2R/IL-2 mutant mice is associated with impaired intestinal T lymphopoiesis. *Gastroenterology.* 2000;118:880-891.
33. Stallmach A, Wittig B, Giese T, et al. Protection of trinitrobenzene suflonic acid-induced colitis by interleukin 2-IgG2b fusion protein in mice. *Gastroenterology.* 1999;117:866-876.
34. Kronenberg M, Cheroutre H. Do mucosal T cells prevent intestinal inflammation? *Gastroenterology.* 2000;118:974-977.
35. Maes B, Vanrenterghem Y. Anti-interleukin-2 receptor monoclonal antibodies in renal transplantation. *Nephrol Dial Transplant.* 1999;14:2824-2826.
36. Chapman TM, Keating GM. Basiliximab: a review of its use in induction therapy in renal transplantation. *Drugs.* 2003;63:2803-2835.
37. Vincenti F, Kirkman R, Light S, et al. Interleukin-2-receptor blockade with daclizumab to prevent acute rejection in renal transplantation. *N Engl J Med.* 1998;338:161-165.
38. Savo AM, Book BK, Henson S, Hakimi J, Pescovitz MD. Daclizumab rapidly saturates interleukin-2-a (CD25) on lymph node lymphocytes in children. *Transplant Proc.* 1999;31:1182-1183.
39. Van Assche G, Dalle I, Noman M, et al. A pilot study on the use of the humanized anti interleukin-2 receptor antibody daclizumab in active ulcerative colitis. *Am J Gastroenterol.* 2003;98:369-376.
40. Van Assche G, Sandborn WJ, Feagan BG, et al. Daclizumab, a humanized monoclonal antibody to the interleukin-2 receptor (CD25), for the treatment of moderately to severely active ulcerative colitis: A randomised, double-blind, placebo-controlled, dose-ranging trial. *Gut.* 2006;55:1568-1574.
41. Creed TJ, Norman MR, Probert CS, et al. Basiliximab (anti-CD25) in combination with steroids may be an effective new treatment for steroid-resistant ulcerative colitis. *Aliment Pharmacol Ther.* 2003;18(1):65-75.
42. Cole MS, Stellrecht KE, Shi JD, et al. HuM291, a humanized anti-CD3 antibody, is immunosuppressive to T cells while exhibiting reduced mitogenicity in vitro. *Transplantation.* 1999;68:563-571.
43. Carpenter PA, Appelbaum FR, Corey L, et al. A humanized non-FcR-binding anti-CD3 antibody, visilizumab, for treatment of steroid-refractory acute graft-versus-host disease. *Blood.* 2002;99(8):2712-2719.
44. Plevy S, Salzberg B, Reguiero M, et al. A humanized anti-CD3 monoclonal antibody, visilizumab, for the treatment of severe steroid-refractory ulcerative colitis: preliminary results of a phase I study [abstract]. *Gastroenterology.* 2003,124:A7.

45. Plevy S, Salzberg B, Hommes D, et al. A humanized anti-CD3 monoclonal antibody, visilizumab, for the treatment of severe steroid-refractory ulcerative colitis: Results of a phase I study [abstract]. *Gastroenterology.* 2004;126:A75.
46. Brod SA, Marshall GD Jr, Henninger EM, et al. Interferon-β 1b treatment decreases tumor necrosis factor-alpha and increases interleukin-6 production in multiple sclerosis. *Neurology.* 1996;46:1633-1638.
47. Kaser A, Molnar C, Tilg H. Differential regulation of interleukin 4 and interleukin 13 production by interferon-alpha. *Cytokine.* 1998;10:75-81.
48. Cottone M, Magliocco A, Trallori G, et al. Clinical course of inflammatory bowel disease during treatment with interferon for associated chronic active hepatitis. *Ital J Gastroenterol.* 1995;27(1):3-4.
49. Musch E, Andus T, Malek M. Induction and maintenance of clinical remission by interferon-beta in patients with steroid-refractory active ulcerative colitis-an open long-term pilot trial. *Aliment Pharmacol Ther.* 2002;16(7):1233-1239.
50. Nikolaus S, Rutgeerts P, Fedorak R, et al. Interferon beta-1a in ulcerative colitis: A placebo controlled, randomised, dose escalating study [Erratum in: *Gut.* 2003;52(11):1657.]. *Gut.* 2003;52(9):1286-1290.
51. Musch E, Raedler A, Andus T. A phase II placebo-controlled, randomized, multicenter study to evaluate efficiency and safety of interferon beta-1a in patients with ulcerative colitis [abstract]. *Gastroenterology.* 2002;122:A431.
52. Sumer N, Palabiyikoglu M. Induction of remission by interferon alpha in patients with chronic active ulcerative colitis. *Eur J Gastroenterol Hepatol.* 1995;7:597-602.
53. Madsen SM, Schlichting P, Davidsen B, et al. An open-labeled, randomized study comparing systemic interferon-alpha-2A and prednisolone enemas in the treatment of left-sided ulcerative colitis. *Am J Gastroenterol.* 2001;96(6):1807-1815.
54. Tilg H, Vogelsang H, Ludwiczek O, et al. A randomised placebo controlled trial of pegylated interferon alpha in active ulcerative colitis. *Gut.* 2003;52(12):1728-1733.
55. Beck PL, Podolsky DK. Growth factors in inflammatory bowel disease. *Inflamm Bowel Dis.* 1999;5(1):44-60.
56. Sandborn WJ, Sands BE, Wolf DC, et al. Repifermin (keratinocyte growth factor-2) for the treatment of active ulcerative colitis: a randomized, double-blind, placebo-controlled, dose-escalation trial. *Aliment Pharmacol Ther.* 2003;17(11):1355-1364.
57. Sinha A, Nightingale J, West KP, Berlanga-Acosta J, Playford RJ. Epidermal growth factor enemas with oral mesalamine for mild-to-moderate left-sided ulcerative colitis or proctitis. *N Engl J Med.* 2003;349(4):350-357.

25

Novel Nonbiologic Therapy for Ulcerative Colitis

William J. Sandborn, MD

A variety of novel nonbiologic treatments have been evaluated for the medical treatment of patients with ulcerative colitis. This chapter will review the results from clinical trials that assessed the efficacy of novel nonbiologic medications for this treatment indication.

MYCOPHENOLATE MOFETIL

Mycophenolate mofetil is an ester prodrug of mycophenolic acid, the active moiety that gives the drug its immunosuppressive properties.[1] Mycophenolic acid decreases *de-novo* synthesis of guanosine nucleotides by reversible inhibition of inosine monophosphate dehydrogenase. This drug has a directed action against T and B lymphocytes, because they depend on the de novo synthesis of purines for proliferation.[1]

A small controlled trial reported that mycophenolate mofetil 15 mg/kg/d had similar efficacy as AZA 2.5 mg/kg/d in patients with chronically active Crohn's disease (CD).[2] In contrast, a small controlled trial of mycophenolate mofetil 20 mg/kg/d versus AZA 2.0 mg/kg/d in patients with chronically active ulcerative colitis (UC) demonstrated a superior outcome with AZA.[3] Similarly, an uncontrolled study did not report a benefit with mycophenolate in patients with UC.[4] Based on the currently available evidence, patients with UC should not be treated with mycophenolate mofetil.

TACROLIMUS

Tacrolimus (FK506) is a macrolide antibiotic that belongs to the calcineurin inhibitor class of drugs. Tacrolimus exerts immunosuppressive effects by inhibiting the production of IL-2 by T helper cells.[5,6]

Small uncontrolled case series have suggested that tacrolimus may be beneficial in patients with refractory ulcerative colitis.[7-13] A small controlled trial reported that oral tacrolimus is effective in patients with severe UC who fail IV corticosteroids.[14] Tacrolimus was dosed orally to achieve target blood levels of 5 to 10 ng/ml or 10 to 15 ng/ml. Both doses were superior to placebo, but the best results were observed in the patients who achieved target blood levels of 10 to 15 ng/ml. There is currently less experience with tacrolimus than with cyclosporine or infliximab in this patient group, but it appears that tacrolimus is a therapeutic alternative in this clinical setting.

NICOTINE

Epidemiology studies have demonstrated that nonsmokers are at increased risk of developing UC.[15] There are multiple potential mechanistic explanations for this beneficial effect.[16] Two placebo-controlled trials of transdermal nicotine patches reported that the highest tolerated dose of nicotine (up to 25 mg/24 hours and 22 mg/24 hours, respectively) was effective in patients with active UC.[17,18] A controlled trial of transdermal nicotine at the highest tolerated dose (up to 25 mg/16 hours) showed equivalence to prednisolone for active ulcerative colitis.[19] A controlled trial of transdermal nicotine (15 mg/24 hours) was superior to oral mesalamine for active left-sided colitis refractory to rectal mesalamine.[20] A controlled trial using a lower dose of transdermal nicotine (15 mg/16 hours) for maintenance of remission was negative.[21] Two uncontrolled studies of nicotine enemas for active distal UC reported a beneficial

Lichtenstein GR, ed.
Ulcerative Colitis: The Complete Guide to Medical Management (pp. 273-282)

clinical effect and a reduction in both blood concentrations of nicotine (by first-pass hepatic metabolism of nicotine) and side effects.[22,23] Side effects from transdermal nicotine occur frequently and include contact dermatitis, nausea, vomiting, headaches, sleep disturbance, diaphoresis, tremor, and lightheadedness.[16-19,21]

HEPARIN

IBD has been associated with a hypercoagulable state, and heparin has been proposed as a potential therapy in UC both for its anticoagulant and anti-inflammatory effects.[24] Five uncontrolled trials have suggested that both intravenous and subcutaneous heparin may be of benefit in patients with active UC.[25-29] A placebo-controlled trial of subcutaneous porcine heparin 10,000 units 2 to 3 times daily in patients with active UC reported a response rate of 42% for the heparin group and 19% for the placebo group.[30] In a small comparative trial in patients with severely active ulcerative colitis or Crohn's colitis, IV heparin had a similar response to IV corticosteroids.[31] In contrast, in a larger comparative trial, IV heparin was less effective than IV corticosteroids and was associated with more bleeding complications.[32]

Uncontrolled studies of low molecular weight heparin (both enoxaparin and nadroparin) suggested benefit in patients with active ulcerative colitis.[33-35] A placebo-controlled trial of low molecular weight heparin (tinzaparin) failed to demonstrate efficacy.[36]

SHORT CHAIN FATTY ACIDS

Luminal n-butyrate and other short chain fatty acids (SCFAs) produced by bacterial carbohydrate fermentation are the major luminal source of energy for colonocytes, and colonocytes from patients with UC may have reduced capacity to oxidize SCFAs.[37] Two small and poorly designed controlled trials suggested that SCFA enemas may be beneficial for active distal UC.[38,39] Subsequently, 4 placebo-controlled trials with larger sample sizes have been conducted.[40-43] Two of 2 studies comparing butyrate enemas to placebo[40,41] and 2 of 3 studies comparing SCFA enemas to placebo[41-43] failed to demonstrate efficacy in patients with active left-sided UC. A 60 g oat bran diet raised fecal butyrate concentrations in a controlled trial in patients with active UC, but the implication of this physiologic endpoint for clinical efficacy is unclear.[44] A placebo-controlled trial of essential fatty acid supplementation failed to demonstrate efficacy for maintenance of remission in patients with UC.[45] Another placebo-controlled trial of an oral supplement enriched with fish oil, soluble fiber, and antioxidants failed to demonstrate efficacy for inducing remission but did demonstrate a steroid-sparing benefit.[46]

FISH OIL

Fish oil (eicosapentaenoic acid and docosahexaenoic acid) inhibits 5-lipoxygenase and other enzymes involved in arachidonate metabolism of leukotriene B4. Leukotriene B4 is a chemoattractant for polymorphonuclear leukocytes. Mucosal and rectal dialysate concentrations of leukotriene B4 correlate with disease activity. A small placebo-controlled trial suggested that fish oil may be of benefit in patients with active UC.[47] However, 4 subsequent placebo-controlled trials did not demonstrate clinical efficacy of fish oil compared with placebo in patients with active UC[48-50] or for maintenance of remission.[51] A controlled trial comparing sulfasalazine and fish oil also failed to demonstrate efficacy for fish oil.[52] These negative clinical results were observed in spite of the finding that fish oil did result in a significant decrease in colonic concentrations of leukotriene B_4.[48]

ANTIBIOTICS

Given the attractive but unsubstantiated hypothesis that UC may be a specific infectious colitis, studies evaluating treatment with antibiotics were logical. A controlled trial of oral tobramycin in patients with mild to moderately active UC demonstrated short-term induction efficacy, but there was no maintenance benefit.[53,54] Small comparative trials demonstrated that metronidazole was less effective than sulfasalazine for the treatment of active ulcerative colitis, but suggested that metronidazole might have a maintenance benefit.[55,56] One of two placebo-controlled trials of oral ciprofloxacin in patients with active ulcerative colitis demonstrated efficacy.[57,58] Controlled trials of oral vancomycin,[59] IV metronidazole,[60] IV tobramycin and metronidazole,[61] and IV ciprofloxacin[62] in patients with severely active UC demonstrated no clinical benefit compared with placebo. Uncontrolled trials suggested that the nonabsorbable antibiotic rifaximin may be of benefit in patients with active UC.[63-65] A small placebo-controlled trial did not show a clear benefit.[66] Based on the nearly uniform negative outcome of these studies, antibiotics have no role in the treatment of UC except in the case of a documented or suspected coexisting infection with a specific infectious organism.

ZILEUTON AND OTHER LEUKOTRIENE INHIBITORS

Initial studies suggested that compounds acting to inhibit 5-lipoxygenase might be of benefit in patients with UC.[67,68] However, larger controlled trials with adequate sample sizes were negative.[69-72] The Merck compound MK-591 (Whitehouse Station, NJ) resulted in a significant decrease in colonic luminal concentrations of leukotriene B4, but did not demonstrate clinical efficacy when compared with placebo in patients with mild to moderately active UC.[69] There was a trend toward clinical benefit for Zileuton compared with placebo in patients with mild to moderately active UC, but the results did not reach statistical significance.[70,71] Zileuton was less effective than 5-aminosalicylic 1.6 g/d and similar to placebo for maintaining remission in patients with UC.[72]

Ridogrel inhibits thromboxane synthase. A pilot study indicated that ridogrel reduced colonic mucosal thromboxane B_2 release in patients with UC.[73] Subsequently, 2 large controlled trials failed to demonstrate efficacy of ridogrel in patients with active UC.[74]

ALLOPURINOL

The xanthine oxidase inhibitor allopurinol inhibits oxygen free radical formation and has been proposed as a treatment for UC. A placebo-controlled trial failed to demonstrate efficacy of allopurinol combined with mesalamine as compared to mesalamine alone for maintaining remission in patients with UC.[75]

BISMUTH

Bismuth compounds have both antidiarrheal and antibacterial properties. Uncontrolled studies of bismuth subsalicylate enemas[76] and tripotassium dicitrato bismuth enemas[77] suggested benefit in patients with mild to moderately active distal UC. These observations were confirmed by a small controlled trial comparing bismuth citrate enemas to 5-aminosalicylic enemas that demonstrated equivalence in patients with mild to moderately active distal UC.[78] Systemic absorption of bismuth after rectal administration was minimal.

LIDOCAINE/ROPIVACAINE

Topical anesthetic agents including both lidocaine and ropivacaine may have anti-inflammatory effects. Uncontrolled studies of 2% lidocaine enemas[79,80] and ropivacaine gel enemas[81] have been reported to be of benefit in patients with mild to moderately active distal UC. A placebo-controlled trial of ropivacaine enemas in this same patient population has been completed, but to date the results have not been made available. Systemic absorption of these agents after rectal administration is minimal.[82,83]

ROSIGLITAZONE

Rosiglitazone (peroxisome proliferator-activated receptor gamma [PPARγ] ligand) is used for the treatment of diabetes. Recent data have demonstrated that PPARγ is reduced in patients with UC, and animal models have suggested benefit under treatment with PPARγ ligand therapy. In a pilot study, 15 patients with active ulcerative colitis were treated with rosiglitazone 4 mg twice a day for 12 weeks.[84] Clinical response was observed in 54% of patients, clinical remission in 27%, and endoscopic remission in 20%. A placebo-controlled trial demonstrated efficacy of rosiglitazone over placebo.[85]

LEVAMISOLE

Levamisole is an antihelmintic agent. Levamisole also has immunostimulatory properties and is used as an adjuvant therapy with 5-fluorouracil for the treatment of colorectal cancer. Placebo-controlled trials of levamisole in patients with active UC and with UC in remission failed to demonstrate efficacy.[86,87]

DISODIUM CROMOGLYCATE

Disodium cromoglycate is a mast-cell stabilizer that is used to treat allergic diseases. A small randomized pilot study indicated a possible benefit in patients with UC.[88] Subsequently, larger controlled trials in patients with active UC[90] and patients with UC in remission[90-92] failed to demonstrate efficacy.

OCTREOTIDE

The intestinal somatostatin content is reduced in patients with UC, and in vitro somatostatin diminishes the activity of intestinal lymphocytes.[93] A placebo-controlled trial of subcutaneous octreotide failed to demonstrate efficacy in patients with ulcerative colitis.[94]

ZINC

Zinc has been demonstrated to decrease in vitro peripheral blood natural killer activity in patients with UC.[95] The results of our study show a long-lasting effect of in vivo zinc administration, which decreased peripheral blood natural killer cell activity in IBD. A controlled trial of zinc failed to demonstrate efficacy for the treatment of active UC.[96]

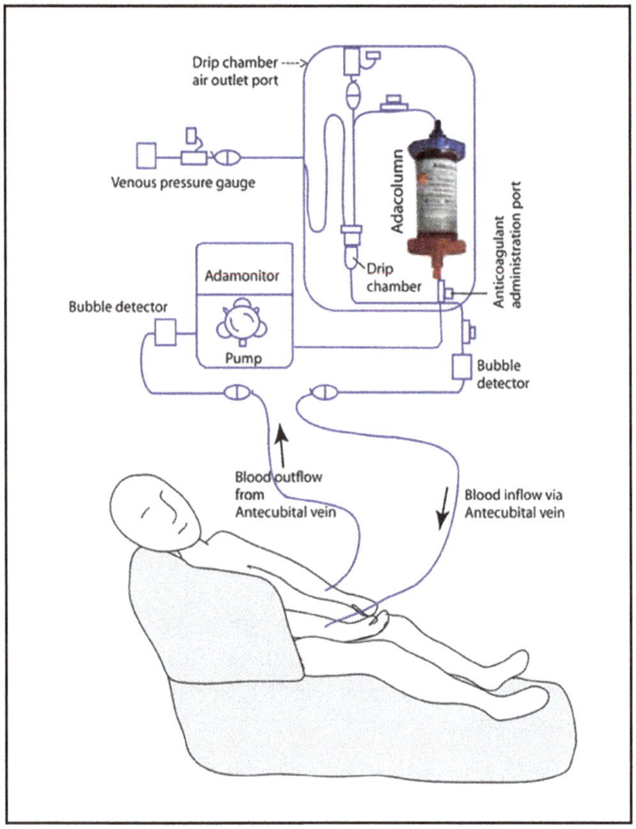

FIGURE 25-1. Adacolumn circuit: an outline of the extracorporeal circulation through the Adacolumn device. (Reprinted with permission from Katz S. Leukocytapheresis: an "out-of-body" experience in inflammatory bowel disease. *Gastroenterol Hepatol.* 2006;2:906-913.)

APHERESIS

Apheresis is a method of extracorporeally removing cells from the circulatory system. Simple centrifugation has been used to remove leukocyte components; however, the use of fibers or columns to remove specific components from whole blood results in the removal of up to 4 times as many white blood cells and may, therefore, result in a greater therapeutic effect. Two types of selective apheresis filters have been investigated for the treatment of UC in Japan and Europe. Whole venous blood is perfused through an adsorption column. In the first method, Cellsorba FX (Asahi Medical, Tokyo, Japan), the column contains a filter composed of nonwoven polyester fibers that removes granulocytes, monocytes, lymphocytes, and some platelets. In the second method, Adacolumn (Japan Immunoresearch Laboratories Co, Ltd, Takasaki, Japan), the column is packed with cellulose acetate beads that remove activated granulocytes and monocytes (but not lymphocytes or platelets; Figure 25-1).

Uncontrolled pilot studies of simple centrifugation apheresis suggested that apheresis might be of clinical benefit in patients with steroid-resistant active UC.[97-99]

Uncontrolled pilot studies in patients with active UC have suggested that Cellsorba apheresis may be of clinical benefit for inducing and maintaining response and remission and for steroid sparing.[100-105] A pilot study in pediatric patients with active UC was also encouraging.[106] An uncontrolled pilot study with another nonwoven polyester fiber selective apheresis filter called Finecell in patients with active UC yielded similar results.[107] Subsequently, a nonblinded, multicenter trial comparing Cellsorba apheresis as an adjunct to the current treatment regimen (including prednisone) with high-dose prednisone in patients with active UC was performed.[108] Patients treated with Cellsorba apheresis were reported to have greater clinical benefit, greater decreases in clinical and endoscopic activity, greater steroid sparing, and fewer adverse events than patients treated with high doses of prednisone. These data are difficult to interpret because of the lack of blinding and the absence of a sham apheresis control group. Sham-controlled trials of Cellsorba apheresis are needed.

Uncontrolled pilot studies have suggested that Adacolumn apheresis may be of clinical benefit for inducing response and remission in patients with active UC and for steroid sparing in patients with steroid-dependent disease.[101,109-117] A nonblinded, multicenter trial comparing Adacolumn apheresis as an adjunct to continuing prednisolone therapy with conventional therapy, including increasing the prednisolone dose in patients with active ulcerative colitis, was performed.[118] Patients treated with Adacolumn apheresis were reported to have greater rates of response and remission and fewer adverse events than patients treated with high doses of prednisolone. These data are difficult to interpret because of the lack of blinding and the absence of a sham apheresis control group. Two nonblinded trials comparing once-weekly and twice-weekly Adacolumn apheresis in patients with active UC have suggested that twice-weekly apheresis induction therapy may induce remission more rapidly.[119,120] A sham-controlled trial of Adacolumn apheresis in patients with active UC has now been completed and shows relative lack of efficacy.[121]

ALOE VERA

Aloe vera has been claimed to have anti-inflammatory effects. A small placebo-controlled trial of oral aloe vera gel was performed in 44 patients with active ulcerative colitis.[122] Clinical remission and response occurred more commonly in aloe vera-treated patients, but the results were not statistically significant, and there were no differences from placebo in improvement in endoscopic inflammation.

HYDROXYCHLOROQUINE AND CHLOROQUINE

The 4-aminoquinolines hydroxychloroquine and chloroquine exert anti-inflammatory and immunomodulatory effects in vitro, possibly through lysosomal stabilization.[123] These agents are effective for the treatment of rheumatoid arthritis. An uncontrolled study failed to demonstrate efficacy of hydroxychloroquine in patients with active UC refractory to oral corticosteroids.[124] A blinded, controlled trial in 40 patients with active UC showed similar efficacy for induction of partial and complete remission with sulfasalazine and chloroquine.[125] This study was not powered to formally determine noninferiority, and thus the results are not definitive.

PROBIOTIC THERAPY WITH *E. COLI NISSLE* 1917, *TRICHURIS SUIS*, AND *SACCHAROMYCES BOULARDII*

Probiotic bacteria may be of benefit in patients with ulcerative colitis. Two pilot controlled studies have reported that *E. coli Nissle* 1917 might be equivalent to mesalamine for maintaining remission in patients with ulcerative colitis.[126,127] However, these trials were not statistically powered to demonstrate noninferiority (equivalence). Subsequently, an adequately powered noninferiority trial was performed that demonstrated equivalence between *E. coli Nissle* 1917 and mesalamine.[128]

Helminths induce mucosal T cells to make Th2 and regulatory cytokines.[129] Helminth-induced mucosal IL-4, TGFbeta, and IL-10 likely are part of the protective process. Helminths affect pathways of innate immunity like TLR4 expression and function. Worms also induce various regulatory-type T cell subsets in the gut that limit effector T cell growth and function. These effects of helminths might have therapeutic effects in patients with ulcerative colitis. A pilot study reported that the helminth *Trichuris suis* might be beneficial in patients with active ulcerative colitis.[130] A subsequent small placebo-controlled trial demonstrated efficacy for inducing clinical response but not remission in active UC.[131]

The nonpathogenic yeast *Saccharomyces boulardii* has been used to treat *Clostridium difficile* colitis. *S. boulardii* acts as a shuttle liberating effective enzymes, proteins, and trophic factors during its intestinal transit, which improves host immune defenses, digestion, and absorption of nutrients.[132] In addition, during its intestinal transit *S. boulardii* secretes polyamines (mainly spermine and spermidine that regulate gene expression and protein synthesis) and traps T cells in mesenteric lymph nodes.[132,133] An uncontrolled pilot study suggested that *S. boulardii* might be of benefit in patients with active UC.[134] A placebo-controlled trial is needed to confirm these preliminary observations.

DEHYDROEPIANDROSTERONE

Dehydroepiandrosterone (DHEA) is a steroid hormone with a variety of in vitro activities including inhibition of NFKβ, IL-6, IL-12, and PPARα. DHEA is effective for the treatment of systemic lupus erythematosus. A pilot study suggested that DHEA might be of clinical benefit for inducing response and remission in patients with active UC.[135] A placebo-controlled trial of DHEA in patients with CD is ongoing.

PROTEASE INHIBITION WITH THE TRYPTASE INHIBITOR APC2059

Inhibition of tryptase and other protease inhibitors could prevent mast cell degranulation in gut mucosa with subsequent release of inflammatory mediators. Uncontrolled pilot studies of APC2059 (a highly specific tryptase inhibitor) and the Bowman Birk protein (a soybean extract with more broad protease inhibitor activity) showed modest clinical activity in patients with active UC.[136,137] No large placebo-controlled trials have been performed.

CONCLUSION

A wide variety of nonbiologic novel agents have been evaluated for the treatment of UC. Tacrolimus is effective for induction of remission in patients with severe steroid-refractory UC. Transdermal nicotine is effective for induction of response in patients with active UC, and the probiotic *E. coli Nissle* 1917 is as effective as mesalamine for maintaining remission. A large sham-controlled trial of the Adacolumn apheresis device has been completed but the results are not yet available. A majority of other novel treatment agents evaluated to date have failed to demonstrate efficacy for induction and/or maintenance therapy in patients with UC. In the future, it is likely that small-molecule nonbiologic molecules directed against specific targets like TNFα and other proinflammatory cytokines will be developed that will be highly effective for the treatment of UC.

REFERENCES

1. Lipsky JJ. Mycophenolate mofetil. *Lancet.* 1996;348:1357-1359.
2. Neurath MF, Wanitschke R, Peters M, Krummenauer F, Meyer zum Buschenfelde KH, Schlaak JF. Randomised trial of mycophenolate mofetil versus azathioprine for treatment of chronic active Crohn's disease. *Gut.* 1999;44:625-628.
3. Orth T, Peters M, Schlaak JF, et al. Mycophenolate mofetil versus azathioprine in patients with chronic active ulcerative colitis: a 12-month pilot study. *Am J Gastroenterol.* 2000;95:1201-1207.
4. Fellermann K, Steffen M, Stein J, et al. Mycophenolate mofetil: Lack of efficacy in chronic active inflammatory bowel disease. *Aliment Pharmacol Ther.* 2000;14:171-176.
5. Liu J, Farmer JD Jr, Lane WS, Friedman J, Weissman I, Schreiber SL. Calcineurin is a common target of cyclophilin-cyclosporin A and FKBP- FK506 complexes. *Cell.* 1991;66:807-815.
6. Flanagan WM, Corthesy B, Bram RJ, Crabtree GR. Nuclear association of a T-cell transcription factor blocked by FK-506 and cyclosporin A. *Nature.* 1991;352:803-807.
7. Bousvaros A, Wang A, Leichtner AM. Tacrolimus (FK-506) treatment of fulminant colitis in a child. *J Pediatr Gastroenterol Nutr.* 1996;23:329-333.
8. Bousvaros A, Kirschner BS, Werlin SL, et al. Oral tacrolimus treatment of severe colitis in children. *J Pediatr.* 2000;137:794-799.
9. Fellermann K, Ludwig D, Stahl M, David-Walek T, Stange EF. Steroid-unresponsive acute attacks of inflammatory bowel disease: Immunomodulation by tacrolimus (FK506). *Am J Gastroenterol.* 1998;93:1860-1866.
10. Fellermann K, Tanko Z, Herrlinger KR, et al. Response of refractory colitis to intravenous or oral tacrolimus (FK506) [see comment]. *Inflamm Bowel Dis.* 2002;8:317-324.
11. Baumgart DC, Wiedenmann B, Dignass AU. Rescue therapy with tacrolimus is effective in patients with severe and refractory inflammatory bowel disease. *Aliment Pharmacol Ther.* 2003;17:1273-1281.
12. Hogenauer C, Wenzl HH, Hinterleitner TA, Petritsch W. Effect of oral tacrolimus (FK 506) on steroid-refractory moderate/severe ulcerative colitis. *Aliment Pharmacol Ther.* 2003;18:415-423.
13. Baumgart DC, Pintoffl JP, Sturm A, Wiedenmann B, Dignass AU. Tacrolimus is safe and effective in patients with severe steroid-refractory or steroid-dependent inflammatory bowel disease: a long-term follow-up. *Am J Gastroenterol.* 2006;101:1048-1056.
14. Ogata H, Matsui T, Nakamura M, et al. A randomised dose finding study of oral tacrolimus (FK506) therapy in refractory ulcerative colitis [see comment]. *Gut.* 2006;55:1255-1262.
15. Calkins BM. A meta-analysis of the role of smoking in inflammatory bowel disease. *Dig Dis Sci.* 1989;34:1841-1854.
16. Sandborn WJ. Nicotine therapy for ulcerative colitis: a review of rationale, mechanisms, pharmacology, and clinical results. *Am J Gastroenterol.* 1999;94:1161-1171.
17. Pullan RD, Rhodes J, Ganesh S, et al. Transdermal nicotine for active ulcerative colitis [see comment]. *N Engl J Med.* 1994;330:811-815.
18. Sandborn WJ, Tremaine WJ, Offord KP, et al. Transdermal nicotine for mildly to moderately active ulcerative colitis: a randomized, double-blind, placebo-controlled trial. *Ann Intern Med.* 1997;126:364-371.
19. Thomas GA, Rhodes J, Ragunath K, et al. Transdermal nicotine compared with oral prednisolone therapy for active ulcerative colitis. *Eur J Gastroenterol Hepatol.* 1996;8:769-776.
20. Guslandi M, Frego R, Viale E, Testoni PA. Distal ulcerative colitis refractory to rectal mesalamine: role of transdermal nicotine versus oral mesalamine. *Can J Gastroenterol.* 2002;16:293-296.
21. Thomas GA, Rhodes J, Mani V, et al. Transdermal nicotine as maintenance therapy for ulcerative colitis. *N Engl J Med.* 1995;332:988-992.
22. Sandborn WJ, Tremaine WJ, Leighton JA, et al. Nicotine tartrate liquid enemas for mildly to moderately active left-sided ulcerative colitis unresponsive to first-line therapy: a pilot study. *Aliment Pharmacol Ther.* 1997;11:663-671.
23. Green JT, Thomas GA, Rhodes J, et al. Nicotine enemas for active ulcerative colitis: a pilot study. *Aliment Pharmacol Ther.* 1997;11:859-863.
24. Korzenik JR. IBD: A vascular disorder? The case for heparin therapy. *Inflamm Bowel Dis.* 1997;3:87-94.
25. Gaffney PR, O'Leary JJ, Doyle CT, et al. Response to heparin in patients with ulcerative colitis. *Lancet.* 1991;337:238-239.
26. Gaffney PR, Doyle CT, Gaffney A, Hogan J, Hayes DP, Annis P. Paradoxical response to heparin in 10 patients with ulcerative colitis. *Am J Gastroenterol.* 1995;90:220-223.
27. Folwaczny C, Fricke H, Endres S, Hartmann G, Jochum M, Loeschke K. Anti-inflammatory properties of unfractioned heparin in patients with highly active ulcerative colitis: A pilot study. *Am J Gastroenterol.* 1997;92:911-912.
28. Folwaczny C, Wiebecke B, Loeschke K. Unfractioned heparin in the therapy of patients with highly active inflammatory bowel disease. *Am J Gastroenterol.* 1999;94:1551-1555.
29. Evans RC, Wong VS, Morris AI, Rhodes JM. Treatment of corticosteroid-resistant ulcerative colitis with heparin: a report of 16 cases. *Aliment Pharmacol Ther.* 1997;11:1037-1040.
30. Korzenik JR. Heparin: an emerging counterintuitive therapy for inflammatory bowel disease. *Current Treatment Options in Gastroenterology.* 2000;3:95-98.
31. Ang YS, Mahmud N, White B, et al. Randomized comparison of unfractionated heparin with corticosteroids in severe active inflammatory bowel disease. *Aliment Pharmacol Ther.* 2000;14:1015-1022.
32. Panes J, Esteve M, Cabre E, et al. Comparison of heparin and steroids in the treatment of moderate and severe ulcerative colitis [see comment]. *Gastroenterology.* 2000;119:903-908.
33. Torkvist L, Thorlacius H, Sjoqvist U, et al. Low molecular weight heparin as adjuvant therapy in active ulcerative colitis. *Aliment Pharmacol Ther.* 1999;13:1323-1328.
34. Dotan I, Hallak A, Arber N, et al. Low-dose low-molecular weight heparin (enoxaparin) is effective as adjuvant treatment in active ulcerative colitis: an open trial. *Dig Dis Sci.* 2001;46:2239-2244.
35. Vrij AA, Jansen JM, Schoon EJ, de Bruine A, Hemker HC, Stockbrugger RW. Low molecular weight heparin treatment in steroid-refractory ulcerative colitis: clinical outcome and influence on mucosal capillary thrombi. *Scand J Gastroenterol.* 2001;(Suppl):41-47.
36. Bloom S, Kiilerich S, Lassen MR, et al. Low molecular weight heparin (tinzaparin) vs. placebo in the treatment of mild to moderately active ulcerative colitis. *Aliment Pharmacol Ther.* 2004;19:871-878.
37. Roediger WE. The colonic epithelium in ulcerative colitis: an energy-deficiency disease? *Lancet.* 1980;2:712-715.
38. Scheppach W, Sommer H, Kirchner T, et al. Effect of butyrate enemas on the colonic mucosa in distal ulcerative colitis [see comment]. *Gastroenterology.* 1992;103:51-56.
39. Senagore AJ, MacKeigan JM, Scheider M, Ebrom JS. Short-chain fatty acid enemas: a cost-effective alternative in the treatment of nonspecific proctosigmoiditis [see comment]. *Dis Colon Rectum.* 1992;35:923-927.
40. Steinhart AH, Hiruki T, Brzezinski A, Baker JP. Treatment of left-sided ulcerative colitis with butyrate enemas: a controlled trial. *Aliment Pharmacol Ther.* 1996;10:729-736.

41. Scheppach W. Treatment of distal ulcerative colitis with short-chain fatty acid enemas: a placebo-controlled trial. German-Austrian SCFA Study Group. *Dig Dis Sci.* 1996;41:2254-2259.
42. Breuer RI, Soergel KH, Lashner BA, et al. Short chain fatty acid rectal irrigation for left-sided ulcerative colitis: a randomised, placebo controlled trial. *Gut.* 1997;40:485-491.
43. Vernia P, Marcheggiano A, Caprilli R, et al. Short-chain fatty acid topical treatment in distal ulcerative colitis. *Aliment Pharmacol Ther.* 1995;9:309-313.
44. Hallert C, Bjorck I, Nyman M, Pousette A, Granno C, Svensson H. Increasing fecal butyrate in ulcerative colitis patients by diet: controlled pilot study. *Inflamm Bowel Dis.* 2003;9:116-121.
45. Middleton SJ, Naylor S, Woolner J, Hunter JO. A double-blind, randomized, placebo-controlled trial of essential fatty acid supplementation in the maintenance of remission of ulcerative colitis. *Aliment Pharmacol Ther.* 2002;16:1131-1135.
46. Seidner DL, Lashner BA, Brzezinski A, et al. An oral supplement enriched with fish oil, soluble fiber, and antioxidants for corticosteroid sparing in ulcerative colitis: a randomized, controlled trial. *Clin Gastroenterol Hepatol.* 2005;3:358-369.
47. Aslan A, Triadafilopoulos G. Fish oil fatty acid supplementation in active ulcerative colitis: a double-blind, placebo-controlled, crossover study. *Am J Gastroenterol.* 1992;87:432-437.
48. Stenson WF, Cort D, Rodgers J, et al. Dietary supplementation with fish oil in ulcerative colitis [see comment]. *Ann Intern Med.* 1992;116:609-614.
49. Hawthorne AB, Daneshmend TK, Hawkey CJ, et al. Treatment of ulcerative colitis with fish oil supplementation: a prospective 12 month randomised controlled trial. *Gut.* 1992;33:922-928.
50. Greenfield SM, Green AT, Teare JP, et al. A randomized controlled study of evening primrose oil and fish oil in ulcerative colitis. *Aliment Pharmacol Ther.* 1993;7:159-166.
51. Loeschke K, Ueberschaer B, Pietsch A, et al. n-3 fatty acids only delay early relapse of ulcerative colitis in remission. *Dig Dis Sci.* 1996;41:2087-2094.
52. Dichi I, Frenhane P, Dichi JB, et al. Comparison of omega-3 fatty acids and sulfasalazine in ulcerative colitis. *Nutrition.* 2000;16:87-90.
53. Burke DA, Axon AT, Clayden SA, Dixon MF, Johnston D, Lacey RW. The efficacy of tobramycin in the treatment of ulcerative colitis. *Aliment Pharmacol Ther.* 1990;4:123-129.
54. Lobo AJ, Burke DA, Sobala GM, Axon AT. Oral tobramycin in ulcerative colitis: Effect on maintenance of remission. *Aliment Pharmacol Ther.* 1993;7:155-158.
55. Gilat T, Suissa A, Leichtman G, et al. A comparative study of metronidazole and sulfasalazine in active, not severe, ulcerative colitis: an Israeli multicenter trial. *J Clin Gastroenterol.* 1987;9:415-417.
56. Gilat T, Leichtman G, Delpre G, Eshchar J, Bar Meir S, Fireman Z. A comparison of metronidazole and sulfasalazine in the maintenance of remission in patients with ulcerative colitis. *J Clin Gastroenterol.* 1989;11:392-395.
57. Mantzaris GJ, Archavlis E, Christoforidis P, et al. A prospective randomized controlled trial of oral ciprofloxacin in acute ulcerative colitis. *Am J Gastroenterol.* 1997;92:454-456.
58. Turunen UM, Farkkila MA, Hakala K, et al. Long-term treatment of ulcerative colitis with ciprofloxacin: a prospective, double-blind, placebo-controlled study [see comment]. *Gastroenterology.* 1998;115:1072-1078.
59. Dickinson RJ, O'Connor HJ, Pinder I, Hamilton I, Johnston D, Axon AT. Double blind controlled trial of oral vancomycin as adjunctive treatment in acute exacerbations of idiopathic colitis. *Gut.* 1985;26:1380-1384.
60. Chapman RW, Selby WS, Jewell DP. Controlled trial of intravenous metronidazole as an adjunct to corticosteroids in severe ulcerative colitis. *Gut.* 1986;27:1210-1212.
61. Mantzaris GJ, Hatzis A, Kontogiannis P, Triadaphyllou G. Intravenous tobramycin and metronidazole as an adjunct to corticosteroids in acute, severe ulcerative colitis. *Am J Gastroenterol.* 1994;89:43-46.
62. Mantzaris GJ, Petraki K, Archavlis E, et al. A prospective randomized controlled trial of intravenous ciprofloxacin as an adjunct to corticosteroids in acute, severe ulcerative colitis. *Scand J Gastroenterol.* 2001;36:971-974.
63. Riegler G, Russo MI, Carratu R, Ferrieri A. Considerazioni clinico-terapeutiche sul trattamento di disturbi addominali aspecifici in pazienti affetti da rettocolite ulcerosa in fase di quiescenza: note preliminari della terapia con Rifaximina. *Rivista Europea Per Le Scienze Mediche e Farmacologiche.* 1992;14:9-14.
64. Pinto A, Borruto G, Dell' Anna A, Turco L, Ferrieri A. An open, uncontrolled trial of oral rifaximin, a non-absorbable antibiotic, in inflammatory bowel disease refractory to conventional therapy. *Eur J Clin Res.* 1997;9:217-224.
65. Lukas M, Konecny M, Zboril V. Rifaximin in patients with mild to moderate activity of ulcerative colitis: an open label study. *Gastroenterology.* 2002;122:A-434.
66. Gionchetti P, Rizzello F, Ferrieri A, et al. Rifaximin in patients with moderate or severe ulcerative colitis refractory to steroid-treatment: A double-blind, placebo-controlled trial. *Dig Dis Sci.* 1999;44:1220-1221.
67. Laursen LS, Naesdal J, Bukhave K, Lauritsen K, Rask-Madsen J. Selective 5-lipoxygenase inhibition in ulcerative colitis. *Lancet.* 1990;335:683-685.
68. Hillingso J, Kjeldsen J, Laursen LS, et al. Blockade of leukotriene production by a single oral dose of MK-0591 in active ulcerative colitis. *Clin Pharmacol Ther.* 1995;57:335-341.
69. Roberts WG, Simon TJ, Berlin RG, et al. Leukotrienes in ulcerative colitis: Results of a multicenter trial of a leukotriene biosynthesis inhibitor, MK-591. *Gastroenterology.* 1997;112:725-732.
70. Laursen LS, Lauritsen K, Bukhavr K, et al. Selective 5-lipoxygenase inhibition by zileuton in the treatment of relapsing ulcerative colitis. A randomized double blind placebo controlled multicenter trial. *Eur J Gastroenterol Hepatol.* 1994;6:209-215.
71. Peppercorn MA, Das K, Elson C, et al. Zileuton, a 5-lipoxygenase inhibitor in the treatment of active ulcerative colitis: a double-blind placebo controlled trial. *Gastroenterology.* 1994;106:A751.
72. Hawkey CJ, Dube LM, Rountree LV, Linnen PJ, Lancaster JF. A trial of zileuton versus mesalazine or placebo in the maintenance of remission of ulcerative colitis. The European Zileuton Study Group for Ulcerative Colitis. *Gastroenterology.* 1997;112:718-724.
73. Casellas F, Papo M, Guarner F, et al. Effects of thromboxane synthase inhibition on in vivo release of inflammatory mediators in chronic ulcerative colitis. *Eur J Gastroenterol Hepatol.* 1995;7:221-226.
74. Tytgat GN, Van Nueten L, Van De Velde I, Joslyn A, Hanauer SB. Efficacy and safety of oral ridogrel in the treatment of ulcerative colitis: two multicentre, randomized, double-blind studies. *Aliment Pharmacol Ther.* 2002;16:87-99.
75. Jarnerot G, Strom M, Danielsson A, et al. Allopurinol in addition to 5-aminosalicylic acid based drugs for the maintenance treatment of ulcerative colitis. *Aliment Pharmacol Ther.* 2000;14:1159-1162.
76. Ryder SD, Walker RJ, Jones H, Rhodes JM. Rectal bismuth subsalicylate as therapy for ulcerative colitis. *Aliment Pharmacol Ther.* 1990;4:333-338.
77. Srivastava ED, Swift GL, Wilkinson S, Williams GT, Evans BK, Rhodes J. Tripotassium dicitrato bismuthate enemas in the treatment of ulcerative proctitis. *Aliment Pharmacol Ther.* 1990;4:577-581.

78. Pullan RD, Ganesh S, Mani V, et al. Comparison of bismuth citrate and 5-aminosalicylic acid enemas in distal ulcerative colitis: a controlled trial. *Gut.* 1993;34:676-679.
79. Bjorck S, Dahlstrom A, Ahlman H. Topical treatment of ulcerative proctitis with lidocaine. *Scand J Gastroenterol.* 1989;24:1061-1072.
80. Bjorck S, Dahlstrom A, Johansson L, Ahlman H. Treatment of the mucosa with local anaesthetics in ulcerative colitis. *Agents & Actions.* 1992;C60-C72.
81. Arlander E, Ost A, Stahlberg D, Lofberg R. Ropivacaine gel in active distal ulcerative colitis and proctitis: a pharmacokinetic and exploratory clinical study. *Aliment Pharmacol Ther.* 1996;10:73-81.
82. Arlander E, Sjovall J, Sorstad J, Norsten-Hoog C, Gustafsson LL. Rectal ropivacaine is absorbed proportionally to the dose, with low intraindividual variability. *Br J Clin Pharmacol.* 2003;55:14-22.
83. Arlander E, Cederlund T, Mare K. No volume effect on retrograde colonic spread of rectally-administered ropivacaine gel. *Aliment Pharmacol Ther.* 2003;18:655-660.
84. Lewis JD, Lichtenstein GR, Stein RB, et al. An open-label trial of the PPAR-gamma ligand rosiglitazone for active ulcerative colitis. *Am J Gastroenterol.* 2001;96:3323-3328.
85. Lewis JD, Lichtenstein GR, Deren JJ, et al. Rosiglitazone for active ulcerative colitis: a randomized placebo-controlled trial. *Gastroenterology.* 2008;134(3):688-695.
86. Hermanowicz A, Nowak A, Gajos L. Controlled therapeutic trial of levamisole and sulphasalazine in acute ulcerative colitis. *Gut.* 1984;25:S34-S38.
87. Hermanowicz A, Sliwinski Z, Nowak A, Gajos L. The effect of levamisole on the maintenance of remission of ulcerative colitis: a 2-year double-blind study. *Scand J Gastroenterol.* 1987;22:367-371.
88. Mani V, Lloyd G, Green FH, Fox H, Turnberg LA. Treatment of ulcerative colitis with oral disodium cromoglycate: a double-blind controlled trial. *Lancet.* 1976;1:439-441.
89. Buckell NA, Gould SR, Day DW, Lennard-Jones JE, Edwards AM. Controlled trial of disodium cromoglycate in chronic persistent ulcerative colitis. *Gut.* 1978;19:1140-1143.
90. Binder V, Elsborg L, Greibe J, et al. Disodium cromoglycate in the treatment of ulcerative colitis and Crohn's disease. *Gut.* 1981;22:55-60.
91. Willoughby CP, Heyworth MF, Piris J, Truelove SC. Comparison of disodium cromoglycate and sulphasalazine as maintenance therapy for ulcerative colitis. *Lancet.* 1979;1:119-122.
92. Whorwell PJ, Whorwell GM, Bamforth J, et al. A double-blind controlled trial of the effect of sodium cromoglycate in preventing relapse in ulcerative colitis. *Postgrad Med J.* 1981;57:436-438.
93. Fais S, Annibale B, Boirivant M, Santoro A, Pallone F, Delle Fave G. Effects of somatostatin on human intestinal lamina propria lymphocytes: modulation of lymphocyte activation. *J Neuroimmunol.* 1991;31:211-219.
94. van Bergeijk JD, Wilson JH, Nielsen OH, et al. Octreotide in patients with active ulcerative colitis treated with high dose corticosteroids (OPUS 1). *Eur J Gastroenterol Hepatol.* 2002;14:243-248.
95. Van de Wal Y, Van der Sluys Veer A, Verspaget HW, et al. Effect of zinc therapy on natural killer cell activity in inflammatory bowel disease. *Aliment Pharmacol Ther.* 1993;7:281-286.
96. Dronfield MW, Malone JD, Langman MJ. Zinc in ulcerative colitis: A therapeutic trial and report on plasma levels. *Gut.* 1977;18:33-36.
97. Ayabe T, Ashida T, Taniguchi M, et al. A pilot study of centrifugal leukocyte apheresis for corticosteroid-resistant active ulcerative colitis [see comment]. *Intern Med.* 1997;36:322-326.
98. Ayabe T, Ashida T, Kohgo Y. Centrifugal leukocyte apheresis for ulcerative colitis. *Therapeutic Apheresis.* 1998;2:125-128.
99. Kohgo Y, Hibi H, Chiba T, et al, and the Study Group for Alternative Therapies in Ulcerative Colitis P. Leukocyte apheresis using a centrifugal cell separator in refractory ulcerative colitis: a multicenter open label trial. *Therapeutic Apheresis.* 2002;6:255-260.
100. Sawada K, Ohnishi K, Fukui S, et al. Leukocytapheresis therapy, performed with leukocyte removal filter, for inflammatory bowel disease. *J Gastroenterol.* 1995;30:322-329.
101. Sawada K, Ohnishi K, Kosaka T, et al. Leukocytapheresis with leukocyte removal filter as new therapy for ulcerative colitis. *Therapeutic Apheresis.* 1997;1:207-211.
102. Yajima T, Takaishi H, Kanai T, et al. Predictive factors of response to leukocytapheresis therapy for ulcerative colitis. *Therapeutic Apheresis.* 1998;2:115-119.
103. Jo Y, Matsumoto T, Mibu R, Iida M. Addition of leukocytapheresis to steroid therapy: is it beneficial in recurrence of moderate-to-severe ulcerative colitis? *Dis Colon Rectum.* 2003;46:S3-S9.
104. Sasaki M, Tsujikawa T, Fujiyama Y, Bamba T. Leukocytapheresis therapy for severe ulcerative colitis. *Therapeutic Apheresis.* 1998;2:101-104.
105. Kawamura A, Saitoh M, Yonekawa M, et al. New technique of leukocytapheresis by the use of nonwoven polyester fiber filter for inflammatory bowel disease. *Therapeutic Apheresis.* 1999;3:334-337.
106. Tomomasa T, Kobayashi A, Kaneko H, et al. Granulocyte adsorptive apheresis for pediatric patients with ulcerative colitis. *Dig Dis Sci.* 2003;48:750-754.
107. Sakata H, Kawamura N, Horie T, et al. Successful treatment of ulcerative colitis with leukocytapheresis using non-woven polyester filter. *Therapeutic Apheresis & Dialysis.* 2003;7:536-539.
108. Sawada K, Muto T, Shimoyama T, et al. Multicenter randomized controlled trial for the treatment of ulcerative colitis with a leukocytapheresis column. *Current Pharmaceutical Design.* 2003;9:307-321.
109. Rembacken BJ, Newbould HE, Richards SJ, et al. Granulocyte apheresis in inflammatory bowel disease: Possible mechanisms of effect. *Therapeutic Apheresis.* 1998;2:93-96.
110. Sands BE, Sandborn WJ, Wolf DC, et al. Pilot study of the safety and efficacy of granulocyte/monocyte adsorption apheresis with adacolumn in patients with inflammatory bowel disease. *Am J Gastroenterol.* 2004;99:S263-S264.
111. Naganuma M, Funakoshi S, Sakuraba A, et al. Granulocytapheresis is useful as an alternative therapy in patients with steroid-refractory or -dependent ulcerative colitis. *Inflamma Bowel Dis.* 2004;10:251-257.
112. Hanai H, Watanabe F, Saniabadi AR, Matsushitai I, Takeuchi K, Iida T. Therapeutic efficacy of granulocyte and monocyte adsorption apheresis in severe active ulcerative colitis. *Dig Dis Sci.* 2002;47:2349-5233.
113. Hanai H, Watanabe F, Takeuchi K, et al. Leukocyte adsorptive apheresis for the treatment of active ulcerative colitis: a prospective, uncontrolled, pilot study. *Clin Gastroenterol Hepatol.* 2003;1:28-35.
114. Hanai H, Watanabe F, Yamada M, et al. Adsorptive granulocyte and monocyte apheresis versus prednisolone in patients with corticosteroid-dependent moderately severe ulcerative colitis. *Digestion.* 2004;70:36-44.
115. Kanke K, Nakano M, Hiraishi H, Terano A. Clinical evaluation of granulocyte/monocyte apheresis therapy for active ulcerative colitis [see comment]. *Dig Liver Dis.* 2004;36:811-817.

116. Suzuki Y, Yoshimura N, Saniabadi AR, Saito Y. Selective granulocyte and monocyte adsorptive apheresis as a first-line treatment for steroid naive patients with active ulcerative colitis: a prospective uncontrolled study. *Dig Dis Sci.* 2004;49:565-571.
117. Yamamoto T, Umegae S, Kitagawa T, et al. Granulocyte and monocyte adsorptive apheresis in the treatment of active distal ulcerative colitis: a prospective, pilot study. *Aliment Pharmacol Ther.* 2004;20:783-792.
118. Shimoyama T, Sawada K, Hiwatashi N, et al. Safety and efficacy of granulocyte and monocyte adsorption apheresis in patients with active ulcerative colitis: a multicenter study. *Journal of Clinical Apheresis.* 2001;16:1-9.
119. Sakuraba A, Naganuma M, Hibi T, Ishu H. Intensive therapy of granulocyte and mottocyte adsorption apheresis induces rapid remission in patients with ulcerative colitis. *Gastroenterology.* 2003;124(Suppl S):A522.
120. Sakuraba A, Inoue N, Kohgo Y, et al. A multicenter randomized controlled trial between weekly and semiweekly treatment of granulocyte and monocyte adsorption apheresis therapy. *Gastroenterology.* 2005;128(Suppl 2):A585.
121. Sands BE, Sandborn WJ, Feagan B, et al. A randomized, double-blind, sham-controlled study of granulocyte/monocyte apheresis for active ulcerative colitis. *Gastroenterology.* 2008;135(2):400-409.
122. Langmead L, Feakins RM, Goldthorpe S, et al. Randomized, double-blind, placebo-controlled trial of oral aloe vera gel for active ulcerative colitis. *Aliment Pharmacol Ther.* 2004;19:739-747.
123. Fox RI. Mechanism of action of hydroxychloroquine as an antirheumatic drug. *Seminars in Arthritis & Rheumatism.* 1993;23:82-91.
124. Mayer L, Turtel P, Present D. Effect of hydroxychloroquine in the treatment of active ulcerative colitis: results of the open label phase of the controlled trial. *Gastroenterology.* 1991;100:A230.
125. Goenka MK, Kochhar R, Tandia B, Mehta SK. Chloroquine for mild to moderately active ulcerative colitis: comparison with sulfasalazine. *Am J Gastroenterol.* 1996;91:917-921.
126. Kruis W, Schutz E, Fric P, Fixa B, Judmaier G, Stolte M. Double-blind comparison of an oral *Escherichia coli* preparation and mesalazine in maintaining remission of ulcerative colitis. *Aliment Pharmacol Ther.* 1997;11:853-858.
127. Rembacken BJ, Snelling AM, Hawkey PM, Chalmers DM, Axon AT. Non-pathogenic *Escherichia coli* versus mesalazine for the treatment of ulcerative colitis: a randomised trial. *Lancet.* 1999;354:635-639.
128. Kruis W, Fric P, Pokrotnieks J, et al. Maintaining remission of ulcerative colitis with the probiotic *Escherichia coli* Nissle 1917 is as effective as with standard mesalazine. *Gut.* 2004;53:1617-1623.
129. Weinstock JV. Helminths and mucosal immune modulation. *Ann NY Acad Sci.* 2006;1072:356-364.
130. Summers RW, Elliott DE, Qadir K, Urban JF Jr, Thompson R, Weinstock JV. Trichuris suis seems to be safe and possibly effective in the treatment of inflammatory bowel disease. *Am J Gastroenterol.* 2003;98:2034-2041.
131. Summers RW, Elliott DE, Urban JF Jr, Thompson RA, Weinstock JV. Trichuris suis therapy for active ulcerative colitis. A randomized controlled trial. *Gastroenterology.* 2005;(In Press).
132. Buts JP, De Keyser N. Effects of *Saccharomyces boulardii* on intestinal mucosa. *Dig Dis Sci.* 2006;51:1485-1492.
133. Dalmasso G, Cottrez F, Imbert V, et al. *Saccharomyces boulardii* inhibits inflammatory bowel disease by trapping T cells in mesenteric lymph nodes. *Gastroenterology.* 2006;131:1812-1825.
134. Guslandi M, Giollo P, Testoni PA. A pilot trial of *Saccharomyces boulardii* in ulcerative colitis. *Eur J Gastroenterol Hepatol.* 2003;15:697-698.
135. Andus T, Klebl F, Rogler G, Bregenzer N, Scholmerich J, Straub RH. Patients with refractory Crohn's disease or ulcerative colitis respond to dehydroepiandrosterone: a pilot study. *Aliment Pharmacol Ther.* 2003;17:409-414.
136. Tremaine WJ, Brzezinski A, Katz JA, et al, Group AUCS. Treatment of mildly to moderately active ulcerative colitis with a tryptase inhibitor (APC 2059): An open-label pilot study. *Aliment Pharmacol Ther.* 2002;16:407-413.
137. Lichtenstein GR, Deren J, Katz S, Kennedy A, Ware J. The Bowman Birk protease inhibitor: a novel therapy for treatment of patients with active ulcerative colitis. *Gastroenterology.* 2002;122:A-60.

SECTION III

SPECIFIC CLINICAL PRESENTATIONS

26

Medical Management of Severe Ulcerative Colitis

Niraj Jani, MD and Miguel Regueiro, MD

The majority of patients with ulcerative colitis (UC) are managed with oral or topical 5-aminosalicylates and corticosteroids and do not require hospitalization. Patients who have extensive mucosal inflammation on colonoscopy and persistent symptoms of diarrhea and bleeding despite these medications are defined as severe UC. This chapter will review the medications currently available for severe UC as well as those under investigation and provide the authors' approach to the management of this condition.

INITIAL EVALUATION

The initial evaluation of patients with severe UC includes a careful history and physical exam, laboratory studies for complete blood count, electrolyte and renal profile, erythrocyte sedimentation rate (ESR), stool for salmonella, shigella, campylobacter, *E. coli* 0157:H7, ova and parasites, *Clostridium difficile* toxin, and (if abdominal pain is present) an abdominal x-ray and/or an abdominal and pelvic CT scan in select patients to exclude toxic megacolon or perforation. There are many different disease activity indices that have been used in patients with UC. None of these indices have been validated. One of the commonly used indices, the Truelove and Witts' DAI, defines severe colitis as greater than 6 bowel movements/24 hours and at least one of the following: blood in the stool, temperature greater than 37.8°C, pulse greater than 90/min, hemoglobin less than 10.0 mg/L, and doubling of the ESR/CRP level (Table 26-1).[1] When a patient presents with the aforementioned signs and symptoms, a limited flexible sigmoidoscopy with minimal air insufflation may be safely performed and may confirm the diagnosis of UC (Figure 26-1) and exclude the presence of other factors or disease states that can simulate active UC. Specifically, biopsies may be taken for cytomegalovirus, which has been associated with exacerbation of UC (Figure 26-2).[2] A full colonoscopy or barium studies are generally not warranted and may precipitate toxic megacolon.[3] Keeping a patient on IV nutrition is not necessarily beneficial, and feeding a patient with severe colitis may afford some of the trophic effects of nutrients, which may be beneficial.[4]

MEDICATIONS FOR SEVERE ULCERATIVE COLITIS

Corticosteroids

Corticosteroids are potent anti-inflammatory and immunosuppressive agents that inhibit the production of arachidonic acid, alter leukocyte function, and decrease the expression of proinflammatory cytokines, eg, IL-1, IL-2, IL-4, IL-5, IL-6, IL-8, and interferon-γ.[5-9] Most patients who experience an exacerbation of UC will respond to oral corticosteroids, eg, prednisone (40 to 60 mg/d). The landmark study by Truelove and Witts in 1954 reported an overall remission rate of 40% in patients treated with oral cortisone (100 mg/d for 6 weeks); patients with mild disease achieved a higher remission rate (75%) than those with severe disease (31%).[1] Patients who continue to experience symptoms of severe UC despite adequate oral corticosteroids require admission to the hospital for IV treatment (Table 26-2).

Lichtenstein GR, ed.
Ulcerative Colitis: The Complete Guide to Medical Management (pp. 285-292)

TABLE 26-1

CRITERIA FOR CLASSIFICATION OF SEVERITY OF ULCERATIVE COLITIS

	Severe	Mild
Diarrhea	≥6 times in 24 hours	≤4 times in 24 hours
Blood in stool	Obvious	None or slight
Fever	>37.8°C	Normal
Pulse	≥90/min	Normal
Anemia	Hb ≤100 g/L	No
ESR, CRP	≥Doubled	Normal

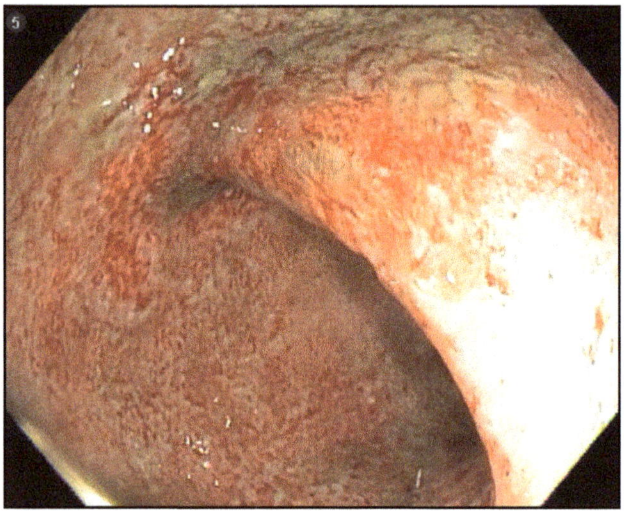

FIGURE 26-1. Colonoscopic photo from a patient with severe ulcerative colitis failing oral corticosteroids and 5-ASA. (Courtesy of Douglas Weine, MD.)

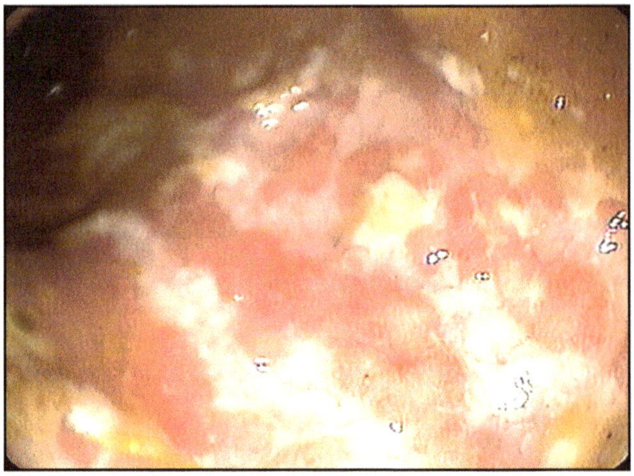

FIGURE 26-2. Colonoscopic photo from a patient with panulcerative colitis presenting with worsening bloody diarrhea. (Courtesy of Ellen Scherl, MD, and Douglas Weine, MD.)

Intravenous corticosteroids remain the first-line therapy for patients with severe UC failing oral corticosteroids. In one of the earliest published reports of IV corticosteroids for severe UC, 36/49 (73%) patients who received IV prednisolone (0.75 to 1.0 mg/kg/d) had a complete response and were able to maintain that response (in the short-term) with oral prednisolone 10 to 15 mg four times per day and sulfasalazine.[10] In an open-label trial by Sood et al, dexamethasone pulse therapy has also been demonstrated to be effective for treatment of patients with severe UC.[11] Fourteen patients were treated with dexamethasone (100 mg daily infusion) for 3 days, and by day 15, 93% achieved a clinical remission that was sustained in the majority (79%) of patients at day 60. Subsequently, there have been numerous studies confirming the efficacy of IV corticosteroids for severe UC, albeit at varying doses, duration of therapy, and corticosteroid preparation. Although there is perceived to be a dose-response phenomenon with corticosteroids, there are limited data to support exceeding a daily dose of 48 mg of methylprednisolone (or equivalent dose in another glucocorticosteroid). To date, there are no controlled trials that have compared once-daily corticosteroid dosing with multiple or continuous infusion dosing for the treatment of severe UC. There is no clear pharmacologic data to support that one regimen is preferred to the other.

It has been the author's experience that most patients with severe UC will respond to IV methylprednisolone 48 mg/d. Patients who are heavier than 100 kg may require a higher daily dose, eg, 60 mg/d. A meta-analysis by Turner et al suggests that doses of greater than 60 mg/day are not associated with additional benefit.[13] Whether methylprednisolone is initiated as a single daily dose, divided doses, or a continuous IV drip is arbitrary. Typically, we initiate once-daily methylprednisolone; however, if the patient has shown no sign of improvement within 2 to 3 days, we will convert to continuous infusion. This practice has not been tested in a prospective randomized fashion. Although IV methylprednisolone is our corticosteroid of choice, equivalent dosing of comparable corticosteroids is acceptable, eg, hydrocortisone 300 mg/d. The benefits of IV corticosteroids for the treatment of severe UC are clear; however, the risks must be weighed. The short- and long-term side effects from corticosteroids have been previously described and are well-reported.[12,14,15]

Cyclosporine

Cyclosporine is an immunosuppressive macrolide that inhibits the production of IL-2 by activated T lymphocytes, and downregulates the synthesis of other inflammatory cytokines (IL-3, IL-4, TNFα, and IFNγ).[16–18] Historically, (prior to the era of infliximab) patients who have not responded to 7 to 10 days of IV corticosteroids have had one of two choices: either a total proctocolectomy or IV

TABLE 26-2

INTRAVENOUS MEDICATIONS FOR THE TREATMENT OF SEVERE ULCERATIVE COLITIS

MEDICATION	DOSE/FREQUENCY	EVIDENCE-BASED DATA SUPPORTING EFFICACY IN SEVERE UC
Methylprednisolone	40 to 60 mg/d	+
Hydrocortisone	300 to 400 mg/d	+
Cyclosporine	2 to 4 mg/kg/d	+
Azathioprine	20 to 40 mg/kg/d	+/-
Infliximab	5 mg/kg, 1 to 3 infusions	+/-
		May be most effective in patients with steroid-responsive UC
Basiliximab	40 mg/single dose	Preliminary data positive
Visilizumab	10 to 15 mg/d on 2 consecutive days	Preliminary data positive

cyclosporine. Overall, results from 20 different uncontrolled trials have shown that approximately 60% to 90% of patients with severe UC are spared urgent colectomy.[18,19] In the only placebo-controlled trial by Lichtiger and Present, 9 of 11 patients treated with cyclosporine 4 mg/kg/d showed improvement at day 7 compared to none of the placebo patients.[20] Intravenous cyclosporine (4 mg/kg/d) was also found to be as effective as methylprednisolone (40 mg/d) in the acute management of severe UC.[21] Van Assche and colleagues evaluated a lower dose of cyclosporine for severe UC. In this noninferiority study, 73 patients with severe UC were randomized to receive cyclosporine 2 mg/kg dose or 4 mg/kg.[22] There was no difference in clinical response rates between the 2 mg/kg and 4 mg/kg doses. This study was underpowered to detect a difference; however, there was no trend observed favoring any specific therapy.

Patients who respond to 7 days of IV cyclosporine are switched to oral cyclosporine and an immunomodulator, such as AZA or 6-MP. Despite the encouraging short-term response to cyclosporine, the long-term effects of cyclosporine therapy are less than favorable. After 6 to 8 months, 44% of patients generally relapse, and 30% to 50% may require surgery.[23,24] Arts et al studied the long-term outcome of IV cyclosporine treatment in 86 patients and found that 84% had a favorable response by day 9, but by day 178, 25% required colectomy and 3% had died of opportunistic infections.[25,26] A long-term follow-up study by Cohen et al suggests that patients who have failed treatment with AZA/6-MP and are treated with cyclosporine plus continued AZA/6-MP have worse outcomes than those who are naïve to AZA/6-MP and receive cyclosporine plus 6-MP/AZA.[27] Furthermore, data from a retrospective cohort study by Moskovitz et al suggest that while cyclosporine shows efficacy in the short- to medium-term treatment of severe UC, 88% of patients in the study required colectomy at 7 years.[28] In this study, azathioprine-naive patients had better outcomes with 59% of those already receiving azathioprine requiring colectomy compared with 31% of those starting azathioprine concurrently with cyclosporine therapy ($P<0.05$).

Patients started on cyclosporine need careful monitoring for potential drug-related toxicity. Although cyclosporine whole blood levels do not correlate with clinical efficacy, trough levels should be maintained between 200 and 400 ng/mL. It should be emphasized that there are 3 separate assays available to measure trough levels of cyclosporine A. These methods are a monoclonal assay, a polyclonal assay, and use of high-pressure liquid chromatography. Patients with a serum cholesterol level less than 120 mg/dL are at increased risk of developing seizures due to an increased level of freely circulating cyclosporine. Serious opportunistic infections, eg, *Pneumocystis carinii* pneumonia (PCP) or cytomegalovirus have been reported in 10% to 15% of patients being treated with cyclosporine.[26] Patients receiving cyclosporine should begin PCP prophylaxis with trimethoprim/sulfamethoxazole (Bactrim) one double-strength tablet 3 times weekly. The most common side effects of cyclosporine, occurring in up to 50% of patients, include nausea, vomiting, hepatotoxicity, nephrotoxicity, hypertension, and paresthesias.[26,29]

It is considered appropriate to contemplate use of cyclosporine therapy in patients who have failed to respond to 7 days of adequate doses of IV corticosteroids. Patients with known renal insufficiency, active infection(s), uncontrolled hypertension, or a known seizure disorder are not appropriate candidates for use of cyclosporine. Generally, cyclosporine is not administered to patients with a serum cholesterol less than 120 mg/dL. The standard dose at which cyclosporine is initiated is 4 mg/kg/d, and in patients who are intolerant, ie, nausea, vomiting, we decrease the dose to 2 mg/kg/d. Data from a randomized, double-blind comparison study suggest that 4 mg/kg IV cyclosporine provides no additional clinical benefit over 2 mg/kg.[23] We monitor the trough level and decrease the cyclosporine dose if the level is >350 ng/mL. Patients who respond to 5 to 7 days of IV cyclosporine are converted to oral corticosteroids and 8 mg/kg/d of oral cyclosporine (Neoral Sandimmune; Novartis). AZA (2.0 to 2.5 mg/kg/d) or 6-MP (1.0 to 1.5 mg/kg/d) and *Pneumocystis* pneumonia prophylaxis (as mentioned previously) is also initiated. Over the subsequent 3 to 6 months, the corticosteroids are tapered, and by 6 months, the cyclosporine is discontinued. Patients require surgery if they have not responded to IV cyclosporine or relapse within 6 months of starting oral cyclosporine. There is also a possibility of using infliximab in patients who have had an adequate washout period from cyclosporine. However, a recent study shows increased risk of adverse events with use of cyclosporine in combination with infliximab, regardless of which agent is initiated first.[30] This study showed that salvage therapy (switching from either cyclosporine or infliximab) was effective in approximately 30% of patients. Serious adverse events were found in 16% of patients treated with cyclosporine first, including one death from *E. coli* sepsis. In addition, there is a case report of an immunoblast developing in a patient who had received quadruple immunosuppression including long-term cyclosporine and 1 dose of infliximab.[31]

Azathioprine

AZA and 6-MP are routinely administered for the maintenance of remission of steroid- or cyclosporine-induced remission in patients with severe UC. The role of these agents in the acute management of severe UC is limited, primarily due to the fact that clinical efficacy is not achieved for 3 to 6 months. One small open-label study suggests that IV AZA may be of benefit in the acute management of severe UC.[32] In this study, 5 of 9 patients with severe steroid-refractory UC who received IV AZA (20 to 40 mg/kg) followed by oral AZA (2.0 mg/kg/d) had a clinical response and avoided colectomy. In a randomized, placebo-controlled study by Sood et al, AZA was determined to have no effect in achieving remission in patients with severe UC when given in combination with prednisolone, but was linked to a lower proportion of relapses compared with placebo.[33] In a small head-to-head trial of AZA versus sulfasalazine, Sood et al found that the 2 agents had comparable relapse rates but that there was a trend toward earlier treatment failure with AZA.[34] Although further evaluation is needed to confirm the efficacy of IV AZA in severe UC, this approach may offer an alternative to hospitalized patients with steroid-refractory UC. Currently, it is not our practice to administer IV AZA to patients with severe UC.

Infliximab

TNFα is a proinflammatory cytokine that is upregulated in UC. Infliximab is a chimeric anti-TNFα monoclonal antibody that effectively induces and maintains remission in patients with inflammatory and fistulizing CD. Infliximab is currently approved by the FDA for the treatment of moderate to severe UC.[35] Several small studies have evaluated the role of infliximab in the treatment of severe, steroid-refractory UC. In a double-blind, placebo-controlled pilot study, Sands et al evaluated the efficacy of a single infusion of infliximab (5 to 20 mg/kg) in 11 patients with UC refractory to IV corticosteroid treatment.[36] Fifty percent of the 8 patients who received infliximab improved by 2 weeks, while none in the placebo group improved. There was a 25% relapse rate by 10 weeks; however, it should be stressed that all patients only received a single infusion of infliximab. In an open-label study by Chey et al, 8 patients with severe UC refractory to medical therapy and scheduled for colectomy received a single infusion of infliximab 5 mg/kg.[37] All 8 patients (100%) responded to the single infusion of infliximab and maintained the response 16 weeks later. In an uncontrolled, retrospective study by Su et al, 27 patients with UC were treated with infliximab; 24 patients were defined as severely active.[38] Twelve patients (44%) had a complete remission, 6 (22%) had a partial response, and 9 (34%) did not respond to infliximab. Eighteen of 19 relapses were successfully treated with a reinfusion of infliximab. Upon stratification for prior steroid response, steroid-refractory patients were much less likely to respond to infliximab than steroid-responsive patients. In another open-label experience by Gornet et al, 19 patients with steroid-refractory UC were treated with infliximab 5 mg/kg at weeks 0, 2, and 6.[39] The majority of patients (66%) had a response by day 7 and 42% were in remission at 1 month. In an underpowered, randomized, placebo-controlled trial on infliximab for the treatment of moderate to severe steroid-resistant UC by Probert et al, 22 patients received infliximab (5 mg/kg) or placebo at weeks 0 and 2.[40] There was no difference in remission rates between the placebo or infliximab groups at weeks 2 or 6 (30% versus 39%, 6 weeks). An open-label infusion (10 mg/kg) was given to 20 patients who had ongoing symptoms at 6 weeks, with only 4 of the patients responding.[40] The majority of patients in all of these trials experienced minimal to no adverse events, with the most frequent being infusion reactions, nausea, headaches, and mild upper respiratory-type symptoms, as has been reported in prior experience.[41]

Infliximab is now indicated for the treatment of moderate to severe UC. FDA approval was based on 2 randomized, double-blind, placebo-controlled studies that showed that patients with moderately to severely active UC treated with infliximab at weeks 0, 2, and 6, and every 8 weeks thereafter, were more likely to have a clinical response at weeks 8, 30, and 54 than those receiving placebo.[35] Generally, patients who are failing IV corticosteroids and do not respond to an infusion of infliximab require a total proctocolectomy. It is not advisable to administer cyclosporine to a patient who has failed infliximab given the long duration of efficacy of infliximab, and conversely do not give infliximab to cyclosporine nonresponders.[30]

INVESTIGATIONAL THERAPIES FOR SEVERE ULCERATIVE COLITIS

Agents that have been or are currently under investigation for the management of severe UC include tacrolimus, basiliximab, and visilizumab. These agents are not approved by the FDA and should be considered experimental therapy.

TACROLIMUS

Tacrolimus, similar to cyclosporine, is a macrolide immunosuppressant that downregulates lymphocyte activation and proliferation and is used in the prophylaxis against organ rejection in patients receiving allogeneic liver, kidney, or heart transplants. While the exact mechanism of action of this agent is unknown, it appears that tacrolimus inhibits IL-2 synthesis through the calcineurin pathway. Experimental evidence suggests that tacrolimus binds to an intracellular protein, FKBP-12, creating a complex of tacrolimus-FKBP-12, calcium, calmodulin, and calcineurin that inhibits phosphatase activity. This effect may prevent the dephosphorylation and translocation of nuclear factors of activated T cells, which are believed to initiate gene transcription for the formation of lymphokines.[42-44] Tacrolimus is 10- to 100-fold more potent than cyclosporine in inhibiting lymphocyte activation in vitro and has been used to prevent organ rejection. In an open-label study by Hogenauer et al, 9 patients with moderate to severe steroid-refractory UC received oral tacrolimus (0.15 mg/kg/d) for 12 weeks.[45] All of the patients had a clinical response by 2 weeks with 6/9 (67%) maintaining remission by 12 weeks. Ultimately 3/9 (33%) patients underwent colectomy by 21 months despite the initial response. One patient developed severe thrombocytopenia with intestinal bleeding, and another patient had anemia and leukopenia. Other side effects noted were mild renal impairment, paresthesias, alopecia, and hypomagnesemia. Another study reported less favorable results with less than 50% initial response rate and colectomy rate of 34%.[46] Furthermore, a randomized, placebo-controlled study by Ogata et al showed a dose-dependent efficacy of tacrolimus in the induction of remission in patients with refractory UC.[47] The optimal dose range in this study was 10 to 15 ng/mL for 2 weeks. The study involved 63 patients with refractory, active UC who were randomized to high-dose tacrolimus (10 to 15 ng/mL), low dose-tacrolimus (5 to 10 ng/mL), or placebo. The high-dose group showed a significantly greater rate of improvement in DAI score (68.4% versus 10% of the placebo group; $P<0.001$). In addition, 20% of patients in the high-dose group achieved clinical remission, and 78.9% had mucosal healing. A range of immunosuppressives have also been used in the treatment of uveitis. Specifically, cyclosporine and sirolimus (rapamycin) have been used for their anti-inflammatory effects. Cyclosporine, tacrolimus, and sirolimus are all similar anti-inflammatories that inhibit T cell function and have recently been described as steroid-sparing agents in the treatment of uveitis (intraocular inflammation).[44,48,49] Anti-TNFα agents have also been used for the treatment of uveitis. There are novel agents that work through either inhibition of T cells or neutralization of TNFα that are helpful in UC and other anti-inflammatory disorders.

BASILIXIMAB

Basiliximab is a chimeric monoclonal antibody that binds to CD25, which is required for high-affinity binding IL-2 to the IL-2 receptor (IL-2R). Basiliximab forms a complex with IL-2R, preventing binding of IL-2 and hence inhibiting T cell proliferation.[50] There are data to support higher levels of IL-2 in patients with steroid-refractory UC, and basiliximab may be used to increase the efficacy of steroids.[51,52] In an open-label, uncontrolled trial, 10 patients with steroid-refractory active UC received a single IV bolus of 40 mg of basiliximab.[53] At 8 weeks, 90% of the patients achieved clinical remission, with 11 patients requiring colectomy. After 24 weeks, 7/9 (78%) of the patients remained in clinical remission, and 5 patients were able to discontinue steroids. Adverse events included paresthesias, photosensitivity, lethargy, and pyrexia. A more recent study showed that 10 of 20 (50%) patients given a single 40-mg dose of basiliximab plus steroid therapy achieved clinical remission in 10 weeks. Remission was achieved in 7 of 13 patients in the study with moderate disease and 3 of 7 patients with severe disease. At 24 weeks, 13 of 20 (65%) patients were in clinical remission. Five patients later required colectomy, and 1 patient required rescue cyclosporine. Treatment was described as well tolerated, with 2 patients developing herpes zoster.[54]

VISILIZUMAB

Visilizumab is a humanized anti-CD3 monoclonal antibody characterized by a mutated IgG2 isotype with a lack of binding to Fc gamma-receptors. It has the ability to induce apoptosis selectively in activated T cells and has been studied in treating graft versus host disease.[55] A recent phase I study evaluated the efficacy of visilizumab in 32 patients with severe steroid-refractory UC.[56] After failing to improve with 5 days of IV corticosteroids, patients were given 2 days of visilizumab (10 to 15 µg/kg). At 30 days, 84% of patients showed clinical response, 41% achieved clinical remission, and 44% achieved endoscopic remission. The most common adverse event was a self-limited cytokine release syndrome (ie, nausea, arthralgias, and chills), which was reported in 100% and 83% of patients in the 15- and 10-µg/kg dose groups, respectively. A study by Targan et al found that Epstein Barr virus (EBV) titers rose with T cell depletion in patients with steroid-refractory ulcerative colitis treated with visilizumab, but fell to baseline as T cells returned.[57] More recently, it has been announced that the manufacturer (Protein Design Labs, Fremont, CA) has elected to stop further development of this compound for treatment of IBD.

CONCLUSION

There are limited medical options for the treatment of patients with severe UC not improving on oral corticosteroids and 5-ASA. Gastroenterologists with experience in treating such patients will have varied medication preferences. The following guidelines represent the authors' approach to the treatment of patients with severe UC (Figure 26-3).

Patients admitted to the hospital with severe UC receive IV fluid and electrolyte resuscitation. IV methylprednisolone 48 to 60 mg/d is administered in divided doses or as a continuous "drip." In the event a patient has not received 5-ASA as an outpatient, these medications are not initiated until the patient has responded to the IV steroids. There is a rare, but well-described paradoxical exacerbation of UC in a small percentage of patients starting 5-ASA.[58] Otherwise, the 5-ASA agents are generally stopped upon admission to the hospital and restarted when the patient begins to respond to IV therapy and is tolerating an oral diet. Patients may remain on enteral feeding unless there is concern of toxic megacolon or perforation. We generally feed patients with severe UC a low-fat diet and restrict dairy products and caffeinated/carbonated beverages. In certain cases, we will restrict enteral feeding for purposes of patient comfort, ie, to decrease the number of bowel movements that result from eating; however, the primary treatment of patients with severe colitis (keeping them NPO) has not been demonstrated to be effective. Patients who respond to IV corticosteroids are converted to an equivalent dose of oral corticosteroid, and the 5-ASA agent is restarted at a dose of more than 4 g/d. Oral AZA (2.0 to 2.5 mg/kg/d) or 6-MP (1.0 to 1.5 mg/kg/d) is started prior to discharge from the hospital after assessing the genotype or enzyme activity (preferable) of thiopurine methyl transferase (TPMT).

At our institution, patients who do not respond to 5 to 7 days of IV corticosteroids are treated with cyclosporine or infliximab, or undergo a total proctocolectomy. Certain patients may also be eligible for novel research therapies that are administered through investigational protocols.

REFERENCES

1. Truelove SC, Witts LJ. Cortisone in ulcerative colitis: preliminary report on a therapeutic trial. *Br Med J.* 1954;2:375-378.
2. Rachima C, Maoz E, Apter S, et al. CMV associated with ulcerative colitis in immunocompetent individuals. *Postgrad Med J.* 1998;74:486-489.
3. Regueiro M, Peppercorn M. Inflammatory bowel disease. In: Tayor M, ed. *Gastrointestinal Emergencies.* 2nd ed. Philadelphia, PA: Williams and Wilkins; 1997:599-625.
4. Lichtiger S. Cyclosporine for severe ulcerative colitis: pro. *Inflamm Bowel Dis.* 2009;15(1):141-142.
5. Brattsan R, Linden M. Cytokine modulation by glucocorticoids: mechanisms and actions in cellular studies. *Aliment Pharmacol Ther.* 1996;10:81-92.
6. Goppelt-Streube M. Molecular mechanisms involved in the regulation of prostaglandin biosynthesis by glucocorticoids. *Biochem Pharmacol.* 1997;53:1389-1395.
7. Goulding N, Euzger H, Butt S, et al. Novel pathways for glucocorticoid effects on neutrophils in chronic inflammation. *Inflamm Res.* 1998;47:S158-S165.
8. Hawkey C, Truelove S. Effect of prednisolone on prostaglandin synthesis by rectal mucosa ulcerative colitis: investigation by laminar flow bioassay and radioimmunoassay. *Gut.* 1981;22:190-193.
9. Swartz S, Dluhy R. Corticosteroids: clinical pharmacology and therapeutic use. *Drug.* 1978;16:238-255.
10. Truelove SC, Jewell DP. Intensive intravenous regimen for severe attacks of ulcerative colitis. *Lancet.* 1974;1:1067-1070.
11. Sood A, Midha V, Sood N, et al. A prospective, open-label trial assessing dexamethasone pulse therapy in moderate to severe ulcerative colitis. *J Clin Gastroenterol.* 2002;35:328-331.
12. Hanauer SB, Stathopoulous G. Risk-benefit assessment of drugs used in treatment of inflammatory bowel disease. *Drug Safe.* 1991;6:192-219.
13. Turner D, Walsh CM, Steinhart AH, Griffiths AM. Response to corticosteroids in severe ulcerative colitis: a systematic review of the literature and a meta-regression. *Clin Gastroenterol Hepatol.* 2007;5(1):103-110.
14. Hanauer SB. Drug therapy: inflammatory bowel disease. *N Engl J Med.* 1996;334:841-848.
15. Hanauer SB, Meyers S, Sachar D. The pharmacology of anti-inflammatory drugs in inflammatory bowel disease. In: Kirsner J, Shorter R, eds. *Inflammatory Bowel Disease.* 4th ed. Baltimore, MD: Williams and Wilkins; 1995:643-663.
16. Di Pavoda F. Pharmacology of cyclosporine (Sandimmune): pharmacologic effects on immune function: in vitro studies. *Pharmacol Rev.* 1989;41:373-405.
17. Langford C, et al. Use of cytotoxic agents and cyclosporine in the treatment of autoimmune disease. *Ann Intern Med.* 1998;129:49-58.
18. Sandborn W. A critical review of cyclosporine therapy in inflammatory bowel disease. *Inflamm Bowel Dis.* 1995;1:48-63.
19. Cohen R, Stein R, Hanauer S. Intravenous cyclosporine in ulcerative colitis: a five-year experience. *Am J Gastroenterol.* 1999;94:1587-1592.

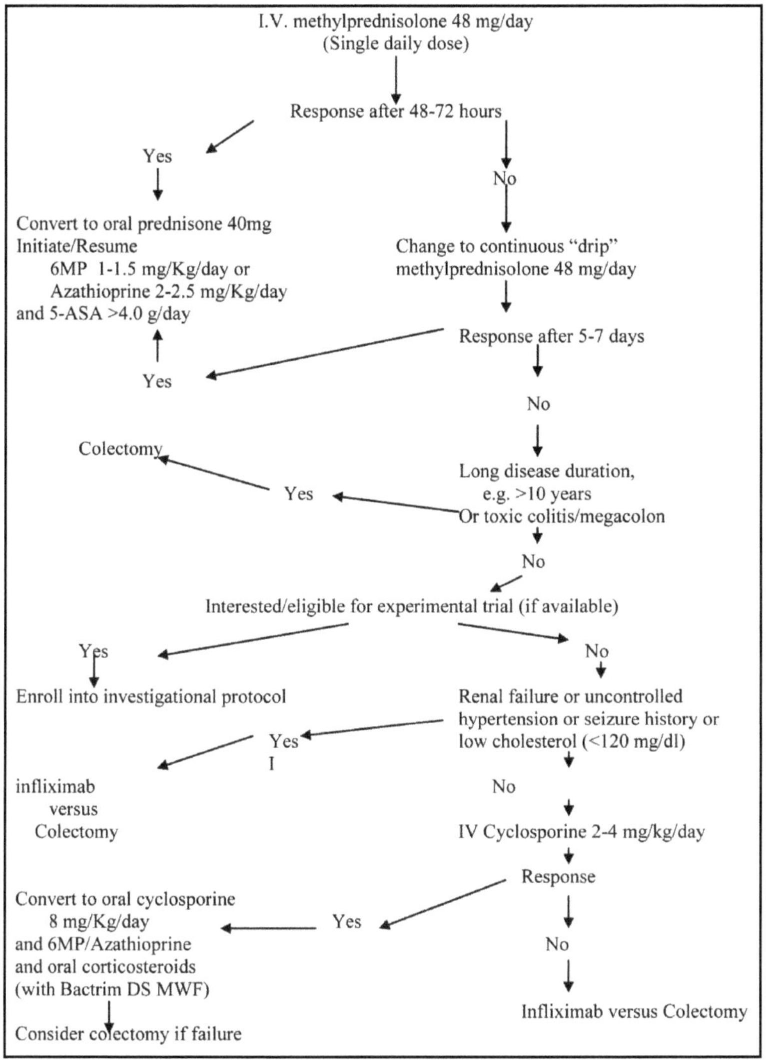

FIGURE 26-3. Proposed treatment algorithm for management of patients with severe ulcerative colitis admitted to the hospital.

20. Lichtiger S, Present DH, Kornbluth A, et al. Cyclosporine in severe ulcerative colitis refractory to steroid therapy. *N Engl J Med.* 1994;330:1841-1845.
21. D'Haens G, Lemmens L, Geboes K, et al. Intravenous cyclosporine versus intravenous corticosteroids as single therapy for severe attacks of ulcerative colitis. *Gastroenterology.* 2001;120:1323-1329.
22. Van Assche G, D'Haens G, Noman M, et al. Randomized, double-blind comparison of 4 mg/kg versus 2 mg/kg intravenous cyclosporine in severe ulcerative colitis. *Gastroenterology.* 2003;125:1025-1031.
23. Rayner C, McCormack G, Emmanuel A, et al. Long-term results of low-dose intravenous cyclosporin for acute severe ulcerative colitis. *Aliment Pharmacol Ther.* 2003;18:303-308.
24. Arts J, D'Haens G, Zeegers M, et al. Long-term outcome of treatment with intravenous cyclosporine in patients with severe ulcerative colitis. *Inflamm Bowel Dis.* 2004;10:73-78.
25. Quan V, Saunders B, Hicks B, et al. Cyclosporin treatment for ulcerative colitis complicated by fatal *Pneumocystis carinii* pneumonia. *BMJ.* 1997;314:363-364.
26. Stein R, Cohen R, Hanauer S. Complications during cyclosporine therapy for inflammatory bowel disease. *Gastroenterology.* 1997;112:A1096.
27. Cohen RD, Stein R, Hanauer SB. Intravenous cyclosporin in ulcerative colitis: a five-year experience. *Am J Gastroenterol.* 1999;94(6):1587-1592.
28. Moskovitz DN, Van Assche G, Maenhout B, et al. Incidence of colectomy during long-term follow-up after cyclosporine-induced remission of severe ulcerative colitis. *Clin Gastroenterol Hepatol.* 2006;4(6):760-765.
29. Sternthal M, George J, Kornbluth A, et al. Toxicity associated with the use of cyclosporine in patients with inflammatory bowel disease. *Gastroenterology.* 1996;110:A109.
30. Maser EA, Deconda D, Lichtiger S, Ullman T, Present DH, Kornbluth A. Cyclosporine and infliximab as rescue therapy for each other in patients with steroid-refractory ulcerative colitis. *Clin Gastroenterol Hepatol.* 2008;6:1112-1116.
31. Schwartz LK, Kim MK, Coleman M, Lichtiger S, Chadburn A, Scherl E. Case report: lymphoma arising in an ileal pouch anal anastomosis after immunomodulatory therapy for inflammatory bowel disease. *Clin Gastroenterol Hepatol.* 2006;4(8):1030-1034.
32. Mahadevan U, Tremaine WJ, Johnson T. Intravenous azathioprine in severe ulcerative colitis: a pilot study. *Am J Gastroenterol.* 2000;95:3463-3468.
33. Sood A, Midha V, Sood N, Kaushal V. Role of azathioprine in severe ulcerative colitis: one-year, placebo-controlled, randomized trial. *Indian J Gastroenterol.* 2000;19(1):14-16.
34. Sood A, Midha V, Sood N, Avasthi G. Azathioprine versus sulfasalazine in maintenance of remission in severe ulcerative colitis. *Indian J Gastroenterol.* 2003;22:79-81.

35. Rutgeerts P, Sandborn WJ, Feagan BG, et al. Infliximab for induction and maintenance therapy for ulcerative colitis. *N Engl J Med.* 2005;353:2462-2476.
36. Sands B, Tremaine W, Sandborn W, et al. Infliximab in the treatment of severe, steroid-refractory ulcerative colitis: a pilot study. *Inflamm Bowel Dis.* 2001;7:83-88.
37. Chey W, Hussain A, Ryan C, et al. Infliximab for refractory ulcerative colitis. *Am J Gastroenterol.* 2001;96(8):2373-2381.
38. Su C, Salzberg B, Lewis J, et al. Efficacy of anti-tumor necrosis factor therapy in patients with ulcerative colitis. *Am J Gastroenterol.* 2002;97:2577-2584.
39. Gornet JM, Couve S, Hassani Z, et al. Infliximab for refractory ulcerative colitis or indeterminate colitis: an open-label multicentre study. *Aliment Pharmacol Ther.* 2003;18:175-181.
40. Probert CS, Hearing SD, Schreiber S, et al. Infliximab in moderately severe glucocorticoid resistant ulcerative colitis: a randomized controlled trial. *Gut.* 2003;52:998-1002.
41. Rutgeerts P, Van Assche G, Vermeire S, et al. Optimizing anti-TNF treatment in inflammatory bowel disease. *Gastroenterology.* 2004;126:1593-1610.
42. Prograf (tacrolimus capsules) [package insert]. Deerfield, IL: Astellas Pharma US, Inc; 2008.
43. Yin M, Ochs RS. Mechanism for the paradoxical inhibition and stimulation of calcineurin by the immunosuppresive drug tacrolimus (FK506). *Arch Biochem Biophys.* 2003;419:207-213.
44. Sandborn WJ, Present DH, Isaacs KL, et al. Tacrolimus for the treatment of fistulas in patients with Crohn's disease: a randomized, placebo-controlled trial. *Gastroenterology.* 2003;125(2):380-388.
45. Hogenauer C, Wenzl HH, Hinterleitner TA, et al. Effect of oral tacrolimus (FK 506) on steroid-refractory moderate/severe ulcerative colitis. *Aliment Pharmacol Ther.* 2003;18:415-423.
46. Fellerman K, Tanko Z, Herrlinger KR, et al. Response of refractory colitis to intravenous or oral tacrolimus (FK 506). *Inflamm Bowel Dis.* 2002;8:317-324.
47. Ogata H, Matsui T, Nakamura M, et al. A randomised dose finding study of oral tacrolimus (FK506) therapy in refractory ulcerative colitis. *Gut.* 2006;55:1255-1262.
48. Flanagan WM, Corthésy B, Bram RJ, Crabtree GR. Nuclear association of a T-cell transcription factor blocked by FK-506 and cyclosporin A. *Nature.* 1991;352:803-807.
49. Hess AD. Mechanisms of action of cyclosporine: considerations for the treatment of autoimmune diseases. *Clin Immunol Immunopathol.* 1993;68:220-228.
50. Kovarik JM, Rawlings E, Sweny P, et al. Prolonged immunosuppressive effect and minimal immunogenicity from chimeric (CD 25) monoclonal antibody SDZ CHI 621 in renal transplantation. *Transplant Proc.* 1996;28:913-914.
51. Walker K, Potter J, House A. Interleukin-2 synthesis in the presence of steroids: a model of steroid resistance. *Clin Exp Immunol.* 1987;68:162-167.
52. Kam J, Szefler S, Surs W, et al. Combination of IL-2 and IL-4 reduced glucocorticoid receptor binding affinity and T-cell response to glucocorticoids. *J Immunol.* 1993;151:3460-3466.
53. Creed TJ, Norman MR, Probert CS, et al. Basiliximab (anti-CD25) in combination with steroids may be an effective new treatment for steroid-resistant ulcerative colitis. *Aliment Pharmacol Ther.* 2003;18:65-75.
54. Creed TJ, Probert CS, Norman MN, et al. Basiliximab for the treatment of steroid-resistant ulcerative colitis: further experience in moderate and severe disease. *Aliment Pharmacol Ther.* 2006;23:1435-1442.
55. Carpenter PA, Appelbaum FR, Corey L, et al. A humanized non-FcR-binding anti-CD3 antibody, visilizumab, for treatment of steroid-refractory acute graft-versus-host disease. *Blood.* 2002;99:2712-2719.
56. Plevy S, Salzberg B, van Assche G, et al. A phase I study of visilzumab, a humanized anti-CD3 monoclonal antibody in severe steroid-refractory ulcerative colitis. *Gastroenterol.* 2007;1333:1414-1422.
57. Targan SR, Salzberg BA, Mayer L, et al. A phase I-II study: multiple dose levels of visilizumab are well tolerated and produce rapid and sustained improvement in ulcerative colitis patients refractory to treatment with IV steroids (ivsr-Uc) [abstract 493]. *Gastroenterology.* 2005;128(Suppl 2):A-75.
58. Schwartz AG, Targan SR, Saxon A, et al. Sulfasalazine-induced exacerbation of ulcerative colitis. *N Engl J Med.* 1982;306:409-412.

Medical Management of Toxic Megacolon in the Patient With Ulcerative Colitis

27

Robynne Chutkan, MD and Nabil Toubia, MD

INTRODUCTION

Toxic megacolon is an infrequent but potentially fatal complication of inflammatory bowel disease (IBD). It was first recognized as a clinical entity by Marshak et al[1] in 1950, with the term *toxic megacolon* coined by Roth et al in 1959.[2] It is defined as segmental or total colonic distention of 6 cm or more in the setting of acute colitis associated with signs and symptoms of systemic toxicity.[3,4] Other conditions predisposing to toxic megacolon have been reported since its initial description in patients with ulcerative colitis (UC) and include Crohn's disease,[5,6] pseudomembranous colitis (PMC),[7-11] infectious colitis,[12-22] and ischemic colitis.[23,24]

IBD continues to be the most common cause leading to toxic megacolon. Given the associated high morbidity and mortality, early recognition and management of toxic megacolon are of utmost importance. Abdominal imaging, using either plain abdominal films or abdominal CT scan, has improved its recognition and diagnosis and helped identify potential candidates for early surgical intervention. Colonoscopy is relatively contraindicated due to the high rate of complications.

The standard medical approach to treatment of toxic megacolon has not changed substantially over the past 3 decades and continues to focus on treatment directed at the underlying cause of colitis in addition to general supportive measures. Early in the course of the disease, it is crucial to exclude superimposed infection such as *Clostridium difficile*[25] and cytomegalovirus (CMV) infection [26] as potential exacerbating factors because the choice of medications and therapy would differ significantly if these are present. Medications such as opiates, antidiarrheals, and anticholinergics, which can worsen the condition, should be avoided. Colonic decompression techniques as well as positional changes ("barrel rolling") may be considered in the medical management of this condition.[27-29] Recognizing progressive, complicated disease that constitutes an indication for surgical intervention is an integral part of the medical management of patients with toxic megacolon.

Epidemiology

The precise incidence of toxic megacolon complicating UC is difficult to determine and varies in the literature, but has been estimated at 1% to 2.5%.[6] Most of the reported data are generated from tertiary medical centers that care for individuals with more severe forms of colitis. One such study reported an incidence of 17% in patients admitted with severe UC,[30] although in patients admitted with less severe UC, the incidence was 6.4%.[31] Data from a private practice setting revealed an incidence of 17% among patients with UC followed over 15 years.[32] Greenstein et al reported a 10% incidence of toxic megacolon in patients with ulcerative colitis admitted to the hospital.[33] The data were collected over 19 years and involved 1236 IBD patients. Other investigators have reported an incidence of up to 28% in patients requiring surgical treatment for IBD.[34]

Summarizing the above, it appears that the incidence of toxic megacolon varies between 1% and 6% in all hospitalized UC patients and 10% to 20% for those

Lichtenstein GR, ed.
Ulcerative Colitis: The Complete Guide to Medical Management (pp. 293-298)

admitted with fulminant disease. Factors linked to an increased risk of developing toxic megacolon include premature discontinuation of IBD medications, intake of precipitating medications, invasive procedures, and superimposed enteric infections.

NATURAL HISTORY

Toxic megacolon may be the first manifestation of IBD in about 30% of patients[35] and can present at any time during the course of the disease as an acute exacerbation of chronic disease. There is no predilection for either gender or any specific age group. Morbidity and mortality rates from toxic megacolon have been extensively documented over the past 5 decades and vary between the medical and surgical literature. There also exist variations according to the date of the reported literature, with older literature reporting higher mortality rates. More recent reports suggest a decline in both surgical and medical mortality, likely related to increased recognition, intensive support, and therapy in a multidisciplinary setting as well as early surgical intervention and improved postoperative care.

A comprehensive review of the early literature revealed an overall mortality of 19% from toxic megacolon.[36] Mortality was higher in the medically managed patients—27% compared to 19.5% in the surgical group. Perforation represented the single most important determinant of mortality, reaching 41% in those patients found to have colonic perforations versus 8.5% for those without colonic perforation. This has been demonstrated in several other studies.[33,37-39] Conversely, more recent evidence suggests much lower rates with reports from the European Collaborative Study on Inflammatory Bowel Disease (EC-IBD) showing less than 0.2% mortality rate in UC over a 4-year follow-up.[39] This is likely a reflection of earlier recognition of complicated disease and parallels the increased trend in the use of immunosuppressive therapy following an acute attack. In the era predating anti-metabolite therapy, long-term follow-up studies revealed a high percentage of patients requiring surgical therapy following their initial medical therapy for toxic megacolon.[33] In a study from the Mayo clinic, 29% of patients had recurrent fulminant colitis or toxic megacolon, and 47% of the patients treated medically eventually required surgery despite successful initial medical management.[40] The extent of the inflammation did not seem to affect the mortality from the disease but did influence its incidence because patients with universal colitis are more likely to progress to fulminant disease than those with limited distal colitis.[41]

PATHOGENESIS

The exact pathogenic mechanisms leading to colonic dilatation and systemic toxicity in severe colitis still remain uncertain. Several hypotheses have been postulated:

- Direct extension of inflammation into the smooth muscle layer of the colonic wall leading to its dysfunction, relaxation, and subsequent dilation
- Defective smooth muscle contraction and poor response to normal kinetic stimuli
- Release of inhibitory soluble mediators perpetuated by inflammatory cytokines
- Release into the circulation of cytokines and bacterial antigens across the injured colonic wall culminating in systemic toxicity.

The most plausible mechanism leading to toxic dilatation is probably multifactorial, resulting from a combination of several events that are concomitantly at play.

Correlation between the depth of the ulcerative process and the degree of dilatation has been shown in a study by Buckell et al[42] leading to the conclusion that the spread of inflammation to the deeper layer of the colonic wall has a considerable effect on the development of toxic megacolon.[41] Damage to the submucosal and myenteric plexuses was proposed as a potential etiology for colonic dilatation through disruption of normal neurogenic stimuli.[43]

However, this was not a universal finding, with some pathologic studies showing preserved neural plexuses.[44-46] Smooth muscular dysfunction in patients with UC resulting from poor colonic response to biochemical stimuli mediated by vasoactive intestinal polypeptide (VIP), substance P, neurotensin, and leukotrienes has also been reported.[47-51] The role of IL-1B, an inflammatory cytokine, was highlighted in a recent study showing increased levels of IL-1B in the muscularis propria of patients with UC.[52] Those levels were compared to controls taken from normal margins of colon cancer resection specimens. Higher levels of IL-1B correlated with diminished smooth muscular contractility in UC specimens. The same effect was reproduced in the normal muscle following addition of higher concentrations of IL-1B. The IL-1B treated cells also showed an increased concentration of hydrogen peroxide. Moreover, the addition of a hydrogen peroxide scavenger negated the effects of IL-1B on the treated cells, suggesting that hydrogen peroxide might be a mediator of colonic dysmotility induced by higher levels of inflammatory cytokines.

Nitric oxide, a known inhibitor of smooth muscle contraction, has also been studied as a potential agent in the development of toxic megacolon.[53] Mourelle et al analyzed nitric oxide synthase activity and levels in resected colon specimens taken from patients with toxic megacolon.[54] These were compared to levels obtained from specimens of patients with nontoxic ulcerative colitis and colonic neoplasm. A higher level of nitric oxide synthase activity was found in toxic megacolon specimens, leading the authors to conclude that nitric oxide might be closely involved in the pathogenesis of this syndrome. Other experimental studies showed a decrease in the levels of nitric oxide synthase in rat colons after oral decontamination using nonabsorbable broad-spectrum antibiotics. Contractility of the colonic muscle as well as intracolonic pressure improved following the pharmacologic blockade of nitric oxide synthase activity.[55]

Other investigators have proposed an alternative neuronal reflex mechanism in addition to the local factors, leading to dilation in other segments of the GI tract.[30] Small bowel and stomach distention heralded the development of toxic megacolon and multisystem organ failure in their study. The authors suggested that the activation of intestinal extrinsic inhibitory reflexes mediated through the neuronal long and short reflexes occurred following biochemical activation at the local colonic level.

The systemic toxicity may also be related to the inflammatory involvement across the colonic wall and through the serosa, resulting in free or sealed microperforations. Surgical specimens commonly show inflammation involving the full thickness of the colonic wall.[43,45,56] With the mucosa now denuded and the natural barrier disrupted, bacterial toxins and antigens can invade and promote the release of cytokines leading to fever, leukocytosis, multisystem organ failure, and shock.[30,41]

CLINICAL MANIFESTATIONS AND DIAGNOSIS

The task of establishing the diagnosis and instituting appropriate, safe, and effective therapy can be challenging to a clinician faced with a new patient with no prior history of IBD. As previously discussed, some referral centers have reported the presence of toxic megacolon in initial presentation of IBD in up to one-third of patients.

In a previously undiagnosed IBD patient, it is essential to obtain a thorough medical history and search for clues that hint at the diagnosis of IBD. Subtle signs and symptoms that are often missed or overlooked by the patient can lead the clinician to the correct diagnosis. These may include a family history of IBD, a history of intermittent bloody diarrhea, perianal disease, aphthous ulcerations, anemia of unexplained etiology, as well as extraintestinal manifestations such as arthritis, uveitis, episcleritis, sclerosing cholangitis, erythema nodosum, or pyoderma gangrenosum. In this subgroup of patients, it is crucial to rule out enteric infection as a potential etiology. Careful inquiry into recent travel, HIV status, and exposure to enteric pathogens as well as antibiotics is essential. Stool cultures for common bacterial infections including *Campylobacter*, *Shigella*, *Salmonella*, *Clostridium difficile* toxin, and ova and parasites should be part of the initial evaluation.

TABLE 27-1

DIAGNOSTIC CRITERIA FOR ESTABLISHING THE DIAGNOSIS OF TOXIC MEGACOLON

At least three of the following:

- Fever >38°C (101.5°F)
- Heart rate >120/minute
- Neutrophilic leukocytosis >10.500/ L
- Anemia

In addition to the above, at least one of the following:

- Dehydration
- Altered consciousness
- Electrolyte imbalances
- Hypotension

In patients with a known diagnosis of IBD, toxic megacolon often follows an acute and severe flare of the underlying disease, usually within 7 to 10 days of symptom onset. Many IBD patients would have already been started on steroid therapy at that point. Initiating steroids in a patient with no prior IBD diagnosis can be risky, particularly if an infectious etiology is overlooked.

The first task in the clinical decision-making is to recognize the syndrome of toxic megacolon and its underlying etiology. The diagnosis of toxic megacolon is made based on clinical and radiographic evidence (Table 27-1). The most commonly adopted clinical criteria for diagnosing toxic megacolon were originally formulated by Jalan et al.[3] They include any 3 of either fever >101.5°F, heart rate >120 beats/minute, white blood cell count >10,500 mm, or anemia, in addition to one of the following criteria: dehydration, mental status changes, electrolyte imbalances, and hypotension. One should be highly suspicious of toxic megacolon in all UC patients with worsening abdominal distention and tenderness, particularly when it is combined with a decrease in diarrhea. Tachycardia, fever, hypotension, and altered consciousness are not uncommon signs. Physical examination may demonstrate increased tympani on abdominal percussion, as well as diminished bowel sounds. Biochemical abnormalities are often encountered and should be monitored daily. These include hypokalemia, metabolic alkalosis, hypomagnesemia, hypophosphatemia, hypocalcemia, and hypoalbuminemia. Some of these abnormalities, such as hypokalemia and hypomagnesemia, have a negative effect on smooth muscle contractility, lead to worsening colonic dilatation, and should be aggressively corrected. An elevated white blood cell count with a left shift is a frequent finding, although leukocytosis is nonspecific and could signal perforation or may become pronounced following steroid therapy. Once established, steroid therapy can potentially mask some of the physical signs of perforation. Anemia may be present in patients with toxic megacolon due to either chronic disease or acute blood loss. Hematocrit levels should be monitored and transfusion therapy initiated when clinically indicated.

Abdominal imaging is essential to establish the diagnosis of toxic megacolon and to rule out perforation. Flat and upright abdominal films are generally readily available, simple to obtain, and offer a significant amount of information. Dilatation in any segment of the colon of 6 cm or more is suggestive of the diagnosis. The transverse colon is the most common site of dilatation due to its anatomic location. Its superior and anterior location tends to trap air preferentially when patients are in the supine position.[57] If the patient remains in this position, further air accumulation and distention in the same segment will ensue. Rolling the patient to the prone position tends to redistribute the air to other segments of the colon. That observation has led to the therapeutic application of patient repositioning techniques. Evidence of proximal small bowel and gastric dilatation has been shown in several studies to have additional prognostic value and is worth looking for on abdominal imaging. Patients with these findings are more likely to progress to toxic megacolon and multiple organ failure.[58] The plain abdominal film can also offer details about the extent of mucosal involvement in about 80% of cases.[59] Other features such as absence of the haustral pattern, presence of nodular and polypoid luminal projections, and a scalloped contour of the large bowel[60] may also be demonstrated on the abdominal film. Once the diagnosis of toxic megacolon is established, daily abdominal films are crucial in the follow-up of disease progression or resolution.

Computer tomography (CT) scanning is being more frequently used in clinical practice, especially in the setting of IBD. However, CT imaging has not been extensively studied in the setting of UC-induced toxic megacolon. Although more expensive, CT scans are more sensitive at detecting small perforations not seen on plain abdominal films and provide more information about abscess and fistula formation. Moreover, in a retrospective study by Imbriaco and Balthazar,[61] CT scan was better than conventional abdominal imaging at evaluating the length and severity of colitis as well as in identifying presence of dilatation, particularly in fluid-filled colonic segments. In that series, the investigators looked at 18 patients with confirmed clinical diagnoses of toxic megacolon and included 12 patients with pseudomembranous colitis, 4 with UC, and 2 with CMV. Findings on CT scan were nonspecific in suggesting a particular etiology for toxic megacolon and were nonpredictive of the clinical response to conservative therapy. Nevertheless, CT scan was able to detect abdominal complications missed by clinical exam and plain abdominal films in 22% of the cases. Only 1 of the 4 patients found to have extraintestinal complications survived, indicating the need to image patients earlier for clinically unsuspected complications. Interestingly, pylephlebitis, also known as ascending septic thrombophlebitis—an apparently under-reported and serious complication of intra-abdominal inflammation—was found in 13% of patients in that series. The role of CT scan needs to be further evaluated prospectively to determine its prognostic role in the setting of toxic megacolon.

High-resolution abdominal ultrasonography (HRUS) has also been suggested as a potential tool for investigating severe colitis and toxic megacolon. In a study by Arienti et al, HRUS suggested the development of disease when thinning of the large bowel wall was encountered, as opposed to the usual thickening found in the setting of mild to moderate colitis.[62] Furthermore, HRUS correlated closely with other imaging modalities in accurately diagnosing extensive colitis and activity level. Further assessment and standardization of this technology in toxic megacolon needs to be undertaken to confirm its usefulness in clinical practice.

Limited flexible sigmoidoscopy and mucosal biopsy with minimal insufflation done by an experienced endoscopist can be particularly helpful, especially when faced with a patient with no known history of IBD or when the underlying diagnosis is in question. The biopsies may differentiate between infectious causes such as pseudomembranous colitis (associated with *Clostridium difficile*) and CMV. Extreme caution has to be exercised during the procedure, given the increased risk of perforation. One should probably obtain a CT scan with IV and nonbarium-based oral contrast prior to performing the limited sigmoidoscopy because the CT scan may provide information about the condition of the proximal colon and exclude other abdominal complications such as perforation and abscess formation.

MEDICAL MANAGEMENT

There is no controlled evidence supporting the use of different medical regimens in toxic megacolon. Current recommendations and practice rely on retrospective data and expert opinion, and the decision to go to surgery should be individualized based on the overall clinical picture of the patient. Hospitalization and surgical consultation, as well as nothing by mouth, are mandatory. Nasogastric tubes or long intestinal tubes are useful for decompression purposes. Narcotics, antidiarrheals, and anticholinergic medications should be strictly avoided. Daily blood work and abdominal films, as well as aggressive correction of fluid and electrolyte abnormalities, are essential. Rolling maneuvers where the bed is flattened and the patient rolls over into a prone position for 10 to 15 minutes every 2 to 3 hours may be helpful.

There is no evidence to support total parenteral nutrition as a therapeutic modality in the patient with toxic megacolon, although it may play a role in the nutritionally depleted patient with an expected prolonged course and surgery that appears likely. Prophylactic antisecretory therapy to prevent gastric stress-related mucosal ulceration and prophylaxis against deep venous thrombosis, given the increased risk of pulmonary embolism in patients with toxic megacolon, are often instituted. Broad-spectrum antibiotics are often used to reduce the risk of septic complications and potential perforation. No controlled trials exist documenting the efficacy of antibiotics, but, given the high risk for perforation, experts recommend adjunctive broad-spectrum antibiotics. Bacteremia can be present in 25% of patients with toxic megacolon even in the absence of overt perforation. IV steroids using either hydrocortisone 100 mg IV every 8 hours or 300 mg continuously are the mainstay of therapy once an infectious etiology has been excluded. Methylprednisolone 60 mg daily in divided doses or corticotropin (ACTH) 40 units every 8 hours for steroid-naïve patients have historically been used, but have no advantage over IV hydrocortisone.[3,41,63] The effectiveness of these agents in patients with toxic megacolon is demonstrated by a clinical series by Jalan,[3] reporting mortality in 9 out of 10 patients treated supportively for toxic megacolon as compared to only one-third of those treated with steroids. The aminosalicylates have no role in the therapy of toxic megacolon. Cyclosporine has not been adequately studied in the setting of toxic megacolon, although its benefit for severe refractory UC is well-documented.[64] There is one report of successful infliximab use for toxic megacolon from Hyderabad, India,[65] and one report of successful tacrolimus use from Germany.[66] Hyperbaric oxygen therapy has also been reported as a potential therapy.[67]

Medical therapy is considered successful when signs of toxicity are reduced, fluid and transfusion requirements decrease, abdominal and colonic dilatation begin to resolve, and labs improve. If persistent fever or abdominal pain is present, then perforation and abscess need to be excluded. Any of the prior findings are clear indications for surgery. Massive hemorrhage, increasing signs of toxicity, and progression of colonic dilatation are indications for urgent operation. Surgical studies recommend colectomy following 48 to 72 hours of unsuccessful medical therapy.[3] Other experts recommend continuation of medical therapy for up to 7 to 10 days if the patient appears to be clinically stable or improving, despite persistent megacolon.

REFERENCES

1. Marshak RH, Lester LJ, Friedman AI. Megacolon: a complication of ulcerative colitis. *Gastroenterology.* 1950;16:768-772.
2. Roth JLA, Valdes-Dapnea A, Stein GN, Bockus HL. Toxic megacolon in ulcerative colitis. *Gastroenterology.* 1959;37:239.
3. Jalan K, Sircus W, Card WI, et al. An experience of ulcerative colitis. I. Toxic dilation in 55 cases. *Gastroenterology.* 1969;57:68-82.
4. Fazio VW. Toxic megacolon in ulcerative colitis and Crohn's colitis. *Clin Gastroenterol.* 1980;9:389-407.
5. Schachter H, Goldstein MJ, Kirsner JB. Toxic dilation complicating Crohn's disease of the colon. *Gastroenterology.* 1967;5:136-140.
6. Greico MB, Bordan DL, Geiss AC, et al. Toxic megacolon complicating Crohn's colitis. *Ann Surg.* 1980;191:75-80.
7. Agnifili A, Gola P, Marino M, et al. The role and timing of surgery in the treatment of pseudomembranous colitis: a case complicated by toxic megacolon. *Hepato-Gastroenterology.* 1994;41:394-396.
8. Brown CH, Ferrante WA, Davis WD Jr. Toxic dilation of the colon complicating pseudomembranous enterocolitis. *Am J Dig Dis.* 1968;13:813.
9. Bradley SJ, Weaver DW, Maxwell NP, et al. Surgical management of pseudomembranous colitis. *Am Surg.* 1988;54:329-332.
10. Cone JB, Wetzel W. Toxic megacolon secondary to pseudomembranous colitis. *Dis Colon Rectum.* 1982;25:478-482.
11. Hoogland T, Cooperman AM, Farmer RG, et al. Toxic megacolon-unusual complication of pseudomembranous colitis. *Clevel Clin Q.* 1977;44:149-155.
12. Anderson JB, Tanner AH, Brodribb AJ. Toxic megacolon due to *Campylobacter* colitis. *Int J Colorect Dis.* 1986;1:58-59.
13. Bellary SV, Isaacs P. Toxic megacolon (TM) due to Salmonella. *J Clin Gastroenterol.* 1990;12:605-607.
14. Ciftci AO, Karnak I, Senocak ME, et al. Spectrum of complicated intestinal amebiasis through resected specimens: incidence and outcome. *J Pediatr Surg.* 1999;34:1369-1373.
15. Deppisch LM, Crans CA. Salmonellosis: a cause of toxic megacolon. *J Clin Gastoenterol.* 1990;12:483-485.
16. Greenstein AJ, Greenstein RJ, Sachar DB. Toxic dilatation in amebic colitis: successful treatment without colectomy. *Am J Surg.* 1980;139:456-458.
17. Jackson TL Jr, Young RL, Thompson JS, et al. Toxic megacolon associated with *Campylobacter jejuni* colitis. *Am J Gastroenterol.* 1999;94:280-282.
18. Kalkay MN, Ayanian ZS, Lehaf EA, et al. *Campylobacter*-induced toxic megacolon. *Am J Gastoenterol.* 1983;78:557-559.
19. Mendonca HL, Vieta JO, Korelitz BI. Perforation of the colon in unsuspected amebic colitis: report of two cases. *Dis Colon Rectum.* 1977;20:149-153.
20. Schneider A, Runzi M, Peitgen K, et al. *Campylobacter jejuni*-induced severe colitis: a rare cause of toxic megacolon. *Z Gastroenterol.* 2000;38:307-309.
21. Upadhyay AK, Neely JA. Toxic megacolon and perforation caused by Shigella. *Br J Surg.* 1989;76:1217.
22. Wilson AP, Ridgway GL, Sarner M, et al. Toxic dilatation of the colon in *Shigellosis. Br Med J.* 1990;301:1325-1326.
23. Markoglou C, Avgerinos A, Mitrakou M, et al. Toxic megacolon secondary to acute ischemic colitis. *Hepato-Gastroenterology.* 1993;40:188-190.
24. Robertson RH, McDowell HA Jr, Jander HP, et al. Toxic megacolon due to ischemic enterocolitis associated with retroperitoneal fibrosis. *Gastroenterology.* 1980;78:585-591.
25. Garcia-Osogobio S, Takahashi T, Gamboa-Dominguez A, et al. Toxic pseudomembranous colitis in a patient with ulcerative colitis. *Inflamm Bowel Dis.* 2000;6:188-190.

26. Cooper HS, Raffensper EC, Jonas L, et al. Cytomegalovirus inclusions in patients with ulcerative colitis and toxic dilatation requiring colonic resection. *Gastroenterology.* 1977;72:1253-1256.
27. Kramer P, Wittenberg J. Colonic gas distribution in toxic megacolon. *Gastoenterology.* 1981;80:433-437.
28. Panos MZ, Wood MJ, Asquith P. Toxic megacolon: the knee-elbow position relieves bowel distention. *Gut.* 1993;34:1726-1727.
29. Present DH. The knee-elbow position relieves distension [letter]. *Gut.* 1994;35:1150.
30. Caprilli R, Latella G, Vernia P, et al. Multiple organ dysfunction in ulcerative colitis. *Am J Gastroenterol.* 2000;95:1258-1262.
31. Latella G, Vernia P, Viscido A, et al. GI distension in severe ulcerative colitis. *Am J Gastroenterol.* 2002;97:1169-1175.
32. Danovitch SH. Fulminant colitis and toxic megacolon. *Gastroenterology Clin North Am.* 1989;18:73-82.
33. Greenstein AJ, Sachar DB, Gibas A, et al. Outcome of toxic dilation in ulcerative and Crohn's colitis. *J Clin Gastroenterol.* 1985;7:137-143.
34. Brooke BN, Sampson PA. An indication for surgery in acute ulcerative colitis. *Lancet.* 1964;2:1272.
35. Adams JT. Toxic dilatation of the colon: a surgical disease. *Arch Surg.* 1973;106:678-682.
36. Strauss RJ, Flint GW, Platt N, et al. The surgical management of toxic dilatation of the colon: a report of 28 cases and review of the literature. *Ann Surg.* 1976;184:682-688.
37. Roys G, Kaplan MS, Juler GL. Surgical management of toxic megacolon. *Am J Gastroenterol.* 1977;68:161-166.
38. Binder SC, Patterson JF, Glotzer DJ. Toxic megacolon in ulcerative colitis. *Gastoenterology.* 1974;66:909-915.
39. Witte J, Shivananda S, Lennard-Jones JE, et al. Disease outcome in inflammatory bowel disease: mortality, morbidity and therapeutic management of a 796-person inception cohort in the European Collaborative Study on Inflammatory Bowel Disease (EC-IBD). *Scand J Gastroenterol.* 2000;35:1272-1277.
40. Grant CS, Dozois RR. Toxic megacolon: Ultimate fate of patients after successful medical management. *Am J Surg.* 1984;147:106-110.
41. Present DH. Toxic megacolon. *Med Clin North Am.* 1993;77:1129-1148.
42. Buckell N, Williams GT, Bartram CI, et al. Depth of ulceration in acute colitis: correlation with outcome and clinical and radiological features. *Gastoenterology.* 1980;79:19-25.
43. Smith FW, Law DH, Nickel WF Jr, Slesenger MH. Fulminant ulcerative colitis with toxic dilatation of the colon: medical and surgical management of eleven cases with observations regarding etiology. *Gastoenterology.* 1962;42:233.
44. McInerny GT, Sauer WG, Baggenstross AH, et al. Fulminating ulcerative colitis with marked colonic dilation: a clinicopathologic study. *Gastroenterology.* 1962;42:244-257.
45. Norland CC, Kirsner JB. Toxic dilatation of the colon (toxic megacolon): etiology, treatment, and prognosis in 42 patients. *Medicine.* 1969;48:229-250.
46. Prohaska JV, Greer D, Ryan JF. Acute dilatation of the colon in ulcerative colitis. *Arch Surg.* 1964;89:24-30.
47. Snape WJ, Willams R, Hyman PE. Defect in colonic smooth muscle contraction in patients with ulcerative colitis. *Am J Physiol.* 1991;261:G987-G991.
48. Spriggs E, Code C, Bargen Ja, et al. Motility of the pelvic colon and rectum of normal persons and patients with ulcerative colitis. *Gastroenterology.* 1951;19:480-490.
49. Koch TR, Camey JA, Go VL, et al. Spontaneous contractions and some electrophysiologic properties of circular muscle from normal sigmoid colon and ulcerative colitis. *Gastroenterology.* 1988;95:77-84.
50. Snape WJ, Kao HW. Role of inflammatory mediators in colonic smooth muscle function in ulcerative colitis. *Dig Dis Sci.* 1988;33:65S-70S.
51. Pons L, Droy-lefaix MT, Bueno L. Leukotriene D4 participates in colonic transit disturbances induced by intracolonic administration of trinitrobenzene sulfonic acid in rats. *Gastroenterology.* 1992;102:149-156.
52. Vrees MD, Pricolo VE, Potenti FM, et al. Abnormal motility in patients with ulcerative colitis: the role of inflammatory cytokines. *Arch Surg.* 2002;137:439-445.
53. Tomita R, Tanjoh K. Tole of nitric oxide in the colon of patients with ulcerative colitis. *World J Surg.* 1998;22:88-91.
54. Mourelle M, Casellas F, Guarner F, et al. Induction of nitric oxide synthase in colonic smooth muscle from patients with toxic megacolon. *Gastroenterology.* 1995;109:1497-1502.
55. Mourelle M, Vilaseca J, Guarner F, et al. Toxic dilatation of colon in a rat model of colitis is linked to an inducible form of nitric oxide synthase. *Am J Physiol.* 1996;270:G425-G430.
56. Meyers S, Janowitz HD. Systemic corticosteroids therapy of ulcerative colitis. *Gastroenterology.* 1985;89:1189-1191.
57. Kramer P, Wittenberg J. Colonic gas distribution in toxic megacolon. *Gastroenterology.* 1981;80:433-437.
58. Caprilli R, Vernia P, Latella G, et al. Early recognition of toxic megacolon. *J Clin Gastoenterol.* 1987;9:160-164.
59. Prantera C, Lorenzetti R, Cerro P, et al. The plain abdominal film accurately estimates extent of active ulcerative colitis. *J Clin Gastroenterol.* 1991;13:231-234.
60. Halpert RD. Toxic dilation of the colon. *Radiol Clin North Am.* 1987;25:147-154.
61. Imbriaco M, Balthazar E. Toxic megacolon: role of CT in evaluation and detection of complications. *Clinical Imaging.* 2001;25:349-354.
62. Arienti V, Campieri M, Boriani L, et al. Management of severe ulcerative colitis with the help of high resolution ultrasonography. *Am J Gastroenterol.* 1996;91:2163-2169.
63. Rosenberg W, Ireland A, Jewell DP. High-dose methylprednisolone in the treatment of active ulcerative colitis. *J Clin Gastroenterol.* 1990;12:40-41.
64. Lichtiger S, Present DH, Kornbluth A, et al. Cyclosporine in severe ulcerative colitis refractory to steroid therapy. *N Engl J Med.* 1994;330:1841-1845.
65. Siram PV, Reddy KS, Rao GV, Santosh D, Reddy DN. Infliximab in the treatment of ulcerative colitis with toxic megacolon. *Indian J Gastroenterol.* 2004;23:22-23.
66. Pascu M, Muller AR, Wiedenmann B, Dignass AU. Rescue therapy with tacrolimus in a patient with toxic megacolon. *Int J Colorectal Dis.* 2003;18:271-275.
67. Kuroki K, Masuda A, Uehara H, et al. A new treatment for toxic megacolon. *Lancet.* 1998;352:782.
68. Welfare MR, Barton JR, Cobden I. Hyperbaric oxygen for toxic megacolon. *Lancet.* 1999;353:70-71.

28

Medical Management of Ulcerative Proctitis

Philip B. Miner Jr, MD

Dramatic changes have occurred in the understanding and management of inflammatory bowel disease (IBD) during the past decade; however, ulcerative proctitis has been ignored with regard to careful assessment of the causes of proctitis and specific treatment. The factors related to the interaction of luminal contents with the gastrointestinal immune system are beginning to be unraveled, which should enable improvement in management. Biologic therapy is coming of age, and dozens of new "silver bullet" compounds are being developed to treat both Crohn's disease and ulcerative colitis, but little has been done to study ulcerative proctitis. The principal reason for this neglect is the assumption that ulcerative proctitis simply represents a short version of ulcerative colitis, but this is probably incorrect.

Pathophysiology and Diagnosis

Inflammation and Extent of Disease

It is generally accepted that ulcerative proctitis involves the distal 15 to 20 cm of colon and always involves the junction of the anal canal and the rectum. It is often taught that left-sided ulcerative colitis is an extension of ulcerative proctitis; however, the area with the most severe inflammation in left-sided ulcerative colitis is the sigmoid colon, and the rectum often is less inflamed and may appear nearly normal.[1,2] Prior to the advent of flexible endoscopy, the explanation for less active inflammation in the rectum was that the "rectal sparing" was due to topical rectal therapy. During the development of mesalamine derivatives to treat ulcerative colitis, it became clear that the rectum has less inflammation than the sigmoid colon in left-sided ulcerative colitis but was always inflamed in ulcerative proctitis. Treatment response also distinguishes the 2 disorders as well as the importance of maintenance treatment. The distinction between these 2 disorders helps explain the different clinical courses of these 2 entities.

From a practical perspective, the advent of videoendoscopy permits frequent assessment of the degree of mucosal inflammation and response to therapy as well as provides an opportunity to biopsy the mucosa for histologic evaluation. Endoscopic evaluation is essential to the management of ulcerative proctitis as it permits the assessment of the severity and extent of mucosal inflammation. Biopsies are easily obtainable and play an important role in distinguishing the severity and nature of the inflammation. In ulcerative proctitis, the laboratory evaluation is often normal, and the only method to assess disease severity is history, physical examination, and videoendoscopy with biopsy. During the initial evaluation, laboratory assessment is essential (Table 28-1) in order to exclude a treatable infectious cause of colitis and to assess the immunologic pressure on the patient in terms of inflammation and metabolic homeostasis. Stool studies for enteric pathogens, parasites, *Clostridium difficile*, leukocytes, eosinophils, and Charcot-Leyden crystals provide support for idiopathic colonic inflammation as well as directing management. Identifying a specific cause of proctitis is important as specific therapy may be possible. Diagnostic considerations are presented in Table 28-2.

Lichtenstein GR, ed.
Ulcerative Colitis: The Complete Guide to Medical Management (pp. 299-306)

TABLE 28-1

POTENTIAL CAUSES OF RECTAL INFLAMMATION INCLUDED IN THE DIFFERENTIAL DIAGNOSIS OF ULCERATIVE PROCTITIS

Idiopathic ulcerative proctitis
Crohn's proctitis
Solitary rectal ulcer syndrome
Ischemia
Traumatic injury
Enemas
Anal intercourse
Radiation
Gynecologic cancer
Prostate cancer
Enteric infection
Campylobacter jejuni
Amebiasis
Yersinia enterocolitica
Clostridium difficile
Systemic infection
Syphilis
Tuberculosis
Histoplasmosis
Herpes
Bechet's syndrome
Medications
Ergotamine
Gold
Estrogens

TABLE 28-2

INITIAL EVALUATION OF A PATIENT WITH SUSPECTED ULCERATIVE PROCTITIS

History and physical examination
Laboratory
• Blood tests
Complete blood count with differential
Erythrocyte sedimentation rate
Comprehensive metabolic profile (electrolytes, calcium, albumen, tests of liver function)
C-reactive protein
• Stool tests
Blood
Fecal leukocytes, eosinophils, Charcot-Leyden crystals
Clostridium difficile toxin
Cultures for enteric pathogens
Ova and parasite evaluation
• Visualizing the colonic mucosa
Rigid proctosigmoidoscopy with biopsy (unsedated)
Flexible sigmoidoscopy to the splenic flexure with biopsy (unsedated)
Colonoscopy to the cecum with biopsies (sedated)

IMPORTANCE OF HISTOLOGY

During the initial stage of evaluation, mucosal biopsies should be obtained in order to determine the chronicity of disease and to exclude other causes of colitis. The principal alternative diagnosis that needs to be considered in the first attack of ulcerative proctitis is enteric infection. The endoscopic appearance is indistinguishable from idiopathic ulcerative colitis, but the microscopic changes are more acute and the mucosal atrophy and the crypt changes of chronic colitis (crypt distortion [ie, crypt branching]) are absent. Documentation of a specific organism should be sought; however, even in well-recognized infectious colitis, an isolated organism can be identified less than half the time.[3] Acute self-limited colitis (ASLC) generally involves most of the colon and may last for several months. Isolated rectal involvement is possible. The long-term prognosis is excellent with no chronic disease issues that need to be considered. For the consultant, it is often impossible to reconstruct the initial illness. Long-term remission following an acute attack raises the possibility of ASLC and supports a trial period of management without maintenance therapy. *Clostridium difficile* may masquerade as chronic colitis or may cause relapse of symptomatic disease. The characteristic "explosive volcano" seen microscopically is a useful histologic marker of this infectious colitis. *Clostridium difficile* commonly begins in the right colon and often excludes the rectum and thus is an unusual cause of proctitis.[4] All patients with distinct ulceration of the rectum require biopsies to exclude solitary rectal ulcer syndrome (SRUS). SRUS has a pathognomonic histologic picture of disrupted submucosal muscle fibers (fibromuscular obliteration of the lamina propria). SRUS is an ischemic lesion that does not respond to the immunosuppressive treatment offered for IBD and requires special attention to the physiology of defecation to prevent the internal prolapse of rectal mucosal into the anal canal.

Anorectal Physiology in Health and With Inflammation

The complex physiology of the anorectum is adversely influenced by inflammation with increased sensitivity to sensation and an amplification of reflex muscular responses stimulated by stool in the rectum. Tenesmus is the sensation of incomplete evacuation of the rectum or nonproductive straining to defecate. It occurs when rectal contraction is accompanied by internal anal sphincter relaxation.[5,6]

In the presence of inflammation, there is sensitivity to lower-than-normal volumes of balloon distention and exaggerated relaxation of the internal anal sphincter.[5,6] The sensations accompanying this response are perceived rectal fullness, urgency to defecate, and a sense of incomplete evacuation. Occasionally, tenesmus continues when visible inflammation is no longer present. When this occurs, treatment for microscopic inflammation or pharmacologic manipulation of rectal contractility and IAS relaxation improves these symptoms.[5,6] In addition to the influence of rectal inflammation on anorectal physiology, proctitis and left-sided ulcerative colitis change the physiology of the normal-appearing proximal colon. This was recognized as early as 1962 when Lennard-Jones et al[7] described proximal constipation in patients with left-sided ulcerative colitis. Other studies support the concept of inhibition of stool movement proximal to the line of demarcation of disease.[8] The changes in motility have important implications for topical rectal therapy.

DIAGNOSIS

By definition, proctitis is inflammation of the rectum, and the symptoms that accompany the disease are related to the consequences of rectal inflammation. The initial evaluation plan is delineated in Table 28-2. The symptoms include a sense of urgency to defecate, frequency of attempted defecation, tenesmus, and blood and mucous with or without formed stool elements. Because of the limited extent of the disease, systemic symptoms are usually absent. Visible inflammation defines the disease and ideally is obtained by video endoscopy, which establishes the anal verge as the beginning of the inflammation and normal mucosa occurring with intubation of the sigmoid colon. Biopsies help define the disease further and should demonstrate chronic colitis. Laboratory changes reflect the severity and extent of mucosal inflammation; therefore, laboratory studies are usually normal. Essentially, the diagnosis of proctitis is a clinical diagnosis that is supported by the lack of evidence of an alternative explanation for rectal inflammation. The differential diagnosis of proctitis is summarized in Table 28-1. Exploration of the differential diagnosis depends on the clinical history and suspicion of specific diseases.

With relapsing disease or unremitting symptoms despite aggressive treatment, extension of disease from proctitis to left-sided ulcerative colitis or pancolitis should be considered. Several epidemiologic studies have been published demonstrating extension of disease in a significant number of patients with proctitis. In a study of 1116 patients from a referral practice database, Farmer et al reported a 46% extension rate from ulcerative proctitis to more extensive disease.[9] This percentage is higher than community studies, but emphasizes the need to consider extension of disease in patients with poor control of their symptoms.[10]

SPECIFIC TREATMENT OF MUCOSAL INFLAMMATION

Aminosalicylates

The aminosalicylates are the backbone of the treatment of ulcerative colitis and proctitis.[11-14] The efficacy of sulfasalazine in the treatment of IBD was suspected in the 1940s and verified in the 1950s with confirmation of value in maintenance of remission documented in 1964. With the understanding of the efficacy of the 5-aminosalicylate acid (5-ASA) portion of sulfasalazine in the treatment of ulcerative colitis in 1977, numerous derivatives and formulations have been developed, investigated, and marketed (Table 28-3). The impaired motility of the colon proximal to the line of demarcation of active disease decreases the amount of orally administered mesalamine in contact with the inflamed mucosa.[15] During an acute relapse, rectal suppositories or enemas have the advantage of excellent contact with the inflamed mucosa whereas the oral drugs are distributed in the stool and dwell in the normal section of the colon.[16] 5-ASA drugs are considered very safe, although there are patients who are sensitive to 5-ASA and develop a chemical colitis manifested by edematous and often ulcerated mucosa that appears similar to Crohn's colitis. In a careful evaluation of patients with indisputable mesalamine sensitivity, it has been demonstrated that a specific serologic marker or specific histologic finding is not present in individuals with mesalamine toxicity.[17] If mesalamine sensitivity is suspected, discontinue the mesalamine drug for 72 hours. If symptomatic improvement occurs, this withdrawal trial supports mesalamine sensitivity.

For patients with ulcerative proctitis, conservative maintenance management with mesalamine follows the guidelines that have been established for ulcerative colitis.[18-20] Primary therapy with mesalamine suppositories is favored. The direct rectal application of a 1000-mg mesalamine suppository provides a concentrated dose to the distal 15 to 20 cm of the colon that is superior to rectal mesalamine concentrations with oral medications. Because the rectum effectively moves a liquid enema out of the rectum and into

TABLE 28-3

AVAILABLE AMINOSALICYLATES

Product	Preparation	Dose
Rectal		
ROWASA	Enema	4 g nightly
CANASA	Suppository	1000 mg
		1000 mg qd to bid
Oral		
Bacterial Azoreductase Dependent		
Sulfasalazine		500 mg; up to 4 g qd
Dipentum	Olsalazine	250 mg; up to 2 g qd
Colazal	Balsalazide	750 mg; up to 6.75 g qd (2.4 g 5-ASA)
Delayed-Release		
Pentasa	Mesalamine (ethylcellulose microgranules)	250 mg; up to 4 g qd
		500 mg; up to 4 g qd
Asacol	Mesalamine (Eudragit-S)	400 mg; up to 4.8 g qd
Apriso	Mesalamine	375 mg, 1.5 g daily qd
Lialda	Mesalamine	1.2 g up to 4.8 g qd

the proximal sigmoid and descending colon, the concentration of mesalamine delivered to the rectum with a suppository may actually be higher than the dose provided by a 4-g mesalamine enema. An acceptable initial treatment for ulcerative proctitis begins with a 1000-mg mesalamine suppository once a day until remission is achieved. The management protocol for maintenance of remission of ulcerative proctitis is weakly "evidence based" as the data for long-term daily treatment with mesalamine to maintain remission are sparse.[18,19] It is reasonable to continue mesalamine with at least one-half of the dose required to establish a remission. An acceptable alternative is to taper the mesalamine and wait for a symptomatic relapse. Some individuals, however, have critiqued this latter approach, noting that these patients may predispose themselves to subsequent flares given that medication is not continued. It is also unknown if these patients subsequently develop more extensive disease in their colons. Each relapse should be retreated, and if the interval between relapses is short, then continuous maintenance is recommended.

Because of the predominance of left-sided disease, the combination of oral and topical aminosalicylates is useful in inducing and maintaining remission.[21,22] A study by Safdi et al elegantly suggests that topical mesalamine is more effective than oral mesalamine in left-sided UC, but that the combination of 2.4 g of oral mesalamine and mesalamine enemas is linked to earlier and more complete cessation of rectal bleeding.[21] A study by D'Albasio et al demonstrated that the combination of 1.6 g of oral mesalamine with twice-weekly mesalamine enemas was linked to higher rates of maintenance of remission compared to oral therapy alone in patients with UC (61% versus 31%, respectively).[22] Topical mesalamine (enemas and suppositories) is effective in maintaining remission in patients with distal colitis even when used as infrequently as twice per week.[23] In another study, Biddle et al established that 75% (9 of 12) of patients randomized to receive mesalamine enemas remained in remission at 1 year, whereas 85% (11 of 13) of patients on placebo had relapsed by 16 weeks.[24] Similarly, mesalamine suppositories maintained long-term remission in patients with ulcerative proctitis. By 12 and 24 months, respectively, 86% and 89% of placebo-treated patients had relapsed, compared with 32% and 46% of patients treated with mesalamine suppositories. A meta-analysis established that, in patients with left-sided UC and ulcerative proctitis, topical mesalamine showed greater efficacy and fewer side effects than oral therapies and topical steroids.[25]

Campieri et al demonstrated that mesalamine suppositories were effective in inducing remission in patients with ulcerative proctitis (distal colitis up to 20 cm).[26] In that study, 74% of patients receiving mesalamine suppositories (1.5 g) achieved clinical remission at 4 weeks, compared with only 39% of patients receiving placebo.

Glucocorticoids

The general immunosuppression caused by glucocorticoids often induces symptomatic remission in patients with ulcerative proctitis. However, avoiding glucocorticoid therapy has become the mantra of the gastroenterologist caring for IBD patients. Many questions focus on the medical cost of the short-term benefit of steroids in terms of changing the character of disease and the iatrogenic medical complications that arise from steroid use. Glucocorticoids follow mesalamine in the "induction of remission" treatment algorithm. Their use should be accompanied by a strategy to minimize the cumulative systemic exposure to steroids. Topical rectal therapy applies the steroid dose to the area of the inflammation with the same distribution characteristics demonstrated for mesalamine suppositories and enemas. The inflamed mucosa poorly absorbs steroids, and systemic glucocorticoid effects are least likely with topical rectal therapy with limited colonic distribution (ie, suppositories rather than enemas). As the mucosa heals, glucocorticoid absorption improves, and systemic effects of steroids may occur.

Systemic steroids are rarely indicated in ulcerative proctitis; however, seasonal or infectious relapses can be linked to high numbers of eosinophils, which may be determined by increased numbers of fecal eosinophils,[27,28] Charcot-Leyden crystals in the stool, or with biopsy evidence of eosinophilic mucosal migration. When eosinophils are implicated in the symptomatic relapse of disease, high-dose, short-term steroids are often effective.[29] The diurnal variation of eosinophil function often provides a useful clinical clue that eosinophil activation is related to the current flare of colitis.[30] Eosinophils are most active between 11 pm and 2 am; thus, a patient with dominant colitis symptoms during this time likely has active eosinophils that should be modulated.[30] Eosinophils are usually sensitive to high plasma levels of steroids; thus, an intravenous dose of steroids (eg, Solu-Medrol 60 mg IV) or a rapidly tapering daily dose of oral steroids (eg, 60, 50, 40, 30, 20, 10 mg of prednisone) may induce a durable remission lasting weeks, months, or until a new stimulus activates the colitis. Even without documented eosinophilic activation of a colitis flare, an excellent clinical response to the first 48 hours of systemic steroids suggests eosinophils are pivotal in the current flare of the disease, and a short course of steroids may be all that is required for inducing remission. Lessons from the Tryptophan-Eosinophil-Myalgia syndrome include the recognition that approximately 15% of eosinophils are resistant to steroids, making this subgroup of patients difficult to manage. If a patient has one severe flare within 1 year or 2 or more flares within 1 year mandating more than 3 months of continuous steroids to control a relapse, immunomodulation therapy should be considered as *there is no place in the treatment of IBD for maintenance steroids.*[31,32] A recent American Gastroenterological Association position paper recommends the use of steroids as initial treatment in moderate-to-severe Crohn's disease and ulcerative colitis but not as maintenance therapy.[32]

Early in the development of budesonide, an enema formulation was determined to be beneficial[33-35]; however, budesonide is only commercially available in the United States as an ileal release form for Crohn's disease. The theoretical advantage of budesonide revolves around the efficient first-pass hepatic clearance of this steroid from the portal blood. This should decrease the systemic availability of the steroid and permit local steroid suppression of the disease without systemic toxicity. It is unfortunate that further studies were not conducted with topical rectal budesonide; however, approximately 15% of the blood flow from the distal colon escapes the portal system, increasing the amount of drug that may be available in the systemic circulation. Resurgence in interest in topical rectal administration of budesonide may provide another option for the long-term management of ulcerative proctitis.

Immunomodulation

Occasionally, refractory proctitis requires daily treatment with more potent immunologically active agents. Immunomodulation with 6-mercaptopurine (6-MP) or azathioprine (AZA) has become the standard of practice in the management of patients with difficult Crohn's disease. Initial concerns about the toxicity of these drugs have become less of an issue than the toxicity of chronic steroid use. The experience in patients with Crohn's disease led to the management of pancolitis with 6-MP/AZA. Success with ulcerative colitis management has permitted the expansion of the patients suitable for treatment to those with relatively refractory left-sided ulcerative colitis. When instituting therapy with AZA or 6-MP, it is possible to initiate therapy with a low dose and work up to the target dose or begin therapy at the target dose initially. Recent guidelines and the FDA have suggested that thiopurine methyltransferase be measured prior to initiation of therapy to exclude those patients who have low enzyme activity or who are homozygous mutant in this enzyme.[32] If a low dose is initially used, one can begin with 50-mg 6-MP and increase the dose to as high as 1.5 mg/kg in 25-mg increments until there is control of the disease or emerging toxicity. Most of the toxicity occurs in the first few months of treatment, and blood tests are followed carefully for leukopenia, abnormal aminotransferase levels, and pancreatitis. Methotrexate (25 mg intramuscularly [IM] once a week) may also be used to induce remission in patients with active Crohn's disease (Crohn's colitis), but many responsive patients have only a short period before a methotrexate-resistant relapse occurs. There are no controlled data, however, to support the use of methotrexate in patients with ulcerative colitis. Once symptomatic control is achieved, the dose may be lowered to 15 mg IM a week. The American Gastroenterology Association recommends that patients treated with methotrexate undergo routine laboratory work-up, including complete blood counts and liver-associated laboratory chemistries. Patients with persistently abnormal liver-associated chemistries should either discontinue therapy with methotrexate or undergo liver biopsy, the association recommends.[32]

OTHER TREATMENT

Numerous new drugs are being evaluated for use in ulcerative colitis. Each compound in development is being directed at a specific area of the gastrointestinal immune system. None of these drugs has crossed the registration hurdle of the FDA, but several new drugs should be available in the next few years. Heparin was briefly advocated for management of refractory ulcerative colitis, but a recent properly conducted trial with low molecular weight heparin failed to demonstrate therapeutic benefit.[36] Short-chain fatty acid enemas are not commercially available but have been reported to improve left-sided colitis.[37] These reports lack proper controls and numbers of patients. ICAM-1 antisense enemas (Alicaforsen) were reported to induce remission as often as mesalamine enemas with the benefit of prolonged remission.[38] Properly controlled trials are in progress to determine the initial response to ICAM-1 antisense enemas (Alicaforsen) and to assess the durability of the response. Epidermal growth factor enemas have also been shown to be effective in treating left-sided ulcerative colitis in a small double-blind study.[39] Ciprofloxacin and metronidazole are commonly used in patients with Crohn's disease for their effects on the immune system. Metronidazole failed to improve ulcerative colitis in a controlled trial, and the value of metronidazole in patients with left-sided ulcerative colitis is limited to the treatment of infectious colitis (eg, *Clostridium difficile)*.[40] Emerging interest in probiotics raises a new area for the management of IBD based on inducing changes in the relationship between the luminal environment and the mucosal immune system. Probiotics are an intriguing area of therapeutic development.

Surgical Intervention

Occasionally, the symptoms of ulcerative proctitis or steroid toxicity may be so severe that colectomy may be considered. The proper intervention is a total colectomy. Recently, the success of total proctocolectomy and ileal pouch anal anastomosis (IPAA) construction has been reported for patients with refractory left-sided ulcerative colitis,[41] which may be extrapolated to ulcerative proctitis if surgical intervention is unavoidable.

MODIFYING SYMPTOMS

Controlling mucosal inflammation is the cornerstone of management of ulcerative proctitis. Proper management also includes attention to the symptoms of the disease. In general, the diarrhea of ulcerative proctitis has little to do with the accelerated passage of digested material through the colon as the diarrhea occurs due to mucosal inflammation with blood, fluid, and colonic spasm contributing to the symptoms. For this reason and the inhibition of proximal colonic motility occurring as a result of rectal inflammation described earlier, antidiarrheal agents are not only ineffective, but they may increase the symptoms. Oral fiber supplementation with psyllium (Metamucil, Procter & Gamble, Cincinnati, OH) has been used effectively in ulcerative proctitis although the mechanism of action is not well understood. Improved symptoms may be related to the ability of psyllium to modulate colonic fluid, which will increase the fluid in desiccated stool proximal to the line of demarcation of disease and also absorb any excessive fluid in the lumen. Recent attention to the effects of the luminal environment on colonic inflammation offers another possible mechanism of action as psyllium may dilute luminal contents and reduce the concentration of any proteins, chemicals, or toxins that might play a role in activating the mucosal immune system.

Perineal dermatitis presents with perineal itching, pain, and occasionally bleeding. The attempt to maintain perineal hygiene in the presence of diarrhea often leads to physical trauma from the perineum-related cleansing. Patients should be instructed in proper perineal hygiene, including gentle cleansing following a stool and with bathing. The perineum should not be scrubbed, but gently flooded with water and patted dry (not rubbed) with the use of a hair dryer to evaporate the residual moisture. Care should be taken not to burn the skin. A barrier can be gently applied to protect the skin from the acidic stool contents, which remove the protective oils and injure the skin. I recommend Balneol (Solvay Pharmaceuticals, Marietta, GA), although recently I have been using a 3.3% concentration of cholestyramine in white petroleum, which is formulated locally and provides considerable symptomatic relief. In addition to the diarrheal stools, spontaneous relaxation of the internal anal sphincter occurs commonly with rectal inflammation.[5,6] The IAS relaxation is associated with small amounts of rectal mucus leakage, which damages the skin through the same mechanism. Because histamine is related to normal IAS relaxation, antihistamines are useful in decreasing the perineal soiling and injury.[42]

Tenesmus occurs with rectal contraction and IAS relaxation. In IBD patients, tenesmus is related to rectal inflammation and often improves with control of rectal inflammation. Antihistamines decrease rectal spasm and restore the physiologic integrity of the anal sphincter complex. Topical rectal therapy can be initiated to control the tenesmus, or antihistamines can be used to change the anorectal dynamics and improve this troublesome symptom.[43]

REFRACTORY DISEASE

Patients who fail to respond to treatment should be re-evaluated in order to determine whether the initial diagnosis is correct or whether there has been extension of the disease to include a larger proportion of the colon. Unrecognized problems may include infection, solitary rectal ulcer syndrome, ischemic colitis, Crohn's colitis, concurrent irritable bowel syndrome, drug-induced colitis, or mesalamine sensitivity. Mesalamine sensitivity may occur at any time in the course of treatment. Cases where documentation of sensitivity to mesalamine is present benefit from withdrawing the drug and observing symptomatic improvement. In our series, this was followed by a mesalamine enema challenge and repeat assessment of symptoms and endoscopic appearance.[44] The response to withdrawal is dramatic and usually occurs within 72 hours. Because little is lost by discontinuing the mesalamine treatment for this brief period, suspected mesalamine sensitivity should be tested by withdrawing mesalamine and reassessing the symptoms. Reassessment should include physical examination, laboratory tests including stool cultures with an assessment for *Clostridium difficile*, visualizing the mucosa by flexible sigmoidoscopy, or colonoscopy with biopsy evaluation.

CONCLUSION

Ulcerative proctitis can respond to topical mesalamine for both induction and maintenance of remission. However, because some proctitis patients will extend to either left-sided or universal ulcerative colitis, it is wise to discuss adding oral mesalamine to topical mesalamine treatment.[10] Studies have shown that topical 5-ASAs are more effective in controlling proctitis and proctosigmoiditis than steroids alone, and topical 5-ASAs can be helpful in maintaining remission. Because patients may have difficulty retaining suppositories or enemas, steroid foams may be helpful in inducing remission. Proctitis has not been associated with an increased risk of dysplasia or colorectal cancer. However, proctitis can extend to left-sided and universal colitis, and, therefore, one needs to be vigilant in dysplasia and cancer screening when patients have extended. It is argued that if a patient extends to left-sided or universal colitis, screening colonoscopy should be started at the time of the diagnosis of proctitis, not from the time the patient extended (again the argument being that it is difficult to determine when the patient extended). While most patients with proctitis have mild to moderate disease, some patients will have refractory disease, and in those patients the entire spectrum of therapy for universal colitis needs to be used. This includes IV steroids, cyclosporine, and in select patients infliximab or surgery. In conclusion, proctitis spans the spectrum of mild, moderate, and severe disease and is capable of extending to left-sided or universal ulcerative colitis at which time it confers an increased risk of dysplasia and colorectal cancer. However, if proctitis stays limited to the distal 15 to 20 cm, there is no increased risk of dysplasia or cancer.

REFERENCES

1. Carbonnel F, Lavergne A, Lémann M, et al. Colonoscopy of acute colitis: a safe and reliable tool for assessment of severity. *Dig Dis Sci.* 1994;39:1550-1557.
2. Rajwal SR, Puntis JW, McClean P, et al. Endoscopic rectal sparing in children with untreated ulcerative colitis. *J Pediatr Gastroenterol Nutr.* 2004;38:66-69.
3. Jewkes J, Larson HE, Price AB, Sanderson PJ, Davies HA. Aetiology of acute diarrhea in adults. *Gut.* 1981;22:388-392.
4. Cimolai N. Anaerobic infections. In: Cimolai N, ed. *Laboratory Diagnosis of Bacterial Infections.* New York, NY: Marcel Dekker, Inc; 2001:713.
5. Rao SS, Read NW, Davison PA, Bannister JJ, Holdsworth CD. Anorectal sensitivity and responses to rectal distention in patients with ulcerative colitis. *Gastroenterology.* 1987;93(6):1270-1275.
6. Rao SS, Holdsworth CD, Read NW. Symptoms and stool patterns in patients with ulcerative colitis. *Gut.* 1988;29(3):342-345.
7. Lennard-Jones JE, Langman MJ, Jones FA. Faecal stasis in proctocolitis. *Gut.* 1962;3(4):301-305.
8. Cowan GO, Das KM, Eastwood MA. Further studies of sulphasalazine metabolism in the treatment of ulcerative colitis. *Br J Med.* 1977;2:1057-1059.
9. Farmer RG, Easley KA, Rankin GB. Clinical patterns, natural history and progression of ulcerative colitis: a long-term follow-up of 1116 patients. *Dig Dis Sci.* 1993;38:1137.
10. Langholz E, Munkholm P, Davidsen M, Nielsen OH, Binder V. Changes in extent of ulcerative colitis: a study on the course and prognostic factors. *Scand J Gastroenterol.* 1996;31(3):260-266.
11. Vecchi M, Saibeni S, Devani M, Rondonotti E, De Franchis R. Review article: diagnosis, monitoring and treatment of distal colitis. *Aliment Pharmacol Ther.* 2003;17(Suppl 2):2-6.

12. Gisbert JP, Gomollon F, Mate J, Pajares JM. Role of 5-aminosalicylic acid (5-ASA) in treatment of inflammatory bowel disease: a systematic review. *Dig Dis Sci.* 2002;47:471-488.
13. Frieri G, Pimpo MT, Palumbo GC, et al. Rectal and colonic mesalazine concentration in ulcerative colitis; oral versus oral plus topical treatment. *Aliment Pharmcol Ther.* 1999;13:1413-1417.
14. Cohen RD, Woseth DM, Thisted RA, Hanauer SB. A meta-analysis and overview of the literature on treatment options for left-sided ulcerative colitis and ulcerative proctitis. *Am J Gastroenterol.* 2000;95:1263-1276.
15. Hebden JM, Blackshaw PE, Perkins AC, Wilson CG, Spiller RC. Limited exposure of the healthy distal colon to orally-dosed formulation is further exaggerated in active left-sided ulcerative colitis. *Aliment Pharmcol Ther.* 2000;14:155-161.
16. Gionchetti P, Rizzello F, Venture A, et al. Comparison of oral with rectal mesalazine in the treatment of ulcerative proctitis. *Dis Colon Rectum.* 1998;41:93-97.
17. Sturgeon JB, Bhatia P, Hermans D, Miner PB Jr. Exacerbation of chronic ulcerative colitis with mesalamine. *Gastroenterology.* 1995;108:1889-1893.
18. Marteau P, Crand J, Foucault M, Rambaud JC. Use of mesalazine slow release suppositories 1 g three times per week to maintain remission of ulcerative proctitis: a randomized double blind placebo controlled multicenter study. *Gut.* 1998;42:195-199.
19. d'Albasio G, Paoluzi P, Campieri M, et al. Maintenance treatment of ulcerative proctitis with mesalazine suppositories: a double-blind placebo-controlled trial. The Italian IBD Study Group. *Am J Gastroenterol.* 1998;93:799-803.
20. Pica R, Paoluzi OA, Iacopini F, et al. Oral mesalamine (5-ASA) treatment may protect against proximal extension of mucosal inflammation in ulcerative proctitis. *Inflamm Bowel Dis.* 2004; 10:731-736.
21. Safdi M, DeMicco M, Sninsky C, et al. A double-blind comparison of oral versus rectal mesalamine versus combination therapy in the treatment of distal ulcerative colitis. *Am J Gastroenterol.* 1997;92(10):1867-1871.
22. D'Albasio G, Pacini F, Camarri E, et al. Combined therapy with 5-aminosalicylic acid tablets and enemas for maintaining remission in ulcerative colitis: a randomized double-blind study. *Am J Gastroenterol.* 1997;92(7):1143-1147.
23. Hanauer S, Good LI, Goodman MW, et al. Long-term use of mesalamine (Rowasa) suppositories in remission maintenance of ulcerative proctitis. *Am J Gastroenterol.* 2000;95(7):1749-1754.
24. Biddle WL, Greenberger NJ, Swan JT, McPhee MS, Miner PB Jr. 5-aminosalicylic acid enemas: effective agent in maintaining remission in left-sided ulcerative colitis. *Gastroenterology.* 1988;94(4):1075-1079.
25. Cohen RD, Woseth DM, Thisted RA, Hanauer SB. A meta-analysis and overview of the literature on treatment options for left-sided ulcerative colitis and ulcerative proctitis. *Am J Gastroenterol.* 2000;95(5):1263-1276.
26. Campieri M, DeFranchis R, Bianchi Porro G, Ranzi T, Brunetti G, Barbara L. Mesalazine (5-aminosalicylic acid) suppositories in the treatment of ulcerative proctitis or distal proctosigmoiditis: a randomized controlled trial. *Scand J Gastroenterol.* 1990;25(7): 663-668.
27. Jeziorska M, Haboubi N, Schofield P, Woolley DE. Distribution and activation of eosinophils in inflammatory bowel disease using an improved immunohistochemical technique. *J Pathol.* 2001;194(4):484-492.
28. Carvalho ATP, Elia CCS, de Souza HSP, et al. Immunohistochemical study of intestinal eosinophils in inflammatory bowel disease. *J Clin Gastroenterol.* 2003;36:120-125.
29. Sangfelt P, Carlson M, Thörn M, Lööf L, Raab Y. Neutrophil and eosinophil granule proteins as markers of response to local prednisolone treatment in distal ulcerative colitis and proctitis. *Am J Gastroenterol.* 2001;96(4):1085-1090.
30. Miner PB. Seeing red in inflammatory bowel disease: the eosinophil at center stage? *Inflamm Bowel Dis.* 2006;10(3):329-330.
31. Lichtenstein GR, Hanauer SB, Sandborn WJ; Practice Parameters Committee of American College of Gastroenterology. Management of Crohn's disease in adults. *Am J Gastroenterol.* 2009;104(2): 465-483.
32. Lichtenstein GR, Abreu MT, Cohen R, Tremaine W; American Gastroenterological Association. American Gastroenterological Association Institute medical position statement on corticosteroids, immunomodulators, and infliximab in inflammatory bowel disease. *Gastroenterology.* 2006;130(3):935-939.
33. Bar-Meir S, Fidder HH, Faszczyk M, et al; International Budesonide Study Group. Budesonide foam versus hydrocortisone acetate foam in the treatment of active ulcerative proctosigmoiditis. *Dis Colon Rectum.* 2003;46:929-936.
34. Danielsson A, Edsbacker S, Lofberg R, et al. Pharmacokinetics of budesonide enema in patients with distal ulcerative colitis or proctitis. *Aliment Pharmacol Ther.* 1993;7:401-407.
35. Hanauer SB, Robinson M, Pruitt R, et al. Budesonide enema for the treatment of active, distal ulcerative colitis and proctitis: a dose-ranging study. US Budesonide enema study group. *Gastroenterology.* 1998;115:525-532.
36. Chande N, McDonald JW, Macdonald JK. Unfractionated or low-molecular weight heparin for induction of remission in ulcerative colitis. *Cochrane Database Syst Rev.* 2008;(2):CD006774.
37. Breuer RI, Soergel KH, Lashner BA, et al. Short chain fatty acid rectal irrigation for left-sided ulcerative colitis: a randomised, placebo controlled trial. *Gut.* 1997;40(4):485-491.
38. Miner PB Jr, Wedel MK, Xia S, Baker BF. Safety and efficacy of two dose formulations of alicaforsen enema compared with mesalazine enema for treatment of mild to moderate left-sided ulcerative colitis: a randomized, double-blind, active-controlled trial. *Aliment Pharmacol Ther.* 2006;23(10):1403-1413.
39. Sinha A, Nightingale J, West KP, Berlanga-Acosta J, Playford RJ. Epidermal growth factor enemas with oral mesalamine for mild-to-moderate left-sided ulcerative colitis or proctitis. *N Engl J Med.* 2003;349:395-397.
40. Kelly CP, LaMont JT. Clostridium difficile: more difficult than ever. *N Engl J Med.* 2008;359(18):1932-1940.
41. Hassan I, Horgan AF, Nivatvongs S, Harrington J, Larson DR. Outcome of patients undergoing ileal pouch-anal anastomosis for left-sided chronic ulcerative colitis. *J Gastrointest Surg.* 2003;7:567-571.
42. Burleigh DE, D'Mello A. Neural and pharmacologic factors affecting motility of the internal anal sphincter. *Gastroenterology.* 1983;84(2):409-417.
43. Griffin MG, Miner PB. Refractory distal colitis: explanations and options. *Aliment Pharmacol Ther.* 1996;10:39-48.
44. Sturgeon JB, Bhatia P, Hermens D, Miner PB Jr. Exacerbation of chronic ulcerative colitis with mesalamine. *Gastroenterology.* 1995;108(6):1889-1893.

29

Medical Therapy of Left-Sided Ulcerative Colitis

Douglas B. Haghighi, DMD, MD and Bret A. Lashner, MD, MPH

Left-sided ulcerative colitis (UC) is not a distinct entity, but a less extensive form of pancolitis. Therefore, the epidemiologic and genetic characteristics are thought to be analogous. However, the rate of colorectal cancer seems to be proportional to the extent of disease. The primary treatment that has been used for left-sided disease is topical 5-ASA agents. In patients who do not respond to topical therapy, oral 5-ASA agents of differing delivery methods to the distal bowel can be used. There is much debate pertaining to the clinical superiority of the aforementioned oral 5-ASA agents.

Incidence and Prevalence

The incidence and prevalence of left-sided disease in UC is difficult to quantify because no epidemiologic studies have been conducted that consider that particular subset of patients with the disease. The current data pertain only to the overall incidence and prevalence of the disease. The highest incidence of UC is seen in the northern hemisphere, notably the United States, Canada, Scandinavia, Israel, and Northern Europe. Depending on the demographic area studied, the annual incidence of UC ranges from 0.5 to 6.3/100,000.[1,2] The prevalence of UC ranges from 10 to 70/100,000, but was noted to be as high as 169 per 100,000 in an Israeli study.[3] Studies in the United Kingdom and the United States have demonstrated that the disease does not predilect to a particular gender. However, Caucasians are at an increased risk of developing UC versus non-Caucasians.[4] Interestingly, a study from the United Kingdom reported that first-generation Asian migrants developed UC at the same rate as native Europeans within one generation, which would point to an environmental exposure as a possible factor in developing the disease.[5] Additional evidence for an environmental cause for UC, especially from an exposure at a young age, is the extreme variability in mortality among birth cohorts.[6]

Genetic Susceptibility

It is not known if patients with left-sided UC have any different genetic predisposition from those with more extensive disease. However, several studies have evaluated the overall genetic susceptibility of UC in certain ethnic groups. In Israel, Ashkenazi Jews who are of Eastern European descent have a nearly 6 times higher risk of developing the disease versus Sephardic Jews, who have Spanish, African, and Middle Eastern backgrounds, despite analogous environmental exposures. Moreover, as many as 20% of UC patients have a first- or second-degree relative who is afflicted with the disease. The relative risk for a first-degree relative of an ulcerative colitis patient to develop the disease is 5.1.[7] The patients who manifest the human leukocyte antigen-B27 are more likely to develop ankylosing spondylitis and uveitis.[1]

The perinuclear antineutrophil cytoplasmic antibodies (p-ANCA) have also been associated with ulcerative colitis. One study noted that 75% manifest p-ANCAs.[8] Jewish patients with the disease have a high rate of being p-ANCA positive and developing primary sclerosing cholangitis (PSC). Also, a positive test for p-ANCA may differentiate between ulcerative colitis and Crohn's disease as well as aid in the diagnosis of indeterminate colitis. P-ANCAs may be a predictor of chronic pouchitis because they were

Lichtenstein GR, ed.
Ulcerative Colitis: The Complete Guide to Medical Management (pp. 307-318)

observed in 100% of patients with chronic pouchitis and 50% of patients with a pouch but no pouchitis.[9]

Several studies have alluded to specific mutations, which would represent linkages to ulcerative colitis. The chromosomes involved include 1, 3, 4, 6, 7, 10, 12, 16, and 22.[10,11]

ENVIRONMENTAL FACTORS

Current smokers are not as likely to develop UC compared to community-based nonsmoking controls. Moreover, former smokers are more likely to develop the disease when compared to controls.[12,13] Former smokers, when compared to nonsmokers, are diagnosed at a younger age and have a greater degree of active disease at the time of diagnosis.[14] The above information is complicated by the fact that passive smoking exposure in nonsmoking children increases risk of the development of UC when compared to community-based controls.[15] Nicotine, in the form of a transdermal patch or as chewing gum, has successfully treated UC, especially in former smokers, by a mechanism that has yet to be elucidated.[16,17] Nicotine addiction may occur if therapy lasts longer than 8 weeks, and maintenance therapy with nicotine patches is not effective.[18]

There are several other potential studied risk factors for ulcerative colitis. Three cohort studies have demonstrated possible harmful effects of oral contraceptive use on the development of UC, but these findings could not be supported by a case-control study of incident cases and community-based controls.[19] A case-control study noted that a high intake of mono- and polyunsaturated fat, as well as vitamin B6, has been shown to be associated with the development of UC.[20] Finally, a meta-analysis of 13 case-control studies involving 2270 UC patients demonstrated that appendectomy reduced the risk of developing the disease by 69%.[21] The reason for this association is unclear. There are presently no data that specifically evaluate whether left-sided disease is modified with any of these risk factors.

CLINICAL FEATURES

The typical presentation of a UC patient includes rectal bleeding, diarrhea, tenesmus, and abdominal pain. Criteria developed by Truelove and Witts in 1955 has been used to classify the severity of the disease as either mild, moderate, or severe.[22] Patients who have mild disease have 4 or fewer bowel movements per day, small amounts of blood in their stool, a normal sedimentation rate, with no fever, tachycardia, or anemia. Those who are classified as severe have more than 6 bowel movements per day, have anemia, tachycardia, and fever, with a sedimentation rate more than 30. Patients with moderate disease activity fall in between mild and severe disease. Patients who are considered "toxic" with fulminant colitis are febrile, tachycardic, commonly have greater than 10 bowel movements per day with bleeding, and have abdominal tenderness and distension. Also, these patients have radiologic evidence of bowel wall edema with possible dilation. Patients with left-sided disease have numerous trips to the washroom to pass small amounts of blood and mucous and have tenesmus.

Because patients with moderate disease (according to Truelove and Witts index of disease activity[22]) have a wide variability. Such a classification of disease activity is inadequate for clinical trials where objective and sensitive measures of disease activity are required. A combination of endoscopic, histologic, and symptom score usually is preferred in clinical trials. Numerous objective markers of inflammation including measurement of the ESR, orosomucoid levels, CRP, leukocyte and platelet count, neopterin, IL-8, indium-labeled white blood cell scanning, and fecal alpha-1-antitrypsin determinations have been investigated as markers of disease activity; but none is as sensitive as the history, physical examination, and colonoscopy.[23]

ESTABLISHING THE DIAGNOSIS

IBD patients who are experiencing abdominal pain and/or diarrhea may be suffering from an exacerbation of their disease, a superimposed viral infection like CMV, or irritable bowel syndrome-like manifestations of IBD. Visualization of the colonic mucosa is invaluable in establishing the diagnosis of ulcerative colitis. Colonoscopy with biopsy for histological analysis can correctly differentiate ulcerative colitis from Crohn's colitis, as well as from other colonic diseases in 85% to 90% of the patients. The remaining 10% to 15% will be classified as indeterminate colitis. Of note, greater than half of those patients with indeterminate colitis eventually will be diagnosed with Crohn's colitis.[24]

Colonoscopy to establish the diagnosis should not be performed in patients with severe disease due to the increased risk for bowel perforation. The necessary information can be obtained by flexible sigmoidoscopy in an unprepared colon and with minimal air insufflation.

Recently, fecal lactoferrin had been used to differentiate inflammatory from noninflammatory conditions. Kane and co-workers[25] from the University of Chicago, the Mayo Clinic, and Children's Hospital in Boston studied 104 CD patients, 80 UC patients, 31 IBS patients, and 56 health controls. Fecal lactoferrin was markedly elevated in active CD and active UC. All other groups had relatively low levels. For detecting active inflammation, fecal lactoferrin had a sensitivity of 90% and a specificity of 100%.

Fecal lactoferrin is inexpensive and readily available for use in clinical practice. With the excellent sensitivity and specificity as reported above, it could be a very important first-line test to distinguish among symptomatic IBD patients who are candidates for further testing to assess extent and severity of disease and for anti-inflammatory therapy.

ASSESSING THE EXTENT OF DISEASE: LEFT-SIDED DISEASE VERSUS PANCOLITIS

Untreated UC usually involves the rectal mucosa and extends proximally in a continuous fashion. To adequately determine the extent of disease, it is important to perform a colonoscopy that defines the extent of the disease. Radiology is rarely employed for this reason as it underestimates the true extent of the disease and does not allow for biopsies to be obtained.

Unlike CD, the extent of disease in ulcerative colitis is the principal variable in elucidating the prognosis. In a series of 1116 patients, 46% had endoscopic proctosigmoiditis, 17% had left-sided disease (to the splenic flexure), and 37% had pancolitis at the time of presentation.[26] Patients presenting with pancolitis were more likely to develop refractory symptoms, toxic megacolon, malignancy, extraintestinal manifestations, and require surgery. On follow-up, more than half of the patients with limited disease advanced to more extensive disease. Another series demonstrated that of 1736 patients with ulcerative colitis, nearly 20% were diagnosed with ulcerative proctitis at presentation.[27] Also, in 27% of the patients, extension of disease was noted: 16% to the sigmoid colon, 7% to the splenic flexure, and extensive disease in just under 5%. The estimated risk of disease extension to the sigmoid colon or to the splenic flexure is 20% at 5 years and 54% at 10 years. The risk of extension beyond the splenic flexure is 10% at 10 years. The risk is further increased by being a nonsmoker, having three or more relapses a year, as well as receiving immunosuppressives or systemic steroids. Based on this information, repeated examinations may be necessary to confirm that the disease has not advanced proximally, which would alter prognosis.

COMPLICATIONS

Cholestatic liver disease is the most common hepatic abnormality of IBD and is approximately 3 times more common in UC than in CD.[28] Approximately 5% of UC patients will develop cholestasis, most commonly pericholangitis. Only 1% to 2% of UC patients will develop PSC, a cholestatic liver disease diagnosed by the appearance of extrahepatic and intrahepatic strictures on a cholangiogram. PSC usually is a consequence of pancolitis and is seen less often in left-sided disease. Pericholangitis usually does not progress to cirrhosis, but PSC can progress and may require liver transplantation. Rarely, PSC patients will develop cholangiocarcinoma. Cholestatic liver disease in UC is a risk factor for colorectal cancer and dysplasia.[29] Treatment of bowel symptoms, even total proctocolectomy, does not influence the course of cholestatic liver disease. Fatty infiltration of the liver, chronic active hepatitis, amyloidosis, and drug-induced liver disease (from steroids, AZA, 6-MP, or sulfasalazine) are other reported hepatic manifestations of IBD.

Erythema nodosum, present in up to 3% of patients, is characterized by raised tender erythematous nodules, typically appearing on the extremities. Pyoderma gangrenosum, a rare ulcerating and necrotic lesion, seen in both CD and UC represents an extraintestinal manifestation of vasculitis. Healing is prolonged and usually requires immunosuppressive therapy with steroids, 6-MP or AZA, oral antibiotics for superinfection, and steroid injections for indurated margins. Cyclosporine or infliximab have been successful in cases refractory to steroids, AZA, and/or 6-MP.

Arthritis of IBD is usually nonerosive, mono or pauciarticular, and asymmetric. The large joints are most often affected, and there is no synovial destruction. Arthritis more often affects females, exhibits no subcutaneous nodules, and correlates with disease activity.

Ocular symptoms and signs of IBD include blurred vision, eye pain, photophobia, inflammatory cells in the anterior chamber, and keratic precipitates. Patients with uveitis often have HLA-B27, while patients with episcleritis and iritis usually do not.

There may be a small increase in mortality associated with UC. This increase is likely secondary to either surgical complications or cardiovascular catastrophes. Among 1160 UC patients identified between 1962 and 1987 and followed to 1997, Winther et al reported that 261 patients had died.[30] Compared to the general Danish population, the standardized mortality ratio for ulcerative colitis patients was 1.05 (95% confidence interval [CI] 0.92 to 1.19). Twenty-five (9.6%) deaths were caused by complications of ulcerative colitis, mostly from postoperative infectious and cardiovascular complications. The highest mortality was seen in patients diagnosed after age 50 who required surgery. The standardized mortality ratio for colorectal cancer was 1.49 (95% CI 0.47 to 2.82). Overall cancer mortality was diminished in ulcerative colitis patients (SMR 0.70, 95% CI 0.52 to 0.93), likely due to non-smoking effects in this population.[30] Card and colleagues used a large UK database to examine IBD mortality.[31] The relative risk of death was 1.44 (95% CI 1.31 to 1.58) for ulcerative colitis and 1.73 (95% CI 1.54 to 1.96) for CD. Risks were highest in UC patients aged 40 to 59 (relative risk 1.79) and Crohn's patients aged 20 to 39 (relative risk 3.82). Surgical complications can be minimized by avoiding steroids whenever possible and recommending surgery earlier in the course of disease if appropriate (ie, operating before toxic megacolon develops). Cardiovascular complications can be minimized through aggressive control of disease activity and aggressive use of programs of cigarette smoking cessation. It is also reassuring to note that cancer surveillance strategies may be working by reducing cancer-related mortality.

COLORECTAL CANCER

Over the course of the disease, colorectal cancer is expected to occur in nearly 6% and be the cause of death in approximately 3% of UC patients with extensive disease. Colorectal cancer incidence and mortality rates seem to be decreasing and are approaching the rates of populations unaffected by IBD.[32] However, the risk of colorectal cancer in UC patients is elevated and has been estimated to be more than 4 times what is expected among age- and gender-matched controls.[33] Most of the studies conducted to evaluate cancer in UC are done on patients with pancolitis. The risk in patients with left-sided disease appears to be lower.

The colorectal cancer risk in UC increases with increasing extent and duration of disease, older age at symptom onset, and cholestatic liver disease.[34] High-risk patients, such as those with disease proximal to splenic flexure of more than 7 years, should be enrolled in surveillance programs where colonoscopies with multiple biopsies are performed every 1 to 3 years, depending on the individual risk. The screening interval should decrease as the duration of disease increases.[35] Surveillance should be performed in patients with left-sided disease, but because the risk is lower, it can be done less often.[34-38] The risk of colorectal cancer in left-sided colitis may be delayed but, over time, it equals that of universal colitis.[39] The American College of Gastroenterology guidelines recommend examinations every 1 to 2 years for the first decade after screening in patients with both left-sided and extensive UC.[40,41] Recent studies have suggested that cancer incidence may not actually rise over time, and the need to intensify surveillance after 20 years is disputed.[42] However, this may reflect increased surveillance. New evidence suggests that the risk of colon cancer may be decreased in patients with persistently quiescent disease, but again this may reflect continued surveillance in this population. It is unclear whether surveillance requirements may be reduced to every 5 years in patients with quiescent UC.[43]

The finding of the premalignant lesions of low-grade dysplasia and high-grade dysplasia should prompt action of some sort, such as colectomy or more intensive surveillance. Because the natural history of patients found to have low-grade dysplasia was thought to be relatively benign, intensive surveillance rather than colectomy usually was recommended to these patients.

A cohort study on 46 UC patients found to have low-grade dysplasia in flat mucosa during a surveillance colonoscopy demonstrated that, over time, 14 (30%) patients progressed to more advanced neoplasia (high-grade dysplasia or cancer). Seven patients developed colorectal cancer (2 stage I, 2 stage II, and 3 stage III). Survival curves demonstrated that the rate of progression was 53% at 5 years and 80% at 10 years. Among the 35 patients who had intensive surveillance after the initial finding of low-grade dysplasia, 4 developed cancer, and 5 developed high-grade dysplasia. Even in the 11 patients who had colectomy for low-grade dysplasia, 2 had cancer, and 1 had high-grade dysplasia in the colectomy specimen.[44]

When total proctocolectomy in ulcerative colitis is performed for the detection of dysplasia, there is associated with it a decreased quality of life, even if an IPAA is created. Typically, IPAA patients have 4 to 6 soft bowel movements daily as well as risks of incontinence, impotence, and pouchitis. For this reason, colectomy is reserved for patients with the highest risk of mortality from colorectal cancer. There is no controversy in recommending colectomy for patients who are found to have high-grade dysplasia or colorectal cancer. The progression of patients with low-grade dysplasia to more advanced pathology has not been known until now, but was not felt to be high enough to warrant colectomy with the resultant decreased quality of life. The previous study demonstrates that intensive surveillance in patients found to have low-grade dysplasia is not an acceptable strategy. The risk of cancer is too high. If confirmed by experienced pathologists, the finding of low-grade dysplasia in flat mucosa should prompt a recommendation for total colectomy in ulcerative colitis patients.

As noted previously, performing cancer surveillance via colonoscopy can minimize cancer mortality by recommending colectomy in patients who develop dysplasia. Unfortunately, surveillance programs generally have failed to influence mortality. Improvement in mortality rates will come as cancer surveillance techniques improve. Chromoendoscopy represents an easy, readily available technique that could be an important advance. Kiesslich and colleagues used chromoendoscopy in a randomized clinical trial of 165 ulcerative colitis patients.[45] In this study, 81 had conventional colonoscopic surveillance, and 84 had chromoendoscopy (0.1% methylene blue staining of the mucosa prior to biopsy) with more directed biopsy. Dysplasia was detected in 32 (38%) patients with chromoendoscopy and in 10 (12%) patients with conventional endoscopy (P=0.003). Other similar techniques are now undergoing evaluation in surveillance of patients with UC, including narrow band imaging and confocal microscopy.

Matsumoto and colleagues from Japan reported similar success with chromoendoscopy.[46] In 57 patients who had 117 surveillance examinations over an 8-year period, 20 patients with low-grade dysplasia and 8 patients with high-grade dysplasia were identified. Most of these dysplastic lesions were seen in flat mucosa, and the 49% rate of dysplasia detection is much higher than any rate from cancer surveillance programs, which usually is less than 10%.

Currently, research is being done to optimize the understanding of cancer biology and to determine whether intermediate markers of malignancy provide a more objective, accurate, sensitive, specific, and clinically useful marker than dysplasia. Candidate markers include DNA aneuploidy detected by flow cytometry and suppressor gene (particularly p53) mutations and loss of heterozygosity detected either immunohistochemically or with polymerase chain reaction techniques.[47-49]

Another area of controversy in ulcerative colitis and neoplasia is in regard to dysplasia-associated lesions or masses, the so-called DALM lesion. Distinguishing a DALM from an adenoma or a pseudopolyp may be impossible, but is vital in determining appropriate therapy. Typically, DALMs are elevated and have the nodular appearance of a sessile adenoma.[50] DALMs are thought to carry a poor prognosis and should prompt consideration for a colectomy. Two series of patients with DALMs did not have colectomy and did not develop cancer at a follow-up of 42 and 49 months.[51,52] However, in one of these studies, further review was performed at 82 months, and 1 in 24 patients developed adenocarcinoma and required colectomy.[53] To be safe, polypoid lesions with dysplasia in an area never affected with colitis (ie, a right-sided polyp in a patient with left-sided disease) in patients over the age of 50 years are the only lesions that should be considered adenomas and should be treated with polypectomy. Polypoid lesions with dysplasia in an area previously affected with colitis or in a younger person should be considered DALMs and treated with colectomy.[52] Patients with a stricture that cannot be traversed or adequately biopsied should have a colectomy as a result of the high risk of cancer or dysplasia in the stricture.[54]

CHEMOPREVENTION

Therapy for colorectal cancer is not always effective. Therefore, strategies for chemoprevention, when effective, should strongly be considered in IBD patients. For sporadic colorectal cancer, nonsteroidal anti-inflammatory drugs, folic acid, and calcium have been shown to be effective chemopreventive agents, largely from epidemiologic studies. In IBD patients, 5-ASA, folic acid, and ursodeoxycholic acid have been studied.

There have been 7 epidemiologic studies and a meta-analysis looking at 5-ASA as a chemopreventive agent.[55-62] The evidence is weak, but because 5-ASA also is effective in maintaining remission, these agents should be recommended for regular long-term use with at least 2 g/d. Three epidemiologic studies have studied folic acid with respect to chemoprevention.[63-65] Once again, the evidence is weak, but because folic acid is inexpensive, safe, and recommended for prevention of atherosclerotic heart disease, it too should be recommended for long-term use in IBD patients. There have been 2 studies, 1 epidemiologic and 1 randomized clinical trial, looking at ursodeoxycholic acid for cancer chemoprevention in IBD patients with PSC.[66,67] Both studies showed effectiveness, and ursodeoxycholic acid should be used in PSC patients for both cancer chemoprevention and for its effect on liver function. A third study, which was a cohort study, could not demonstrate such an effect.[68]

MANAGEMENT OF COLITIS

The general principles of medical therapy in UC, whether it is for distal disease or pancolitis, are to induce remission of the disease, maintain it, and prevent the extraintestinal manifestations of the disease, which were noted above.[69] Initially, a patient with UC should be counseled on dietary modifications and supplements to optimize their nutrition status, which will be outlined later. Medical therapy for distal disease or extensive disease should be instituted in a step-wise fashion. The spectrum of medical treatment in UC begins with 5-ASA agents (topical/oral), then progresses to steroids (oral/IV) and finally to immunosuppressive therapy. The initial therapy for extensive disease is an oral 5-ASA agent, and if the patient does not respond, then topical 5-ASA therapy is added. When juxtaposed to the treatment of extensive disease, initial therapy for left-sided disease is topical 5-ASA, and if the patient does not respond, then an oral 5-ASA agent is used to supplement therapy.

Therapy for patients with mild or moderate disease flare should include supportive therapy with fluids, anticholinergics, and antidiarrheals. However, antidiarrheals in patients with severely active disease could precipitate toxic megacolon. Supportive therapy allows the naturally remitting feature of UC to occur. Indeed, approximately one-third of the patients given placebo in randomized clinical trials achieve remission. Diet recommendations should include a multivitamin supplement. Complete bowel rest with total parental nutrition is not effective as primary therapy for UC patients.

Dietary supplements may be helpful. Eicosapentaenoic acid (fish oil) competes with arachidonic acid for metabolism by 5-lipoxygenase to produce leukotriene B5, a much less potent proinflammatory cytokine than arachidonic acid metabolite leukotriene B4. High doses of oral fish oil can treat UC and enable patients to reduce steroid intake.[70,71] However, extremely high doses cause odoriferous side effects, which limits the patient acceptance and use of such therapy.

Short-chain fatty-acids (acetate, butyrate, and propriate), which are products of colonic bacteria metabolism of dietary fiber, are fuel sources preferred by the colonic mucosa over glucose and ketone bodies. Short-chain fatty-acid enemas may be useful in patients with moderately active proctosigmoiditis, especially those refractory to more conventional therapy.[72,73] Oral butyrate coated in pH-dependent soluble polymer targeted for colonic delivery when combined with oral 5-ASA improves symptoms in UC better than 5-ASA alone.[74]

Administration of a nonpathogenic strain of *Escherichia coli* (*E. coli Nissle* 1917) was as effective as 5-ASA in maintaining remission in patients with ulcerative colitis.[75] Such a finding suggests that favorably altering the colonic flora with a probiotic may negate the "proinflammatory" effects of as-yet unidentified pathogenic bacteria.

AMINOSALICYLATES

For the past 50 years, sulfasalazine, the combination of sulfapyridine and 5-ASA, has been available for use in ulcerative colitis. 5-ASA is the therapeutically active ingredient that is released when colonic bacteria cleave a diazo bond with sulfapyridine. 5-ASA interferes with both the cyclo-oxygenase and 5-lipoxygenase pathways of arachidonic acid metabolism, as well as free-radical scavenging. Sulfasalazine given in divided doses of 2 to 4 g/d usually is helpful for treating mildly to moderately active UC and for maintaining remission.[76] Sulfasalazine is a competitive inhibitor of folic acid absorption (it inhibits the enzyme folate conjugase in the jejunum), and an oral supplement of folate is needed in patients so treated.[64]

Up to half of patients are allergic to or intolerant of sulfasalazine, especially at high doses, primarily to the sulfapyridine moiety of the medication. 5-ASA can be delivered directly to the patients with similar effectiveness by using newer, but more expensive, preparations:

- Topical
  - Rowasa enemas (Solvay, Marrietta, GA)
- Oral preparations
  - Olsalazine (Dipentum Celltech)
  - Resin-coated mesalamine (Asacol, Procter & Gamble, Cincinnati, OH)
  - Ethylcellulose-coated 5-ASA beads (Pentasa, Shire, Florence, NY)
- Multimatrix (MMX) mesalamine (Lialda, Shire, Wayne, PA)
- Delayed- and extended-release mesalamine (Apriso)
- Balsalazide (Colazal)

Olsalazine consists of two 5-ASA molecules linked by a diazo bond that requires cleavage from colonic bacteria. Although effective, a secretory diarrhea in 10% of patients limits its usefulness.[77] The frequency of diarrhea from Dipentum can be diminished by taking the medication with food. All of these compounds can both induce and maintain remission. Recently, Lialda (a delayed-release MMX mesalamine preparation) has been shown to be effective with once-daily dosing and is approved for use in UC.[78,79] Apriso (granulated mesalamine) 1.5 g/d (releasing at a pH of >6) in a delayed and extended capsule has been shown to maintain remission in mild to moderate UC.[80,81]

Balsalazide (Colazal, Salix, Raleigh, NC) is 5-ASA attached via a diazo bond to an inert carrier molecule. Theoretically, 5-ASA products with a diazo bond delivery system should have an advantage over the resin-coated agents in regard to drug delivery to the distal colon and therefore efficacy in treating left-sided disease. Over the past several years, there have been several studies comparing the efficacy of balsalazide to mesalamine in inducing remission of left-sided UC. The results of these studies have yielded conflicting results. A randomized placebo-controlled study from England compared balsalazide 6.75 mg to mesalamine 2.4 mg with the primary endpoint being the proportion of patients in complete remission, defined as patient score of none/mild and endoscopy score of 0 to 1. At the end of 3 months, 62% of patients taking balsalazide achieved remission compared to 37% who were administered mesalamine. Moreover, 48% of the patients taking balsalazide had adverse effects compared to 71% for the group prescribed mesalamine.[82] However, these results should be interpreted appropriately, given that the formulation of mesalamine in the United Kingdom is reported to release less than 80% of a comparable dose manufactured in the United States.[83]

Another randomized clinical UK study from 2002 compared balsalazide 6.75 g to mesalamine 2.5 g with the primary endpoint as a patient functional assessment in regard to rectal bleeding with the secondary endpoint being time to remission, proportion in complete remission, and improvement in sigmoidoscopic score. No significant difference was demonstrated in the primary endpoint with remission occurring in 46% of the balsalazide group and 44% of those taking mesalamine. Also, none of the secondary endpoints demonstrated a significant difference.[84] A third randomized clinical study conducted in the United States in 2002 examined the dose-response of balsalazide (2.25 and 6.75 mg) and mesalamine 2.4 mg in inducing remission in mild to moderate UC patients. The primary endpoint was the improvement in rectal bleeding plus at least one other variable that included a physician assessment, abdominal pain, stool frequency, improvement with sigmoidoscopy, and patient functional assessment at 8 weeks. The secondary endpoints included the measurement of patients who achieved complete remission, had an improved biopsy score, and had improved quality of life with a decrease in adverse outcomes. The primary endpoints were not met in this study. However, balsalazide at a dosage of 6.75 mg led to a statistically significant difference versus lower balsalazide dosage.[85] A new formulation of balsalazide (containing 1.1 g per tablet) allows for bid dosing—3.3 g tablets twice a day—for induction of remission in mild to moderate UC.[86]

Despite the theoretical advantage of balsalazide over mesalamine in treating left-sided UC, there is no clear clinical advantage. Therefore, topical 5-ASA therapy should be the first-line therapy for inducing remission in left-sided UC, followed by an oral 5-ASA if the patient does not respond favorably. The ultimate goal of therapy is to maintain remission with the oral 5-ASA agent, which induces reversal of disease, and to try to avoid corticosteroid use because of the many side effects. Currently, no trial has examined the use of mesalamine in the treatment of left-sided colitis versus pancolitis as a primary endpoint. All studies that have assessed mesalamine in the treatment of left-sided colitis to date are post-hoc analyses.

Because of the predominance of left-sided disease, the combination of oral and topical aminosalicylates is critical in inducing and maintaining remission.[90,91] A study by Safdi et al elegantly suggests that topical mesalamine is more effective than oral in left-sided UC, but that the combination of 2.4 g of oral mesalamine and mesalamine enemas is linked to earlier and more complete cessation of rectal bleeding.[90] A study by D'Albasio et al demonstrated that the combination of 1.6 g of oral mesalamine with twice-weekly mesalamine enemas was linked to higher rates of maintenance of remission compared to oral therapy alone in patients with UC (61% versus 31%, respectively).[91] Topical mesalamine (enemas and suppositories) is effective in maintaining remission in patients with distal colitis even when used as infrequently as twice per week.[92] In another study, Biddle et al established that 75% (9 of 12) of patients randomized to receive mesalamine enemas remained in remission at 1 year, whereas 85% (11 of 13) of patients on placebo had relapsed by 16 weeks.[93] Similarly, mesalamine suppositories maintained long-term remission in patients with ulcerative proctitis.[92] By 12 and 24 months, respectively, 86% and 89% of placebo-treated patients had relapsed, compared with 32% and 46% of patients treated with mesalamine suppositories. A meta-analysis established that, in patients with left-sided UC and ulcerative proctitis, topical mesalamine showed greater efficacy and fewer side effects than oral therapies and topical steroids.[94]

Campieri et al demonstrated that mesalamine suppositories were effective in inducing remission in patients with ulcerative proctitis (distal colitis up to 20 cm).[95] In that study, 74% of patients receiving mesalamine suppositories (1.5 g) achieved clinical remission at 4 weeks, compared with only 39% of patients receiving placebo.

CORTICOSTEROIDS

Oral, IV, or topical steroids are very effective for treating active ulcerative colitis through inhibition of phospholipase A2 and the subsequent decrease in the levels of leukotrienes. There is no difference in outcome if steroids are given on a continuous basis or given as a "pulse."[87] Prolonged prednisone administration, though, is limited by its side effects. Budesonide, a steroid analog, is 90% inactivated by the liver during the first pass. The compound is modified by packaging with ethylcellulose beads and eudrigit-L, ensuring small bowel and colonic effects before it is absorbed and inactivated. However, it is most efficacious in the terminal ileum and right colon and is not a first-line agent for left-sided disease. Budesonide has fewer adverse effects than prednisone.[88,89] Due to adrenal suppression, long-term use for its maintenance is not recommended.

IMMUNOSUPPRESSIVES

6-MP and its S-imidazole precursor, AZA, are purine ring analogs that interfere with DNA replication in rapidly dividing cells, such as lymphocytes and macrophages. These drugs are safe and effective, have different adverse effects from corticosteroids, and can be considered "steroid-sparing." Approximately 10% of patients require discontinuation for reversible marrow suppression, about 3% will experience acute pancreatitis, and 1% will develop allergy characterized by abdominal pain, fever, and rash. Both AZA and 6-MP at daily doses of 50 to 100 mg are effective maintenance therapy in UC, enabling patients to avoid long-term use of corticosteroids.[96,97] The duration of therapy before clinical response is observed can be longer than 3 months. Because of this delay in response, adjusting the dose according to response may not be appropriate. Some have suggested that the dose of immunosuppressives be increased until mild leukopenia develops because patients treated to leukopenia have a faster and more complete response.[98] Metabolite levels of 6-TG, the active metabolite, and 6-MMP, the toxic metabolite, can be determined to identify the dose that will find the narrow window between toxicity and effectiveness.[99]

Cyclosporine is a cyclic polypeptide that is used extensively as an immunosuppressive agent in organ transplantation. It inhibits (IL-2) gene transcription and thereby reduces activation of lymphocytes, mostly T helper cells. Cyclosporine binds to lipoproteins and requires bile salts for absorption. It is metabolized and inactivated by hepatic cytochrome p450 activity. Nephrotoxicity, hepatotoxicity, hypertrichosis, gingival hyperplasia, tremors, paresthesias, seizures, and lymphoproliferative disorders are the most common adverse effects. High-dose IV cyclosporine can initiate a quick response and successfully delay colectomy in up to 80% of patients with severely active UC.[100] The long-term success of avoiding a colectomy is 50% or less. Responders, though, have a superior quality of life than patients who require surgery.[101] Once remission is induced with IV cyclosporine, patients should be maintained on oral cyclosporine for at least 6 months as prednisone is tapered and AZA or 6-MP becomes effective.[102] There are no data specifically evaluating cyclosporine for left-sided UC.

Infliximab, a chimeric anti-TNFα antibody, has been approved for treatment of ulcerative colitis, regardless of extent of disease, based on the ACT 1 and ACT 2 trials.[103] These 2 randomized clinical trials studied a combined 768 patients followed for 46 weeks (ACT 1) or 22 weeks (ACT 2) and found that more than 60% of patients given infliximab responded to therapy compared to less than 40% of placebo-treated patients. Besides being effective, long-term infliximab use was tolerated well in this study. The anti-inflammatory cytokines IL-10 and IL-11 have not been approved for UC.

NONADHERENCE TO MEDICAL THERAPY

Nonadherence to medications for chronic diseases is an important and often ignored problem. In ulcerative colitis patients taking 5-ASA chronically, nonadherence has been measured as high as 60%.[104] Recognizing the factors responsible for nonadherence and addressing these factors could lead to better adherence and better clinical outcomes. Sewitch and colleagues from Montreal, Quebec, measured non-adherence among 153 IBD patients.[104] Nonadherence was seen in 41% and was mostly unintentional (81%). Nonadherence was predicted by disease in remission, new patient status, and shorter disease duration.

Certainly, it is in the patient's best interest to take medications. There are certain steps a physician can do to improve the likelihood of adherence, including the following:

- Stress the importance of medication to maintain remission
- Establish an interactive, long-term relationship with a patient
- Minimize cost
- Make the dosing schedule as convenient at possible

Reducing the frequency of administration of medication is certain to improve adherence to therapy. Some medications, though, lose effectiveness if the dosing frequency is reduced. Mesalamine may be one medication that requires multiple doses a day because it is a medicine that acts topically before it is excreted.

In a small, randomized clinical trial, UC patients in remission on mesalamine were given either once-daily dosing (N = 12) or conventional 2 or 3 times daily dosing 5-ASA (N = 10).[105] At 6 months, one patient in each group relapsed, and adherence was higher in the once-daily dosing (90% versus 76%, P=0.07). Also, patients were more often satisfied with once-daily dosing (83% versus 60%, P=0.18).[105]

While the differences in this small, randomized clinical trial were not statistically significant, it is clear and intuitive that patients are more adherent to medications and more often satisfied with their medical regimen with once-daily dosing.

CONCLUSION

Despite there being no epidemiologic or genetic studies specifically evaluating left-sided ulcerative colitis, it is likely the results would be analogous to those of pancolitis. The risk of cancer is proportional to extent of the disease, and therefore left-sided colitis patients are at lower risk of cancer than patients with pancolitis. First-line therapy in left-sided colitis is topical or oral 5-ASA agents. Studies evaluating the efficacy of oral 5-ASA agents that have differing drug delivery mechanisms have demonstrated minor clinical differences. Once-daily therapy, though, is sure to improve adherence. If patients do not respond to the 5-ASA class of medications, steroids, immunosuppressives, and biologic agents are then used, respectively, in a stepwise fashion to treat left-sided disease.

REFERENCES

1. Sandler RS. Epidemiology of inflammatory bowel disease. In: Targan SR, Shanahan F, eds. *Inflammatory Bowel Disease: from Bench to Bedside.* Baltimore, MD: Williams & Wilkin; 1994.
2. Loftus EV Jr, Silverstein MD, Sandborn WJ, Tremaine WJ, Harmsen WS, Zinsmeister AR. Ulcerative colitis in Olmsted County, Minnesota, 1940-1993: incidence, prevalence, and survival. *Gut.* 2000;46:336-343.
3. Niv Y, Abuksis G, Fraser GM. Epidemiology of ulcerative colitis in Israel: A survey of Israeli kibbutz settlements. *Am J Gastroenterol.* 2000;95:693-698.
4. Hassan K, Cowan FJ, Jenkins HR. The incidence of childhood inflammatory bowel disease in Wales. *Eur J Epidemiol.* 1999;149: 916-924.
5. Carr I, Mayberry JF. The effects of migration on ulcerative colitis: a three-year prospective study among Europeans and first- and second-generation South Asians in Leicester (1991-1994). *Am J Gastroenterol.* 1999;94:2918-2922.
6. Delco F, Sonnenberg A. Birth-cohort phenomenon in the time trends of mortality from ulcerative colitis. *Am J Epidemiol.* 1999;149: 350-366.

7. Orholm M, Fonager K, Sorensen HT. Risk of ulcerative colitis and Crohn's disease among offspring of patients with ulcerative chronic inflammatory bowel disease. *Am J Gastroenterol.* 1999;94:323-608.
8. Yang H, Rotter JI, Toyoda H, et al. Ulcerative colitis: A genetically heterogenous disorder defined by genetic (HLA class II) and subclinical (antineutrophil cytoplasmic antibodies) markers. *J Clin Invest.* 1999;92:1080-1084.
9. Sandborn WJ, Landers CJ, Tremaine WJ, Targan SR. Antineutrophil cytoplasmic antibody correlates with chronic pouchitis after ileal pouch-anal anstomosis. *Am J Gastroenterol.* 1995;90:740-747.
10. Van heel DA, Santsangi J, Carey AH, Jewell DP. Inflammatory bowel disease: progress toward a gene. *Can J Gastroenterol.* 2000;14:207-218.
11. Trachtenberg EA, Yang H, Hayes E, et al. HLA class II haplotype associated with inflammatory bowel disease in Jewish (Ashkenasi) and non-Jewish Caucasian populations. *Hum Immunol.* 2000;61: 326-333.
12. Sandborn WJ. Nicotene therapy for ulcerative colitis: a review of rationale, mechanisms, pharmacology, and clinical results. *Am J Gastroenterol.* 1999;94:1161-1171.
13. Reif S, Lavy A, Keter D, et al. Lack of association between smoking and Crohn's disease but unusual association with ulcerative in Jewish patients in Israel: a multicenter study. *Am J Gastroenterol.* 2000;95:474-478.
14. Reigler G, Tartaglione MT, Carratu R, et al. Age related clinical severity at diagnosis in 1705 patients with ulcerative colitis: a study by GISC. *Dig Dis Sci.* 2000;45:462-465.
15. Lashner BA, Shaheen MJ, Hanuaer SB, Kirschner BS. Passive smoking is associated with an increased risk of developing inflammatory bowel disease in children. *Am J Gastroenterol.* 1993;88:336-359.
16. Lashner BA, Hanauer SB, Silversteen MD. Testing nicotine gum for ulcerative colitis patients: experience with single-patient trials. *Dig Dis Sci.* 1990;35:827-835.
17. Pullan RD, Rhodes J, Ganesh S, et al. Transdermal nicotine for active ulcerative colitis. *N Engl J Med.* 1994;330:811-815.
18. Thomas GAO, Rhodes J, Mani V, et al. Transdermal nicotine maintenance therapy for ulcerative colitis. *N Engl J Med.* 1995;332: 984-992.
19. Lashner BA, Kane SV, Hanauer SB. Lack of association between oral contraceptives and ulcerative colitis. *Gastroenterology.* 1990;99:1032-1036.
20. Geerling BJ, Bagnelie PC, Badart-Smook A, Russel MG, Stockbrugger RW, Brummer RJ. Diet as a risk factor for the development of ulcerative colitis. *Am J Gastroenterol.* 1994;94:3258-3262.
21. Koutroubakis IE, Vlachinikolis IG. Appendectomy and the development of ulcerative colitis: results of a meta-analysis of published case control studies. *Am J Gastroenterol.* 2000;95:171-176.
22. Truelove SC, Witts LJ. Cortisone in ulcerative colitis: final report on a therapeutic trial. *BMJ.* 1955;2:1041-1048.
23. Nielson OH, Vainer B, Madsen SM, Seidelin JB, Heegaard NH. Established and emerging biological activity markers of inflammatory bowel disease. *Am J Gastroenterol.* 2000;95:359-367.
24. Kirschner JB. Problems in the differentiation of ulcerative colitis and Crohn's disease of the colon. *Gastroenterology.* 1975;68:187-191.
25. Kane SV, Sandborn WJ, Rufo PA, et al. Fecal lactoferrin is a sensitive and specific marker in identifying intestinal inflammation. *Am J Gastroenterol.* 2003;98:1309-1314.
26. Farmer RG, Easly KA, Rankin GB. Clinical patterns, natural history, and progression of ulcerative colitis: a long term follow-up of 1,116 patients. *Dig Dis Sci.* 1993;38:1137-1146.
27. Meucci G, Vecchi M, Astegiano M, et al. The natural history of ulcerative proctitis: a multicenter, retrospective study. *Am J Gastroenterol.* 2000;95:469-473.
28. Ponsioen CI, Tytgan GN. Primary sclerosing cholangitis: a clinical review. *Am J Gastoenterol.* 1998;93:515-523.
29. Shetty K, Rybicki L, Brzezinsnki A, Carey WD, Lashner BA. The risk of dysplasia in ulcerative colitis patients with primary sclerosing cholangitis. *Am J Gastroenterol.* 1994;94:1643-1649.
30. Winther KV, Jess T, Langholz E, Munkholm P, Binder V. Survival and cause-specific mortality in ulcerative colitis: follow-up of a population-based cohort in Copenhagen county. *Gastroenterology.* 2003;125:1576-1582.
31. Card T, Hubbard R, Logan RFA. Mortality in IBD: a population-based study. *Gastroenterology.* 2003;125:1583-1590.
32. Langholz E, Munkholm P, Davidsen M, Binder V. Colorectal cancer risk and mortality in patients with ulcerative colitis. *Gastroenterology.* 1992;103:1444-1451.
33. Karlen P, Lofberg R, Brostrem O, Leijonmark CE, Hellers G, Persson PG. Increased risk of ulcerative colitis: a population based study. *Am J Gastroenterol.* 1999;94:1047-1092.
34. Lashner BA, Hannauer SB, Silverstein MD. Optimal timing of colonoscopy to screen for cancer in ulcerative colitis. *Ann Intern Med.* 1998;108:274-278.
35. Provenzale D, Kowdley KV, Arora S, Wong JB. Prophylactic colectomy for the surveillance for chronic ulcerative colitis? A decision analysis. *Gastroenterology.* 1995;109:1188-1196.
36. Eaden JA, Ward BA, Mayberry JF. How gastroenterologists screen for colonic cancer for chronic ulcerative colitis: an analysis of performance. *Gastrointest Endosc.* 2000;51:123-128.
37. Delco F, Sonnenberg A. A decision analysis of surveillance for colorectal cancer in ulcerative colitis. *Gut.* 2000;46:500-506.
38. Rubin CE, Haggitt RC, Burma GC, et al. DNA aneuploidy in colonic biopsies predicts future development of dysplasia in ulcerative colitis. *Gastroenterology.* 1992;103:1611-1620.
39. Sachar DB, Greenstein AJ. Cancer risk in left-sided colitis. *Gastroenterology.* 1991;101(5):1457-1458.
40. Kornbluth A, Sachar DB; Practice Parameters Committee of the American College of Gastroenterology. Ulcerative colitis practice guidelines in adults (update): American College of Gastroenterology, Practice Parameters Committee. *Am J Gastroenterol.* 2004;99(7):1371-1385.
41. Itzkowitz SH, Present DH. Crohn's and Colitis Foundation of America Colon Cancer in IBD Study Group. Consensus conference: Colorectal cancer screening and surveillance in inflammatory bowel disease. *Inflamm Bowel Dis.* 2005;11(3):314-321.
42. Rutter MD, Saunders BP, Wilkinson KH, et al. Thirty-year analysis of a colonoscopic surveillance program for neoplasia in ulcerative colitis. *Gastroenterology.* 2006;130(4):1030-1038.
43. Rutter M, Saunders B, Wilkinson K, et al. Severity of inflammation is a risk factor for colorectal neoplasia in ulcerative colitis. *Gastroenterology.* 2004;126(2):451-459.
44. Ullman T, Croog V, Harz N, Sachar D, Iktowitz S. Progression of flat low grade dysplasia to advanced neoplasia in patient with ulcerative colitis. *Gastroenterology.* 2003;1245:1311-1319.
45. Kiesslich R, Fritsch J, Holtman M, et al. Methylene blue-aided chromoendoscopy for the detection of intraepithelial neoplasia and colon cancer in ulcerative colitis. *Gastroenterology.* 2003;124:880-888.
46. Matsumoto T, Nakamura S, Jo Y, Yao T, Ida M. Chromoendoscopy might improve diagnostic accuracy in cancer surveillance for ulcerative colitis. *Am J Gastroenterol.* 2003;98:1827-1833.
47. Brentall TA, Crispin DA, Rabinovitch PS, et al. Mutations in P53 gene: An early marker of neoplastic progression in ulcerative colitis. *Gastroenterology.* 1994;107:369-378.
48. Lashner BA, Shapiro BD, Husain A, Goldblum JR. Evaluation of the usefulness of testing for the p53 mutations in colorectal

cancer surveillance for ulcerative colitis. *Am J Gastroenterol.* 1999; 94:456-462.

49. Blackstone MO, Riddell RH, Rogers BHG, Levin B. Dysplasia-associated lesion or mass (DALM) detected by colonoscopy in long-standing ulcerative colitis: an indication for colectomy. *Gastroenterology.* 1981;80:366-374.
50. Engelsgjred M, Farraye FA, Odze RD. Polypectomy may be adequate treatment for adenoma-like dysplastic lesions in chronic ulcerative colitis. *Gastroenterology.* 1999;117:1288-1294.
51. Rubin PH, Friedman S, Harpaz N, et al. Colonoscopic polypectomy in chronic colitis: conservative management after endoscopic resection of dysplastic polyps. *Gastroenterology.* 1999;117: 1295-1300.
52. Odze RD. Adenomas and adenoma-like DALMs in chronic ulcerative colitis: a clinical, pathological, and molecular review. *Am J Gastroenterol.* 1994;94:1746-1750.
53. Odze RD, Farraye FA, Hecht JL, Hornick JL. Long-term follow-up after polypectomy treatment for adenoma-like dysplastic lesions in ulcerative colitis. *Clin Gastroenterol Hepatol.* 2004;2:534-541.
54. Lashner BA, Turner BC, Bostwick DG, Frank PH, Hanauer SB. Dysplasia and cancer complicating strictures in ulcerative colitis. *Dig Dis Sci.* 1990;35:349-352.
55. Pinczowski D, Ekbom A, Baron J, et al. Risk factors for colorectal cancer in patients with ulcerative colitis. *Gastroenterology.* 1994;117-120.
56. Lindberg BU, Broome U, Persson B. Proximal colorectal dysplasia or cancer in ulcerative colitis. *Dis Colon Rectum.* 2001;44:77-85.
57. Moody GA, Jayanthi V, Probert CS, et al. Long term therapy with sulfasalazine protects against colorectal cancer in ulcerative colitis. *Eur J Gastroenterol Hepatol.* 1996;8:1179-1183.
58. Eaden J, Abrams K, Ekbom A, et al. Colorectal cancer prevention ulcerative colitis *Aliment Pharmacol Ther.* 2000;14:145-153.
59. Bernstein CN, et al. Does the use of 5-aminosalicylic acid in inflammatory bowel disease prevent the development of colorectal cancer? *Am J Gastroenterol.* 2003;98:27484-27488.
60. Rubin DR, LoSavio A, Yadron N, et al. Aminosalicylate therapy in the prevention of dysplasia and colorectal cancer in ulcerative colitis. *Clin Gastroenterol Hepatol.* 2006;4:1346-1350.
61. Van Staa TP, Card T, Logan RF, Leufkens HG. 5-aminosalicylate use and colorectal cancer risk in inflammatory bowel disease: a large epidemiologic study. *Gut.* 2005;54:1573-1578.
62. Velayos FS, Terdiman JP, Walsh JM. Effect of 5-aminosalicylate use on colorectal cancer and dysplasia risk: a systematic review and meta-analysis of observational studies. *Am J Gastroenterol.* 2005;100:1345-1353.
63. Lashner BA. Effect of folate supplementation on the incidence of dysplasia and cancer in ulcerative colitis. *Gastroenterology.* 1989;97:255-259.
64. Lasher BA. Red blood cell folate is associated with the development of dysplasia and cancer in ulcerative colitis. *J Cancer Res Clin Oncol.* 1993;119:549-54.
65. Lashner BA, Provencher KS, Seidner DL, et al. The effect of folic acid on the risk for cancer or dysplasia in ulcerative colitis. *Gastroenterology.* 1997;112:29-32.
66. Tung BY, Emond MJ, Haggitt RC, et al. Ursodiol use is associated with lower prevalence of colonic neoplasia in patients with ulcerative colitis and primary sclerosing cholangitis. *Ann Intern Med.* 2001;134:89-95.
67. Pardi DS, Loftus EV Jr, Kremers WK, et al. Ursodeoxycholic acid as a chemopreventive agent in patients with ulcerative colitis and primary sclerosing cholangitis. *Gastroenterology.* 2003;124:889-893.
68. Wolf JM, Rybicki LA, Lashner BA. The impact of ursodeoxycholic acid on cancer, dysplasia, and mortality in ulcerative colitis patients with primary sclerosing cholangitis. *Aliment Pharmacol Ther.* 2005;22:783-788.
69. Kornbluth A, Sachar DB. Ulcerative colitis practice guidelines in adults (update): American College of Gastroenterology, Practice Parameters Committee. *Am J Gastroenterol.* 2004;99:1371-1385.
70. Stenson WF, Cort D, Rodgers J, et al. Dietary supplementation with fish oil in ulcerative colitis. *Ann Intern Med.* 1992;116:609-614.
71. Belluzi A, Boschi S, Brignola C, Munari A, Cariani G, Miglio F. Polyunsaturated fatty acids and inflammatory bowel disease. *Am J Clin Nutr.* 2000;71:339S-342S.
72. Sheppach W, Sommer H, Kirschner T, et al. Effect of butyrate enemas on the colonic mucosa in the distal ulcerative colitis. *Gastroenterology.* 1992;116:609-614.
73. Breuer RI, Soergel KH, Lashner BA, et al. Short chain fatty acid rectal irrigation for left sided ulcerative colitis: a randomized placebo-controlled trial. *Gut.* 1997;40:485-491.
74. Vernia P, Monteleone G, Grandinetti G, et al. Combined oral sodium butyrate and mesalazine treatment compared to oral mesalazine alone in ulcerative colitis: randomized, double-blind, placebo-controlled pilot study. *Dig Dis Sci.* 2000;45:976-981.
75. Rembacken BJ, Snelling AM, Hawkey PM, Chalmers DM, Axon AT. Non-pathogenic *Escherichia coli* versus mesalazine for the treatment of ulcerative colitis: A randomized trial. *Lancet.* 1999;354:635-639.
76. Brzezinski A, Rankin GB, Seidner DL, Lashner BA. 5-aminosalicylic acid in inflammatory bowel disease: old and new preparations. *Cleve Clin J Med.* 1995;62:317-323.
77. Meyers S, Sachar DB, Present DH, Janowitz HD. Olsalazine sodium in the treatment of ulcerative colitis among patients intolerant of sulfasalazine: a prospective, randomized, placebo-controlled, double-blind, dose-ranging clinical trial. *Gastroenterology.* 1987;93: 1255-1262.
78. Kamm MA, Sandborn WJ, Gassull M, et al. Once-daily, high-concentration MMX mesalamine in active ulcerative colitis. *Gastroenterology.* 2007;132:66-75.
79. Lichtenstein GR, Kamm MA, Boddu P, et al. Effect of once- or twice-daily MMX mesalamine (SPD476) for the induction of remission of mild to moderately active ulcerative colitis. *Clin Gastroenterol Hepatol.* 2007;5:95-102.
80. Kruis W, Kiudelis G, Racz I, et al. Once-daily versus three-times-daily mesalazine granules in active ulcerative colitis: a double-blind, double-dummy, randomised non-inferiority trial. *Gut.* 2008;doi:10.1136.
81. Lichtenstein G, Merchant K, Shaw A, Yuan J, Bortey E, Forbes W. Once-daily 1.5-g granulated mesalamine effectively maintains remission in patients with ulcerative colitis who switch from different 5-ASA formulations. *Am J Gastroenterol.* 2008;13(Suppl 1): s429-S430.
82. Green JRB, Lobo AJ, Holdsworth CD, et al. Balsalazide is more effective and better tolerated than mesalamine in the treatment of acute ulcerative colitis. *Gastroenterology.* 1998;114:15-22.
83. Haghighi D, Lashner B. Left-sided ulcerative colitis. *Gastroenterol Clin North Am.* 2004;33(2):271-284.
84. Pruitt R, Hanson J, Safdi M, et al. Balsalazide is superior to mesalamine in the time to improvement of signs and symptoms of acute mild-to-moderate ulcerative colitis. *Am J Gastroenterol.* 2002;97:3077-2941.
85. Levine D, Riff D, Pruitt R, et al. A randomized, double blind, dose-response comparison of balsalazide (6.75 g), balsalazide (2.25 g), and mesalamine (2.4 g) in the treatment of active, mild to moderate ulcerative colitis. *Am J Gastroenterol.* 2002;97:1398-1407.
86. Bosworth BP, Pruitt RE, Gordon GL, et al. Balsalazide tablets 3.3 g twice daily improves signs and symptoms of mild to moderate ulcerative colitis [abstract T1152]. *Gastroenterology.* 2008;134 (Suppl 1):A495.
87. Oshitani N, Matsumoto T, Jinno Y, et al. Prediction of short-term outcome for patients with active ulcerative colitis. *Dig Dis Sci.* 2000;45:982-986.

88. Rutgeerts P, Lofberg R, Malchow H, et al. A comparison of budesonide with prednisolone for active Crohn's disease. *N Engl J Med.* 1994;331:842-845.
89. Greenberg GF, Feagon BG, Martin F, et al. Oral budesonide for active Crohn's disease. *N Engl J Med.* 1994;331:836-841.
90. Safdi M, DeMicco M, Sninsky C, et al. A double-blind comparison of oral versus rectal mesalamine versus combination therapy in the treatment of distal ulcerative colitis. *Am J Gastroenterol.* 1997;92(10):1867-1871.
91. D'Albasio G, Pacini F, Camarri E, et al. Combined therapy with 5-aminosalicylic acid tablets and enemas for maintaining remission in ulcerative colitis: a randomized double-blind study. *Am J Gastroenterol.* 1997;92(7):1143-1147.
92. Hanauer S, Good LI, Goodman MW, et al. Long-term use of mesalamine (Rowasa) suppositories in remission maintenance of ulcerative proctitis. *Am J Gastroenterol.* 2000;95(7):1749-1754.
93. Biddle WL, Greenberger NJ, Swan JT, McPhee MS, Miner PB Jr. 5-aminosalicylic acid enemas: effective agent in maintaining remission in left-sided ulcerative colitis. *Gastroenterology.* 1988;94(4):1075-1079.
94. Cohen RD, Woseth DM, Thisted RA, Hanauer SB. A meta-analysis and overview of the literature on treatment options for left-sided ulcerative colitis and ulcerative proctitis. *Am J Gastroenterol.* 2000;95(5):1263-1276.
95. Campieri M, DeFranchis R, Bianchi Porro G, Ranzi T, Brunetti G, Barbara L. Mesalazine (5-aminosalicylic acid) suppositories in the treatment of ulcerative proctitis or distal proctosigmoiditis: a randomized controlled trial. *Scand J Gastroenterol.* 1990;25(7): 663-668.
96. Present DH. 6-Mercaptopurine and other immunosuppressive agents in the treatment of Crohn's disease and ulcerative colitis. *Gastroenterol Clin North Am.* 1989;18:57-72.
97. Hawthorne AB, Logan RFA, Hawkey CJ. Randomized controlled trial of azathioprine withdrawal in ulcerative colitis. *BMJ.* 1992;305:20-22.
98. Colonna T, Korelitz BI. The role leukopenia in the 6-mercaptopurine-induced remission of refractory Crohn's disease. *Am J Gastroenterol.* 1994;89:362-366.
99. Dubinsky MC, Lamothe S, Yang HY, et al. Pharmacogenomics and metabolite measurement for 6-mercaptopurine therapy in inflammatory bowel disease. *Gastroenterology.* 2000;118:705-713.
100. Lichtiger S, Present DH, Kornbluth A, et al. Cyclosporine in severe ulcerative colitis refractory to steroid therapy. *N Engl J Med.* 1994;330:1841-1845.
101. Cohen RD, Brodsky AL, Hanauer SB. A comparison of the quality of life in patients with severe ulcerative colitis after total colectomy versus medical treatment with intravenous cyclosporine. *Inflamm Bowel Dis.* 1999;5:1-10.
102. Kornbluth A, Present DH, Lichtiger S, Hanauer SB. Cyclosporine for severe ulcerative colitis: a user's guide. *Am J Gastroenterol.* 1997;92:1424-1428.
103. Rutgeerts P, Sandborn WJ, Feagan BG, et al. Infliximab for induction and maintenance therapy for ulcerative *N Engl J Med.* 2005,353:2462-2476.
104. Sewitch MJ, Abahamowicz M, Barkum A, et al. Patient nonadherence to medication in inflammatory bowel disease. *Am J Gastroenterol.* 2003;98:1535-1544.
105. Kane S, Huo D, Magnanti K. A pilot study of once daily versus conventional dosing mesalamine for maintenance of ulcerative colitis. *Clin Gastroenterol Hepatol.* 2003;1:170-173.

30 Management of Refractory Ulcerative Colitis

Edward V. Loftus Jr, MD; Ellen J. Scherl, MD, FACP, AGAF;
and Melissa H. Rosen, MD

Most patients with ulcerative colitis (UC) fortunately are able to maintain their disease in remission or a near-remission state with 5-ASA agents alone, or, in some cases, with no medications at all. A longitudinal study of the course of disease activity in a population-based inception cohort of UC patients from Copenhagen County, Denmark, highlighted this point.[1] Very few patients over the long term remained completely relapse-free (18% after 5 years) or continuously active (1% after 5 years). Most patients experienced an intermittently relapsing course of disease. However, in any given year, approximately 50% of patients experienced a relapse.[1]

Thus, UC is a condition characterized by relapses interspersed with periods of disease remission. Aminosalicylates or corticosteroids may control many of these relapses; however, some disease exacerbations will be seemingly refractory to such therapy. More intensive medical therapy, and sometimes even surgery, may be required. Among Copenhagen County UC patients, the cumulative risk of colectomy, which was almost always performed for disease activity, was 9% in the first year after diagnosis and about 1% thereafter, such that the 10-year risk was about 24% and the 20-year risk about 30%.[2]

In this chapter, medical therapies to manage the moderately active steroid-dependent, moderately active steroid-refractory, and severely active UC patient will be reviewed.

Treatment of the Moderate Steroid-Dependent or Steroid-Refractory Patient

Natural History of Response to Corticosteroids

The "natural history" of response to a first course of corticosteroids was examined in a population-based inception cohort of UC patients from Olmsted County, Minnesota. All 63 patients were diagnosed with UC between 1970 and 1993, and they were county residents at the time of diagnosis.[3] Information on clinical response to the first course of corticosteroids administered for UC was based on review of all available medical records. The short-term, 30-day response to corticosteroids was high at 84% (complete response in 54% and partial response in 30%).[3] However, the long-term response was less impressive—by the end of 1 year, only 49% were in remission off corticosteroids, 22% were steroid-dependent, and 29% had undergone colectomy. Although this study has weaknesses, including its observational nature and the fact that much of the follow-up occurred in the "pre-immunosuppressive era," it highlights the point that UC patients who are active enough to require corticosteroids are at high risk for steroid dependency as well as proctocolectomy.[3] Therefore, patients should be aggressively transitioned to

Lichtenstein GR, ed.
Ulcerative Colitis: The Complete Guide to Medical Management (pp. 319-330)

steroid-sparing agents, such as purine analogs, at the first hint of steroid dependency.

Molecular Mechanisms of Steroid Resistance

The mechanisms for steroid resistance in UC at the cellular level are being actively investigated.[4] Normally, corticosteroids exert significant antiproliferative effects on lymphocytes, but peripheral lymphocytes obtained from patients hospitalized for severe colitis who had not responded to corticosteroids seemed to be resistant to these effects.[5] This resistance at the cellular level may be due to a number of factors, including levels of drug-pumping proteins, abnormalities in the glucocorticoid receptor, and the level of activation of inflammatory intracellular signalers such as nuclear factor kappa beta (NFKB).[4]

The multi-drug resistance gene (MDR1) produces a protein known as p-glycoprotein 170, which serves as a drug efflux pump and actively expels corticosteroids and other drugs from the cytoplasm.[6] MDR1 appears to be overexpressed in the peripheral blood lymphocytes of UC patients who require surgery for medically refractory disease.[7] Conversely, blocking the protein made by MDR1 results in higher intracellular levels of steroids and cyclosporine.[8] Overexpression of MDR1 may play a role in drug resistance in other conditions such as rheumatoid arthritis and epilepsy.[4] It turns out that MDR1 is only one of many cellular detoxification genes with downregulated expression in the colon of UC patients, and this may be explained by a loss of expression of the transcription factor pregnane X receptor.[9]

Perhaps changes in the number or function of glucocorticoid receptors influences steroid-responsiveness in UC. In one study of 23 UC patients, a transcriptionally inactive form of messenger ribonucleic acid (mRNA) for the human glucocorticoid receptor (hGRβ) was present in the peripheral blood lymphocytes of 9% of steroid-responsive patients and 83% of steroid-resistant patients.[10] However, some have speculated that hGRβ is induced by proinflammatory cytokines and that the differences observed are due to chronic inflammation (in other words an effect, not a cause).[4]

Finally, it may be that transcription factors such as NFKB are constitutively overexpressed in the intestinal tissue of drug-resistant inflammatory bowel disease (IBD) patients, resulting in the production of numerous proinflammatory mediators, which appear to not only inhibit hGRβ transcription but also compete with corticosteroids for nuclear DNA receptors.[11,12]

General Management Principles of the Steroid-Dependent or Steroid-Refractory Ulcerative Colitis Patient

It is always worthwhile to take a step back and reassess the entire clinical scenario when faced with a steroid-dependent or steroid-refractory UC patient. Is the diagnosis of UC secure? Is there an additional diagnosis (eg, IBS[13] or celiac disease)? Is the patient compliant with all prescribed medications? Between 40% and 60% of IBD patients are not adherent with their prescribed medical regimens,[14,15] and patients with recurrent disease are more likely to be noncompliant than those who remain in remission.[16] However, the prevalence of nonadherence in steroid-dependent or steroid-refractory UC patients is unknown. Does the patient have 5-ASA hypersensitivity colitis? Both sulfasalazine and non-sulfa aminosalicylate medications have been associated with a paradoxical worsening of colitis symptoms.[17,18] If corticosteroids are started concomitantly with aminosalicylates, the hypersensitivity may be blunted or partially treated by the steroids, resulting in a "steroid-dependent" presentation.[18] A short trial of 5-ASA cessation may be in order. Is the patient taking a nonsteroidal anti-inflammatory drug (NSAID)? Some studies suggest that concomitant use of NSAIDs results in exacerbation of IBD,[19,20] but the data are conflicting.[21,22] A recent systematic review of the topic concluded that the evidence for a link between NSAIDs and IBD flares was weak.[23] Likewise, there is no consensus as to whether the cyclooxygenase-2 inhibitors (celecoxib, rofecoxib, and valdecoxib) increase the risk of relapse in quiescent IBD patients.[24-27] A recent preliminary report of a randomized trial of celecoxib 200 mg twice daily versus placebo in quiescent UC showed that disease activity in the celecoxib-treated patients was similar to that of placebo-treated patients at the end of the 14-day study.[28]

Purine Analogs (6-Mercaptopurine and Azathioprine)

The most common indication for purine analog therapy in UC is steroid dependency. In contrast to the situation in CD, where numerous trials and meta-analyses demonstrate efficacy of purine analogs for a number of indications, the evidence base for employing these therapies in UC is weaker. At least 9 randomized, controlled trials of AZA for various indications in UC have been performed.[29-37]

The first published trial could not demonstrate that AZA 2.5 mg/kg/d was superior to placebo for the treatment of active UC.[29] While it could be argued that the duration of the induction trial was only 1 month, considerably shorter than the recognized interval between initiation of treatment and onset of full clinical response, even at the end of the 6-month maintenance study, there was no significant difference between treatment groups.[29] A 6-month placebo-controlled trial of AZA 1.5 mg/kg/d for maintenance of remission in 30 UC patients showed significant benefit, with an absolute treatment difference of almost 50%.[31] Another trial published the same year compared AZA 2.5 mg/kg/d with sulfasalazine for treatment of active UC and concluded that the treatments were equivalent in efficacy.[30] However, the small sample size (n = 20) suggests the trial was likely underpowered to detect true differences in efficacy between the treatments.[30] Kirk and colleagues studied AZA 2.0 to 2.5 mg/kg/d in 44 patients with active UC and saw improvement in disease activity scores and lower cumulative steroid doses in the patients receiving active drug.[32] However, remission rates in the 2 groups were not compared.

Perhaps the best evidence in support of the use of purine analogs in UC comes from a double-blind, placebo-controlled study of AZA for maintenance of remission in UC.[33] All 79 patients had been on AZA for at least 6 months prior to randomization. They were stratified by activity to either remission (n = 67) or stable low-grade or steroid-dependent disease (n = 12). They were then randomized to either continuation of AZA at the same dose (median, 100 mg/d) or placebo and were followed for 1 year. At the end of the study, the relapse rate was 36% in the AZA group and 59% in the placebo group.[33] In the subgroup with low-grade activity or steroid-dependent disease, no benefit could be demonstrated, but the sample size of this group was quite small.

A series of randomized trials of AZA for UC, some with methodological flaws, have recently been reported.[34-36,38] In a randomized, open-label, placebo-controlled trial from India, 83 steroid-dependent patients received either AZA (2 mg/kg/d) or placebo in addition to sulfasalazine and prednisolone, and corticosteroids were tapered over 3 to 4 months and followed for 12 months.[34] Although remission rates were no different, the relapse rate in the AZA-treated patients was lower. In a randomized, single-blind, controlled trial from Milan, 52 steroid-dependent UC patients received either AZA 2 mg/kg/d or 5-ASA 3.2 g/d for 6 months.[38] Treatment success, defined as clinical and endoscopic remission off steroids, was achieved in 58% of AZA-treated and only 26% of 5-ASA-treated patients. In an Indian trial, 35 newly diagnosed UC patients with severe activity were randomized to receive either sulfasalazine plus AZA or sulfasalazine monotherapy, and were followed for 1 year.[35] Both treatment groups also received an initial course of steroids to induce remission. The relapse rate was significantly higher in the patients receiving sulfasalazine monotherapy (56% versus 24% in the combination therapy group).[35] Finally, a small randomized, open-label, controlled trial of AZA (2.5 mg/kg/d) or sulfasalazine (6 g/d) in 25 newly diagnosed UC patients showed no difference in relapse rates at the end of the 18-month trial.[36]

The results of randomized, controlled trials of AZA therapy in UC were recently synthesized and published in the Japanese literature.[39] Full details of this article were not available, but according to the abstract, the results of 4 trials were pooled. The pooled odds ratio of response to therapy was not significantly elevated for induction of remission, but was 2.3 (95% confidence interval [CI] 1.3 to 4.0) for maintenance of remission.[39] In other words, AZA-treated patients were twice as likely to remain in remission than placebo-treated patients. The number needed to treat to prevent one additional recurrence was 6 patients. Although the pooled odds ratio of adverse events was 2.3, this was not statistically significant.[39] In addition to randomized trials, a number of uncontrolled trials or observational studies suggest a benefit of purine analogs for refractory UC,[40-46] with remission rates in the 50% to 70% range.

The optimal dose of purine analogs in refractory UC has not been rigorously studied, but it has been assumed that it is similar to the optimal dose used in Crohn's disease (ie, 2.0 to 2.5 mg/kg/d assuming normal thiopurine methyltransferase metabolism). One small observational study examined the outcome of AZA dose escalation from a median of 2.0 mg/kg to a median of 2.7 mg/kg daily in 16 UC patients with chronic active disease or recurrent flares.[47] In 4 patients (25%), a clinical response was achieved, but 5 patients (31%) developed dose-limiting side effects, and 7 (44%) did not respond.[47]

Should patients who improve on purine analogs be continued on 5-ASA therapy? On the one hand, several observational studies suggest that prolonged use of 5-ASA therapy might result in a lower risk of colorectal dysplasia or cancer.[48] On the other hand, combination therapy may result in a potentially important drug interaction resulting in inhibition of thiopurine methyltransferase resulting in leukopenia.[49] A recent study compared the efficacy of AZA monotherapy (2.2 mg/kg) and combination therapy with AZA and olsalazine (500 mg tid) for maintenance of remission in 70 steroid-dependent UC patients.[37] Remission rates at the end of the 2-year study were similar (81% monotherapy versus 82% combination therapy). Patients on combination therapy experienced more adverse events (diarrhea, leukopenia), incurred higher cost, and had poorer compliance than those on monotherapy.[37] Additional studies with similar design and larger numbers will need to be performed to definitively answer the question of purine monotherapy versus combination therapy with 5-ASA.

METHOTREXATE

Unlike the case in Crohn's disease, there is little evidence proving a benefit for methotrexate in refractory ulcerative colitis. In an open-label study of parenteral methotrexate (25 mg weekly) in 7 UC patients, initial symptomatic improvement was noted in all but 2, while a more prolonged response was seen in 3 patients.[50] However, endoscopic and/or histologic improvement was not observed. In another uncontrolled study, 8 refractory UC patients received oral methotrexate 15 mg weekly, and 3 patients had a partial clinical response.[51] The mean daily prednisone dose decreased from 26 mg at study start to 12.7 mg at week 18, but complete withdrawal of corticosteroids was not possible. By the end of the 18-week study, all but one had discontinued the drug due to adverse events or lack of efficacy.[51] In another uncontrolled study, parenteral methotrexate 12.5 mg weekly in those intolerant of or not responsive to AZA was administered to 10 steroid-dependent UC patients.[52] Six patients responded completely, and 4 had a partial response.[52] A retrospective review of the experience with methotrexate for IBD at the John Radcliffe Hospital suggested a remission rate of approximately 60% in those remaining on the drug for at least 3 months.[53]

In an Israeli multicenter study, 67 UC patients with active disease despite corticosteroids and/or immunosuppressives were randomized to receive either methotrexate 12.5 mg by mouth once weekly or placebo once weekly.[54] The study authors failed to see significant differences in remission rates (47% to 49%) and time to remission in the 2 treatment groups. However, it has been speculated that perhaps the dosage was too low or the route of oral administration was incorrect.[55] In a trial of therapies for steroid-dependent IBD, 34 UC patients on corticosteroids were randomized to 6-MP 1.5 mg/kg/d, methotrexate 15 mg by mouth weekly, or mesalamine 3 g/d and were followed for 30 weeks.[56] Those patients achieving remission in the first part of the study were followed for an additional 76 weeks for maintenance of remission. In the first part of the study, 79% of those on 6-MP, 58% of the methotrexate-treated patients, and 25% of the mesalamine arm achieved remission and tapered off corticosteroids.[56] In the second study phase, remission off steroids was maintained in 64% of the 6-MP group, 14% of the methotrexate group, and none of the mesalamine group. The authors concluded that methotrexate might be efficacious for induction of remission in steroid-dependent UC, but that its efficacy for maintenance of remission in this group of patients was weak at best.[56]

At this point in time, it is difficult to place methotrexate in the usual treatment algorithm for refractory UC given the results of the trial by Oren and colleagues.[54] However, the study by Maté-Jiménez and colleagues,[56] and some of the uncontrolled data,[50-53] suggest that select UC patients with steroid-dependent disease might benefit from the drug. In clinical scenarios where other treatment alternatives are not appealing or are being refused by the patient, methotrexate could be considered.

Cummings et al in 2005[57] published a chart review on patients treated with oral methotrexate at the inflammatory bowel disease clinics of Oxford and Wycombe General Hospital in the UK and concluded that oral methotrexate at 20 mg weekly was moderately effective in steroid-dependent or refractory UC patients. The study involved 42 patients with ulcerative colitis (either steroid refractory or steroid dependent) who were given azathioprine and developed intolerance to the medication (31/42) or remained medically refractory to it (11/42). The mean dose of methotrexate was approximately 20 mg orally per week for a period of 30 weeks. Remission was achieved in 42% of the patients, defined as complete withdrawal of steroids for more than 3 months and response (good, partial, or failure of response). There was a good response in 54% and partial response in 18%. Side effects occurred in 23% of patients with 10% stopping treatment.

A recent retrospective study evaluated 32 patients with UC of whom 72% were intolerant and 28% were unresponsive 6-MP or thiopurine.[58] An induction dose of methotrexate 25 mg/week was given either orally (20 patients) or intramuscularly (12 patients), and a maintenance dose of 20 mg/week was given for an average of 1 year. Clinical response was achieved in 68% of UC patients comprising 7 out of 9 (78%) patients in the 6-MP/azathioprine refractory group and nearly two-thirds (15 out of 23) of patients in the intolerant group. Steroid withdrawal occurred in 7 out of 19 patients. Although the numbers are small, there was no difference in clinical response between the oral and intramuscular administration groups. Adverse events occurred in 17.4% of patients and required discontinuation in 8.3%. Generally, 25 mg/week oral or intramuscular methotrexate was effective and well-tolerated in UC.

There appears to be an emerging role for methotrexate in UC, especially in the 6-MP/azathioprine refractory or intolerant population. Cases of UC and indeterminant colitis are not cured by ileal pouch-anal anastomosis and therefore may require maintenance immunomodulator therapy. A re-evaluation of the role of methotrexate in treating UC is needed. Larger randomized controlled trials evaluating both steroid-free remission and mucosal healing in both thiopurine naïve and thiopurine intolerant/refractory UC patients are warranted. While waiting for randomized controlled trials, we may consider the role of methotrexate 25 mg/week intramuscularly with replacement folic acid 1 to 5 mg per day in 6-MP naïve or experienced UC patients.

INFLIXIMAB

Numerous open-label, uncontrolled studies have reported the use of infliximab for various indications in UC, including steroid dependency, steroid resistance, and severe acute colitis.[59-73] The short-term response rates in these studies range from 20% to 100%, while responses over the long-term range from 12% to 70%. In a recently published review of the literature, the clinical response to infliximab was stratified by indication.[74] The median short-term response rate was 77%, and the median long-term response rate was 45%. It appeared that, in general, pediatric patients were more likely to clinically respond than adult patients, and UC patients with steroid-refractory disease were less likely to respond than those with steroid-dependent disease.[74]

In the first randomized, controlled trial of 11 UC patients hospitalized for severe, steroid-refractory disease, 50% of infliximab-treated patients and none of the placebo-treated patients responded (ie, avoided colectomy, steroid dose increase, and cyclosporine).[75] Probert and colleagues performed a randomized trial of 2 infusions of infliximab 5 mg/kg or placebo in 43 patients with moderately severe steroid-refractory UC.[76] At the end of the 6-week study, endoscopic remission rates were 13% in the infliximab group and 5% in the placebo group, and clinical remission rates were 39% and 30%, respectively. These small differences were not significantly different statistically, but the authors acknowledged that their study was powered to detect a 51% absolute difference in remission rates and may have been underpowered to detect smaller differences.[76] In the third study, randomized and controlled but only single-blinded, the investigators randomized 13 UC patients hospitalized for acute severe colitis (not yet deemed steroid-responsive or steroid-refractory) to infliximab 5 mg/kg IV at 0, 2, and 6 weeks or prednisolone 1.5 mg/kg intravenously daily for 2 weeks, 1 mg/kg/d for 1 week, followed by a taper.[77] Treatment success was defined as a more than 5 point decrease in a modified Truelove-Witts activity score and avoidance of colectomy and steroid dose increase. Response rates were 83% in the infliximab group and 86% in the prednisolone group.[77] The authors concluded that infliximab may be effective in the treatment of acute colitis. Finally, a preliminary report from a randomized, placebo-controlled trial of infliximab in acute severe colitis indicated that the 90-day colectomy rate was significantly lower in infliximab-treated patients (29%) versus placebo-treated patients (67%; $P=0.017$).[78]

Infliximab is now indicated for the treatment of moderate to severe UC. FDA approval was based on 2 randomized, double-blind, placebo-controlled studies that showed that patients with moderately to severely active UC treated with infliximab at weeks 0, 2, and 6, and every 8 weeks thereafter, were more likely to have a clinical response at weeks 8, 30, and 54 than those receiving placebo.[79] Patients considered for infliximab were on varying doses of corticosteroids with less than 40% of patients in all groups considered to be corticosteroid-refractory. Additionally, patients were included if there was documented lack of efficacy or intolerance to at least 1 treatment, and in ACT 2, this may mean 5-ASA therapy alone. The mean Mayo score was 8.4, suggesting that infliximab may be more appropriate for moderate steroid-dependent UC rather than severe refractory UC.

MYCOPHENOLATE MOFETIL

Mycophenolate mofetil is most commonly employed as immunosuppressive therapy following renal or cardiac transplantation. The results of its use in uncontrolled studies in refractory UC have been quite mixed.[80,81] In an unblinded but randomized trial comparing mycophenolate mofetil 20 mg/kg/d to AZA 2 mg/kg/d in chronic active UC, all 24 patients received a tapering course of corticosteroids initially and were followed for 1 year.[82] At the end of the study, 100% of the AZA group versus 88% of the mycophenolate group had achieved and maintained remission, and at earlier time points, the remission rates were consistently higher in the AZA group. The median decreases in the disease activity score from baseline were not significantly different.[82] In addition to infectious complications, such as the ones described in this trial, another adverse event that has been described is an atypical colitis characterized by colonic ulcers and lower gastrointestinal hemorrhage.[83] For all of these reasons, mycophenolate is rarely utilized in the treatment of refractory UC; however, it could be used judiciously in selected patients.

TACROLIMUS

A randomized, placebo-controlled study by Ogata et al showed a dose-dependent efficacy of tacrolimus in the induction of remission in patients with refractory UC.[84] The study involved 63 patients with refractory active UC who were randomized to high-dose tacrolimus (10 to 15 ng/mL), low-dose tacrolimus (5 to 10 ng/mL), or placebo. The high-dose group showed a significantly greater rate of improvement in DAI score (68.4% versus 10% of the placebo group; $P<0.001$). In addition, 20% of patients in the high-dose group achieved clinical remission, and 78.9% had mucosal healing. The optimal dose range in this study was 10 to 15 ng/mL for 2 weeks.

General Management Principles of the Severe Acute Colitis Patient

Exacerbation of colitis severe enough to warrant hospitalization or even surgery is a common clinical problem, especially in the first year after diagnosis of UC. Population-based studies from Norway and Sweden suggest that the cumulative colectomy rate for UC in the first year after diagnosis is 8% to 9%.[2,85] Severe colitis is usually defined by the Truelove and Witts criteria: 6 or more bloody stools daily, temperature greater than 37.5°C, pulse greater than 90 beats per minute, hemoglobin less than 10.5 g/dL, and sedimentation rate of greater than 30 mm/hr.[86] Historically, severe colitis was associated with significant morbidity and mortality,[87] but early recognition of severity and appropriate initiation of either medical or surgical therapy have reduced mortality to less than 2%.[88-92]

Infectious agents that may have either triggered a new case of UC or have resulted in an exacerbation of existing UC must be identified and treated. *Clostridium difficile* toxin can be recovered from the stool in up to 15% to 20% of patients hospitalized with UC exacerbations, although its role as a true trigger remains somewhat controversial.[93-95] Nevertheless, it should be treated with metronidazole or oral vancomycin. There are scattered reports of bacterial pathogens such as *Shigella*, *Salmonella*, and *Campylobacter* resulting in UC exacerbations. A less recognized infectious trigger in some patients is cytomegalovirus (CMV). This has been highlighted in several case series.[96-98] These studies suggest that the prevalence of CMV superinfection in severe, steroid-resistant UC might be as high as 39%.[96] Recognition of CMV superinfection can substantially reduce colectomy rates in these patients. The diagnosis is typically made with biopsy—the pathologist should be asked to specifically look for cytomegalic inclusion bodies and perform immunohistochemical stains for CMV if necessary. Treatment consists of withdrawal of immunosuppression and initiation of IV ganciclovir.

If the patient with severe acute colitis has not improved after 5 to 7 days of corticosteroid therapy, a decision needs to be made regarding colectomy or more intensive medical therapy (ie, IV cyclosporine, tacrolimus, or infliximab).

CORTICOSTEROIDS

The dose of corticosteroid employed for severe UC varies across studies. Typically, intravenous methylprednisolone at a dosage ranging from 40 mg/d to approximately 1 mg/kg/d (or the equivalent dose if another corticosteroid is used) is administered as part of the "Oxford regimen."[99] The evidence that higher doses of IV corticosteroids are beneficial in this setting is conflicting. A recent open-label, uncontrolled study from India indicated that "pulse therapy" with dexamethasone at 100 mg/d (the equivalent of 530 mg of methylprednisolone) for 3 days, not followed by additional IV or oral corticosteroids, resulted in clinical remission within 15 days in all but one of 14 patients.[100] However, this finding remains unconfirmed. Hydrocortisone enemas may help reduce tenesmus and urgency.

AZATHIOPRINE

In a small open-label pilot study, 9 UC patients hospitalized with severe acute colitis who were refractory to at least 7 days of IV corticosteroids received an IV loading dose of AZA, between 20 and 40 mg/kg body weight.[101] This was followed by initiation of oral AZA at 2.0 mg/kg/d, and corticosteroids were tapered in the responders. Five patients (56%) avoided colectomy and were able to taper off corticosteroids over the next 3 months, and 3 (33%) were in clinical remission at this point.[101] Further confirmatory data are needed, however, before recommending this route of administering AZA in the setting of the hospitalized UC patient.

CYCLOSPORINE

Cyclosporine is a peptide with selective inhibition of various aspects of cellular and humoral immunity. The availability of this drug revolutionized the management of solid-organ transplant recipients. An open-label, uncontrolled trial of IV cyclosporine 4 mg/kg/d in severe steroid-refractory UC strongly suggested efficacy, with a median response time of 5 to 6 days and a short-term avoidance of colectomy in 73%.[102] The first randomized trial of cyclosporine for acute severe UC unresponsive to parenteral corticosteroids was reported soon thereafter.[103] In this study, 20 steroid-refractory patients hospitalized with severe UC received either cyclosporine 4 mg/kg/d or placebo as a continuous infusion for 14 days.[103] Responders then received oral cyclosporine 8 mg/kg/d. Nine patients (82%) responded to cyclosporine, avoiding colectomy in the short term, while none of the 9 placebo-treated patients responded. Response was maintained at 6 months in approximately one-half of the initial responders. Furthermore, all 5 patients in the placebo arm who were given open-label cyclosporine responded.[103]

In a randomized trial of 30 patients with severe acute UC refractory to oral steroids or AZA, IV cyclosporine 4 mg/kg/d monotherapy was compared to IV methylprednisolone 40 mg/d.[104] The response rate at 8 days was 64% in the cyclosporine group versus 53% in the steroid group.[104] Nonresponders received combination cyclosporine and methylprednisolone, and 40% responded. Responders in both groups received a tapering dose of oral corticosteroids, oral cyclosporine 8 mg/kg/d for 3 months, and oral AZA 2 to 2.5 mg/kg/d. At the end of 1 year, 78% of the initial cyclosporine responders were in remission versus only 37% of the initial steroid responders.[104] No major toxicities were observed. This trial suggested that cyclosporine monotherapy was as effective as IV methylprednisolone in this patient subgroup. However, the study was not formally powered as an equivalence study, and a type II error (failure to detect a significant difference in treatments) is a possibility here.

A third randomized trial compared cyclosporine monotherapy (4 mg/kg/d continuous infusion) to cyclosporine plus prednisolone 1 mg/kg/d in 30 patients with severe steroid-refractory UC.[105] Response rates after 2 weeks were 67% in the cyclosporine monotherapy group and 93% in the combination therapy group, suggesting that combination therapy with cyclosporine and corticosteroids may be more effective than cyclosporine alone.[105] Approximately one-fourth of patients experienced adverse events including paresthesias, hypertension, and mild renal insufficiency.

The largest randomized trial of cyclosporine for this indication compared 2 doses: a 2 mg/kg/d infusion versus a 4 mg/kg/d dose.[106] Response rates after 8 days were similar (83% and 82%), and there was a trend toward a higher incidence of hypertension in the high-dose group (24% versus 9% in the low-dose group).[106] The authors concluded that high-dose therapy conferred no advantage over a 2 mg/kg/d dose.

These 4 trials unequivocally demonstrate the short-term efficacy of IV cyclosporine in the setting of severe acute colitis, and this has been corroborated by numerous uncontrolled trials and case series.[107-123] The short-term avoidance of colectomy in most of these studies ranges from 56% to 92%. However, the probability of requiring colectomy following cyclosporine rescue therapy increases, and most series report that only 30% to 60% of patients avoid colectomy over the next 3 to 5 years. Longer-term data of up to 7 years demonstrate a colectomy avoidance rate as low as 12%[124] up to 58%,[125] indicating the difficulty of maintaining remission. Several studies demonstrated that a transition from cyclosporine to AZA or 6-MP was associated with a higher likelihood of avoiding colectomy.[109,113,115,122] Conversely, patients already on a purine analog prior to initiation of cyclosporine were more likely to undergo colectomy, with one study significant for a colectomy rate of 88% within 1 year of the start of IV cyclosporine.[124] Patients taking immunomodulator therapy prior to initiation of cyclosporine may represent a group of patients with more severe refractory disease who may not benefit from cyclosporine treatment.

It is our practice to start a purine analog when the patient is dismissed from the hospital and to continue oral cyclosporine for at least 3 months to allow for the full onset of effect of the purine analog. Thus, patients are managed for a time period on "transplant-level" triple immunosuppressive therapy and require prophylaxis for *Pneumocystis jirovecii* (formerly *Pneumocystis carinii*).[126]

Adverse events have been reported following cyclosporine rescue therapy, including paresthesias, hypertrichosis, hypertension, tremor, renal insufficiency, electrolyte abnormalities, seizure, and infection, some of which have been fatal.[127] Thus, the risks of cyclosporine therapy must be weighed against the benefits on a case-by-case basis, and patients who undergo this course of treatment should be followed carefully and instructed to have a low threshold to seek medical attention. Where cyclosporine therapy will fit into our treatment algorithm for UC with the advent of infliximab use for this indication remains to be determined.

Historically, cyclosporine has been the only option for colectomy avoidance in patients with steroid-refractory UC. Despite the introduction of new medications for UC, the colectomy rate has remained stable at 27% over the past 3 decades, excluding the infliximab data.[128] The advent of infliximab questions its role in steroid-refractory severe UC. The ACT 1 and ACT 2 trials were randomized, double-blind, placebo-controlled studies demonstrating that patients with moderate to severe UC were more likely to have a clinical response to infliximab versus placebo. Corticosteroid dosing was not standardized prior to randomization, and the majority of patients in these studies were not considered to be steroid-refractory with less than 40% of all patients noted to be steroid-refractory. The authors of the ACT 1 and ACT 2 trials suggest that all patients with medically refractory UC should be offered both colectomy and infliximab as treatment options.[79] Further studies to evaluate the role of infliximab in steroid-refractory UC and the impact on colectomy avoidance are warranted.

In patients who fail infliximab therapy and require colectomy, some studies have demonstrated an increase in infectious complications after ileal pouch anal-anastomosis (IPAA). One prospective study found an increase in anastomotic leaks and infectious complications in the infliximab group.[129] In contrast, another study found no increase in postoperative complications in the infliximab-treated group.[130] The use of infliximab in patients with steroid-refractory severe UC remains to be defined.

There is little evidence for combining cyclosporine and infliximab in steroid-refractory UC patients. In patients with severe UC who have failed either cyclosporine or infliximab, Maser et al studied the use of switching therapy to infliximab for cyclosporine first failures or switching to cyclosporine for infliximab first failures.[131] Remission rates with switch/salvage therapy occurred in only one-third of patients and had limited duration. Furthermore, there was an increased risk of serious infectious complications if salvage therapy occurred within a month of stopping or switching therapy. Serious adverse events were noted in 16% of patients, including one death from gram-negative *E. coli* sepsis in a patient treated with infliximab 1 day after cyclosporine cessation. Switch/salvage therapy with either infliximab or cyclosporine is not recommended unless the washout period is greater than 1 month.

TACROLIMUS

Tacrolimus is most commonly utilized for immunosuppression following solid-organ transplantation. Although it has low oral bioavailability like cyclosporine, it has the theoretical advantage of not requiring bile or noninflamed bowel for absorption and, therefore, might be easier to administer orally than cyclosporine. There are no randomized trials of tacrolimus in refractory UC. A number of uncontrolled experiences, however, suggest a benefit in some patients.[132-137] In a pediatric case series, 14 patients with severe steroid-refractory colitis (10 UC, 2 Crohn's, 2 indeterminate) were treated with 0.1 mg/kg by mouth twice daily in conjunction with a tapering course of steroids followed by purine analog therapy.[133] The 2-week response rate was 69%, but an additional 4 patients required colectomy after discharge from the hospital, such that the survival free of colectomy at the end of 1 year was 38%.[133] In an experience from Lubeck, Germany, patients with steroid-refractory UC or indeterminate colitis, only some of whom were hospitalized, received either continuous infusion with 0.01 to 0.02 mg/kg/d for up to 14 days followed by 0.1 to 0.2 mg/kg/d by mouth or oral treatment alone.[134] The short-term response (avoidance of colectomy) was high at 92%; however, in patients with complete 2-year follow-up, the colectomy rate was 50%.[134] In another German case series, 23 patients with severe acute steroid-dependent or steroid-refractory UC were treated with oral tacrolimus 0.1 mg/kg/d in 2 divided doses followed by dose titration to therapeutic levels.[137] The median duration of treatment with tacrolimus was 12 months. Ninety-six percent of patients responded in the short term, and overall 74% of the UC patients treated went into a remission for at least 8 weeks. Significant reduction or discontinuation of corticosteroids was possible in 83% of patients.[137] After a median follow-up of 18 months, colectomy was avoided in 20 UC patients (87%). In an Austrian case series of 9 moderate to severe steroid-refractory UC patients who received oral tacrolimus 0.15 mg/kg/d, 67% were in complete remission at 3 months. After a mean follow-up of 1 year, colectomy was avoided in two-thirds.[136] In UC patients in whom other medical or surgical therapies are not attractive, tacrolimus may be a viable option.

CONCLUSION

Medically refractory UC can be difficult to manage. Steroid dependence and resistance are not uncommon and may be due to abnormally high expression of drug-pumping proteins such as p-glycoprotein 170 (product of MDR1 gene), increased activation of intracellular signalers such as NFKB, or abnormalities in the glucocorticoid receptor. Factors producing a "refractory" picture, such as medical nonadherence, coexistent IBS, 5-ASA hypersensitivity, NSAID use, and superinfection with cytomegalovirus or *Clostridium difficile*, should be excluded. There is reasonably good evidence to warrant a trial of AZA or 6-MP in the moderate steroid-resistant or steroid-dependent patient. The evidence for methotrexate is weak at best. Infliximab may be considered part of the medical armamentarium in select patients with moderate to severe UC.

Patients with severe acute colitis should be hospitalized and undergo stool studies and a flexible sigmoidoscopy with biopsies to rule out superinfection, receive IV corticosteroids, and be followed carefully for the development of toxic megacolon. For those severe patients not responding to corticosteroids, judicious use of cyclosporine (and possibly tacrolimus) may be beneficial. The challenge is whether to consider initiation of therapy with infliximab in the steroid-refractory patient as the role of infliximab in severe UC remains controversial. In the patient with severe refractory UC, colectomy must always be discussed as a therapeutic option.

REFERENCES

1. Langholz E, Munkholm P, Davidsen M, Binder V. Course of ulcerative colitis: analysis of changes in disease activity over years. *Gastroenterology.* 1994;107:3-11.
2. Langholz E, Munkholm P, Davidsen M, Binder V. Colorectal cancer risk and mortality in patients with ulcerative colitis. *Gastroenterology.* 1992;103:1444-1451.
3. Faubion WA, Loftus EV, Harmsen WS, Zinsmeister AR, Sandborn WJ. The natural history of corticosteroid therapy for inflammatory bowel disease: a population-based study. *Gastroenterology.* 2001;121:255-260.
4. Farrell RJ, Kelleher D. Glucocorticoid resistance in inflammatory bowel disease. *J Endocrinol.* 2003;178:339-346.
5. Hearing SD, Norman M, Probert CS, Haslam N, Dayan CM. Predicting therapeutic outcome in severe ulcerative colitis by measuring in vitro steroid sensitivity of proliferating peripheral blood lymphocytes. *Gut.* 1999;45:382-388.
6. Ho GT, Moodie FM, Satsangi J. Multidrug resistance 1 gene (P-glycoprotein 170): an important determinant in gastrointestinal disease? *Gut.* 2003;52:759-766.
7. Farrell RJ, Murphy A, Long A, et al. High multidrug resistance (P-glycoprotein 170) expression in inflammatory bowel disease patients who fail medical therapy. *Gastroenterology.* 2000;118:279-288.
8. Farrell RJ, Menconi MJ, Keates AC, Kelly CP. P-glycoprotein-170 inhibition significantly reduces cortisol and cyclosporin efflux from human intestinal epithelial cells and T lymphocytes. *Aliment Pharmacol Ther.* 2002;16:1021-1031.
9. Langmann T, Moehle C, Mauerer R, et al. Loss of detoxification in inflammatory bowel disease: dysregulation of pregnane X receptor target genes. *Gastroenterology.* 2004;127:26-40.
10. Honda M, Orii F, Ayabe T, et al. Expression of glucocorticoid receptor beta in lymphocytes of patients with glucocorticoid-resistant ulcerative colitis. *Gastroenterology.* 2000;118:859-866.
11. Bantel H, Domschke W, Schulze-Osthoff K, Kaskas B, Gregor M. Abnormal activation of transcription factor NF-kappaB involved in steroid resistance in chronic inflammatory bowel disease. *Am J Gastroenterol.* 2000;95:1845-1846.
12. Bantel H, Schmitz ML, Raible A, Gregor M, Schulze-Osthoff K. Critical role of NF-kappaB and stress-activated protein kinases in steroid unresponsiveness. *FASEB J.* 2002;16:1832-1834.
13. Sachar DB. Ten common errors in the management of inflammatory bowel disease. *Inflamm Bowel Dis.* 2003;9:205-209.
14. Kane SV, Cohen RD, Aikens JE, Hanauer SB. Prevalence of nonadherence with maintenance mesalamine in quiescent ulcerative colitis. *Am J Gastroenterol.* 2001;96:2929-2933.
15. Sewitch MJ, Abrahamowicz M, Barkun A, et al. Patient nonadherence to medication in inflammatory bowel disease. *Am J Gastroenterol.* 2003;98:1535-1544.
16. Kane S, Huo DZ, Aikens J, Hanauer S. Medication nonadherence and the outcomes of patients with quiescent ulcerative colitis. *Am J Med.* 2003;114:39-43.
17. Schwartz AG, Targan SR, Saxon A, Weinstein WM. Sulfasalazine-induced exacerbation of ulcerative colitis. *N Engl J Med.* 1982;306:409-412.
18. Sturgeon JB, Bhatia P, Hermens D, Miner PB Jr. Exacerbation of chronic ulcerative colitis with mesalamine. *Gastroenterology.* 1995;108:1889-1893.

19. Evans JMM, McMahon AD, Murray FE, McDevitt DG, Macdonald TM. Non-steroidal anti-inflammatory drugs are associated with emergency admission to hospital for colitis due to inflammatory bowel disease. *Gut.* 1997;40:619-622.
20. Felder JB, Korelitz BI, Rajapakse R, Schwarz S, Horatagis AP, Gleim G. Effects of nonsteroidal anti-inflammatory drugs on inflammatory bowel disease: a case-control study. *Am J Gastroenterol.* 2000;95:1949-1954.
21. Bonner GF, Walczak M, Kitchen L, Bayona M. Tolerance of nonsteroidal anti-inflammatory drugs in patients with inflammatory bowel disease. *Am J Gastroenterol.* 2000;95:1946-1948.
22. Bonner GF, Fakhri A, Vennamaneni SR. A long-term cohort study of nonsteroidal anti-inflammatory drug use and disease activity in outpatients with inflammatory bowel disease. *Inflamm Bowel Dis.* 2004;10:751-757.
23. Forrest K, Symmons D, Foster P. Systematic review: is ingestion of paracetamol or non-steroidal anti-inflammatory drugs associated with exacerbations of inflammatory bowel disease? *Aliment Pharmacol Ther.* 2004;20:1035-1043.
24. Mahadevan U, Loftus EV, Tremaine WJ, Sandborn WJ. Safety of selective cyclooxygenase-2 inhibitors in inflammatory bowel disease. *Am J Gastroenterol.* 2002;97:910-914.
25. Reinisch W, Miehsler W, Dejaco C, et al. An open-label trial of the selective cyclooxygenase-2 inhibitor, rofecoxib, in inflammatory bowel disease-associated peripheral arthritis and arthralgia. *Aliment Pharmacol Ther.* 2003;17:1371-1380.
26. Biancone L, Tosti C, Geremia A, et al. Rofecoxib and early relapse of inflammatory bowel disease: an open-label trial. *Aliment Pharmacol Ther.* 2004;19:755-764.
27. Matuk R, Crawford J, Abreu MT, Targan SR, Vasiliauskas EA, Papadakis KA. The spectrum of gastrointestinal toxicity and effect on disease activity of selective cyclooxygenase-2 inhibitors in patients with inflammatory bowel disease. *Inflamm Bowel Dis.* 2004;10:352-356.
28. Sandborn WJ, Stenson WF, Brynskov J, Steidle G, Robbins J. Safety of celecoxib in patients with ulcerative colitis in remission: a randomized, double-blind, placebo-controlled study [abstract]. *Am J Gastroenterol.* 2004;99:S257-S258.
29. Jewell DP, Truelove SC. Azathioprine in ulcerative colitis: final report on controlled therapeutic trial. *Br Med J.* 1974;4: 627-630.
30. Caprilli R, Carratu R, Babbini M. Double-blind comparison of the effectiveness of azathioprine and sulfasalazine in idiopathic proctocolitis: preliminary report. *Am J Dig Dis.* 1975;20:115-120.
31. Rosenberg JL, Wall AJ, Levin B, Binder HJ, Kirsner JB. A controlled trial of azathioprine in the management of chronic ulcerative colitis. *Gastroenterology.* 1975;69:96-99.
32. Kirk AP, Lennard-Jones JE. Controlled trial of azathioprine in chronic ulcerative colitis. *Br Med J Clin Res Ed.* 1982;284:1291-1292.
33. Hawthorne AB, Logan RF, Hawkey CJ, et al. Randomised controlled trial of azathioprine withdrawal in ulcerative colitis. *BMJ.* 1992;305:20-22.
34. Sood A, Midha V, Sood N, Kaushal V. Role of azathioprine in severe ulcerative colitis: one-year, placebo-controlled, randomized trial. *Ind J Gastroenterol.* 2000;19:14-16.
35. Sood A, Kaushal V, Midha V, Bhatia KL, Sood N, Malhotra V. The beneficial effect of azathioprine on maintenance of remission in severe ulcerative colitis. *J Gastroenterol.* 2002;37:270-274.
36. Sood A, Midha V, Sood N, Avasthi G. Azathioprine versus sulfasalazine in maintenance of remission in severe ulcerative colitis. *Ind J Gastroenterol.* 2003;22:79-81.
37. Mantzaris GJ, Sfakianakis M, Archavlis E, et al. A prospective randomized observer-blind 2-year trial of azathioprine monotherapy versus azathioprine and olsalazine for the maintenance of remission of steroid-dependent ulcerative colitis. *Am J Gastroenterol.* 2004;99:1122-1128.
38. Ardizzone S, Samolvico F, Bollani S, Imbesi V, Colombo E, Bianchi Porro G. Azathioprine is more effective than oral 5-ASA in the treatment of steroid-dependent ulcerative colitis (Abstr.). *Gastroenterology.* 2001;120:A127.
39. Ohno K, Masunaga Y, Ogawa R, Hashiguchi M, Ogata H. A systematic review of the clinical effectiveness of azathioprine in patients with ulcerative colitis. *Yakugaku Zasshi J Pharmaceut Soc Japan.* 2004;124:555-560.
40. Lobo AJ, Foster PN, Burke DA, Johnston D, Axon AT. The role of azathioprine in the management of ulcerative colitis. *Dis Colon Rectum.* 1990;33:374-377.
41. Steinhart AH, Baker JP, Brzezinski A, Prokipchuk EJ. Azathioprine therapy in chronic ulcerative colitis. *J Clin Gastroenterol.* 1990;12:271-275.
42. George J, Present DH, Pou R, Bodian C, Rubin PH. The long-term outcome of ulcerative colitis treated with 6-mercaptopurine. *Am J Gastroenterol.* 1996;91:1711-1714.
43. Ardizzone S, Molteni P, Imbesi V, Bollani S, Bianchi Porro G. Azathioprine in steroid-resistant and steroid-dependent ulcerative colitis. *J Clin Gastroenterol.* 1997;25:330-333.
44. Fraser AG, Orchard TR, Jewell DP. The efficacy of azathioprine for the treatment of inflammatory bowel disease: a 30 year review. *Gut.* 2002;50:485-489.
45. Lobel EZ, Korelitz BI, Xuereb MA, Panagopoulos G. A search for the optimal duration of treatment with 6-mercaptopurine for ulcerative colitis. *Am J Gastroenterol.* 2004;99:462-465.
46. Lopez-Sanroman A, Bermejo F, Carrera E, Garcia-Plaza A. Efficacy and safety of thiopurinic immunomodulators (azathioprine and mercaptopurine) in steroid-dependent ulcerative colitis. *Aliment Pharmacol Ther.* 2004;20:161-166.
47. Rayner CK, Hart AL, Hayward CMM, Emmanuel AV, Kamm MA. Azathioprine dose escalation in inflammatory bowel disease. *Aliment Pharmacol Ther.* 2004;20:65-71.
48. Velayos FS, Walsh JME, Terdiman JP. Effect of 5-aminosalicylate use on colorectal cancer and dysplasia risk in ulcerative colitis: A meta-analysis (Abstr.). *Gastroenterology.* 2004;126:A20.
49. Lowry PW, Franklin CL, Weaver AL, et al. Leukopenia resulting from a drug interaction between azathioprine or 6-mercaptopurine and mesalamine, sulphasalazine, or balsalazide. *Gut.* 2001;49:656-664.
50. Kozarek RA, Patterson DJ, Gelfand MD, Botoman VA, Ball TJ, Wilske KR. Methotrexate induces clinical and histologic remission in patients with refractory inflammatory bowel disease. *Ann Intern Med.* 1989;110:353-356.
51. Baron TH, Truss CD, Elson CO. Low-dose oral methotrexate in refractory inflammatory bowel disease. *Dig Dis Sci.* 1993;38:1851-1856.
52. Paoluzi OA, Pica R, Marcheggiano A, et al. Azathioprine or methotrexate in the treatment of patients with steroid-dependent or steroid-resistant ulcerative colitis: results of an open-label study on efficacy and tolerability in inducing and maintaining remission. *Aliment Pharmacol Ther.* 2002;16:1751-1759.
53. Fraser AG, Morton D, McGovern D, Travis S, Jewell DP. The efficacy of methotrexate for maintaining remission in inflammatory bowel disease. *Aliment Pharmacol Ther.* 2002;16:693-697.
54. Oren R, Arber N, Odes S, et al. Methotrexate in chronic active ulcerative colitis: a double-blind, randomized, Israeli multicenter trial. *Gastroenterology.* 1996;110:1416-1421.
55. Kozarek RA. Methotrexate and ulcerative colitis: wrong drug? Wrong dose? Or wrong disease? *Gastroenterology.* 1996;110:1652-166.

56. Maté-Jiménez J, Hermida C, Cantero-Perona J, Moreno-Otero R. 6-Mercaptopurine or methotrexate added to prednisone induces and maintains remission in steroid-dependent inflammatory bowel disease. *Eur J Gastroenterol Hepatol.* 2000;12:1227-1233.
57. Cummings JR, Herrlinger KR, Travis SP, Gorard DA, McIntyre AS, Jewell DP. Oral methotrexate in ulcerative colitis. *Aliment Pharmacol Ther.* 2005;21(4):385-389.
58. Wahed M, Louis-Auguste JR, Baxter LM, et al. Efficacy of methotrexate in Crohn's disease and ulcerative colitis patients unresponsive or intolerant to azathioprine/mercaptopurine. *Aliment Pharmacol Ther.* 2009;30(6):614-620.
59. Chey WY. Infliximab for patients with refractory ulcerative colitis. *Inflamm Bowel Dis.* 2001;7:S30-S33.
60. Chey WY, Hussain A, Ryan C, Potter GD, Shah A. Infliximab for refractory ulcerative colitis. *Am J Gastroenterol.* 2001;96:2373-2381.
61. Kaser A, Mairinger T, Vogel W, Tilg H. Infliximab in severe steroid-refractory ulcerative colitis: a pilot study. *Wien Klin Woch.* 2001;113:930-933.
62. Actis GC, Bruno M, Pinna-Pintor M, Rossini FP, Rizzetto M. Infliximab for treatment of steroid-refractory ulcerative colitis. *Dig Liver Dis.* 2002;34:631-634.
63. Kohn A, Prantera C, Pera A, Cosintino R, Sostegni R, Daperno M. Anti-tumour necrosis factor alpha (Infliximab) in the treatment of severe ulcerative colitis: Result of an open study on 13 patients. *Dig Liver Dis.* 2002;34:626-630.
64. Mamula P, Markowitz JE, Brown KA, Hurd LB, Piccoli DA, Baldassano RN. Infliximab as a novel therapy for pediatric ulcerative colitis. *J Pediatr Gastroenterol Nutr.* 2002;34:307-311.
65. Su CY, Salzberg BA, Lewis JD, et al. Efficacy of anti-tumor necrosis factor therapy in patients with ulcerative colitis. *Am J Gastroenterol.* 2002;97:2577-2584.
66. Gornet JM, Couve S, Hassani Z, et al. Infliximab for refractory ulcerative colitis or indeterminate colitis: an open-label multicentre study. *Aliment Pharmacol Ther.* 2003;18:175-181.
67. Lam ECS, Bailey RJ. Infliximab salvage therapy after cyclosporine in an acute flare of chronic ulcerative colitis. *Can J Gastroenterol.* 2003;17:198-200.
68. Papadakis KA, Treyzon L, Abreu MT, Fleshner PR, Targan SR, Vasiliauskas EA. Infliximab in the treatment of medically refractory indeterminate colitis. *Aliment Pharmacol Ther.* 2003;18:741-747.
69. Armuzzi A, De Pascalis B, Lupascu A, et al. Infliximab in the treatment of steroid-dependent ulcerative colitis. *Eur Rev Med Pharmacol Sci.* 2004;8:231-233.
70. Bermejo F, Lopez-Sanroman A, Hinojosa J, Castro L, Jurado C, Gomez-Belda AB. Infliximab induces clinical, endoscopic and histological responses in refractory ulcerative colitis. *Rev Esp Enferm Dig.* 2004;96:94-97.
71. Jimenez JM. Infliximab in the treatment of severe ulcerative colitis. *Rev Esp Enferm Dig.* 2004;96:89-93.
72. Kohn A, Prantera C, Pera A, Cosintino R, Sostegni R, Daperno M. Infliximab in the treatment of severe ulcerative colitis: a follow-up study. *Eur Rev Med Pharmacol Sci.* 2004;8:235-237.
73. Mamula P, Markowitz JE, Cohen LJ, von Allmen D, Baldassano RN. Infliximab in pediatric ulcerative colitis: two-year follow-up. *J Pediatr Gastroenterol Nutr.* 2004;38:298-301.
74. Rossetti S, Actis GC, Fadda M, Rizzetto M, Palmo A. The use of the anti-tumour necrosis factor monoclonal antibody-infliximab-to treat ulcerative colitis: implications and trends beyond the available data. *Dig Liver Dis.* 2004;36:426-431.
75. Sands BE, Tremaine WJ, Sandborn WJ, et al. Infliximab in the treatment of severe, steroid-refractory ulcerative colitis: a pilot study. *Inflamm Bowel Dis.* 2001;7:83-88.
76. Probert CSJ, Hearing SD, Schreiber S, et al. Infliximab in moderately severe glucocorticoid resistant ulcerative colitis: a randomised controlled trial. *Gut.* 2003;52:998-1002.
77. Ochsenkuhn T, Sackmann M, Goke B. Infliximab for acute, not steroid-refractory ulcerative colitis: a randomized pilot study. *Eur J Gastroenterol Hepatol.* 2004;16:1167-1171.
78. Järnerot G, Hertervig E, Friis-Liby I, et al. Infliximab as rescue therapy in severe to moderately severe ulcerative colitis: a randomized, placebo-controlled study. *Gastroenterology.* 2005;128(7):1805-1811.
79. Rutgeerts P, Sandborn WJ, Feagan BG, et al. Infliximab for induction and maintenance therapy for ulcerative colitis. *N Engl J Med.* 2005;353(23):2462-2476.
80. Fellermann K, Steffen M, Stein J, et al. Mycophenolate mofetil: lack of efficacy in chronic active inflammatory bowel disease. *Aliment Pharmacol Ther.* 2000;14:171-176.
81. Ford AC, Towler RJ, Moayyedi P, Chalmers DM, Axon ATR. Mycophenolate mofetil in refractory inflammatory bowel disease. *Aliment Pharmacol Ther.* 2003;17:1365-1369.
82. Orth T, Peters M, Schlaak JF, et al. Mycophenolate mofetil versus azathioprine in patients with chronic active ulcerative colitis: a 12-month pilot study. *Am J Gastroenterol.* 2000;95:1201-1207.
83. Skelly MM, Logan RF, Jenkins D, Mahida YR, Hawkey CJ. Toxicity of mycophenolate mofetil in patients with inflammatory bowel disease. *Inflamm Bowel Dis.* 2002;8:93-97.
84. Ogata H, Matsui T, Nakamura M, et al. A randomised dose finding study of oral tacrolimus (FK506) therapy in refractory ulcerative colitis. *Gut.* 2006;55(9):1255-1262.
85. Moum B, Ekbom A, Vatn MH, et al. Clinical course during the 1st year after diagnosis in ulcerative colitis and Crohn's disease: results of a large, prospective population-based study in southeastern Norway, 1990-93. *Scand J Gastroenterol.* 1997;32:1005-1012.
86. Truelove SC, Witts LJ. Cortisone in ulcerative colitis: final report on a therapeutic trial. *Br Med J.* 1955;2:1041-1048.
87. Edwards FE, Truelove SC. The course and prognosis of ulcerative colitis: short term prognosis. *Gut.* 1963;4:299-308.
88. Travis SP, Farrant JM, Ricketts C, et al. Predicting outcome in severe ulcerative colitis. *Gut.* 1996;38:905-910.
89. Carbonnel F, Gargouri D, Lemann M, et al. Predictive factors of outcome of intensive intravenous treatment for attacks of ulcerative colitis. *Aliment Pharmacol Ther.* 2000;14:273-279.
90. Ho GT, Mowat C, Goddard CJR, et al. Predicting the outcome of severe ulcerative colitis: development of a novel risk score to aid early selection of patients for second-line medical therapy or surgery. *Aliment Pharmacol Ther.* 2004;19:1079-1087.
91. Daperno M, Sostegni R, Scaglione N, et al. Outcome of a conservative approach in severe ulcerative colitis. *Dig Liver Dis.* 2004;36:21-28.
92. Benazzato L, D'Inca R, Grigoletto F, et al. Prognosis of severe attacks in ulcerative colitis: effect of intensive medical treatment. *Dig Liver Dis.* 2004;36:461-466.
93. Meyers S, Mayer L, Bottone E, Desmond E, Janowitz HD. Occurrence of *Clostridium difficile* toxin during the course of inflammatory bowel disease. *Gastroenterology.* 1981;80:697-670.
94. Meyer AM, Ramzan NN, Loftus EV Jr, Heigh RI, Leighton JA. The diagnostic yield of stool pathogen studies during relapses of inflammatory bowel disease. *J Clin Gastroenterol.* 2004;38:772-775.
95. Boetticher NC, Pardi DS, Loftus EV, Sandborn WJ. *Clostridium difficile* infection in ulcerative colitis (Abstr.). *Am J Gastroenterol.* 2004;99:S261.
96. Cottone M, Pietrosi G, Martorana G, et al. Prevalence of cytomegalovirus infection in severe refractory ulcerative and Crohn's colitis. *Am J Gastroenterol.* 2001;96:773-775.

97. Criscuoli V, Casa A, Orlando A, et al. Severe acute colitis associated with CMV: a prevalence study. *Dig Liver Dis.* 2004;36:818-820.
98. Loftus EV Jr. Hunting for the owl's eye in acute severe colitis: the role of cytomegalovirus. *Dig Liver Dis.* 2004;36:803-805.
99. Truelove SC, Jewell DP. Intensive intravenous regimen for severe attacks of ulcerative colitis. *Lancet.* 1974;1:1067-1070.
100. Sood A, Midha V, Sood N, Awasthi G. A prospective, open-label trial assessing dexamethasone pulse therapy in moderate to severe ulcerative colitis. *J Clin Gastroenterol.* 2002;35:328-331.
101. Mahadevan U, Tremaine WJ, Johnson T, et al. Intravenous azathioprine in severe ulcerative colitis: a pilot study. *Am J Gastroenterol.* 2000;95:3463-3468.
102. Lichtiger S, Present DH. Preliminary report: cyclosporin in treatment of severe active ulcerative colitis. *Lancet.* 1990;336:16-19.
103. Lichtiger S, Present DH, Kornbluth A, et al. Cyclosporine in severe ulcerative colitis refractory to steroid therapy. *N Engl J Med.* 1994;330:1841-1845.
104. D'Haens G, Lemmens L, Geboes K, et al. Intravenous cyclosporine versus intravenous corticosteroids as single therapy for severe attacks of ulcerative colitis. *Gastroenterology.* 2001;120:1323-1329.
105. Svanoni F, Bonassi U, Bagnolo F, Caporuscio S. Effectiveness of cyclosporine A (CsA) in the treatment of active refractory ulcerative colitis (UC) (Abstr.). *Gastroenterology.* 1998;114:A1096.
106. Van Assche G, D'Haens G, Noman M, et al. Randomized, double-blind comparison of 4 mg/kg versus 2 mg/kg intravenous cyclosporine in severe ulcerative colitis. *Gastroenterology.* 2003;125:1025-1031.
107. Actis GC, Ottobrelli A, Pera A, et al. Continuously infused cyclosporine at low dose is sufficient to avoid emergency colectomy in acute attacks of ulcerative colitis without the need for high-dose steroids. *J Clin Gastroenterol.* 1993;17:10-13.
108. Carbonnel F, Boruchowicz A, Duclos B, et al. Intravenous cyclosporine in attacks of ulcerative colitis: short-term and long-term responses. *Dig Dis Sci.* 1996;41:2471-2476.
109. Fernandez-Banares F, Bertran X, Esteve-Comas M, et al. Azathioprine is useful in maintaining long-term remission induced by intravenous cyclosporine in steroid-refractory severe ulcerative colitis. *Am J Gastroenterol.* 1996;91:2498-2499.
110. Van Gossum A, Schmit A, Adler M, et al. Short- and long-term efficacy of cyclosporin administration in patients with acute severe ulcerative colitis: Belgian IBD Group. *Acta Gastroenterol Belg.* 1997;60:197-200.
111. Hyde GM, Thillainayagam AV, Jewell DP. Intravenous cyclosporin as rescue therapy in severe ulcerative colitis: time for a reappraisal? *Eur J Gastroenterol Hepatol.* 1998;10:411-413.
112. Wenzl HH, Petritsch W, Aichbickler BW, Hinterleitner TA, Fleischmann G, Krejs GJ. Short-term efficacy and long-term outcome of cyclosporine treatment in patients with severe ulcerative colitis. *Z Gastroenterol.* 1998;36:287-293.
113. Yoon C, Kornbluth A, George J, et al. Is cyclosporine as effective in chronic ulcerative colitis as in severe ulcerative colitis? [abstract]. *Gastroenterology.* 1998;114:A1120-A1121.
114. Stack WA, Long RG, Hawkey CJ. Short- and long-term outcome of patients treated with cyclosporin for severe acute ulcerative colitis. *Aliment Pharmacol Ther.* 1998;12:973-978.
115. Cohen RD, Stein R, Hanauer SB. Intravenous cyclosporin in ulcerative colitis: a five-year experience. *Am J Gastroenterol.* 1999;94:1587-1592.
116. Hermida-Rodriguez C, Perona JC, Garcia-Valriberas R, Garcia JMP, Mate-Jimenez J. High-dose intravenous cyclosporine in steroid-refractory attacks of inflammatory bowel disease. *Hepatogastroenterology.* 1999;46:2265-2268.
117. Actis GC. Cyclosporin for steroid-refractory ulcerative colitis. *Am J Gastroenterol.* 2000;95:830.
118. Rowe FA, Walker JH, Karp LC, Vasiliauskas EA, Plevy SE, Targan SR. Factors predictive of response to cyclosporin treatment for severe, steroid-resistant ulcerative colitis. *Am J Gastroenterol.* 2000;95:2000-2008.
119. Naftali T, Novis B, Pomeranz I, et al. Cyclosporin for severe ulcerative colitis. *Isr Med Assoc J.* 2000;2:588-591.
120. Chiba T, Orii S, Shitomi T, et al. Effects of cyclosporine in steroid-refractory severe acute ulcerative colitis. *J Clin Gastroenterol.* 2002;34:101-103.
121. Campbell S, Ghosh S. Combination immunomodulatory therapy with cyclosporine and azathioprine in corticosteroid-resistant severe ulcerative colitis: the Edinburgh experience of outcome. *Dig Liver Dis.* 2003;35:546-551.
122. Danalioglu A, Kaymakoglu S, Mungan Z, et al. Cyclosporin for severe ulcerative colitis attacks. *Hepatogastroenterology.* 2003;50.
123. Arts J, D'Haens G, Zeegers M, et al. Long-term outcome of treatment with intravenous cyclosporin in patients with severe ulcerative colitis. *Inflamm Bowel Dis.* 2004;10:73-78.
124. Moskovitz DN, Van Assche G, Maenhout B, et al. Incidence of colectomy during long-term follow-up after cyclosporine-induced remission of severe ulcerative colitis. *Clin Gastroenterol Hepatol.* 2006;4(6):760-765.
125. Campbell S, Travis S, Jewell D. Ciclosporin use in acute ulcerative colitis: a long-term experience. *Eur J Gastroenterol Hepatol.* 2005;17(1):79-84.
126. Poppers DM, Scherl EJ. Prophylaxis against *Pneumocystis pneumonia* in patients with inflammatory bowel disease: toward a standard of care. *Inflamm Bowel Dis.* 2008;14(1):106-113.
127. Sandborn WJ. A critical review of cyclosporine therapy in inflammatory bowel disease. *Inflamm Bowel Dis.* 1995;1:48-63.
128. Fellermann K, Ludwig D, Stahl M, David-Walek T, Stange EF. Steroid-unresponsive acute attacks of inflammatory bowel disease: Immunomodulation by tacrolimus (FK506). *Am J Gastroenterol.* 1998;93:1860-1866.
129. Long MD, Plevy SE. Poorly responsive ulcerative colitis in the hospital. *Clin Gastroenterol Hepatol.* 2009;7(6):635-640.
130. Selvasekar CR, Cima RR, Larson DW, et al. Effect of infliximab on short-term complications in patients undergoing operation for chronic ulcerative colitis. *J Am Coll Surg.* 2007;204(5):956-962.
131. Kunitake H, Hodin R, Shellito PC, Sands BE, Korzenik J, Bordeianou L. Perioperative treatment with infliximab in patients with Crohn's disease and ulcerative colitis is not associated with an increased rate of postoperative complications. *J Gastrointest Surg.* 2008;12(10):1730-1736.
132. Maser EA, Deconda D, Lichtiger S, Ullman T, Present DH, Kornbluth A. Cyclosporine and infliximab as rescue therapy for each other in patients with steroid-refractory ulcerative colitis. *Clin Gastroenterol Hepatol.* 2008;6(10):1112-1126.
133. Bousvaros A, Kirschner BS, Werlin SL, et al. Oral tacrolimus treatment of severe colitis in children. *J Pediatr.* 2000;137:794-799.
134. Fellermann K, Tanko T, Herrlinger KR, et al. Response of refractory colitis to intravenous or oral tacrolimus (FK506). *Inflamm Bowel Dis.* 2002;8:317-324.
135. Pascu M, Muller HP, Muller AR, Wiedenmann B, Dignass AU. Rescue therapy with tacrolimus in a patient with toxic megacolon. *Intl J Colorectal Dis.* 2003;18:271-275.
136. Hogenauer C, Wenzl HH, Hinterleitner TA, Petritsch W. Effect of oral tacrolimus (FK 506) on steroid-refractory moderate/severe ulcerative colitis. *Aliment Pharmacol Ther.* 2003;18:415-423.

137. Baumgart DC, Wiedenmann B, Dignass AU. Rescue therapy with tacrolimus is effective in patients with severe and refractory inflammatory bowel disease. *Aliment Pharmacol Ther.* 2003;17:1273-1281.

31

Pseudointractability of Inflammatory Bowel Disease

Mansour A. Parsi, MD and Jean-Paul Achkar, MD

The inflammatory bowel diseases, ulcerative colitis and Crohn's disease (CD), are chronic medical conditions for which there are increasing numbers of efficacious medical therapies. However, some patients with inflammatory bowel disease (IBD), either on initial presentation or at some point during their subsequent disease course, develop symptoms that do not respond to conventional medical therapies. These patients are typically classified as having intractable or refractory disease and may go on to receive alternative medical therapies, including investigational agents, or may be referred for surgery. It is estimated that up to 30% of ulcerative colitis patients and up to 70% of CD patients will require surgery, most commonly for refractory disease, at some point in their disease course.[1] With the advent of the ileal pouch-anal anastomosis procedure, surgery for ulcerative colitis no longer requires a permanent ileostomy. Although most ulcerative colitis patients who undergo colectomy with ileal pouch-anal anastomosis do very well, there is an increasing recognition of long-term sequelae of this surgery as discussed later in this chapter. Surgery for CD, on the other hand, is usually only a temporizing intervention with clinical recurrence rates as high as 76% at 15 years following initial surgery.[2]

It is important to be aware, however, that some IBD patients who do not respond to conventional medical therapy may not truly have intractable or refractory IBD as the reason for their nonresponse. Factors such as incorrect diagnosis, aggravating factors, a superimposed condition with symptoms that mimic those of IBD (such as irritable bowel syndrome), or less-than-adequate medical therapy can lead to what is referred to as "pseudointractable" disease. There are several possible reasons for pseudointractability in IBD as outlined in Figure 31-1.

In this chapter, we will focus on the factors or conditions that the astute clinician should keep in mind regarding pseudointractable disease when dealing with a patient who has what appears to be difficult-to-control IBD.

Misdiagnosis

Before proceeding with alternative medical therapies or surgery for what appears to be intractable disease, it is important to confirm the diagnosis of IBD, especially in recently diagnosed patients. It is always important to maintain an awareness that presenting symptoms may be due to an illness that can mimic the symptoms of IBD such as gastrointestinal infection, complications of diverticular disease, neoplastic disease, systemic processes, functional disorders such as irritable bowel syndrome, lactose intolerance, celiac disease, or bacterial overgrowth.[3] In this section, we will focus on diseases other than IBD that can present with ileal or colonic inflammation.

Diseases That Cause Ileitis

Gastrointestinal infections can mimic the symptoms and the endoscopic appearance of CD and UC. Infectious entities that can be confused with ileocecal CD include *Yersinia enterocolitica*, tuberculosis, cytomegalovirus infection, and histoplasmosis. These infections can present with right lower quadrant pain, fever, and diarrhea. Endoscopy may demonstrate changes similar to those seen in CD, including aphthous lesions, ulcerations, and mucosal edema in the terminal ileum, cecum, and the ascending colon.

Lichtenstein GR, ed.
Ulcerative Colitis: The Complete Guide to Medical Management (pp 331-340)

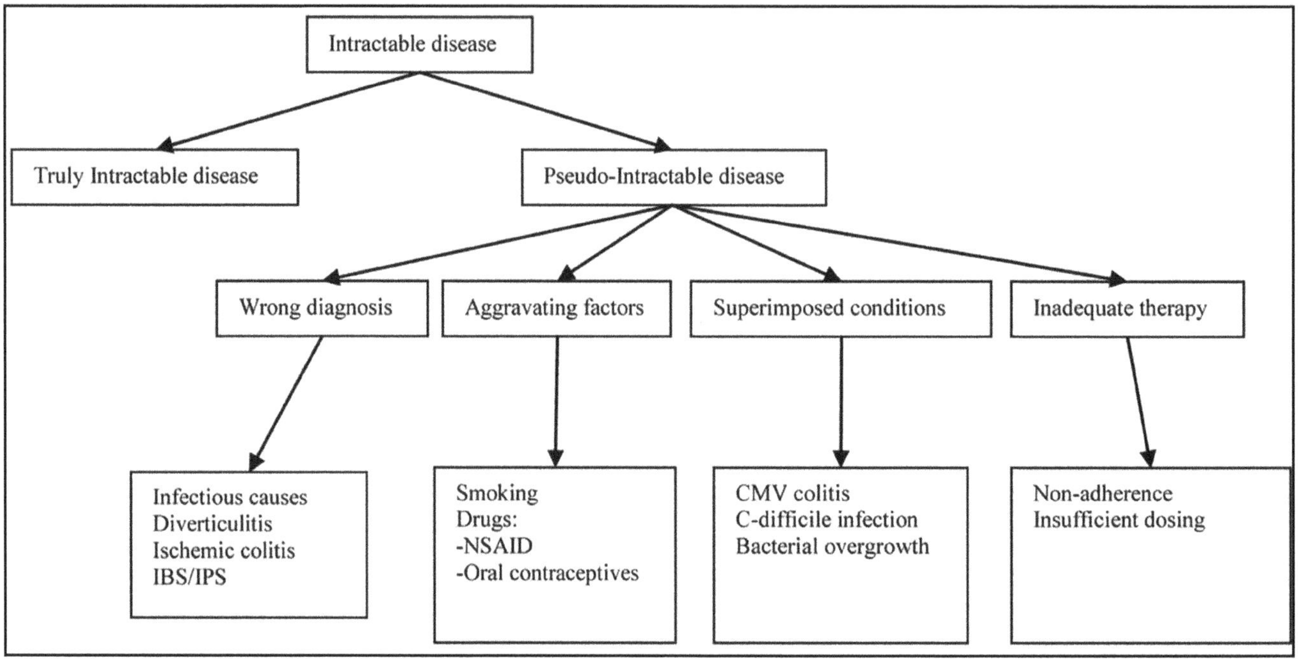

FIGURE 31-1. Causes of pseudointractability in IBD.

Yersinia enterocolitica is a food-borne infection that can lead to symptoms of abdominal pain, diarrhea, and fever along with extraintestinal symptoms of arthritis, erythema nodosum, and aphthous stomatitis.[4-6] Intestinal tuberculosis is rare in the United States but should be considered in at-risk populations such as individuals who are immunosuppressed or incarcerated. Tuberculosis of the gastrointestinal tract most commonly affects the ileocecal region, is not always associated with pulmonary disease (some report that up to 50% do not have pulmonary involvement but have gastrointestinal involvement), and can present with fistula or abscess formation and perforation.[7-10] Cytomegalovirus infection occurs mostly in immunocompromised patients and is discussed further below.[11] Gastrointestinal histoplasmosis usually occurs with disseminated infection, and predominant terminal ileal disease is found in one-third of cases.[12]

Other conditions that can cause ileitis and mimic CD include neoplastic processes such as carcinoid tumors and non-Hodgkin's lymphoma; systemic diseases leading to vasculitis such as systemic lupus erythematosus and Behçet's disease; and inflammatory processes involving the right lower quadrant such as appendicitis, pelvic inflammatory disease, and tubo-ovarian abscess.

Diseases That Cause Colitis

Invasive infections that affect the colon such as *Shigella*, *Salmonella*, *Campylobacter jejuni*, enteroinvasive *Escherichia coli*, and amebiasis can mimic UC or Crohn's colitis with symptoms of bloody diarrhea and abdominal cramping and endoscopic changes of mucosal edema, erosions, and superficial ulcerations.[13] Bacterial infections such as *Shigella* and *Salmonella* typically run a short-term course that is complete within 2 weeks, and therefore, in the acute setting, a diagnosis of IBD should not be made until an infection has been ruled out. In such situations, microbiological studies of stool are important, and mucosal biopsies can help in the differential diagnosis. Typical histologic changes seen in acute infectious colitis include predominant neutrophil accumulation in the lamina propria and crypts and mononuclear cells in the upper third of the lamina propria.[14] In contrast, typical changes of IBD include chronic features such as crypt branching (crypt distortion) and basal plasmacytosis.[14] Amebic colitis, on the other hand, can present more gradually with several weeks of symptoms, including diarrhea, abdominal pain, bloody stools, and weight loss.[15] Fulminant colitis and perforation can develop, especially in patients receiving corticosteroids, immunocompromised patients, and pregnant women. This infection, caused by the parasite *Entamoeba histolytica*, should be suspected in travelers to or immigrants from endemic areas such as Central and South America, Africa, and Asia.[15]

The clinical presentation of ulcerative colitis or Crohn's colitis can be mimicked by a number of other entities affecting the colon, including radiation colitis, ischemic colitis, and complications of diverticular disease. A detailed history and review of risk factors should raise appropriate awareness for radiation and ischemic colitis, and colonic mucosal biopsies can show typical histologic changes in such cases.[14]

Complications of diverticular disease should especially be considered in individuals over the age of 60 because of the high prevalence of diverticulosis in this age group. Diverticulitis can mimic segmental colonic CD, especially when presenting with associated complications of fistula or abscess formation. In addition, histologic changes of diverticulitis can include transmural inflammation and granuloma formation, which can make differentiation from CD difficult.[16] It is also important to keep in mind that diverticulitis can develop superimposed on underlying quiescent IBD in older individuals. Clinically and radiographically, it can be very difficult to distinguish between diverticulitis and active CD in such situations. In addition, it is important to be aware of a less common but increasingly recognized complication of diverticular disease, which is segmental colitis in the region of diverticulosis.[16-19] This condition most commonly affects the sigmoid colon, and patients typically present with rectal bleeding, altered bowel habits (diarrhea or constipation alternating with diarrhea), and abdominal pain.[16-19] Endoscopy reveals erythema, patchy mucosal hemorrhage, granularity, and exudates adjacent to multiple diverticular orifices. Histologic findings can be similar to those seen in CD. These patients have been reported to respond to therapy with 5aminosalicylates.[17,19]

Finally, when approaching the nonresponding patient with inflammatory disease of the colon, it is important to differentiate between ulcerative colitis and CD because both the medical and surgical therapies of these disorders can differ. Several findings such as sparing of the rectum, patchy colonic inflammation, the presence of perianal disease, the occurrence of internal fistulas, or the finding of noncaseating granulomas on biopsy are suggestive of CD in this setting. However, there are several factors that can make it difficult to distinguish between ulcerative colitis and Crohn's colitis even if one of these findings is present. For example, topical therapies for IBD can lead to rectal sparing while oral or systemic therapies can cause patchy healing. Furthermore, inflammation in the periappendiceal region is frequently seen in patients with left-sided ulcerative colitis[20] and should not be considered as a skip lesion of Crohn's. The finding of granulomas is suggestive of CD but can also be due to superimposed infectious processes or can be caused by crypt rupture and extruded mucin occurring in either ulcerative colitis or CD.[14] Intubation of the terminal ileum during colonoscopy[21] and evaluation of the small bowel with either a small bowel series or capsule endoscopy can yield important information in such situations. Serologic assays that attempt to distinguish between UC and Crohn's may be of some help. Perinuclear antineutrophic cytoplasmic antibodies are found in 50% to 65% of ulcerative colitis patients while anti-*Saccharomyces cerevisiae* antibodies, anti-outer membrane porin C IgA antibody, and anti-I2 are found in subsets of patients with CD.[13]

AGGRAVATING FACTORS

Smoking

It has been well-established that there is a connection between IBD and cigarette smoking.[22-34] However, smoking has opposing effects on ulcerative colitis and CD. Ulcerative colitis appears to be a disease of nonsmokers. Former smokers are at the highest risk for developing ulcerative colitis, while current smokers have the lowest risk.[24-30] It is felt that the nicotine in tobacco cigarettes may have a preventive influence on ulcerative colitis, and nicotine patches have been used with mixed results to treat patients with this disease.[35,36] Smoking also seems to have an impact on the course of ulcerative colitis.[37-39] Among smokers with ulcerative colitis who stop smoking, the severity of the disease worsens after smoking cessation as demonstrated by an increase in the disease activity and the more frequent need for immunosuppressive therapy.[39] Therefore, in ulcerative colitis patients with previously quiescent disease whose symptoms suddenly worsen, it is important to inquire about recent changes in smoking habits. These patients may need increasing doses of medications or addition of an immunomodulator to their treatment regimen.

Cigarette smoking has an opposite effect on CD.[32-34] Current or former smokers have a higher risk of developing CD compared to patients who never smoked. In siblings with similar genetic susceptibility for IBD, smokers tend to develop CD while nonsmokers develop UC.[40] This association seems to be valid also for second-hand smoking as well.[41] Crohn's disease patients who smoke have an increased number of relapses, increased risk of postoperative recurrence, and an increased need for aggressive immunosuppressive therapy.[42-45] Smoking has also been shown to negatively affect response to treatment with infliximab in patients with CD.[46,47] Therefore, although all patients should be encouraged to quit smoking, particular efforts should be directed to smokers with CD who are not responding to medical therapy. It has been shown that CD patients who quit smoking note fewer exacerbations and require less corticosteroids or immunosuppressive therapy to control symptoms compared with patients who continue to smoke.[48]

Nonsteroidal Anti-Inflammatory Drugs

Nonsteroidal anti-inflammatory drugs are among the most commonly used medications throughout the world. In the United States alone, an estimated 15 to

20 million people are long-term users of NSAIDs.[49] Peripheral arthritis or arthralgias are common extraintestinal manifestations in IBD, occurring in up to 25% of patients. Therefore, many patients with IBD invariably seek over-the-counter NSAID preparations because they are widely available and easy to attain. Some physicians may also prescribe these agents without realizing the potential risk of exacerbating the underlying IBD.

NSAIDs have long been known to induce ulceration in the stomach and duodenum, can lead to increased permeability of the small intestine, and cause occult blood loss.[50,51] It has also been shown that NSAIDs can have deleterious effects on small bowel and colonic mucosa.[52-56] Specifically, NSAIDs have been shown to cause ulceration and strictures in the jejunum, ileum, and colon, sometimes with life-threatening complications.[57] The clinical manifestations of NSAID-associated small and large bowel tract toxicity include diarrhea, abdominal pain, blood and protein loss, colitis, and perforation.

In addition, although there are conflicting results, several studies suggest that NSAIDs are associated with exacerbations of IBD.[58-65] Studies have also shown a higher-than-expected use of NSAIDs among patients admitted to the hospital for flares of IBD.[66] However, it is important to note that no prospective controlled trials evaluating the effects of NSAID use in IBD have been performed. A recent preliminary report of a randomized trial of celecoxib 200 mg twice daily versus placebo in quiescent ulcerative colitis showed that disease activity in the celecoxib-treated patients was similar to that of placebo-treated patients at the end of the 14-day study.[67] The means by which NSAIDs may aggravate underlying IBD is not completely clear, but a mechanism similar to that of NSAID-induced enterocolitis is possible and may involve the arachidonic acid metabolism pathways. The formation of prostaglandins, which have a cytoprotective role in the gastrointestinal tract, is inhibited by NSAIDs. NSAIDs also cause increased gut permeability, which may disrupt the intestinal protective barrier, allowing mucosal exposure to luminal substances, which in turn may lead to an inflammatory reaction and worsening of IBD.

IBD patients who are refractory to medical therapy should be carefully asked about their use of over-the-counter medications with a focus on NSAID use. Often, it is helpful to specifically run through a list of several of these preparations and to also ask patients what they take if they develop a headache or joint pains.

Based on the issues presented above, we would recommend that, when possible, non-NSAID analgesics such as acetaminophen should be used first when symptoms warrant use of medications for pain relief in patients with IBD. When an extraintestinal manifestation such as arthritis is the presenting problem, treatment of the underlying IBD should be emphasized and use of NSAIDs discouraged if possible. In cases where NSAIDs are required, use of cyclooxygenase-2 inhibitors may offer a better option.[68]

Oral Contraceptives

In addition to NSAIDs, certain other drugs such as gold[69-71] and oral contraceptives have been suggested to cause a clinical picture resembling IBD. While there have been some case reports of acute colitis associated with isotretinoin,[72] a more recent population-based, case-control study concluded that there is no association between isotretinoin and IBD.[73] In terms of oral contraceptives, there are conflicting reports in the literature regarding the effects of these agents on the risk of development of IBD.[74-79] Several studies have suggested an increased risk of IBD in women taking oral contraceptives,[74-77] while others have failed to show such an association.[78,79] There are also conflicting results on whether oral contraceptive use modifies the course of existing IBD as demonstrated by differing results from 2 cohort studies.[44,79] Timmer et al found that prior or current use of oral contraceptives increased the risk of relapse threefold in women with quiescent CD (hazard ratio 3.0, 95% confidence interval 1.5 to 5.9).[44] Cosnes et al, on the other hand, found no increased risk for CD relapse among contraceptive users.[79] Based on the existing literature, stopping or avoiding contraceptive pills in women who develop IBD or who are refractory to medical therapy is not justified. However, if the symptoms of IBD begin shortly after initiation of oral contraceptives and the disease does not respond to standard therapy, stopping the oral contraceptives can be considered.

SUPERIMPOSED CONDITIONS

Cytomegalovirus Infection

Cytomegalovirus (CMV) is a well-recognized cause of infection in immunosuppressed patients such as those with acquired immunodeficiency syndrome (AIDS), transplant recipients, and cancer patients receiving chemotherapy.[80] Gastrointestinal infection with CMV is usually due to reactivation of latent virus and can affect any part of the intestinal tract.[81] When CMV affects the small intestine or colon, its presentation can mimic CD and UC with endoscopic and radiographic changes consisting of ulcerations, erosions, and mucosal hemorrhage and clinical complications of perforation and toxic megacolon.

CMV infection has also been described as a superimposed condition in patients with IBD and can be a cause for relapse, a more severe disease course, or pseudo-intractability to medical therapy.[83-88] Patients with IBD are at a higher risk for CMV infection due to several factors, including the frequent use of corticosteroids and immunomodulators, tropism of CMV for sites of inflammation, and altered immunity in malnourished IBD patients. CMV tends to localize to the colon in patients with IBD, although disseminated disease has been reported. Endoscopic findings of CMV infection can range from normal-appearing mucosa to the more typical findings of mucosal erosion or ulceration, which can be impossible to distinguish from active IBD. Histopathologic examination may reveal cytomegalic cells, which are larger than surrounding cells and often contain an intranuclear inclusion that is eccentrically placed and surrounded by a clear halo, giving it an "owl's eye" appearance. CMV-infected cells are usually confined to the areas of mucosal ulceration but may also be found in macroscopically normal-appearing mucosa.

The incidence of gastrointestinal CMV infection in IBD patients has been reported to range from 0.5% to 4%. Kaufman et al reviewed 93 cases of gastrointestinal CMV infection, most of which occurred in patients with AIDS. However, 11 patients had ulcerative colitis, and 11 had CD, accounting for a prevalence of 4.6% in UC and 0.8% in CD patients.[83] In another report, among 1895 patient hospital admissions for IBD exacerbations, 10 patients were diagnosed as having superimposed CMV infection for a prevalence of 0.53%.[88] Treatment with ganciclovir and withdrawal of immunosuppressive treatment resulted in gradual improvement and induction of remission of the underlying IBD in most patients.

Importantly, the true incidence of CMV infection in IBD may be underestimated because the reported studies are mostly retrospective, and diagnostic evaluations for CMV frequently were not pursued in many patients presenting with IBD flares. In a prospective study from Italy, among 62 patients with severe colitis (55 with ulcerative colitis and 7 with CD), 19 patients (30%) were resistant to intravenous steroids and bowel rest.[89] In all of them, rectal biopsies were obtained by flexible proctoscopy and examined for cytomegalovirus infection. Buffy coat preparation on leukocytes was also performed to detect systemic infection. In 7 (5 with ulcerative colitis and 2 with CD) out of 19 (36%) patients with refractory disease, CMV was diagnosed in the rectal biopsy specimens as well as by buffy coat preparation. Five of these patients went into remission after antiviral treatment.[89]

Therefore, in patients with IBD colitis who are refractory to medical therapy and who fail to respond to intravenously administered steroids, searching for CMV infection by performing a flexible sigmoidoscopy with biopsies, CMV serology, or serum DNA PCR prior to treatment with potent immunosuppressive agents, such as cyclosporine or surgery, is indicated. In cases where CMV infection is diagnosed, treatment of the infection by systemic antiviral therapy often leads to the remission of the underlying symptoms.

Clostridium difficile Infection

Clostridium difficile (*C. difficile*) is one of the most common hospital-acquired infections and is a frequent cause of morbidity and mortality among elderly hospitalized patients. It usually colonizes the human intestinal tract after the normal gut flora has been altered by antibiotic therapy. Several studies have reported an association between superimposed *C. difficile* infection and exacerbations of IBD.[90-93] The prevalence of infection with this organism among IBD patients with flares may be as high as 20% to 30%.[93,94] The reason for this association is not entirely clear. It may be that the frequent hospitalizations and exposure to antibiotics of patients with IBD places them at increased risk for the infection. Other factors, however, are likely to be involved because *C. difficile* infection may be detected in IBD outpatients even in the absence of recent antibiotic use.[93]

In patients with refractory IBD, especially those with colonic involvement, testing for *C. difficile* infection should be considered. The best diagnostic test is the assay for *C. difficile* toxins in stool.[95,96] It is important to test for both *C. difficile* toxins A and B because single toxin assays fail to detect a substantial number of infections in IBD patients.[96] Endoscopy, if performed, may demonstrate findings ranging from normal to patchy or diffuse colitis with or without pseudomembranes. Treatment consists of oral metronidazole or vancomycin or intravenous metronidazole in those unable to take oral medication.[97] Rifaximin has also been used to treat patients with *C. difficile*.[98,99]

Bacterial Overgrowth

Bacterial overgrowth syndrome (primarily involving the small intestine) occurs when the normally low bacterial colonization in the upper gastrointestinal tract significantly increases. Small bowel bacterial overgrowth is often associated with anatomic abnormalities of the gastrointestinal tract, abnormalities of intestinal motility, or defects of intestinal mucosal surface and immune defense mechanisms. Patients with CD often have one or more of these abnormalities such as strictures, fistulas, and mucosal defects and thus are at increased risk of developing bacterial overgrowth. Small bowel bacterial overgrowth is being increasingly recognized in patients with CD, which may partly explain why some of these patients respond clinically to broad-spectrum antibiotics.[100-103]

In patients with CD who fail to respond to optimal medical therapy and who continue to have symptoms such as diarrhea, abdominal cramping, and bloating, bacterial overgrowth should be considered, especially when there is no evidence of ongoing active CD. The gold standard for the diagnosis of bacterial overgrowth has traditionally been the demonstration of excessive bacterial concentrations in a jejunal aspirate, which can be performed during endoscopy or by fluoroscopy with jejunal intubation. Other diagnostic tests such as 14C-d-xylose breath test and hydrogen breath test are noninvasive and are more easily done to document bacterial overgrowth, but may be difficult to interpret in patients with fistulas.

Sometimes, it is more practical to empirically treat the patient with broad-spectrum antibiotics.

Irritable Bowel Syndrome

IBD and irritable bowel syndrome are 2 chronic conditions that can present with similar symptoms such as diarrhea and abdominal pain but have very different underlying pathophysiologies. It is important to be aware that irritable bowel syndrome can occur superimposed on underlying IBD, leading to symptoms that do not respond to therapies aimed at treating IBD. Clinically, it can be difficult to differentiate between these 2 conditions especially in the absence of rectal bleeding and systemic illness. However, endoscopies with biopsies and radiographic studies usually enable the clinician to determine if there is evidence of active IBD. Recently, measurement of fecal lactoferrin, a protein found in the secondary granules of the polymorphonuclear leukocytes, has been suggested as being able to distinguish IBD from irritable bowel syndrome, noninvasively, with high sensitivity and specificity.[104]

INADEQUATE THERAPY

Nonadherence

Adherence is the *degree to which a patient follows a prescribed treatment regimen.* In studies of patient behavior, only about half of those who leave a physician's office with a prescription take the drug as directed. Adherence decreases when the drug regimen is complex, inconvenient, expensive, of long duration, unpleasant to administer, has adverse effects, or requires lifestyle alterations. Regimens should therefore be simplified and matched to the patient's schedules where possible.

The prevalence of nonadherence to medical regimens for IBD has been reported to range from 40% to 60%.[105,106] Adherence rates for infliximab appear to be higher (<90%), according to data on 1185 infliximab infusions scheduled for 274 patients.[107] Lack of adherence has been associated with relapse among ulcerative colitis patients previously in remission.[108] Because even the best treatment plan fails without patient compliance, nonadherence to the recommended medical regimen should be ruled out in all refractory patients. Direct questioning of the patients may at times clarify the issue, but in selected situations, where the suspicion for nonadherence remains high, urinary salicylate levels and erythrocyte 6-thioguanine nucleotide levels can serve as surrogate markers for determining compliance to 5-ASA agents and purine analogs, respectively.[109-111] Recognizing nonadherence and adopting strategies to optimize patient compliance are important components in the management of IBD patients.

Insufficient Dosing

Before labeling a patient's disease as truly intractable, the dosage of medications used to treat IBD should be fully optimized. Studies in ulcerative colitis have shown that 5-aminosalicylic acid compounds demonstrate a dose-response effect and therefore increasing the daily dose of these drugs may increase response in those not adequately controlled with lower doses.[112,113] One study, for example, included 87 patients with mildly to moderately active ulcerative colitis who were randomly assigned to receive mesalamine at a dose of 1.6 g or 4.8 g per day or placebo for 6 weeks.[113] Response was assessed by clinical assessment and proctosigmoidoscopy. Patients receiving 4.8 g per day of mesalamine had a significantly higher complete response compared to those treated with 1.6 g per day. Based on similar results in several studies showing a dose-related response for induction of remission and possibly for maintenance of remission in ulcerative colitis, it is important to maximize dosing of 5-aminosalicylic acid agents before determining that a patient with ulcerative colitis is not responding to this class of agents.

Corticosteroids have long been known to be effective in inducing remission of active IBD, but dosing should be optimized, and these agents should not be used for maintenance of remission.[114] Prednisone doses between 40 and 60 mg daily may be required for induction of remission in active IBD.[112] We recommend starting at the 40-mg dose and using the 60-mg dose in patients who do not optimally respond. Budesonide is a newer glucocorticoid that has high affinity for the glucocorticoid receptor but low systemic activity due to extensive first-pass metabolism in the liver.[114] In the United States, budesonide is available in an oral controlled-release form that is effective for active ileal and right colonic CD. The starting dose should be 9 mg daily, and if response to this dose of budesonide is incomplete, switching to oral prednisone is appropriate as studies have suggested somewhat lower efficacy compared to conventional corticosteroids.[115] Hospitalized patients with severe CD or UC should be treated with intravenous steroids such as methylprednisolone (32 to 60 mg daily) or hydrocortisone (300 mg daily) either in divided doses or as a continuous infusion.[112] The initial steroid dose should be maintained for a short period until significant clinical improvement is observed, followed by a slow taper over several weeks.

Immunomodulatory drugs, such as azathioprine and 6-mercaptopurine, have been shown to be efficacious in IBD and to exert a steroid-sparing effect. A common problem seen in pseudorefractory cases of IBD is underdosing of these agents due to concerns for potential toxicity. In patients with normal thiopurine methyltransferase enzyme activity or genotype, dosing should be maximized at 1 to 1.5 mg/kg daily for 6-mercaptopurine or 2 to 2.5 mg/kg daily for azathioprine with regular monitoring of cell blood counts. Measurement of 6-thioguanine nucleotide metabolites can be helpful to assess adherence.[116]

PSEUDOINTRACTABILITY IN PATIENTS WITH ILEAL POUCH-ANAL ANASTOMOSIS

Total proctocolectomy with ileal pouch-anal anastomosis has become the surgical procedure of choice in patients with ulcerative colitis with either dysplasia or disease refractory to medical therapy.[117-119] The most common long-term complication of ileal pouch-anal anastomosis in patients with underlying ulcerative colitis is pouchitis, an inflammatory process of the ileal reservoir (pouch).[120-122] Studies have shown that as many as 24% to 46% of patients with ulcerative colitis develop at least one episode of pouchitis within 10 years after surgery.[122,123]

The most frequently reported symptoms of pouchitis are increased stool frequency, fecal urgency, abdominal cramping, and pelvic discomfort. However, these symptoms are nonspecific and can be due to other inflammatory conditions such as inflammation of the rectal cuff (cuffitis), undiagnosed CD, or noninflammatory conditions such as irritable pouch syndrome.[124-129] Therefore, pouchitis should ideally be diagnosed by pouch endoscopy with biopsies in symptomatic patients.[130] In clinical practice, however, patients often are diagnosed as having pouchitis based on symptoms alone and are treated empirically with antibiotics. Although patients with symptoms of pouchitis may respond favorably to broad-spectrum antibiotic therapy, this approach may not be ideal because patients without pouchitis will be unnecessarily exposed to antibiotics and have delays in a correct diagnosis.[128]

In patients with presumed pouchitis who do not respond to antibiotic therapy, other diagnoses such as CD of the pouch, rectal cuff inflammation, or irritable pouch syndrome should be investigated. This is best done by a pouch endoscopy with examination of the afferent limb and biopsies. Rectal cuff inflammation can be diagnosed easily by pouch endoscopy and can be treated with topical therapies. Making the diagnosis of CD in a patient who has undergone an ileal pouch for presumed ulcerative colitis can be challenging. In a recent study, the finding of afferent limb ulceration on pouch endoscopy was shown to be associated with a diagnosis of CD in patients not using NSAIDs.[131] In that study, other endoscopic and histologic findings in the pouch or afferent limb did not help differentiate between ulcerative colitis and CD. If CD is suspected, a small bowel follow-through may detect disease proximal to the pouch and confirm the diagnosis.[132] Alternatively, the use of computed tomography enterography or magnetic resonance imaging enterography has been proposed as an alternative method to visualize the small bowel.

Further diagnostic tests may become necessary to exclude other diagnoses. Infectious etiologies can be investigated by stool sampling and pouch biopsy. Several cases documenting CMV infection of the pouch in patients who had "refractory" pouchitis have been described, and treatment with ganciclovir led to resolution of symptoms.[133,134]

Patients who have ongoing symptoms with a normal pouch endoscopy and biopsies may suffer from a functional disorder of the pouch termed irritable pouch syndrome.[128,129] These patients often show increased visceral sensitivity to balloon dilatation of their pouch compared to individuals with normal pouches.[135] In a recent study, fecal lactoferrin was shown to be able to distinguish irritable pouch syndrome from pouchitis, cuffitis, or CD with a high sensitivity and specificity and thus help with diagnosis of this group of patients.[129] In patients with irritable pouch syndrome, treatment strategies similar to those used in irritable bowel syndrome such as antidiarrheals, anticholinergics, and antidepressants may be beneficial.

CONCLUSION

It is important to keep in mind that some IBD patients who do not respond to conventional medical therapies may not truly have refractory IBD as the reason for their nonresponse, but instead have "pseudointractable" disease. The clinician must consider possibilities such as an incorrect diagnosis, a superimposed condition that can present with symptoms that mimic those of IBD, aggravating factors, or the fact that the patient may be on less-than-adequate medical therapy in such situations.

REFERENCES

1. Sachar DB. Indications for surgery in inflammatory bowel disease: a gastroenterologist's opinion. In: Kirsner JB, ed. *Inflammatory Bowel Disease*. Philadelphia, PA: WB Saunders Company; 2000: 611-615.
2. Achkar JP, Hanauer SB. Medical therapy to reduce postoperative Crohn's disease recurrence. *Am J Gastroenterol.* 2000;95:1139-1146.
3. Lichtenstein GR, Hanauer SB, Sandborn WJ; Practice Parameters Committee of American College of Gastroenterology. Management of Crohn's disease in adults. *Am J Gastroenterol.* 2009;104(2): 465-483.
4. Macfarlane PI, Miller V. *Yersinia enterocolitica* mimicking Crohn's disease. *J Pediatr Gastroenterol Nutr.* 1986;5:671.
5. Sandler M, Girdwood AH, Kottler RE, Marks IN. Terminal ileitis due to *Yersinia enterocolitica*: a case report and review of the literature. *S Afr Med J.* 1982;62:573-576.
6. Vantrappen G, Agg HO, Ponette E, et al. *Yersinia enteritis* and enterocolitis: gastroenterological aspects. *Gastroenterology.* 1977;72:220-227.
7. Arnold C, Moradpour D, Blum HE. Tuberculous colitis mimicking Crohn's disease. *Am J Gastroenterol.* 1998;93:2294229-6.

8. Horvath KD, Whelan RL. Intestinal tuberculosis: return of an old disease. *Am J Gastroenterol.* 1998;93:692-696.
9. Gan HT, Chen YQ, Bu H, Yang XY. Differentiation between intestinal tuberculosis and Crohn's disease in endoscopic biopsy specimens by polymerase chain reaction. *Am J Gastroenterol.* 2002;97:1446-1451.
10. Pulimood AB, Ramakrishna BS, Kurian G, et al. Endoscopic mucosal biopsies are useful in distinguishing granulomatous colitis due to Crohn's disease from tuberculosis. *Gut.* 1999;45:537-541.
11. Caroline DF, Hilpert PL, Russin VL. CMV colitis mimicking Crohn's disease in a patient with acquired immune deficiency syndrome (AIDS). *Can Assoc Radiol J.* 1987;38:227-228.
12. Cappell MS, Mandell W, Grimes MM, Neu HC. Gastrointestinal histoplasmosis. *Dig Dis Sci.* 1988;33:353-360.
13. Sands BE. From symptom to diagnosis: clinical distinctions among various forms of intestinal inflammation. *Gastroenterology.* 2004;126:1518-1532.
14. Carpenter HA, Talley NJ. The importance of clinicopathologic correlation in the diagnosis of inflammatory conditions of the colon: histological patterns with clinical implications. *Am J Gastroenterol.* 2000;95:878-896.
15. Stanley SL. Amoebiasis. *Lancet.* 2003;361:1025-1034.
16. Shepherd NA. Diverticular disease and chronic idiopathic inflammatory bowel disease: associations and masquerades. *Gut.* 1996;38:801-802.
17. Peppercorn MA. Drug-responsive chronic segmental colitis associated with diverticula: a clinical syndrome in the elderly. *Am J Gastroenterol.* 1992;87:609-612.
18. Gledhill A, Dixon MF. Crohn's-like reaction in diverticular disease. *Gut.* 1998;42:392-395.
19. Imperiali G, Meucci G, Alvisi C, et al. Segmental colitis associated with diverticula: a prospective study. *Am J Gastroenterol.* 2000;95:1014-106.
20. D'Haens, Geboes K, Peeters M, et al. Patchy cecal inflammation associated with distal ulcerative colitis: a prospective endoscopic study. *Am J Gastroenterol.* 1997;92:1275-1279.
21. Geboes K, Ectors N, D'Haens G, Rutgeerts P. Is ileoscopy with biopsy worthwhile in patients presenting with symptoms of inflammatory bowel disease. *Am J Gastroenterol.* 1998;93:201-206.
22. Harries AD, Baird A, Rhodes J. Non-smoking: a feature of ulcerative colitis. *BMJ.* 1982;284:706.
23. Jick H, Walker AM. Cigarette smoking and ulcerative colitis. *N Engl J Med.* 1983;308:261-263.
24. Logan RF, Edmond M, Somerville KW, Langman MJ. Smoking and ulcerative colitis. *BMJ.* 1984;288:751-753.
25. Thornton JR, Emmett PM, Heaton KW. Smoking, sugar, and inflammatory bowel disease. *BMJ.* 1985;290:1786-1787.
26. Tobin MV, Logan RF, Langman MJ, McConnell RB, Gilmore IT. Cigarette smoking and inflammatory bowel disease. *Gastroenterology.* 1987;93:316-321.
27. Benoni C, Nilsson A. Smoking habits in patients with inflammatory bowel disease: a case-control study. *Scand J Gastroenterol.* 1987;22:1130-1136.
28. Boyko EJ, Koepsell TD, Perera DR, Inui TS. Risk of ulcerative colitis among former and current cigarette smokers. *N Engl J Med.* 1987;316:707-710.
29. Lindberg E, Tysk C, Andersson K, Jarnerot G. Smoking and inflammatory bowel disease: a case control study. *Gut.* 1988;29:352-357.
30. Silverstein MD, Lashner BA, Hanauer SB. Cigarette smoking and ulcerative colitis: a case-control study. *Mayo Clin Proc.* 1994;69:425-429.
31. Persson PG, Ahlbom A, Hellers G. Inflammatory bowel disease and tobacco smoke: a case-control study. *Gut.* 1990;31:1377-1381.
32. Calkins BM. A meta-analysis of the role of smoking in inflammatory bowel disease. *Dig Dis Sci.* 1989;34:1841-1854.
33. Somerville KW, Logan RF, Edmond M, Langman MJ. Smoking and Crohn's disease. *BMJ.* 1984;289:954-956.
34. Silverstein MD, Lashner BA, Hanauer SB, Evans AA, Kirsner JB. Cigarette smoking in Crohn's disease. *Am J Gastroenterol.* 1989;84:31-33.
35. Pullan RD, Rhodes J, Ganesh S, et al. Transdermal nicotine for active ulcerative colitis. *N Engl J Med.* 1994;330:811-815.
36. Sandborn WJ, Tremaine WJ, Offord KP, et al. Transdermal nicotine for mildly to moderately active ulcerative colitis: a randomized, double-blind, placebo-controlled trial. *Ann Intern Med.* 1997;126:364-371.
37. Boyko EJ, Perera DR, Koepsell TD, Keane EM, Inui TS. Effects of cigarette smoking on the clinical course of ulcerative colitis. *Scand J Gastroenterol.* 1988;23:1147-1152.
38. Rudra T, Motley R, Rhodes J. Does smoking improve colitis? *Scand J Gastroenterol Suppl.* 1989;170:61-63.
39. Beaugerie L, Massot N, Carbonnel F, Cattan S, Gendre JP, Cosnes J. Impact of cessation of smoking on the course of ulcerative colitis. *Am J Gastroenterol.* 2001;96:2113-2116.
40. Bridger S, Lee JC, Bjarnason I, Jones JE, Macpherson AJ. In siblings with similar genetic susceptibility for inflammatory bowel disease, smokers tend to develop Crohn's disease and non-smokers develop ulcerative colitis. *Gut.* 2002;51:21-25.
41. Sandler RS, Sandler DP, McDonnell CW, Wurzelmann JI. Childhood exposure to environmental tobacco smoke and the risk of ulcerative colitis. *Am J Epidemiol.* 1992;135:603-608.
42. Sutherland LR, Ramcharan S, Bryant H, Fick G. Effect of cigarette smoking on recurrence of Crohn's disease. *Gastroenterology.* 1990;98:1123-1128.
43. Breuer-Katschinski BD, Hollander N, Goebell H. Effect of cigarette smoking on the course of Crohn's disease. *Eur J Gastroenterol Hepatol.* 1996;8:225-228.
44. Timmer A, Sutherland LR, Martin F. Oral contraceptive use and smoking are risk factors for relapse in Crohn's disease. *Gastroenterology.* 1998;114:1143-1150.
45. Cosnes J, Carbonnel F, Carrat F, Beaugerie L, Cattan S, Gendre J. Effects of current and former cigarette smoking on the clinical course of Crohn's disease. *Aliment Pharmacol Ther.* 1999;13:1403-1411.
46. Parsi MA, Achkar JP, Richardson S, et al. Predictors of response to infliximab in patients with Crohn's disease. *Gastroenterology.* 2002;123:707-713.
47. Arnott ID, McNeill G, Satsangi J. An analysis of factors influencing short-term and sustained response to infliximab treatment for Crohn's disease. *Aliment Pharmacol Ther.* 2003;17(12):1451-1457.
48. Cosnes J, Beaugerie L, Carbonnel F, Gendre JP. Smoking cessation and the course of Crohn's disease: an intervention study. *Gastroenterology.* 2001;120:1093-1099.
49. Fennerty MB. NSAID-related gastrointestinal injury: evidence-based approach to a preventable complication. *Postgrad Med.* 2001;110:87-94.
50. Bjarnason I, Williams P, So A, et al. Intestinal permeability and inflammation in rheumatic arthritis: effects of non-steroidal anti-inflammatory drugs. *Lancet.* 1984;2:1171-1174.
51. Bjarnason I, Zanelli G, Smith T, et al. Non-steroidal anti-inflammatory drug induced intestinal inflammation in humans. *Gastroenterology.* 1987;93:480-489.
52. Bjarnason I, Smethurst P, Fenn CG, et al. NSAID small bowel injury and cytoprotection. *Dig Dis Sci.* 1989;34:407-411.
53. Bjarnason I, Hayllar J, Macpherson AJ, et al. Side effects of nonsteroidal anti-inflammatory drugs on the small and large intestine in humans. *Gastroenterology.* 1993;104:1832-1847.
54. Davies NM. Toxicity of non-steroidal anti-inflammatory drugs in the large intestine. *Dis Colon Rectum.* 1995;38:1311-1321.

55. Gibson GR, Whitacre EB, Ricotti CA. Colitis induced by non-steroidal anti-inflammatory drugs. *Arch Intern Med.* 1992;152:625-632.
56. Gleeson M, Ramsay D, Hutchinson S, et al. Colitis associated with non-steroidal anti-inflammatory drugs. *Lancet.* 1994;344:1028.
57. Aabakken L, Osnes M. Nonsteroidal anti-inflammatory drug induced disease in the distal ileum and large bowel. *Scand J Gastroenterol.* 1989;24(suppl 163):48-55.
58. Kaufmann HJ, Taubin HL. Nonsteroidal anti-inflammatory drugs activate quiescent inflammatory bowel disease. *Ann Intern Med.* 1987;107:513-516.
59. Rampton DS, Sladen GE. Relapse of ulcerative proctocolitis during treatment with non-steroidal anti-inflammatory drugs. *Postgrad Med J.* 1981;57:297-299.
60. Walt RP, Hawkey CJ, Langman MJS. Colitis associated with non-steroidal anti-inflammatory drugs. *Br Med J.* 1984;288:238.
61. Rampton DS, McNeil NI, Sarner M. Analgesic ingestion and other factors preceding relapse in ulcerative colitis. *Gut.* 1983;24:187-189.
62. Rutherford D, Stockdill G, Hamer-Hodges DW, et al. Proctocolitis induced by salicylate. *Br Med J.* 1984;288:794.
63. Chakraborty TK, Bhatia D, Heading RC, et al. Salicylate induced exacerbation of ulcerative colitis. *Gut.* 1987;28:613-615.
64. Gibson GR, Whitacre EB, Ricotti CA. Colitis induced by non-steroidal anti-inflammatory drugs. *Arch Intern Med.* 1992;152:625-632.
65. Felder JB, Korelitz BI, Rajapakse R, Schwarz S, Horatagis AP, Gleim G. Effects of nonsteroidal anti-inflammatory drugs on inflammatory bowel disease: a case-control study. *Am J Gastroenterol.* 2000;95:1949-1954.
66. Evans JMM, McMahon AD, Murray FE, et al. Non-steroidal anti-inflammatory drugs are associated with emergency admission to hospital for colitis due to inflammatory bowel disease. *Gut.* 1997;40:619-622.
67. Sandborn WJ, Stenson WF, Brynskov J, Steidle G, Robbins J. Safety of celecoxib in patients with ulcerative colitis in remission: a randomized, double-blind, placebo-controlled study (abstract). *Am J Gastroenterol.* 2004;99:S257-S258.
68. Mahadevan U, Loftus EV, Tremaine WJ, Sandborn WJ. Safety of selective cyclooxygenase-2 inhibitors in inflammatory bowel disease. *Am J Gastroenterol.* 2002;97:910-914.
69. Nisar M, Winfield J. Gold induced colitis and hepatic toxicity in a patient with rheumatoid arthritis. *J Rheumatol.* 1994;21:938-939.
70. Kirkham B, Wedderburn L, MacFarlane DG. Gold-induced colitis. *Br J Rheumatol.* 1989;28:272-273.
71. Vessey M, Jewell D, Smith A, Yeates D, McPherson K. Chronic inflammatory bowel disease, cigarette smoking, and use of oral contraceptives: findings in a large cohort study of women of childbearing age. *BMJ.* 1986;292:1101-1103.
72. Martin P, Manley PN, Depew WT, Blakeman JM. Isotretinoin-associated proctosigmoiditis. *Gastroenterology.* 1987;93:606-609.
73. Bernstein CN, Nugent Z, Longobardi T, Blanchard JF. Isotretinoin is not associated with inflammatory bowel disease: a population-based case-control study. *Am J Gastroenterol.* 2009;July 21 [e pub ahead of print].
74. Logan RF, Kay CR. Oral contraception, smoking and inflammatory bowel disease: findings in the Royal College of General Practitioners Oral Contraception Study. *Int J Epidemiol.* 1989;18:105-107.
75. Lesko SM, Kaufman DW, Rosenberg L, et al. Evidence for an increased risk of Crohn's disease in oral contraceptive users. *Gastroenterology.* 1985;89:1046-1049.
76. Godet PG, May GR, Sutherland LR. Meta-analysis of the role of oral contraceptive agents in inflammatory bowel disease. *Gut.* 1995;37:668-673.
77. Lashner BA, Kane SV, Hanauer SB. Lack of association between oral contraceptive use and Crohn's disease: a community-based matched case-control study. *Gastroenterology.* 1989;97:1442-1447.
78. Lashner BA, Kane SV, Hanauer SB. Lack of association between oral contraceptive use and ulcerative colitis. *Gastroenterology.* 1990;99:1032-1036.
79. Cosnes J, Carbonnel F, Carrat F, Beaugerie L, Gendre JP. Oral contraceptive use and the clinical course of Crohn's disease: a prospective cohort study. *Gut.* 1999;45:218-222.
80. Goodgame RW. Gastrointestinal cytomegalovirus disease. *Ann Intern Med.* 1993;119:924-935.
81. Cooper HS, Raffensperger EC, Jonas L, Fitts WT. Cytomegalovirus inclusions in patients with ulcerative colitis and toxic dilation requiring colonic resection. *Gastroenterology.* 1977;72:1253-1256.
82. Berk T, Gordon SJ, Choi HY, Cooper HS. Cytomegalovirus infection of the colon: a possible role in exacerbations of inflammatory bowel disease. *Am J Gastroenterol.* 1985;80:355-360.
83. KaufmanHS,KahnAC,Iacobuzio-DonahueC,et al.Cytomegaloviral enterocolitis: Clinical associations and outcome. *Dis Colon Rectum.* 1999;42:24-30.
84. Eyre-Brook IA, Dundas S. Incidence and clinical significance of colonic cytomegalovirus infection in idiopathic inflammatory bowel disease requiring colectomy. *Gut.* 1986;27:1419-1425.
85. Farmer GW, Vincent MM, Fuccillo DA, et al. Viral investigations in ulcerative colitis and regional enteritis. *Gastroenterology.* 1973;65:8-18.
86. Loftus EV, Alexander GL, Carpenter HA. Cytomegalovirus as an exacerbating factor in ulcerative colitis. *J Clin Gastroenterol.* 1994;19:306-309.
87. Vega R, Bertran X, Menacho M, et al. Cytomegalovirus infection in patients with inflammatory bowel disease. *Am J Gastroenterol.* 1999;94:1053-1056.
88. Papadakis KA, Tung JK, Binder SW, et al. Outcome of cytomegalovirus infections in patients with inflammatory bowel disease. *Am J Gastroenterol.* 2001;96:2137-2142.
89. Cottone M, Pietrosi G, Martorana G, et al. Prevalence of cytomegalovirus infection in severe refractory ulcerative and Crohn's colitis. *Am J Gastroenterol.* 2001;96:773-775.
90. Farrell RJ, LaMont JT. Pathogenesis and clinical manifestations of *Clostridium difficile* diarrhea and colitis. *Curr Top Microbiol Immunol.* 2000;250:109-125.
91. Bolton RP, Sherriff RJ, Read AE. Clostridium difficile associated diarrhea: a role in inflammatory bowel disease? *Lancet.* 1980;1:383-384.
92. Trnka YM, LaMont JT. Association of *Clostridium difficile* toxin with symptomatic relapse of chronic inflammatory bowel disease. *Gastroenterology.* 1981;80:693-696.
93. Greenfield C, Aguilar Ramirez JR, Pounder RE, et al. Clostridium difficile and inflammatory bowel disease. *Gut.* 1983;24:713-717.
94. Meyer AM, Ramzan NN, Loftus EV, et al. The diagnostic yield of stool studies during relapses of inflammatory bowel disease. *Gastroenterology.* 2002;122(4 Suppl 1):A-219.
95. Cleary RK. *Clostridium difficile*-associated diarrhea and colitis: clinical manifestations, diagnosis, and treatment. *Dis Colon Rectum.* 1998;41:1435-1449.
96. Markowitz JE, Brown KA, Mamula P, Drott HR, Piccoli DA, Baldassano RN. Failure of single-toxin assays to detect *Clostridium difficile* infection in pediatric inflammatory bowel disease. *Am J Gastroenterol.* 2001;96:2688-2690.
97. Cleary RK. *Clostridium difficile*-associated diarrhea and colitis: clinical manifestations, diagnosis, and treatment. *Dis Colon Rectum.* 1998;41:1435-1449.
98. Garey KW, Salazar M, Shah D, Rodrigue R, DuPont HL. Rifamycin antibiotics for treatment of *Clostridium difficile*-associated diarrhea. *Ann Pharmacother.* 2008;42:827-835.

99. Garey KW, Jiang Z-D, Bellard A, DuPont HL. Rifaximin in treatment of recurrent *Clostridium difficile*-associated diarrhea: an uncontrolled pilot study. *J Clin Gastroenterol.* 2009;43(1):91-92
100. Rhodes JM, Middleton T, Jewell DP. The lactulose breath test as a diagnostic test for small bowel bacterial overgrowth. *Scand J Gastroenterol.* 1979;14:333-336.
101. Catiglione F, Del Vecchio Blanco G, Rispo A, et al. Orocecal transit time and bacterial overgrowth in patients with Crohn's disease. *J Clin Gastroenterol.* 2000;31:63-66.
102. Mishkin D, Boston FM, Blank D, Yalovsky M, Mishkin S. The glucose breath test: a diagnostic test for small bowel strictures in Crohn's disease. *Dig Dis Sci.* 2002;47:489-494.
103. Funayama Y, Sasaki I, Naito H, et al. Monitoring and antibacterial treatment for postoperative bacterial overgrowth in Crohn's disease. *Dis Colon Rectum.* 1999;42:1072-1077.
104. Kane SV, Sandborn WJ, Rufo PA, et al. Fecal lactoferrin is a sensitive and specific marker in identifying intestinal inflammation. *Am J Gastroenterol.* 2003;98:1309-1314.
105. Kane S, Cohen RD, Aikens JE, Hanauer SB. Prevalence of nonadherence with maintenance mesalamine in quiescent ulcerative colitis. *Am J Gastroenterol.* 2001;96:2929-2933.
106. van Hees PA, van Tongeren JH. Compliance to therapy in patients on a maintenance dose of sulfasalazine. *J Clin Gastroenterol.* 1982;4: 333-336.
107. Kane S, Dixon L. Adherence rates with infliximab therapy in Crohn's disease. *Aliment Pharmacol Ther.* 2006;24(7):1099-1103.
108. Kane S, Huo D, Aikens J, Hanauer S. Medication nonadherence and the outcomes of patients with quiescent ulcerative colitis. *Am J Med.* 2003;114:39-43.
109. Shaw IS, Jobson BA, Silverman D, et al. Is your patient taking the medicine? A simple assay to measure compliance with 5-aminosalicylic acid-containing compounds. *Aliment Pharmacol Ther.* 2002;16:2053-2059.
110. Aithal GP, Hoffmann BJ. Steering azathioprine safely: lessons from pharmacogenetics. *Am J Gastroenterol.* 2001;96:3202-3203.
111. Dubinsky MC, Lamothe S, Yang HY, et al. Pharmacogenomics and metabolite measurement for 6-mercaptopurine therapy in inflammatory bowel disease. *Gastroenterology.* 2000;118:705-713.
112. Kornbluth A, Sachar DB. Ulcerative colitis practice guidelines in adults (update): American College of Gastroenterology, Practice Parameters Committee. *Am J Gastroenterol.* 2004;99:1371-1385.
113. Schroeder KW, Tremaine WJ, Ilstrup DM. Coated oral 5-aminosalicylic acid therapy for mildly to moderately active ulcerative colitis: a randomized study. *N Engl J Med.* 1987;317:1625-1629.
114. Katz JA. Treatment of inflammatory bowel disease with corticosteroids. *Gastroenterol Clin N Am.* 2004;33:171-189.
115. Kane SV, Schoenfeld P, Sandborn WJ, et al. Systematic review: the effectiveness of budesonide therapy for Crohn's disease. *Aliment Pharmacol Ther.* 2002;16:1509-1517.
116. Lichtenstein GR. Use of laboratory testing to guide 6-mercaptopurine/azathioprine therapy. *Gastroenterology.* 2004;127:1558-1564.
117. Parks AG, Nicholls RJ. Proctocolectomy without ileostomy for ulcerative colitis. *Br Med J.* 1978;2:85-88.
118. Pemberton JH, Kelly KA, Beart RW Jr, Dozois RR, Wolff BG, Ilstrup DM. Ileal pouch-anal anastomosis for chronic ulcerative colitis: long-term results. *Ann Surg.* 1987;206:504-513.
119. Nicholls RJ, Moskowitz RL, Shepherd NA. Restorative proctocolectomy with ileal reservoir. *Br J Surg.* 1985;72:S76-S79.
120. Zuccaro G Jr, Fazio VW, Church JM, Lavery IC, Ruderman WB, Farmer RG. Pouch ileitis. *Dig Dis Sci.* 1989;34:1505-1510.
121. Sandborn WJ. Pouchitis following ileal pouch-anal anastomosis: definition, pathogenesis, and treatment. *Gastroenterology.* 1994;107:1856-1860.
122. Fazio VW, Ziv Y, Church JM, et al. Ileal pouch-anal anastomoses complications and function in 1005 patients. *Ann Surg.* 1995;222:120-127.
123. Penna C, Dozois R, Tremaine W, et al. Pouchitis after ileal pouch-anal anastomosis for ulcerative colitis occurs with increased frequency in patients with associated primary sclerosing cholangitis. *Gut.* 1996;38:234-239.
124. Lavery IC, Sirimarco MT, Ziv Y, Fazio VW. Anal canal inflammation after ileal pouch-anal anastomosis: the need for treatment. *Dis Colon Rectum.* 1995;38:803-806.
125. Thompson-Fawcett MW, Mortensen NJ, Warren BF. "Cuffitis" and inflammatory changes in the columnar cuff, anal transitional zone, and ileal reservoir after stapled pouch-anal anastomosis. *Dis Colon Rectum.* 1999;42:348-355.
126. De Oca J, Sanchez-Santos R, Rague JM, et al. Long-term results of ileal pouch-anal anastomosis in Crohn's disease. *Inflamm Bowel Dis.* 2003;9:171-175.
127. Peyregne V, Francois Y, Gilly FN, Descos JL, Flourie B, Vignal J. Outcome of ileal pouch after secondary diagnosis of Crohn's disease. *Int J Colorectal Dis.* 2000;15:49-53.
128. Shen B, Achkar JP, Lashner BA, et al. Irritable pouch syndrome: a new category of diagnosis for symptomatic patients with ileal pouch-anal anastomosis. *Am J Gastroenterol.* 2002;97:972-977.
129. Parsi MA, Shen B, Achkar JP, et al. Fecal lactoferrin for diagnosis of symptomatic patients with ileal pouch-anal anastomosis. *Gastroenterology.* 2004;126:1280-1286.
130. Shen B, Achkar JP, Lashner BA, et al. Endoscopic and histologic evaluation together with symptom assessment are required to diagnose pouchitis. *Gastroenterology.* 2001;121:261-267.
131. Wolf JM, Achkar JP, Lashner BA, et al. Afferent limb ulcers predict Crohn's disease in patients with ileal pouch-anal anastomosis. *Gastroenterology.* 2004;126:1686-1691.
132. Mahadevan U, Sandborn WJ. Diagnosis and management of pouchitis. *Gastroenterology.* 2003;124:1636-1650.
133. Moonka D, Furth EE, MacDermott RP, Lichtenstein GR. Pouchitis associated with primary cytomegalovirus infection. *Am J Gastroenterol.* 1998;93:264-266.
134. Munoz-Juarez M, Pemberton JH, Sandborn WJ, Tremaine WJ, Dozois RR. Misdiagnosis of specific cytomegalovirus infection of the ileoanal pouch as refractory idiopathic chronic pouchitis: report of two cases. *Dis Colon Rectum.* 1999;42:117-120.
135. Shen B, Sanmiguel C, Parsi MA, et al. Irritable pouch syndrome is characterized by visceral hypersensitivity and poor quality of life score [abstract]. *Gastroenterology.* 2004;126:A-124.

32

Medical Management of Extraintestinal Manifestations of Ulcerative Colitis

Lloyd Mayer, MD and Robert Pittman, MD

The inflammatory bowel diseases (IBDs) are a group of intestinal disorders with specific features that share the potential to become systemic. The systemic nature of these conditions is best exemplified by the presence of extraintestinal manifestations. Physicians who care for patients with IBD are frequently confronted with symptoms of these manifestations, and often these can be worse than the underlying bowel disease. These disorders can be difficult to manage and responsible for considerable morbidity and mortality.

Extraintestinal manifestations of IBD have been reported to affect a wide variety of organ systems. Most commonly, the skin, joints, eyes, and biliary tract are affected. As our understanding of IBD as a systemic disorder evolves, the attention paid to extraintestinal manifestations increases. As such, other organ systems, such as the hematologic, pulmonary, and circulatory systems, are being included under the umbrella of extraintestinal manifestations. Because the number of extraintestinal manifestations is increasing, it is becoming more challenging to classify these disorders.

Traditionally, extraintestinal manifestations have been grouped according to the affected organ system. An alternative classification focuses on the relationship of the extraintestinal manifestation to the underlying bowel disease; that is, some extraintestinal manifestations occur concurrent with flares of IBD, while others occur and progress independently of the underlying bowel disease (Table 32-1). The former extraintestinal manifestations improve with treatment of the bowel inflammation, while the latter do not respond to such therapy. There are others that are a consequence of the disease (eg, hydronephrosis, renal calculi, amyloidosis) and are in a different category altogether. Lastly, it is important to recognize that the consequences of the different therapies (eg, corticosteroids and surgery) used to treat IBD can have manifestations of their own (eg, nutritional deficiency, osteoporosis, osteonecrosis), and this should be recognized quickly by the treating physician so as not to think that the problem is related to the underlying bowel disease.

A comprehensive review of all extraintestinal manifestations for both Crohn's disease (CD) and ulcerative colitis (UC) is beyond the scope of this review. As such, the extraintestinal manifestations most commonly associated with UC will be reviewed here. In certain instances, there is considerable overlap with respect to the association of a particular disorder with both UC and CD.

The Epidemiology of Extraintestinal Manifestations

The prevalence of extraintestinal manifestations reported in the literature varies depending on the population that is studied and the specific diseases that are considered. The lifetime risk of any extraintestinal manifestation in a patient with IBD is about 21% to 36%.[1-5] Arthritis is the most common extraintestinal manifestation seen. When peripheral arthritis is excluded, the reported prevalence of extraintestinal diseases is about 16% in one study[3] and 6% in another study with stricter inclusion criteria.[6] It is estimated that 80% of the cases of extraintestinal manifestations occur after the onset of UC symptoms. Concurrent development of colitis and extraintestinal manifestations occurs in 10% of cases, and the remaining 10% occur prior to the onset of clinical disease.[6,7] Some extraintestinal manifestations are present in both CD and UC, most frequently in patients who have evidence of colonic pathology,

Lichtenstein GR, ed.
Ulcerative Colitis: The Complete Guide to Medical Management (pp 341-364)

TABLE 32-1

CLASSIFICATION OF COMMON EXTRAINTESTINAL MANIFESTATIONS BY DISEASE ACTIVITY

BEFORE/CONCOMITANT WITH ACTIVE INFLAMMATION	INDEPENDENT OF ACTIVE INFLAMMATION
Peripheral arthritis (type I)	Pyoderma gangrenosum
Erythema nodosum	Primary sclerosing cholangitis
Aphthous ulcers	Uveitis
Episcleritis/iritis	Ankylosing spondylitis/sacroiliitis
	Peripheral arthritis (type II)

irrespective of the particular type of IBD.[5] Furthermore, there is a statistically significant increased risk of multiple extraintestinal manifestations in a patient with a single extraintestinal manifestation.[1]

PATHOGENESIS OF EXTRAINTESTINAL DISEASES

Although the association of extraintestinal manifestations with UC and CD has been recognized for many years,[8,9] there is still no definitive explanation for this occurrence or the predilection of certain patients to manifest these symptoms. The extraintestinal manifestations are largely inflammatory in nature, much like the underlying bowel diseases. This observation would support a common pathophysiologic mechanism. However, such mechanisms have escaped characterization. The variable relationships to the severity of colitis and response to proctocolectomy suggest a complex interaction of different biological processes. Despite many studies aimed at defining the link between IBD and extraintestinal manifestations, the pathophysiology of extraintestinal manifestations remains poorly defined. In addition, studies to define which extraintestinal manifestations are particularly associated with UC as opposed to CD are inconclusive. For the most part, extraintestinal manifestations are more common in patients with colitis, whether the underlying disease is UC or CD.

IBD is thought to reflect the interplay of genetic, environmental, and immunologic factors. These also play a role in the development of extraintestinal manifestations. A study examining familial IBD showed that affected parent-child pairs were concordant for extraintestinal manifestations in 70.1%, and siblings were concordant for extraintestinal manifestations in 83.8%.[10] Moreover, the finding that extraintestinal manifestations can be clustered within a single patient supports the notion that a common pathophysiologic mechanism is involved in all of them. A multivariate analysis of 535 patients with UC reported that cigarette smoking and appendectomy were independent factors associated with dermatologic and axial skeleton disorders.[11]

An immunologic mechanism, related to the colon, seems the most likely cause of extraintestinal manifestations. The theory that IBD itself is a result of dysregulation of mucosal immune responses, coupled with the observation that other immune-mediated inflammatory diseases are clustered in patients with IBD, supports this notion.[12] Greenstein et al reported a 42% incidence of extraintestinal manifestations in patients with colonic disease compared to a 23% incidence in patients with isolated small bowel disease.[5] In the literature, antibodies to human tropomyosin 5 have been shown to bind to colonocytes and activate the complement pathway in patients with UC.[13-15] Interestingly, epitopes recognized by these autoantibodies are shared amongst colon, biliary, and skin epithelia.[16] It has also been shown that the interplay between the mucosal immune system and luminal flora are responsible for not only intestinal manifestations of IBD, but also extraintestinal manifestations.[17,18]

The genetics of extraintestinal manifestations have been studied as well. Numerous studies have examined the role of HLA class II genes in UC. The results of these studies are somewhat mixed, likely due to heterogeneity between the populations studied and methodological differences in study design.[19-22] Nevertheless, there seems to be an association with certain HLA alleles and disease behavior, particularly with respect to extraintestinal manifestations. In a study of UC patients undergoing surgery,[23] the DRB1*0103 allele showed a statistically significant association with extraintestinal manifestations overall and with arthritis, aphthous ulcers, and uveitis in particular.

MEDICAL MANAGEMENT OF COMMON EXTRAINTESTINAL MANIFESTATIONS

Clinical trials aimed at management of extraintestinal manifestations are limited due to the relatively small number of patients affected at any given center. Proposed pathogenetic mechanisms have led to the application of directed therapies, although the experience with these approaches is minimal. Case series from IBD referral centers have reported a variety of therapies for extraintestinal manifestations, and such studies remain the cornerstone of evidence for managing these complications. In many instances, studies have not separated UC patients from CD patients, so much of the evidence applies to IBD patients in general.

Role of Proctocolectomy

The definitive surgical therapy for UC is restorative proctocolectomy and IPAA. The impact of this surgery on extraintestinal manifestations is variable. Those extraintestinal manifestations that parallel colitis activity are cured with this surgical procedure. The other extraintestinal manifestations, however, can remain or even occur after surgery. One retrospective series showed that ocular manifestations and primary sclerosing cholangitis were unaffected by surgery. The presence of a rectal remnant or ileal reservoir did not affect the evolution of the extraintestinal manifestation.[24] In addition, the presence of extraintestinal manifestations is a significant risk factor for the development of pouchitis in patients with UC undergoing IPAA.[25]

EXTRAINTESTINAL DISEASES RELATED TO COLITIS ACTIVITY

Erythema Nodosum

Erythema nodosum (EN) is the most common cutaneous manifestation of IBD. Most of the literature reports a greater association with UC as opposed to CD. Reported rates are between 0.9% and 4%,[5,26] with women affected more frequently.[3,26] EN typically affects the extensor surfaces of the extremities, especially the pretibial area. The condition consists of painful red or violet nodules 1 to 5 cm in diameter that usually appear just prior to or simultaneously with bowel inflammation (Figure 32-1).

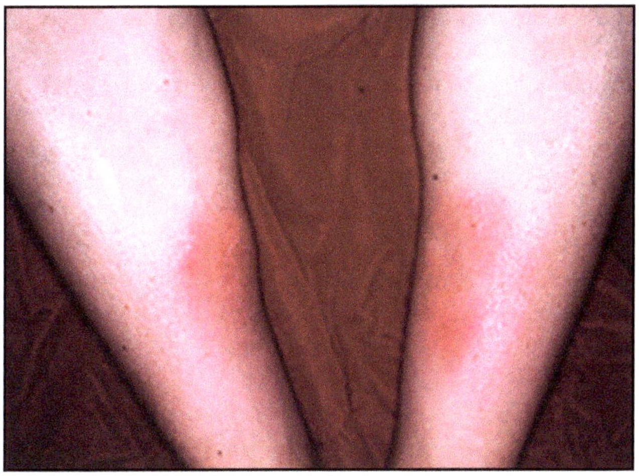

FIGURE 32-1. Erythema nodosum affecting both lower extremities of a patient with ulcerative colitis. (Courtesy of Mark Lebwohl, MD, New York, NY.)

EN is seen in a number of other systemic disorders as well. However, when one encounters a case of EN, evidence of IBD should be sought because the cutaneous symptoms can predate colonic symptoms. Because only 10% of colitis-associated EN occurs in the absence of bowel inflammation, other causes of EN should be considered. Common causes, other than colitis, for this manifestation include sarcoidosis, post-streptococcal infection, and medications, especially oral contraceptives.

Biopsies of these lesions show a focal panniculitis, but the clinical presentation of this disorder is usually sufficient to make the diagnosis. It is not unusual for peripheral arthritis to accompany EN. Erythema nodosum involving the skin overlying a joint can be mistaken for arthritis. The pathogenesis of this condition remains unknown. In addition to the proposed mechanisms described previously (see the section on Pathogenesis of Extraintestinal Diseases), there is some evidence to suggest that the risk of developing EN is associated with a polymorphism in the TNFα gene.[27]

The skin lesions usually respond to treatment of the colitis or resolve spontaneously and regress within 3 months without any evidence of scarring.[28] Therefore, symptomatic relief is the aim of therapy in the typical cases. Although NSAIDs are effective in treating this condition, their use should be weighed carefully given the possibility of inducing a flare of the underlying bowel disease.[29,30] As such, alternative analgesics such as acetaminophen and opiates should be utilized. Most patients have a single episode, although 30% of patients will have recurrence of this disorder.

There are refractory cases that can last for months. Usually, these cases respond to systemic corticosteroids or immunomodulators, although these interventions are based primarily on anecdotal evidence. It is reasonable to biopsy the lesions for histological confirmation prior to initiating immunosuppressive therapy. Potassium iodide, an agent used by dermatologists for more than a century, has been reported to be effective in treating this condition, although the side effect profile is significant and the mechanism of action is not understood.[31] Newer biologic agents, including infliximab, have been reported to be successful in the pediatric population.[32] This observation is intriguing given the described polymorphism in the TNFα gene, although anti-TNFα therapies are significantly more effective in CD than UC.

Aphthous Stomatitis

Aphthous stomatitis is a common manifestation of colitis and can be a source of significant discomfort. The reported prevalence is approximately 30%.[5] This entity is more common in CD than in UC and may precede or accompany a flare or the onset of disease. The lesions consist of aphthous ulcers in the buccal mucosa, gingiva, and tongue. It is unusual for these lesions to affect the tonsils and oropharynx. The differential diagnosis of these lesions is extensive and includes trauma, malignancy, infections (HSV, TB, syphilis), Behçet's disease, and side effects of medications. Aphthous ulceration is a reported side effect of methotrexate, which can be used to treat CD.[33] The exact pathogenesis of these lesions remains unclear. Proposed mechanisms are similar to those for IBD in general. In addition, this manifestation seems to be associated with the presence of uveitis, EN, and arthritis.

Therapy directed at these lesions is targeted at limiting the immune response and providing analgesia, while concurrently treating the underlying bowel inflammation. Topical steroids in the form of sprays or mouthwash are the mainstay of treatment. Examples include betamethasone valerate mouthwash, triamcinolone mouthwash, budesonide spray, and beclomethasone spray. Others have suggested using steroid preparations designed for the treatment of asthma, but spraying the medications onto the buccal mucosa.[34] In addition, topical analgesics such as lidocaine rinse and sucralfate suspension can be used. Thalidomide is used with great efficacy outside of the United States, and infliximab is similarly effective. Other systemic therapy is used primarily to treat the bowel disease and may accelerate the healing of oral lesions.

Type I Peripheral Arthritis

The prevalence of the form of peripheral arthritis that parallels disease activity is estimated to be 12.8% to 23%,[35,36] thereby making this the most common extraintestinal manifestation of IBD. Peripheral arthritis occurs more often in CD than in UC. The estimated incidence of peripheral arthropathy in UC is between 5% and 10%.[37] Orchard et al have proposed a classification scheme that includes 2 categories. Type I arthritis describes the more common entity of pauciarticular synovitis that parallels bowel disease activity. In addition, patients with peripheral arthralgias in the absence of acute synovial inflammation, about 5.3%, are usually placed in this group. When only patients with clinical evidence of joint inflammation are included in the analysis, the prevalence of type I arthritis in UC approaches 4%.[37] Type II arthritis refers to a polyarticular synovitis that can occur and progress independently of the underlying IBD (discussed later). There has been criticism of this classification system due to the lumping of patients with arthralgias only into type I arthritis, when a distinct pathogenetic mechanism may be responsible for the heterogeneity in phenotype.[38]

The pathophysiology of colitis-associated arthritis is thought to be due to both genetic factors and enteric bacteria. There is an association with HLA-B27, HLA-B35, and HLA-DRB0103 and type I arthritis.[39-41] Because type I arthritis flares in concert with bowel disease, it is likely that luminal antigens are important in the pathogenesis of this manifestation, similar to what is seen in reactive arthritis associated with infectious colitis. However, the data supporting this mechanism in UC are not convincing.

Type I arthropathy affects 5 or fewer joints, one of which is weight bearing. The knee is the most commonly affected site, followed by the hips and ankles. The arthritis is acute and migratory, and typically flares with the underlying bowel disease, although it can manifest just prior to the onset of bowel symptoms. The condition is self-limited for most patients, with 90% of the cases resolving by 6 months[42]; recurrence rates are 25% to 40%. Long-term consequences of this type of arthritis are minimal. Joint deformities do not occur, and radiographs usually show effusions and soft tissue edema.

On physical examination, the joints may appear hot or swollen. If only 1 or 2 joints are affected, arthrocentesis should be performed to rule out septic arthritis and crystal disease. In addition, EN overlying the joint should be considered, especially if there is no joint effusion. The synovial fluid typically reflects a sterile inflammatory effusion, with a neutrophilic predominance.[35,43]

Similar to the management of EN, the primary aim of therapy for type I arthritis is analgesia. Usually, the symptoms will improve as the underlying bowel inflammation improves. NSAIDs should be used with caution in patients with active bowel disease, although some clinicians successfully use these agents. Data exist demonstrating the adverse impact of NSAIDs on the small intestine and colon.[44] In the setting of IBD, the data are mixed with respect to adverse events and association with flares requiring hospital admission.[30,45,46] Acetaminophen-based analgesics are often an adequate substitute. However, patients frequently prefer NSAIDs to acetaminophen for arthritic symptoms.[47,48] The cyclo-oxygenase 2 (COX-2) inhibitors may play a role in treatment here as well. Despite initial reports of COX-2 inhibitors exacerbating IBD,[49] more recent retrospective and prospective studies examining the toxicity of COX-2 inhibitors in IBD suggest that there is effective relief of arthritis symptoms without an increase in severe adverse events.[50,51] In addition, resting the joint and placing a splint on the affected area are appropriate adjuncts to medical therapy.

Other agents have specific anti-inflammatory properties and can be used in more difficult cases. The sulfapyridine moiety of sulfasalazine has been shown to be anti-arthritic.[52] If patients are taking a different 5-ASA-based agent for their colitis, it is reasonable to switch them to sulfasalazine. The dose needs to be titrated up to a goal of 4 g/d. Other aminosalicylates do not control synovial inflammation unless they control the underlying bowel inflammation. If the patient is taking systemic corticosteroids for colitis, there is usually a treatment effect on the arthritis. For the patient who is not on systemic steroids, but is not responding to analgesics and/or sulfasalazine, intra-articular injection of steroids (eg, methylprednisolone) and local anesthetics

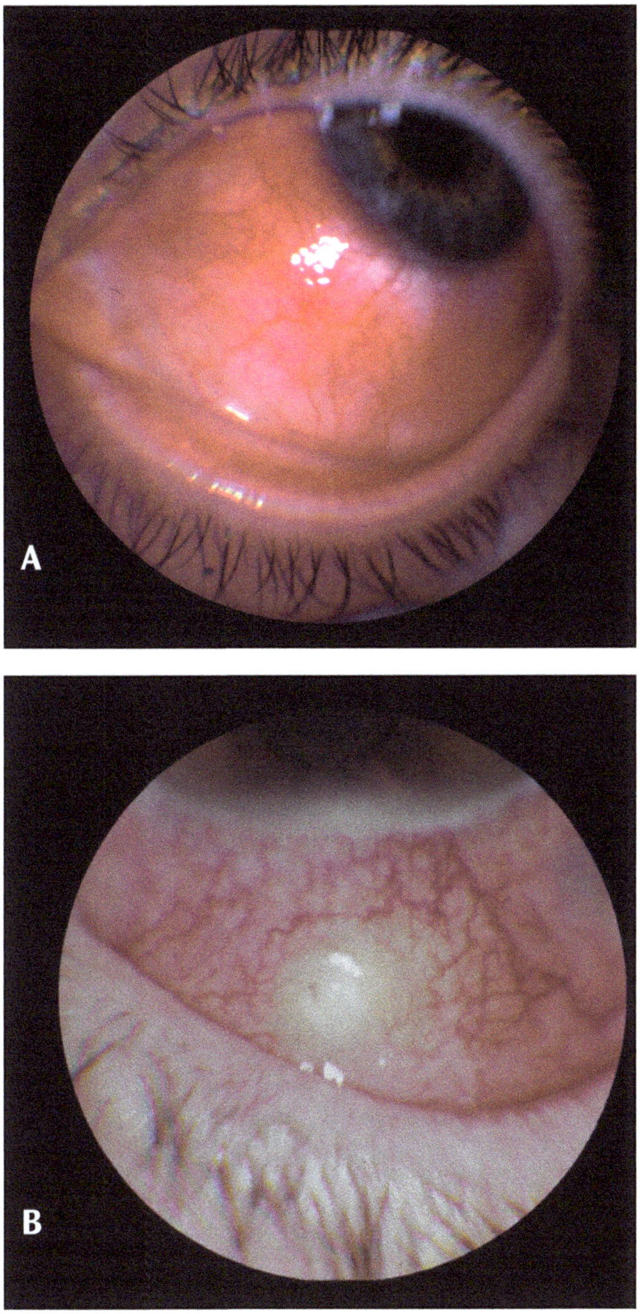

FIGURE 32-2. Ocular manifestations of inflammatory bowel disease. (A) Episcleritis demonstrated by diffuse erythema of the eye with intervening white sclera. (B) Scleritis demonstrated by pronounced injection of the ocular blood vessels, intervening pink sclera, and nodule formation. (Courtesy of Alan Friedman, MD, New York, NY.)

(eg, lidocaine) are an option. Once remission is induced, sulfasalazine is the most appropriate 5-ASA-based maintenance therapy for a patient with a history of arthritis.

Episcleritis and Scleritis

The episclera is the layer just below the conjunctiva. Episcleritis occurs in 2% to 5% of patients with IBD.[53] The condition may be asymptomatic or manifest as burning and itching in one or both eyes. The eyes are red and injected on examination. The intervening sclera remains white (Figure 32-2A).[54] Unlike conjunctivitis, pain is common in this disorder. However, vision loss, photophobia, or papillary abnormalities on exam would suggest a different diagnosis. Therapy is directed at treating the bowel disease, although specific therapy for ocular symptoms is appropriate according to the patient's level of discomfort. Episcleritis usually resolves with resolution of bowel inflammation. Ophthalmic corticosteroid preparations, such as decadron phosphate, and cool compresses are also helpful. If symptoms persist beyond these measures, systemic NSAIDs can be used, albeit with the caveat that bowel symptoms may worsen. In the CD literature, infliximab has been reported to effectively treat episcleritis.[55]

Scleritis implies inflammation of the layer immediately below the episclera. In scleritis, pain is a more predominant feature. The eye appears red, and the intervening sclera is not white, but pink (Figure 32-2B). In addition, subconjunctival hemorrhage is present. The potential consequences of scleritis are more severe than in episcleritis. Sometimes, the posterior eye can become affected and cause retinal detachment or damage to the optic nerve.[56] Treatment is the same as listed previously for episcleritis, although the timing of therapy must be sooner and an urgent referral to an ophthalmologist is necessary.

EXTRAINTESTINAL DISEASES NOT RELATED TO COLITIS ACTIVITY

Pyoderma Gangrenosum

Pyoderma gangrenosum (PG) is more closely associated with UC than CD.[5,26] The prevalence rates in the IBD literature range from 0.5% to 5%.[3,5,36,57] Conversely, about one-third to one-half of patients with PG have IBD.[58] Although less common than EN, PG typically is more troublesome with respect to patient discomfort and response to treatment. In general, PG does not parallel colitis activity, but it has been reported to do so in a number of cases.[59]

The lesions are most commonly seen in patients 30 to 50 years old. The initial lesion is that of an annular erythema that evolves into a fluctuant nodule. Eventually, the lesion expands peripherally and ulcerates (Figure 32-3). The edge of the ulcer is violaceous and raised. Pustules may be seen on the rim of the ulcer.[60] The lesions most typically occur on the trunk and extremities, although reports of the lesions affecting essentially every part of the body have been reported. PG exhibits pathergy; often, lesions are either induced or worsened by trauma. As such, biopsy should be reserved for cases in which a histologic diagnosis is necessary.

TABLE 32-2

SUMMARY OF EIMS THAT PARALLEL BOWEL INFLAMMATION

Condition	Natural History	Goals of Therapy	Therapeutic Agents
Erythema nodosum	Painful, nodular lesions on trunk and extremity; non-scarring; can precede bowel inflammation	Analgesia	Acetaminophen NSAIDs/COX-2 antagonist* Corticosteroids# Immunomodulators# Infliximab#
Aphthous stomatitis	Painful, persistent oral ulcers; lesions typically resolve with induction of remission of IBD	Analgesia	Topical steroid mouthwash/spray Viscous lidocaine
Type I arthritis	Migratory large joint pain without development of permanent deformity; symptoms typically resolve with resolution of IBD but may persist	Analgesia	Acetaminophen NSAIDs/COX-2 antagonist* Sulfasalazine Corticosteroids Systemic Intra-articular
Episcleritis/scleritis	Pain without vision loss; symptoms resolve with resolution of IBD	Relief of symptoms Urgent referral to ophthalmologist for scleritis	Ophthalmologic steroids NSAIDs/COX-2 antagonist* Cool compresses

*NSAIDs should be used cautiously because they can exacerbate bowel inflammation.
#For refractory cases.

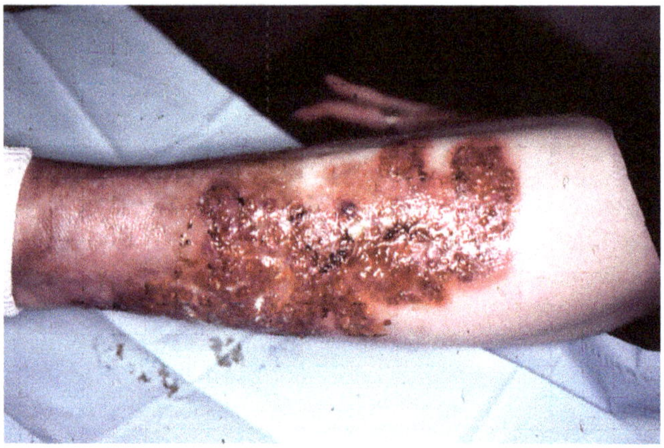

FIGURE 32-3. Pyoderma gangrenosum demonstrated by irregularly bordered necrotic lesion, with pustules affecting the lower extremity. (Courtesy of Mark Lebwohl, MD, New York, NY.)

The histopathology of PG shows a central zone of necrotizing suppurative inflammation and peripheral vascular reaction defined by perivascular and intramural lymphocytic infiltrates with a peripheral neutrophilic component, usually with fibrinoid necrosis.[61] The absence of leukocytoclastic vasculitis and negative cultures and special stains for infectious organisms support the diagnosis of PG. The initial pathogenetic event is perivascular deposition of immunoglobulins, complement, and fibrin. It has been proposed that there is cross-reactivity among autoantibodies directed at luminal antigens that also recognize cytokeratin 18, implying involvement of cell, humoral, and complement-mediated immune responses.[62] As such, dysregulated immunity appears to be central to the disease pathogenesis and remains the target of most therapeutic agents (Table 32-3).

A dermatology consultation is helpful in managing cases of PG. Wound care is a necessary component in the therapy of the lesions. Debridement and hydrocolloid dressings are options for local therapy.[63,64] The role of wound care is primarily to prevent superinfection and relieve pain. Topical antibiotics are not encouraged as they have no proven efficacy; if infection is present, systemic antibiotics are necessary.

In addition, topical agents can be directed at altering the local immune response and preventing bacterial superinfection. Immune-directed topical agents include intralesional injection of corticosteroids[63] and intralesional cyclosporine A.[65] Topical tacrolimus used to treat peristomal lesions in patients with CD showed complete resolution and re-epithelialization of skin within 2 weeks.[66] In addition, this

TABLE 32-3

SUMMARY OF PYODERMA GANGRENOSUM

Clinical Course	Goals of Therapy	Therapeutic Agents
Painful, ulcerating, persistent lesions on trunk and extremities	Wound healing	Débridement Hydrocolloid dressings Antibiotics* Surgery#
Pathergy		
Course is independent of underlying bowel inflammation	Local immune suppression	Intralesional steroids Intralesional cyclosporine A Topical tacrolimus
	Systemic immune suppression	IV/oral corticosteroids IV/oral cyclosporine A Oral tacrolimus Mycophenolate mofetil Thalidomide Infliximab

*Antibiotics are indicated if superinfection is present; usually systemic preparations are required.

#Surgery should be used sparingly, after healing has been initiated given the presence of pathergy.

agent is effective in the treatment of pyoderma lesions either alone or in combination with systemic therapy.[67-69]

Systemic therapy is used in cases where topical approaches are not effective. The primary systemic therapy used to be corticosteroids, either orally or intravenously. The doses required are high (prednisone 40 to 120 mg/d). If one is able to taper, a maintenance course of steroids is usually required.[63,64,70] IV steroids are reserved for refractory cases. In instances when the pyoderma seems to parallel the colitis, the skin lesions can respond to treatment of the underlying bowel inflammation, although therapy may need to be more intense and protracted. Dapsone (100 to 200 mg/d) can be a useful adjunct to steroid therapy.

Cyclosporine A is another systemic immunosuppressive agent that is effective in treating PG. A retrospective study of 11 steroid-refractory patients who were treated with IV cyclosporine (4 mg/kg/d) and subsequently changed to oral maintenance therapy (4 to 7 mg/kg/d) reported complete healing of lesions in all patients with a mean time to response of 4.5 days and mean time to healing of 1.4 months.[71] Careful attention to side effects including hypertension, neurotoxicity, and renal insufficiency is warranted. Oral tacrolimus (0.3 mg/kg/d) is an immunosuppressive macrolide antibiotic that has been shown to successfully treat PG.[72] Side effects include nephrotoxicity, diabetes mellitus, and neurotoxicity. Mycophenolate mofetil is effective in refractory cases when used in conjunction with other agents; the dose is started at 500 mg twice daily and is increased to 1 g twice daily. The other agents are continued until healing of the lesion is appreciated and are then tapered slowly.[73] However, controlled trials are needed to confirm the effectiveness of these agents. The experience with immunomodulators such as AZA and 6-MP has not been encouraging.[74] Their role is primarily as an adjunct to other therapies, particularly infliximab.

Anti-TNFα agents have been shown to be particularly useful in refractory cases and more recently have been considered the treatment of choice. Thalidomide has demonstrated efficacy in multiple case studies, but no clinical trials exist.[75-77] There are emerging data that support the use of infliximab for refractory cases of pyoderma lesions on the trunk, extremities, and peristomal region. Prompt responses to either single or multiple infusions were seen.[78-81] Responders may require maintenance infliximab, and all should be placed on concurrent immunomodulators. A prospective study of infliximab for IBD-associated PG is required to confirm efficacy in this context.

Due to the occurrence of pathergy, surgical therapy for pyoderma should be a last resort. Some reports of successful surgical debridement and allograft skin flaps after systemic immunomodulatory therapy exist.[82] However, long-term wound stabilization is obtained only through control of the systemic and local inflammatory process.

In refractory cases, total proctocolectomy can be considered; however, regression of the lesions is not guaranteed. In addition, new lesions may occur after colectomy.[83] Peristomal lesions are typical in this case and

TABLE 32-4

SUMMARY OF TYPE II ARTHRITIS

CLINICAL COURSE	GOALS OF THERAPY	THERAPEUTIC AGENTS
Persistent arthritis of multiple joints, especially small joints	Analgesia	Acetaminophen NSAIDs/COX-2 antagonist* Joint rest/splinting
Risk of permanent deformity Course is independent of underlying bowel inflammation	Preservation of joint	Sulfasalazine Systemic corticosteroids Immunomodulators# Methotrexate 6-MP Infliximab

*NSAIDs should be used cautiously because they can exacerbate bowel inflammation.
#Methotrexate is the preferred immunomodulator; close attention to side effects is necessary.

need to be treated in the same manner as lesions on the extremities.[84,85]

TYPE II PERIPHERAL ARTHRITIS

Type II peripheral arthritis is less common than type I and is reportedly present in 2.5% of patients with UC.[37] This arthritis differs from type I in a number of ways. Type II arthritis does not parallel colitis activity and can occur and progress independent of the underlying bowel inflammation. Type II arthritis is associated with HLA-B44.[41]

In addition, the course of type II arthritis is longer than type I, typically lasting for months or years (Table 32-4). Clinical presentation reflects polyarticular, symmetrical involvement that is similar to the findings in rheumatoid arthritis. Smaller, non-weight bearing joints are typically involved. However, the patients are seronegative for rheumatoid factor, and joint destruction is not common.

The prolonged course and the independence from colitis activity of type II arthritis can make management challenging. Again, as in type I arthritis, symptomatic relief is the goal, as permanent joint destruction is not part of the pathology. The use of analgesics, either NSAIDs, COX-2 inhibitors, or acetaminophen, is similar to the strategies outlined above in the discussion of type I arthritis. There is more latitude with the use of NSAIDs in this condition as colitis can be quiescent in the setting of joint inflammation. Also, joint rest and splinting can be tried, although the greater number of joints affected and the nature of the small joints affected makes this a difficult therapy to administer. For similar reasons, intra-articular injection of corticosteroids is not practical.

If relief does not occur with the above measures, sulfasalazine can be tried. The optimal dose is 4 g/d. Patients who remain symptomatic can attempt a trial of systemic corticosteroids, such as prednisolone 15 mg/d. A strategy for tapering the steroids, such as starting an immunomodulator, should be initiated at this time. Given the prolonged course of this disease, the use of maintenance steroids is correlated with a significant side effect profile and should be avoided.

There are no controlled trials examining the role of immunomodulators such as 6-MP, AZA, and methotrexate in the treatment of type II arthritis. However, given the success of these agents in rheumatoid arthritis and IBD, it is not unreasonable to extrapolate their utility to the context of type II arthritis. Most clinicians prefer methotrexate in this setting, by either oral or subcutaneous route. Side effects of methotrexate, including oral ulceration and hepatotoxicity, must be considered when choosing an immunomodulator. If methotrexate is preferred, the dose is given weekly and titrated to symptomatic relief or a maximum dose of 25 mg per week. The dosing is the same for oral and subcutaneous administration. 6-MP and AZA are usually started at 50 mg/d and are titrated up to a dose of 1.5 mg/kg or 2.5 mg/kg, respectively. Close attention to side effects, especially leukopenia, is necessary.

Last, newer biologic therapies can be used in refractory cases. Anti-TNFα agents, such as infliximab and etanercept, have been shown to be efficacious in rheumatoid arthritis and ankylosing spondylitis (AS).[86,87] Moreover, a cohort of patients with CD-related arthralgias and arthritis were prospectively treated with infliximab with encouraging results.[88] The use of infliximab for this indication requires further study. See chapters on infliximab for dosing details and precautions.

Axial Arthropathies

Two axial arthropathies have been described in IBD: isolated sacroiliitis and AS. The two conditions comprise a spectrum of seronegative axial arthropathies in patients with IBD. Isolated sacroiliitis refers to inflammatory changes in the sacroiliac joint, whereas AS implies spinal column involvement in the setting of sacroiliitis. The current thinking is that a small percentage of patients with sacroiliitis will progress to the more debilitating condition, AS.

Ankylosing spondylitis is more common in UC than CD and is seen in Crohn's colitis more frequently than in ileitis.[6] It affects fewer patients than type I peripheral arthritis. The reported rates of AS in UC vary from 1.6% to 7%.[3,26]

Sacroiliitis is more common than AS. The prevalence of this entity is difficult to determine as many patients with IBD have radiographic evidence of sacroiliitis in the absence of symptoms. The sensitivity of the diagnostic test used will affect the prevalence of this condition. Reported rates are 4% to 18% with radiography[89-91] and in excess of 50% with scintigraphic bone scans.[92]

There is sizeable literature on the pathogenesis of AS. Current theories implicate an interaction between the patient's MHC class I alleles and bacterial antigens. HLA-B27 is present in about 90% of patients with idiopathic AS.[93,94] In contrast, the HLA-B27 allele is present in 25% to 50% of patients with IBD-associated AS. However, only half of the patients with both IBD and the HLA-B27 allele develop AS.[91,95,96] In the CD literature, there are conflicting studies examining the role of HLA-B27 in isolated sacroiliitis.[97,98] Both studies to date only analyzed small numbers of patients and contained heterogenous populations.

It is suspected that the role of HLA-B27 in this disorder centers around the presentation of an enteric bacterial antigen to CD 8^+ T cells that subsequently cause joint inflammation. A variety of bacterial antigens have been studied without clear identification of a unique, responsible organism. There are mixed data in both the IBD-associated AS and idiopathic AS literature regarding *Klebsiella* species as the causative organism.[99] One possible rationale for the lower prevalence of HLA-B27 in IBD-associated AS when compared to the idiopathic form is that intestinal inflammation augments bacterial translocation from the gut to the vasculature in the spine and sacroiliac joints. Therefore, it is presumed that a larger amount of antigen is presented in the setting of colitis. If this is true, then HLA-B27 can be considered a risk factor for antigen presentation at lower concentrations of antigen, whereas other HLA alleles exhibit similar properties in the presence of higher antigenic burdens.[100]

Animal models have demonstrated a putative role for bacteria in the pathogenesis of AS. HLA-B27 transgenic rats, when reared in a sterile environment, are free of colitis and joint pathology but quickly develop these conditions when normal bacteria are introduced.[18,101]

The role of bacterial antigens is particularly intriguing in that, unlike postenteric reactive arthritis, progression of disease is independent of the underlying bowel inflammation. Indeed, there is a relationship between gut and joint inflammation. Bacteroides species have been shown to be promoters of joint inflammation and colitis in animal models.[18] One study reported a 68% prevalence of ileocolitis in patients with spondyloarthropathies.[102,103] It should be noted, however, that many of these patients were on NSAIDs, which may contribute to increased bacterial translocation and the pathologic findings. Follow-up data suggest that patients with persistent gut inflammation failed to resolve their pain and mobility symptoms, and 3% to 4% of the patients in this study eventually developed IBD with a preponderant Crohn's phenotype.[104] Perhaps the predilection for the sacroiliac joints in colitis is related to the proximity of rectal veins to the targeted joint.

Clinically, it can be difficult to differentiate sacroiliitis and AS from more typical back pain that may be coincident in a patient with IBD.[37] The symptoms of this arthropathy are independent of colitis symptoms and often predate a diagnosis of inflammatory bowel disease. Any complaint of back pain, chest wall pain, limited mobility, or buttock pain should prompt an evaluation for axial arthropathy. The axial arthropathies tend to occur in younger patients, are associated with morning stiffness, and symptomatically improve with movement. Typical musculoskeletal back pain typically occurs in older patients, gets more troublesome as the day progresses, and is relieved by rest. Physical examination should evaluate anterior lumbar flexion (modified Schober test), lateral flexion, and chest expansion. Concurrent management with a rheumatologist is imperative. A variety of radiologic studies can be used to evaluate the patient with pain and limited mobility. Currently, plain radiographs (Figure 32-4) and magnetic resonance imaging of the lumbosacral spine are the preferred modalities among clinicians, although computed tomography and nuclear scans are also diagnostic.

Most patients with sacroiliitis are asymptomatic and do not progress to AS (Table 32-5). No studies have evaluated the rate of progression from radiographic disease to clinical disease. Therefore, therapy is directed at relief of symptoms, and there is no role for screening for this disorder in patients with colitis other than by history. In addition, there is no role for checking for the HLA-B27 allele with the intent of risk stratification. The low rate of progression to AS coupled with the large percentage of IBD patients with the HLA-B27 allele who do not develop AS supports this practice.

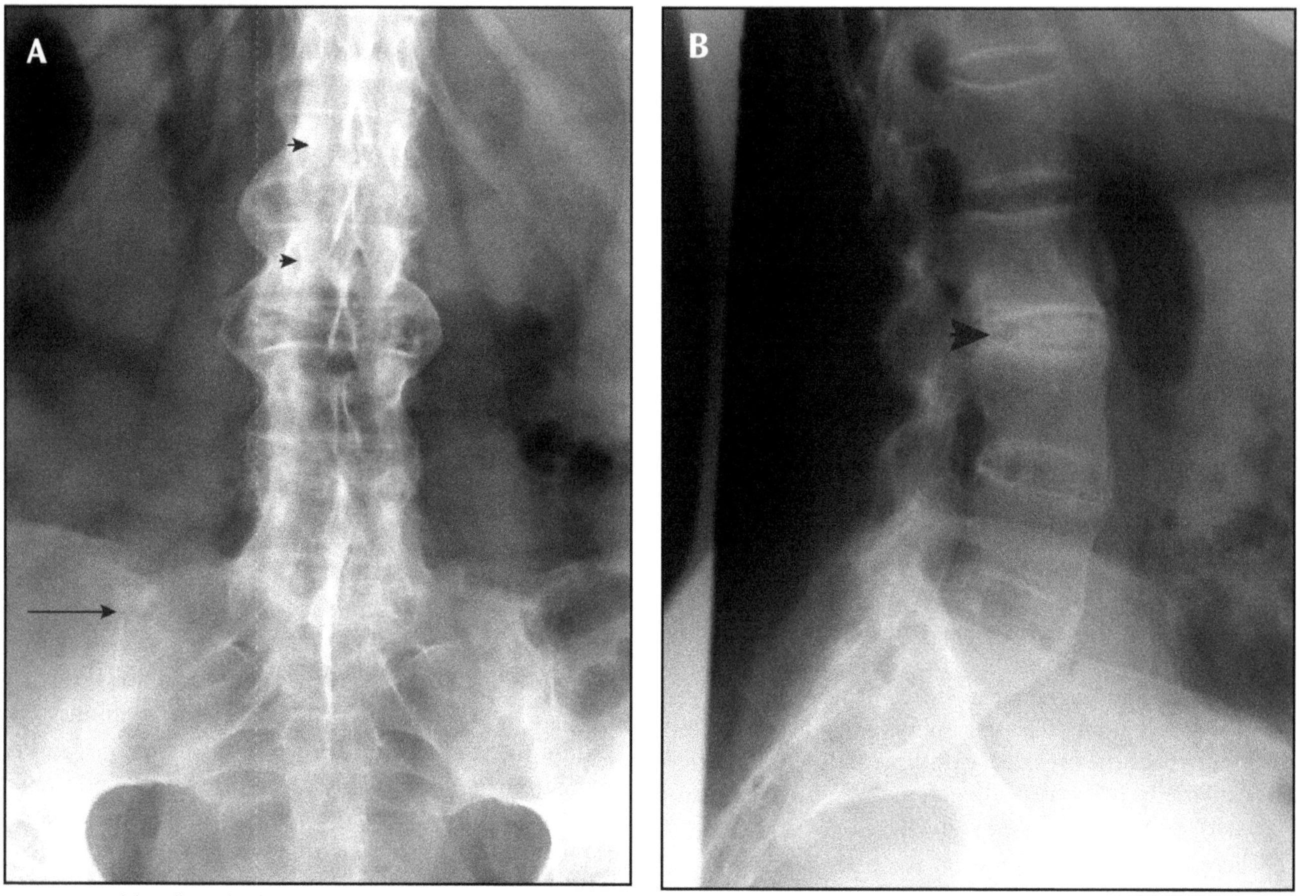

FIGURE 32-4. Plain radiographs of the lumbar spine and sacrum demonstrating advanced ankylosing spondylitis. (A) Anterior/posterior view with fusion of the sacroiliac joints (arrows), disc calcification (arrow heads), and fusion of the vertebral bodies (bamboo spine). (B) Lateral view demonstrating disc calcifications (arrow heads), fusion of the facet joints, and calcification of the anterior longitudinal and posterior longitudinal ligaments. (Courtesy of George Hermann, MD, New York, NY.)

TABLE 32-5

SUMMARY OF SACROILIITIS AND ANKYLOSING SPONDYLITIS

Clinical Course	Goals of Therapy	Therapeutic Agents
Sacroiliitis usually asymptomatic	Analgesia and increased mobility	NSAIDs/COX-2 antagonist*
Ankylosing spondylitis with back stiffness and decreased range of motion; improves with exercise		Physical therapy
Risk of permanent spinal deformity	Preservation of joint	
		Sulfasalazine
Course is independent of underlying bowel inflammation		Methotrexate
		Infliximab
		Bisphosphonates

*NSAIDs should be used cautiously because they can exacerbate bowel inflammation.

Similar to peripheral arthritis, the management of these conditions is directed at relief of symptoms. However, unlike the peripheral arthritides that are seen in the setting of UC, the spondyloarthropathies can cause permanent joint deformity and disability. Thus, there is a role for disease-modifying antirheumatic drugs that may temper the progression of this disease. The rheumatologic literature is extensive with regard to treatment of AS and sacroiliitis. Many gastroenterologists will extrapolate these data and apply them to their patients with colitis. Most studies are on patients with AS; there are no controlled trials looking at therapy for isolated sacroiliitis.

The issues relating to NSAIDs for symptomatic relief are similar to those described above for arthritis. Both NSAIDs and COX-2 inhibitors are effective in relieving symptoms, although there are no randomized trials of this therapy in colitis patients.

In addition, physical therapy has been studied as a treatment modality and is considered an important part of the treatment regimen in patients with limited mobility. Physical therapy can be prescribed in the form of a home exercise program or therapy with a physiatrist or licensed physical therapist. One study looking at the efficacy of home exercise reported a statistically significant difference in favor of group exercise, and another showed a positive trend with respect to improvement in function.[105,106] A Cochrane review of three trials found a 50% reduction in pain and stiffness in patients treated with a group therapy program compared to patients given a home exercise program.[107]

Sulfasalazine has been used with some success in patients with chronic spondyloarthropathies.[108,109] Sulfasalazine may act by directly decreasing intra-articular inflammation or by helping to heal underlying colitis, thereby reducing mucosal permeability to foreign antigens and modifying responses to the gut flora.

There are limited data demonstrating the benefit of sulfasalazine in treatment of inflammatory exacerbations of AS. A treatment response should be seen within the first 2 to 3 months.[110,111] In very chronic cases, the response is not different from placebo when spinal mobility is the endpoint examined. A 1-year, long-term, placebo-controlled study aimed at examining the role of sulfasalazine in slowing the progression of AS showed no evidence for the retardation of the spinal process in AS.[112]

Sulfasalazine should be considered in a patient with early disease, especially if there is concurrent peripheral arthritis. If the patient tolerates and responds to the treatment, the dose could be tapered over 6 months and eventually discontinued. If the patient relapses, a new course can be instituted. The goal dose is 2 to 3 g/d and should be titrated up by 500 mg every week.

The side effect profile of sulfasalazine is significant. Although there are reports of greater than one-third of patients experiencing side effects,[113] many clinicians feel that this number is an overestimate. The enteric-coated formulation ameliorates many of the abdominal side effects but increases the cost of treatment significantly. Common side effects include nausea, headache, and rash. Patients should be monitored periodically for hepatotoxicity and leukopenia. The drug should not be given to patients with glucose-6-phosphate dehydrogenase deficiency.

Methotrexate has been evaluated in patients who are refractory to NSAIDs.[114] At a weekly dose of 12.5 mg, 53% of patients responded by clinical parameters but there was no benefit with respect to spinal mobility. Similar to the sulfasalazine studies, the patients with peripheral arthritis were the most likely to respond.

Anti-TNFα agents have been studied in AS. A small study evaluated the efficacy of etanercept and showed an 80% response at the primary endpoint versus 30% in the placebo group.[115] Open-label studies of infliximab have demonstrated a rapid clinical and biochemical response in AS.[116,117] Subsequently, infliximab was shown in a multicenter, placebo-controlled trial of NSAID-refractory AS to achieve a rapid clinical response in greater than 50% of patients in the treatment arm.[118] In addition, patients were able to come off of NSAIDs. Similar to the dosing schedule for CD and rheumatoid arthritis, infliximab should be administered every 6 to 8 weeks in order to minimize adverse effects and maintain efficacy. Thalidomide was studied in a heterogenous group of patients who were refractory to other medications, including methotrexate. The study showed an improvement with respect to mobility, but the study was too small to draw any specific conclusions.

Bisphosphonate therapy has been examined in AS. The rationale here relates to the finding of increased bone turnover in the spine. In addition, there are data showing that bisphosphonates suppress proinflammatory cytokines such as IL-1, TNFα, and IL-6, and demonstrate anti-inflammatory properties in arthritic conditions.[119] Monthly IV infusions of pamidronate 60 mg have been shown, in 2 small studies, to have a trend toward effectiveness.[120,121] There needs to be further study of this agent in AS. It may have a role in treating patients who do not respond to infliximab.

The IL-1 receptor antagonist anakinra is also a potential therapy in AS. Preliminary data from an efficacy study not only showed clinical improvement, but also demonstrated regression of lesions by magnetic resonance.[122]

Complementary medicines are sought in many patients with AS. There are studies published showing effects of certain therapies; however, the ability to compare these to allopathic studies is limited. Chiropractic care has been reportedly effective in case reports.[123]

Uveitis

The reported prevalence of uveitis in UC is 3% to 5%.[6] The pathogenesis of uveitis is not completely understood, but associations with HLA-B27 and cross-reactivity of antibodies to colonic antigens with anterior and posterior chamber proteins has been shown.[124] In addition, the homing of peripheral leukocytes to the ocular tissue and the interaction of endothelial adhesion molecules with these cells is deranged so that inflammatory cells infiltrate the eye in patients with IBD.[125]

Uveitis implies inflammation of the vascular lining of the eye. When the inflammation is located anterior to the lens, it is termed anterior uveitis and affects the iris and ciliary body. Posterior uveitis implies inflammatory

TABLE 32-6

SUMMARY OF UVEITIS

Clinical Course	Goals of Therapy	Therapeutic Agents
Red, painful eye Photophobia: Vision threatening condition	Reduce intraocular inflammation and preserve vision	Ophthalmologic corticosteroids –Topical –Intraocular
Course is independent of underlying bowel inflammation	Urgent referral to ophthalmologist is indicated	Cycloplegic agents Systemic corticosteroids NSAIDs* Immunomodulators

*NSAIDs should be used cautiously because they can exacerbate bowel inflammation.

changes in the structures of the posterior chamber of the eye, namely the vitreous, choroid, and retina. The clinical features of anterior uveitis include pain, blurred vision, and photophobia (Table 32-6). On examination, the pupil may be miotic contrary to the dilated pupil that is seen in acute-angle glaucoma. Redness extends from the limbus outward with the most intense erythema juxtaposed to the iris (ciliary flush). Evidence of inflammatory cells in the anterior chamber, called a hypopyon, can be seen. Light reflexes are likely to be sluggish.[126] In contrast, visual loss implies posterior uveitis and/or retinitis, and immediate referral to an ophthalmologist is indicated. Often, there is associated arthritis and EN, as mentioned previously. Because it is possible to develop uveitis prior to the onset of bowel disease or in periods of remission, ocular symptoms should be addressed during routine follow-up of colitis patients.

Similar to episcleritis and scleritis, ophthalmologic preparations of corticosteroids, either topical or intraocular, are the mainstays of therapy. In addition, cycloplegics may be used to limit the development of long-term complications and reduce pain. Frequently, systemic therapy is required for more difficult cases. It has been suggested that if the bowel is inflamed, systemic therapy is required in order to achieve resolution of the ocular inflammation.[127] A group in Massachusetts reported success with a step-up approach to therapy where patients who failed systemic corticosteroids received systemic NSAIDs, immunomodulators, and cytotoxic therapy.[128] Colectomy has been beneficial in a few cases, although a case of uveitis after total proctocolectomy has been reported.[129] The experience with infliximab to treat uveitis is limited to CD. Prolonged uveitis can lead to intraocular adhesions and the development of glaucoma.

Primary Sclerosing Cholangitis

Primary sclerosing cholangitis (PSC) is a chronic progressive cholestatic disorder that affects both intrahepatic and extrahepatic bile ducts. The pathologic consequences of this condition include ongoing inflammation, obliteration, and fibrosis of the bile ducts. The disease impacts both quality of life and hepatocellular function, ultimately causing portal hypertension, cirrhosis, and end-stage liver disease (Table 32-7). PSC is currently recognized as the fourth most common indication for liver transplantation.[130] Most cases of PSC in the United States and Europe are associated with IBD, but the behavior of PSC is not affected by the concurrent diagnosis of IBD. PSC develops independently of colitis, and the diagnosis of IBD is frequently made after the diagnosis of PSC. The colitis can be relatively mild with respect to both symptoms and histology. Medical therapy directed at IBD and proctocolectomy do not impact the course of PSC. In addition, PSC confers an augmented risk of cholangiocarcinoma and colorectal cancer in patients with colitis, thus there is a need for more aggressive screening for colonic dysplasia.

Based on data from multiple studies, the prevalence of PSC in UC ranges from 2.4% to 7.4%.[12,131-135] The reported rates vary depending on the method used to diagnose the disorder. The incidence of PSC is increasing, perhaps in part due to screening of IBD patients with periodic liver function tests. Data support the notion that PSC is seen much more commonly in UC compared to CD.[136] About 75% of patients with PSC also have chronic UC. Approximately 4% of patients with IBD will develop PSC.[131] There are no reported cases of PSC in patients with isolated small bowel CD. Roughly 70% of these patients are men. In the non-IBD population, PSC is more common in women.[137] The mean

TABLE 32-7

SUMMARY OF PRIMARY SCLEROSING CHOLANGITIS

Clinical Course	Goals of Therapy	Therapeutic Agents
Indolent cholestatic process with development of cirrhosis, portal hypertension, and liver failure	Symptom control Pruritus	Bile-acid resins Antihistamines Opioid antagonists Plasmapheresis
Symptomatic complications include pruritus, cholangitis, metabolic bone disease	Bone disease	Bisphosphonates Calcium supplementation Vitamin D supplementation
Significantly increased risk of colorectal adenocarcinoma and cholangiocarcinoma	Fat-soluble vitamin deficiency	Supplementation of vitamins A, D, E, and K
Progression of disease is independent of underlying bowel inflammation	Cholangitis	Antibiotics, bowel rest Endoscopic dilation of dominant stricture if present
Common indication for liver transplantation	Control of hepatic fibrosis	Ursodeoxycholic acid Budesonide* AZA/6-MP Methotrexate Colchicine

*Systemic corticosteroids are not recommended for this chronic, indolent condition with associated metabolic bone disease.

age at diagnosis is 40 years.[138] Reported prevalence rates of cholangiocarcinoma in patients with PSC are between 10% and 30%. The concurrent diagnosis of PSC in patients with UC confers an estimated risk of colorectal cancer that approaches 50% after 25 years of disease.

The precise pathogenesis of PSC is unknown. Current theories suggest dysfunction of both host immune and non-immune mechanisms. Like other extraintestinal manifestations, normal intestinal flora and their metabolites are implicated in the pathogenesis.[139] Investigators examining surgical specimens from patients undergoing colectomy have proposed that the inflamed colon leads to increased permeability. By this notion, bacteria or bacterial toxins gain access to the portal circulation and may be responsible for the development of PSC.[140,141] The role of abnormal bile acids produced by luminal flora has been examined, and no significant conclusions were drawn.[142,143] The lack of a predominance of severe colitis in patients with PSC questions the reliability of these hypotheses. An animal model of PSC has led to the suggestion that bacterial peptides that are produced in the inflamed colon lead to histologic features of PSC, although the translation of these studies to human subjects has been unsuccessful.[144] In addition, there seems to be a genetic component that contributes to the pathogenesis of PSC.[145,146] Investigators have noted a familial clustering of cases and an association with HLA haplotypes and TNFα polymorphisms.[147-149] Similarly, immune-mediated mechanisms have been examined without any distinct conclusion with respect to pathogenesis. A variety of immune system abnormalities, including hypergammaglobulinemia and autoantibodies, are seen in patients with PSC.[150,151] Moreover, common epitopes between human colonic mucosa and biliary mucosa have been reported.[16] Nevertheless, the exact biological mechanism that leads to PSC remains unknown.

The clinical course of PSC is variable. Many patients are asymptomatic at the time of diagnosis but have biochemical evidence of cholestasis, most commonly elevation of serum alkaline phosphatase. Patients can remain asymptomatic for many years. However, symptoms do not necessarily correlate with the severity of disease, and disease does not progress at a uniform rate in all patients. In most patients, the presence of symptoms such as fatigue, weight loss, jaundice, and pruritus suggests advanced disease. Jaundice with fevers and chills are typical of bacterial cholangitis and may be the result of a dominant stricture in the extrahepatic biliary tree. Also, malabsorption of fats and fat-soluble vitamins can occur, leading to weight loss and bone disease. The median survival is estimated to be 10 to 15 years from diagnosis.[152,153] Patients who are symptomatic at diagnosis have a shortened survival compared to those who are asymptomatic at the time of diagnosis.[154]

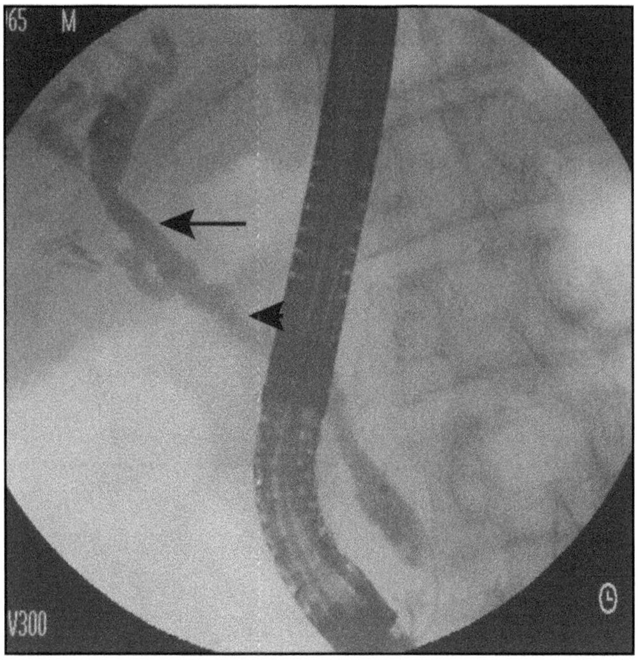

FIGURE 32-5. Endoscopic cholangiogram demonstrating PSC. The extrahepatic bile ducts have an irregular contour due to multiple strictures (arrow head) with intervening dilated segments (arrow). (Courtesy of David Jaffe, MD, New York, NY.)

The diagnosis of PSC can be difficult. Secondary sclerosing cholangitis must first be excluded. Currently, most cases are diagnosed by routine screening with liver function tests in patients with IBD. Typically, an elevated serum alkaline phosphatase may be the only abnormality in the early course of the disease. However, elevated transaminases and bilirubin and hypoalbuminemia can be seen. As a general rule, autoantibodies occur less frequently than in other types of autoimmune liver disease. A serum antimitochondrial antibody should be assayed so that primary biliary cirrhosis is excluded, as this entity can have an identical presentation. Hypergammaglobulinemia and pANCA positivity are frequently seen.[155] Data suggest that a positive pANCA is present in 30% to 80% of PSC patients.[156] As alluded to above, HLA testing is not of significant value. As in other hepatic disorders, serum ceruloplasmin and urinary copper can serve as a marker of impairment in biliary excretion.

Cholangiography is the confirmatory test for PSC. Endoscopic retrograde cholangiopancreatography (ERCP) is the gold standard diagnostic test for PSC, although magnetic resonance cholangiopancreatography (MRCP) is becoming more sensitive and specific for diagnosing this entity. The major criticism of MRCP is its inability to image subtle abnormalities in the intrahepatic ducts and within the walls of the extrahepatic ducts. A recent study comparing MRCP to ERCP in PSC, however, reports 88% sensitivity and 99% specificity for MRCP, although the findings that led to the diagnosis were different between the two modalities.[157] Percutaneous approaches are reserved for cases where ERCP is unsuccessful. Typical features of PSC on cholangiography include diffuse or segmental stenoses of the intrahepatic or extrahepatic bile ducts, with subsequent dilatation of the duct proximal to the stenosis (Figure 32-5). The intervening segments of normal or dilated bile duct in diffuse strictures produce a beaded appearance that is classic for PSC. Dominant strictures of the larger bile ducts are seen in only 7% of patients.[158]

The role of liver biopsy in PSC is limited. Definitive diagnosis is not possible by histology, and cholangiography is a necessary adjunct. There is a significant sampling error associated with percutaneous liver biopsy in patients with early disease. Infrequently, the onion-skin lesion is identified, which is the most characteristic histologic sign of PSC (Figure 32-6).[159] Biopsy is useful in grading the severity of the disease and following the progression of a patient's disease. A histologic scoring system from 1 through 4 has been established and is based on the extent of disease.[160] The lower scores reflect a predominance of immune cells, particularly lymphocytes, whereas the higher scores describe bridging fibrosis and cirrhosis.

The only definitive management for PSC is liver transplantation. Medical therapies, however, are frequently employed to slow the progression of disease and manage the associated complications. The indolent nature of the disease makes studying the efficacy of any agents specifically directed at treating PSC difficult. Currently, there are no drugs that have been shown to alter the natural history of the disease. Nevertheless, various agents, including choleretic, immunosuppressive, and antifibrotic drugs have been tried.

Ursodeoxycholic acid (UDCA) is a 7B-epimer of chenodeoxycholic acid that is a hydrophilic bile acid with choleretic, hepatoprotective, and immunomodulatory properties. The increased concentration of hydrophilic bile acids that results with UDCA therapy is thought to be less toxic to cholangiocytes,[161] although the consistency of this finding has been questioned.[162] UDCA has also been described as a choleretic agent by improving canalicular transport and stimulating secretion of toxic bile acids.[163-165] There have been a total of 7 controlled trials with UDCA in PSC.[166-172] Most of the studies have demonstrated an effect on biochemical markers, including alkaline phosphatase, transaminases, albumin, and bilirubin, but effects on histological progression could not be demonstrated. A Cochrane review of 6 of these trials noted that they are all of limited methodological quality. UDCA did not significantly reduce the risk of death, requirement for transplantation, varices, ascites, and encephalopathy. In addition, there was no impact on histologic or cholangiographic features.[173] There is some preliminary evidence that high-dose UDCA (20 to 30 mg/kg/d) is effective in altering histological progression and cholangiographic appearance and may improve mortality.[174,175] Despite the lack of convincing evidence, many

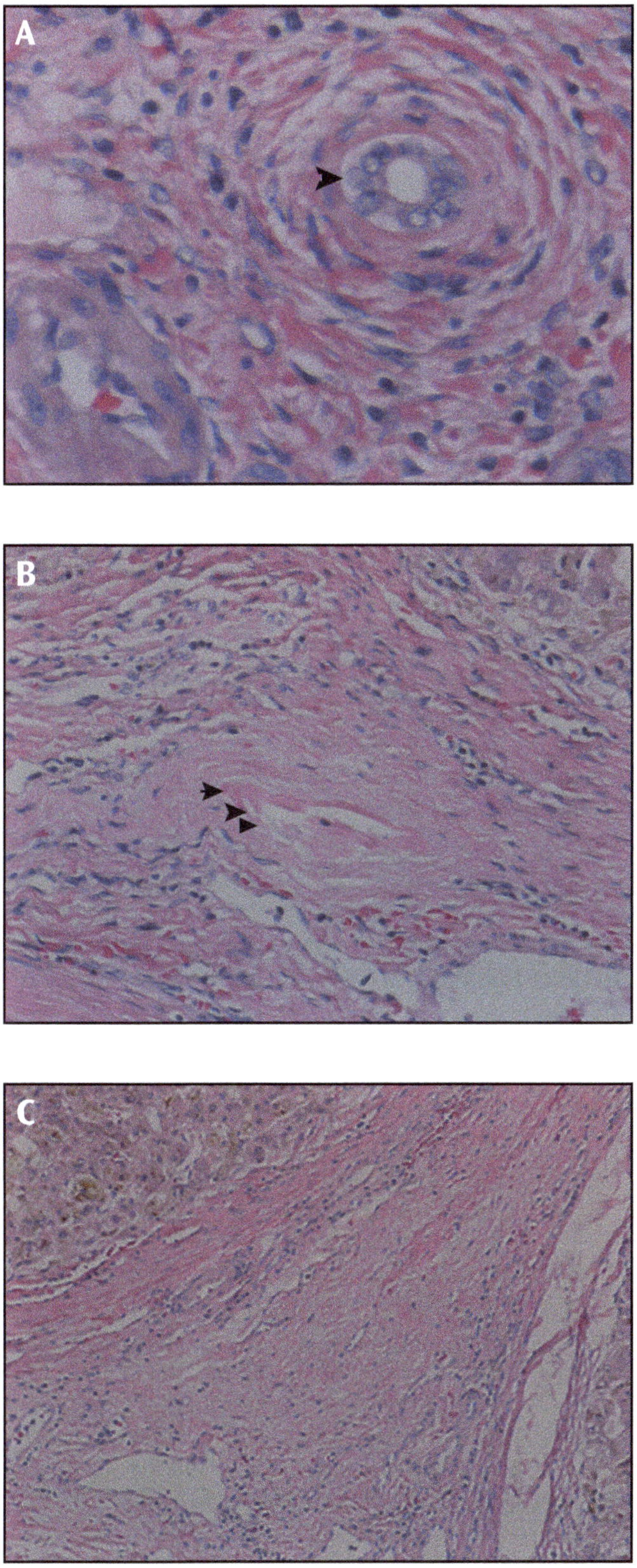

FIGURE 32-6. Histology of PSC. (A) Onion-skin lesion consisting of inflammatory infiltrate surrounding a bile duct (arrow heads) as seen with early disease. (B) Advanced lesion with fibrosis of bile duct (arrow heads). (C) End stage PSC as demonstrated by cirrhosis with nodule formation and bridging fibrosis; the bile ducts are completely destroyed, and the hepatic lobules contain brown deposits of bile consistent with cholestasis. (Courtesy of M. Isabel Fiel, MD, New York, NY.)

clinicians place patients on UDCA given its limited side effect profile and high degree of tolerability.

Another use for UDCA that has been studied is that of chemoprevention of colon cancer. As mentioned above, the risk of colorectal cancer in patients with both IBD and PSC is greater than that of patients with isolated UC. The mechanism of action for cancer chemoprevention is unknown, although 3 hypotheses have been proposed. UDCA decreases the concentration of deoxycholic acid in the colon.[176] Deoxycholic acid has been shown to be cytotoxic to colonic epithelial cells, to induce hyperproliferation of these cells, and has been implicated in carcinogenesis.[177] In addition, it blocks pathways of cell-cycle regulation that are perturbed in UC and CRC,[178] and it may act as an antioxidant to stabilize mitochondrial membranes.[179] A study of 59 patients with UC and PSC showed a statistically significant decreased risk of dysplasia in the UDCA-treated group compared to controls not taking UDCA.[180] UDCA seemed to be most protective in the subgroup of patients with high-grade dysplasia. Although promising, this single study has been criticized for a number of reasons, including not being placebo-controlled, having a small number of subjects, and heterogeneity between the groups with respect to duration of disease and age at diagnosis.[181]

Immunosuppressive and antifibrotic agents either alone or in combination with each other or UDCA have also been studied. Corticosteroids have been studied in short-term studies and are not practical for treating a chronic, indolent disease like PSC given their multiple side effects, particularly bone disease. This consideration is particularly important in the PSC population, as they are already at increased risk for bone disease due to their underlying liver disease.[182] In contrast, budesonide has limited systemic side effects and may be appropriate. This agent has been studied alone and in combination with UDCA. A study of 21 patients with PSC treated with 9 mg/d of budesonide for 1 year found no impact on the degree of fibrosis or stage of disease.[183] Moreover, significant worsening of osteoporosis was noted. A combination study of budesonide and UDCA versus prednisone and UDCA showed a mild short-term benefit of normalizing liver function tests and symptoms for the prednisone group and no benefit for the budesonide group.[184]

A case series from Germany of 15 patients with PSC treated with AZA, prednisolone, and UDCA for a median time of 41 months reported encouraging results.[185] Patients who did not respond initially to UDCA monotherapy had improvement in liver function tests after the addition of immunomodulators. In addition, 6 patients had histologic improvement on biopsy. The data for methotrexate are mixed. In an uncontrolled trial of 10 patients, methotrexate improved liver function tests and histologic score,[186] but a more rigorous follow-up study of methotrexate failed to show a survival benefit.[187] Similarly, tacrolimus has been shown to only improve liver enzymes.[188] Cyclosporine failed to show a benefit in symptoms, liver function tests, or survival.[189]

Antifibrotic and hepatoprotective agents that have been studied include colchicine, pentoxifylline, and D-Penicillamine. Colchicine is presumed to have antifibrotic properties due to its interference in collagen secretion. Colchicine alone, or in combination with corticosteroids, has not been shown to be of significant benefit.[190,191] The study examining the combination regimen reported a trend toward improved survival, but the number of patients was small and the treatment group was compared to historical controls. Penicillamine and pirfenidone both lack benefit and are associated with considerable toxicity.[192,193] Despite the lack of promising results with antifibrotic therapy, the current trends in the field appear to recognize the need to study these agents in combination.

Medical and endoscopic therapy has also been employed to manage symptoms. The major symptoms are pruritus, fatigue, bone disease, and steatorrhea. Symptoms related to mechanical obstruction of biliary flow include cholangitis and stone formation. The mechanism of pruritus in cholestasis is not due to bile acid deposition in the skin.[194] Rather, it has been shown that pruritus is largely mediated by central endogenous opioid receptors.[195] Although UDCA is used by many practitioners, there are no controlled trials evaluating its use for this symptom. The primary therapies for management of itching associated with PSC are bile-acid resins. Careful attention to the dosing schedule of these agents is necessary, as they will interfere with the absorption of other medications if given simultaneously. Cholestyramine (12 to 16 g/d) is effective in patients provided that enough bile is being excreted into the intestine.[196] Usually, symptoms begin to abate a few days after starting therapy. For patients who are unable to tolerate cholestyramine, colestipol hydrochloride can be used. Second-line agents for pruritus include rifampin (300 mg/d),[197] phenobarbital,[198] and antihistamines. The effectiveness of these agents has been established; however, large studies do not exist. Evening administration can help mitigate side effects. Opioid antagonists, such as naloxone[199] and naltrexone,[200] have been shown to be well-tolerated and effective in patients with cholestatic jaundice and pruritus. The agents, however, remain reserved for patients who are refractory to other agents. Last, refractory pruritus can be treated with plasmapheresis.[201]

The bone disease associated with PSC is primarily osteoporosis. The precise pathogenetic mechanism of the osteoporosis is unknown. It does not seem to be due to vitamin D deficiency, as most patients have normal serum levels of both 25-hydroxyvitamin D and 1,25-hydroxyvitamin D. All therapy for bone disease in PSC is extrapolated from the primary biliary cirrhosis literature, and no controlled trials exist. It is reasonable to try standard osteoporosis therapy including calcium supplementation, vitamin D, and bisphosphonates.[202] One study suggests that alendronate is the most effective bisphosphate in the setting of cholestatic liver disease.[203] Patients must be educated on how to take bisphosphonates, as the development of esophagitis in a patient with portal hypertension and esophageal varices can be catastrophic.

If liver disease is advanced, fat malabsorption and steatorrhea can occur. There is no established therapy for steatorrhea associated with cholestasis. Dietary manipulations can be attempted, although the effectiveness is likely to be limited. It is reasonable to rule out pancreatic insufficiency and celiac disease, as these entities are rarely associated with PSC.[204,205] Fat-soluble vitamins are frequently deficient and should be supplemented. Vitamin A deficiency is the most common, followed by vitamins D and E.[206] Vitamin K deficiency is usually less pronounced, unless disease is very advanced.

Bacterial cholangitis occurs in patients with PSC and a dominant extrahepatic biliary stricture, as well as in patients with advanced disease and no dominant stricture. Cholangitis usually presents as abdominal pain, fever, and vomiting. The course is generally more benign than ascending cholangitis from biliary obstruction related to stones. The mainstay of treatment is antimicrobials with broad gram-negative coverage and good penetration into the bile, such as ciprofloxacin.

In the setting of a dominant stricture, which occurs in 7% to 20% of patients with PSC, endoscopic therapy alone and in concert with medical therapy has been studied. Dominant strictures can account for most of the symptoms and hyperbilirubinemia in many patients with PSC. In addition, these strictures can lead to the formation of choledocholithiasis. Endoscopic dilation is the preferred method of treating these strictures. This therapy is associated with fewer episodes of cholangitis and improvement of cholangiographic findings and liver enzymes.[207] Endoscopic therapy in addition to UDCA was shown to prolong transplant-free survival vs untreated controls.[208] Stenting is not necessary and is associated with increased complication rates. Surgical treatment of dominant strictures is discouraged in the era of liver transplantation.

Last, cholangiocarcinoma is a particularly troublesome problem. Cholangiocarcinoma can be very difficult to diagnose and frequently is found in explanted livers. Brush cytology has a poor diagnostic yield, approximating 30%. Serum tumor markers such as CA 19-9 and carcinoembryonic antigen are not useful for detecting early disease.[209] Traditional treatment of cholangiocarcinoma with chemotherapy, radiotherapy, and resection, in addition to liver transplantation, is not encouraging.[210] Given the difficulty in diagnosing this lesion, screening programs are not advocated.

Referral to a transplant hepatologist is appropriate when the patient develops a complication of portal hypertension, such as varices or ascites. In addition, an episode of cholangitis, intractable pruritus, and weight loss should prompt a transplant evaluation and work-up.

PULMONARY MANIFESTATIONS

Pulmonary manifestations of IBD are becoming recognized with increasing frequency. The literature, mostly case reports and case series, describes many cases of both subclinical and active pulmonary disease. However, pulmonary manifestations are much less common than the extraintestinal manifestations discussed previously.

The pulmonary extraintestinal manifestations can be grouped into 2 broad categories: drug-related (see following) and drug-unrelated. The latter consists of airway disease, vasculitis, and interstitial lung disease. Pulmonary vasculitis associated with IBD is similar to that seen in Wegener's granulomatosis. Inflammation has been reported to affect each part of the respiratory tract from the trachea to the bronchioles. Bronchiectasis is the most commonly reported airway abnormality. The interstitial diseases include bronchiolitis obliterans with organizing pneumonia, fibrosing alveolitis, and eosinophilic pneumonia.[211]

The precise incidence of pulmonary extraintestinal manifestations is unknown. Subclinical disease, defined largely by abnormal pulmonary function tests, is reported in about 40% to 60% of IBD patients.[211-213] Airway disease and vasculitis appears more commonly in UC, whereas interstitial disease occurs more in CD. Abnormal carbon monoxide diffusion capacity is seen more commonly in IBD patients, although airway dysfunction is also described. The bowel inflammation tends to precede the onset of pulmonary symptoms. In addition, the pulmonary disease does not parallel the underlying bowel inflammation. Patients with more severe IBD symptoms, however, have greater derangement of pulmonary function.

The pathogenesis of pulmonary manifestations is unknown as well. Overlap syndromes between IBD and sarcoidosis or Wegener's granulomatosis raise the possibility of a common spectrum of disease with predominant intestinal or pulmonary symptoms respectively. No studies have reliably demonstrated a common genetic mutation, infectious organism, or autoantibody in patients with IBD and pulmonary disease. Like some of the more common extraintestinal manifestations, patients with pulmonary disease have other concomitant extraintestinal manifestations (eg, arthritis, uveitis), suggesting a common pathophysiologic mechanism.[214]

Patients usually present with symptoms of cough (dry or productive), pleuritic chest pain, and dyspnea. Potential causative culprit medications, such as sulfasalazine and mesalamine, should be discontinued. If symptoms persist, blood tests, particularly for antineutrophil cytoplasmic antibodies and angiotensin converting enzyme, should be performed as well as skin testing for tuberculosis exposure and sputum analysis if a productive cough is present. In addition, a chest radiograph or high-resolution computed tomography scan is indicated. Patients with advanced disease should be referred to a pulmonologist for spirometry and diffusion capacity testing.

Treatment for IBD-associated pulmonary manifestations is directed at addressing the pulmonary process, not the underlying bowel inflammation. Corticosteroids are used for most pulmonary inflammatory lesions. Due to the relative rarity of these extraintestinal manifestations, no trials exist for specific agents. Colectomy has never been shown to be a curative treatment of IBD-associated pulmonary disease.

HEMATOLOGIC MANIFESTATIONS

Hematologic extraintestinal manifestations include anemia and thrombophilic disorders. In the context of IBD, anemia is most commonly due to either iron deficiency alone or in combination with anemia of chronic disease. Other etiologies of anemia, such as hemolysis, drug-induced bone marrow suppression, and vitamin B12 and folate deficiency, also occur.

ANEMIA

The overall prevalence estimates for anemia in IBD ranges from 8% to 73%.[215] There does not appear to be a difference in prevalence between UC and CD. Anemia is responsible for a significant impact on quality of life and should be considered an important aspect of caring for the patient with IBD. The mechanism of iron deficiency in patients with IBD is multifactorial. Patients often have either overt or occult chronic blood loss. In addition, gastrointestinal symptoms can limit the quantity of iron intake, and malabsorption may be present. The presence of chronic inflammation, with consequent bone marrow sequestration of iron further exacerbates the anemia.

Therapy for IBD-associated anemia should be directed at the presumptive pathogenesis of the disorder. Once diagnosed as such, iron deficiency can be treated with supplementation. Oral supplements can be tried, although frequently they are ineffective or poorly tolerated. More recently, IV iron preparations have been shown to increase mean hemoglobin levels. Parenteral iron in combination with recombinant erythropoietin has been shown to improve mean hemoglobin concentration and improve quality of life.[216,217]

Autoimmune hemolytic anemia has been described in patients with UC and CD. The frequency of this extraintestinal manifestation is low, with sporadic case reports and small case series comprising the literature. The estimated prevalence is between 0.5% and 2%.[218,219] This entity is more common in women.[221] This anemia is Coombs positive. Interestingly, up to 2% of patients with UC will have a positive Coombs test without evidence of hemolysis.[219] The presumptive pathogenetic mechanism is that the diseased colon allows for absorption of antigens that generate antibodies that cross-react with red cells.[222] Hemolytic anemia starts either at the time of diagnosis of colitis or afterward. There are conflicting reports on whether hemolysis parallels disease activity,[218,223,224] although recent data suggest that severe colitis is more commonly associated.[219] Initial therapy for hemolysis associated with colitis is corticosteroids. If unsuccessful, immunomodulators can be started. For refractory cases, splenectomy has been successful with or without concurrent proctocolectomy, depending on the degree of colonic involvement.[218,219]

Thrombophilia

IBD confers up to a threefold greater risk of venous thromboembolism than in age-matched controls.[225,226] Descriptions of both arterial and venous thromboembolism associated with IBD exist, with an incidence ranging between 1% and 8%.[226-229] Although the risk of venous thromboembolism is increased in those patients who have had surgical procedures, many patients with IBD and inactive disease can develop venous thrombosis.[230] In addition, the incidence of venous thrombosis in IBD is greater than in other inflammatory diseases and other bowel diseases.[231] The risk remains after controlling for confounding variables like oral contraceptive use, number of pregnancies, prior surgery, and smoking. The overall risk of thromboembolism in IBD increases with advancing age.

The precise pathogenesis of thrombophilia in IBD remains unknown. The systemic inflammatory response leads to a variety of changes that impact on thrombogenesis. In IBD, a number of alterations in the prothrombotic and antithrombotic regulatory molecules have been described. Elevated levels of anticardiolipin antibodies,[228] fibrinogen, and factor VIII[230] have been reported. In addition, impaired fibrinolysis due to poor release of tissue plasminogen activator or high plasminogen activator inhibitor has been seen in IBD.[231] Also, free protein S deficiency[232] and elevated factor VII coagulant activity, lipoprotein (a), and fibrinogen have been reported in both CD and UC.[233] Despite these associations, no study has correlated a direct link between any of these laboratory findings and increased rate of thromboembolism for this patient population.

An association between factor V Leiden mutation and ulcerative colitis was described,[234] but this finding could not be confirmed by other investigators, for either CD or UC.[235,236] A more recent study found that APC resistance is not associated with IBD, but, when present, it increases the risk of thromboembolism.[227] Subsequent studies failed to demonstrate an association between IBD and any of the most frequent hereditary prothrombotic conditions (ie, factor V Leiden, methylene tetrahydrofolate reductase, and prothrombin gene mutations).[237-239]

The presentation of thrombosis in IBD is usually peripheral venous thrombosis. However, there are reports of cerebrovascular and sagittal sinus thromboses.[240] In the postoperative state, mesenteric venous thrombosis can occur.[241]

Therapy for thrombosis in IBD is anticoagulation with unfractionated or low-molecular weight heparin or warfarin. Hospitalized IBD patients without evidence of thrombosis should receive thromboembolism prophylaxis with either subcutaneous heparin or compression boots. There is no role for testing IBD patients for underlying hypercoagulable states prior to the development of clinical thrombosis.

Drug-Induced Extraintestinal Manifestations

When suspecting extraintestinal manifestations, a careful medication history needs to be obtained. Many of the therapeutic agents used for IBD have side effects that can mimic extraintestinal manifestations. For example, there are reports of hemolysis[242,243] and eosinophilic pneumonia[214] related to sulfasalazine and mesalamine. Pulmonary and hepatic side effects of methotrexate are well-established. Infliximab has been linked to a lupus-like syndrome with antinuclear antibodies.[244] The diagnosis of a drug-induced extraintestinal manifestation is confirmed by resolution of the symptoms upon withdrawal of the offending agent.

Conclusion

Extraintestinal manifestations of UC are a significant source of morbidity. For the most part, the pathogenesis of these conditions is unknown, and the risk factors for their development in an individual remain to be identified. As such, management can be especially challenging. The therapeutic options for these conditions are expanding as newer agents that target the dysregulated immune system in IBD are developed.

REFERENCES

1. Rankin GB, Watts HD, Melnyk CS, et al. National Cooperative Crohn's Disease Study: extraintestinal manifestation and perianal complications. *Gastroenterology.* 1979;77:914-920.
2. Farmer RG, Hawk WA, Turnbull RB Jr. Clinical patterns in Crohn's disease: a statistical study of 615 cases. *Gastroenterology.* 1975;68:627-635.
3. Monsen U, Sorstad J, Hellers G, et al. Extracolonic diagnoses in ulcerative colitis: An epidemiological study. *Am J Gastroenterol.* 1990;85:711-716.
4. Veloso FT, Carvalho J, Magro F. Immmune-related systemic manifestations of inflammatory bowel disease: a prospective study of 792 patients. *J Clin Gastroenterol.* 1996;23:29-34.
5. Greenstein AJ, Janowitz HD, Sachar DB. The extra-intestinal complications of Crohn's disease and ulcerative colitis: a study of 700 patients. *Medicine.* 1976;55:401-412.
6. Bernstein CN, Blanchard JF, Rawsthorne P, Yu N. The prevalence of extraintestinal diseases in inflammatory bowel disease: a population-based study. *Am J Gastroenterol.* 2001;96:1116-1122.
7. Levine JB. Extraintestinal manifestations of inflammatory bowel diseases. In: Kirsner JB. *Inflammatory Bowel Disease.* 5th ed. Philadelphia: WB Saunders Co; 2000:397-409.
8. Bargen JA, Barker NW. Consequences and sequellae of chronic ulcerative colitis. *Ann Intern Med.* 1929;3:335-352.
9. Crohn BB. Ocular lesions complicating ulcerative colitis. *Am J Med Sci.* 1925;169:260-267.
10. Satsangi J, Grootscholten C, Holt H, et al. Clinical patterns of familial inflammatory bowel disease. *Gut.* 1996;38:738-741.
11. Manguso F, Sanges M, Staiano T, Gargiulo S, et al. Cigarette smoking and appendectomy are risk factors for extraintestinal manifestations in ulcerative colitis. *Am J Gastroenterol.* 2004;99(2): 327-334.
12. Snook JA, de Silva HJ, Jewell DP. The association of autoimmune disorders with inflammatory bowel disease. *QJM.* 1989;72: 835-840.
13. Das KM, Sakamaki S, Vecchi M, Diamond B. The production and characterization of monoclonal antibodies to a human colonic antigen associated with ulcerative colitis: cellular localization of the antigen by using the monoclonal antibody. *J Immunol.* 1987;139:77-84.
14. Biancone L, Mandal A, Yang H, et al. Production of immunoglobulin G and G1 antibodies to cytoskeletal protein by lamina propria cells in ulcerative colitis. *Gastroenterology.* 1995;109:3-12.
15. Geng X, Biancone L, Dai HH, et al. Tropomyosin isoforms in intestinal mucosa: Production of autoantibodies to tropomyosin isoforms in ulcerative colitis. *Gastroenterology.* 1998;114:912-922.
16. Das KM, Vecchi M, Sakamaki S. A shared and unique epitope(s) on human colon, skin, and biliary epithelium detected by a monoclonal antibody. *Gastroenterology.* 1990;98:464-469.
17. Sartor RB. Review article: how relevant to human inflammatory bowel disease are current animal models of intestinal inflammation? *Aliment Pharmacol Ther.* 1997;11(suppl 3):89-96.
18. Rath HC, Herfarth HH, Ikeda JS, et al. Normal luminal bacteria, especially *Bacteroides* species, mediate chronic colitis, gastritis, and arthritis in HLA-B27/human beta2 microglobulin transgenic rats. *J Clin Invest.* 1996;98:945-953.
19. Duerr RH, Neigut DA. Molecularly defined HLA-DR2 alleles in UC and an anti-neutrophil cytoplasmic antibody-positive subgroup. *Gastroenterology.* 1995;108:423-427.
20. Toyoda H, Wang SJ, Yang H, et al. Distinct association of HLA Class II genes with inflammatory bowel disease. *Gastroenterology.* 1993;104:741-748.
21. Asakura H, Tsuchiya M, Aiso S, et al. Association of the human leukocyte DR2 antigen with Japanese ulcerative colitis. *Gastroenterology.* 1982;82:413-418.
22. Satsangi J, Welsh KI, Bunce M, et al. Contribution of genes of the major histocompatibility complex to susceptibility and disease phenotype in inflammatory bowel disease. *Lancet.* 1996;347:1212-1217.
23. Roussomoustakaki M, Satsangi J, Welsh K, et al. Genetic markers may predict disease behavior in patients with ulcerative colitis. *Gastroenterology.* 1997;112:1845-1853.
24. Goudet P, Dozois RR, Kelly KA, Ilstrup DM, Phillips SF. Characteristics and evolution of extraintestinal manifestation associated with ulcerative colitis after proctocolectomy. *Dig Surg.* 2001;18:51-55.
25. Hata K, Watanabe T, Shinozaki M, Nagawa H. Patients with extraintestinal manifestations have a higher risk of developing pouchitis in ulcerative colitis a multivariate analysis. *Scand J Gastroenterol.* 2003;38:1055-1058.
26. Mir-Madjlessi SH, Taylor JS, Farmer RG. Clinical course and evaluation of erythema nodosum and pyoderma gangrenosum in chronic ulcerative colitis: a study of 42 patients. *Am J Gastroenterol.* 1985;80:615-620.
27. Orchard TR, Ahmad T, Welsh KI, Jewell DP. Extra-intestinal manifestations of inflammatory bowel disease and polymorphisms in the TNF-alpha gene: further evidence for phenotype determining genes in the MHC region on chromosome 6. *Gastroenterology.* 2001;120:2320.
28. Orchard TR, Chua C, Cheng H, Jewell DP. Clinical features of erythema nodosum (EN) and uveitis associated with inflammatory bowel disease. *Gastroenterology.* 2000;118:755.
29. Felder JB, Korelitz BI, Rajapakse R, Schwarz S, Horatagis AP, Gleim G. Effects of nonsteroidal anti-inflammatory drugs on inflammatory bowel disease: a case-control study. *Am J Gastroenterol.* 2000;95:1949-1954.
30. Evans JM, McMahon AD, Murray FE, McDevitt DG, MacDonald TM. Non-steroidal anti-inflammatory drugs are associated with emergency admission to hospital for colitis due to inflammatory bowel disease. *Gut.* 1997;40:619-622.
31. Marshall JK, Irvine EJ. Successful therapy of refractory erythema nodosum associated with Crohn's disease using potassium iodide. *Can J Gastroenterol.* 1997;11:501-502.
32. Kugathasan S, Miranda A, Nocton J, Drolet BA, Raasch C, Binion DG. Dermatologic manifestations of Crohn's disease in children: response to infliximab. *J Pediatr Gastroenterol Nutr.* 2003;37(2):150-154.
33. Bauer J, Fartasch M, Schuler G, et al. Ulcerative stomatitis as clinical clue to inadvertent methotrexate overdose. *Hautarzt.* 1999;50: 670-673.
34. Orchard TR, Jewell DP. Extraintestinal manifestations: Skin, joints, and mucocutaneous manifestations. In: Kirsner JB, Sartor RB, Sandborn WJ, eds. *Inflammatory Bowel Disease.* 6th ed. Philadelphia: WB Saunders Co; 2004:658-672.
35. Weiner SR, Clarke J, Taggart NA, Utsinger PD. Rheumatic manifestations of inflammatory bowel disease. *Semin Arth Rheum.* 1991;20:353-366.
36. Dekker-Saeys BJ, Meuwissen SGM, Van Den Berg-Loonen EM, et al. Prevalence of peripheral arthritis, sacroiliitis, and ankylosing spondylitis in patients suffering from inflammatory bowel disease. *Ann Rheum Dis.* 1978;37:36-41.
37. Orchard TR, Wordsworth BP, Jewell DP. Peripheral arthropathies in inflammatory bowel disease: their articular distribution and natural history. *Gut.* 1998;42:387-391.
38. Brynskov J, Binder V. Arthritis and the gut. *Eur J Gastroenterol Hepatol.* 1999;11:997-999.

39. Roussomoustakaki M, Satsangi J, Welsh KI, et al. Genetic markers may predict disease behavior in patients with ulcerative colitis. *Gastroenterology.* 1997;112:1645-1653.
40. Orchard TR, Dhar A, Simmons JD, Vaughan R, Welsh KI, Jewell DP. MHC class I chain-like gene A (MICA) and its associations with inflammatory bowel disease and peripheral arthropathy. *Clin Exp Immunol.* 2001;126:437-440.
41. Orchard TR, Thiyagasraja S, Welsh KI, Wordsworth BP, Hill Gaston JS, Jewell DP. Clinical phenotype is related to HLA genotype in the peripheral arthropathies of inflammatory bowel disease. *Gastroenterology.* 2000;118:274-278.
42. Wordsworth P. Arthritis and inflammatory bowel disease. *Curr Rheumatol Rep.* 2000;2:87.
43. Gravallese EM, Kantrowitz FG. Arthritic manifestations of inflammatory bowel disease. *Am J Gastroenterol.* 1988;83:703.
44. Lang J, Price AB, Levi AJ, Burke M, Gumpel JM, Bjarnason I. Diaphragm disease: pathology of disease of the small intestine induced by non-steroidal anti-inflammatory drugs. *J Clin Pathol.* 1988;41:516-526.
45. Felder JB, Korelitz BI, Rajapakse R, Scwarz S, Horatagis AP, Gleim G. Effects of nonsteroidal anti-inflammatory drugs on inflammatory bowel disease: a case-control study. *Am J Gastroenterol.* 2000;95:1859-1861.
46. Bonner GF, Walczak M, Kitchen L, Bayona M. Tolerance of nonsteroidal anti-inflammatory drugs in patients with inflammatory bowel disease. *Am J Gastroenterol.* 2000;95:1946-1948.
47. Wolfe F, Zhao S, Lane N. Preference for nonsteroidal anti-inflammatory drugs over acetaminophen by rheumatic disease patients: a survey of 1,799 patients with osteoarthritis, rheumatoid arthritis, and fibromyalgia. *Arthritis Rheum.* 2000;43:378-385.
48. Pincus T, Swearingen C, Cummin P, et al. Preference for nonsteroidal anti-inflammatory drugs versus acetaminophen and concomitant use of both types of drugs in patients with osteoarthirits. *J Rheumatol.* 2000;27:1020-1027.
49. Bonner GF. Exacerbation of inflammatory bowel disease associated with use of celecoxib. *Am J Gastroenterol.* 2001;96:1306-1308.
50. Mahadevan U, Loftus EV Jr, Tremaine WJ, Sandborn WJ. Safety of selective cyclooxygenase-2 inhibitors in inflammatory bowel disease. *Am J Gastroenterol.* 2002;97:910-914.
51. Reinisch W, Miehsler W, Dejaco C, et al. An open-label trial of the selective cyclo-oxygenase-2 inhibitor, rofecoxib, in inflammatory bowel disease-associated peripheral arthritis and arthralgia. *Aliment Pharmacol Ther.* 2003;17:1371-1380.
52. Kirsner JB, Shorter RG. Recent developments in "nonspecific" inflammatory bowel disease (first of two parts). *N Engl J Med.* 1982;306:775.
53. Petrelli EA, McKinley M, Troncale FJ. Ocular manifestations of inflammatory bowel disease. *Ann Ophthalmol.* 1982;14:356.
54. Leibowitz HM. The red eye. *N Engl J Med.* 2000;343:345-351.
55. Finkelstein W. Treatment of acute episcleritis associated with Crohn's disease with infliximab. *Am J Gastoenterol.* 2002;97:S152.
56. Mintz R, Feller ER, Bahr RL, Shah SA. Ocular manifestations of inflammatory bowel disease. *Inflamm Bowel Dis.* 2004;10:135-139.
57. Basler RSW. Ulcerative colitis and the skin. *Med Clin North Am.* 1980;64:941-954.
58. Stenson WF. Inflammatory bowel diseases. In: Yamada T, ed. *The Textbook of Gastroenterology.* Philadelphia, PA: Lippincott Williams & Wilkins; 1999:1775-1839.
59. Thornton JR, Teague RJ, Low-Bier TS, et al. *Pyoderma gangrenosum* in ulcerative colitis. *Gut.* 1980;21:247-248.
60. Brunsting LA, Goeckerman WH, O'Leary PA. *Pyoderma gangrenosum*: clinical and experimental observations in five cases occurring in adults. *Arch Dermatol.* 1930;22:655.
61. Crowson AN, Magro C, Mihm MC Jr. *Pyoderma gangrenosum*: a review. *J Cutan Pathol.* 2003;30:97-107.
62. Magro CM, Crowson AN. Sterile neutrophilic folliculitis with perifollicular vasculopathy: a distinctive cutaneous reaction pattern reflecting systemic disease. *J Cutan Pathol.* 1998;25:215.
63. Chow RKP, Ho VC. Treatment of *Pyoderma gangrenosum. J Am Acad Dermatol.* 1996;34:1047.
64. Powell FC, Su WPD, Perry HO. *Pyoderma gangrenosum*: classification and management. *J Am Acad Dermatol.* 1996; 34:395.
65. Mrowictz U, Christophers E. Clearing of *Pyoderma gangrenosum* by intralesional cyclosporine A [letter]. *Br J Dermatol.* 1991;125:499.
66. Khurrum Baig M, Marquez H, Noguerass JJ, et al. Topical tacrolimus (FK 506) in the treatment of recalcitrant parastomal *Pyoderma gangrenosum* associated with Crohn's disease: report of two cases. *Colorectal Dis.* 2004;6:250-253.
67. Richter-Hintz D, Schuppe H-C, Homey B, et al. Topical tacrolimus (FK 506) is effective in the treatment of *pyoderma gangrenosum. J Am Acad Dermatol.* 2000;42:304.
68. Schuppe H-C, Homey B, Assmann T, et al. Topical tacrolimus for *Pyoderma gangrenosum. Lancet.* 1998;351:832.
69. Jolles S, Niclasse S, Benson E. Combination oral and topical tacrolimus in therapy-resistant *Pyoderma gangrenosum. Br J Dermatol.* 1998;140:564-565.
70. Wines N, Wines M, Ryman W. Understanding *Pyoderma gangrenosum*: a review. *Med General Med.* 2001;27:6.
71. Friedman S, Marion JF, Scherl E, Rubin PH, Present DH. Intravenous cyclosporine in refractory *Pyoderma gangrenosum* complicating inflammatory bowel disease. *Inflamm Bowel Dis.* 2001;7:1-7.
72. Abu Elmagd K, Jegasothy BV, Ackerman CD, et al. Efficacy of FK 506 in the treatment of recalcitrant *Pyoderma gangrenosum. Transplant Proc.* 1991;23:3328-3329.
73. Nousari HC, Lynch W, Anhalt GJ. The effectiveness of mycophenolate mofetil in refractory *Pyoderma gangrenosum. Arch Dermatol.* 1998;134:1509-1511.
74. Breathbach SM, Wells GC, Valdimarsson H. Idiopathic *Pyoderma gangrenosum* and impaired lymphocyte function: failure of aziothioprine and corticosteroid therapy. *Br J Dermatol.* 1981;104:567.
75. Federman GL, Federman DG. Recalcitrant pyoderma gangrenosum treated with thalidomide. *Mayo Clin Proc.* 2000;75:842-844.
76. Farrell AM, Black MM, Bracka A, Bunker CB. *Pyoderma gangrenosum* of the penis. *Br J Dermatol.* 1998;138:337-340.
77. Moraes M, Russo G. Thalidomide and its dermatologic uses. *Am J Med Sci.* 2001;321:321.
78. Tan MH, Gordon M, Lebwohl O, George J, Lebwohl MG. Improvement of *Pyoderma gangrenosum* and psoriasis associated with Crohn's disease with anti-tumor necrosis factor monoclonal antibody. *Arch Dermatol.* 2001;137:930-933.
79. Hong JJ, Merel NJ, Hanauer SB. Treatment of *Pyoderma gangrenosum* complicating Crohn's disease with infliximab. *Gastroenterology.* 2001;120:A621(Abstr. 3143).
80. Sapienza MS, Cohen S, DiMarino AJ. Improvement of *Pyoderma gangrenosum* after infliximab treatment for fistulizing Crohn's disease. *Am J Gastroenterol.* 2001;96:S307(Abstr. 972).
81. Ljung T, Staun M, Grove O, et al. *Pyoderma gangrenosum* associated with Crohn's disease: Effect of TNF-alpha blockade with infliximab. *Scand J Gastroenterol.* 2002;37:1108-1110.
82. Rozen SM, Nahabedian MY, Manson PN. Management strategies for *Pyoderma gangrenosum*: case studies and review of the literature. *Ann Plast Surg.* 2001;47:310-315.
83. Cox NH, Peebles-Brown DA, MacKie RM. *Pyoderma gangrenosum* occurring 10 years after proctocolectomy for ulcerative colitis. *Br J Hosp Med.* 1986;36:363.
84. Hughes AP, Jackson JM, Callen JP. Clinical features and treatment of peristomal *Pyoderma gangrenosum. JAMA.* 2000;284:1546-1548.
85. Keltz M, Lebwohl M, Bishop S. Periostomal *Pyoderma gangrenosum. J Am Acad Dermatol.* 1992;27:360-364.

86. Feldmann M, Maini RN. Anti-TNF alpha therapy of rheumatoid arthritis: what have we learned? *Annu Rev Immunol.* 2001;19: 163-196.
87. Keyser FD, Mielants H, Veys EM. Current use of biologicals for the treatment of spondyloarthropathies. *Expert Opin Pharmacother.* 2001;2:85-93.
88. Herfath H, Obermeier F, Andus T, et al. Improvement of arthritis and arthralgia after treatment with infliximab (Remicade) in a German prospective, open-label, multicenter trial in refractory Crohn's disease. *Am J Gastroenterol.* 2002;97(10):2688-2690.
89. Haslock I, Wright V. The muculo-skeletal complications of Crohn's disease. *Medicine.* 1973;52:217-225.
90. Moll JMH, Haslock I, Macrea IF, Wright V. Association between ankylosing spondylitis, psoriatic arthritis, Reiter's disease, the intestinal arthropathies and Behcet's syndrome. *Medicine.* 1974;53:343-364.
91. Dekker-Saeys BJ, Meuwissen SGM, Van Den Berg-Loonen EM, et al. Clinical characteristics and results of histocompatibility typing (HLA B27) in 50 patients with both ankylosing spondylitis and inflammatory bowel disease. *Ann Rheum Dis.* 1978;37:36-41.
92. Davis P, Thomson A, Lentle B. Quantitative sacroiliac scintigraphy in patients with Crohn's disease. *Arthritis Rheum.* 1978;21:234-237.
93. Brown MA, Pile KD, Kennedy LG, et al. HLA class I associations of anykylosing spondylitis in the white population in the United Kingdom. *Ann Rheum Dis.* 1996;55:268-270.
94. Brewerton D, Caffrey M, Hart F, James D, Nichols A, Sturrock R. Ankylosing spondylitis and HLA-27. *Lancet.* 1973;i:904-907.
95. Brewerton D, Caffery M, Nicholls A, Walters D, James D. HLA-27 and arthropathies associated with UC and psoriasis. *Lancet.* 1974;i:956-958.
96. Mallas EG, Mackintosh P, Asquith P, Cooke WT. Histocompatibility antigens in inflammatory bowel disease: their clinical significance and their association with arthropathy with special reference to HLA-B27 (W27). *Gut.* 1976;17:906-910.
97. Orchard TR, Holt H, Bradley L, et al. Prevalence of sacroiliitis in CD, and its correlation with clinical, radiologic and genotypic parameters. *Gastroenterology.* 2002;122:W1298.
98. Steer S, Jones H, Hibbert J, et al. Low back pain, sacroiliitis, and the relationship with HLA-B27 in CD. *J Rheumatol.* 2003;30:518-522.
99. Ebringer A. Ankylosing spondylitis is caused by *Klebsiella.* Evidence from immunogenetic, microbiologic, and serologic studies. *Rheum Dis Clin North Am.* 1992;18:105-121.
100. Smale S, Natt RS, Orchard TR, Russell AS, Bjarnason I. Inflammatory bowel disease and spondyloarthropathy. *Arthritis Rheum.* 2001;44:2728-2736.
101. Taurog JD, Richardson JA, Croft JT, et al. The germ-free state prevents development of gut and joint inflammation in HLA B27 transgenic rats. *J Exp Med.* 1994;180:2359-2364.
102. Mielants H, Veys E, Vos MD, et al. The evolution of spondyloarthropathies in relation to gut histology. I. Clinical Aspects. *J Rheumatol.* 1995;22:2266-2272.
103. Mielants H, Veys E, Culvelier C, et al. The evolution of spondyloarthropathies in relation to gut histology. II. Histological aspects. *J Rheumatol.* 1995;22:2273-2278.
104. Mielants H, Veys E, Culvelier C, et al. The evolution of spondyloarthropathies in relation to gut histology. III. Relation between gut and joint. *J Rheumatol.* 1995;22:2279-2284.
105. Analay Y, Ozcan E, Karan A, Diracoglu D, Aydin R. The effectiveness of intensive group exercise on patients with ankylosing spondylitis. *Clin Rehabil.* 2003;17:631-636.
106. Sweeney S, Taylor G, Calin A. The effect of a home based exercise intervention package on outcome in ankylosing spondylitis: a randomized controlled trial. *J Rheumatol.* 2002;29:763-766.
107. Dagfinrud H, Hagen K. Physiotherapy interventions for ankylosing spondylitis. *Cochrane Database Syst Rev.* 2001;4:CD002822.
108. Dougados M, Maetzel A, Mijiyawa M, et al. Evaluation of sulphasalazine in the treatment of spondyloarthropathies. *Ann Rheum Dis.* 1992;51:955.
109. Mielants H, Veys EM, Joos R. Sulphasalazine (Salazopyrin) in the treatment of enterogenic reactive synovitis and ankylosing spondylitis with peripheral arthritis. *Clin Rheumatol.* 1986;5:80.
110. Dougados M, van den Linden S, Leirisalo-Repo M, et al. Sulfasalazine in the treatment of spondylarthropathy: a randomized, multicenter, double-blind, placebo-controlled study. *Arthritis Rheum.* 1995;38:618.
111. Nissila M, Lehtinen K, Leirisalo-Repo M, et al. Sulfasalazine in the treatment of ankylosing spondylitis: a 26-week placebo-controlled clinical trial. *Arthritis Rheum.* 1988;31:1111.
112. Taylor HG, Beswick EJ, Dawes PT. Sulphasalazine in ankylosing spondylitis: a radiological, clinical and laboratory assessment. *Clin Rheumatol.* 1991;10:43.
113. Gran JT, Husby G. Ankylosing spondylitis: current drug treatment. *Drugs.* 1992;44:585.
114. Sampaio-Barros PD, Costallat LT, Bertolo MB, Neto JF, Samara AM. Methotrexate in the treatment of ankylosing spondylitis. *Scand J Rheumatol.* 2000;29(3):160-162.
115. Gorman JD, Sack KE, Davis JC Jr. Treatment of ankylosing spondylitis by inhibition of tumor necrosis factor alpha. *N Engl J Med.* 2002;346:1349-1356.
116. Van den Bosch F, Kruithof E, Baeten D, DeKeyser F, Mielants H, Veys EM. Effects of a loading dose regimen of three infusions of chimeric monoclonal antibody to tumour necrosis factor alpha (infliximab) in spondyloarthropathy: an open pilot study. *Ann Rheum Dis.* 2000;59:428-433.
117. Brandt J, Haibel H, Cornely D, et al. Successful treatment of active ankylosing spondylitis with the anti-tumor necrosis factor alpha monoclonal antibody infliximab. *Arthritis Rheum.* 2000;43:1346-1352.
118. Braun J, Brandt J, Listing J, et al. Treatment of active ankylosing spondylitis with infliximab: a randomized controlled multicentre trial. *Lancet.* 2002;359:1187-1193.
119. Pennanen N, Lapinjoki S, Urtti A, Monkkonen J. Effect of liposomal and free bisphosphonates on the IL-1 beta, IL-6 and TNF alpha secretion from RAW 264 cells in vitro. *Pharm Res.* 1995;12: 916-922.
120. Haibel H, Bandt J, Rudwaleit M, Soerensen H, Sleper J, Braun J. Treatment of active ankylosing spondylitis with pamidronate. *Rheumatology.* 2003;42:1018-1020.
121. Maksymowych WP, Jhangri GS, Fitzgerald AA, et al. A six-month randomized, controlled, double-blind, dose-response comparison of intravenous pamidronate (60 mg versus 10 mg) in the treatment of nonsteroidal anti-inflammatory drug-refractory ankylosing spondylitis. *Arthritis Rheum.* 2002;46:766-773.
122. Tan AL, Marzo-Ortega H, O'Connor P, Fraser A, Emery P, McGonagle DG. Efficacy of anakinra in active ankylosing spondylitis: a clinical and magnetic resonance imaging study. *Ann Rheum Dis.* 2004; Apr 5 (article not yet available in print).
123. Rose KA, Kim WS. The effect of chiropractic care for a 30-year-old male with advanced ankylosing spondylitis: a time series case report. *J Manipulative Physiol Ther.* 2003;26:E1.
124. Orchard TR, Chua CN, Ahmad T, Cheng H, Welsh KI, Jewell DP. Uveitis and erythema nodosum in inflammatory bowel disease: clinical features and the role of HLA genes. *Gastroenterology.* 2002;123:714-718.
125. Salmi M, Jalkanen S. Endothelial ligands and homing of mucosal leukocytes in extraintestinal manifestations of inflammatory bowel disease. *Inflamm Bowel Dis.* 1998;4:149-156.

126. Mintz R, Feller ER, Bahr RL, Shah SA. Ocular manifestations of inflammatory bowel disease. *Inflamm Bowel Dis.* 2004;10:135-139.
127. Present DH. Extraintestinal manifestations. *Mt. Sinai J Med.* 1983;50:126.
128. Soukiasian SH, Foster CS, Raizman MB. Treatment strategies for scleritis and uveitis associated with inflammatory bowel disease. *Am J Ophthalmol.* 1994;118:601-611.
129. Baiocco PJ, Gorman BD, Korelitz BI. Uveitis occurring after colectomy and ileal-rectal sleeve anastomosis for ulcerative colitis. *Dig Dis Sci.* 1984;29:570-572.
130. Primary liver disease of liver transplant recipients, 1991 and 1992. *UNOS Update.* 1993;9(8):27-29.
131. Schrumpf E, Elgjo K, Fausa O, et al. Sclerosing cholangitis in ulcerative colitis. *Scand J Gastroenterol.* 1980;15:689-697.
132. Shepherd HA, Selby WS, Chapman RWG, et al. Ulcerative colitis and persistent liver dysfunction. *Quart J Med.* 1989;52:503-513.
133. Olsson R, Danielsson A, Jarnerot G, et al. Prevalence of primary sclerosing cholangitis in patients with ulcerative colitis. *Gastroenterology.* 1991;100:1319-1323.
134. Schrumpf E, Fausa O, Kolmannskog F, et al. Sclerosing cholangitis in ulcerative colitis: a follow-up study. *Scand J Gastroenterol.* 1982;17:33-39.
135. Rasmussen HH, Fallingborg J, Mortensen PB, et al. Primary sclerosing cholangitis in patients with ulcerative colitis. *Scand J Gastroenterol.* 1992;27:732-736.
136. Rabinowitz M, Gavaler JS, Schade RR, et al. Does primary sclerosing cholangitis occurring in association with inflammatory bowel disease differ from that occurring in the absence of inflammatory bowel disease: a study of sixty-six subjects. *Hepatology.* 1990;11:7-11.
137. Rabinowitz M, Gavaler JS, Schade RR, et al. Does primary sclerosing cholangitis occurring in association with inflammatory bowel disease differ from that occurring in the absence of inflammatory bowel disease: a study of 66 subjects. *Hepatology.* 1990;11:7-11.
138. Lindor K, Wiesner R, LaRusso N. Recent advances in the management of primary sclerosing cholangitis. *Semin Liver Dis.* 1987;7:322-327.
139. Lee Y-M, Kaplan MM. Primary sclerosing cholangitis. *N Engl J Med.* 1995;332:924-933.
140. Palmer KR, Duerden BJ, Holdworth CD. Bacteriological and endotoxin studies in cases of ulcerative colitis submitted to surgery. *Gut.* 1980;21:851-854.
141. Eade MN, Brook BN. Portal bacteremia in cases of ulcerative colitis submitted to colectomy. *Lancet.* 1969;1:1008-1009.
142. Dew MJ, van Berge Henegouwen GP, Huybregts AWM, et al. Hepatotoxic effect of bile acids in inflammatory bowel disease. *Gastroenterology.* 1980;78:1393-1401.
143. Holzbach RT, Marsh ME, Freedman MR, et al. Portal vein bile acids in patients with severe inflammatory bowel disease. *Gut.* 1980;21:428-435.
144. Hobson CH, Butt TJ, Ferry DM, et al. Enterohepatic circulation of bacterial chemotactic peptide in rats with experimental colitis. *Gastroenterology.* 1988;94:1006-1013.
145. Jorge AD, Esley C, Ahumada J. Family incidence of primary sclerosing cholangitis associated with immunological diseases. *Endoscopy.* 1987;19:114-117.
146. Quigley EMM, LaRusso NF, Ludwig J, et al. Familial occurrence of primary sclerosing cholangitis and ulcerative colitis. *Gastroenterology.* 1983;85:1160-1165.
147. Schrumpf E, Fausa O, Forre O, et al. HLA antigens and immunoregulatory T cells in ulcerative colitis associated with hepatobiliary disease. *Scand J Gastroenterol.* 1982;17:187-191.
148. Olerup O, Olsson R, Hultcrantz R, et al. HLA-DR and HLA-DQ are not markers for rapid disease progression in primary sclerosing cholangitis. *Gastroenterology.* 1995;108:870-878.
149. Mitchell SA, Grove J, Spurkland A, et al. Association of the tumour necrosis factor A-308 but not the interleukin 10-627 promoter polymorphism with genetic susceptibility to primary sclerosing cholangitis. *Gut.* 2001;49:288-294.
150. Zauli D, Schrumpf E, Crespi C, et al. An autoantibody profile in primary sclerosing cholangitis. *J Hepatol.* 1987;5:14-18.
151. Angulo P, Peter JB, Gershwin ME, et al. Serum autoantibodies in patients with primary sclerosing cholangitis. *J Hepatol.* 1999;32:182-187.
152. Broome U, Olsson R, Loof L, et al. Natural history and prognostic factors in 305 Swedish patients with primary sclerosing cholangitis. *Gut.* 1996;38:610-615.
153. Farrant JM, Hayllar KM, Wilkinson M, et al. Natural history and prognostic variable in primary sclerosing cholangitis. *Gastroenterology.* 1991;100:1710-1717.
154. Wiesner RH, Grambsch PM, Dickson ER, et al. Primary sclerosing cholangitis: natural history, prognostic factors and survival analysis. *Hepatology.* 1989;10:430-436.
155. Menon K, Wiesner R. Etiology and natural history of primary sclerosing cholangitis. *J Hepat Pancreat Surg.* 1999;6:343-351.
156. Duerr RH, Targan SR, Landers CJ, et al. Anti-neutrophil cytoplasmic antibodies: a link between primary sclerosing cholangitis and ulcerative colitis. *Gastroenterology.* 1991;100:1385-1391.
157. Textor HJ, Flacke S, Pauleit D, et al. Three-dimensional magnetic resonance cholangiopancreatography with respiratory triggering in the diagnosis of primary sclerosing cholangitis: comparison with endoscopic retrograde cholangiography. *Endoscopy.* 2002;34:984-990.
158. Kaya M, Petersen BT, Angulo P, Lindor KD. Balloon dilatation compared to stenting of dominant strictures in primary sclerosing cholangitis. *Gastroenterology.* 2000;111:34A.
159. Wiesner RH. Current concepts in primary sclerosing cholangitis. *Mayo Clin Proc.* 1994;69:969-982.
160. Ludwig J, Barham SS, LaRusso NF, et al. Morphologic features of chronic hepatitis associated with primary sclerosing cholangitis and chronic ulcerative colitis. *Hepatology.* 1981;1:632-640.
161. Lazaridis KN, Gores GJ, Lindor KD. Ursodeoxycholic acid mechanisms of action and clinical use in haptobiliary disorders. *J Hepatol.* 2001;35:134-146.
162. Beuers U, Spengler U, Zwiebel FM, Pauletzki J, Fischer S, Paumgartner G. Effect of ursodeoxychoic acid on the kinetics of the major hydrophobic bile acids in health and in chronic cholestatic liver disease. *Hepatology.* 1992;15:603-608.
163. Beuers U, Nathanson MH, Isales CM, Boyer JL. Tauroursodeoxycholic acid stimulates hepatocellular exocytosis and mobilizes extracellular Ca++ mechanisms defective in cholestasis. *J Clin Invest.* 1993;92:2984-2993.
164. Beuers U, Throckmorton DC, Anderson MS, et al. Tauroursodeoxycholic acid activates protein kinase C in isolated rat hepatocytes. *Gastroenterology.* 1996;110:1553-1563.
165. Beuers U, Bilzer M, Chittattu A, et al. Tauroursodeoxycholic acid inserts the apical conjugate export pump, Mrp2, into canalicular membranes and stimulates organic anion secretion by protein kinase C-dependent mechanisms in cholestatic rat liver. *Hepatology.* 2001;33:1206-1216.
166. Beuers U, Spengler U, Kruis W, et al. Ursodeoxycholic acid for treatment of primary sclerosing cholangitis: A placebo-controlled trial. *Hepatology.* 1992;16:707-714.
167. Lo S, Hermann R, Chapman RW, et al. Ursodeoxycholic acid in primary sclerosing cholangitis: a double-blind placebo controlled trial [Abstract]. *Hepatology.* 1992;16:92A.
168. Van Thiel DH, Wright HI, Gavaler JS. Ursodeoxycholic acid therapy for primary sclerosing cholangitis: preliminary report of a randomized controlled trial [Abstract]. *Hepatology.* 1992;16:62A.

169. Stiehl A, Walker S, Stiehl L, Rudolph G, Hofmann WJ, Theilmann L. Effect of ursodeoxycholic acid on liver and bile duct disease in primary sclerosing cholangitis: a 3-year pilot study with a placebo-controlled study period. *J Hepatol.* 1994;20:57-64.
170. DeMaria N, Colantoni A, Rosenbloom E, Van Thiel DH. Ursodeoxycholic acid does not improve the clinical course of primary sclerosing cholangitis over a 2-year period. *Hepatogastroenterology.* 1996;43:1472-1479.
171. Lindor KD. Ursodiol for primary sclerosing cholangitis. Mayo Primary Sclerosing Cholangitis-Ursodeoxycholic Acid Study Group. *N Engl J Med.* 1997;336:691-695.
172. Van Hoogstraten HJ, Wolfhagen FH, van de Meeberg PC, et al. Ursodeoxycholic acid therapy for primary sclerosing cholangitis: results of a 2-year randomized controlled trial to evaluate single versus multiple daily doses. *J Hepatol.* 1998;29:417-423.
173. Chen W, Gluud C. Bile acids for primary sclerosing cholangitis. *Cochrane Database Syst Rev.* 2003;(2):CD003626.
174. Harnois DM, Angulo P, Jorgensen RA, Larusso NF, Lindor KD. High-dose ursodeoxycholic acid as a therapy for patients with primary sclerosing cholangitis. *Am J Gastroenterol.* 2001;96:1558-1562.
175. Mitchell SA, Bansi DS, Hunt N, Von Bergmann K, Fleming KA, Chapman RW. A preliminary trial of high-dose ursodeoxycholic acid in primary sclerosing cholangitis. *Gastroenterology.* 2001;12:900-907.
176. Martinez JD, Stratagoules ED, LaRue JM, et al. Different bile acids exhibit distinct biological effects: the tumor promoter deoxycholic acid induces apoptosis and the chemopreventive agent ursodeoxycholic acid inhibits cell proliferation. *Nutr Cancer.* 1998;31:111-118.
177. Nagengast FM, Grubben MJ, van Munster IP. Role of bile acids in colorectal carcinogenesis. *Eur J Cancer.* 1995;31A:1067-1070.
178. Ochsenkuhn T, Bayerdorffer E, Meining A, et al. Colonic mucosal proliferation is related to serum deoxycholic acid levels. *Cancer.* 1999;85:1664-1669.
179. Rodrigues CM, Kren BT, Steer CJ, Setchell KD. The site-specific delivery of ursodeoxycholic acid to the rat colon by sulfate conjugation. *Gastroenterology.* 1995;109:1835-1844.
180. Tung BY, Emond MJ, Haggitt RC, et al. Ursodiol use is associated with lower prevalence of colonic neoplasia in patients with ulcerative colitis and primary sclerosing cholangitis. *Ann Intern Med.* 2001;134;89-95.
181. Croog VJ, Ullman TA, Itzkowitz SH. Chemoprevention of colorectal cancer in ulcerative colitis. *Int J Colorectal Dis.* 2003;18:392-400.
182. Angulo P, Therneau TM, Jorgensen A, et al. Bone disease in patients with primary sclerosing cholangitis: prevalence, severity and prediction of progression. *J Hepatol.* 1998;29:729-735.
183. Angulo P, Batts KP, Jorgensen RA, LaRusso NA, Lindor KD. Oral budesonide in the treatment of primary sclerosing cholangitis. *Am J Gastroenterol.* 2000;95:2333-2337.
184. Van Hoogstraten HJ, Vleggaar FP, Boland GJ, et al. Budesonide or prednisone in combination with ursodeoxycholic acid in primary sclerosing cholangitis: a randomized double-blind pilot study. *Am J Gastroenterol.* 2000;95:2015-2022.
185. Schramm C, Schirmacher P, Helmreich-Becker I, Gerken G, zum Buschenfelde KH, Lohse AW. Combined therapy with azathioprine, prednisolone, and ursodiol in patients with primary sclerosing cholangitis: a case series. *Ann Intern Med.* 1999;131:943-946.
186. Knox TA, Kaplan MM. Treatment of primary sclerosing cholangitis with oral methotrexate. *Am J Gastroenterol.* 1991;86:546-552.
187. Knox TA, Kaplan MM. A double-blind controlled trial of oral-pulse methotrexate therapy in the treatment of primary sclerosing cholangitis. *Gastroenterology.* 1994;106:494-499.
188. Van Thiel DH, Carroll P, Abu-Elmagd K, et al. Tacrolimus (FK 506), a treatment for primary sclerosing cholangitis: results of an open-label preliminary trial. *Am J Gastroenterol.* 1995;90:455-459.
189. Wiesner R, Steiner B, LaRusso N, et al. A controlled clinical trial evaluating cyclosporine in the treatment of primary sclerosing cholangitis. *Hepatology.* 1991;14:63A.
190. Olsson R, Broome U, Danielsson A, et al. Colchicine treatment of primary sclerosing cholangitis. *Gastroenterology.* 1995;108:1199-1203.
191. Lindor KD, Wiesner RH, Colwell LJ, et al. The combination of prednisone and colchicines in patients with primary sclerosing cholangitis. *Am J Gastroenterol.* 1991;86:57-61.
192. LaRusso NF, Wiesner RH, Ludwig J, et al. Prospective trial of penicillamine in primary sclerosing cholangitis. *Gastroenterology.* 1988;95:1036-1042.
193. Angulo P, MacCarty RL, Sylvestre PB, et al. Pirfenidone in the treatment of primary sclerosing cholangitis. *Dig Dis Sci.* 2002;47:157-161.
194. Ghent CN. Pruritus of cholestasis is related to effects of bile salts on liver, not the skin. *Am J Gastroenterol.* 1987;82:117-118.
195. Jones EA, Bergasa NV. The pruritus of cholestasis and the opioid system. *JAMA.* 1992;268:3359-3362.
196. Datta D, Sherlock S. Treatment of pruritus of obstructive jaundice with cholestyramine. *Br Med J.* 1963;1:216-219.
197. Bachs L, Pares A, Elena M, et al. Effects of long-term rifampicin administration in primary biliary cirrhosis. *Gastroenterology.* 1992;102:2077-2080.
198. Bloomer JR, Boyer JL. Phenobarbital effects in cholestatic liver diseases. *Ann Intern Med.* 1975;82:310-317.
199. Bergasa NV, Talbot TL, Alling DW, et al. Effects of naloxone infusions in patients with the pruritus of cholestasis: a double-blind, randomized, controlled trial. *Ann Intern Med.* 1995;123:161-167.
200. Wolfhagen FH, Sternieri E, Hop WC, et al. Oral naltrexone treatment for cholestatic pruritus: A double-blind, placebo-controlled study. *Gastroenterology.* 1997;113:1264-1269.
201. Cohen LB, Ambinder EP, Wolke AM, et al. Role of plasmapheresis in primary biliary cirrhosis. *Gut.* 1985;26:291-4.
202. Crippin JS, Jorgensen RA, Dickson ER, et al. Hepatic osteodystrophy in primary biliary cirrhosis: Effects of medical treatment. *Am J Gastroenterol.* 1994;89:47-50.
203. Pares A, Guanaben N, Inmaculada R, et al. Aledronate is more effective than etidronate for increasing bone mass in osteopenic patients with primary biliary cirrhosis. *Hepatology.* 1999;30:1245A.
204. Borkje B, Vetvik K, Odegaard S, et al. Chronic pancreatitis in patients with sclerosing cholangitis and ulcerative colitis. *Scand J Gastroenterol.* 1985;3:539-542.
205. Hay JE, Wiesner RH, Shorter RG, et al. Primary sclerosing cholangitis and celiac disease: a novel association. *Ann Intern Med.* 1988;109:713-717.
206. Jorgensen RA, Lindor KD, Sartin JS, et al. Serum lipid and fat-soluble vitamin levels in primary sclerosing cholangitis. *J Clin Gastroenterol.* 1995;20:215-219.

207. Kaya M, Petersen BT, Angulo P, et al. Balloon dilatation compared to stenting of dominant strictures in primary sclerosing cholangitis. *Am J Gastroenterol.* 2001;96(4):1059-1066.
208. Stiehl A, Rudolph G, Sauer P, et al. Efficacy of ursodeoxycholic acid treatment and endoscopic dilation of major duct stenoses in primary sclerosing cholangitis: an 8-year prospective study. *J Hepatol.* 1997;26:560-566.
209. Nichols JC, Gores GJ, LaRusso NF, et al. Diagnostic role of serum CA 19-9 for cholangiocarcinoma in patients with primary sclerosing cholangitis. *Mayo Clin Proc.* 1993;68:874-879.
210. Marsh JW Jr, Shunzaburo I, Makowka L, et al. Orthotopic liver transplantation for primary sclerosing cholangitis. *Ann Surg.* 1988;207:21-25.
211. Marvisi M, Borrello PD, Brianti M, et al. Changes in the carbon monoxide diffusion capacity of the lung in ulcerative colitis. *Eur Respir J.* 2000;16:965-968.
212. Herrlinger KR, Noftz MK, Dalhoff K, et al. Alterations in pulmonary function in inflammatory bowel disease are frequent and persist during remission. *Am J Gastroenterol.* 2002;97:377-381.
213. Kuzela L, Vavrecka A, Prikazska M, et al. Pulmonary complications in patients with inflammatory bowel disease. *Hepatogastroenterology.* 1999;46:1714-1719.
214. Storch I, Sachar D, Katz S. Pulmonary manifestations of inflammatory bowel disease. *Inflamm Bowel Dis.* 2003;9:104-115.
215. Wilson A, Reyes E, Ofman J. Prevalence and outcomes of anemia in inflammatory bowel disease: a systematic review of the literature. *Am J Med.* 2004;116(7A):44S-49S.
216. Schreiber S, Howaldt S, Schnoor M, et al. Recombinant erythropoietin for the treatment of anemia in inflammatory bowel disease. *N Engl J Med.* 1996;334:619-623.
217. Gasche C, Dejaco C, Waldhoer T, et al. Intravenous iron and erythropoietin for anemia associated with Crohn's disease: A randomized, controlled trial. *Ann Intern Med.* 1997;126:782-787.
218. Gumaste V, Greenstein AJ, Meyers R, Sachar DB. Coombs-positive autoimmune hemolytic anemia in ulcerative colitis. *Dig Dis Sci.* 1989;34:1457-1461.
219. Giannadaki E, Potamianos S, Roussomoustakaki M, Kyriakou D, Fragkiadakis N, Manousos ON. Autoimmune hemolytic anemia and positive Coombs test associated with ulcerative colitis. *Am J Gastroenterol.* 1997;92:1872-1874.
220. Hochman JA. Autoimmune hemolytic anemia associated with Crohn's disease. *Inflamm Bowel Dis.* 2002;8:98-100.
221. Manousos ON, Giannadaki E, Mouzas I, et al. Ulcerative colitis is as common in Crete as in Northern Europe: a 5 year prospective study. *Eur J Gastroenterol Hepatol.* 1996;8:893-898.
222. Yates P, Macht LM, Williams NA, et al. Red cell autoantibody production by colonic mononuclear cells from a patient with ulcerative colitis and autoimmune haemolytic anaemia. *Br J Haematol.* 1992;82:753-756.
223. Shashaty GG, Rath CE, Britt J. Autoimmune hemolytic anemia associated with ulcerative colitis. *Am J Hematol.* 1977;3:199-208.
224. Tavarela VF, Fraga J, Carvalho J, et al. Autoimmune hemolytic anemia in ulcerative colitis: A case report with review of the literature. *J Clin Gastroenterol.* 1991;13:445-447.
225. Miehsler W, Reinisch W, Valic E, et al. Is inflammatory bowel disease an independent and disease specific risk factor for thromboembolism? *Gut.* 2004;53:542-548.
226. Bernstein CN, Blanchard JF, Houston DS, Wajda A. The incidence of deep venous thrombosis and pulmonary embolism among patients with inflammatory bowel disease: a population-based cohort study. *Thromb Haemost.* 2001;85:430-434.
227. Novacek G, Miehsler W, Kapiotis S, et al. Thromboembolism and resistance to activated protein C in patients with inflammatory bowel disease. *Dig Dis Sci.* 1999;94:8685-8690.
228. Aichbichler B, Petritsch W, Reight G, et al. Anti-cardiolipin antibodies in patients with inflammatory bowel disease. *Dig Dis Sci.* 1999;44:852-856.
229. Koutroubakis I. Role of thrombotic vascular risk factors in inflammatory bowel disease. *Dig Dis.* 2000;18:161-167.
230. Talbot R, Hepell J, Dozois R, et al. Vascular complications of inflammatory bowel disease. *Mayo Clin Proc.* 1986;61:140-145.
231. Conlan MG, Haire WD, Burnett DA. Prothrombotic abnormalities in inflammatory bowel disease. *Dig Dis Sci.* 1989;34:1089-1093.
232. Aadland E, Odegaard OR, Roseth A, Try K. Free protein S deficiency in patients with Crohn's disease. *Scand J Gastroenterol.* 1994;29:333-335.
233. Hudson M, Chitolie A, Hutton RA, Smith MS, Pounder RE, Wakefield AJ. Thrombotic vascular risk factors in inflammatory bowel disease. *Gut.* 1996;38:733-737.
234. Probert CSJ, Haslam N, Aslam S, et al. Is factor V Leiden associated with inflammatory bowel disease? *Gut.* 1997;41:A36.
235. Jackson LM, O'Gorman PJ, O'Connell J, et al. Thrombosis in inflammatory bowel disease: clinical setting, procoagulant profile and factor V Leiden. *Q J Med.* 1997;90:183-188.
236. Levine A, Lahav J, Zahavi I, et al. Activated protein C resistance in pediatric inflammatory bowel disease. *J Ped Gastroenterol Nutrition.* 1998;26:172-174.
237. Vecchi M, Sacchi E, Saibeni S, et al. Inflammatory bowel diseases are not associated with major hereditary conditions predisposing to thrombosis. *Dig Dis Sci.* 2000;45:1465-1469.
238. Helio T, Wartiovaara U, Halme L, et al. Arg506Gln factor V mutation and Val34Leu factor XIII polymorphism in Finnish patients with inflammatory bowel disease. *Scand J Gastroenterol.* 1999;34:170-174.
239. Heneghan MA, Cleary B, Murray M, O'Gorman TA, McCarthy CF. Activated protein C resistance, thrombophilia, and inflammatory bowel disease. *Dig Dis Sci.* 1998;43:1356-1361.
240. Johns DR. Cerebrovascular complications of inflammatory bowel disease. *Am J Gastroenterol.* 1991;86:367-370.
241. Fichera A, Cicchiello LA, Mendelson DS, Greenstein AJ, Heimann TM. Superior mesenteric vein thrombosis after colectomy for inflammatory bowel disease: a not uncommon cause of postoperative acute abdominal pain. *Dis Colon Rectum.* 2003;46:643-648.
242. Van Hees PA, van Elferen LW, van Rossum JM, van Tongeren JH. Hemolysis during salicylazosulfapyridine therapy. *Am J Gastroenterol.* 1978;70:501-505.
243. Teplitsky V, Virag I, Halabe A. Immune complex haemolytic anaemia associated with sulfasalazine. *BMJ.* 2000;320:1113.
244. Vermeire S, Noman M, Van Assche G, et al. Autoimmunity associated with anti-tumor necrosis factor alpha treatment in Crohn's disease: a prospective cohort study. *Gastroenterology.* 2003;125:32-39.

33

Nicotine and Inflammatory Bowel Disease

Truc T. Trinh, MD; Richard S. Bloomfeld, MD, MS; and Stephen J. Bickston, MD, AGAF

Cigarette smoking is one of the most significant environmental factors implicated in both ulcerative colitis (UC) and Crohn's disease (CD). Epidemiological and clinical observations have firmly established the dual effects of smoking on UC and CD. Tobacco smoking is negatively associated with the development of UC (lower risk of developing UC in current smokers) and positively (higher risk of developing CD in current smokers) associated with the development of CD. These contrasting effects of smoking on the risk of developing each disease and the clinical course further support the distinction between these 2 major forms of inflammatory bowel disease (IBD). The mechanisms underlying the discrepancy of effects of cigarette smoking on UC and CD remain elusive, although several causal factors have been implicated. This chapter will review the current literature on cigarette smoking and IBD, including historical perspectives, clinical associations of smoking with each IBD phenotype (UC and CD), proposed mechanisms of actions, and therapeutic implications, specifically in UC.

Cigarette Smoking and Ulcerative Colitis

Ulcerative colitis is generally a disease of nonsmokers and ex-smokers. This negative association between UC and smoking was first reported by Harries and colleagues in 1982.[1] Numerous case reports and epidemiological studies in different countries have confirmed this strong association.[2-13] Although the overall calculated relative risks vary among case-control studies, they consistently document a lower risk of UC in current smokers compared to lifelong nonsmokers (Figure 33-1A). The beneficial effects of smoking appear suspended, however, as former smokers not only lose their protection against the disease, but have an even higher risk for developing UC than lifetime nonsmokers.[5-9,11,12,14-17] Representative relative risks reported in most studies for former smokers, nonsmokers, and current smokers are 2.5, 1.0, and 0.6, respectively.[6-8,18]

A meta-analysis of 9 comparable case-control studies of UC calculated a lifetime relative risk to nonsmokers of 2.9 (2.6 to 3.2) compared to current smokers.[15] Pooled odds ratio (OR) for current smokers compared to lifetime nonsmokers was 0.41 (0.34 to 0.48), whereas the pooled OR for ex-smokers to nonsmokers was 1.64 (1.36 to 1.98), confirming the additional increased risk conferred by former smoking status above baseline nonsmoking (Figure 33-1B). Several studies also found a dose-dependent correlation, with a decreasing risk of UC with increasing current levels of smoking compared to nonsmoking.[2,3,6-8] In former smokers, this trend was reversed, with increasing risk associated with increasing prior level of usage.[3,7,8] Taken together, these studies strongly indicate that both lifelong nonsmoking and, more importantly, former smoking are significant risk factors for UC. The dosage relationship further strengthens the case for the protective effects of smoking on colitis.

The inverse relationship between smoking and UC has been confirmed in population-based cohort studies and also in family-based studies. Penny et al[19] investigated the prevalence of UC and CD among 17,700 Mormons (a predominantly nonsmoking population) and found a fivefold increased incidence of UC over the general population. Tysk et al[20] reviewed 56 epidemiological studies in Sweden from 1930 to 1990. They found a shift from an earlier female

Lichtenstein GR, ed.
Ulcerative Colitis: The Complete Guide to Medical Management (pp 365-380)

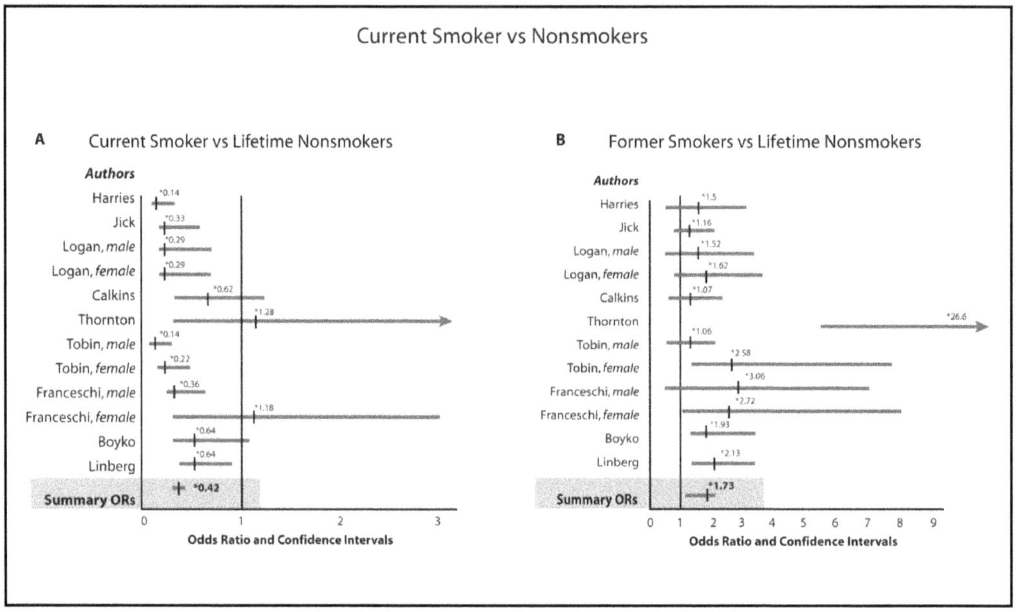

FIGURE 33-1. Individual and summary odds ratios (with 95% confidence intervals) of lifetime risk of ulcerative colitis in current smokers compared with lifetime nonsmokers (panel A) and in former smokers versus lifetime nonsmokers (panel B). (Reproduced with permission from Calkins BM. A meta-analysis of the role of smoking in inflammatory bowel disease. *Dig Dis Sci.* 1989;34:1841-1845.)

predominance of UC to later male predominance over this 60-year span. During this same interval, reciprocal changes in smoking pattern between the sexes have been observed, with an increase in women smokers relative to men.

Within a similar genetic susceptibility background, smoking status generally dictates the IBD phenotype, where nonsmokers develop UC and smokers develop CD.[21-23] In one study of 89 sibling pairs discordant for smoking status at diagnosis, 23 were also discordant for IBD phenotype. In 21 of these 23 discordant pairs, CD developed in the smoking and UC developed in the nonsmoking sibling.[21] A Danish study of twins discordant for smoking also confirmed that smoking status was an important determinant on the IBD phenotype.[22]

The relationship between smoking *duration* and UC is less clear. One group has directly evaluated this.[7] No significant trend was noted between duration of smoking and the risk of UC once adjustments were made for confounding factors (multivariate RR for duration ≥15 years = 1.3). Several groups have also addressed the temporal relationship between disease onset and smoking cessation.[6-8,24] Motley et al[24] reported the highest risk within the first 3 years (particularly the first year) of smoking cessation; others also reported an increased risk period remaining beyond 10 years.[7,8] Although these studies differ with respect to the duration that a former smoker continues to be at risk for UC, they all show an increased risk among former smokers.

Several studies have also documented the inverse relationship between smoking and another UC-related disease, primary sclerosing cholangitis (PSC).[25-27] This protective effect was observed in smokers with and without IBD, suggesting a systemic rather than local beneficial effect (ie, colonic).[25-27]

EFFECTS OF SMOKING ON ULCERATIVE COLITIS CLINICAL COURSE

Not only do current smokers have a relative protection against developing UC, they also appear to have a milder disease course. Approximately 45% of intermittent smokers who resume smoking note improvement of their symptoms.[28] Disease exacerbations, hospitalizations, requirements for steroids or other immunomodulatory therapies, and colectomy rates are generally lower for smokers compared to nonsmokers.[6,29] A meta-analysis reported an average OR of 0.57 (0.38 to 0.85) for total colectomy in current smokers compared to nonsmokers with UC (Figure 33-2).[6,29-33] One study also suggested smoking as a protective modifying factor in UC-associated colon cancer.[34] Finally, the incidence of pouchitis after proctocolectomy in UC is lower in current smokers than nonsmokers.[35,36]

Former smokers with UC appear to have a worse clinical course compared to lifelong nonsmokers.[6] In one representative study, cessation of smoking was associated with an increased rate of hospitalization and need for steroids or immunomodulatory therapies during the first year.[37] The risk of colectomy within this timeframe was not increased.[37]

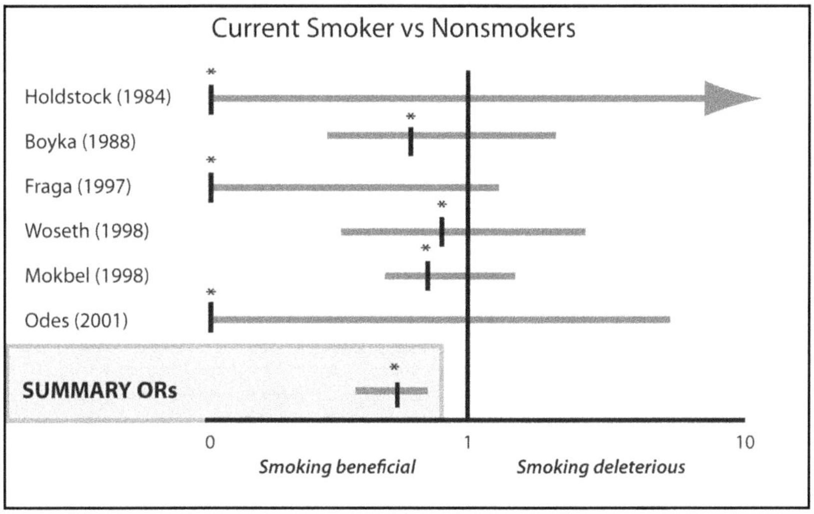

FIGURE 33-2. Individual and summary odds ratios (with 95% confidence intervals) for colectomy rates in current smokers versus nonsmokers with ulcerative colitis. (Reprinted from Cosnes J. Tobacco and IBD: relevance in the understanding of disease mechanisms and clinical practice. *Best Pract Res Clin Gastroenterol. 2004*;18:481-486 with permission from Elsevier.)

SMOKING AND CROHN'S DISEASE

In contrast to its protective effects in UC, smoking exerts permissive effects on the development of CD.[3,7,8,38-40] A meta-analysis of 7 studies reported pooled ORs of 2.0 (1.65 to 2.47) for current smokers and 1.83 (1.33 to 2.51) for ex-smokers compared to lifetime nonsmokers (Figure 33-3).[15] The risk for CD is greatest in the first 4 years of smoking cessation and least after 10 years of cessation.[7,15] Three studies included in the former meta-analysis evaluated the dose relationship between current smoking and CD; however, their findings were inconclusive.[6-8] Others have found a positive dose-dependent effect, with higher doses (>15 cigarettes/day) associated with more harmful effects and daily doses rather than cumulative consumption being important.[41]

EFFECTS OF SMOKING ON THE CLINICAL COURSE OF CROHN'S DISEASE

Smoking has adverse effects on clinical and surgical outcomes in CD.[42-46] At any given point, compared to nonsmokers, current smokers are 50% more likely to have disease exacerbation independent of age, gender, disease duration, or concurrent therapy.[41] They are also more likely to require steroids or other immunotherapies.[41,47] Active smokers are also at increased risk for surgery during the course of their disease.[45,48]

Smoking is associated with specific disease phenotypes, which may also explain the observed increase in surgical risk. Current smoking is preferentially associated with ileal disease, whereas nonsmoking is positively associated with colonic disease.[5,47,48] Additionally, those with exclusive colonic disease are less sensitive to the harmful effects of smoking. Patients with CD who continue to smoke are more likely to develop fibrostenotic or penetrating forms of the disease.[49,50]

Disease course after surgery is significantly worsened by continued smoking. Cottone et al[42] followed 182 CD patients over a 20-year period and found that the cumulative risks of all recurrence endpoints (endoscopic, clinical, and surgical) were significantly increased for current smokers compared to nonsmokers. Interestingly, patients who had stopped smoking at least 1 year before surgery had outcomes similar to the nonsmoking group.[42] The increased risk of postsurgical recurrence in active smokers is confirmed by several studies (Figure 33-4).[42-46] A recent retrospective study of 267 patients with ileocolonic CD requiring surgery found that active smoking significantly increases the risk for both reoperation and the necessity for multiple operations.[51] Postsurgical symptomatic recurrence was particularly increased in heavier (>15 cigarettes/day) compared to lighter smokers and in female smokers compared to female nonsmokers.[42,46]

Fortunately, not only does smoking cessation decrease the risk of developing CD, it also markedly improves the clinical course. Disease activity in ex-smokers is significantly reduced compared to smokers and is similar to that of nonsmokers. Endoscopic and clinical disease recurrence after surgery in this population approximates the rates in nonsmokers after 1 year of smoking cessation.[42,52] A prospective study following 59 patients with CD who quit smoking during an intervention program found that after 1 year of cessation, disease exacerbation, medical therapies, and surgical needs were similar in ex-smokers and nonsmokers, with both being lower than continued smokers (Figure 33-5).[52]

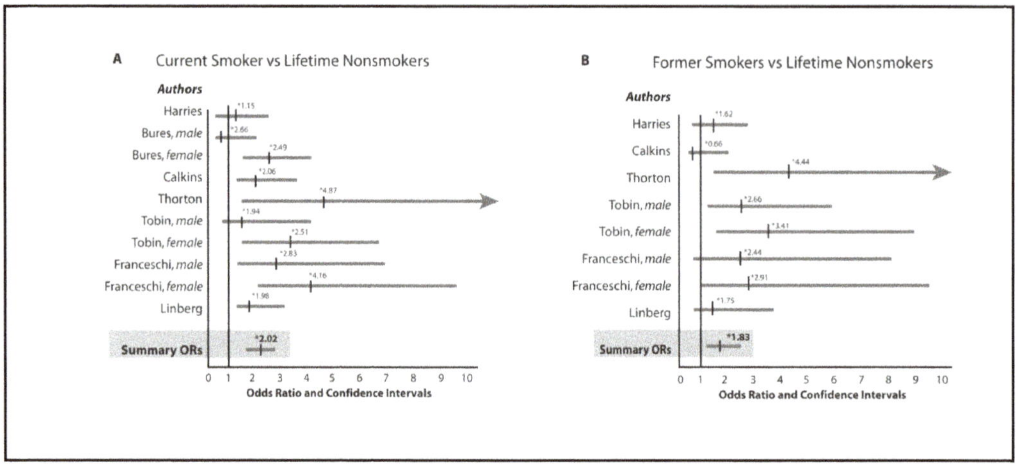

FIGURE 33-3. Individual and summary odds ratios and 95% confidence intervals for seven studies included in a meta-analysis of lifetime risk of Crohn's disease in current smokers compared with lifetime nonsmokers (panel A) and in former smokers with lifetime nonsmokers (panel B). (Reproduced with permission from Calkins BM. A meta-analysis of the role of smoking in inflammatory bowel disease. *Dig Dis Sci.* 1989;34:1841-1845.)

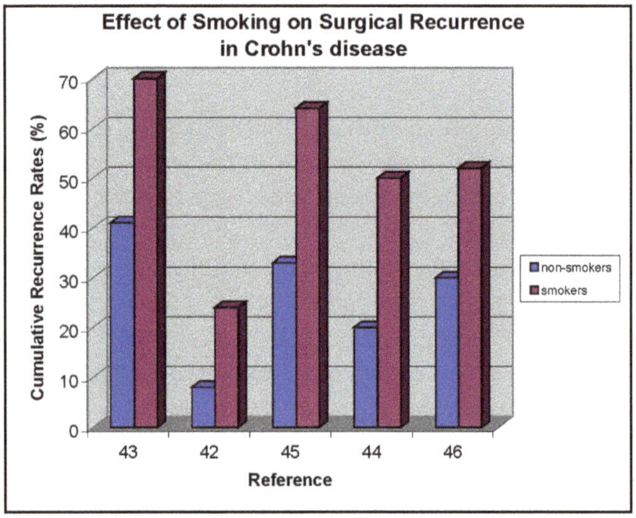

FIGURE 33-4. Effects of smoking on cumulative re-operation rates in Crohn's disease in 5 studies; $P<0.01$ in smokers compared to nonsmokers in all studies.

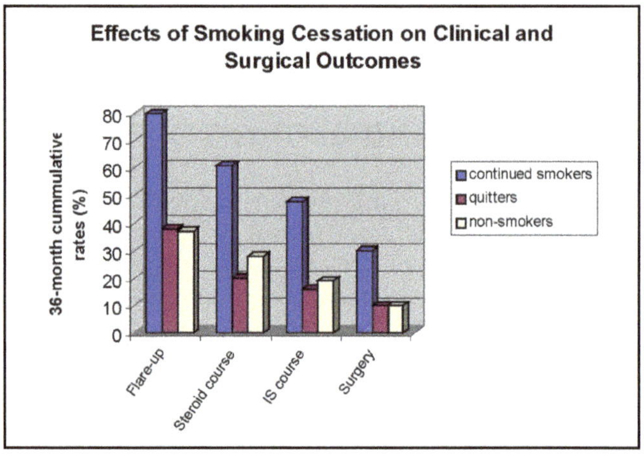

FIGURE 33-5. Respective 36-month cumulative rates (%) of exacerbations, steroid course, immunosuppressive therapy (IS) and surgery in patients with Crohn's disease who quit smoking compared to continued smokers, non-smokers and matched controls. (Reprinted from Cosnes J. Tobacco and IBD: relevance in the understanding of disease mechanisms and clinical practice. *Best Pract Res Clin Gastroenterol. 2004*;18:481-486 with permission from Elsevier.)

SMOKING AND PATIENT SUBGROUPS

GENDER

Gender differences may influence the effects of smoking on both UC and CD.[24,53,54] In UC, Motley et al[24] reported that in men, smoking may delay disease onset. On average, male ex-smokers presented with disease 17 years later than nonsmokers. This finding was not seen in women. Men, but not women, with UC who continue to smoke also experienced improvement in their health-related quality of life compared to nonsmokers.[55] Cosnes et al[53] evaluated the relationship between smoking status, gender, and disease course in 1784 patients with IBD. They confirmed the dichotomous effects of smoking in colitis: beneficial in UC, but permissive in CD. The authors also concluded that gender modulates the disease course in both UC and CD. Men with UC who smoke not only have a delayed onset of disease, but also have an improved clinical course if they continue to smoke. This difference was less marked in women with UC. In contrast, in CD, the detrimental effects of smoking are more prominent in women than in men. Women who smoke develop earlier and more severe disease than their nonsmoking counterparts. These differential effects of smoking on CD were not significant in the 2 male cohorts. It appears that women are more sensitive to the damaging effects of smoking, whereas men are more likely to benefit from its protective effects.

Potential confounding factors contributing to this gender difference in both forms of colitis have been proposed, including concomitant oral contraceptive use (OCP), variations in smoking habit or style, and hormonal interactions. In CD, some studies have reported disease exacerbation with concomitant OCP use and worsened clinical course with prior use,[56,57] while OCP use does not appear to increase the risk or alter the disease course in UC.[58,59] In the study by Cosnes et al,[53] although OCP use was associated with smoking status in both forms of colitis, no differences in medical or surgical therapies were seen in OCP users versus nonusers regardless of smoking status. Subtle differences in smoking styles may also contribute to the gender-specific effects of smoking. One group observed a greater relative exposure to smoke versus nicotine in women smokers, partly due to consumption of more "light" or filter cigarettes.[60] This may be relevant because several studies suggest the protective mechanisms are mediated through nicotine, while the detrimental effects are due to other tobacco components.[61,62] A synergistic interaction between smoking and estrogen on the immune system has also been hypothesized. Specifically, smoking may potentiate estrogen's effects on cytokine dysregulation and T and B cell interactions. This proinflammatory role of estrogen has been proposed in other autoimmune diseases, such as systemic lupus erythematosus, where there is a female predilection.[63]

ETHNICITY

Three large studies in the Israeli Jewish population[64] have failed to confirm the positive association between smoking and CD, suggesting that ethnic or geographic factors may be involved.[14,65,66] The largest of these studies included patients in 4 different regions of the country and found no association in any of the areas.[14] However, both this study and that of Fich et al did find the usual inverse association of smoking and UC.[14,66] The explanation for this discrepant finding in CD remains speculative. The lack of association of CD and smoking in the Jewish population may be largely due to overriding genetic factors.[67,68] Twin and other family-based studies have found a stronger genetic susceptibility in CD than UC.[69,70] Epidemiologic studies have consistently reported an overall higher prevalence of CD in the Jewish population. Conversely, in UC, where environmental factors may be more influential than genetics, the usual association with smoking is still observed.

PASSIVE SMOKING AND INFLAMMATORY BOWEL DISEASE

The relationship between passive smoking and IBD is inconclusive. In one study, adults exposed to second-hand smoke as children were half as likely to develop UC later in life.[10] Another study found that passive smoking exposure at birth was associated with increased risks of both IBD phenotypes.[71] A Swedish study reported an increased risk of CD but not UC in individuals exposed to secondhand smoke as children.[48] Finally, an Israeli study of adult IBD patients found no significant differences in passive smoking exposure between IBD and control patients, although UC patients did appear to have lowers level of exposure on quantitative analysis.[72]

POSSIBLE MECHANISMS OF ACTION

The mechanisms underlying the dichotomous effects of smoking on CD and UC remain unclear. Further elucidation of these mechanisms is complicated by the variability of smoking effects based on gender and ethnicity, the lack of an optimal animal model, and the complexity of tobacco smoke constituents. Factors considered to be important include immune system effects, eicosanoid effects, intestinal motility, colonic mucous production, gut permeability, and colonic blood flow.

IMMUNE SYSTEM

Cigarette smoking alters innate and adaptive immune responses. Macrophages in smokers exhibit a functionally impaired ability to kill intracellular bacteria.[73,74] Similarly, the adaptive immune response, including both cellular and humoral pathways, is down-regulated in healthy smoking controls.[74,75] In vitro studies have reported that both smoking and nicotine decrease the production of several proinflammatory cytokines, specifically IL-1β, IL-2, IL-8, IL-10, and TNFα, peripherally in blood mononuclear cells and locally within colonic tissues from controls and UC patients.[76-80] In vivo studies have also shown a similar reduction in these cytokines in colonic mucosa from healthy mice and patients with UC when exposed to either smoking or nicotine.[80-82] Smokers with active IBD have significantly lower concentrations of mucosal IL-1β and IL-8 than nonsmokers.[78,80] Another study found that in patients with active UC, transdermal nicotine up to 22 mg daily for 4 weeks reduces mucosal IL-8 levels without any significant effects on other cytokines or mucin gene expression.[82]

OTHER INFLAMMATORY PATHWAYS

Both smoking and nicotine may also affect eicosanoid-mediated inflammatory pathways. One study reported lower levels of various eicosanoids in the colonic mucosa of smokers compared to healthy controls.[83] In rabbits treated with subcutaneous nicotine, rectal mucosal eicosanoid levels were reduced compared to the untreated group.[84] Nicotine also has important neuroimmune effects that may be pertinent in intestinal inflammation.[85-87] Nicotine can interact with nicotinic receptors along the hypothalamic-pituitary-adrenal axis (HPA) to modulate ACTH and endogenous corticosteroid production. In addition, the immunosuppressive effects of smoking/nicotine may be mediated through the autonomic nervous system, independent of the HPA axis, as demonstrated in studies with adrenalectomized animals.[88]

TABLE 33-1

ANIMAL MODELS OF THE EFFECTS OF SMOKING ON INTESTINAL INFLAMMATION

Model (Reference)	Agent	Findings
DNBS colitis (rat) *(100)*	Cigarette smoke	• Decreased colonic damage • Decreased LTB_4, NOS • No increase in TNFα, IL-1β, IL-6
DNBS colitis (rat) *(99)*	Cigarette smoke + Hexamethonium	• Increased colonic damage and MPO activity • Neutralization of smoking-related harmful effects
TNBS colitis (rat) *(61)*	Cigarette smoke + LTB_4 antagonist	• Increased colonic damage and MPO activity • Increase ROM production
DNBS colitis (rat) *(102)*	Nicotine 5-20 μg/mL Nicotine 5 μg/mL Nicotine (5-20 μg/mL) + Hexamethonium	• Reduced colonic damage and MPO activity • Enhanced colonic inflammation and MPO activity • Abolished beneficial effects of nicotine, increased MPO activity
TNBS colitis (rat) *(98)*	Nicotine 2.5-250 μg/mL	• Dose-dependent effects: decreased colonic damage at low dose, increased at high dose • No effects on NOS, PGE_2, IL-1, increased LTB_4
Iodoacetamide jejunitis (rat) *(103)*	Nicotine 12.5-250 μg/mL	• Increased jejunal damage, decreased PGE_2, NOS
Iodoacetamide colitis (rat) *(103)*	Nicotine 12.5-250 μg/mL	• Decreased colonic damage, increased microcirculation
Jejunitis and colitis IL-10 KO mice *(62)*	Nicotine 12.5 μg/mL	• Increased jejunal injury, amelioration of colonic injury accompanied by local induction of somatostatin and ITF mRNA
IL-10 KO mice (bone marrow macrophages) *(101)*	Carbon monoxide	• Inhibition of IL-12 production induced by LPS • No effect on IL-6, TNFα, NO

Abbreviations: DNBS, di-nitrobenzene sulfonic acid; LTB4, leukotriene B4; MPO, myloperoxidase; NOS, nitric oxide synthase; ROM, reactive oxygen metabolites; TNBS, trinitrobenzene sulfonic acid: IL-10 KO, IL-10 knock-out: ITF, intestinal trefoil factor

Adapted from Cosnes J. Tobacco and IBD: relevance in the understanding of disease mechanisms and clinical practice. *Best Pract Clin Gastroenterol.* 2004;18:481-496.

Other Effects: Intestinal Motility, Mucous Production, Gut Permeability, and Blood Flow

Patients with UC treated with nicotine patches often report that defecation urgency is the earliest symptom to improve. This is likely related to a delay in gastrointestinal motility[89] or a decrease in rectal blood flow.[90] Intraluminally administered nicotine has been shown in vivo to relax smooth muscle tone and contractile activity in the distal colon primarily through the release of nitric oxide.[91]

Alterations in colonic mucous production have been seen in patients with active UC.[92] Although in vitro studies initially observed increased mucous production in smokers

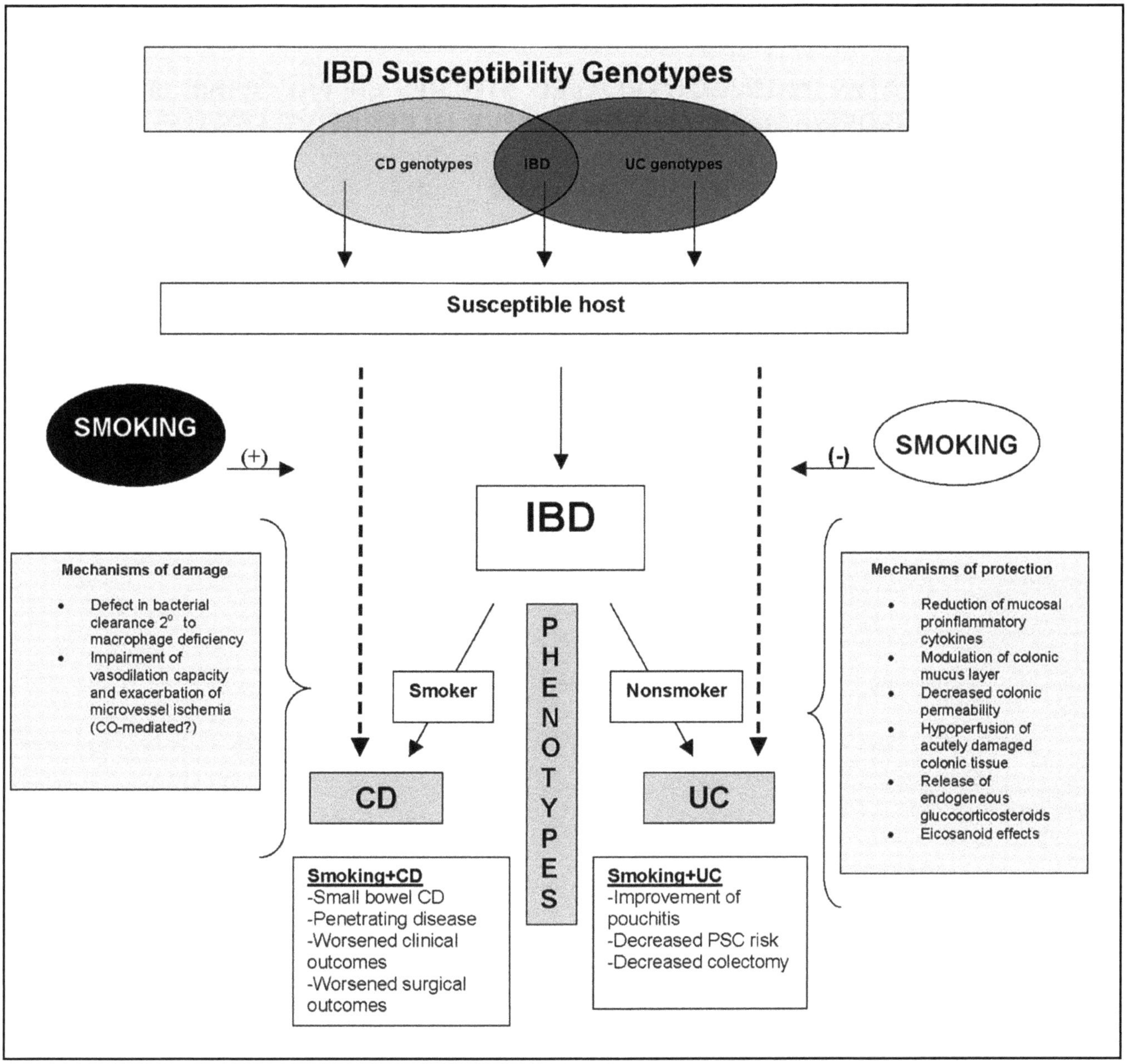

FIGURE 33-6. A schematic representation of permissive effects of smoking on CD pathogenesis (+) and protective effects on UC (-) and influences on IBD phenotypes and clinical course. (+) denotes permissive, (-) denotes protective effects.

with UC compared to healthy smokers,[93] in vivo studies on rabbits as well as humans were inconclusive and failed to show that the beneficial effects of smoking/nicotine relate to its effects on colonic mucous production.[94]

The effects of smoking on intestinal permeability have also been evaluated, albeit, with conflicting conclusions. Early studies observed increased gut permeability in UC patients compared to healthy controls and decreased gut permeability in healthy controls who smoke.[95] Subsequent studies did not find any differences in gut permeability between smokers with UC and nonsmokers with UC.[96]

Finally, the effects of smoking on mucosal blood flow have been studied in detail. Smoking produces a transient reduction in rectal blood flow. One study reported that rectal blood flow was significantly increased in patients with UC compared to controls.[90] Smoking may normalize this. Conversely, in CD, changes in the bowel wall microvasculature similar to ischemia have been observed.[97] It is possible that the effects of smoking on mucosal blood flow would exacerbate a situation in which ischemia is already present.

Animal Models

Despite the lack of an ideal animal model for the divergent effects of smoking and nicotine on CD and UC, much insight has been gained from various experimental models of intestinal inflammation (Table 33-1).[61,62,98-103] For example, in trinitrobenzene sulfonic acid (TNBS)-induced

TABLE 33-2

RESPONSE RATES IN UNCONTROLLED STUDIES OF NICOTINE GUM OR TRANSDERMAL PATCH FOR ACTIVE ULCERATIVE COLITIS

Reference (Citation)	Smoking status	N	Response (%)	Type	Dose	Duration
Roberts (13)	Former	1	100%	Gum	4 mg x 5/d	24 wk
Perera 123)	Combined	11	27%	Gum	4 mg x 5/d	8 wk
Watson (125)	Former	1	100%	Gum	NA	4 y
Srivastava (126)	Combined	18	78%	Patch	22 mg/24 h	4 wk
Guslandi (124)	Former	2	50%	Patch	15 mg/24 h	5 wk
	Never	1	100%	Patch	15 mg/24 h	5 wk
Guslandi (109)	Former	6	100%	Patch	15 mg/24 h	5 wk
	Never	4	25%	Patch	15 mg/ 24 h	5 wk

Adapted from Sandborn WJ. Notice therapy for ulcerative colitis: a review of rationale, mechanisms, pharmacology, and clinical results. *Am J Gastroenterol.* 1999;94(5):1161-1171.

colitis in rats, a model more similar to human CD than UC, several authors have independently found a biphasic effect of chronic nicotine exposure.[61,98,99] In these studies, lower nicotine doses (2.5 to 25 μg/mL) were protective in the colon while higher doses (250 μg/mL) were harmful. These effects were abrograted by the nicotinic ganglionic blocker hexamethonium, suggesting a nicotine-specific effect. Two studies have assessed the regional effects of nicotine on the small versus large intestine, using various models that mimic human CD.[62,103] The first evaluated the effects of nicotine on iodoacetamide-induced jejunitis versus colitis and found that chronic low-dose nicotine administration was protective in the colon, but exacerbated jejunal damage.[103] Other regional differences were reported. In the jejunum, nicotine-induced damage was accompanied by decreased PGE2 production and increased NOS activity without effects on the microcirculation, whereas in the colon, enhancement of the microcirculation was observed without changes in NOS activity. The second study using IL-10 -/- knockout mice, a genetically-derived model of human CD, also found clear differences in regional responses to low-dose nicotine (12.5 μg/mL) with aggravation of jejunal injury and improvement of colitis.[62] In this study, the amelioration of colitis was accompanied by the induction of local mucosal-protective factors. Taken together, these observations recapitulate some of the features of smoking and human IBD, where the effects are modulated by dose of nicotine or other smoke agent, duration of exposure, and target organ studied.

Summary

It is unlikely that smoking and its constituents modulate intestinal inflammation by exerting a direct effect on mediators in the inflammatory pathway. If this were the case, both CD and UC should benefit from smoking and nicotine. It is possible that the dual effects of smoking on these 2 disease processes are secondary to its action on entirely different mechanisms rather than a common pathway. A conceptual framework for understanding the effects of smoking in IBD would appropriately include its causal role in disease pathogenesis and protection and its modifier role in influencing the specific IBD phenotype and the overall clinical course and severity (Figure 33-6).

TABLE 33-3

RESULT OF SIX CONTROLLED TRIALS OF NICOTINE GUM OR TRANSDERMAL PATCH FOR ULCERATIVE COLITIS

Reference (Citation)	Therapy Groups (N)	Response (%)	*P*	Indication	Type	Dose	Duration
Lashner *(104)*	Nicotine (7)	43%		Active	Gum	2 mg x	2 wk
	Placebo (7)	0%				5-7/d	
Pullan *(105)*	Nicotine (35)	49%	0.03	Active	Patch	25 mg/24 h	6 wk
	Placebo (37)	24%					
Sandborn *(106)*	Nicotine (31)	39%	0.01	Active	Patch	22 mg/24 h	4 wk
	Placebo (33)	9%					
Thomas *(107)*	Nicotine (19)	20%	0.08	Active	Patch	25 mg/16 h	6 wk
	Prednisolone (24)	45%					
Guslandi *(127)*	Nicotine (21)	71%		Active	Patch	15 mg/24 h	5 wk
	Prednisone (17)	88%					
Thomas *(108)*	Nicotine (40)	45%	0.28	Remission	Patch	15 mg/16 h	26 wk
	Placebo (40)	50%					

Adapted from Sandborn WJ. Nicotine therapy for ulcerative colitis: a review of rationale, mechanisms, pharmacology, and clinical results. *Am J Gastroenterol.* 1999;94(5):1161-1171.

THERAPEUTIC IMPLICATIONS IN INFLAMMATORY BOWEL DISEASE

The compelling evidence of the protective role of smoking in UC has led to several therapeutic trials testing nicotine as the active moiety.[104-112] This section will briefly discuss the pharmacology of several nicotine-based therapies, with particular focus on nicotine gum, transdermal patches, and topically administered enemas. The findings of several clinical trials for active and maintenance UC will be reviewed. Finally, therapeutic implications and areas for future investigation will be discussed.

PHARMACOLOGY OF NICOTINE GUM, TRANSDERMAL PATCHES, AND NICOTINE ENEMAS

Nicotine is rapidly metabolized in the liver by the cytochrome P450 pathway.[113,114] Its major metabolites, cotinine and nicotine-N-oxide, are pharmacologically inactive.[113] Due to an effective first-pass hepatic metabolism, oral administration results in a bioavailability of only 20% to 44%.[115] Transdermal patches, which effectively bypass hepatic metabolism, have a mean bioavailability of 75% to 90% compared to an IV administration.[116] Nicotine enemas result in the lowest bioavailability (15% to 25% depending on formulation), providing a theoretically reduced side effect profile.[115] Delayed-release oral capsules of 3- and 6-mg nicotine tartrate delivered to the ileocolon have reported bioavailabilities of 41% and 42%, respectively.[117]

Polacrilex gum containing 4 mg of nicotine results in theoretical peak blood nicotine levels that are roughly equivalent to two-thirds that observed with cigarettes and smokeless tobacco.[118] Actual nicotine absorption delivered by chewing gum is inconsistent due to individual variations in dosing schedule, chewing duration and intensity, saliva production affecting pH-dependent absorption, and relative levels of nicotine swallowed or retained in the mouth, an important factor determining the extent of first-pass hepatic metabolism.[64] Transdermal nicotine patches offer a more reliable dose-delivery vehicle, whereby amount absorbed and steady-state plasma levels are directly proportional to the nicotine dose and duration of application.[119] A 30-mg patch delivers a maximal dose of 22 mg of nicotine and corresponds to peak and trough plasma nicotine levels equal to two-thirds the level observed with smoking.[119]

Unfortunately, both nicotine gum and patches are commonly associated with systemic side effects, particularly in nonsmokers, limiting their widespread application. This led to trials of topically administered nicotine as enemas or delayed-release oral capsule formulations. The potential advantage of these 2 modalities is to provide clinical benefits while markedly decreasing systemic bioavailability and the associated side effects.[111,112,120,121]

Trials of Nicotine Gum and Transdermal Patches

The efficacy of nicotine therapy in UC was first noted in uncontrolled trials (Table 33-2).[13,109,122-126] Initial studies of nicotine gum reported differences in ex-smokers and nonsmokers, where gum given as 4 mg at 5 to 7 sticks a day was beneficial in smokers with active colitis, but was not helpful and was poorly tolerated in nonsmokers with active disease.[13,123,125] Similarly, several uncontrolled studies of nicotine transdermal patches at doses of 15 mg/24 h and 30 mg/24 h reported a beneficial effect in active steroid-dependent UC.[109,124,126] Again, better response was seen in the former smoking versus the nonsmoking group, who generally tolerated nicotine therapy poorly.

Subsequently, 6 controlled trials of nicotine gum and transdermal therapy in UC have been performed (summarized in Table 33-3). Five evaluated the use of nicotine in active UC,[104-107,127] while one addressed the efficacy of nicotine in maintaining remission.[108] Two were randomized, placebo-controlled trials of the efficacy of transdermal nicotine therapy in mild to moderate UC.[105,106] In the first, Pullan et al randomized 72 patients with active left-sided UC to 15 to 25 mg/d of nicotine as tolerated or placebo for 6 weeks.[105] Demographics of both groups were similar, including the number of ex-smokers and nonsmokers represented. All patients were maintained on their usual medications (mesalamine in all, and low-dose prednisone in 12). The serum nicotine and cotinine concentrations were equivalent to one-third of the values of those who smoked 20 cigarettes per day. Seventeen of the 35 patients in the nicotine group had complete remission as compared to 9 of the 37 in the placebo group (*P*=0.03). The nicotine group also had greater improvement of clinical grade of colitis (*P*<0.001), histologic grade (*P*=0.03), and several other disease activity indices (*P*<0.05). However, side effects were also greater in the treatment group compared to placebo (*P*=0.002). Most frequently reported side effects included nausea, lightheadedness, headache, and contact dermatitis.

TABLE 33-4

RESPONSE IN TWO UNCONTROLLED STUDIES OF NICOTINE ENEMAS FOR ACTIVE LEFT-SIDED ULCERATIVE COLITIS

Reference (Citation)	N	Response (%)	Enema Dose	Duration
Sandborn *(120)*	7	71%	6 mg/d	4 wk
Green *(121)*	22	73%	4 mg/d	4 wk

Adapted from Sandborn WJ. Nicotine therapy for ulcerative colitis: A review of rationale, mechanisms, pharmacology, and clinical results. *Am J Gastroenterol.* 1999;94(5):1161-1171.

The most recent randomized double-blind placebo-controlled trial by Sandborn et al included 64 nonsmoking patients with mild to moderate active UC randomized to ≤22 mg transdermal nicotine (11 mg for 1 week and titrated to highest tolerated thereafter) versus placebo for 4 weeks.[106] Similar to the previous study by Pullan et al, maintenance medications (5-ASA products, oral steroids) were continued. After 4 weeks, 12 of 31 patients in the nicotine treatment group had clinical improvement compared to 3 of 33 in the placebo group (*P*=0.007). Compared to the placebo group, a significant number of adverse reactions were associated with the nicotine treatment (77% versus 30%), with 13% requiring discontinuation because of severe side effects.

Thomas et al[107] compared the efficacy of transdermal nicotine patches (n = 19) at the highest tolerated dose (25 mg/16 hr, average 20 mg) with prednisolone (n = 24) at 15 mg/d in active UC for a 6-week duration. No significant differences in remission rate were noted between the nicotine group and the steroid group, although there was a trend toward the prednisolone group being superior (45% versus 20%, *P*=0.08). The prednisolone group also had a higher response rate and lower side effect profile. Of note, all patients were withdrawn from mesalamine at day 10 of this study. Another randomized, controlled trial of 38 patients with active UC comparing transdermal nicotine therapy (15 mg/d) to prednisone (30 mg/d) tapered over 5 weeks also found no significant differences between the 2 groups, although a trend favoring the steroid group was again observed (*P*=0.05).[127] In this study, patients who maintained remission were subsequently treated with mesalamine and were followed for 6 months. Interestingly, the steroid-induced remission group had significantly more relapses than the nicotine-induced remission group.

Uncontrolled studies have evaluated other potential therapeutic roles of nicotine.[109,128] Guslandi et al[128] followed 30 patients brought into remission with mesalamine (2 g/d) and either oral prednisone (30 mg x 1 week, with subsequent taper) or transdermal nicotine (15 mg/d). After 12 months, 14 of 15 patients initially treated with mesalamine/prednisone relapsed compared to 7 of 15 patients in the mesalamine/nicotine group (P=0.007). In a recent study of 30 patients with active left-sided UC refractory to mesalamine enemas (4 g), the addition of 15 mg transdermal nicotine was superior to the addition of oral mesalamine in inducing remission (12/15 versus 5/15, P=0.027).[129] Taken together, these studies suggest that transdermal nicotine is effective in active UC at least as an adjunctive therapy. It is not clear, however, whether this is secondary to a synergistic effect of nicotine with other concomitant therapies or whether nicotine as monotherapy would also be effective.

In contrast to its efficacy as induction therapy for active UC, transdermal nicotine therapy does not appear to be effective for maintenance of remission. Only one study has addressed this question in a controlled trial.[108] Here, patients in remission were either treated with low-dose nicotine patch (15 mg/16 h) or placebo and followed for 6 months. All patients were on mesalamine during initiation of the study; however, once target nicotine dose was achieved, this was discontinued. After 6 months, 14 in the nicotine group and 17 in the placebo group relapsed (P=0.28). There are at least 2 explanations for the lack of difference. First, similar to steroids, nicotine may have a role in inducing but not maintaining remission. Alternatively, the lack of efficacy may have reflected suboptimal nicotine dosing or a sample size too small to detect a difference.

Alternative and Future Nicotine Therapies

Despite the efficacy of nicotine gum and transdermal patches in active UC, their widespread use is limited by intolerable side effects, particularly in nonsmokers. Approaches to improving the tolerability of nicotine therapy include altered drug delivery systems and the use of nicotinic receptor agonists.

Topically administered nicotine via colonic enemas or delayed-release oral formulations offers the potential advantage of maximizing local benefits (ie, at the colon) while minimizing associated side effects secondary to lower systemic bioavailability. In pharmacokinetic studies, a standard enema preparation achieves a mean maximum serum nicotine concentration of 2 to 3 ng/mL, with essentially undetectable levels after 3 to 8 hours.[115] For 3- and 6-mg delayed-release oral formulations, the mean maximum concentrations are roughly 7.3 ng/mL and 10 ng/mL, respectively. These levels are clearly lower than those seen in active smokers with UC (mean trough level 11 ng/mL) and those reported in the clinical trials with therapeutic doses of transdermal nicotine (mean trough of 8.2 ng/mL[105] and 11.3 ng/mL[106]).

These pharmacokinetic observations led to 2 open protocol pilot studies of the efficacy of nicotine enemas in active left-sided UC (Table 33-4). Both studies demonstrated clinical and endoscopic improvement. In the first study by Sandborn et al,[120] 10 patients with active left-sided UC unresponsive to 5-ASAs were treated with nicotine tartrate liquid enemas (3 mg/100 mL at 1 week then 6 mg/100 mL for 3 weeks). Five of 7 (71%) patients demonstrated a significant decrease in clinical activity and endoscopic inflammation. However, in this study 3 of 7 patients could not retain the enema. The second open study by Green et al[112] included 22 nonsmoking patients with active distal colitis treated with 6 mg/100 mL nicotine carbomer liquid enemas for 4 weeks. Patients were kept on constant doses of their pretreatment medications (prednisone in 8, mesalamine in 16) for 1 month before the trial and during the study. Sixteen of the 17 patients who completed the study had improvement in their clinical scores; 10 of 17 had endoscopic and histologic improvement. Three of the 17 achieved a full remission. Pooled data from both studies demonstrate an approximately 85% clinical response. In contrast to the transdermal nicotine therapies, minimal side effects were reported. However, obvious disadvantages of these topical therapies include difficulty of retaining tartrate enemas and utility limited to distal colitis.

A novel approach to nicotine therapy includes nicotinic receptor agonists. The nicotine receptors as a class are complex. They belong to a set of gene families that include alpha and beta subunits. The alpha subunits may function as homo-oligomers or combine with beta subunits.[130] At this time, the physiology of nicotinic receptor subtypes in the gastrointestinal tract has not been fully elucidated, but this is a fertile area for research, as it appears that different subtypes have differential expression and properties in the intestine.[131] In mice, deficiency of the nicotinic acetylcholine receptor β-4 subunit is associated with intestinal autonomic dysfunction.[132] In fact, nicotinic receptors with β-4 subunits predominate in the autonomic nervous system and are likely responsible for the nicotine-associated tachycardia and hypertension.[133] As our understanding of the receptor physiology evolves, candidate molecules may be developed that provide the benefits seen with smoking and current forms of nicotine therapies while minimizing the side effects. One promising agonist, metanicotine (TC 2403, formerly RJR-2403), a selective agonist of $\alpha_4\beta_2$ nicotinic receptors, has minimal activity at nicotinic receptors containing the β-4 subunit and is currently undergoing phase 2 investigation for the treatment of active UC.[134]

Side Effects of Nicotine therapy

Both the potential short- and long-term adverse effects of nicotine therapy limit its widespread application in clinical practice. Nicotine is a potent neuroactive compound and interacts with both central and autonomic nervous systems via nicotinic acetylcholine receptors.[135] Immediate physiologic actions of nicotine include tachycardia, increased blood pressure, and increased alertness secondary to CNS stimulation.[135] These effects often lead to undesirable side effects seen with nicotine therapy, particularly in nonsmokers. In a 4-week placebo-controlled trial of transdermal nicotine 22 mg/24 h, the overall incidence of adverse effects in the nicotine group was 77% compared to 30% for the placebo group.[106] Most frequently reported side effects include contact dermatitis, dizziness, nausea, headaches, and sleep disturbances. Because tolerance to nicotine develops rapidly, a widely used strategy in nonsmokers is to start therapy at low dose with subsequent dose escalation over days to weeks.[122,136]

Although the long-term health risks of smoking are well-established, this has been less clearly established for nicotine. Addiction, cardiovascular risks, and carcinogenesis are among the feared consequences of nicotine therapy. Studies suggest nicotine addiction does not occur with standard transdermal therapy. Nicotine addiction results from a rapid rise in plasma nicotine level with subsequent central nervous system (CNS) stimulation, as seen in smoking. In contrast, transdermal nicotine therapy results in a gradual rise in plasma levels to approximately two-thirds the level achieved with smoking.[137,138] In the 6-month trial of transdermal nicotine therapy for maintenance UC, nicotine addiction was not observed.[108] The effects of nicotine on atherogenesis and cardiovascular risk are not well-established. Although animal studies suggest nicotine may accelerate atherosclerosis, data are lacking in human studies.[139,140] A 26-week study of transdermal nicotine for maintenance of UC reported lower plasma levels of fibrinogen in the treatment group than placebo, and no differences in other parameters of platelet activation, serum lipids, or endothelial injury.[139] Finally, the association with nicotine and cancer is also inconclusive. Nicotine itself is not a carcinogen, but is a precursor to one of the carcinogens in tobacco smoke, N-nitrosamines.[141] Whether non-tobacco sources of nicotine are converted to these carcinogenic byproducts is unknown.[142]

CONCLUSIONS AND FUTURE DIRECTIONS

The compelling evidence for the negative effects of smoking in CD is now firmly established. Smoking cessation should be a major therapeutic goal in the management of CD, particularly in young women and patients with ileal disease. The beneficial effects of smoking on UC are also equally validated. However, because of the health risks associated with smoking and the availability of other treatments, it is unlikely that cigarette smoking will become standard therapy for UC. Whether nicotine replacement therapy offers equivalent benefits to smoking remains to be seen, although available data show only modest benefits when used as adjunctive therapy in mild to moderate active disease. Further studies are warranted to address appropriate therapeutic and side-effect dose response for smoking and nicotine. Comparative trials of nicotine monotherapy with other approved therapies are also needed. Controlled studies with therapeutic doses of nicotine for maintenance in UC will also be helpful. Finally, the therapeutic role of nicotine for specific clinical indications should be formally evaluated in ex-smokers with UC, pouchitis after colectomy or IPAA in PSC, and in Crohn's colitis.

Smoking continues to be one of the strongest environmental modifiers in both CD and UC. Properly studied, this can advance our understanding of these diseases. The underlying mechanisms of benefit and harm require further clarification, with particular attention to the interaction with genetic factors, such as the NOD2/CARD15 genotype. The advances in sophisticated animal models of IBD, together with the substantial progress in our understanding of the genetics of IBD, are reasons for optimism that as nicotine compounds are developed and refined, novel therapies for disease treatment and modification will become available to our patients.

REFERENCES

1. Harries AD, Baird A, Rhodes J. Non-smoking: a feature of ulcerative colitis. *Br Med J.* 1982;284:706.
2. Jick H, Walker AM. Cigarette smoking and ulcerative colitis. *N Engl J Med.* 1983;308:261-263.
3. Tobin MV, Logan RFA, Langman MJS, McConnel RB, Gilmore IT. Cigarette smoking and inflammatory bowel disease. *Gastroenterology.* 1987;93:316-321.
4. Nakamura Y, Larbarthe D. A case-control study of ulcerative colitis with relation to smoking habits and alcohol consumption in Japan. *Am J Epidem.* 1994;140:902-911.
5. Benoni C, Nilsson A. Smoking habits in patients with inflammatory bowel disease. *Gastroenterology.* 1987;22:1130-1136.
6. Boyko EJ, Koepsell TD, Perera DR, Inui TS. Risk of ulcerative colitis among former and current smokers. *N Engl J Med.* 1987;316: 707-710.
7. Franceschi S, Panza E, La Vecchia C, Parazzini F, Decarli A, Bianchi PG. Non-specific inflammatory bowel disease and smoking. *Am J Epidemiol.* 1987;125:445-452.
8. Lindberg E, Tysk C, Anderson K, et al. Smoking and inflammatory bowel disease. *Gut.* 1988;29:352-357.
9. Lorusso D, Leo S, Misciagna G, Guerra V. Cigarette smoking and ulcerative colitis: A case control study. *Hepatogastroenterol.* 1989;36:202-204.
10. Sandler RS, Sandler DP, McDonnell CW, et al. Childhood exposure to environmental tobacco smoke and the risk of ulcerative colitis. *Am J Epidemiol.* 1992;135:603-608.

11. Silverstein MD, Lashner BA, Hanauer SB. Cigarette smoking and ulcerative colitis: a case control study. *Mayo Clin Proc.* 1994;69:425-429.
12. Logan RFA, Edmond M, Somerville KW, Langman MJS. Smoking and ulcerative colitis. *BMJ.* 1984;288:751-753.
13. Roberts CJ, Diggle R. Non-smoking and ulcerative colitis. *BMJ.* 1982;285:440.
14. Reif S, Lavy A, Keter D, et al. Lack of association between smoking and Crohn's disease but the usual association with ulcerative colitis in Jewish patients in Israel: a multicenter study. *Am J Gastroenterol.* 2000;95:474-478.
15. Calkins BM. A meta-analysis of the role of smoking in inflammatory bowel disease. *Dig Dis Sci.* 1989;34:1841-1854.
16. Rubin DT, Hanauer SB. Smoking and inflammatory bowel disease. *Eur J Gastroenterol Hepatol.* 2000;12:855-862.
17. Motley RJ, Rhodes J, Kay S, et al. Late presentation of ulcerative colitis in ex-smokers. *Int J Colorectal Dis.* 1988;3:171-175.
18. Perrson PG, Alhlbom A, Hellers G. Inflammatory bowel disease and tobacco smoke: a case-control study. *Gut.* 1990;31:1377-1381.
19. Penny WJ, Penny E, Mayberery JF, et al. Prevalence of inflammatory bowel disease amongst Mormoms in Britain and Ireland. *Soc Sci Med.* 1985;21:287-290.
20. Tysk C, Jarnerot G. Has smoking changed the epidemiology of ulcerative colitis? *Scand J Gastroenterol.* 1992;27:508-512.
21. Bridger S, Lee JC, Bjarnason I, et al. In siblings with similar genetic susceptibility for inflammatory bowel disease, smokers tend to develop Crohn's disease and non-smokers develop ulcerative colitis. *Gut.* 2002;51:21-25.
22. Orholm M, Binder V, Sorensen TI, et al. Concordance of inflammatory bowel disease among Danish twins: results of a nationwide study. *Scand J Gastroenterol.* 2000;35:1075-1081.
23. Lee JC, Lennard-Jones JE. Inflammatory bowel disease in 67 families each with three or more affected first-degree relatives. *Gastroenterology.* 1996;111:587-596.
24. Motley RJ, Rhodes J, Ford GA, et al. Time relationship between cessation of smoking and onset of ulcerative colitis. *Digestion.* 1987;37:125-127.
25. Mitchell SA, Thyssen M, Orchard TR, et al. Cigarette smoking, appendectomy, and tonsillectomy as risk factors for the development of primary sclerosing cholangitis: a case control study. *Gut.* 2002;51:567-573.
26. van Erpecum KJ, Smits SM, van de Meeberg PC, et al. Risk of primary sclerosing cholangitis is associated with nonsmoking behavior. *Gastroenterology.* 1996;110:1503-1506.
27. Loftus EV, Sandborn WJ, Tremaine WJ, et al. Primary sclerosing cholangitis is associated with nonsmoking: a case-control study. *Gastroenterology.* 1996;110:1494-1502.
28. Rudra T, Motley RJ, Rhodes J. Does smoking improve colitis? *Scand J Gastroenterol.* 1989;170(Suppl):61-63.
29. Mokbel M, Carbonnel F, Beaugerie L, et al. Effect of smoking on the long-term course of ulcerative colitis. *Gastroenterologie Clinique et Biologique.* 1998;22:858-862.
30. Holdstock G, Savage D, Harman M, et al. Should patients with inflammatory bowel disease smoke? *Brit Med J (Cl Res).* 1984;288:362.
31. Fraga XF, Vergara M, Medina C, et al. Effects of smoking on the presentation and clinical course of ulcerative colitis. *Eur J Gastroenterol Hepatol.* 1997;9:683-687.
32. Woseth DM, Hanauer SB. Influence of smoking history on disease course in ulcerative colitis. *Gastroenterology.* 1998;114:A1116.
33. Odes Hs, Fich A, Reif S, et al. Effects of current cigarette smoking on clinical course of Crohn's disease and ulcerative colitis. *Dig Dis Sci.* 2001;46:1717-1721.
34. Pinczowski D, Ekborn A, Baron J, et al. Risk factors for colorectal cancer in patients with ulcerative colitis: a case-control study. *Gastroenterology.* 1994;107:117-120.
35. Merrett MN, Mortensen N, Kettlewe M, et al. Smoking may prevent pouchitis in patients with restorative proctocolectomy for ulcerative colitis. *Gut.* 1996;38:362-364.
36. Stahlberg D, Gullberg K, Liljeqvist L, et al. Pouchitis following pelvic pouch operation for ulcerative colitis: incidence, cumulative risk, and risk factors. *Dis Col Rect.* 1996;39:1012-1018.
37. Beugerie L, Massot N, Carbonnel F, et al. Impact of cessation of smoking on the course of ulcerative colitis. *Am J Gastroenterol.* 2001;96.
38. Harries AD, Baird A, Rhodes J. Non-smoking: a feature of ulcerative colitis. *BMJ.* 1982;284:706.
39. Silverstein MD, Lashner BA, Hanauer SB, Evans AA, Kirsner JB. Cigarette smoking in Crohn's disease. *Am J Gastroenterol.* 1989;84:31-33.
40. Somerville KW, Logan RFA, Edmond M, Langman MJS. Smoking and Crohn's disease. *BMJ.* 1984;289:954-956.
41. Cosnes J, Carbonnel F, Carrat F, et al. Effects of current and former cigarette smoking on the clinical course of Crohn's disease. *Aliment Pharmacol Ther.* 1999;13:1403-1411.
42. Cottone M, Rosselli M, Orlando A, et al. Smoking habits and recurrence in Crohn's disease. *Gastroenterology.* 1994;106:643-648.
43. Sutherland LR, Ramcharan S, Bryant H, Fick G. Effect of cigarette smoking on recurrence of Crohn's disease. *Gastroenterology.* 1990;98:1123-1128.
44. Moskovitz D, McLeod R, Greenberg G, et al. Operative and environmental risk factors for recurrence of Crohn's disease. *Int J Colorectal Dis.* 1999;14:224-226.
45. Breuer-Katschinski BD, Hollander N, Goebelll H. Effect of cigarette smoking on the clinical course of Crohn's disease. *Eur J Gastroenterol Hepatol.* 1996;8s:225-228.
46. Yamamoto T, Keighley MRB. Smoking and disease recurrence after operation for Crohn's disease. *Br J Surg.* 2000;87:388-404.
47. Russel MG, Volovics A, Schoon EJ, et al. Inflammatory bowel disease: Is there any relation between smoking status and disease presentation? *Inflamm Bowel Dis.* 1998;4:182-186.
48. Lindberg E, Jamerot G, Hultfeldt B. Smoking in Crohn's disease: effect on localization and clinical course. *Gut.* 1992;33:779-782.
49. Picco MF, Bayless TM. Tobacco consumption and disease duration are associated with fistulizing and stricturing behaviors in the first years of Crohn's disease. *Am J Gastroenterol.* 2003;98:363-368.
50. Louis E, Michel V, Hugot JP, et al. Early development of stricturing or penetrating pattern in Crohn's disease is influenced by disease location, number of flares, and smoking but not by NOD2/CARD15 genotype. *Gut.* 2003;52:552-557.
51. Ryan WR, Allan RN, Yamamoto T, et al. Crohn's disease patients who quit smoking have a reduced risk of reoperation for recurrence. *Am J Surg.* 2004;187:219-225.
52. Cosnes J, Beaugerie L, Carbonnel F, Gendre J-P. Smoking cessation and the course of Crohn's disease: an intervention study. *Gastroenterology.* 2001;120:1093-1099.
53. Cosnes J, Nion-Larmurier I, Afchain P, Beugerie L, Gendre J-P. Gender differences in the response of colitis to smoking. *Clin Gastroenterol Hepatol.* 2004;2:41-48.
54. Bjornsson S, Johannsson JH. Inflammatory bowel disease in Iceland, 1990-1994: a prospective, nationwide, epidemiological study. *Eur J Gastroenterol Hepatol.* 2000;12:31-38.
55. Russel MG, Nieman FH, Bergers JM, et al. Cigarette smoking and quality of life in patients with inflammatory bowel disease. *Eur J Gastroenterol.* 1996;8:1075-1081.

56. Godet PG, May GR, Sutherland LR. Meta-analysis of the role of oral contraceptive agents in inflammatory bowel disease. *Gut.* 1995;37:668-673.
57. Timmer A, Sutherland LR, Martin F. Oral contraceptive use and smoking are risk factors for relapse in Crohn's disease. The Canadian Mesalamine for Remission of Crohn's Disease Study Group. *Gastroenterology.* 1998;114:1143-1150.
58. Russel MG, Engels LG, Muris JW, et al. Modern life in the epidemiology of inflammatory bowel disease: a case-control study with special emphasis on nutritional factors. *Eur J Gastroenterol Hepatol.* 1998;10:243-249.
59. Bitton A, Peppercorn MA, Antonioli DA, et al. Clinical, biological, and histologic parameters as predictors of relapse in ulcerative colitis. *Gastroenterology.* 2001;120:13-20.
60. Zeman MV, Hiraki L, Sellers EM. Gender differences in tobacco smoking: higher relative exposure to smoke than nicotine in women. *J Womens Health Gend Based Med.* 2002;11:147-153.
61. Guo X, Ko JK, Mei QB, Cho CH. Aggravating effect of cigarette smoke exposure on experimental colitis is associated with leukotriene B(4) and reactive oxygen metabolites. *Digestion.* 2001;63:180-187.
62. Eliakim R, Fan QX, Babyatsky MW. Chronic nicotine administration differentially alters jejunal and colonic inflammation in interleukin-10 deficient mice. *Eur J Gastroenterol Hepatol.* 2002;14:607-614.
63. Rider V, Abdou NI. Gender differences in autoimmunity: Molecular basis for estrogen effects in systemic lupus erythematosus. *Int Immunopharmacol.* 2001:1009-1024.
64. Benowitz NL, Peyton J, Sanapridi C. Determination of nicotine intake while chewing polacrilex gum. *Clin Pharmacol Ther.* 1987;41:467-473.
65. Reif S, Klein I, Arber N, et al. Lack of association between smoking and inflammatory bowel disease in Jewish patients in Israel. *Gastroenterology.* 1995;108:1683-1687.
66. Fich A, Eliakim R, Sperber AD, et al. The association between smoking and inflammatory bowel disease among Israeli Jewish patients. *Inflamm Bowel Dis.* 1997;3:6-9.
67. Yang H, McElree C, Roth MP, et al. Familial empiric risks of inflammatory bowel disease: differences between Jews and non-Jews. *Gut.* 1993;34:517-524.
68. Rose JD, Roberts GM, Williams G, et al. Cardiff Crohn's disease jubilee. The incidence over 50 years. *Gut.* 1988;29:346-351.
69. Tysk C, Lindberg C, Jarnerot G, et al. Ulcerative colitis and Crohn's disease in an unselected population of monozygotic and dizygotic twins: A study of heritability and the influence of smoking. *Gut.* 1988;20:990-996.
70. Gilat T, Hacohen D, Lilos P, et al. Childhood factors in ulcerative colitis and Crohn's disease: an international cooperative study. *Scand J Gastroenterol.* 1987;22:1009-1024.
71. Lashner BA, Shaheen NJ, Hanauer SB, Kirschner BS. Passive smoking is associated with an increased risk of developing inflammatory bowel disease in children. *Am J Gastroenterol.* 1993;88:356-359.
72. Eliakim R, Reif S, Lavy A, et al. Passive smoking in patients with inflammatory bowel disease: an Israeli multicentre case-control study. *Eur J Gastroenterol Hepatol.* 2000;12:975-979.
73. Beutler B. The complex regulation and biology of TNF. *Oncogenesis.* 1990;2:9-18.
74. Holt PG, Keast D. Environmentally induced changes in immunological function: acute and chronic effects of inhalation of tobacco smoke and other atmospheric contaminants in man and experimental animals. *Bacteriol Rev.* 1977;41:205-216.
75. Miller LG, Goldstein G, Murphy M, et al. Reversible alterations in immuoregulaltory T cells in smoking. *Chest.* 1982;6:527-529.
76. Madretsma GS, Donze GJ, Van Dijk JP, et al. Nicotine inhibits the in vitro production of interleukin 2 and tumor necrosis factor-a by human mononuclear cells. *Immunopharmacology.* 1996;35:47-51.
77. Madretsma S, Wolters LM, Van Dijk JP, et al. In-vivo effect of nicotine in cytokine production by human nonadherent mononuclear cells. *Eur J Gastroenterol Hepatol.* 1996;8:1017-1020.
78. Bhatti MA, Hodgson HJ. Peripheral blood pro-inflammatory cytokine profile in active inflammatory bowel disease (IBD) differs between smokers and non-smokers. *Gut.* 1997;40(suppl):A24.
79. Bhatti MA, Hodgson HJ. Nicotine downregulates IL-8 production and tissue expression in inflammatory bowel disease. *Gastroenterology.* 1997;112:A934.
80. Sher ME, Bank S, Greenber R, et al. The influence of cigarette smoking on cytokine levels in inflammatory bowel disease. *Am J Gastroenterol.* 1996;91:1981.
81. Van Dijk JP, Meissen MA, Brouwer JJ, et al. Transdermal nicotine inhibits interleukin-2 synthesis by mononuclear cells derived from healthy volunteers. *Eur J Clin Invest.* 1998;28.
82. Louvet B, Busine MP, Desmeumaux P, et al. Transdermal nicotine decreases mucosal IL-8 expression but has no effect on mucin gene expression in ulcerative colitis. *Gastroenterology.* 1998;114:A1028.
83. Motley RJ, Rhodes J, Williams G, et al. Smoking, eicosanoids and ulcerative colitis. *J Pharmacy Pharmacol.* 1990;42:288-289.
84. Zijlstr FJ, Srivastava ED, Rhodes M, et al. Effect of nicotine on rectal mucus and mucosal eicosanoids. *Gut.* 1994;35.
85. Sopori M. Effects of cigarette smoke on the immune system. *Nat Rev Immunol.* 2002;2:372-377.
86. Wilkins JN, Carlson HE, Van Vunakis H, et al. Nicotine from cigarette smoking increases circulating levels of cortisol, growth hormones, and prolactin in male chronic smokers. *Pyschopharm.* 1992;78:305-308.
87. Sternberg EM, Chrousos GP, Wilder RL, Gold PW. The stress response and the regulation of inflammatory disease. *Ann Intern Med.* 1992;117(10):854-866.
88. Singh SP, Kalra R, Puttfarcken P, et al. Acute and chronic nicotine exposures modulate the immune system through different pathways. *Toxicol Appl Pharmacol.* 2000;164:65-72.
89. Scott AM, Kellow JE, Eckersley GM, et al. Cigarette smoking and nicotine delay postprandial mouth-cecum transit time. *Dig Dis Sci.* 1992;37:1544-1547.
90. Srivasta ED, Russell MA, Feyerabend C, et al. Effects of ulcerative colitis and smoking on rectal blood flow. *Gut.* 1990;31:1021-1024.
91. Green JT, McKirdy HC, Rhodes J, et al. Intraluminal nicotine reduces smooth muscle tone and contractile activity in the distal large bowel. *Eur J Gastrenterol Hepatol.* 1999;11:1299-1303.
92. Podolsky D, Isselbacher KJ. Glycoprotein composition of colonic mucus. *Gastroenterology.* 1984;87:991-998.
93. Cope GF, Heatley RV, Kelleher J. Smoking and colonic mucus in ulcerative colitis. *Br Med J.* 1986;293:481.
94. Ryder SD, Raouf AH, Parker N, Walker RJ, Rhodes JM. Abnormal mucosal glycoprotein synthesis in inflammatory bowel diseases is not related to cigarette smoking. *Digestion.* 1995;56:370-376.
95. Prytz H, Benoni C, Tagesson C. Does smoking tighten the gut? *Scand J Gastroenterol.* 1989;24:1084-1088.
96. Benoni C, Prytz H. Effects of smoking on the urine excretion of oral ^{51}CR EDTA in ulcerative colitis. *Gut.* 1998;42:656-658.
97. Wakefield AJ, Sankey EA, Dhillon AP, et al. Granulomatous vasculitis in Crohn's disease. *Gastroenterology.* 1991;100:1279-1287.
98. Eliakim R, Karmeli F, Rachmilewitz D, et al. Effect of chronic nicotine administration on trinitrobenzene sulphonic acid-induced colitis. *Eur J Gastrenterol Hepatol.* 1998;10:1013-1019.
99. Galeazzi F, Blennerhassett PA, Qiu B, et al. Cigarette smoke aggravates experimental colitis in rats. *Gastroenterology.* 1999;117:A1065.

100. Ko JK, Sham NF, Guo X, et al. Beneficial intervention of experimental colitis by passive cigarette smoking through the modulation of cytokines in rats. *J Invest Med.* 2001;49:21-29.
101. Hegazi R, Rao KN, Mayle A, Sepulveda AR, Otterbein LE, Plevy SE. Carbon monoxide ameliorates chronic murine colitis through a heme oxygenase 1-dependent pathway. *J Exp Med.* 2005;202(12):1703-1713.
102. Qiu B, Deng YK, Galeazzi F, Collins S. Neural involvement in the bivalent action of nicotine on experimental colitis in rats. *Gastroenterology.* 1997;112:A1065.
103. Eliakim R, Karmeli F, Cohen P. Dual effects of chronic nicotine administration augmentation of jejunitis and amelioration of colitis induced by iodoacetamide in rats. *Int J Colorectal Dis.* 2001;16:14-21.
104. Lashner BA, Hanauer SB, Silverstein MD. Testing nicotine gum for ulcerative colitis patients: experience with single-patient trials. *Dig Dis Sci.* 1990;35:827-832.
105. Pullan RD, Rhodes J, Ganesh S, et al. Trandermal nicotine for active ulcerative colitis. *N Engl J Med.* 1994;330:811-815.
106. Sandborn WJ, Tremaine WJ, Offord KP, et al. Transdermal nicotine for mildly to moderately active ulcerative colitis: a randomized double-blind, placebo-controlled trial. *Ann Intern Med.* 1997;126:364-371.
107. Thomas GAO, Rhodes J, Ragunath, et al. Transdermal nicotine compared with oral prednisolone therapy for active ulcerative colitis. *Eur J Gastroenterol.* 1996;8:769-776.
108. Thomas GAO, Rhodes J, Mani V, et al. Transdermal nicotine as maintenance therapy for ulcerative colitis. *N Engl J Med.* 1995;332:988-992.
109. Guslandi M, Tittobello A. Pilot trial of nicotine patches as an alternative to corticosteroids in ulcerative colitis. *J Gastroenterol.* 1996;31:627-629.
110. Green JT, Evans BK, Rhodes J, et al. An oral formulation of nicotine for release and absorption in the colon: its development and pharmacokinetics. *Br J Clin Pharmacol.* 1999;48:485-493.
111. Green JT, Thomas GAO, Rhodes J, et al. Pharmacokinetics of nicotine carbomer enema: a new treatment modality for ulcerative colitis. *Clin Pharmacol Ther.* 1997;61:340-348.
112. Green J, Thomas GAO, Rhodes J, et al. Nicotine enemas for active ulcerative colitis: a pilot study. *Aliment Pharmacol Ther.* 1997;11:859-863.
113. Benowitz NL, Kut F, Jacob P, et al. Cotinine disposition and effects. *Clin Pharmacol Ther.* 1983;34:604-611.
114. Kyerematen GA, Vessell ES. Metabolism of nicotine. *Drug Metab Rev.* 1991;23:3-41.
115. Zins BJ, Sandborn WJ, Mays DC, et al. Pharmacokinetics of nicotine tartrate after single-dose liquid enema, oral, and intravenous administration. *J Clin Pharmacol.* 1997;37:426-436.
116. Mulligan SC, Masterson JG, Devane JG, et al. Clinical and pharmacokinetic properties of a transdermal nicotine patch. *Clin Pharmacol Ther.* 1990:331-337.
117. Compton RF, Sandborn WJ, Lawson GM, et al. A dose-ranging pharmacokinetic study of nicotine tartrate following single-dose delayed-release oral and intravenous administration. *Aliment Pharmacol Ther.* 1997;11:865-874.
118. Benowitz NL, Porchet H, Sheiner L, et al. Nicotine absorption and cardiovascular effects with smokeless tobacco use: comparison with cigarettes and nicotine gum. *Clin Pharmacol Ther.* 1988;44:23-28.
119. Bannon YB, Corish J, Corrigan OI, et al. Transdermal delivery of nicotine in normal human volunteers: a single and multiple dose study. *Eur J Clin Pharmacol.* 1989;37:285-296.
120. Sandborn WJ, Tremaine WJ, Leighton JA. Nicotine tartrate liquid enemas for mildly to moderately active left-sided ulcerative colitis unresponsive to first-line therapy. *Aliment Pharmacol Ther.* 1997;11:663-671.
121. Green, JT, Thomas GAO, Rhodes J, et al. Nicotine enemas for active ulcerative colitis: a pilot study. *Aliment Pharmacol Ther.* 1997;11:859-863.
122. Sandborn WJ. Nicotine therapy for ulcerative colitis: A review of rationale, mechanisms, pharmacology, and clinical results. *Am J Gastroenterol.* 1999;94:1161-1171.
123. Perera DR, Janeway CM, Feld A, et al. Smoking and ulcerative colitis. *Br Med J.* 1984;288:1533.
124. Guslandi M, Tittobello A. Steroid-sparing effect of transdermal nicotine in ulcerative colitis. *J Clin Gastroenterol.* 1994;18:347-350.
125. Watson JP, Lewis RA. Ulcerative colitis responsive to smoking and to nicotine chewing gum in a patient with a1 antitrypsin deficiency. *Respir Med.* 1995;89:635-636.
126. Srivastava ED, Russel MA, Feyerabend C, et al. Transdermal nicotine in active ulcerative colitis. *Eur J Gastroenterol Hepatol.* 1991;3:815-818.
127. Guslandi M, Tittobello A. Outcome of ulcerative colitis after treatment with transdermal nicotine. *Eur J Gastroenterol.* 1998;10:513-515.
128. Guslandi M. Long-term effects of a single course of nicotine treatment in acute ulcerative colitis: remission maintenance in a 12-month follow-up study. *Int J Colorectal Dis.* 1999;14:261-262.
129. Guslandi M, Frego R, Viale E, et al. Distal ulcerative colitis refractory to rectal mesalamine: role of transdermal nicotine versus oral mesalamine. *Can J Gastroenterol.* 2002;16:293-296.
130. Papke R. The kinetic properties of neuronal nicotine receptors: genetic basis of functional diversity. *Prog Neurobiol.* 1993;41:509-531.
131. Zhou X, Ren J, Brown E, et al. Pharmacologic properties of nicotinic acetylcholine receptors expressed by guinea pig small intestinal myenteric neurons. *J Pharmacol Exp Ther.* 2002;302:889-897.
132. Wang N, Orr-Urtreger A, Chapman J, et al. Deficiency of nicotine acetylcholine receptor B_4 subunit causes autonomic cardiac and intestinal dysfunction. *Molecular Pharmacol.* 2003;63:574-580.
133. Bencherif M, Schmitt JD. Targeting neuronal nicotinic receptors: a path to new therapies. *Curr Drug Targets CNS Neurol Disord.* 2002;1:349-357.
134. Papke R, Webster J, Lipiello P, et al. The activation and inhibition of human nicotinic acetylcholine receptors by RJR-2403 indicate a selectivity for the alpha4beta2 receptor subtype. *J Neurochem.* 2000;75:204-216.
135. Benowitz NL. Pharmacologic aspects of cigarette smoking and nicotine addiction. *N Engl J Med.* 1988;319:1318-1330.
136. Porchet H, Benowitz NL, Scheiner LB. Pharmacodynamic model for tolerance: application to nicotine. *J Pharmacol Exp Ther.* 1988;244:231-236.
137. Benowitz NL, Henningfield JE. Establishing a nicotine threshold for addiction: the implications for tobacco regulation. *N Engl J Med.* 1994;331:123-125.
138. Henningfield JE, Keenan R. Nicotine delivery kinetics and abuse liability. *J Consult Clin Psychiatry.* 1993;61:743-750.
139. Thomas GAO, Davies SV, Rhodes J, et al. Is transdermal nicotine associated with cardiovascular risk? *J R Coll Physicians Lond.* 1995;29:392-396.
140. Benowitz NL. The role of nicotine in smoking-related cardiovascular disease. *Prevent Med.* 1997;26:1422-1431.
141. Carmella SG, Borukhova A, Desai D, et al. Evidence for endogenous formation of tobacco-specific nitrosamines in rats treated with tobacco alkaloids and sodium nitrite. *Carcinogenesis.* 1997;18:587-592.
142. Hecht SS, Hoffman D. The relevance of tobacco-specific nitrosamines to human cancer. *Cancer Surveys.* 1989;8:273-294.

34

Management of Steroid-Refractory and Steroid-Dependent Severe Ulcerative Colitis

Jesse A. Green, MD, FACG and Richard P. MacDermott, MD, FACG

INTRODUCTION

Glucocorticosteroids continue to be an important therapy for patients with severe ulcerative colitis (UC).[1,2] The onset of action of steroids in responders is rapid (usually within 48 hours), and they often are very effective, with response rates approaching 70% to 80%.[1,2] However, steroids are associated with many common and potentially severe side effects. Furthermore, those patients who either fail to respond to steroids or who have lost their response to steroids[3] pose a common clinical challenge in which the risks and benefits of the available medical options (immunomodulators and biologics) and the surgical options (colectomy with IPAA) must be carefully weighed and considered by both patient and physician. It will be the purpose of this chapter to review our current approach to the steroid-refractory and steroid-dependent ulcerative colitis patient, who has either chronic severe (moderate to severe) or acute severe (fulminant) ulcerative colitis.

Definition of Steroid-Refractory and Steroid-Dependent Ulcerative Colitis

While it is common practice to treat patients with steroids for at least 6 months before determining a patient to have steroid-refractory UC, there is no well-accepted clear definition of steroid-dependent disease. Feagan et al defines steroid-dependent disease as that which does not respond to more than 3 months of treatment with steroids.[4]

Therefore, in chronic, steroid-dependent, moderate to severe UC, even though the UC is inactive on therapeutic doses of steroids, the disease flares either at low doses or relapses shortly after discontinuation of steroids, and the patient is unable to successfully discontinue the steroids. Chronic, moderate to severe UC patients who are both steroid-refractory and steroid-dependent have severe active UC, which is both unresponsive to high-dose steroids and which worsens when attempting to taper the steroids.

OVERALL APPROACH TO THE STEROID-REFRACTORY AND STEROID-DEPENDENT ULCERATIVE COLITIS PATIENT

It is critical to make an overall assessment of the patient before adding new medications to his or her current medical regimen. We must ask several important questions. First, does the patient have chronic severe (moderate to severe) or acute severe (fulminant) UC? While the chronic severe (moderate to severe) patient can be treated as an outpatient, the acute severe (fulminant) patient needs to be immediately hospitalized. Second, does the patient have either significant blood work abnormalities or findings consistent with toxic (fulminant) disease on abdominal imaging studies, which might require emergent care? Third, have all other possible causes of bloody diarrhea been excluded? A limited, cautious sigmoidoscopic or colonoscopic exam (performed only in the absence of contraindications) with biopsies and samples for culture may provide critically important information on whether or not there is another cause that could explain the steroid-refractory and steroid-dependent disease course in the acutely or chronically ill UC patient. Important causes of bloody diarrhea to consider include *Clostridium difficile*, hemorrhagic

Lichtenstein GR, ed.
Ulcerative Colitis: The Complete Guide to Medical Management (pp 381-392)

E. coli 0157:H7, *Salmonella*, *Shigella*, *Campylobacter*, cytomegalovirus (CMV), Amebiasis, NSAIDs, Crohn's colitis, ischemic colitis, and radiation colitis. CMV has all too often been overlooked in many cases of severe steroid-refractory and steroid-dependent UC, and it is therefore of particular importance to have mucosal biopsies examined carefully by an expert pathologist for evidence of CMV.[5]

Fourth, is the current extent and severity of the UC known and documented? If not, this may be another reason for a limited, cautious sigmoidoscopic or colonoscopic exam initially, followed by a complete exam after the patient has stabilized. Fifth, has the patient lost significant amounts of weight and/or is the patient malnourished? If so, the patient may require nutritional repletion either with total parenteral nutrition or enteral hyperalimentation prior to giving a malnourished and already immunocompromised patient immunomodulators and biologics. Sixth, are there any extraintestinal manifestations or complications that might influence the choice of therapeutic regimens? For example, the presence of pyoderma gangrenosum or ankylosing spondylitis would be an additional argument to initiate therapy with infliximab, while the presence of ocular inflammation would necessitate an immediate referral to an ophthalmologist prior to embarking on further therapy. Seventh, have the basic approaches to the short-term and long-term side effects of steroids been addressed in the patient? For example, has the patient had a DEXA scan and been placed on appropriate osteoporosis prevention strategies? In addition, does the patient have elevated blood sugars or hemoglobin A1C levels; does the patient have hypertension; has the patient seen an ophthalmologist for glaucoma and cataract screening; and has the patient had problems with mood, personality, or sleep disorders?

Eighth, does the patient understand UC and all of the therapeutic options available? Educational literature and books from the Crohn's and Colitis Foundation of America (www.CCFA.org) can be very helpful. Finally, how stable is the patient's psychological and family support at this time? If the patient is to experience long-term success in coping with severe UC, stable emotional and family support is crucial. Having the patient and other family members work with social workers, psychologists, and psychiatrists can be very helpful as the individual attempts to deal with his or her medical issues.

MECHANISMS OF STEROID RESISTANCE

Glucocorticoids exert their anti-inflammatory effect primarily through inhibition of the gene promoter regions for proinflammatory cytokines, chemokines, and adhesion molecules. This effect occurs by inhibition of the activity of intracellular transcription factors (eg, nuclear factor kB; NF-kB) that promote gene activation.[6] Reduced numbers of glucocorticoid receptors (GCRs), decreased GCR binding affinity, and/or poor DNA binding affinity for GCR, are possible causes of dysfunction at the level of the glucocorticoid receptor, which could lead to impaired glucocorticoid signaling and subsequent steroid resistance in IBD.[6] It is also possible that the excessive production of proinflammatory mediators overwhelms the effects of steroids, resulting in inhibition of glucocorticoid receptor transcriptional activity, with subsequent decreased affinity of the steroid-receptor complex for intracellular ligands.[6] Another possible explanation is that T cell proliferation is relatively resistant to glucocorticoid inhibition in steroid-resistant ulcerative colitis patients.

Multidrug resistance (MDR) has been described in neoplastic cells developing cross-resistance to a wide range of cytotoxic agents following exposure to only one cytotoxic agent. Interestingly, peripheral blood lymphocytes and colonic mucosal cells in steroid-refractory IBD patients exhibit overexpression of MDR1, which may lead to decreased cytoplasmic glucocorticoid concentrations caused by increased P-glycoprotein-mediated efflux of glucocorticoid from the cells.[7] In addition, a MDR1 polymorphism has been found to be associated with IBD.[7] Experimentally, in vitro analysis of T lymphocyte steroid resistance has been demonstrated in preliminary studies to possibly be a predictor of whether or not a patient may respond to steroid therapy.[7] Therefore, it is possible that in the future, we may have objective tests that are capable of identifying those patients who have an increased likelihood of developing steroid resistance.

CLINICAL ASSESSMENT OF DISEASE ACTIVITY

Prior to embarking upon a particular course of therapy for the patient with steroid-refractory and/or steroid-dependent UC, it is important to assess disease activity. This permits the clinician to discern whether there is sufficient time to try medical therapy prior to emergency colectomy. In a study of 56 clinical features, 4 were found to yield the greatest predictive value: maximum daily body temperature, maximum daily pulse rate, bowel frequency, and plasma albumin.[9] In particular, stool frequency (more than 8 per day) and elevated body temperature (>38°C) were highly predictive of the need for colectomy during that hospital admission.[9] Subsequently, elevated CRP was also found to be an important predictive factor of severity.[10] Other prognostic indicators of severity include a severe initial episode and extensive UC,[2,3] as well as 3 or more distended small bowel loops on the initial plain abdominal film.[11]

Clinical observations and laboratory findings can be helpful when deciding whether to commit the patient to additional medical therapy with immunomodulators or biologics as opposed to colectomy for the steroid-refractory and steroid-dependent UC patient. The very severe or fulminant UC patient with multiple major laboratory abnormalities should be strongly encouraged to have a colectomy. Clinical observations and laboratory findings can also help to facilitate the distinction between underlying IBS symptoms vs symptoms due to inflammation in the chronic severe (moderate to severe) steroid-refractory patient. For example, if the patient's symptoms suggest IBS and alarm features are absent, we do not need to immediately institute immunomodulators or biologics, but rather should assess the patient's response to symptom-based antispasmodic and antidiarrheal therapy.[12]

ANTIBIOTICS, FISH OIL, AND NICOTINE IN THE PATIENT WITH CHRONIC SEVERE (MODERATE TO SEVERE) STEROID-REFRACTORY AND STEROID-DEPENDENT ULCERATIVE COLITIS

A pilot study of 7 inpatients, who failed to respond to 1 week of IV steroid therapy, demonstrated a response to broad-spectrum triple-drug antibiotic therapy using ampicillin, gentamicin, and metronidazole, with clinical improvement documented in all 7 patients by resolution of diarrhea and rectal bleeding; defervescence; and normalization of leukocytosis and bandemia.[13] An initial trial of tobramycin in UC demonstrated that treatment with oral tobramycin improved the short-term outcome of patients with acute UC.[14] However, a small underpowered, randomized, prospective controlled trial of tobramycin and metronidazole in patients with acute, severe UC revealed no difference in the response rates of the treatment vs placebo groups.[15] A benefit of rifaximin in UC in a small prospective, controlled trial has been reported, but has not been conclusively demonstrated, and rifaximin will need further evaluation in large double-blind, randomized studies.[16]

In the chronic severe (moderate to severe) steroid-refractory UC patient, fish oils containing eicosapentaenoic acid may be of benefit.[17-19] These lipids were initially noted to attenuate colitis in experimental animal models. Fish oils have been postulated to maintain mucosal membrane integrity and/or suppress the inflammatory response. Diets replete with omega-3 fatty acids have been shown to reduce human blood monocyte TNFα production, as well as the production of proinflammatory mediators such as leukotriene B4. Controlled trials of omega-3 fatty acids in chronic severe (moderate to severe) steroid-refractory UC patients have demonstrated a significant reduction in disease activity compared to controls.[17-19] In addition, omega-3 fatty acids have been shown to reduce rectal leukotriene B4 levels by shunting the leukotriene pathway to produce leukotriene B5 preferentially and less leukotriene B4. Leukotriene B5 has less chemoattractant activity to polymorphonuclear leukocytes. This lowered leukotriene B4 level allows patients to reduce their steroid dose.[18] Limitations to the use of fish oil have included the high dose, which must be used (9 g/d); the "fishy" odor that can emanate from some patients; and its unpleasant taste at times. Fish oil has not been shown to maintain remission in ulcerative colitis.

It has been observed that the onset of UC can be associated with smoking cessation in some patients (see Chapter 33) and that resumption of smoking in some of those patients can occasionally be an effective treatment strategy. Investigators have therefore examined nicotine as a therapeutic approach for steroid-refractory and steroid-dependent UC. The potential mechanism of action for nicotine in refractory UC has been thought to include suppression of cellular and humoral immunity and inhibition of leukotriene B4-modulated inflammation.[20] Controlled trials have demonstrated efficacy for transdermal nicotine in patients with steroid-refractory and steroid-dependent UC.[21,22] While the side effects of the nicotine patch have been tolerated in former smokers, the side effects in nonsmokers have often been troublesome, including nausea, vomiting, dizziness, tachycardia, central nervous system (CNS) stimulation, and hypertension. Although nicotine enemas have not been found to be efficacious for active UC,[23] the development of alternative strategies for delivering nicotine to the inflamed mucosa in the steroid-refractory and/or -dependent UC patient may provide future approaches to make nicotine treatment more tolerable by reducing some of the nicotine side effects.

In summary, the clinical trial data available to date fail to convincingly support a role for antibiotic therapy in chronic severe (moderate to severe) steroid-refractory and steroid-dependent UC. In selected patients, fish oil and/or nicotine may represent reasonable approaches to help reduce the steroid dose. These approaches may be particularly important in patients who are poor surgical candidates or those who wish to avoid colectomy. However, patients need to be told in advance about potential side effects, particularly with respect to the use of nicotine patches.

6-MERCAPTOPURINE/AZA IN THE PATIENT WITH CHRONIC SEVERE (MODERATE TO SEVERE) STEROID-REFRACTORY AND STEROID-DEPENDENT ULCERATIVE COLITIS

6-MP (Purinethol) and AZA (Imuran, Azasan) have both been successfully used for many years in patients with chronic severe (moderate to severe) UC who are steroid-refractory and steroid-dependent. Both 6-MP and AZA have been shown to be effective by inducing remission, improving overall symptoms, and allowing the dose of steroids to be reduced.[24-27] 6-MP and AZA also are both effective in maintaining remission in patients who have had their remission induced by 6-MP or AZA.[25,28]

During the last 3 decades, several controlled trials of AZA in UC have supported their use for induction of remission and also for maintenance of remission.[29-38] AZA was observed to be as effective as sulfasalazine in proctocolitis, in a study conducted over only a 3-month study period.[30] A placebo-controlled study by Sood et al found that AZA had no effect in achieving remission in patients with severe UC when given in combination with prednisolone, but was linked to a lower proportion of relapses compared with placebo.[31] A retrospective chart review of 105 patients concluded that 6-MP is an effective and safe alternative for chronic severe (moderate to severe) steroid-refractory UC patients.[31] This contrasted with results from an earlier study using AZA in UC, which did not demonstrate that AZA could prevent relapse after 12 months of treatment.[32] In evaluating the effectiveness of AZA for maintaining remission, chronic severe (moderate to severe) steroid-refractory UC patients, who were in remission for 2 months on a median dose of 100 mg of AZA, were randomized to receive either continued AZA or placebo.[33] Patients who continued on the AZA had a 1-year relapse rate of 36%, while those on placebo had a higher relapse rate of 59% (P=0.04), which demonstrated the ability of AZA to serve as maintenance therapy for AZA-responsive UC.[33] In another study, 6-MP induced remission in 65% of chronic severe (moderate to severe) steroid-refractory ulcerative colitis patients within 40 weeks, and when the patients discontinued 6-MP, there was a very high relapse rate of 87%.[31] Acute severe (fulminant) ulcerative colitis patients who were in remission induced by intravenous cyclosporine for steroid-refractory severe UC, have been shown to have their remission maintained on AZA.[34] Finally, both AZA and 6-MP have been found to be effective as steroid-sparing agents in patients with chronic severe (moderate to severe) steroid-refractory and steroid-dependent ulcerative colitis.[35-38]

6-MP and AZA pose toxicity concerns of their own, which have been categorized as 1) allergic-type, dose-independent (eg, fever, rash, pancreatitis) and 2) nonallergic, dose- and metabolism-dependent (eg, thrombocytopenia, leukopenia, hepatitis, malignancy).[29] Reversible short-term side effects, due to 6-MP or AZA, have been noted in up to 10% of patients and include fever, rash, nausea, and headaches.[39] Pancreatitis occurs in 2% to 4% of patients on 6-MP or AZA, and the patient should never be restarted on either medication.[39] The development of opportunistic infections in patients on immunomodulators plus steroids should be watched for carefully, because both medications suppress the immune system.

Bone marrow suppression and mild hepatitis (transaminitis) can be reversed by lowering the 6-MP or AZA dosage. The need for close monitoring of the complete blood count (CBC) (eg, every 1 to 2 weeks initially then every 3 months indefinitely) has been clearly demonstrated.[40] AZA is a prodrug that is enzymatically converted to 6-MP, which is then converted to the active moiety, 6-thioguanine (6-TG). This nucleotide is a purine analog that inhibits the synthesis of DNA, RNA, and protein.[41,42] 6-MP is also metabolized to several other metabolites including 6-methylmercaptopurine (6-MMP).[41,42] Thiopurine methyltransferase (TPMT) is the primary enzyme responsible for catalyzing these reactions.[41,42] The levels of 6-TG and 6-MMP depend upon the variations of the genetic polymorphisms of TPMT in each individual patient.[41,42] Levels of erythrocyte 6-TG and 6-MMP correlate with toxicity.[41,42] TPMT deficiency causes AZA or 6-MP to be preferentially metabolized toward the excessive production of 6-TG nucleotides, which results in leukopenia.[41,42] However, adequate 6-TG levels correlate with 6-MP or AZA efficacy in ulcerative colitis. Monitoring of 6-TG levels can guide dose adjustments of 6-MP or AZA in order to optimize the likelihood of a therapeutic response. In nonresponding UC patients, in whom nonadherence is suspected, low or absent metabolite concentrations may be helpful to differentiate UC patients who are not taking their medications from those who do not respond to 6-MP or AZA.[41,42] Hepatotoxicity is correlated with elevated 6-MMP levels.[41,42] The positive and negative predictive value of 6-MMP regarding hepatotoxicity remain largely unexplored in any controlled fashion. Therefore, the bone marrow and liver toxicity associated with 6-MP and AZA is related to TPMT activity and subsequent levels of 6-TG and 6-MMP. Although the toxicities are reversible by discontinuing or lowering the dose of 6-MP or AZA, this would result in a lowering of the 6-TG levels needed to achieve treatment of the ulcerative colitis.

Intermediate TPMT enzyme activity has been observed in up to 11% of the population, with 0.3% having low activity.[41,42] It is possible that detection of very low or absent TPMT activity prior to introducing therapy can help avert potentially life-threatening bone marrow toxicity. Therefore, when starting UC patients on 6-MP or AZA therapy, determining TPMT genotype or phenotype may predict the likelihood of toxicity because patients with low TPMT activity are at increased risk of experiencing myelosuppression.[41,42] Based on controlled trials in IBD, 1.0 to 1.5 mg/kg/d doses of 6-MP and 2.0 to 2.5 mg/kg/d doses of AZA appear to be efficacious. Although the traditional approach is to begin at a 50 mg/d dose and increase based on clinical and laboratory criteria, the alternative now available is to obtain a baseline TPMT level to identify patients with low or absent activity. Those patients with normal TPMT enzymes can be started on higher initial doses of 6-MP or AZA, while those patients with intermediate TPMT enzyme levels (as has been suggested by some but not all investigators) and/or activity should be started on a very low dose of 6-MP or AZA.[41,42] In patients with absent or low TPMT enzyme activity, 6-MP or AZA should be avoided altogether due to the high risk of severe, sometimes fatal myelosuppression.[41,42] If the patient responds well clinically, then frequent monitoring for therapeutic 6-TG levels does not seem warranted. However, if questions arise regarding efficacy or toxicity, then assessing 6-TG and 6-MMP levels may be helpful. Regardless, monthly CBC and liver tests every 3 months should be obtained as long as the patient is on 6-MP or AZA.

Concern has been raised regarding the potential risk of lymphoma in IBD patients treated with 6-MP or AZA.[39,43] The use of immunomodulators in Epstein-Barr virus (EBV) positive IBD patients may increase the likelihood of developing lymphoma.[43] EBV-positive lymphomas have been described in IBD patients receiving 6-MP or AZA.[44] Some IBD patients with EBV-positive lymphoma can be successfully treated by 6-MP or AZA withdrawal.[44] A meta-analysis that evaluated 6 studies in patients with Crohn's disease who were treated with 6-MP or AZA revealed 11 lymphomas versus an expected number of 2.71 and concluded that 6-MP or AZA use in IBD is associated with a fourfold increase in the incidence of lymphoma in IBD patients.[45] This demonstrated that there was 1 lymphoma per 2000 patient-years of follow-up versus 1 lymphoma in approximately 8000 patient-years of follow-up in patients with Crohn's who did not have 6-MP/AZA exposure. The risk in this study could be either due to the medications themselves or the disease activity. It is difficult to distinguish among these. Ultimately, the decision to use 6-MP or AZA must be considered carefully, by weighing the risks and benefits for the individual patient.

Therefore, in summary, either 6-MP or AZA are very appropriate for consideration in chronic severe (moderate to severe) steroid-refractory UC patients who have failed to respond to steroids or patients who are dependent on steroids. At this time, there does not appear to be proven additional clinical benefit when adding 5-ASA products to AZA for maintenance of remission in steroid-dependent ulcerative colitis patients.[46] 6-MP or AZA, unlike 5-ASA agents and steroids, often take 4 to 6 months to demonstrate their full effect. Therefore, 6-MP or AZA should only be initiated in chronic severe (moderate to severe) steroid-refractory UC patients who can endure an additional 4 to 6 months of their disease activity as well as the cumulative steroid side effects. Once a desired therapeutic effect is achieved, 6-MP or AZA is usually continued for 3 to 4 years. There are some individuals who advocate consideration for slight dose reduction at that point for long-term maintenance, whereas others do not follow this practice. Given the lack of any prospective data on this topic, this remains an area of controversy. Acute severe (fulminant) UC patients are not candidates for 6-MP or AZA, but rather require hospitalization for IV steroids and IV antibiotics.[47]

INFLIXIMAB IN THE PATIENT WITH CHRONIC SEVERE (MODERATE TO SEVERE) STEROID-REFRACTORY AND STEROID-DEPENDENT ULCERATIVE COLITIS

The use of infliximab in chronic severe (moderate to severe) steroid-refractory ulcerative colitis was initially studied in 11 patients.[48] Patients received either placebo, infliximab at 5 mg/kg, infliximab at 10 mg/kg, or infliximab at 20 mg/kg.[48] Fifty percent (4 of 8) of patients who received infliximab were considered treatment successes at 2 weeks, in comparison to none of the 3 who received placebo.[48] In patients who received infliximab, improvement in ESR, CRP, and IL-6 correlated with a clinical response.[48] Five of 6 infliximab-treated patients who underwent sigmoidoscopic evaluations had improvement. These results suggested that infliximab administered at 5, 10, or 20 mg/kg/d was tolerated well and might provide clinical benefit to patients with chronic severe (moderate to severe) steroid-refractory UC. In an uncontrolled study, a clinical response was observed in 88% to 100% of infliximab-treated patients with chronic severe (moderate to severe) steroid-refractory UC refractory to conventional therapy.[49] It has also been observed that patients with UC who are refractory to corticosteroids are less likely to respond to infliximab.[50]

The ACT 1 and ACT 2 multicenter, clinical trials have demonstrated the benefit of infliximab in chronic, severe (moderate to severe) steroid-refractory UC patients.[51] UC patients who received infliximab at 0, 2, and 6 weeks in the ACT 1 trial had a 69% (5 mg/kg) and 61% (10 mg/kg) clinical response rate after 8 weeks, compared with a placebo clinical response rate of 37%.[51] UC patients in the ACT 2 trial had a 64% (5 mg/kg) and 69% (10 mg/kg) clinical response rate after 8 weeks, compared with a placebo clinical response rate of 29%.[51] At week 54 in the ACT 1 trial, the clinical response rates were 45% (5 mg/kg), 44% (10 mg/kg), and 20% (placebo); and the clinical remission rates were 35% (5 mg/kg), 34% (10 mg/kg), and 17% for the placebo group.[51] Infliximab, therefore, is an important therapeutic option in patients with chronic, severe (moderate to severe) steroid-refractory UC.[47-51]

The development of primary and disseminated tuberculosis in infliximab-treated patients was the first major infection and significant side effect observed secondary to infliximab. Additional major infections observed in patients treated with infliximab have included pneumonia, sepsis, urinary tract infections, abscesses, and peritonitis. Systemic fungal infections, including coccidioidomycosis, aspergillosis, histoplasmosis, candidiasis, and *Pneumocystis jiroveci* pneumonia, have also been described in patients treated with infliximab. Many of these infections occurred in patients receiving concurrent immunosuppressives, including corticosteroids, AZA, 6-MP, or methotrexate. The increased risk of infection associated with all of these immunosuppressive agents is well-recognized. Furthermore, it has been demonstrated that the use of corticosteroids, whether alone or in conjunction with immunomodulators, increases the risk of postoperative infectious complications in patients undergoing surgery for IBD.[52] Therefore, chronic severe (moderate to severe) steroid-refractory UC patients being treated with infliximab should be completely tapered off of steroids as rapidly as possible in order to help further decrease the risk of opportunistic infections.[53-55] Kunitake et al found preoperative treatment with infliximab was not associated with an increased rate of cumulative postoperative complications in 413 consecutive patients with IBD undergoing abdominal surgery.[53] In contrast, a prospective study by Selvasekar et al found that patients with chronic ulcerative colitis who were treated with infliximab before undergoing IPAA have a nearly threefold increased risk of postoperative pouch-related and infectious complications.[55] Furthermore, a study by Schluender et al showed no increase in preoperative complications with infliximab alone, but did find a high rate of complications among patients using both infliximab and cyclosporine A before colectomy in refractory UC.[54]

NOVEL INVESTIGATIONAL AGENTS IN THE PATIENT WITH CHRONIC SEVERE (MODERATE TO SEVERE) STEROID-REFRACTORY AND STEROID-DEPENDENT ULCERATIVE COLITIS

A number of new agents are currently being evaluated for patients with chronic severe (moderate to severe) steroid-refractory UC. RDP-58 is a D-amino acid decapeptide that inhibits the transcription, translation, and production of TNFα, IL-2, IL-12, and gamma-interferon.[56] The D-amino acid configuration renders the agent resistant to protease degradation, thus tempering its potential toxicity. In a randomized, double-blind, placebo-controlled study, the treatment success rate was higher in patients receiving either the 200 mg/kg (71%) or 300 mg/kg (72%) dose of RDP-58 compared to placebo (43%).[57] In addition, the 200-mg and 300-mg RDP-58 groups also demonstrated improvement in histological scores in comparison with placebo.[57,58]

MLN-02 is a humanized monoclonal antibody that targets leukocytes expressing α4β7 integrins, resulting in inhibition of the migration of leukocytes into the inflamed mucosa.[59] In a study of MLN-02, 181 patients with chronic, moderately active steroid-refractory UC were randomized to receive 6 weeks of MLN-02 at 0.5 mg/kg, 2 mg/kg or placebo. The rates of clinical response and clinical remission were significantly higher in both treatment arms versus placebo.[59] The mean duration of response was approximately 90 days.[59] However, due to the development of progressive multifocal leukoencephalopathy in patients enrolled in clinical trials investigating natalizumab, which is a different monoclonal anti-adhesion molecule, trials of MLN-02 and other adhesion molecule inhibitors in IBD have currently been halted until all potential safety concerns can be addressed.[60]

Visilizumab (HuM291; a humanized anti-CD3 monoclonal antibody) given intravenously to severe, steroid-refractory ulcerative colitis patients led to a rapid improvement by day 15, with 84% of the patients in remission at day 30.[61] Seventy percent of patients given visilizumab 10 mcg/kg/d and 75% of patients given visilizumab 15 mcg/kg/d infusions on days 1 and 2 were in endoscopic remission on day 30.[61] After 1 year, 5 out of 8 patients given visilizumab 15 mcg/kg/d infusions on days 1 and 2 remained relapse-free.[61] The patients were all negative for EBV at baseline, but EBV titers rose in most patients, returning to baseline levels concurrent with T cell repopulation. No serious infectious complications were found. If these results could have been confirmed in randomized, double-blinded, placebo-controlled trials, and if major side effects were not seen, visilizumab might have been an important future treatment for steroid-refractory UC patients.[61] A recent decision by Protein Design Labs was made to stop evaluation of visilizumab in patients with IBD.

Epidermal growth factor (EGF) in enema form has shown early promise in a study of 24 patients, who were simultaneously treated with oral 5-ASA.[62] Ten out of 12 patients treated with EGF enemas plus oral 5-ASA achieved remission for the first 4 weeks of the study, and 8 of 12 remained in remission at 12 weeks. However, a theoretical concern pertaining to EGF is its potential to induce neoplasia because an anti-EGF agent has recently been approved for treatment of colorectal carcinoma.

Daclizumab, a humanized monoclonal antibody against the IL-2 receptor, given intravenously (1 mg/kg) twice over a 4-week period, led to a clinical response in 10 patients, with remission seen in 5 patients at 8 weeks.[63]

Finally, the use of helminth ova (Trichuris suis; pig whipworm) has been evaluated in 54 patients in a randomized, double-blind, placebo-controlled, crossover trial.[64] There was improvement in 43.3% of active ulcerative colitis patients treated with Trichuris suis ova, as opposed to 16.7% of patients treated with placebo.[64] Trichuris suis ova, which do not colonize humans, may prove to be an effective therapy in UC in the future.[64]

CYCLOSPORINE IN THE PATIENT WITH ACUTE SEVERE (FULMINANT) STEROID-REFRACTORY ULCERATIVE COLITIS

In patients presenting with acute severe (fulminant) ulcerative colitis requiring hospitalization for IV corticosteroid treatment, up to 75% will exhibit a partial or complete response within 1 week. For the 25% who fail to improve, the major considerations are IV cyclosporine, IV infliximab, and colectomy.[47] Cyclosporine is a rapidly acting immunosuppressant that works by targeting and inhibiting serine/threonine phosphatase calcineurin, which results in decreased T cell activation.[65] IV cyclosporine has been shown to be effective for acute severe (fulminant) UC patients who have not responded to high-dose IV corticosteroids.[65,66] In 20 patients with severe, steroid-refractory UC, cyclosporine (at a dose of 4 mg/kg/d continuously infused over 14 days) induced remission in 9 of 11 treated patients (82%) compared to none of those receiving placebo.[66] In a subsequent underpowered randomized study of 30 patients, 64% of the cyclosporine-treated group responded at 8 days, in contrast to 53% of patients who had been randomized to receive methylprednisolone.[67] In another underpowered, randomized study of 30 patients comparing cyclosporine 4 mg/kg/d alone to cyclosporine plus methylprednisolone, only 67% in the monotherapy group achieved complete remission after 7 days, compared with 93% in the combination therapy group.[68]

Typically, patients are treated at least 7 to 10 days with parenteral corticosteroids prior to embarking on therapy with cyclosporine.[69] IV cyclosporine (2 to 4 mg/kg/d) can induce a rapid remission in approximately 80% of patients.[69] However, 30% to 50% of responders who do not use a concurrent immunomodulator ultimately require colectomy within the first 6 months for persistent symptoms or drug intolerance.[65-72] Therefore, cyclosporine is most commonly used as a "bridge" to beginning 6-MP or AZA.[65-72] Data from a long-term follow-up study by Cohen et al suggests that patients who are naïve to AZA/6-MP upon initiation of cyclosporine plus AZA/6-MP have improved outcomes compared with those who have failed treatment with AZA/6-MP and are then given cyclosporine in addition to continued 6-MP/AZA.[73] If either 6-MP or AZA is used concurrently, the rates for colectomy decrease, and approximately 60% to 70% of those individuals who respond initially will avoid colectomy.[65-72] With the use of 6-MP or AZA after cyclosporine salvage in corticosteroid-resistant patients, several studies have documented excellent long-term responses: 90% remission in one series and 65% complete and 24% partial response in other series.[67,68,71] Therefore, adding 6-MP or AZA within the first month of cyclosporine therapy, with subsequent conversion to long-term immunomodulators without cyclosporine, increases the chances of long-term remission.[65-67]

The possible side effects associated with cyclosporine can be very significant in IBD, and therefore the risks and benefits pertaining to the use of cyclosporine must be carefully weighed and discussed in detail with the patient prior to beginning therapy. The major concern about using cyclosporine is its potential toxicity, including severe, opportunistic infections; nephrotoxicity; hypertension; seizures; peripheral neuropathy; and anaphylaxis. Fatal outcome due to *Pneumocystis carinii* pneumonia (PCP) has been reported in IBD patients receiving cyclosporine. This has prompted the use of PCP prophylaxis with cotrimoxazole or inhaled pentamidine in patients who are using concurrent corticosteroids.[74] Another report documented a 3% colonic perforation and a 3% postoperative death rate in 32 patients who received cyclosporine after failing IV corticosteroids.[75] Blood levels of cyclosporine must be monitored carefully during its administration. Before use of cyclosporine, serum cholesterol should be evaluated because very low levels of cholesterol can predispose to seizures. Cyclosporine is contraindicated during breast-feeding and should be avoided in pregnancy. Occasionally, however, the benefit-to-risk ratio may favor the use of cyclosporine in certain pregnant patients with severe refractory UC for whom surgery is not an option. In a randomized, double-blind, controlled trial, 2 mg/kg of IV cyclosporine has been found to be equivalent to 4 mg/kg of cyclosporine in terms of efficacy for treating severe, steroid-refractory acute UC.[71] Although no differences in adverse effects were observed in the study, it is hypothesized that the lower cyclosporine dose may translate into an improved long-term toxicity profile.[71] In elderly patients, there is a very high risk of opportunistic infections, and therefore the dose of cyclosporine should be reduced.

INFLIXIMAB IN THE PATIENT WITH ACUTE SEVERE (FULMINANT) STEROID-REFRACTORY ULCERATIVE COLITIS

The use of infliximab in hospitalized patients with acute severe or moderately severe ulcerative colitis, who did not respond to high-dose IV steroids, has been examined.[76] Overall, 67% of patients on placebo required colectomy compared with 29% of patients treated with infliximab over a period of 90 days.[76] The best response to infliximab was seen in hospitalized patients with acute moderately severe UC, with none requiring colectomy, compared with 62.5% of the patients receiving placebo.[76] Therefore, in hospitalized patients with acute severe or moderately severe steroid-refractory UC, infliximab has been shown to be effective.[76] It is unclear whether cyclosporine or infliximab should be used first for a patient with acute severe steroid-refractory UC who is potentially facing a colectomy. It should be emphasized, however, that cyclosporine should not be administered to patients who are hospitalized and initially received infliximab, due to the long biologic half-life of this agent and the potential for significant immunosuppression that may ensue.[77] Additional controlled studies will be needed to evaluate this issue. Currently, however, gastroenterologists are very comfortable using infliximab for Crohn's disease, and, therefore, infliximab may be preferred over cyclosporine for patients with acute severe UC, refractory to IV steroids.

USE OF COLECTOMY AS A POTENTIAL CURE FOR THE PATIENT WITH CHRONIC SEVERE (MODERATE TO SEVERE) OR ACUTE SEVERE (FULMINANT) STEROID-REFRACTORY AND STEROID-DEPENDENT ULCERATIVE COLITIS

Colectomy is our only potential cure for the patient with acute or chronic severe steroid-refractory and steroid-dependent UC.[78] Colectomy not only removes the diseased colon and its associated risks but also allows the discontinuation and avoidance of high-dose steroids, 6-MP/AZA, cyclosporine, and/or infliximab, thereby decreasing the risk of opportunistic infections and other side effects due to these medications.[78] The recognized indications for colectomy in ulcerative colitis include 1) toxic megacolon with impending or actual perforation, 2) massive, persistent hemorrhage, 3) fulminant acute colitis nonresponsive to corticosteroid therapy, 4) chronic, steroid-refractory and steroid-dependent ulcerative colitis, 5) presence of dysplasia or carcinoma, and 6) colonic stricture with obstruction or patient desire to have surgery due to significantly impaired quality of life.[78]

For patients with acute, severe steroid-refractory ulcerative colitis, emergency colectomy has long been an important therapeutic alternative, and its efficacy has been well-documented.[78,79] Colectomy also has an important role in patients with chronic, steroid-refractory and steroid-dependent UC.[78,80] Prior to the early 1980s, single-stage proctocolectomy with the creation of a Brooke ileostomy was the surgical procedure of choice for treating UC. Occasional problems with this procedure have included stomal complications, bowel obstruction, genitourinary problems, and sexual dysfunction. A variant of this procedure is subtotal colectomy with creation of a Brooke ileostomy and a rectal Hartmann's pouch. However, the Hartmann's pouch can result in ongoing inflammation and therefore an increased risk of malignancy in the rectal pouch. The Kock continent ileostomy creates a continent pouch and stomal valve, eliminating the need for an external appliance. Unfortunately, the Kock continent ileostomy has had multiple problems, including the frequent occurrence of stomal valve failure plus a high rate of mechanical, functional, and metabolic complications.

The most common surgical procedure for ulcerative colitis has become total proctocolectomy with or without rectoanal mucosal stripping and ileoanal anastomosis (or IPAA).[80-82] Although the remaining anorectal mucosa can be stripped to the dentate line, its musculature is preserved, allowing continence.[80-82] The terminal ileum is sutured to the anus via an end-to-end anastomosis.[80-82] An ileal reservoir (eg, J pouch [more commonly] or S pouch) is created at the ileoanal anastomotic region to improve continence.[80-82] Well-trained surgeons have a low complication rate, and patients tend to prefer the IPAA because of the cosmetic improvements and continence. When performed by experienced surgeons, IPAA has demonstrated excellent efficacy and patient acceptance.[80-82] Recently, laparoscopic surgery has been performed more frequently in patients with UC.[83] Because of a steep learning curve, patients should be referred to laparoscopic surgeons with extensive experience in treating IBD patients.[83] Advantages of laparoscopic surgery in the IBD population include reduced postoperative ileus, reduced pain, and decreased hospital length of stay; disadvantages include its cost, prolonged surgical time, and requirement for technical expertise.[83,84] A recent review of surgical complications that may be encountered in performing an IPAA with a total proctocolectomy is important to place in perspective.[85]

Patients with both chronic UC and primary sclerosing cholangitis (PSC) present an important clinical challenge. Chronic UC patients with PSC are at a much greater risk for colon carcinoma than the non-PSC, chronic UC patient.[86,87] In PSC patients undergoing proctocolectomy with IPAA, an increased incidence of cancer (14% vs 5%) and an increased incidence of dysplasia (40% vs 7%) were found in the resected specimen, compared with resected colons from the non-PSC, chronic UC patient.[88] Therefore, chronic UC patients with PSC have an additional clinical benefit from colectomy, by removing the colon cancer risk.[86,87] The development of portal hypertension predisposes PSC patients with chronic ulcerative colitis to unique complications such as peristomal varices. Comparison of outcomes between chronic, refractory UC patients with PSC who underwent IPAA versus Brooke ileostomy demonstrated significantly fewer bleeding complications in the IPAA group.[86] Although postoperative complications are increased, proctocolectomy with IPAA should be the procedure of choice in PSC patients with chronic ulcerative colitis.[86,87]

When deciding between Brooke ileostomy and IPAA, additional patient factors may favor one procedure over the other. Patients over age 65 may exhibit suboptimal anal sphincter function that could negatively influence IPAA outcomes; obese or tall patients pose anatomic challenges; side effects of long-term steroid use may also increase the risk of IPAA postoperative complications.[88] Because of this, many surgeons prefer to perform the colectomy and then wait 4 to 6 months before making the pouch. This allows the steroids to be tapered and discontinued, thereby leading to better tissue healing when the pouch is formed. Contraindications to IPAA include anal or rectal carcinoma, CD, and anal sphincter dysfunction. In some instances, anorectal manometry may be necessary to further elucidate the status of the patient's sphincter function.[89]

Overall, excellent function has been widely experienced following IPAA despite several physiologic abnormalities that can occur following this surgery.[90] Although external anal sphincter function is maintained well following IPAA, it may take up to 6 to 12 months to recover internal sphincter function, which is frequently difficult and often incomplete. Bacterial overgrowth in the pouch may lead to subtle vitamin B12 deficiency in IPAA patients, and B12 levels should be carefully monitored and replaced as necessary. Rapid pouch filling and impaired evacuation may result in increased stool frequency and fecal incontinence.[91]

Pouch necrosis and sepsis have accounted for some of the more severe, acute complications of IPAA. In one series, sepsis was observed in nearly 7% of a cohort of patients undergoing IPAA for various diagnoses.[92] Although the safety and practicality of repeat IPAA in patients with septic complications had been questioned in the past, recent evidence suggests such pouch salvage is feasible in many of these patients.[93]

In patients followed for up to 10 years postoperatively, there is a 20% to 50% incidence of pouchitis.[94-96] Pouchitis appears to be more common in patients who have had extraintestinal manifestations associated with IBD.[95] Therefore, patients with extraintestinal manifestations should be counseled regarding this increased risk. This is important because the development of pouchitis negatively impacts postoperative quality of life.[96] In UC patients undergoing IPAA, a 1.5 to 2.0 cm in length "columnar cuff" (anal transition zone; ATZ) of diseased columnar epithelium has been reported.[97] "Cuffitis" has been noted to occur in the columnar cuff of IPAA patients and, similar to pouchitis, can also lead to pouch dysfunction.[98]

Pouchitis presents with symptoms of increased diarrhea, abdominal cramping, urgency, tenesmus, incontinence, fever, and very often rectal bleeding. In patients with these symptoms, the evaluation begins by obtaining stool cultures for enteric pathogens and *C. difficile*. Flexible sigmoidoscopy should be performed, looking for friability, edema, granularity, and ulcerations. When infectious pathogens have been ruled out, initial therapy is instituted with antibiotics: metronidazole, ciprofloxacin, tetracycline, or erythromycin. If antibiotic therapy is not successful, trial therapy is undertaken initially with rectal 5-ASA or rectal steroid products, and then oral 5-ASA products, Entocort (controlled ileal release budesonide), prednisone, or, in refractory patients, 6-MP or AZA.

Of major concern has been the demonstration of dysplasia in the anal transitional zone, although this has been infrequent.[99] Nonetheless, IBD surgeons have advocated caution when preserving the anal transitional zone, which will require lifetime surveillance for dysplasia.[100] Therefore, if preservation of the anal transitional zone is undertaken, the patient should be informed that yearly surveillance by flexible sigmoidoscopy and biopsies for dysplasia and rectal/anal cancer will be necessary in the future. Patients with a long-standing IPAA who develop severe, persistent mucosal atrophy appear to be at increased risk for dysplasia of the pouch mucosa.[101] Close endoscopic surveillance has also been advocated in this group of patients.[102] If dysplasia is found on surveillance biopsies, a mucosectomy may be curative and can be performed through a minimally invasive perineal approach.[103]

Sexual dysfunction can occasionally occur postoperatively in men and women.[104] Postoperative ileal pouch vaginal fistulas have been described as well.[105] Accordingly, patients should be counseled about the possibility of sexual dysfunction as part of the preoperative informed consent process. Increased rates of infertility have been documented in women following IPAA.[106,107] This has led to the recommendation that consideration be given to the storage of eggs for later in vitro fertilization by women undergoing IPAA who plan to have children in the future.

Although complications can occur following colectomy and IPAA for acute and chronic steroid-refractory UC, quality of life (QOL) studies have documented very positive outcomes in the overwhelming majority of patients who have undergone such treatment. In a postoperative QOL study of patients undergoing Brooke ileostomy, 97% of patients were glad they underwent the surgery, and 74% led normal, unrestricted lives.[108] Subsequent studies have also documented excellent QOL outcomes in patients undergoing colectomy with IPAA.[109,110] Other investigators have demonstrated improved QOL when comparing IPAA to Brooke ileostomy.[111]

In summary, restorative proctocolectomy with IPAA remains an important therapeutic option in acute or chronic steroid-refractory patients who have failed medical alternatives to glucocorticoids and who favor surgical treatment when weighing the risks and benefits of continued medical versus surgical approaches. The potential complications and side effects of surgery need to be reinforced with the patient who is considering IPAA, but the significantly improved QOL also needs to be discussed with the patient.

Although steroids remain an important therapeutic option for moderate to severe UC, the impact of long-term steroids in the natural history of ulcerative colitis needs to be re-evaluated in the era of increasing utilization of immunosuppression and the availability of biologics. Precise definitions of steroid dose and duration will be helpful as we evaluate the impact of new immunologic therapies and early immunosuppression on old steroid strategies.

REFERENCES

1. Truelove SC, Witts LJ. Cortisone in ulcerative colitis: final report on a therapeutic trial. *Br Med J.* 1955;4956:1590-1593.
2. Jarnerot G, Rolny P, Sandberg-Gertzen H. Intensive intravenous treatment of ulcerative colitis. *Gastroenterology.* 1985;89:1005-1013.
3. Meyers S, Lerer PK, Feuer EJ, et al. Predicting the outcome of corticoid therapy for acute ulcerative colitis: results of a prospective randomized, double-blind clinical trial. *J Clin Gastroenterol.* 1987;9:50-54.
4. Feagan BG, Loftus EV, Kamm MA, et al. Impact of steroid discontinuation on healthcare resource utilization in Crohn's disease. *Am J Gastroenterol.* 2007;102(suppl 2):S445-S446.
5. Vega R, Bertran X, Menacho M, et al. Cytomegalovirus infection in patients with inflammatory bowel disease. *Am J Gastroenterol.* 1999;94:1053-1056.
6. Farrell RJ, Kelleher D. Glucocorticoid resistance in inflammatory bowel disease. *J Endocrinol.* 2003;178:339-346.
7. Maroo S, Farrell RJ. From SNPs to haplotypes: unraveling the role of MDR1 in IBD. *Inflamm Bowel Dis.* 2006;12:74-76.
8. Hearing SD, Norman M, Probert CS, et al. Predicting therapeutic outcome in severe ulcerative colitis by measuring in vitro steroid sensitivity of proliferating peripheral blood lymphocytes. *Gut.* 1999;45:382-388.
9. Lennard-Jones JE, Ritchie JK, Hilder W, Spicer CC. Assessment of severity in colitis: a preliminary study. *Gut.* 1975;16:579-584.
10. Travis SP, Farrant JM, Ricketts C, et al. Predicting outcome in severe ulcerative colitis. *Gut.* 1996;38:905-910.
11. Chew CN, Nolan DJ, Jewell DP. Small bowel gas in severe ulcerative colitis. *Gut.* 1991;32:1535-1537.
12. Sachar DB. Ten common errors in the management of inflammatory bowel disease. *Inflamm Bowel Dis.* 2003;9:205-209.
13. Peppercorn MA. Are antibiotics useful in the management of nontoxic severe ulcerative colitis? *J Clin Gastroenterol.* 1993;17:14-17.
14. Mantzaris GJ, Hatzis A, Kontogiannis P, et al. Intravenous tobramycin and metronidazole as an adjunct to corticosteroids in acute, severe ulcerative colitis. *Am J Gastroenterol.* 1994;89:43-46.
15. Burke DA, Axon AT, Clayden SA, et al. The efficacy of tobramycin in the treatment of ulcerative colitis. *Aliment Pharmacol Ther.* 1990;4:123-129.
16. Thukral C, Travassos WJ, Peppercorn MA. The role of antibiotics in inflammatory bowel disease. *Curr Treat Options Gastroenterol.* 2005;8:223-228.
17. Aslan A, Triadafilopoulos G. Fish oil fatty acid supplementation in active ulcerative colitis: a double-blind, placebo-controlled, crossover study. *Am J Gastroenterol.* 1992;87:432-437.
18. Stenson WF, Cort D, Rodgers J, et al. Dietary supplementation with fish oil in ulcerative colitis. *Ann Intern Med.* 1992;116:609-614.
19. Hawthorne AB, Daneshmend TK, Hawkey CJ, et al. Treatment of ulcerative colitis with fish oil supplementation: a prospective 12 month randomized controlled trial. *Gut.* 1992;33:922-928.
20. Sandborn WJ. Nicotine therapy for ulcerative colitis: a review of rationale, mechanisms, pharmacology, and clinical results. *Am J Gastroenterol.* 1999;94:1161-1171.
21. Pullan RD, Rhodes J, Ganesh S, et al. Transdermal nicotine for active ulcerative colitis. *N Engl J Med.* 1994;330:811-815.
22. Sandborn WJ, Tremaine WJ, Offord KP, et al. Transdermal nicotine for mildly to moderately active ulcerative colitis: a randomized, double-blind placebo-controlled trial. *Ann Intern Med.* 1997;126:364-371.
23. Ingram JR, Thomas GA, Rhodes J, et al. A randomized trial of nicotine enemas for active ulcerative colitis. *Clin Gastroenterol Hepatol.* 2005;3:1107-1114.
24. Nielsen OH, Vainer B, Rask-Madsen J. Review article: the treatment of inflammatory bowel disease with 6-mercaptopurine or AZA. *Aliment Pharmacol Ther.* 2001;15:1699.
25. Ardizzone S, Molteni P, Imbesi V, Bollani S. AZA in steroid-resistant and steroid-dependent ulcerative colitis. *J Clin Gastroenterol.* 1997;25:330.
26. Mantzaris GJ, Sfakianakis M, Archavlis E, et al. A prospective randomized observer-blind 2-year trial of AZA monotherapy versus AZA and olsalazine for the maintenance of remission of steroid-dependent ulcerative colitis. *Am J Gastroenterol.* 2004;99(6):1122-1128.
27. Hawthorne AB, Logan RF, Hawkey CJ, et al. Randomised controlled trial of AZA withdrawal in ulcerative colitis. *BMJ.* 1992;305(6844):20-22.
28. George J, Present DH, Pou R, et al. The long-term outcome of ulcerative colitis treated with 6-mercaptopurine. *Am J Gastroenterol.* 1996;91:1711-1714.
29. Sandborn WJ. A review of immune modifier therapy for inflammatory bowel disease: AZA, 6-mercaptopurine, cyclosporine and methotrexate. *Am J Gastroenterol.* 1996;91:423-433.
30. Caprilli R, Carratu R, Babbini M. Double-blind comparison of the effectiveness of AZA and sulfasalazine in idiopathic proctocolitis. Preliminary report. *Am J Dig Dis.* 1975;20:115-120.
31. Sood A, Midha V, Sood N, Avasthi G. AZA versus sulfasalazine in maintenance of remission in severe ulcerative colitis. *Indian J Gastroenterol.* 2003;22(3):79-81.
32. Jewell DP, Truelove SC. AZA in ulcerative colitis: final report on a controlled therapeutic trial. *Br Med J.* 1974;4:627-630.
33. Hawthorne AB, Logan RF, Hawkey CJ, et al. Randomized controlled trial of AZA withdrawal in ulcerative colitis. *Br Med J.* 1992;305:20-22.
34. Fernandez-Banares F, Bertran X, Esteve-Comas M, et al. AZA is useful in maintaining long-term remission induced by intravenous cyclosporine in steroid-refractory severe ulcerative colitis. *Am J Gastroenterol.* 1996;91:2498-2499.
35. Rosenberg JL, Wall AJ, Levin B, et al. A controlled trial of AZA in the management of chronic ulcerative colitis. *Gastroenterology.* 1975;69:96-99.
36. Kirk AP, Lennard-Jones JE. Controlled trial of AZA in chronic ulcerative colitis. *Br Med J.* 1982;284:1291-1292.
37. Adler DJ, Korelitz BI. The therapeutic efficacy of 6-mercaptopurine in refractory ulcerative colitis. *Am J Gastroenterol.* 1990;85:717-722.
38. Ardizzone S, Molteni F, Imbesi V, et al. AZA in steroid-resistant and steroid-dependent ulcerative colitis. *J Clin Gastroenterol.* 1997;25:330-333.
39. Present DH, Meltzer SJ, Krumholz MP, et al. 6-mercaptopurine in the management of inflammatory bowel disease: short- and long-term toxicity. *Ann Intern Med.* 1989;111:641-649.

40. Connell WR, Kamm MA, Ritchie JK, et al. Bone marrow toxicity caused by AZA in inflammatory bowel disease: 27 years of experience. *Gut.* 1993;34:1081-1085.
41. Dubinsky MC. AZA, 6-mercaptopurine in inflammatory bowel disease: pharmacology, efficacy, and safety. *Clin Gastroenterol Hepatol.* 2004;2:731-743.
42. Gearry RB, Barclay ML. AZA and 6-mercaptopurine pharmacogenetics and metabolite monitoring in inflammatory bowel disease. *J Gastroenterol Hepatol.* 2005;20:1149-1157.
43. Gelb A, Zalusky R. The use of azathiaprine and 6-mercaptopurine (6-MP) as immunosuppressive therapy in inflammatory bowel disease and its role in the etiology of lymphocytic lymphoma. *Am J Gastroenterol.* 1983;78:316.
44. Larvol L, Soule JC, Tourneau A. Reversible lymphoma in the setting of AZA therapy for Crohn's disease. *N Engl J Med.* 1994;331:883-884.
45. Kandiel A, Fraser AG, Korelitz BI, et al. Increased risk of lymphoma among inflammatory bowel disease patients treated with AZA and 6-mercaptopurine. *Gut.* 2005;54:1121-1125.
46. Mantzaris GJ, Sfakianakis M, Archavlis E, et al. A prospective randomized observer-blind 2-year trial of AZA monotherapy versus AZA and olsalazine for the maintenance of remission of steroid-dependent ulcerative colitis. *Am J Gastroenterol.* 2004;99:1122-1128.
47. Cuffari C, Present DH, Bayless TM, et al. Optimizing therapy in patients with pancolitis. *Inflamm Bowel Dis.* 2005;11:937-946.
48. Sands BE, Tremaine WJ, Sandborn WJ, et al. Infliximab in the treatment of severe, steroid-refractory ulcerative colitis: a pilot study. *Inflamm Bowel Dis.* 2001;7:83-88.
49. Chey WY, Hussain A, Ryan C, et al. Infliximab for refractory ulcerative colitis. *Am J Gastroenterol.* 2001;96:2373-2381.
50. Su C, Salzberg BA, Lewis JD, et al. Efficacy of anti-tumor necrosis factor therapy in patients with ulcerative colitis. *Am J Gastroenterol.* 2002;97:2577-2584.
51. Rutgeerts P, Sandborn WJ, Feagan BG, et al. Infliximab for induction and maintenance therapy for ulcerative colitis. *N Engl J Med.* 2005;353:2462-2476.
52. Iyer S, Lahana R, Buelow R. Rational design and development of RDP58. *Curr Pharm Des.* 2002;8:2217-2229.
53. Kunitake H, Hodin R, Shellito PC, Sands BE, Korzenik J, Bordeianou L. Perioperative treatment with infliximab in patients with Crohn's disease and ulcerative colitis is not associated with an increased rate of postoperative complications. *J Gastrointest Surg.* 2008;12(10):1730-1736.
54. Schluender SJ, Ippoliti A, Dubinsky M, et al. Does infliximab influence surgical morbidity of ileal pouch-anal anastomosis in patients with ulcerative colitis? *Dis Colon Rectum.* 2007;50(11):1747-1753.
55. Selvasekar CR, Cima RR, Larson DW, et al. Effect of infliximab on short-term complications in patients undergoing operation for chronic ulcerative colitis. *J Am Coll Surg.* 2007;204(5):956-962.
56. Travis S, Yap LM, Hawkey C, et al. RDP58 is a novel and potentially effective oral therapy for ulcerative colitis. *Inflamm Bowel Dis.* 2005;11:713-719.
57. Feagan BG, Greenberg GR, Wild G. Treatment of ulcerative colitis with a humanized antibody to the alpha4 beta7 integrin. *N Engl J Med.* 2005;352:2499-2507.
58. Travis S, Yap LM, Hawkey C, et al. RDP58 is a novel and potentially effective oral therapy for ulcerative colitis. *Inflamm Bowel Dis.* 2005;11(8):713-719.
59. Van Assche G, Van Ranst M, Sciot R, et al. Progressive multifocal leukoencephalopathy after natalizumab therapy for Crohn's disease. *N Engl J Med.* 2005;353:362-368.
60. Plevy SE, Salzberg BA, Van Assche G, et al. A humanized anti-CD3 monoclonal antibody, visilizumab, for treatment of severe steroid-refractory ulcerative colitis: results of a phase I study. *Gastroenterology.* 2004;126:A75.
61. Sinha A, Nightingale J, West KP, et al. Epidermal growth factor enemas with oral mesalamine for mild-to-moderate left-sided ulcerative colitis or proctitis. *N Engl J Med.* 2003;349:350-357.
62. Van Assche G, Dalle I, Noman M, et al. A pilot study on the use of the humanized anti-interleukin-2 receptor antibody daclizumab in active ulcerative colitis. *Am J Gastroenterol.* 2003;98:369-376.
63. Summers RW, Elliott DE, Urban JF Jr, et al. Trichuris suis therapy for active ulcerative colitis: a randomized controlled trial. *Gastroenterology.* 2005;128:825-832.
64. Loftus CG, Loftus EV Jr, Sandborn WJ. Cyclosporin for refractory ulcerative colitis. *Gut.* 2003;52:172-173.
65. Lichtiger S, Present DH, Kornbluth A, et al. Cyclosporine in severe ulcerative colitis refractory to steroid therapy. *N Engl J Med.* 1994;330:1841-1845.
66. D'Haens G, Lemmens L, Geboes K, et al. Intravenous cyclosporine versus intravenous corticosteroids as single therapy for severe attacks of ulcerative colitis. *Gastroenterology.* 2001;120:1323-1329.
67. Svanoni F, Bonassi U, Bagnolo F, et al. Effectiveness of cyclosporine A in the treatment of active refractory ulcerative colitis. *Gastroenterology.* 1998;114:A1096.
68. Kornbluth A, Present DH, Lichtiger S, et al. Cyclosporin for severe ulcerative colitis: a user's guide. *Am J Gastroenterol.* 1997;92:1424-1428.
69. Aberra FN, Lewis JD, Hass D, Rombeau JL, Osborne B, Lichtenstein GR. Corticosteroids and immunomodulators: postoperative infectious complication risk in inflammatory bowel disease patients. *Gastroenterology.* 2003;125(2):320-327.
70. Kornbluth A. Is there still a role for cyclosporine in the treatment of inflammatory bowel disease: pro argument. *Inflamm Bowel Dis.* 2003;9:194-197.
71. Van Assche G, D'Heans G, Noman M, et al. Randomized, double-blind comparison of 4 mg/kg versus 2 mg/kg intravenous cyclosporine in severe ulcerative colitis. *Gastroenterology.* 2003;125:1025-1031.
72. Cohen RD, Stein R, Hanauer SB. Intravenous cyclosporin in ulcerative colitis: a five year experience. *Am J Gastroenterol.* 1999;94:1587-1592.
73. Cohen RD, Stein R, Hanauer SB. Intravenous cyclosporine in ulcerative colitis: a five-year experience. *Am J Gastroenterol.* 1999;94(6):1587-1592.
74. Fellermann K, Luhmann D, Stange EF. Is there still a role for cyclosporine in the treatment of inflammatory bowel disease? Con argument. *Inflamm Bowel Dis.* 2003;9:198-201.
75. Carbonnel F, Boruchowicz A, Duclos B, et al. Intravenous cyclosporine in attacks of ulcerative colitis: short-term and long-term responses. *Dig Dis Sci.* 1996;41:2471-2476.
76. Jarnerot G, Hertervig E, Friis-Liby I, et al. Infliximab as rescue therapy in severe to moderately severe ulcerative colitis: a randomized, placebo-controlled study. *Gastroenterology.* 2005;128:1805-1811.
77. Maser EA, Deconda D, Lichtiger S, Ullman T, Present DH, Kornbluth A. Cyclosporine and infliximab as rescue therapy for each other in patients with steroid-refractory ulcerative colitis. *Clin Gastroenterol Hepatol.* 2008;6(10):1112-1116.
78. Cohen JL, Strong SA, Hyman NH, et al. Practice parameters for the surgical treatment of ulcerative colitis. *Dis Colon Rectum.* 2005;48:1997-2009.
79. Block GE, Moossa AR, Simonowitz D, et al. Emergency colectomy for inflammatory bowel disease. *Surgery.* 1977;82:531-536.
80. Pemberton JH, Kelly KA, Beart RW Jr, et al. Ileal pouch-anal anastomosis for chronic ulcerative colitis: long-term results. *Ann Surg.* 1987;206:504-513.

81. Becker JM, Raymond JL. Ileal pouch-anal anastomosis. A single surgeon's experience with 100 consecutive cases. *Ann Surg.* 1986;204:375-383.
82. Meagher AP, Farouk R, Dozois RR, et al. Ileal pouch-anal anastomosis for chronic ulcerative colitis: complications and long term outcome in 1310 patients. *Br J Surg.* 1998;85:800-803.
83. Ording Olsen K, Juul S, Berndtsson I, Oresland T, Laurberg S. Ulcerative colitis: Female fecundity before diagnosis, during disease, and after surgery compared with a population sample. *Gastroenterology.* 2002;122:15-19.
84. Hueting WE, Buskens E, van der Tweel I, Gooszen HG, van Laarhoven CJ. Results and complications after ileal pouch anal anastomosis: a meta-analysis of 43 observational studies comprising 9,317 patients. *Dig Surg.* 2005;22:69-79.
85. Sardinha TC, Wexner SD. Laparoscopic surgery for inflammatory bowel disease: pros and cons. *World J Surg.* 1998;22:370-374.
86. Kartheuser AH, Dozois RR, LaRusso NF, et al. Comparison of surgical treatment of ulcerative colitis associated with primary sclerosing cholangitis: ileal pouch-anal anastomosis versus brooke ileostomy. *Mayo Clin Proc.* 1996;71:748-756.
87. Gorgun E, Remzi FH, Manilich E, et al. Surgical outcome in patients with primary sclerosing cholangitis undergoing ileal pouch-anal anastomosis: a case-control study. *Surgery.* 2005;138:631-639.
88. Kelly KA, Pemberton JH, Wolff BG, et al. Ileal pouch-anal anastomosis. *Curr Probl Surg.* 1992;29:57-131.
89. Farouk R, Pemberton JH, Wolff BG, et al. Functional outcomes after ileal pouch-anal anastomosis for chronic ulcerative colitis. *Ann Surg.* 2000;231:919-926.
90. Levitt MD, Kuan M. The physiology of ileo-anal pouch function. *Am J Surg.* 1998;176:384-389.
91. Stryker SJ, Kelly KA, Phillips SF, et al. Anal and neorectal function after ileal pouch-anal anastomosis. *Ann Surg.* 1986;203:55-61.
92. Fazio VW, Ziv Y, Church JM, et al. Ileal pouch-anal anastomoses complications and function in 1005 patients. *Ann Surg.* 1995;222:120-127.
93. Fazio VW, Wu JS, Lavery IC. Repeat ileal pouch-anal anastomosis to salvage septic complications of pelvic pouches: clinical outcome and quality of life assessment. *Ann Surg.* 1998;228:588-597.
94. de Silva HJ, de Angelis CP, Soper N, et al. Clinical and functional outcome after restorative proctocolectomy. *Br J Surg.* 1991;78:1039-1044.
95. Lohmuller JL, Pemberton JH, Dozois RR, et al. Pouchitis and extraintestinal manifestations of inflammatory bowel disease after ileal pouch-anal anastomosis. *Ann Surg.* 1990;211:622-627.
96. Pemberton JH. The problem with pouchitis. *Gastroenterology.* 1993;104:1209-1211.
97. Thompson-Fawcett MW, Warren BF, Mortensen NJ. A new look at the anal transitional zone with reference to restorative proctocolectomy and the columnar cuff. *Br J Surg.* 1998;85:1517-1521.
98. Thompson-Fawcett MW, Mortensen NJ, Warren BF. "Cuffitis" and inflammatory changes in the columnar cuff, anal transitional zone, and ileal reservoir after stapled pouch-anal anastomosis. *Dis Colon Rectum.* 1999;42:348-355.
99. Remzi FH, Fazio VW, Delaney CP, et al. Dysplasia of the anal transition zone after ileal pouch-anal anastomosis: results of prospective evaluation after a minimum of ten years. *Dis Colon Rectum.* 2003;46:6-13.
100. Becker JM. Ileal pouch-anal anastomosis: current status and controversies. *Surgery.* 1993;113:599-602.
101. Gullberg K, Stahlberg D, Liljeqvist L, et al. Neoplastic transformation of the pelvic pouch mucosa in patients with ulcerative colitis. *Gastroenterology.* 1997;112:1487-1492.
102. Veress B, Reinholt FP, Lindquist K, et al. Long-term histomorphological surveillance of the pelvic ileal pouch: dysplasia develops in a subgroup of patients. *Gastroenterology.* 1995;109:1090-1097.
103. Fazio VW, Tjandra JJ. Transanal mucosectomy. ileal pouch advancement for anorectal dysplasia or inflammation after restorative proctocolectomy. *Dis Colon Rectum.* 1994;37:1008-1011.
104. Bambrick M, Fazio VW, Hull TL, et al. Sexual function following restorative proctocolectomy in women. *Dis Colon Rectum.* 1996;39:610-614.
105. Wexner SD, Rothenberger DA, Jensen L, et al. Ileal pouch vaginal fistulas: Incidence, etiology, and management. *Dis Colon Rectum.* 1989;32:460-465.
106. Johnson P, Richard C, Ravid A, et al. Female infertility after ileal pouch-anal anastomosis for ulcerative colitis. *Dis Colon Rectum.* 2004;47:1119-1126.
107. Gorgun E, Remzi FH, Goldberg JM. Fertility is reduced after restorative proctocolectomy with ileal pouch anal anastomosis: A study of 300 patients. *Surgery.* 2004;136:795-803.
108. Mcleod RS, Lavery IC, Leatherman JR, et al. Factors affecting quality of life with a conventional ileostomy. *World J Surg.* 1986;10:474-480.
109. Moskovitz DN, Maunder RG, Cohen Z, et al. Coping behavior and social support contribute independently to quality of life after surgery for inflammatory bowel disease. *Dis Colon Rectum.* 2000;43:517-521.
110. Fazio VW, O'Riordain MG, Lavery IC, et al. Long-term functional outcome and quality of life after stapled restorative proctocolectomy. *Ann Surg.* 1999;230:584-586.
111. Kohler LW, Pemberton JH, Zinsmeister AR, et al. Quality of life after proctocolectomy: a comparison of Brooke ileostomy, Kock pouch, and ileal pouch-anal anastomosis. *Gastroenterology.* 1991;101:679-684.

35

Prebiotics and Probiotics in Ulcerative Colitis

Robert M. Penner, BSc, MD, FRCP(C), MSc; Karen L. Madsen, PhD; Massimo Campieri, MD; and Richard N. Fedorak, MD, FRCPC

Bacteria have long been known to act as pathogenic agents, sometimes as mediators of enteric infections. This knowledge has motivated the medical study of bacteria, but research has only recently begun to focus on the complex symbiotic interaction between the mammalian host and native, endogenous, intestinal microflora. With the understanding that inflammatory bowel disease (IBD) represents a derangement of the human relationship with our procaryotic guests has come the opportunity to explore therapies that create or restore a healthy colonic bacterial population. Probiotics, prebiotics, and synbiotics represent the therapeutic options currently under study to achieve this end. Although pre- and probiotics are not currently in widespread use for any clinical IBD indication, they represent an elegant use of research to develop a new and safe method of therapy and deserve attention as very promising therapeutic tools. Their clinical roles, and the evidence to date supporting their use, are the subjects of this chapter.

PROBIOTICS

Background

Experimental evidence for the involvement of enteric flora in the pathogenesis of ulcerative colitis and Crohn's disease has been derived from both animal and human experimentation. The most fundamental evidence is that an enteric flora must be present for disease expression. Animal models of IBD consistently lack this expression when maintained in a germ-free environment, and human inflammation is greatest in the area with the highest concentrations of luminal bacteria. A series of supportive clinical observations have been built on this cornerstone. First is the observation that surgical diversion of the fecal stream from an inflamed bowel segment is associated with disease improvement. Next is the direct demonstration of a proinflammatory fecal flora in IBD patients. This has been achieved through the induction of intestinal inflammation and mucosal ulceration by direct instillation of fecal contents from an inflamed gut into the noninflamed guts of susceptible individuals. Finally, current research supports a clinically useful disease model of IBD as an aberrant interaction between host immunity and intestinal microflora in genetically susceptible individuals.

Enteric bacterial species and strains have widely varying biologic effects on their hosts, and the native flora of IBD sufferers differs from that of healthy controls. To date, research into probiotics has focused primarily on their safety and ability to remain viable while reaching target sites within the body. Recently, a more specific understanding has been gained of how individual bacterial species can mediate IBD expression. By categorizing these actions both mechanistically and by responsible bacterial species, we can potentially develop a pharmacopeia of useful enteric flora.

In theory, there are 2 different, but related, manners in which the addition of probiotics to the crossfire between an enteric immune system and its resident microflora may benefit a patient (Table 35-1). First, the probiotics may simply represent a less harmful alternative to a noxious flora, and thus benefit the host by displacing unwanted guests. This can occur through receptor competition, whereby probiotics compete with microbial

Lichtenstein GR, ed.
Ulcerative Colitis: The Complete Guide to Medical Management (pp 393-404)

TABLE 35-1

MECHANISMS OF PROBIOTICS

Mechanism of Action	Biologic Effect
Enhanced barrier function	• Enhanced epithelial resistance • Enhanced phosphorylation of actinin and occludin in epithelial cells • Upregulation of MUC3 mRNA and mucin secretion • Maintenance of F-actin and transport and enzymatic activity • Enhanced colonic permeability • Enhanced epithelial cell glycosylation
Antibody production	• Enhanced antibody production
Cell-mediated immunity	• Enhanced phagocytic activity
Antigen presentation	• Enhanced natural killer activity • Altered dendritic cell phenotype and function
Cell signaling	• Modulation of NF-κB pathway
Apoptosis	• Prevention of epithelial apoptosis • Induction of immune cell apoptosis
Antioxidative	• Enhanced survival in oxidative environment • Inhibited linoleic acid peroxidation • Scavenge free radicals
Adhesive properties	• Prevention of pathogenic strains from adhering to epithelial cells • Disease-specific adhesion • Strain-specific adhesion
Metabolic processes and transport function	• Formation of short-chain fatty acids • Inhibition of secretion
Antimicrobial	• Production of organic acids • Hydrogen peroxide • Bacteriocins • Reduction of luminal pH
Cytokine production	• Increased proinflammatory and/or decreased proinflammatory
Oral tolerance	• Suppression of humoral and cellular responses

pathogens for a limited number of receptors present on the surface epithelium. It can also occur through probiotic release of antimicrobial factors such as lactic and acetic acid, hydrogen peroxide, and bacteriocins. Second, the probiotics may improve the local immune response by enhancing efficacy of immune responses through immunomodulation, decreasing unnecessary inflammation by induction of T-cell apoptosis, or improving barrier function.

Immunomodulation can be achieved by probiotics because of the dynamic and interactive nature of the relationship between the immune system and bacteria, in which immune cells maintain an awareness of bacteria through constant sampling of their antigens.[1] Bacteria can thus modulate the nature of the immune response by inducing pattern-recognition responses that set intracellular signalling pathways in motion.[2,3] Active constituents of bacteria that manipulate the mucosal immune system include enzymes,[4] secreted protein factors,[5] bacterial formulated peptides such as N-formylmethionine-leucine-phenylalanine (fMLP) and lipopolysaccharide (LPS),[3,6] and peptidoglycan cell wall constituents including the muramyl dipeptide (MDP) MurNAc-L-Ala-D-isoGln,[7,8] gamma-D-glutamyl-meso-diaminopimelic acid (iE-DAP),[9] and bacterial deoxyribonucleic acid (DNA).[10-12]

Unfortunately, several questions remain. It is not yet clear which of the mechanisms are most important to improving IBD phenotype or how they can be best put to therapeutic use. The situation is complicated by the fact that different bacterial strains exert different effects, and combinations of bacteria interact in ways that are not yet well understood. It is for this reason that the probiotic literature is currently in a nascent stage, where a variety of single- and multiple-organism preparations are being studied in a variety of clinical settings.

Pharmacokinetics

The probiotic preparations in the clinical IBD literature vary in terms of their active bacterial strain, their concentration, and their carrier medium. Specifics on pharmacokinetics are thus difficult to extrapolate, but 3 generalizations are important. First, to be effective, probiotic preparations must be dosed in a form that will reach their site of action intact and living. Second, probiotics probably need to be administered continuously, or the host's native enteric flora will return to its baseline. Finally, they must be administered at an adequate dosage to maintain a steady-state intestinal population. Whether or not the native enteric flora must be suppressed with antibiotics before administering probiotics remains controversial. Techniques that have been successfully used in the recent literature to enhance probiotic pharmacokinetics include the use of enteric-coated preparations[13] and specific fermented products known to reach the colon in high concentration.[14]

Most probiotic literature to date focuses on enteral dosing for direct luminal effect, but preliminary evidence suggests that some beneficial probiotic effects can be induced systemically with a subcutaneous preparation.[15]

Adverse Events

The safety of lactobacilli and bifidobacterium have been assessed and published as part of a recent workshop.[16] Because common sources of exposure to probiotics exist in the natural environment, including fermented foodstuffs (eg, yogurt, cheese, and fermented vegetables) and human microflora in the oral cavity, intestine, and vagina, many of the commercial probiotic products have been officially designated as "generally regarded as safe." There is no evidence that deliberately ingested lactobacilli or bifidobacterium pose any risk of infection greater than that associated with commensal strains.

Cases of infection due to probiotics are extremely rare; they are estimated to represent between 0.05% and 0.4% of cases of infective endocarditis or bacteremia.[17,18] During the past 30 years, 180 cases of lactobacillemia have been reported, and 69 cases of infective endocarditis have been attributed to lactobacilli.[16] In an important prospective study from Finland, the marked increase seen in the consumption of probiotics by consumers has not led to an increased rate of opportunistic infection by these same probiotics.[19,20] This study provides reassurance that the introduction of probiotics as therapeutic agents has not, and should not, result in increased rates of human infections. Indeed, most of the rare cases of such infections occur in the case of immunocompromised patients or those with serious underlying disease states.[21-29] Obviously, the provision of probiotics to this group of patients should be approached with caution. While several attempts have been made to evaluate the factors that might predispose such severely ill patients to infection by probiotics,[21,23] statistical analysis is lacking, and the number of cases is too small to permit the drawing of any statistically valid conclusions. Studies done on children have shown that probiotic compounds containing lactobacilli and bifidobacterium are well-tolerated by and safe for this age group.[30-32]

Despite these reassuringly low infection rates for healthy humans, it will still be important to monitor probiotic treatment safety through rigorous identification of infecting organisms. These identifications should be verified by molecular studies, because physiologic characterization alone is insufficient for reliable classification. For new probiotic products where the organism is not present in the traditional diet, a more aggressive safety analysis (one similar to that used for pharmacologic compounds) must be followed. Finally, antibiotic resistance to probiotic bacteria is not a hazard, unless it renders the probiotic untreatable, as in the rare case of infection. In this regard, all strains of such probiotics should be susceptible to a number of major antibiotics, certainly to more than two.

Clinical Trials

Because of the inhomogeneity of preparations used in clinical research, we approach the evidence for probiotic use by clinical indication. A summary of this evidence is presented in Table 35-2 for pouchitis and Table 35-3 for ulcerative colitis.

Therapy for Pouchitis

The first clinical setting in which probiotics demonstrated efficacy was in patients with nonspecific inflammation of their ileal reservoirs following colectomy and ileal pouch-anal anastomosis for ulcerative colitis. This pouchitis is a troublesome problem that occurs in 50% of patients after 10 years. Although it is idiopathic, research reveals reduced counts of lactobacilli and bifidobacterium within the pouch, raising the possibility that an altered enteric flora plays a pathophysiologic role.[33] While the majority of patients with pouchitis respond to treatment with antimicrobial agents, approximately 10% of patients experience recurrent or refractory disease, and it is for these patients that probiotics offer potential benefit.

Maintenance of Antibiotic-Induced Remission of Pouchitis

Two randomized, placebo-controlled trials have assessed maintenance of antibiotic-induced remission with VSL#3 (VSL Pharmaceuticals Inc, Fort Lauderdale, FL). VSL#3 con-

TABLE 35-2

CLINICAL EVIDENCE FOR PROBIOTICS IN POUCHITIS

Disease/Setting	Level of Evidence and Probiotic	N	Duration of Probiotic Treatment	Results	Comments
Pouchitis/maintenance of antibiotic-induced remission	2 RCTs				Level A evidence demonstrating efficacy of VSL#3 for maintenance of antibiotic-induced pouchitis remission. Note, the dose of VSL#3 in the clinical trials was generally higher than that used in clinical practice.
	1) VSL#3[20]	40	9 months	Remission rate of 85% on VSL#3 vs 0% on placebo	
	2) VSL#3[34]	36	12 months	Remission rate of 85% on VSL#3 vs 6% on placebo	
Pouchitis/treatment of active disease	1 RCT (LrGG)[35]	20	3 months	No benefit	No evidence currently supports the use of any probiotic for treatment of acute active pouchitis.
	1 Open-label (Cultura)[36]	10	1 month	50% endoscopic improvement, but no clinical benefit	
Pouchitis/postoperative prevention	1 RCT (VSL#3)[37]	40	12 months	Remission rate 90% after 1 year vs 60% with placebo ($P<0.05$)	Level A evidence: evidence for the use of VSL#3 for postoperative prevention of pouchitis.
	1 Cohort (LrGG)[38]	117	12 months	7% pouchitis over 3 years in treatment group vs 29% in historic controls	

LrGG= Lactobacillus rhamnosus GG

TABLE 35-3

CLINICAL EVIDENCE FOR PROBIOTICS IN ULCERATIVE COLITIS

Disease/Setting	Level of Evidence and Probiotic	N	Duration of Probiotic Treatment	Results	Comments
UC/treatment of active disease	4 RCTs				Authors of 39 suggested equivalence with mesalamine, but placebo-controlled data are not yet adequate to support probiotic efficacy in this setting.
	1) EcN[39]	116	3 months	68% remission; 26% maintained at 1 year on EcN, compared with 75% and 25% on mesalamine (P=ns)	
	2) BM (mesalamine allowed)[14]	20	12 weeks	40% remission at 12 weeks in BM group vs 33% on placebo (P=ns)	
	3) BIS1[40]	18	1 month	No significant clinical differences from placebo	
	4) VSL#3[43]	90	8 weeks	80% remission on balsalazide; 77% on balsalazide+VSL#3; 53% on mesalamine	
	2 Open-label				
	1) SB[41]	25	1 month	68% remission	
	2) VSL#3[42]	32	6 weeks	53% remission	
UC/maintenance of remission	4 RCTs				Results are currently variable between treatment regimens, and placebo-controlled results are not highly supportive. One adequately powered RCT demonstrated equivalence between EcN and mesalamine. General clinical use likely requires further supporting evidence.
	1) EcN[45]	120	12 months	84% maintained remission on EcN; 89% on placebo	
	2) EcN[13]	327	12 months	64% maintained remission on EcN; 66% on mesalamine-statistical equivalence	
	3) EcN[39]	116	12 months	26% maintained at 1 year vs 25% on mesalamine (P=ns)	
	4) BM[47]	21	12 months	73% remission at 12 months in BM group vs 10% in placebo group	
	1 Open-label				
	VSL#3[46]	20	12 months	75% remission at 12 months	

BM = bifidobacterium-fermented milk; SB = Saccharomyces boulardii; BIS1 = Bifidobacterium longum/Synergy 1 tains viable lyophilized bacteria: 4 strains of Lactobacillus (*Lactobacillus casei, Lactobacillus plantarum, Lactobacillus acidophilus, and Lactobacillus delbrueckii* subsp. *Bulgaricus*), 3 strains of Bifidobacterium (*Bifidobacterium longum, Bifidobacterium breve, and Bifidobacterium infantis*), and 1 strain of *Streptococcus salivarius* subsp *thermophilus*. In the first study, Gionchetti et al[20] assessed 40 patients with acute active pouchitis. These patients were in clinical and endoscopic remission (with a score of zero in the clinical and endoscopic portion of the pouchitis disease activity index [PDAI]) after 1 month of antibiotic treatment with ciprofloxacin (1 g/d) plus rifaximin (2 g/d). They were then randomized to receive VSL#3 (6 g/d, containing 5×10^{11} colony forming units per gram) or placebo for 9 months. Of the 20 patients who received placebo, 100% had relapses within the 9-month period. In contrast, 17 of the 20 patients (85%) who received VSL#3 were still in remission with a PDAI of zero (eg, normal) after 9 months ($P<0.001$). Furthermore, 100% of the patients receiving VSL#3 had relapses within 4 months after the VSL#3 treatment was stopped. These dramatic results provided the first conclusive evidence that, given the correct dose and combination, probiotics can play a major therapeutic role in the management of IBD. These authors also demonstrated that in patients treated with VSL#3, fecal concentrations of lactobacilli, bifidobacterium, and *Streptococcus salivarius* increased significantly compared with concentrations present before and after treatment. No changes were identified in concentrations of bacteroides, coliforms, clostridia, enterococci, and total aerobes and anaerobes compared with basal levels. Once the VSL#3 was withdrawn, fecal concentrations of lactobacilli, bifidobacterium, and *Streptococcus salivarius* fell back to basal levels.

In the similar second study at a separate institution by Mimura et al,[34] remission (PDAI ≤2) was again achieved in patients with active pouchitis with 4 weeks of combined metronidazole and ciprofloxacin. Patients were then randomized to receive either VSL#3 (6 g/d, as two 3-g sachets, each containing 3×10^{11} colony forming units) or placebo for 1 year. The only major differences in this study, relative to that of the Gionchetti study outlined above,[20] were that the VSL#3 was given at a lower dose (6×10^{11} vs 3×10^{12} colony forming units daily) and follow-up was 12 months rather than 9 months. Remission was maintained at 1 year in 17 patients (85%) on VSL#3 and in 1 patient (6%) on placebo. Whereas many areas of probiotic research are difficult to interpret because of variable probiotic preparations used by different researchers, these results with the multi-species probiotic mixture (VSL#3) were virtually identical to those of the Gionchetti study. The consistency of these results makes maintenance of antibiotic-induced remission of pouchitis a setting in which the efficacy of probiotics is widely agreed upon. It is important to note, however, that in both of these clinical trials, the quantity of VSL#3 was higher than that used in later studies and in current clinical practice.

ACUTE ACTIVE POUCHITIS

In contrast, Kuisma et al[35] did not demonstrate a therapeutic effect of probiotics in the treatment of acute active pouchitis with a single-strain *Lactobacillus rhamnosus* GG formulation. In this randomized, double-blind, placebo-controlled trial, 44 subjects with acute inflamed pouches (PDAI of approximately 8; range 5 to 13) were randomized to receive *Lactobacillus rhamnosus* GG (4×10^{10} colony forming units [cfu] daily in two equal doses) or placebo for 3 months. No differences were found in the mean pretreatment or post-treatment PDAI scores between the 2 treatment groups. No significant changes were seen in the concentrations of aerobic or anaerobic bacteria in the pouch. However, there was a trend toward higher fecal concentrations of total lactobacilli. Nevertheless, only 40% of study subjects were colonized with *Lactobacillus* GG. The cause of the negative therapeutic effects in this clinical trial with *Lactobacillus rhamnosus* GG remains to be determined.

Laake et al[36] used an open, nonrandomized treatment with patients acting as their own controls. Ten subjects with acute active pouchitis were treated with 500 g of the dairy product Cultura (TINE Dairies BA, Oslo, Norway; 100 g contains 1×10^{10} cfu of both *Lactobacillus acidophilus* and *Bifidobacterium lactis*, 3.2 g protein, 1.5 g fat, and 4.3 g carbohydrate). Cultura provided a daily intake of both lactobacilli and bifidobacterium (5×10^{10} cfu) for 4 weeks. Seven of 10 patients had a reduced endoscopic score (using the endoscopic portion of the PDAI) after intervention and a 50% reduction in median values from 3.0 to 1.5 ($P=0.016$). Interestingly, the histological and laser Doppler flowmetry (LDF) scores, as a measure of inflammation, did not change with probiotic therapy. Thus, it is possible that the improvement in endoscopic score represents the bias of a single observer, nonblinded, endoscopic assessment in an open-label clinical trial. Microbiologic assessment of the pouch confirmed that during the probiotic administration, 80% of patients had an increased number of lactobacilli. However, the differences did not reach statistical significance, and 1 week after the probiotic was stopped, the levels of lactobacilli returned to basal levels. Similar to the study by Kuisma et al,[35] treatment of acute active pouchitis with probiotics did not confer a positive therapeutic effect.

Given the impressive results of probiotics in maintenance of antibiotic-induced pouchitis remission, it is surprising that efficacy could not be demonstrated for treatment of acute active pouchitis. It is possible that pretreatment with antibiotics is necessary for probiotics to exert their full effect, that the different strains of probiotics have differing efficacy, or that multi-species preparations (ie, VSL#3) are required in order to be efficacious.

POSTOPERATIVE PREVENTION OF POUCHITIS

To further examine the impressive clinical effect of VSL#3 in the management of pouchitis, the Italian group of Gionchetti et al[37] extended their observations to the use of VSL#3 in the postoperative prevention of pouchitis. They performed a randomized, double-blind, placebo-controlled trial where VSL#3 (9×10^{11} bacteria per day) or placebo was administered for 12 successive months, beginning within 1 week after ileostomy closure and pouch formation. PDAI was assessed at 1, 3, 6, 9, and 12 months. Of the 20 patients randomized to receive VSL#3, 90% had normal pouch (with a PDAI of 0) after 1 year. In contrast, only 60% of patients randomized to receive placebo were in remission after 1 year ($P<0.05$). Once again, in patients treated with VSL#3, there was no significant change in concentrations of bacteroides, coliforms, clostridia, or enterococci in the pouches compared with the basal levels. In contrast, fecal concentrations of lactobacilli, bifidobacterium, and *Streptococcus thermophilus* were significantly increased compared to concentrations at baseline. In the placebo group, fecal concentrations of all species evaluated remained similar to that before starting treatment.[37]

A second trial of probiotics for postoperative prevention of pouchitis was conducted using *L. rhamnosus* GG,[38] an agent that we have seen was unsuccessful in the treatment of acute pouchitis.[35] In this case-control study of 117 patients, results were more positive. There were 39 consecutive patients who underwent IPAA between 1996 and 2001 who were treated with *Lactobacillus rhamnosus* GG in 350 ml/d of Vifit (Mona, Woerden, Netherlands; 1.4×10^{10} live bacteria) and were compared with the 78 preceding consecutive patients who had received no prophylactic therapy. Cumulative risk of pouchitis over 3 years was 7% in the treatment group and 29% in the historic controls, a difference that was statistically significant and led the authors to recommend routine prophylactic therapy with this agent. Although the groups of patients were similar at baseline, this study was not a randomized, controlled trial and is thus not of the same grade of evidence as the earlier study in acute pouchitis. Nevertheless, it raises the interesting question of whether this single-agent probiotic might be useful for prophylaxis, while ineffective for acute therapy. It should also be remembered that this study used a different preparation of *Lactobacillus rhamnosus* GG than the study by Kuisma et al,[35] one with a slightly lower dose of live bacteria.

With 2 randomized, placebo-controlled clinical trials demonstrating statistical significance for VSL#3 in maintenance of antibiotic-induced remission of pouchitis and 1 demonstrating statistical significance for VSL#3 in prevention of pouchitis following operative pouch construction, there is now Level A evidence for the addition of this combination probiotic mixture to the IBD therapeutic armamentarium. Indeed, from the limited data available to date, it appears that this combination probiotic mixture has a superior therapeutic profile to single probiotic agents; and ongoing clinical trials will need to confirm this early observation. Physicians using VSL#3 in patients with ileoanal pouches need to be vigilant regarding the generally higher doses (between 6×10^{11} and 3×10^{12} colony forming units per day) used in the clinical trials and incorporate these into clinical practice until dose-response studies are completed.

ACUTE ACTIVE ULCERATIVE COLITIS

In 1999, Rembacken et al[39] conducted a single-center, randomized, double-dummy study examining 116 patients with active UC, assessing both treatment of acute active disease and maintenance of remission. Patients were randomized to mesalamine (Asacol; Procter & Gamble Pharmaceuticals, Inc, Egham, Surrey, UK), 1.2 g/d in three divided doses, or non-pathogenic *E. coli* Nissle 1917, 1×10^{11} cfu per day in two divided doses. At entry into the study, all patients were given an initial 1-week course of oral gentamicin (80 mg three times daily) to suppress their native *E. coli* flora. Along with the study probiotic or mesalamine, patients were also permitted to receive treatment with tapering prednisolone for moderate and severe disease and rectal hydrocortisone enemas for proctitis for 3 months to induce remission. After entering into remission, patients were maintained on either mesalamine or *E. coli* for up to 12 months. Forty-four patients (75%) in the mesalamine group and 39 patients (68%) in the *E. coli* group attained remission. The median time to remission was similar in both groups. At the end of 12 months, 25% of patients in the mesalamine group and 26% of patients in the *E. coli* group maintained remission. The median duration of remission was similar in both groups. The authors suggest that treatment with this nonpathogenic *E. coli* has an equivalent effect to mesalamine in maintaining remission. Nevertheless, the study was not powered for equivalence, and the remission rates at 1 year were close to historical placebo rates.

More recently, Kato et al[14] performed a 12-week randomized, placebo-controlled trial of a commercially available bifidobacteria-fermented milk (Yakult, Tokyo, Japan) in 20 active UC patients. In this study, patients were allowed to receive 5-ASA or sulfasalazine, as per usual care, at therapeutic doses of 4 g/d. Clinical remission rates, using the 21-point clinical disease activity index, were 40% in the treatment group and 33% in the placebo group, and response rates (drop in DAI of 3 points) were 70% in the treatment, as compared with 33% in the placebo group (P=ns). There was a significantly greater drop in DAI over 12 weeks in the treatment group than the placebo group ($P<0.05$). Although this study failed to show improved remission rates in the patients on bifidobacterium, it can be seen as promising because both groups were eligible to receive therapeutic doses of 5-ASA, making an additional treatment effect more difficult to detect than in most other probiotic studies.

Additional research on *Bifidobacterium* has been done by Furrie and colleagues,[40] who combined the use of a probiotic and a prebiotic nutrient to enhance activity in vivo. Such combination therapies have been referred to as synbiotics, but have had limited clinical data available until this double-blind, randomized, controlled trial. Eighteen patients with active ulcerative colitis for at least a 1-month duration were randomized to receive either placebo or a combination of *Bifidobacterium longum* (2 x 10^{11} freeze-dried bacteria twice daily) and 6 g twice daily of a fructo-oligosaccharide/inulin mixture (Synergy 1; Orafti, Tienen, Belgium) for 4 weeks. Clinical outcomes were measured using a DAI, bowel habit index, and sigmoidoscopy score. Histological scores and levels of inflammatory markers were also measured before and after treatment. No statistically significant difference was noted between groups in terms of clinical or endoscopic outcomes. Sigmoidoscopy scores decreased during treatment in the synbiotic-treated patients from a mean of 4.5 to 3.1, while scores increased in the placebo group from a mean of 2.6 to 3.2. While these trends would seem to favor the treated patients, it is puzzling that the post-treatment scores were almost identical between groups. Measurements of multiple inflammatory markers were significantly reduced following synbiotic treatment, so the authors suggest that a physiologic effect is likely being observed, which will require larger and longer duration trials to confirm, a conclusion with which we agree.

Guslandi et al[41] studied 25 patients with a clinical flare of their UC of a mild to moderate degree, according to Truelove and Witts' criteria. The patients were on maintenance mesalamine (3 g/d) for at least 3 months. Only patients who had a history of poorly tolerating corticosteroids were permitted to enter the study. In this open-label trial, patients received *Saccharomyces boulardii* (750 mg/d in three divided doses) for 4 weeks while their ongoing mesalamine was continued. DAI, before and after probiotic therapy, was determined by the Rachmilewitz UC activity index; it is calculated on the basis of stool frequency, blood in the stool, general condition, fever, abdominal pain, erythrocyte sedimentation rate, and hemoglobin values. A significant reduction in the UC activity index score was observed at the end of treatment ($P<0.05$), and remission (a DAI score ≤5) was achieved in 17 of 25 patients (68%).[41] Interestingly, the remission rate in this pilot study is remarkably similar to the remission rates described above for *E. coli* Nissle 1917.[39]

Also studying treatment of active UC were Bibloni et al,[42] who conducted a promising uncontrolled, open-label trial of VSL#3 in patients with active mild to moderate UC. Thirty-two patients were treated for a total of 6 weeks at a daily dose of 3.6 x 10^{12} bacteria. Uncontrolled results demonstrated a remission rate of 53% and a response rate of 24%, as measured using the UC DAI.

In a study by Tursi et al[43] comparing balsalazide plus VSL#3 with balsalazide alone or mesalamine alone, the authors suggested superiority of the probiotic-containing regimen, but the trial is difficult to interpret due to questionable statistical methodology.

A recent intriguing study by Borody et al,[44] slightly outside of the true probiotic realm, utilized fecal bacteriotherapy (fecal enemas) in 6 patients. These patients had failed maximum standard therapy for UC, including multiple courses of corticosteroids and immunosuppressive therapy. Fecal enemas were prepared fresh (in normal saline) from healthy adult donors, nominated by the patients, and were administered once daily for 5 consecutive days as enemas (retained for 6 to 8 hours). In addition to the fecal enemas, patients were prescribed a high-fiber diet in attempt to stimulate proliferation of infused bacteria. In a series of case reports, the authors document that these 6 patients were able to withdraw all concurrent UC medication approximately 4 to 6 weeks following completion of the fecal enema therapy. In 1 to 13 years of follow-up, there has been no clinical, colonoscopic, or histologic evidence of UC recurrence in any patient, despite the fact that no maintenance therapy has been used.[44] These results are dramatic and worthy of further investigation both from a pathogenesis, as well as a therapeutic, standpoint.

At the present time, probiotics have only Level B evidence in the treatment of acute UC, in large part because of the limited number of randomized, controlled studies that are investigating diverse agents, all of which may have different efficacies. Ongoing international randomized, placebo-controlled, clinical trials will hopefully clarify the role of probiotics in acute ulcerative colitis.

MAINTENANCE OF REMISSION IN ULCERATIVE COLITIS

In 1997, Kruis et al[45] examined 120 patients with inactive UC. These patients were included in a double-blind, double-dummy study comparing mesalamine (Salofalk; Axcan Pharma Inc, Houdan, France), 1.5 g/d in three divided doses, to an oral preparation of *E. coli* Nissle 1917, 5 x 10^{10} cfu/d as a single dose, for 3 months. Clinical remission was defined by the Rackmilewitz DAI score. Seventeen patients could not be included in the data analysis, and thus, intent-to-treat analysis was based upon results of 103 patients. At the end of 3 months, remission rates were 89% in the mesalamine group and 84% in the *E. coli* Nissle 1917 group ($P=0.12$). The authors concluded that *E. coli* Nissle 1917 was equivalent to mesalamine in maintenance of remission. Nevertheless, it is possible that the dose of mesalamine used was near placebo and the study was not adequately powered for equivalence.

In 2004, Kruis et al[13] published a larger and longer duration follow-up clinical trial than their initial maintenance of remission study. There were 327 patients with ulcerative colitis in medically-induced remission included in this double-blind, randomized, controlled study comparing mesalamine (Salofalk) 1.5 g/d in 3 divided doses to an oral preparation of *E. coli* Nissle 1917, 5 x 10^{10} cfu/d as a single dose, for 12 months. Clinical remission was defined using the Rackmilewitz DAI score. At the end of 12 months, relapse rates were 33.9% in the mesalamine group and 36.4% in the *E. coli* Nissle 1917 group. This study was powered as an equivalence trial adequate to detect a 20% difference in relapse rate, and it demonstrated significant equivalence between *E. coli* Nissle 1917 and mesalamine in the maintenance of remission of UC. The statistical power to detect equivalence adds significantly to the body of work on *E. coli* Nissle 1917. It should be noted, however, that the comparator dose of mesalamine was selected as that in the product monograph, but represents a lower dose than that generally used in clinical practice.

Venturi et al[46] examined 20 patients with UC who were intolerant or allergic to 5-ASA. Patients were in clinical, endoscopic, and histological remission following treatment with corticosteroids for a recent acute flare within the previous 3 months. Patients received open-label VSL#3 (1×10^{12} cfu/d in two divided doses) for 12 months. Patients were assessed clinically every 2 months and assessed endoscopically at 6 and 12 months. In this study, clinical remission was defined as absence of visible blood in the stools and no more than 2 bowel movements per day. Endoscopic remission was defined as a score of 0 in accordance with the Baron's UC index. Fifteen of 20 treated patients (75%) remained in remission at the end or after 12 months of study.[46] Once again, significant concentrations of the probiotics present in the VSL#3 were identified in fecal cultures. However, there were no significant changes in fecal concentration of bacteroides, clostridia, coliforms, or total aerobic and anaerobic bacteria.

Finally, Ishikawa et al[47] conducted a randomized, controlled trial study in 21 patients to examine the effect of bifidobacteria-fermented milk in patients with UC in remission. Patients received fermented milk (Yakult, Yakult Honsha Co, Ltd, Tokyo, Japan) that contained live bifidobacterium (*Bifidobacterium breve* and *Bifidobacterium bifidum*) and *Lactobacillus acidophilus* (1×10^{10} cfu per 100 ml once daily) for 12 months. Remission was defined clinically as any global increase in symptoms. Compliance at the 95% level was limited to 7 out of 11 patients consuming the fermented milk product. At the end of 12 months, clinical remission was seen in 8 out of 11 subjects (73%) taking the fermented milk and in 1 out of 10 subjects (10%) taking placebo.[47] Interestingly, despite this significant difference in clinical remission rates, there were no significant differences in the colonoscopic findings at 1 year. This raises the question as to the validity of the clinical assessment tool used in this trial. Furthermore, there were no differences between the 2 groups in total fecal bacterial counts or in bifidobacterium counts. However, the authors were able to recover (from the feces) the bifidobacterium strains present in the fermented milk. A larger, multicenter study with this probiotic product is currently underway.

The establishment of equivalence between *E. coli* Nissle 1917 and mesalamine is perhaps the most promising clinical trial result in terms of probiotic use for maintenance of remission in ulcerative colitis, but because of the dose-dependence of mesalamine in this disease and the lack of placebo-controlled confirmatory results, we are once again left with a scenario in which clear therapeutic recommendations cannot yet be made.

COLLAGENOUS COLITIS

Although microscopic colitis is a separate entity from ulcerative colitis, the fact that probiotic research is also ongoing in this field deserves mention. There has been considerably less study on the enteric flora in microscopic colitis than in UC or CD, but Tromm et al[48] have carried out an open-label pilot investigation using *E. coli* Nissle 1917 in the treatment of 14 patients with collagenous colitis. They found a decrease in stool frequency in 64% of patients, a promising initial result that warrants further research.

Future Directives

It is clear that intestinal bacteria play a significant role in the pathogenesis of inflammatory bowel disease and that specific strains or combinations of strains can have either pathogenic or beneficial effects. Probiotic bacteria modulate a number of the proinflammatory pathways. Understanding of the mechanisms of action of these probiotic bacteria, especially in the case of IBD, will permit the development of definitive criteria for the selection of probiotic strains useful for clinical application. It will also allow for the determination of optimal doses, timing of administration, and synergistic combinations of bacterial species. The advent of molecular techniques that allow us to quantify, identify, and determine the genomics and proteomics of luminal bacteria and probiotics, will significantly advance this area of research. We will need to determine if the use of a single probiotic, or the use of combinations of probiotics, present the best therapeutic approach. We also need to better investigate dosing and colonization issues. Appropriately designed, randomized, controlled clinical trials have clearly identified a therapeutic role for some probiotics in the case of pouchitis. Nevertheless, the plethora of pilot, open-label, and poorly designed clinical trials, as seen in the cases of UC and CD, can be read as tending to overstate the promise of probiotics. Rigorously designed, controlled, clinical trials must be constructed to investigate issues related to efficacy, dose, duration of use, single or multi-strain formulation, and the concomitant use of prebiotics, synbiotics, and antibiotics.

PREBIOTICS

Background

While the use of probiotics constitutes direct colonization of the intestine with ingested bacteria, prebiotics are an indirect route to the same end. They are dietary substances, generally undigested carbohydrates, which selectively alter the fecal flora in favor of "beneficial" probiotic organisms, most commonly *Lactobacillus* and *Bifidobacterium*. They are theoretically tempting because they are relatively innocuous substances, promote the growth of favorable colonic bacteria, and provide that flora with the building blocks required to produce beneficial substances, such as short-chain fatty acids.[49,50] Early evidence of beneficial effects of probiotics have led at least one author to hypothesize that physiologic lactase deficiency may be a human adaptation designed to allow ingested lactose to act as a prebiotic.[51]

Pharmacokinetics

Because the field of prebiotics is so new, and the preparations used are heterogeneous, discussion of pharmacokinetics in general is impossible at this time.

Adverse Events

Clinical trials of prebiotics have generally found no specific adverse events.[50,52,53] As with any dietary fiber, prebiotics have caused bloating in some patients.[53]

Clinical Trials

As with research in probiotics, the prebiotic literature eludes firm conclusions because of the heterogeneous nature of preparations and settings used for experimentation. Animal data have been promising, however. In 3 separate experiments, fructo-oligosaccharides caused a reduction in TNBS-induced colitis in rats,[54] germinated barley foodstuffs decreased DSS-induced mouse colitis,[55] and lactulose decreased DSS-induced colitis in mice.[56] A limited number of human studies in UC are available.

In 1991, Hallert et al[57] conducted a 4-week randomized, placebo-controlled trial of ispaghula husk for maintenance of remission in 36 patients with clinically and endoscopically quiescent UC. The trial had a 19% dropout rate, and was assessed by per-protocol analysis. Although no primary outcome was defined, the authors used a global score of 8 symptoms, assessed on visual analogue scale, and found decreased symptoms in treated patients as compared with placebo, with 69% of patients on ispaghula improving versus 24% on placebo ($P<0.001$). This study had several weaknesses, not the least of which is that their implied primary outcome was an improvement in symptoms from a clinical remission that is undefined in the study's text. Strictly speaking, it was intended as a study of a bulk-forming agent and preceded common use of the concept of prebiotics in the gastroenterology literature. Nevertheless, this study has been seen by some recent authors as the first preliminary evidence for prebiotic use in ulcerative colitis, on the basis that the study agent can increase fecal concentrations of *Bifidobacterium*.[58]

Based on promising preliminary studies,[59,60] Kanauchi and colleagues conducted 2 multicenter, non-randomized, open trials of germinated barley foodstuff (GBF) in the treatment of active UC. The first study, in 2002,[52] involved 18 patients with mild to moderate disease, as defined by Truelove and Witts criteria, who received either their baseline therapy, mostly 5-ASA or sulfasalazine, or baseline therapy combined with 20 to 30 g of GBF daily. After 4 weeks of therapy, the GBF group had a significantly lower clinical activity index than the baseline therapy group ($P=0.045$), and in a single patient who underwent fecal microflora analysis, there was increased *Bifidobacterium* and *Eubacteria*, with a decrease in bacteroides following therapy.

The Kanauchi group's second study was of similar design, but with longer duration.[50] Twenty-one patients with mild to moderate UC were observed for 24 weeks while on baseline therapy plus GBF (20 to 30 g/d). The authors report significantly improved symptom scores over the course of the trial in the patients receiving GBF. While the paper's abstract describes a significant improvement as compared with a control group, no control group is described (or even mentioned) anywhere in the body of the paper. This inconsistency in reported methodology makes the study difficult to interpret.

Future Directions

Clinical research on prebiotics remains in its infancy. Properly randomized, controlled trials are required in order to define a clinical role, but for now prebiotics can be described as promising, based on very early results and an excellent safety profile.

REFERENCES

1. Kraehenbuhl JP. Mucosa-targeted DNA vaccination. *Trends Immunol.* 2001;22(12):646-648.
2. Akira S, Sato S. Toll-like receptors and their signaling mechanisms. *Scand J Infect Dis.* 2003;35(9):555-562.
3. Yamamoto M, Takeda K, Akira S. TIR domain-containing adaptors define the specificity of TLR signaling. *Mol Immunol.* 2004;40(12):861-868.
4. Di Marzio L, Russo FP, D'Alo S, et al. Apoptotic effects of selected strains of lactic acid bacteria on a human T leukemia cell line are associated with bacterial arginine deiminase and/or sphingomyelinase activities. *Nutr Cancer.* 2001;40(2):185-196.

5. Madsen K, Cornish A, Soper P, et al. Probiotic bacteria enhance murine and human intestinal epithelial barrier function. *Gastroenterology.* 2001;121(3):580-591.
6. Anton P, O'Connell J, O'Connell D, et al. Mucosal subepithelial binding sites for the bacterial chemotactic peptide, formylmethionyl-leucyl-phenylalanine (FMLP). *Gut.* 1998;42(3):374-379.
7. Girardin SE, Travassos LH, Herve M, et al. Peptidoglycan molecular requirements allowing detection by Nod1 and Nod2. *J Biol Chem.* 2003;278(43):41702-41708.
8. Inohara N, Ogura Y, Fontalba A, et al. Host recognition of bacterial muramyl dipeptide mediated through NOD2: implications for Crohn's disease. *J Biol Chem.* 2003;278(8):5509-5512.
9. Chamaillard M, Hashimoto M, Horie Y, et al. An essential role for NOD1 in host recognition of bacterial peptidoglycan containing diaminopimelic acid. *Nat Immunol.* 2003;4(7):702-707.
10. Madsen K, Jijon H, Yeung H, McKaigney C, De Simone C. DNA from probiotic bacteria exerts anti-inflammatory actions on intestinal epithelial cells by inhibition of NF-kB. *Gastroenterology.* 2002;122:A546.
11. Akhtar M, Watson JL, Nazli A, McKay DM. Bacterial DNA evokes epithelial IL-8 production by a MAPK-dependent, NF-kappaB-independent pathway. *FASEB J.* 2003;17(10):1319-1321.
12. Rachmilewitz D, Karmeli F, Takabayashi K, et al. Immunostimulatory DNA ameliorates experimental and spontaneous murine colitis. *Gastroenterology.* 2002;122(5):1428-1441.
13. Kruis W, Fric P, Pokrotnieks J, et al. Maintaining remission of ulcerative colitis with the probiotic *Escherichia coli* Nissle 1917 is as effective as with standard mesalazine. *Gut.* 2004;53(11):1617-1623.
14. Kato K, Mizuno S, Umesaki Y, et al. Randomized placebo-controlled trial assessing the effect of bifidobacteria-fermented milk on active ulcerative colitis. *Aliment Pharmacol Ther.* 2004;20(10):1133-1141.
15. Sheil B, McCarthy J, O'Mahony L, et al. Is the mucosal route of administration essential for probiotic function? Subcutaneous administration is associated with attenuation of murine colitis and arthritis. *Gut.* 2004;53(5):694-700.
16. Borriello SP, Hammes WP, Holzapfel W, et al. Safety of probiotics that contain lactobacilli or bifidobacterium. *Clin Infect Dis.* 2003;36(6):775-780.
17. Gasser F. Safety of lactic-acid bacteria and their occurrence in human clinical infections. *Bulletin de L'Institut Pasteur.* 1994;92:45-67.
18. Saxelin M, Chuang NH, Chassy B, et al. Lactobacilli and bacteremia in southern Finland, 1989-1992. *Clin Infect Dis.* 1996;22(3):564-566.
19. Salminen MK, Tynkkynen S, Rautelin H, et al. Lactobacillus bacteremia during a rapid increase in probiotic use of Lactobacillus rhamnosus GG in Finland. *Clin Infect Dis.* 2002;35(10):1155-1160.
20. Gionchetti P, Rizzello F, Venturi A, et al. Oral bacteriotherapy as maintenance treatment in patients with chronic pouchitis: a double-blind, placebo-controlled trial. *Gastroenterology.* 2000;119(2):305-309.
21. Husni RN, Gordon SM, Washington JA, Longworth DL. Lactobacillus bacteremia and endocarditis: review of 45 cases. *Clin Infect Dis.* 1997;25(5):1048-1055.
22. Wolf BW, Wheeler KB, Ataya DG, Garleb KA. Safety and tolerance of *Lactobacillus reuteri* supplementation to a population infected with the human immunodeficiency virus. *Food Chem Toxicol.* 1998;36(12):1085-1094.
23. Patel R, Cockerill FR, Porayko MK, Osmon DR, Ilstrup DM, Keating MR. Lactobacillemia in liver transplant patients. *Clin Infect Dis.* 1994;18(2):207-212.
24. Antony SJ, Stratton CW, Dummer JS. Lactobacillus bacteremia: description of the clinical course in adult patients without endocarditis. *Clin Infect Dis.* 1996;23(4):773-778.
25. Piarroux R, Millon L, Bardonnet K, Vagner O, Koenig H. Are live saccharomyces yeasts harmful to patients? *Lancet.* 1999;353(9167):1851-1852.
26. Rautio M, Jousimies-Somer H, Kauma H, et al. Liver abscess due to a *Lactobacillus rhamnosus* strain indistinguishable from *L. rhamnosus* strain GG. *Clin Infect Dis.* 1999;28(5):1159-1160.
27. Pletincx M, Legein J, Vandenplas Y. Fungemia with *Saccharomyces boulardii* in a 1-year-old girl with protracted diarrhea. *J Pediatr Gastroenterol Nutr.* 1995;21(1):113-115.
28. Horwitch CA, Furseth HA, Larson AM, Jones TL, Olliffe JF, Spach DH. Lactobacillemia in three patients with AIDS. *Clin Infect Dis.* 1995;21(6):1460-1462.
29. Chomarat M, Espinouse D. *Lactobacillus rhamnosus* septicemia in patients with prolonged aplasia receiving ceftazidime-vancomycin. *Eur J Clin Microbiol Infect Dis.* 1991;10(1):44.
30. Pedone CA, Bernabeu AO, Postaire ER, Bouley CF, Reinert P. The effect of supplementation with milk fermented by *Lactobacillus casei* (strain DN-114 001) on acute diarrhoea in children attending day care centres. *Int J Clin Pract.* 1999;53(3):179-184.
31. Vanderhoof JA, Young RJ. Use of probiotics in childhood gastrointestinal disorders. *J Pediatr Gastroenterol Nutr.* 1998;27(3):323-332.
32. Guandalini S, Pensabene L, Zikri MA, et al. *Lactobacillus* GG administered in oral rehydration solution to children with acute diarrhea: a multicenter European trial. *J Pediatr Gastroenterol Nutr.* 2000;30(1):54-60.
33. Ruseler-van Embden JG, Schouten WR, van Lieshout LM. Pouchitis: Result of microbial imbalance? *Gut.* 1994;35(5):658-664.
34. Mimura T, Rizzello F, Helwig U, et al. Once daily high dose probiotic therapy (VSL#3) for maintaining remission in recurrent or refractory pouchitis. *Gut.* 2004;53(1):108-114.
35. Kuisma J, Mentula S, Jarvinen H, Kahri A, Saxelin M, Farkkila M. Effect of *Lactobacillus rhamnosus* GG on ileal pouch inflammation and microbial flora. *Aliment Pharmacol Ther.* 2003;17:509-515.
36. Laake KO, Line PD, Aabakken L, et al. Assessment of mucosal inflammation and circulation in response to probiotics in patients operated with ileal pouch anal anastomosis for ulcerative colitis. *Scand J Gastroenterol.* 2003;38(4):409-414.
37. Gionchetti P, Rizzello F, Helwig U, et al. Prophylaxis of pouchitis onset with probiotic therapy: a double-blind, placebo-controlled trial. *Gastroenterology.* 2003;124(5):1202-1209.
38. Gosselink MP, Schouten WR, van Lieshout LM, Hop WC, Laman JD, Ruseler-van Embden JG. Delay of the first onset of pouchitis by oral intake of the probiotic strain *Lactobacillus rhamnosus* GG. *Dis Colon Rectum.* 2004;47(6):876-884.
39. Rembacken BJ, Snelling AM, Hawkey PM, Chalmers DM, Axon AT. Non-pathogenic *Escherichia coli* versus mesalazine for the treatment of ulcerative colitis: a randomised trial. *Lancet.* 1999;354(9179):635-639.
40. Furrie E, Macfarlane S, Kennedy A, et al. Synbiotic therapy (*Bifidobacterium longum*/Synergy 1) initiates resolution of inflammation in patients with active ulcerative colitis: a randomised controlled pilot trial. *Gut.* 2005;54(2):242-249.
41. Guslandi M, Giollo P, Testoni PA. A pilot trial of *Saccharomyces boulardii* in ulcerative colitis. *Eur J Gastroenterol Hepatol.* 2003;15(6):697-698.
42. Bibloni R, Fedorak RN, Tannock GW, et al. VSL#3 probiotic-mixture induces remission in patients with active ulcerative colitis. *Am J Gastroenterol.* 2005;100(7):1539-1546.
43. Tursi A, Brandimarte G, Giorgetti GM, Forti G, Modeo ME, Gigliobianco A. Low-dose balsalazide plus a high-potency probiotic preparation is more effective than balsalazide alone or mesalazine in the treatment of acute mild-to-moderate ulcerative colitis. *Med Sci Monit.* 2004;10(11):PI126-131.

44. Borody TJ, Warren EF, Leis S, Surace R, Ashman O. Treatment of ulcerative colitis using fecal bacteriotherapy. *J Clin Gastroenterol.* 2003;37(1):42-47.
45. Kruis W, Schutz E, Fric P, Fixa B, Judmaier G, Stolte M. Double-blind comparison of an oral *Escherichia coli* preparation and mesalazine in maintaining remission of ulcerative colitis. *Aliment Pharmacol Ther.* 1997;11(5):853-858.
46. Venturi A, Gionchetti P, Rizzello F, et al. Impact on the composition of the faecal flora by a new probiotic preparation: preliminary data on maintenance treatment of patients with ulcerative colitis. *Aliment Pharmacol Ther.* 1999;13(8):1103-1108.
47. Ishikawa H, Akedo I, Umesaki Y, Tanaka R, Imaoka A, Otani T. Randomized controlled trial of the effect of bifidobacteria-fermented milk on ulcerative colitis. *J Am Coll Nutr.* 2003;22(1):56-63.
48. Tromm A, Niewerth U, Khoury M, et al. The probiotic *E. coli* strain Nissle 1917 for the treatment of collagenous colitis: first results of an open-label trial. *Z Gastroenterol.* 2004;42(5):365-369.
49. Jacobasch G, Schmiedl D, Kruschewski M, Schmehl K. Dietary resistant starch and chronic inflammatory bowel diseases. *Int J Colorect Dis.* 1999;14(4-5):201-211.
50. Kanauchi O, Mitsuyama K, Homma T, et al. Treatment of ulcerative colitis patients by long-term administration of germinated barley foodstuff: multi-center open trial. *Int J Mol Med.* 2003;12(5):701-704.
51. Szilagyi A. Review article: Lactose: a potential prebiotic. *Aliment Pharmacol Ther.* 2002;16(9):1591-1602.
52. Kanauchi O, Suga T, Tochihara M, et al. Treatment of ulcerative colitis by feeding with germinated barley foodstuff: first report of a multicenter open control trial. *J Gastroenterol.* 2002;37 Suppl 14:67-72.
53. Bamba T, Kanauchi O, Andoh A, Fujiyama Y. A new prebiotic from germinated barley for nutraceutical treatment of ulcerative colitis. *J Gastroenterol Hepatol.* 2002;17(8):818-824.
54. Cherbut C, Michel C, Lecannu G. The prebiotic characteristics of fructooligosaccharides are necessary for reduction of TNBS-induced colitis in rats. *J Nutr.* 2003;133(1):21-27.
55. Kanauchi O, Serizawa I, Araki Y, et al. Germinated barley foodstuff, a prebiotic product, ameliorates inflammation of colitis through modulation of the enteric environment. *J Gastroenterol.* 2003;38(2):134-141.
56. Rumi G, Tsubouchi R, Okayama M, Kato S, Mozsik G, Takeuchi K. Protective effect of lactulose on dextran sulfate sodium-induced colonic inflammation in rats. *Dig Dis Sci.* 2004;49(9):1466-1472.
57. Hallert C, Kaldma M, Petersson BG. Ispaghula husk may relieve gastrointestinal symptoms in ulcerative colitis in remission. *Scand J Gastroenterol.* 1991;26(7):747-750.
58. Sartor RB. Therapeutic manipulation of the enteric microflora in inflammatory bowel diseases: antibiotics, probiotics, and prebiotics. *Gastroenterology.* 2004;126(6):1620-1633.
59. Mitsuyama K, Saiki T, Kanauchi O, et al. Treatment of ulcerative colitis with germinated barley foodstuff feeding: a pilot study. *Aliment Pharmacol Ther.* 1998;12(12):1225-1230.
60. Kanauchi O, Iwanaga T, Mitsuyama K. Germinated barley foodstuff feeding: a novel neutraceutical therapeutic strategy for ulcerative colitis. *Digestion.* 2001;63(Suppl 1):60-67.

36 MANAGEMENT OF ACUTE AND CHRONIC POUCHITIS

James M. Becker, MD, FACS and Arthur F. Stucchi, PhD

Although the majority of patients with chronic ulcerative colitis (UC) can be managed medically, an estimated 30 to 40% will eventually require a total proctocolectomy either to control the refractory nature of their disease or to alleviate the escalating potential for malignancy.[1] Until recently, these patients, many of whom are quite young, were left with a permanent Brooke ileostomy that was poorly accepted by both patients and physicians. In fact, patients often refused or delayed curative proctocolectomy because of their aversion to a Brooke ileostomy. However, the past 3 decades have brought surgical alternatives that have significantly improved the quality of life for these patients.

Proctocolectomy with continent ileostomy, or the Kock pouch,[2] was the first procedure to offer patients an alternative to a Brooke ileostomy, but was fraught with technical complications, poor functional results, and the desire by patients to alleviate any type of permanent ileostomy and was thus largely abandoned. Restorative proctocolectomy was re-introduced some 30 years ago[3-5] after being originally proposed by Ravitch and Sabiston in the late 1940s.[6] Because an inverse relationship was found between ileal compliance and stool frequency in patients after an end-to-end or straight ileoanal anastomosis, surgeons sought to accelerate the process of ileal adaptation to improve function. An important technical advance that greatly decreased stool frequency and increased fecal continence was the surgical construction of an ileal pouch or reservoir proximal to the ileoanal anastomosis.[4] Today, most gastrointestinal surgeons agree that restorative proctocolectomy with ileal pouch-anal anastomosis (IPAA) is the definitive operation for the surgical treatment of patients with chronic UC[7,8] and familial adenomatous polyposis (FAP).[9,10] Refinements in operative technique, postoperative care, and patient education have led to substantially improved outcomes and very high patient satisfaction rates.[11,12] Despite the significant improvement in the health-related quality of life these surgical advances have brought to many of these patients,[13] nonspecific, idiopathic inflammation of the ileal pouch or pouchitis occurs in as many as 1 out of 2 patients who have undergone IPAA for chronic UC. Even though pouchitis has now become the most common late postoperative complication following IPAA in these patients,[14,15] its etiology, treatment, and prevention remain poorly understood.

DEFINITION

Historically, one might classify pouchitis as an iatrogenic syndrome because it never existed prior to the emergence of the surgically created ileal pouch. Nils Kock of Gotteborg, Sweden coined the term "pouchitis" shortly after the introduction of the continent ileostomy in the late 1970s.[16] As mentioned, the term describes a nonspecific inflammation of the ileal reservoir that occurs almost exclusively in patients who have undergone restorative proctocolectomy for chronic UC. Despite the high risk of pouchitis in these patients, a standardized definition as well as algorithms for classification, diagnosis, and clinical management of pouchitis were lacking for years, thus creating difficulties in interpreting data related to the actual incidence and treatment of pouchitis.

While pouchitis has long been defined and often treated based on clinical symptoms alone, it has been known since early on that pouch inflammation included endoscopic

Lichtenstein GR, ed.
Ulcerative Colitis: The Complete Guide to Medical Management (pp 405-432)

and histologic components that played a significant diagnostic role.[17] In order to better define diagnostic criteria, a number of quantitative indices have been proposed by Sandborn,[18] Heuschen et al,[19] and Shen et al,[20] that now enable clinicians to determine the extent and severity of pouchitis based on a triad of criteria, including clinical symptoms along with endoscopic and histologic parameters. While the usefulness of these diagnostic indices in the clinical setting is not always practical, their utility as research tools in objectively quantifying the response to medical therapy is unsurpassed. These standardized reporting criteria will also become increasingly important as information on long-term follow-up and outcomes databases on IPAA patients begin to grow.

As will be discussed in further detail, pouchitis can represent a spectrum of inflammatory and noninflammatory disorders of the ileal pouch,[21] and IPAA patients can present with symptoms that may appear clinically similar to pouchitis. Therefore, before the diagnosis is made and definitive treatment begins, other inflammatory and noninflammatory conditions such as cuffitis, irritable pouch syndrome (IPS), and, most importantly, Crohn's disease must be ruled out.[22]

CLINICAL, ENDOSCOPIC, AND HISTOLOGIC PRESENTATIONS OF POUCHITIS

Clinically, pouchitis can present with any number of symptoms frequently consistent with the patient's prior colitis, including increased stool frequency, watery diarrhea, fecal urgency, incontinence, rectal bleeding, abdominal cramping, low-grade fever, and malaise (Table 36-1).[23] Many of these clinical symptoms are common components of the various pouchitis DAIs.[19,20,24] In some patients, pouchitis can be accompanied by extraintestinal manifestations such as arthralgias, myalgias, erythema nodosum, PSC,[25] and inflammatory eye problems.[26] In fact, patients with preoperative extraintestinal manifestations are likely to experience a higher incidence of pouchitis suggesting an association with the underlying IBD.[25,27,28]

When repeated episodes or chronic clinical symptoms persist, the ileal pouch should be examined by flexible ileal pouchoscopy, as described below, which can also be useful in ruling out other inflammatory and noninflammatory conditions.[22] Endoscopically, the mucosal surface of the normally appearing pouch glistens and has a velvety appearance indicative of normal villi (Figure 36-1A). In sharp contract, the inflamed ileal pouch appears erythematous, edematous, hyperemic, and granular.[24] The mucosa is often friable, may bleed on contact, and a mucous exudate is often visible (Figure 36-1B). Mucosal and submucosal hemorrhaging and superficial, focal ulceration are also present in more severe cases (Figure 36-1C). Occasionally, ulcerations may be found along any of the staple or suture lines within the pouch; however, these are generally not associated with more diffuse pouch inflammation. While these mucosal changes may be irregular and not uniform throughout the pouch, the functional integrity of the entire pouch can be affected including, in some severe cases, the ileum just proximal to the pouch. There may also be a clear line of distinction between the unaffected proximal ileum and the inflamed pouch. Endoscopic appearance alone, however, does not always correlate well with the overall clinical presentation.[29]

When examining the ileal pouch endoscopically, the anatomic location of the mucosal inflammation can be an important diagnostic consideration. Although pouchitis typically presents in the distal portion of the pouch, factors such as pouch configuration, severity, and chronicity can affect the distribution of the inflammation. Inflammation can extend proximally in the more severe and chronic cases; however, this can also be indicative of Crohn's disease. If this anatomic presentation persists following therapy, further diagnostic evaluation, as discussed later, should be considered. Also discussed later in more detail, inflammation occurring distal to the pouch in the area of the anal transition zone may indicate that original colonic mucosa still remains and chronic UC has recurred. Although this generally occurs in patients who have undergone a double-stapled ileal pouch-anal canal anastomosis, any inflammation found between the dentate line and the distal apex of the pouch is suspect and must be biopsied.

Histologically, the majority of functioning ileal pouches typically show some cellular elements of inflammation, even in asymptomatic patients undergoing routine surveillance.[17] To demonstrate this point, we showed in our own studies that myeloperoxidase levels (a biochemical marker for neutrophils) in ileal pouch mucosal biopsies from asymptomatic patients were significantly elevated compared with proximal ileum from the same patient.[30] These data indicate that inflammatory cells, especially neutrophils, commonly infiltrate the lamina propria of the ileal pouch. The underlying signal for this attraction is not yet understood; however, inflammation in the ileal pouch has been characterized by the upregulation of adhesion molecules such as E-selectin and the recruitment of CD15-positive cells, emphasizing the role of neutrophil recruitment and migration in the pathogenesis of pouchitis.[31] Interestingly, we also observed increased neutrophils and myeloperoxidase levels in ileal pouches from patients with FAP who had never experienced an episode of pouchitis.[30]

In more pronounced cases of ileal inflammation, increased numbers of lamina propria and stromal neutrophils, plasmacytoid lymphocytes, and eosinophils are clearly evident (Figure 36-2A). Depending on the severity and chronicity of the inflammation, superficial ulceration, crypt abscesses (Figure 36-2B), and goblet cell depletion can

TABLE 36-1

TRIAD OF CRITERIA USED TO DEFINE AND DIAGNOSE POUCHITIS

CLINICAL SYMPTOMS

- Increased stool frequency
- Watery, sometimes bloody diarrhea
- Urgency, abdominal cramping
- Incontinence and nocturnal leakage
- Symptoms consistent with chronic UC
- Extraintestinal manifestations (arthralgias, myalgias, erythema nodosum)
- Low-grade fever, malaise

ENDOSCOPIC FINDINGS

- Nonspecific inflammation
- Edema
- Erythematous
- Hyperemic and granular
- Mucosal friability
- Mucous exudate
- Mucosal and submucosal hemorrhaging
- Superficial and focal ulceration

HISTOLOGIC FINDINGS

- Mucosal edema
- Lamina propria and stromal polymorphonuclear leukocyte infiltration
- Epithelial degeneration of the villi with neutrophilic and lymphocytic infiltrates
- Stromal vascularity and ulceration
- Villous blunting and atrophy
- Crypt and goblet cell hyperplasia
- Neutrophilic infiltrate of the crypt epithelia
- Stromal infiltrates of plasmacytoid, eosinophils, and neutrophils
- Superficial ulceration, crypt abscesses, and goblet cell depletion

also be observed.[32-34] Even in the setting of these chronic inflammatory infiltrates, the presence of granulomas may not necessarily be indicative of CD. These changes are often associated with architectural alterations such as epithelial degeneration of the villi (Figure 36-2C), villous blunting and atrophy, crypt and goblet cell hyperplasia, as well as the presence of a variety of inflammatory cells (Figure 36-3A through C). Some pathologists feel that these types of architectural changes may represent nonspecific, metaplastic changes, which commonly occur as the pouch adapts its new luminal environment.[35,36]

Interestingly, within weeks following the closure of the temporary diverting ileostomy, frequently performed at the time of IPAA, morphological and architectural changes become apparent in the pouch.[37,38] Various studies have described these morphologic changes of the ileal pouch mucosal architecture, namely villous atrophy and crypt hyperplasia. Lerch et al[39] described total villous atrophy and significant crypt hyperplasia after IPAA and concluded that adaptation of the pouch ileum to its neorectal function results in progressive transformation to a more colonic-like mucosa, a phenomena referred to as colonic metaplasia. They

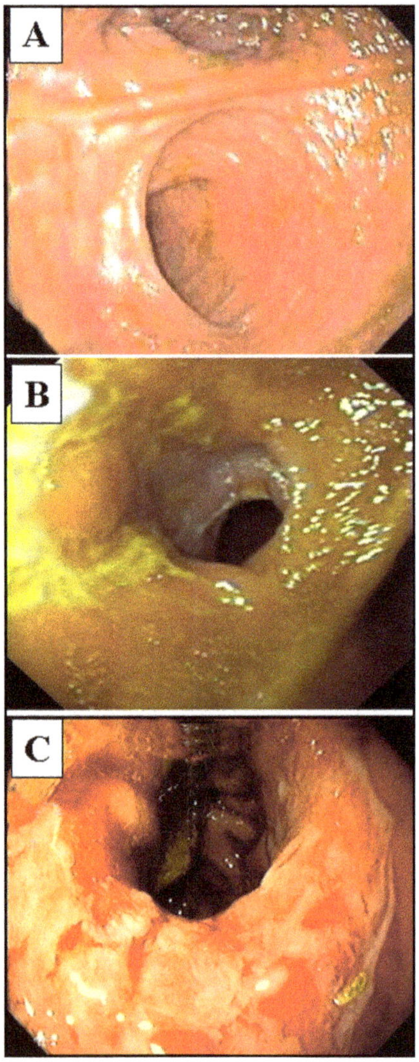

FIGURE 36-1. Endoscopic images of a pelvic ileal J pouch. (A) Normally appearing pouch 5 years after IPAA. The mucosal surface glistens and has a velvety appearance indicative of normal villi. (B) Mild pouchitis. (C) Severely inflamed pouch showing characteristic signs of pouchitis. The mucosal surface appears erythematous and edematous with numerous shallow ulcers and a mucous exudate. Presence of a stricture may be indicative of Crohn's disease.

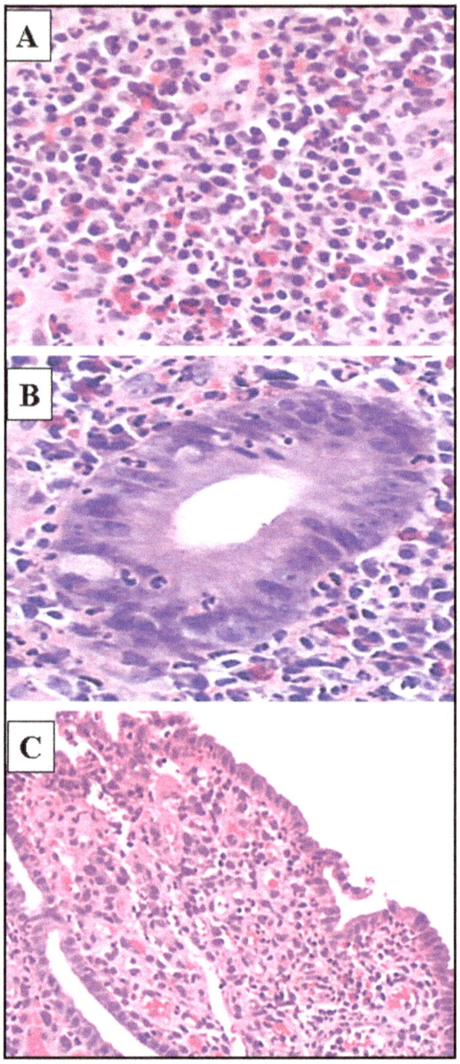

FIGURE 36-2. Photomicrographs of histological sections of ileal pouch mucosa showing (A) Inflammation associated with pouchitis characterized by increased inflammatory cells, primarily neutrophils, eosinophils, and stromal plasma cells; (B) acute cryptitis and increased stromal inflammatory cells; and (C) acute epithelitis and markedly increased vascularity.

described pouch mucosa as nearly indistinguishable from normal colonic mucosal structure and function in which mucin-distended goblet cells and lysozyme containing Paneth's cells were numerous. In similar studies, Shepherd et al[32] also showed that colonic metaplasia was associated with secretory changes that included the presence of more colonic-like sulfomucins and lower concentrations of ileal sialomucins. Nevertheless, others have shown that colonic-like mucosa in the pouch appear to retain some indigenous biochemical and histological characteristics, which include the retention of sucrase-isomaltase activity,[40] secretory-active enteroendocrine cells,[39] and the ability to absorb key nutrients and bile acids.[41] Others have reported metabolic consequences associated with villous atrophy and extent of inflammation in pouch ileum. Patients with subtotal or total villous atrophy had significantly reduced serum levels of albumin, calcium, total cholesterol, triglycerides, and vitamin E, along with reduced absorption rates of bile acids and vitamin B12. Vitamin A, D, and B12 deficiencies were also noted in many of these IPAA patients, prompting these authors to recommend that patients with active chronic inflammation need long-term follow-up with regular ileal pouch surveillance.[42]

It has been hypothesized that the transformation to more colon-like mucosa may prompt the development of "colitis" within the pouch and is a major etiologic factor predisposing the recurrence of mucosal inflammation.[36] However, earlier studies demonstrated that total villous atrophy in the pouch was not a universal finding following IPAA,[40,43] and it was suggested that villous atrophy may be

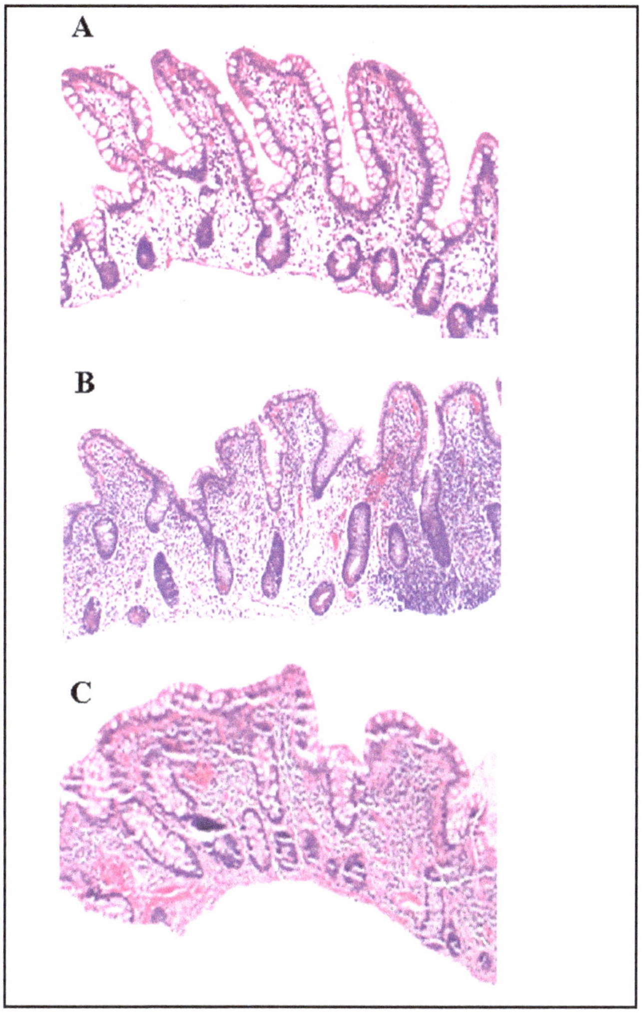

FIGURE 36-3. Photomicrographs of histological sections of ileal pouch mucosa. (A) Nearly normal villous architecture with minimal villous blunting and no histologic abnormality. (B) Biopsy specimen from a patient with acute episodes of moderate pouchitis showing increased vascularity, expansion of the lamina propria by inflammatory cells, acute epithelitis and cryptitis and associated mild to moderate blunting of the villi. (C) Biopsy specimen from a patient with chronic, severe pouchitis showing severe villous blunting with severe atrophy and crypt hyperplasia. (Reprinted from Fruin AB, El-Zammer O, Stucchi AF, et al. Colonic metaplasia in the ileal pouch is associated with inflammation and is not the result of long-term adaptation. *J Gastrointest Surg.* 2003;7:246-254, © with permission from Elsevier Inc.)

transient and more commonly associated with long-standing inflammation.[43] Other studies have not shown such a relationship between mucosal inflammatory changes and villous atrophy.[44]

The contention that ileal pouch mucosa undergoes colonic metaplasia, thus favoring the development of recurrent "colitis" in the pouch, has led to concern over the development of dysplasia and potentially neoplasia in the pouch. Periodic surveillance endoscopy with biopsies has been recommended for all IPAA patients at 5-year intervals to screen for the development of dysplasia,[45] especially in those patients with prior PSC who are more prone to developing pouchitis and mucosal atrophy and have a higher risk of neoplastic transformation.[46]

The results of a study recently reported by our laboratory[47] suggest that the mucosal architectural changes often described as evidence of colonic metaplasia occur primarily in the setting of inflammation and often improve when the inflammation is successfully treated. Moderate architectural changes (Figure 36-3B), severe villous atrophy (Figure 36-3C), and crypt hyperplasia may represent a reparative response to underlying inflammation, as is commonly observed in other inflammatory diseases of the small intestine, such as celiac sprue. Further investigation of the mechanism by which inflammation causes villous atrophy may be relevant to better understanding of pouchitis. Although the risk of dysplasia in ileal pouches up to 20 years after IPAA for chronic UC is uncommon,[48,49] and we have never documented a case in our own series, a recent systematic review of 23 studies with 2040 patients by Scarpa et al[50] provided evidence to the contrary. Thus, periodic surveillance is recommended.

Often, patients are observed with what appears to be moderate inflammatory changes in the pouch such as those described above but exhibit no overt clinical symptoms or vice versa.[29] A significant number of very symptomatic patients with no endoscopic or histologic evidence of pouch inflammation may suffer from a recently described condition known as IPS.[51]

DISEASE CLASSIFICATION

Pouchitis is a very heterogeneous disorder often manifesting in a wide variety of clinical presentations,[21] ranging from an acute therapeutically responsive to a more chronic, relapsing condition and, in fewer cases, to a refractory and therapeutically resistant disease. Pouchitis in patients experiencing these varying manifestations can often be the result of different etiologic or pathophysiologic factors, can have very different clinical courses, respond very differently to similar medications, and have very dissimilar prognoses. For these reasons, clinicians often tend to classify pouchitis based on the frequency of occurrence and recurrence, severity, duration of episodes, and responsiveness to therapy.[52] Patients with acute disease will experience one or more shortened episodes, generally 10 to 14 days, that typically resolve with a 7- to 10-day course or two of antibiotic therapy. Patients with a more chronic syndrome tend to either have more persistent symptoms lasting weeks to months despite therapy or symptoms that respond well to therapy but recur shortly after therapy is discontinued. Patients with refractory disease tend to be symptomatic for long periods of time, often 3 to 4 months or longer, despite aggressive therapy, as discussed later. A small number of these patients will eventually be responsive to long-term treatment; however, a good percentage will remain refractory to medical therapy. This small population of IPAA patients must be carefully screened for other conditions of the ileal pouch that can manifest with symptoms similar to pouchitis, such as infectious pathogens, pelvic sepsis, IPS, cuffitis, CD, as well as other mechanical and functional problems.[53] These patients tend to have the poorest outcomes and are often candidates for pouch diversion, revision, or removal.

INCIDENCE AND CUMULATIVE RISK

In general, the majority of patients undergoing IPAA for chronic UC have a very satisfactory and functional outcome,[11-13,54] despite the fact that 1 out of 2 will develop at least one episode of symptomatic inflammation of the ileal pouch. As previously mentioned, the wide variety of diagnostic criteria utilized to identify this poorly defined clinical entity accounts for considerable variability in the reported incidence. The problem is further compounded by the fact that not all clinical series report complete endoscopic and histologic details or length of follow-up, thus further contributing to the inconsistent interpretation of the actual incidence. However, the recent attempts to gain a better quantitative assessment of the disease[19,20,24] should eventually lead to more standardized reporting and a better estimate of the true incidence.

For all chronic UC patients, pouchitis is not an absolutely certain outcome following IPAA. Based on the current reporting standards, at most, approximately 1 out of 2 of these patients will suffer from at least one episode. The incidence of pouchitis can vary from just 6%[55] to upwards of 58%[56] and 59%[57] in more recent series. As one would expect, the cumulative risk rises significantly as follow-up approaches 10 years, and reports from larger series[58,59] probably give the more reliable indication of the true incidence. In order to gain a better understanding of the incidence rate, we reported the results of a meta-analysis[60] of 17 studies with more than 8300 patients, including our own series of nearly 700 patients, showing the overall incidence rate worldwide was approximately 25%.

Although pouchitis can occur at any time following ileal pouch construction, the greatest overall risk of experiencing the initial episode occurs within the first 2 years after closure of the temporary diverting loop ileostomy. However, a closer look at the risk during this time frame actually shows that the absolute cumulative risk for experiencing a mild to severe episode is highest during the initial 6-month period following ileostomy closure (Figure 36-4A), after which it continues to rise steadily for the next 18 to 36 months before leveling off at around 4 years.[61] Penna et al[28] showed very similar cumulative risk results; however, their study went further in demonstrating the deleterious impact that PSC can have on the cumulative risk of pouchitis. In their study of more than 1000 chronic UC patients having received restorative proctocolectomy, those without preoperative PSC experienced a cumulative incidence of 16%, 23%, 36%, and 45% at 1, 2, 5, and 10 years, respectively. However, in those patients with preoperative PSC, the cumulative risk rose to 22%, 43%, 61%, and 79% at 1, 2, 5, and 10 years, respectively (Figure 36-4B). More than 60% of the patients with PSC experienced repeated episodes of pouchitis compared with only 15% in patients without associated PSC. Aitola et al[25] demonstrated that patients with cholangitis had a significantly more severe and chronic course of inflammation than patients without cholangitis. In their series, at least 1 episode of pouchitis occurred in

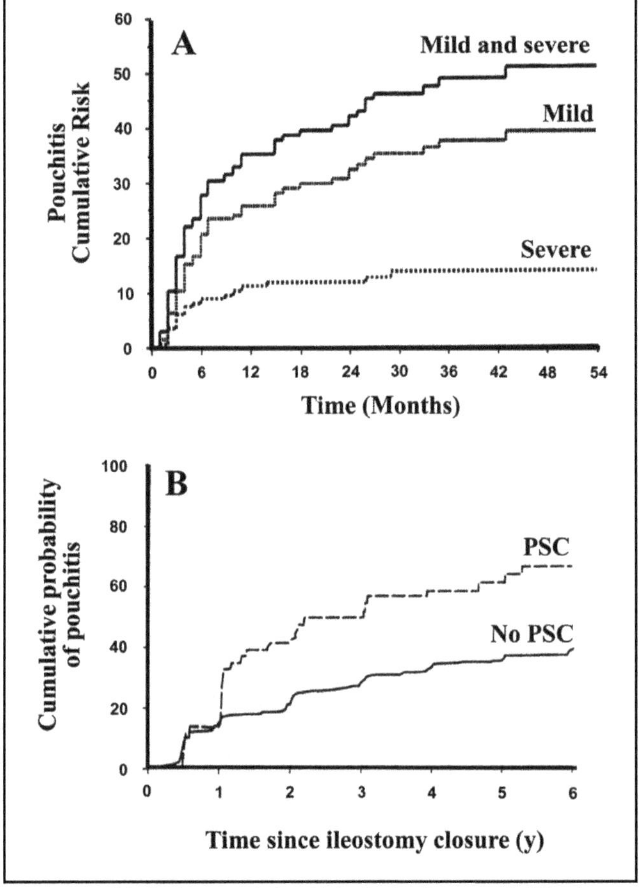

FIGURE 36-4. (A) Absolute cumulative risk for the development of mild and severe pouchitis combined and of mild and severe pouchitis separately. (Reproduced with permission from Springer from Michelassi F, Lee J, Rubin M, et al. Long-term functional results after ileal pouch anal restorative proctocolectomy for ulcerative colitis: A prospective observational study. *Ann Surg.* 2003;238:433-441.) (B) The occurrence of pouchitis estimated as a function of the time after closure of the temporary diverting ileostomy. (Reproduced with permission from the BMJ Publishing Group from Aitola P, Matikainen M, Mattila J, et al. Chronic inflammatory changes in the pouch mucosa are associated with cholangitis found on perioperative liver biopsy specimens at restorative proctocolectomy for ulcerative colitis. *Scand J Gastroenterol.* 1998;33:289-293.)

TABLE 36-2

ILEAL POUCH-ANAL ANASTOMOSIS PATIENT PROFILE, INCIDENCE OF POUCHITIS AND DYSPLASIA

Study Period:	August 1982 to January 2010
Total number of patients:	810
Diagnosis	
Chronic ulcerative colitis (CUC)	708 (88%)
Familial adenomatous polyposis (FAP)	102 (12%)
Age	
Mean	37 yrs
Range	11 to 76 yrs
Male:Female	427:383
Incidence of pouchitis (overall)*	22.2%
CUC—single or acute episode	12.1%
CUC-—multiple or chronic episodes	10.1%
CUC-—refractory	<1%
FAP	0.2%
Incidence of dysplasia	0%

*Follow-up from 590 patients.

30% of the patients without cholangitis, as compared with 90% of the patients with cholangitis. Chronic pouchitis was also more frequent, occurring in 70% of patients in the cholangitis group compared with only 11% in the group without cholangitis. Although the underlying mechanism for this association is not clear, a better understanding of this relationship may give some insight into the pathophysiology of pouchitis.

Interestingly, patients having experienced a single episode of pouchitis within 2 years of their ileostomy closure are nearly two-thirds more likely to suffer subsequent episodes.[62] These patients also tend to have poorer long-term functional results, such as high stool frequency and incontinence even in the absence of clinically active disease, when compared with those patients never having experienced a single episode.[63] While these results suggest that, for some, pouchitis represents a more chronic condition with frequent symptomatic exacerbations, this group only represents a small fraction of the total IPAA patient population.

As indicated earlier, those patients who experience unresolved symptoms for more than 1 month or episodic, but frequent, symptoms for several months are classified as having chronic pouchitis.[14,64] While the frequency of acute pouchitis in most series is reportedly as high as 59%,[57] the incidence of chronic and refractory pouchitis drops considerably. Stahlberg et al[61] reported only a 10% frequency of chronic conditions, while Keranen et al[65] found that only 4.5% of their 291 patients experienced chronic, relapsing episodes of pouchitis. Others have reported the incidence of chronic cases to be as high as 21%[61]; however, the diagnostic criteria amongst these earlier reports vary widely. In our own experience with more than 800 patients who have received IPAA for either chronic UC or FAP (Table 36-2), approximately 22%, all of whom were originally diagnosed with chronic UC, have experienced at least one episode of pouchitis. As noted earlier, pouchitis occurs almost exclusively in patients who have undergone restorative proctocolectomy for chronic UC with either a pelvic pouch or a continent ileostomy and has rarely been documented in patients undergoing the same surgery for FAP. Consistent with these other series, the incidence of pouchitis in FAP patients in our own series is quite low, approximately 0.2%.[66] While nearly one-half of the 22% of our patients with pouchitis have experienced more than one episode, less than 4% of our total patient population has a recurrent problem requiring continuous treatment or maintenance therapy. This figure is in general agreement with those rates recently reported in other large series.[14] In our own experience, an even smaller percentage (<1%) of patients experience unremitting pouchitis that appears refractory to even the most aggressive therapeutic regimens (see Table 36-2). While most of these patients are potential candidates for pouch diversion or excision with conversion to permanent Brooke ileostomy,[66] the final diagnosis for many of the patients often turns out to be CD and not refractory pouchitis. Serologic testing, as discussed below, may be valuable in making this differential diagnosis. Very few pouches are removed for refractory pouchitis,[14] and continued efforts to salvage failed pouches, for whatever reason, should be carefully considered before the decision is made to revert to a permanent ileostomy.[67,68]

RISK FACTORS

Because pouchitis only occurs in about 20% to 50% of all chronic UC patients following IPAA, other determinants clearly must play a role in susceptibility. Numerous factors have been implicated in predisposing IPAA patients to an increased risk of pouchitis; however, some have a more positive relationship to the development of pouchitis than others (Table 36-3). As will be discussed, the literature is clearly divided on many issues. Because pouchitis occurs almost exclusively in patients who have undergone restorative proctocolectomy for chronic UC, it appears that the nature of the original disease may, in fact, be considered the most important risk factor in determining susceptibility.[69] While pouchitis rarely occurs in patients who have undergone similar surgery for FAP, larger series[27,59] have reported that up to 6% to 8% of these patients have experienced at least clinical symptoms. However, the pathophysiologic factors underlying these clinical symptoms may be quite different than those in chronic UC patients.

While pouchitis does not appear to have a proclivity for age or race, the incidence of chronic pouchitis reportedly occurs more often in men.[70] Pouchitis occurs with similar frequency in all pouch configurations (S, J, or W),[69] and the overall incidence is not affected by operative techniques such as one- vs two-stage restorative proctocolectomy[71] or minimally invasive techniques.[72] Interestingly, there have been several reports suggesting that smoking may protect against pouchitis[73,74] as it does for chronic UC[75]; however, the relevant mechanisms responsible for its action are not well understood, and further research is required to establish its therapeutic potential.

As mentioned earlier, patients having either pre- or postoperative PSC have a significantly higher risk for the subsequent development of pouchitis.[61] In addition, patients experiencing pre- and postoperative extraintestinal manifestations other than PSC prior to surgery also have an increased incidence and often severity of pouchitis.[61,76,77] Interestingly, patients who have experienced ankylosing spondylitis or iritis seem to be at an especially high risk.[56] In perhaps one of the larger series to investigate this relationship, a study of 734 patients[27] of whom 91% received IPAA for chronic UC, patients with pre- and postoperative extraintestinal manifestations were shown to have significantly higher rates of pouchitis than did patients without extraintestinal manifestations. Patients with preoperative extraintestinal manifestations had a 39% incidence of at least one episode of pouchitis compared with a 26% incidence in the group without extraintestinal manifestations. Patients who developed extraintestinal manifestations after IPAA experienced a 53% incidence of pouchitis, while those without experienced approximately one-half as many episodes. Interestingly, some patients in this study experienced a temporal relationship between flares of pouchitis and the reappearance of their preoperative extraintestinal manifestations, suggesting that pouchitis may represent a unique recurrence of their IBD or a remanifestation of the original dysregulation of the mucosal immune system that now persists after surgery. Others have noted similar temporal relationships with joint symptoms and pouchitis after IPAA,[78] while other studies suggest that the reappearance of extraintestinal manifestations postoperatively may be indicative of greater risk for the occurrence of refractory pouchitis.[76]

While a number of studies have attempted to correlate the preoperative extent and severity of the original disease to the development of pouchitis, there is no clear consensus. It has been reported that patients with extensive colitis or pancolitis are at higher risk compared with patients who had left-sided disease alone.[79] This finding is supported by our own recent report,[80] showing that the presence of severe colitis that extended into the cecum (severe pancolitis) was significantly associated with the subsequent development of pouchitis. Others studies[81] have shown similar results demonstrating that the gross extent, but not the severity of the original disease, was significantly associated with the subsequent risk of pouchitis. However, in a series of 177 patients who underwent restorative proctocolectomy for chronic UC, those patients with distal colitis experienced a similar likelihood of developing pouchitis as did those patients with more extensive disease.[82] As an interesting caveat to this, as previously mentioned, patients with extraintestinal manifestations prior to IPAA are also at higher risk for pouchitis.[25] However, this is confounded by the fact that these manifestations tend to occur with greater frequency in patients with more extensive disease.

It was originally postulated that patients with extensive disease or pancolitis may experience a certain degree of inflammation in the terminal ileum or "backwash ileitis" that consequently predisposed them to a higher risk of pouchitis. However, much like the data on the extent and severity of preoperative disease, efforts to use the histopathologic

TABLE 36-3

RISK FACTORS FOR POUCHITIS

Risk Factors Predisposing Pouchitis

- Ulcerative colitis
- Pre- and postoperative extraintestinal manifestations
- Primary sclerosing cholangitis
- Pre- or postoperative seropositivity for perinuclear antineutrophil cytoplasmic antibodies (pANCA)*
- Extent of colonic involvement (pancolitis with cecal or appendiceal involvement)*
- Pre- or postoperative pANCA levels
- Backwash ileitis*
- Specific allele for interleukin-1 receptor antagonist
- Prior episodes of pouchitis
- Nonsmoking
- Male gender
- Indeterminate colitis
- Elevated preoperative platelet count
- Preoperative use of steroids
- Duration of follow-up after colectomy
- Portal vein thrombosis after surgery
- Postoperative use of NSAIDs

Risk Factors Not Associated With Pouchitis

- Familial adenomatous polyposis
- Original pouch design (S, W, or J)
- Duration of ulcerative colitis prior to surgery*
- One- or two-stage restorative proctocolectomy
- Postoperative sepsis
- Minimally invasive or laparoscopic techniques
- Fulminant colitis*

* Mixed outcomes in the literature.

status of the preoperative terminal ileum as an indicator of the subsequent risk factor for the development of pouchitis have also been equivocal. In earlier series, both Gustavsson et al[83] and Luukkonen et al[84] concluded that the presence of preoperative architectural and inflammatory changes in the terminal ileum did not predispose patients to the development of pouchitis, and thus does not contraindicate the use of inflamed terminal ileum to construct the ileal pouch. A later series by Schmidt et al[81] did demonstrate that patients who were preoperatively assessed with histopathologic alterations of the terminal ileum, such as villous blunting, appeared to be at a greater risk for the development of pouchitis. However, our own case-control study of 65 chronic UC patients who underwent IPAA, 39 of whom experienced at least one episode of pouchitis, failed to identify any significant histopathologic differences in preoperative ileum between the two groups.[80]

More recent studies have shown unexpected clinical factors associated with an increased risk for acute and chronic pouchitis. For example, the postoperative use of NSAIDs is a risk factor for acute and chronic pouchitis[85] and a number of other pouch disorders as well, prompting the recommendation by Shen et al[86] that the regular use of NSAIDs should be discouraged and that patients may benefit from complete cessation. Patients with indeterminate colitis undergoing IPAA have a higher incidence of chronic pouchitis that may represent persistent immune reactivity to microbial antigens.[87] Okon et al[88] recently showed that the incidence of chronic pouchitis was significantly higher after IPAA in chronic UC patients having thrombocytosis before surgery compared to those having normal platelet counts before surgery. In a more recent prospective multivariate analysis of clinical factors associated with pouchitis after IPAA, Fleshner et al[89] showed that the use of steroids before colectomy and smoking were associated with acute pouchitis. Chronic pouchitis was directly associated with extraintestinal manifestations, elevated platelet counts, and increased length of follow-up, while smoking reduced the incidence of chronic pouchitis. Portal vein thrombi (PVT) are a common finding in the subset of patients who require a CT scan after IPAA.[90] Interestingly, Ball et al[91] recently showed that patients who experience PVT after IPAA have a higher incidence of pouchitis warranting a prospective evaluation of this risk factor.

CAN WE PREDICT SUSCEPTIBILITY?

The question has once again been asked: "Can we immunogenotypically and immunophenotypically profile patients who are at risk for pouchitis?"[92] The identification of clinical, serologic, and histologic markers that would reliably predict susceptibility for pouchitis would be of great interest to surgeons, gastroenterologists, and pathologists. Unfortunately, at the present time, there are no studies that demonstrate a consistent trend for any such marker. However, identifying relevant risk factors may eventually lead to a better understanding of the etiology and pathophysiology of pouchitis, which may facilitate new strategies for treatment and prevention.[92] However, there have been several recent studies that have attempted to gain a better understanding of preoperative histologic, serologic, and genetic markers that might be of potential value in identifying patients who may be at an increased risk.

We recently reported[80] the results of a case-control study from our own series with the objective to determine if there were any histopathologic features unique to the colectomy specimens from patients with chronic UC that may be common to those with an increased risk for the development of pouchitis. The study group consisted of 39 chronic UC patients who had at least one episode of pouchitis during the follow-up period (mean: 57 months, range: 12 to 121 months). There were 26 control patients, all of whom also underwent a total colectomy with IPAA procedure for chronic UC, but did not develop pouchitis during the follow-up period (mean: 78 months, range: 14 to 223 months). Pathologic features from the colectomy specimens that were significantly associated with the subsequent development of pouchitis included early fissuring ulcers in 23% of the pouchitis cases vs 4% of the controls, active inflammation of the appendix in 63% of the pouchitis patients vs 31% of the controls, and appendiceal ulceration in 41% of the pouchitis patients and none in the controls. No significant differences in patient gender, age, or depth or extent of ulceration were identified between the 2 groups. Thus, it appears from this series[80] that there may be several histologic features unique to colectomy specimens from chronic UC patients who have undergone an IPAA procedure and subsequently develop pouchitis, especially appendiceal ulceration, that may be useful in identifying patients at risk.

A number of studies have been undertaken to identify serologic markers that may predict susceptibility to pouchitis. In one of the earlier retrospective studies, Vecchi et al[93] observed an association between patients who underwent IPAA for chronic UC and subsequently developed pouchitis and the presence of perinuclear antineutrophil cytoplasmic antibodies (pANCA) or neutrophil autoantibodies, which are present in a significant percentage of patients with chronic UC.[94] In a similar report shortly thereafter, Sandborn et al[95] examined a series of patients who underwent IPAA for chronic UC with and without chronic pouchitis in order to determine if pANCA may be a useful marker for identifying those patients susceptible to chronic pouchitis. The study showed that all 19 patients with a previous history of chronic UC and chronic pouchitis were positive for pANCA titers, suggesting that this serological marker may identify a genetically distinct subset of chronic UC patients with an increased risk for chronic pouchitis. Despite the potential implications of these early studies, the literature since then has remained mixed on the utility of this particular marker is predicting absolute susceptibility. Although Yang et al[96] confirmed this finding, several other studies[97-99] have subsequently refuted the association between pANCA and pouchitis. Part of the disparity among these earlier studies may be related, in part, to varying diagnostic criteria used to define pouchitis and differences in the methodologies use to measure pANCA titers.

In an attempt to gain a better understanding of the relationship between pANCA and pouchitis, Fleshner et al[100] recently undertook a study in which they systematically stratified preoperative pANCA titers in chronic UC patients undergoing IPAA into those with high, moderate, or low levels, and correlated them with disease outcome. Interestingly, of the nearly two-thirds of the 95 patients who were pANCA-positive before colectomy, only the 10% with the highest pANCA titers (>100 EU/mL) were found to have a significantly higher cumulative risk of developing chronic pouchitis. Unfortunately, once again, there are caveats confounding even this seemingly apparent association. A number of studies have shown that pANCA levels are also increased in chronic UC patients who have PSC.[101,102] As mentioned earlier, chronic UC patients with pre- and post-operative PSC who undergo IPAA have a much greater risk for pouchitis.[61] Although these confounding issues can significantly complicate our understanding of this heterogeneous disorder, they can lead to speculation that there may as yet be an unidentified genotype of patients with chronic UC that has a stronger predilection for pouchitis. Whether pANCA is actually a serologic marker for the subset representative of this genotype remains unclear.[14] Despite studies that suggest its potential utility as a marker of pouchitis risk, there is insufficient evidence at the present time to support the clinical utility and expense of measuring preoperative pANCA titers to identify patients at risk.[103] Conversely, measuring postoperative titers of pANCA and anti-*Saccharomyces cerevisiae* antibodies (ASCA) in patients with refractory pouchitis may play an important role in the differential diagnosis of treatment-resistant patients with unsuspected CD.[23] This was in fact the case in our own cohort of patients where we showed that subjects who were pANCA-/ASCA+ were more likely than those who were pANCA+/ASCA- to have their diagnosis changed to CD postoperatively.[104] These patients were also found to be at increased risk for the development of fistulas postoperatively; however, a larger study is needed to validate these observations.

As mentioned, patients with indeterminate colitis undergoing IPAA have a higher incidence of chronic pouchitis that may represent persistent immune reactivity to microbial antigens.[87] Before undergoing IPAA, patients with indeterminate colitis who have positive antibody reactivity responses to all 3 microbial antigens, oligomannan anti-*Saccharomyces cerevisiae*, outer membrane porin C of *Escherichia coli*, and an antigen (I2) from *Pseudomonas flourescens* (all of which are more commonly associated with CD) have a significantly higher incidence of chronic pouchitis after surgery than those with a negative antibody profile.[87]

Various genetic markers have also been studied in order to gain more insight into their relationship to the incidence of pouchitis. Brett et al[97] investigated whether the presence of the IL-1 receptor antagonist gene (IL-1RA) allele 2, which may be a determinant of susceptibility to chronic UC[105] and several other inflammatory conditions, may be a useful genetic marker to predict the development of pouchitis. They determined the genotypes of the IL-1RA in 28 patients with previous chronic UC and IPAA with no evidence of pouchitis and 25 subjects with previous chronic UC and pouchitis confirmed by strict histologic examination of pouch mucosal biopsy. Interestingly, their results showed that there was an increased frequency of the IL-1RA gene allele 2 in the majority of the patients from the pouchitis group, suggesting that the presence of allele 2 in patients with chronic UC may predispose them to subsequent episodes of pouchitis. IL-1 is a major proinflammatory cytokine that has been implicated in chronic UC.[106] Competitive antagonists that bind to the IL-1 receptor and prevent signal transduction could potentially have significant anti-inflammatory properties.[106] However, expression of the IL-1RA allele 2 gene is associated with decreased levels of IL-1RA,[107] thus exacerbating inflammation. In a more recent study utilizing molecular genetics, Carter et al[105] genotyped 109 chronic UC patients who had undergone colectomy with IPAA for the +2018 single nucleotide polymorphism in the IL-1RA gene, including 82 patients who had been followed prospectively. Their study showed that patients who were IL-RA allele 2 carriers had a significantly increased incidence of pouchitis compared with non-carriers, strongly suggesting that the presence of the IL-RA gene allele 2 identifies patients at risk. These finding make for tempting speculation that antagonists to the IL-1R are potential therapeutic targets.

The utility of other markers expressed in the inflamed colon preoperatively have also been investigated as to whether they may be useful identifiers of susceptibility. One such marker recently examined was human tropomyosin isoform 5 (hTM5), a cytoskeletal protein expressed in normal colonic epithelial cells. An autoimmune response toward hTM5 reportedly occurs in chronic UC.[108] In a prospective longitudinal study of 28 chronic UC patients undergoing IPAA, Biancone et al[109] investigated whether hTM5 expression in the ileum was associated with the subsequent development of pouchitis. Biopsy samples were taken at surgery from the rectum and the newly constructed ileal pouch, and again from the pouch at 6 months after IPAA. As expected, hTM5 expression was strong in all rectal epithelial cells, but not expressed in the ileum. At 6 months after IPAA, the ileum was found to have undergone morphological changes indicative of colonic metaplasia with shortening or reduced number of villi, which were associated with a diffuse hTM5 staining in the epithelial and goblet cells and in the cells lining the crypts and the lumen. The hTM5 score was significantly related to disease activity, leading these authors to conclude that the expression of hTM5 identifies a different pattern of morphological changes in the ileal pouch that may be related to the development of pouchitis.

PATHOPHYSIOLOGY

Despite considerable speculation, the etiology and pathophysiology of this poorly defined clinical entity remains essentially unknown. Infections with enteric pathogens, surgically induced ischemia, and chronic stasis

TABLE 36-4

ETIOLOGIC AND PATHOPHYSIOLOGIC THEORIES OF POUCHITIS

- Stasis or incomplete emptying of the pouch
- Bacterial overgrowth
- Bacterial dysbiosis
- Increased concentrations of secondary bile acids
- Reduced concentrations of short-chain fatty acids
- Enteric pathogens
- Ischemia or reduced mucosal blood flow
- Malabsorption
- Immunologic
- Crohn's disease (unsuspected)

secondary to outflow obstruction can underlie acute episodes of ileal pouch inflammation; however, these factors account for only a small portion of the reported incidences of pouchitis.[110] Although a variety of postulated mechanisms will be discussed, the complexity of pouchitis and the manner in which it presents clinically, ranging from patients with acute antibiotic-responsive episodes to those with a more chronic, relapsing refractory syndrome, suggests that the pathogenesis is multifactorial (Table 36-4). In addition, there are a number of well-documented conditions of the ileal pouch in patients who have undergone IPAA for UC who have symptoms overlapping with pouchitis but have very different etiologies, further complicating the differential diagnosis.[53]

Stasis and Colonic Metaplasia

The closure of the diverting loop ileostomy following IPAA results in a major alteration in the primary function of the terminal ileum. Previously associated with nutrient absorption, the terminal ileal pouch now must adapt to an entirely new role in its function as a neorectum. The storage of feces or stasis within the pouch is a major factor distinguishing a pouch from an end ileostomy.[69] The fact that ileal inflammation does not occur in patients with a Brooke ileostomy certainly implicates stasis in the pathophysiology of pouchitis; however, stasis cannot be the sole factor initiating inflammation because patients having undergone the same operation for FAP presumably have similar degrees of pouch stasis without inflammation.

Not all pouches empty with the same efficiency, although there does not appear to be a relationship between incomplete emptying and the incidence of pouchitis.[111] Nonetheless, while stasis may not be implicated directly in the pathophysiology of pouchitis, it may initiate a cascade of synergistically pathogenic mechanisms that have the potential to signal ileal inflammation. Stasis has been shown to result in bacterial overgrowth and dysbiosis in the functioning pouch.[112] In addition, stasis has been strongly associated with the morphologic and histologic changes in ileal mucosa that accompany the functional transition from ileum to neorectum as previously discussed. Studies in our laboratory in a rat model of IPAA showed that stasis does in fact occur in the ileal pouch and is associated with pouch inflammation and oxidative stress.[113]

Many studies have speculated that architectural transformations occurring in the functioning ileal pouch can predispose to inflammatory changes. As previously discussed, colonic metaplasia occurs to some degree in all functioning ileal pouches,[35] and it is rarely documented either prior to ileostomy closure[32] or in patients with a Brooke ileostomy. The factors that initiate these histological changes are poorly understood; however, it appears that some fecal component coupled with stasis itself initiates these changes because they do not occur until the fecal stream is resumed. Although some histologic abnormalities occur in diverted pouches prior to ileostomy closure,[17] pouchitis rarely occurs, begging the question as to whether these often subtle histologic changes are a prerequisite to inflammation. Similar histologic changes also occur in pouches of FAP patients who rarely experience pouchitis, suggesting that additional mechanisms secondary to fecal insult underlie the occurrence of pouchitis in chronic UC patients. Other predisposing factors initiated by the fecal stream and stasis, discussed later, may play a more pronounced role in the pathophysiology of pouchitis.

Bacterial Overgrowth and Dysbiosis

Even though the underlying pathophysiology of pouchitis is unknown, the fact that clinical symptoms associated with acute episodes of pouchitis respond so well to antibiotics has led investigators to suspect an infectious agent. Nevertheless, despite intensive investigations, no single organism has yet to be identified. However, Gosselink et al[114] recently showed that during episodes of pouchitis, ileal pouch concentrations of several pathogens (eg, *Clostridium perfringens* and hemolytic strains of *E. coli*) increase dramatically. Treatment with metronidazole only eradicated the *C. perfringens*, while treatment with ciprofloxacin eradicated both pathogens, restored normal pouch flora, and was associated with significant relief of symptoms.

Even in the most efficiently functioning pouch, residual volume remains following evacuation.[115] As mentioned, stasis facilitates bacterial overgrowth,[116] which has been implicated in the pathophysiology of pouchitis. The fact that several antibiotics including metronidazole and ciprofloxacin are therapeutic in acute flare-ups and maintenance of remission of pouchitis further supports a pathogenic role for bacteria. Following closure of the loop ileostomy and resumption of the fecal stream, the ileal pouch becomes colonized by large numbers of bacteria indigenous to the colon.[117] Total bacterial counts in the healthy ileal pouch are higher compared with either normal ileum[116] or ileostomy effluent,[69] but significantly lower than those found in normal distal colon. Anaerobes typically predominate the bacterial population of the healthy pouch[114] compared with ileostomy effluent.[118] Studies in our laboratory in a rat model of IPAA also showed that stasis was accompanied by significant bacterial overgrowth.[119]

Although the pathophysiologic implications of bacterial overgrowth in the pouch are unclear, it does appear that the integrity of the pouch environment depends on the stability of the microbial population. Ruseler-van Embden et al[117] demonstrated that bacterial dysbiosis occurs during pouchitis in which the anaerobic population of the pouch was significantly reduced in favor of the aerobes. Of particular note were the reduced numbers of the anaerobes lactobacilli and bifidobacteria. Their study concluded that pouchitis possibly results from instability of the flora in the pouch, which causes an alteration in bacterial homeostasis. Subsequently, protection of the pouch epithelium by the mucous layer becomes affected by increased activity of bacterial-derived enzymes.[117] Others have shown that the total counts for facultatively anaerobic bacteria[120] and intramural aerobic facultative bacterial counts[121] were significantly greater in patients with pouchitis compared with control groups, suggesting that these particular species may play a role in the pathogenesis of pouchitis. More recently, Komanduri et al have shown unique microfloral patterns in patient with pouchitis.[122] Through cloning and sequencing, they showed a persistence of *Fusobacter* and Enteric species associated with the disease state and the absence of specific bacteria, such as *Streptococcus* species, in the inflamed pouch. The authors hypothesize that by demonstrating dysbiosis in the microbial biofilm adherent to the mucosa in pouchitis provides direct evidence of the role of bacteria in the pathogenesis of pouchitis.[122]

Perhaps the more compelling evidence implicating bacterial dysbiosis are the studies by Gionchetti et al,[123] showing that highly concentrated doses of an oral probiotic preparation containing lactobacilli and bifidobacteria (VSL#3) were effective for both the prevention of onset and subsequent flare-ups in patients with chronic pouchitis. Since then, a number of randomized, double-blind, placebo-controlled studies have shown VSL#3 is effective in preventing the onset of acute pouchitis in patients with newly formed ileal pouches and in maintaining remission following antibiotic treatment in patients with refractory or recurrent pouchitis.[124] Although their studies provide very convincing evidence that beneficial probiotic bacteria can decrease relapses of chronic pouchitis after antibiotic treatment, issues such as the optimal dosing and timing of probiotic administration need to be addressed to determine the optimal clinical application. More importantly, determination of the mechanisms by which beneficial bacteria protect mucosal surfaces of the pouch may give investigators valuable insight into the pathogenic role that bacteria play in pouchitis. While factors affecting bacterial homeostasis in the pouch are not completely understood, it is apparent that the maintenance of a stable bacterial ecosystem is integral to a healthy functioning pouch.[124]

Short-Chain Fatty Acids and Glutamine

The bacterial population of the pouch can significantly contribute to functional integrity by producing nutrients key to maintaining optimal epithelial function. Although the pouch ileum undergoes some colon-like architectural changes,[35] it still retains functional properties indigenous to normal ileum, suggesting that the nutritional requirements of these cells may be altered. Hence, if the availability of luminal substrates plays a role in the pathophysiology of pouchitis, they might likely involve either butyrate, an essential nutrient of colonocytes,[125] or L-glutamine, a preferred nutrient of the ileal enterocyte.[126]

In a well-functioning pouch as in the normal colon, anaerobic bacterial fermentation produces short-chain fatty acids (SCFAs), mainly butyrate, propionate, and acetate from certain dietary carbohydrates[127] and undigested dietary fiber.[128] SCFA may be the preferred energy source by ileal epithelia, especially in those instances where colon-like architectural changes have occurred. In addition, SCFAs have been shown to promote sodium and water absorption,[129] suppress enteropathic bacteria, and are integral to the maintenance of optimal luminal pH.[117] Thus, it appears that SCFA may play a role in the functional integrity of the pouch, and reduced concentrations may alter the susceptibility of pouch epithelial cells to inflammation, especially because a number of studies[130-132] have shown that fecal SCFA concentrations are significantly reduced in patients with pouchitis. Earlier attempts to demonstrate the therapeutic efficacy of topical SCFA treatment demonstrated only a slight benefit in ameliorating mucosal inflammation.[133] However, a recent report by Welters et al[134] did show that dietary supplementation with inulin, which ferments to SCFA, led to a reduction of inflammation of pouch mucosa, suggesting that a SCFA deficiency may be implicated in the pathophysiology of pouchitis.

While the SCFA data are equivocal, there are data suggesting that glutamine may play a more important role in protecting intestinal mucosa.[135] Glutamine deficiency is associated with mucosal injury and impaired healing, suggesting that it may be a more critical energy substrate for ileal epithelium.[126] A recent study showed that IPAA resulted in changes in the distribution of glutamine and its metabolites in ileal pouch mucosa, particularly in patients with UC,[136] suggesting that the luminal concentrations of glutamine may be essential for optimal epithelial cell function in the pouch. In a small series, Wischmeyer et al[137] showed that topical glutamine was efficacious in 6 of 10 patients with chronic pouchitis, suggesting a potential role for glutamine deficiency in the pathophysiology of pouchitis. However, further investigation with larger trials is again necessary to confirm their therapeutic efficacy.

Bile Acids

As mentioned, bacterial overgrowth and dysbiosis are implicated in metabolic alterations that may affect pouch function. Among others, bacterial overgrowth, especially by species more indigenous to the colon, may affect bile acid metabolism in the ileal reservoir.[116] Salemans et al[138] subsequently showed that, in patients with IPAA, bile acid reabsorption was impaired. They suggested that bacterial overgrowth leads to deconjugation and dehydroxylation of bile acids resulting in reduced absorption and serum bile acid levels. There are well-documented metabolic consequences following restorative proctocolectomy with IPAA,[139] particularly in the enterohepatic recirculation of bile acids; however, bile acid loss is compensated, and steatorrhea is minimal.[138] However, because Natori et al[140] demonstrated that the fecal output of unconjugated secondary and 7-dehydroxylated bile acids was increased in patients with IPAA compared with output from a terminal ileostomy, this indicates that the conditions in the ileal pouch are sufficiently anaerobic to facilitate the conversion of primary to secondary bile acids. Because the presence of secondary[141] and deconjugated[39] bile acids are cytotoxic to ileal epithelial cells and have been shown to affect water and salt permeability and cell death,[142] they may be a contributing factor in the pathophysiology of pouchitis.

Mucosal Ischemia

Ischemia can be a contributory factor in intestinal inflammation, and surgically induced intestinal ischemia has been shown to cause mucosal inflammation and tissue damage.[143] During the surgical construction of the ileal pouch, secondary mesenteric vessels must be divided to provide adequate length for alleviating mesenteric tension when the J pouch is brought down into the pelvis for the anal anastomosis.[7] Anatomic limitations can sometimes leave tension on arteries and veins supplying the pouch that can potentially lead to ischemia. Ischemic ileitis can be responsible for a series of microvascular and biochemical events that can initiate epithelial cell damage and culminate in necrosis and even cell death.[144] Although surgically induced ischemia is an unlikely pathophysiologic factor underlying pouchitis, several techniques have been utilized to demonstrate that ischemic events do occur in the ileal pouch. Studies have shown that mucosal blood flow to the ileal pouch is compromised[145,146] compared with ileum of patients with an end ileostomy. Interestingly, this occurred more frequently in patients with chronic UC compared with FAP.[147] In addition, more than twice the number of patients with postoperative inflammatory complications showed reduced mucosal blood flow to the pouch, suggesting that subclinical ischemia may exist under certain conditions and contribute to the development of ileal inflammation. Interestingly, intestinal mucosa is relatively low in endogenous antioxidant defenses like catalase, glutathione, and superoxide dismutase, which may make it particularly susceptible to ischemic injury by free radical production.[148,149] However, despite an earlier report[149] showing that the administration of allopurinol, a potent xanthine oxidase inhibitor, significantly improved symptoms in approximately one-half of the patients with chronic pouchitis, a later report refuted these findings and showed that allopurinol did not reduce the risk of a first attack of pouchitis when administered prophylactically.[150] The fact that patients with chronic UC and FAP undergo the same procedure, and the incidence of pouchitis in patients with FAP is extremely low, argues against ischemia as a direct and independent mechanism in the pathophysiology of pouchitis. Nevertheless, this does not rule out mucosal ischemia and hypoxia as a contributor to a multifactorial pathogenic sequence of inflammatory events in a genetically susceptible individual.

Oxidative Stress and Nitric Oxide

Although the pathophysiology of chronic intestinal inflammation is not understood, a growing body of experimental and clinical data suggests that a dysregulated immune response to indigenous bacterial antigens plays a significant role.[151] This uncontrolled activation of the mucosal immune system results in oxidative stress, or the sustained overproduction of reactive oxygen species, oxygen free radicals, and nitric oxide (NO), and has been implicated in part with the intestinal injury and dysfunction associated with chronic intestinal inflammation.[152] Despite a strong relationship with chronic UC, there are few data demonstrating that this pathophysiologic mechanism is associated with ileal pouch inflammation. In one of the few studies to investigate this hypothesis clinically, Levin et al[149] showed that inhibiting the production of oxygen free radicals with allopurinol either terminated an episode of acute pouchitis or prevented pouchitis from recurring in 50% of patients, suggesting a pathogenic role for oxidative stress in ileal pouch inflammation. Our own studies[30] showed that several markers of oxidative stress were significantly elevated in ileal pouch biopsies from patients with pouchitis, indicating that excessive oxygen free radicals are present. Whether this is an epiphenomenon associated with chronic inflammation is unclear, and further studies are needed.

Interestingly, commonly prescribed drugs used to treat pouchitis, including metronidazole,[153] 5-ASA,[154] and bismuth,[155,156] can scavenge free radicals.[157] Although the use of antimicrobials and anti-inflammatories were initially explored based on the assumption that alterations in bacterial flora were responsible for pouchitis, there is now plausible evidence to suggest that the efficacy of these agents may be derived, in part, from their antioxidant properties as well.

Similarly, there is little evidence demonstrating a pathophysiologic role for NO in pouchitis, although a study by Kroesen et al[158] showed that inducible NO synthase (iNOS) expression was positively correlated with clinical severity. These data suggest a pathogenic role for iNOS in the pathophysiology of pouchitis and imply that reducing cytotoxic levels of NO with the topical application of highly selective iNOS inhibitors may represent a novel new approach for the treatment of pouchitis.

Cytokines, Chemokines, Prostaglandins, and Growth Factors

Proinflammatory cytokines and prostaglandins (PG) including IL-1β, IL-6, IL-8, TNFα, PGE_2, and leukotriene B4 (LTB_4) all play pathophysiologic roles in chronic intestinal inflammation.[106] Stimulated inflammatory cells secrete these cytokines which then initiate the production of other inflammatory mediators such as leukotrienes, NO, reactive oxygen species, and platelet activating factor. Hence cytokines can initiate, amplify, and exacerbate mucosal inflammation.

Earlier studies by Patel et al[159] showed that IL-1β, IL-6, IL-8, and TNFα levels were significantly increased in pouchitis and active UC compared with uninflamed pouch and normal controls, and there was a significant correlation between levels of cytokines expressed in pouchitis and active UC. LTB_4 release was also significantly elevated in patients with active pouchitis compared with either normal pouches[160] or pouches in patients with FAP.[161] In later studies, Bulois et al[162] showed that IL-8 mRNA levels were significantly higher in patients with pouchitis while IL-10 levels were unchanged, suggesting that pouchitis is associated with a mucosal imbalance between IL-8 and IL-10. More recently, Helwig et al[163] demonstrated that the expression of IL-8, monocyte chemoattractant protein-1 and 3, and the CXC chemokine IP-10 were significantly higher in pouchitis, all of which were significantly lower after antibiotic treatment. These studies suggest that a similar cascade of proinflammatory cytokines and chemokines is expressed during active pouchitis, raising the question as to whether pouchitis is merely a cytokine-induced reactivation of the immunologic mechanisms similar to those initiating chronic UC. In either event, these data support the importance of cytokines and chemokines in leukocyte recruitment in pouch tissue during acute and perhaps chronic pouchitis.

Transforming growth factor-beta 1 (TGF-β1), a cytokine growth factor also chemotactic for neutrophils, has also been shown to be increased in healthy pouch mucosa[164] as well as in serum from patients with pouchitis,[165] suggesting that TGF-β1 may not only play a role in the adaptive, metaplastic response occurring in the pouch, but also in the acute inflammatory response. Hence, while the enhanced production of proinflammatory cytokines, chemokines, prostaglandins, and leukotrienes in the pathophysiology of pouchitis is still being defined, the therapeutic implications remain speculative. The potential efficacy of anti-cytokines, anti-inflammatory cytokines, cytokine- and chemokine-receptor antagonists, leukotriene synthesis inhibitors, and anti-leukotrienes have far-reaching therapeutic implications in the treatment of pouchitis, especially because these treatments have been successfully utilized in other chronic inflammatory disorders.

Regulatory Neuropeptides

Regulatory neuropeptides, such as substance P (SP), are widely distributed throughout the gastrointestinal tract and are thought to play a key role in motility, secretion, immunoregulation, and inflammation.[166,167] SP is also thought to play a role in IBD.[168] SP is secreted by nerves and inflammatory cells, such as macrophages, eosinophils, lymphocytes, and dendritic cells, and mediates neurogenic inflammation through its interaction with the high affinity neurokinin 1 receptor (NK1-R).[167] Patients with chronic UC have markedly increased colonic levels of SP,[169] NK-1R,[170] and SP immunoreactive nerve fibers.[171] Interestingly, Keranen et al[172] showed that the number and intensity of ileal SP and vasoactive intestinal polypeptide (VIP) immunoreactive nerve fibers were significantly increased in pouchitis compared with ileum from normal pouch, and, despite the resolution of clinical symptoms, these levels remained elevated.[173] Although there have been no studies in humans to date, recent studies in a rat model of IPAA developed in our laboratory showed that a specific NK-1R antagonist was effective in preventing ileal pouch inflammation.[174] The experimental data implicate SP in the pathophysiology of ileal pouch inflammation and suggest that NK-1R antagonists may be of therapeutic value in the management of clinical pouchitis.

Recurrence of Chronic Ulcerative Colitis

Despite an unclear etiology, the fact that the majority of patients with pouchitis were originally diagnosed with chronic UC leaves many investigators with the impression that pouchitis is either a recurrence of the original colitis or the appearance of a new form of IBD. There are several direct lines of evidence to support this premise. There is a remarkable resemblance in the underlying immunologic abnormalities and especially the clinical presentation between chronic, refractory pouchitis and chronic UC.[92] This observation is further supported by the previously mentioned fact that the incidence of pouchitis following IPAA in patients with FAP is extremely low.[175] Patel et al[159] also noted that there are remarkable similarities between the levels of cytokines expressed in pouchitis and active UC. In addition, chronic and refractory pouchitis are often associated with extraintestinal manifestations similar to those accompanying chronic UC, especially if these conditions existed prior to IPAA.[176] As mentioned earlier, the most notable of the extraintestinal manifestations is PSC, which is strongly associated with an increased risk of pouchitis.[28] The prevalence of pANCA is greater in patients with chronic pouchitis compared with patients without pouchitis. In one series, Sandborn et al[95] noted that patients with a previous history of chronic UC and chronic pouchitis were 100% positive for pANCA. Interestingly, like patients with chronic UC, smokers are less likely to develop pouchitis than nonsmokers or former smokers.[73] The mucosal inflammation that characterizes pouchitis bears a notable histological and functional resemblance to colitis, especially in the presence of colonic-like architectural changes. Finally, the presence of RFD9-positive macrophages,[177] remarkably similar cytokine and chemokine expression,[159] similarities in mucins,[178] and increased platelet-activating factor production[179] (all of which are associated with UC) further support the premise that pouchitis may, in fact, represent a recurrence of the original colitis.

Unsuspected Crohn's Disease

Crohn's colitis, either unrecognized at the time of proctocolectomy or diagnosed as indeterminate,[180] represents a very small percentage of patients with chronic or refractory pouchitis.[181] Patients with refractory pouchitis can present with endoscopic and histologic features similar to CD, such as superficial and transmural ulcers, fissures, granulomas, and sometimes fistulae. Fistulas occurring late postoperatively, especially those arising from the pouch, are strongly suggestive of CD, while those occurring within 6 months of the ileostomy closure can be the result of anastomotic dehiscence. These Crohn's-like features can occur in the ileal pouch even in the absence of inflammation in patients with unquestionable chronic UC.[110] Hence, the certain confirmation of this diagnosis often requires careful review of the original colectomy specimen by an experienced gastrointestinal pathologist and perhaps also confirmed by serologic testing.[104]

If CD of the ileal pouch is suspected, the diagnosis can be complicated by differing clinical, endoscopic, radiographic, and histologic presentations. A recent study by Shen et al[182] of 78 patients with CD of the pouch found a range of presentations that included 28 patients with inflammatory, 18 patients with fibrostenotic, and 32 with fistulizing disease of the pouch, with each representing a different clinical phenotype. Each of the 3 phenotypes was associated with different risk factors: inflammatory CD was associated with higher afferent-limb endoscopy scores; fibrostenotic CD was associated with higher afferent-limb and higher cuff endoscopy scores; and fistulizing CD was associated with younger age, female gender, a preoperative diagnosis of indeterminate colitis, and no use of NSAIDs. These results suggest that each of these diseases has a different etiology and disease process and the identification and management of some of the modifiable risk factors may reduce morbidity. A follow-up study by this same group[183] subsequently showed that the predominant symptoms were different in each of the clinical phenotypes of CD of the pouch. Predominant symptoms, as expected, were diarrhea and/or pain in patients with inflammatory CD, obstructive symptoms in patients with fibrostenotic CD, and fistular drainage in those with fistulizing disease. Despite the differing presentations, each of the 3 phenotypes similarly affected health-related quality of life scores. Fistulizing Crohn's disease may be associated with a higher risk for pouch failure.

Diagnostic Algorithms and Treatment

As mentioned earlier, pouch dysfunction can be caused by a number of inflammatory and noninflammatory diseases of the ileal pouch that can mimic pouchitis.[53] Pouchitis clearly encompasses a continuum of clinical symptoms that vary over time, thus making the diagnosis difficult.[21] For example, increased stool frequency is a hallmark of pouchitis; however, infections with *C. difficile* and cytomegalovirus, decreased pouch compliance, pelvic sepsis, and IPS all present with similar symptoms.[184] Historically, the medical management of pouchitis has been primarily empiric and has been predicated more on individual clinical experiences than evidence-based knowledge gained from only a few randomized, placebo-controlled clinical trials that have been published. Antibiotics have been and still are the foundation of treatment, especially for patients with acute episodes. However, for the approximately one-third of patients who experience recurrence[185] and the 10% to 15% who suffer from chronic episodes or unremitting pouchitis, current treatment strategies are inadequate. For these more refractory patients, novel therapeutics are emerging that may not only offer relief[186] and long-term remission,[123,187] but perhaps more importantly may allow investigators to gain further insight into pathophysiologic mechanisms. Table 36-5 lists the current and emerging therapeutic options for treating acute, chronic, and refractory pouchitis. Many anecdotal therapies have not been included in this table.

From our own experience, when an IPAA patient presents with clinical symptoms consistent with pouchitis

TABLE 36-5

TREATMENT OPTIONS FOR POUCHITIS

Acute

- Antibiotics
- Antidiarrheals
- Supplementary fiber
- Steroids, topical

Chronic or Relapsing

- Antibiotics, continuous, combination low dose
- Aminosalicylates, oral or topical
- Steroids, oral or topical
- Immunosuppressives or immune modifiers
- Antifungals
- Bismuth, oral or topical

Chronic Refractory

- Immunosuppressives or immune modifiers
- Biologics, anti-TNFα antibody
- Antibiotic combinations
- Pouch revision or excision

Maintenance and Prophylaxis

- Probiotics
- Immunosuppressives or immune modifiers

Emerging

- Antisense inhibitors
- Other anti-TNFα or other similar biologics

(see Table 36-1), we first establish the clinical course of their presentation. Depending on whether they are acute, chronic, relapsing, or refractory, we utilize a series of differential diagnostic and treatment algorithms that we have developed over the past 20 years to manage these patients.

ACUTE OR EPISODIC POUCHITIS

Antibiotics have been the mainstay of therapy for acute symptoms. A historic review of the literature shows that the most commonly prescribed antibiotics for acute episodes of pouchitis are metronidazole (10 to 20 mg/kg)[188,189] and ciprofloxacin (500 mg bid).[190] Hurst et al[185] showed that nearly 96% of symptomatic patients treated orally with either metronidazole or ciprofloxacin experienced a resolution of symptoms. In a randomized clinical trial designed to compare the effectiveness and side effect profiles of ciprofloxacin and metronidazole for treating acute pouchitis, Shen et al[191] showed that while ciprofloxacin and metronidazole were both effective in treating acute pouchitis, ciprofloxacin produced a greater improvement in symptoms and endoscopy findings. Interestingly, none of the patients who received ciprofloxacin experienced any side effects, whereas approximately one-third of the patients administered metronidazole reported side effects including dyspepsia and nausea among others. Shen's study[191] thus concluded that ciprofloxacin should be the antibiotic of choice for acute episodes of pouchitis. Ciprofloxacin's therapeutic efficacy compared with metronidazole may be due to its effectiveness in restoring normal pouch flora by eradicating pathogens associated with pouchitis such as *C. perfringens* and hemolytic strains of *E. coli*.[114] In an attempt to reduce the side effect profile of oral metronidazole, Nygaard et al[192] administered up to 160 mg/d directly into the ileal reservoir. Although the topical application of small doses of metronidazole relieved symptoms and was tolerated well, even for extended periods, this line of therapy for acute episodes is not optimal. In our own series, oral metronidazole alone (250 mg qid) was shown to reduce overall stool frequency by 55% and nocturnal frequency and leakage by 63% and 82%, respectively. Other antibiotics such as erythromycin, amoxicillin with clavulanic acid, doxycycline, and tetracycline have also been reportedly used with some success, although there have been no randomized or comparative trials suggesting that their efficacy is better than the current standards for acute therapy. The efficacy of antibiotic treatment for acute or episodic pouchitis has also been compared with topical steroids. In a prospective, double-blind, double-dummy, 6-week controlled trial, 26 patients with an active episode of pouchitis either received a budesonide enema (2 mg/100 mL) plus placebo tablets or oral metronidazole (500 mg bid) plus placebo enema.[193] Both drugs were shown to be equally efficacious; however, the budesonide enemas were better tolerated than the oral metronidazole, suggesting that topical steroids could be an alternative treatment for antibiotic-intolerant patients with acute episodes.

As noted earlier, there are a number of diseases of the ileal pouch that present with overlapping pouchitis-like symptoms.[194] As such, not all symptomatic IPAA patients necessarily have pouchitis; therefore, our diagnostic and treatment algorithms for all patients begin with a careful history by an experienced nurse practitioner or a certified wound and ostomy nurse. First-time and acute patients, especially within a year of IPAA, are carefully queried about adequate use of antidiarrheals (loperamide), a high-fiber diet and supplementary fiber (methylcellulose or psyllium), and other factors that may cause similar symptoms. Generally, these patients are monitored for up to a

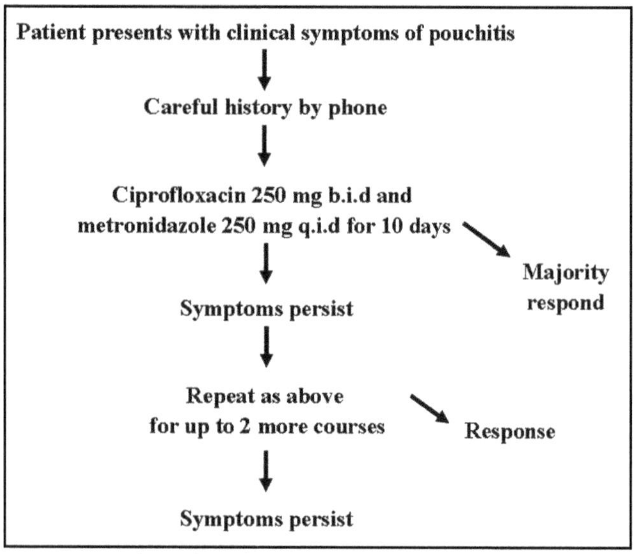

FIGURE 36-5. Diagnostic and treatment algorithm for acute and episodic pouchitis.

week, and, if their symptoms do not resolve, then antibiotic therapy is begun. In our experience,[66] rapid relief is often achieved with a 10-day combination course of the broad-spectrum antibiotics ciprofloxacin (250 mg bid) and metronidazole (250 mg qid; Figure 36-5). A significant portion of these patients experience an improvement in clinical symptoms within several days, especially in stool frequency. Those patients who either do not respond or show partial improvement to this initial trial will undergo at least one more 10-day course at the same dose before further diagnostic evaluation is undertaken. Most patients with acute disease respond favorably to antibiotic therapy; however, on average, about 10% to 15% will experience relapsing episodes that will require a more prolonged course of therapy.[63,195] However, if they initially tolerated the medications well, they will be retreated with the same combination of antibiotics. Although antibiotics at different doses may still be appropriate therapy, patients who do not respond or repeatedly relapse when therapy is discontinued are at a critical diagnostic point of our treatment algorithm.

CHRONIC OR RELAPSING POUCHITIS

Treatment and prevention of chronic or relapsing pouchitis can be a challenging and frustrating task for the practitioner and patient as well. Antibiotics, especially in combination, are certainly still appropriate and effective in treating these patients, many of whom require frequent and often continuous antibiotic treatment with either low maintenance doses or full-dose pulse therapy in order to remain in remission.[196] However, the management of patients with chronic antibiotic-resistant pouchitis can often be the most difficult and is a common cause of either pouch resection or diversion. A number of trials have been carried out using rifaximin, a nonabsorbable broad-spectrum antibiotic, either alone or in combination with other antibiotics for patients with chronic, treatment-resistant pouchitis. Gionchetti et al[197] treated 18 patients with chronic active, treatment-resistant pouchitis orally with rifaximin (1 g bid) in combination with ciprofloxacin (500 mg bid). After 15 days, more than 88% of the patients responded with one-third in complete remission and more than one-half with a clinical improvement. In a later study, Abdelrazeq et al[198] also showed that rifaximin (1 g bid)-ciprofloxacin (500 mg bid) in combination for 2 weeks is safe and effective in chronic active refractory pouchitis and may salvage a significant percentage of at-risk pouches. A smaller, more recent placebo-controlled pilot trial by Isaacs et al[199] showed that 2 of 8 patients (25%) treated with rifaximin alone (400 mg tid) were in clinical remission at week 4 compared to 0 of 9 patients (0%) treated with placebo. The study did show that while rifaximin was well-tolerated, a larger trial would be required to determine if rifaximin is effective for the treatment of active pouchitis.

Others have also reported therapeutic efficacy with prolonged courses of 2 antibiotics in combination for patients with recurrent episodes. Mimura et al[200] reported that 82% of patients administered metronidazole (400 to 500 mg bid) in combination with ciprofloxacin (500 mg bid) for 1 month went into remission. Although there have been reports indicating that a short course of metronidazole alone was effective in patients with chronic pouchitis,[189] our experience indicates that a longer administration of combination therapies is required in order to achieve and maintain remission. If repeated courses of antibiotics are unsuccessful or if patients develop resistance, other therapeutic options should be considered (see Table 36-5). More recently, Shen et al[201] tested the efficacy of a recently approved antibiotic, tinidazole (15 mg/kg/d) in combination with ciprofloxacin (1 g/d), in 16 consecutive chronic UC patients with chronic refractory pouchitis (disease >4 weeks and failure to respond to >4 weeks of single-antibiotic therapy). Compared with mesalamine therapy, patients taking a 4-week course of ciprofloxacin and tinidazole had a significant reduction in the total pouchitis DAI scores and a significant improvement in quality-of-life scores.

Several alternatives, both topical and oral, have been tested in patients with chronic or relapsing pouchitis. Although the scientific reasoning behind these alternatives appeared reasonable, most have shown little clinical utility. These include such treatments at bismuth carbomer foam enemas nightly for 3 weeks, which were shown to be safe but not efficacious for active chronic pouchitis.[202] In a similar but longer trial, however, Gionchetti et al[155] treated 12 patients with antibiotic-resistant chronic pouchitis nightly for 45 days with bismuth carbomer enemas, which were effective in achieving and maintaining remission in 60% of patients. When patients with chronic antibiotic-resistant pouchitis were administered bismuth subsalicylate tablets (2 g/d) for 4 weeks along with their regular antibiotics, nearly 85% responded favorably.[156] Interestingly, nearly one-half of the responders were able to discontinue antibiotic usage over the 4-week period. Other topical agents have also been tested in patients with treatment-resistant chronic pouchitis, including nutrients essential for ileal enterocytes such as butyrate and glutamine, again with little clinical utility. In a randomized clinical trial that was not placebo-controlled, Wischmeyer et al[137] showed only marginal benefit for maintaining remission in 19 patients who were administered either glutamine or butyrate suppositories for 3 weeks.

For patients with chronic or relapsing pouchitis who are either resistant to antibiotics or relapse shortly after antibiotic therapy is discontinued, therapy with oral or topical anti-inflammatory agents and immunomodulators is reasonable and, in some cases, effective, especially given their efficacy for UC.[196] Unfortunately, trials with these agents are limited, often anecdotal, and not well-controlled. In one of the few prospective, double-blind, controlled trials to assess the efficacy of topical corticosteroids, budesonide enemas were shown to be an effective alternative treatment for active pouchitis.[193] A more recent study by Gionchetti et al[203] showed that controlled ileal release oral budesonide (9 mg/d) for 8 weeks also appeared effective in inducing remission in 20 patients with chronic, antibiotic-resistant pouchitis. Others have reported limited efficacy in very small uncontrolled trials with topical anti-inflammatories such as mesalamine[204]; however, there are no randomized, controlled trials of any oral mesalamine agents for the treatment of pouchitis. Reports of other small series have been reviewed using immunosuppressives such as AZA or 6-MP[14] that showed some effectiveness in allowing patients to discontinue steroids and maintain remission for up to 3 years. Shen[196] has also reported that immunosuppressives are effective in antibiotic-resistant patients. Trials with the free radical inhibitor allopurinol showed limited efficacy for treatment[149] and none for prevention,[150] suggesting that free radical injury may not contribute to the pathogenesis of pouchitis. However, studies reported from our own series[30] indicated that pouchitis was associated with significant oxidative stress. Perhaps antioxidants or free radical scavengers other than allopurinol may be more efficacious, but none have been tested to date.

The maintenance of remission between flare-ups has perhaps been one of the more frustrating aspects for patients experiencing chronic, relapsing episodes. Until recently, little could be offered to this 10% to 15% of patients other than the sequential administration of various antibiotics alone or in combination or trial and error with other anti-inflammatories or immunosuppressives. However, the recent advent of probiotics, which appear to play a greater role in the maintenance of remission than in treatment, may offer these patients a viable option.[187] Probiotics are live organisms, in this case bacterium, that are typically indigenous to the gastrointestinal tract in humans. Because it was postulated that inflammation in the pouch may be caused by a microbial imbalance[117] or dysbiosis[112] in the usual pouch flora, there have been attempts to modify the bacterial flora with live nonpathogenic organisms that potentially confer health benefits by improving the microbial balance. An early report by Gionchetti et al[205] was followed up with a randomized, double-blind, placebo-controlled trial of the probiotic formulation VSL#3.[123] In this trial, 40 patients with chronic pouchitis in remission after treatment with antibiotics received either placebo or a 6 g/d oral dose of VSL#3, containing 5 x 10^{11}/g of viable lyophilized bacteria including *lactobacilli*, *bifidobacteria*, and *streptococcus*, for 9 months. Remarkably, 85% of the patients treated with VSL#3 remained in remission for 9 months compared to none of 20 patients who were treated with placebo. Others have subsequently confirmed that oral bacteriotherapy with high-dose probiotics is effective in maintaining antibiotic-introduced remission for up to a year.[187,206] As expected, a significant improvement in quality of life was associated with these extended periods of remission. Thus, preventing relapse of chronic pouchitis by restoring luminal microbial balance with nontoxic, physiologic bacteria is a significant clinical advancement for frustrated patients and physicians alike.[207]

In managing patients suffering from chronic or relapsing episodes of pouchitis, we have developed a diagnostic and treatment algorithm to systematically rule out other confounding clinical possibilities prior to further treatment (Figure 36-6). Patients who do not respond to at least 2 or in some cases 3 courses of the ciprofloxacin and metronidazole regimen described in Figure 36-5 or relapse soon after antibiotic therapy is discontinued will undergo flexible ileal pouchoscopy with biopsies, which many feel is the

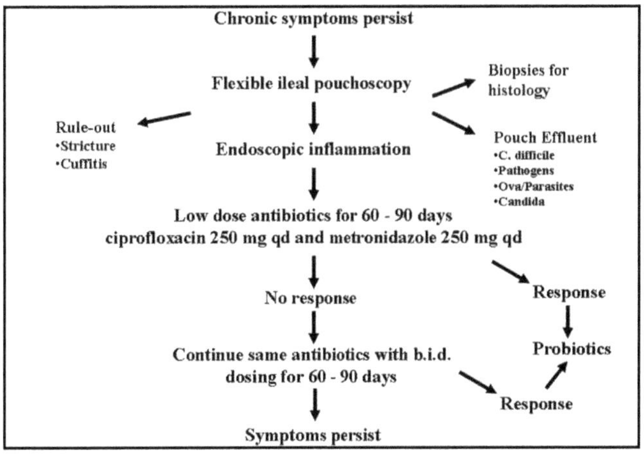

FIGURE 36-6. Diagnostic and treatment algorithm for chronic or relapsing pouchitis.

cornerstone of the differential diagnosis algorithm in these patients. Prior to beginning the endoscopic procedure, a rectal digital exam is performed to rule out ileoanal anastomotic stricture. After passing the scope, the ileum proximal to the pouch and the pouch are closely examined for endoscopic elements of inflammation, as described previously. If inflammation is apparent or suspect, biopsies from all sites are taken. Although endoscopy without biopsy has been a recommended cost-saving strategy,[208] a thorough histologic description can be a critical determinant of diagnosis and a long-term treatment plan for patients with chronic or relapsing pouchitis.

It is also important at this point to carefully examine the rectal cuff or anal transition zone for evidence of retained rectal mucosa, especially in patients known to have undergone a double-stapled anastomosis. Again, if the area is suspect, biopsies should be taken because this mucosa is particularly susceptible to recurrence of residual UC or cuffitis.[209] Cuffitis can be a cause of pouch dysfunction after a double-stapled restorative proctocolectomy and can present with symptoms mimicking pouchitis.[210] If cuffitis is identified, particularly if there is evidence of dysplasia, the retained mucosa is surgically removed by a transanal approach and the pouch advanced and re-anastomosed to the dentate line. However, medical therapy can include local treatment with topical anti-inflammatories including mesalamine and corticosteroids.[196]

Following a thorough exam of the pouch including the blind limb, digital images and mucosal biopsies are obtained from any suspicious or inflamed areas of the pouch as well as from the ileum proximal to the pouch. Before removing the scope, a sample of pouch effluent is collected sterilely to rule out infectious pathogens such a *C. difficile*,[211] parasites, or yeast. Ileal pouch fungal infections are often overlooked and can be a significant cause of pouchitis-like symptoms. We reported[212] a series of 44 patients, of which 20 tested positively for *Candida*. Fourteen of these patients were subsequently treated orally with either fluconazole or topically with nystatin for 5 days. Interestingly, 65% had a clinical response with return of stool frequency to baseline and alleviation of cramping and urgency. After a careful review of the endoscopy and pathology reports, a treatment plan is implemented.

Some of our patients with chronic or recurring episodes of pouchitis require a long-term, low-dose combination antibiotic regimen with ciprofloxacin (250 mg qd) plus metronidazole (250 mg qd) for up to 90 days to achieve a response.[66] The dose will be increased to twice per day in nonresponsive patients, or in other cases that dosing interval is reduced to every other day. Others[14] have reported antibiotic regimens that include anywhere from 500 mg of ciprofloxacin or 250 mg of metronidazole every third day to 500 mg ciprofloxacin twice daily or 250 mg metronidazole 3 times daily in order to achieve or maintain a response. Patients who develop antibiotic resistance may require combination antibiotic therapy or a rotating schedule of 3 or more antibiotics.[14] At this point, patients who either do not respond or relapse frequently, especially when antibiotic therapy is discontinued, are further evaluated.

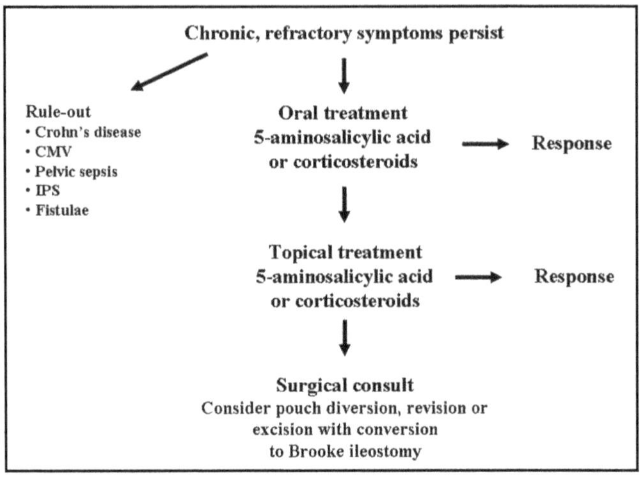

FIGURE 36-7. Diagnostic and treatment algorithm for refractory, treatment-resistant pouchitis.

REFRACTORY POUCHITIS

Severe, idiopathic, refractory pouchitis is rare, occurring in our series in less than 1% of patients (see Table 36-2). At this point, our diagnostic and treatment algorithm for marked, refractory pouchitis (Figure 36-7) will begin to further explore the more atypical possibilities, including several less common but documented viral pathogens such as primary cytomegalovirus (CMV).[213,214] Specific CMV infection of the ileal pouch has been misdiagnosed as idiopathic refractory chronic pouchitis[215]; therefore, it must be ruled out before immune modifier therapy or pouch excision is considered in these patients.

Perhaps the greatest cause for concern in these patients is, of course, Crohn's disease. This diagnosis can be particularly difficult to confirm. Although uncommon, a patient with refractory pouchitis can present with clinical, endoscopic, and pathologic features resembling CD such as complex perianal or pouch fistulizing disease, ileitis proximal to the pouch, or both. In some cases, this can be attributed to a misdiagnosis of the initial colitis or an original diagnosis that was indeterminate. At this point, serology testing is ordered to determine pANCA or ASCA titers. In our own cohort, serologic profiles showed some utility in differentiating between UC and CD and were useful in predicting the development of fistulas postoperatively.[104] In some cases, the original colectomy slides must be re-reviewed by an experienced gastrointestinal pathologist to aid in the differential diagnosis. Generally speaking, the diagnosis of CD in IPAA patients often results in severe morbidity and significant risk of pouch excision. Until recently, these patients could only be treated with standard Crohn's therapies.[216] However, the advent of anti-TNFα antibody therapy (infliximab), which has revolutionized the treatment of CD, has also been shown to benefit IPAA patients who develop Crohn's of the ileal pouch. In one of the earlier studies to report the clinical benefit of anti-TNFα treatment of refractory patients who underwent IPAA for UC and were subsequently diagnosed with CD, Ricart et al[217] reported that 6 of the 7 patients treated with infliximab had a complete response. In a later study of 26 patients with an IPAA and Crohn's-related complications, Colombel et al[218] showed that infliximab was beneficial in both the short- and long-term treatment of these patients and concluded that optimal pouch function requires long-term treatment with infliximab in these patients. Refractory fistulizing disease can occur in the ileal pouch, and although it is not always indicative of CD,[219] infliximab can also be used to treat these patients.[220] In those cases where refractory pouchitis does not seem to reflect underlying CD, there may be a link to other immunologic mechanisms that manifest clinically as extraintestinal complications.

Patients who continue to present with increased stool frequency, urgency, and abdominal pain despite normal endoscopic findings and remain refractory to standard therapy may be experiencing a condition resembling irritable bowel syndrome. Shen et al[51] published an interesting series designed to assess the etiology of bowel symptoms alone using a standard disease activity index.[18] Clinical symptoms, endoscopy, and histology were assessed in 61 consecutive symptomatic patients who underwent IPAA for chronic UC. While one-half of the patients clearly were experiencing pouchitis and 6% had cuffitis, the remaining patients were experiencing clinical symptoms without the typically associated endoscopic or histologic findings. These patients were subsequently defined as suffering from IPS. Nearly 90% of the patients with confirmed pouchitis responded to antibiotic therapy, while the 12 patients with IPS responded to antidiarrheals or anticholinergics, some in combination with antidepressants. Thus, a significant number of symptomatic patients who present clinically with what appears to be pouchitis but do not meet the diagnostic criteria might be classified as suffering from IPS.[51] Parsi et al[221] recently demonstrated that fecal lactoferrin levels can be a sensitive and noninvasive marker to initially evaluate symptomatic patients. Patients with fecal lactoferrin levels below 7 mg/mL did not have pouchitis, while patients with higher levels underwent endoscopy with biopsies to differentiate among different causes of pouch inflammation. Although fecal lactoferrin levels reliably separated patients with IPS from those with pouchitis, cuffitis, or CD with a sensitivity of 100% and specificity of 85%, further studies are needed to better define the role of this test in the management of patients with IPAA.

With regard to emerging therapeutics for patients suffering from chronic, unremitting, or refractory but confirmed pouchitis, Miner et al[186] recently described a novel treatment with a topical formulation of alicaforsen, an antisense inhibitor of intercellular adhesion molecule-1 (ICAM-1). The scientific rationale for this therapy is based on the underlying principle that an increased expression of ICAM-1, in part, mediates the influx of neutrophils, a histologic hallmark of mucosal inflammation. In an open-label, uncontrolled study, 12 patients with chronic, unremitting pouchitis were treated with a 240-mg alicaforsen antisense enema nightly for 6 weeks. Clinical evaluation and endoscopy were performed at baseline and at weeks 3, 6, and 10. Pouchoscopy with biopsy was carried out at baseline and at 6 and 10 weeks. After 6 weeks of treatment, a significant reduction in the clinical symptom and endoscopy subscores was noted. Nearly one-half also had a decrease in the histology subscore. The alicaforsen enemas were well-tolerated, and no serious side effects were noted, perhaps warranting a larger, randomized, placebo-controlled trial. Other promising antisense therapeutics are also under investigation for IBD that may have subsequent implications for the treatment of refractory pouchitis.[222] Other treatments that have employed nutritional agents and dietary supplements such as fibers have shown little benefit[223]; although a randomized, double-blind, crossover study by Welters et al[134] did show that enteral inulin supplementation led to a reduction of inflammation in pouch mucosa. Oral tacrolimus (0.05 mg/kg bid) has recently shown efficacy in the treatment of refractory pouchitis, perhaps warranting a further controlled, long-term evaluation.[224]

More recently, CT and MRI are becoming useful diagnostic aids in difficult cases and can be useful in detecting pouch-related complications such as small-bowel obstruction, pouchitis, leakage, abscess, intramural hematomas, desmoid tumors, or recurrent CD.[225] A recent study by Nadgir et al[226] used MRI to identify the presence of inflammation related to the pouch reservoir in symptomatic patients who present with clinically suspected complicated pouchitis. MRI showed abnormalities consistent with complicated pouchitis in 7 of 9 patients, with findings including pouch wall thickening, abnormal wall enhancement, peripouch fluid collection, sinus and fistula tract formation, lymphadenopathy, and peripouch stranding and fatty proliferation. Such MRI findings in patients with complicated or refractory pouchitis should raise the suspicion of CD and should prompt further investigation. Small bowel involvement using wireless capsule endoscopy may also provide useful diagnostic information in patients with chronic refractory pouchitis. Calabrese et al[227] reported that patients with chronic pouchitis showed diffuse lesions from the duodenum to ileum consisting of aphthae, erosions, erythema, atrophy, cobblestone, and deep/fissural ulcers, suggesting that wireless capsule endoscopy could be useful to show involvement of small bowel in patients with chronic pouchitis.

SURGICAL TREATMENT

At this point in our treatment algorithm, nonresponsive patients with apparently refractory pouchitis, who have either unacceptable pouch function or suspected CD and have not responded to immunomodulators or anti-TNFα therapy, are faced with limited options, including a defunctioning ileostomy with pouch diversion or pouch excision with conversion to permanent ileostomy. Selected patients are carefully counseled at this point to consider pouch revision in lieu of pouch excision, especially if CD has been definitively ruled out. Surgical revision of the pouch is technically feasible using either a transanal approach or a combined abdominoperineal approach with pouch revision and re-anastomosis. Surgical salvage techniques can include completion of the rectal mucosectomy, ileoanal anastomotic strictureplasty, and total pouch reconstruction as viable alternatives to permanent ileostomy. Most series[228] including our own[67] have reported a high success rate of salvage surgery with patients reporting satisfactory outcomes and a substantially increased quality of life. In a more recent series by Dehni et al,[229] 64 patients underwent revisional surgery for complications including sepsis, mechanical dysfunction, residual epithelial cuff, and previous intraoperative difficulties. A combined abdominoperineal approach was used in the majority of cases, and at the 5 year follow-up, 94% of patients had a functional pouch. Although nearly one-half of these patients experienced some degree of day and night incontinence, three-quarters of patients reported an acceptable level of bowel function, and 50% rated their satisfaction with the outcome as good to excellent. A similar series by Tekkis et al[68] also reported favorable outcomes at 5 years; however, they noted that patients undergoing abdominal salvage surgery for septic complications were less likely to have a successful outcome compared with those undergoing the same procedure for nonseptic indications. Although pouch excision with construction of a conventional Brooke ileostomy is the most widely used procedure after unsuccessful salvage surgery, conversion to a continent ileostomy or Kock pouch is a feasible alternative that may be considered in patients motivated to remain continent.[230]

The pouch failure rate in our series, necessitating conversion to permanent Brooke ileostomy, is approximately 2% as compared to the pooled estimate of 6.2% we found when we surveyed the literature.[60] Approximately one-half of these were histologically and/or serologically confirmed to have Crohn's disease. We have had no pouch failures as a direct result of refractory pouchitis. Others have also reported that few pouch failures are the direct result of refractory pouchitis.[185,231] On another note, our low pouch failure rate is due not only to the fact that increased experience decreases the risk of pouch-related complications and improves long-term outcome,[232] but also due to our continued effort to salvage failed pouches. Approximately 60% of the pouches in our series that failed were successfully salvaged, thus avoiding permanent ileostomy.[67]

CONCLUSION

Although the majority of patients with chronic UC who undergo colectomy with IPAA report having a significantly improved quality of life after surgery,[233] pouchitis continues to overshadow the long-term functional results of this sphincter-saving operation. At present, the etiology of pouchitis is unknown; however, the cause is most likely multifactorial and appears to encompass a spectrum of manifestations and diseases.[21] A recent commentary called pouchitis one of the most challenging and disappointing diagnoses faced by gastroenterologists treating patients with IBD.[234] This sentiment is certainly echoed by the many surgeons who follow their IPAA patients.[7] Fortunately, for the majority of IPAA patients, episodes of pouchitis are acute and managed medically; however, the real challenge these authors allude to is managing the small percentage of patients with more chronic or refractory pouchitis. Most series, including our own, show the number of these patients is quite low and should not affect the decision to perform IPAA. Interestingly, as we surpass the 30th anniversary of the revival of IPAA and the numbers of patients with long-term follow-up increases, we are finally beginning to recognize a number of risk factors associated with inflammatory and noninflammatory diseases of the ileal pouch, including pouchitis.[235] These new studies may allow us to better identify high-risk patients before surgery. There are many promising and novel therapeutic approaches for the treatment of refractory pouchitis; and while many are unproven clinically, there is substantial supporting evidence to suggest that many may be efficacious and should be further pursued. However, a better understanding of the etiology of pouchitis can lead to the development of novel therapeutic interventions that may prevent or reduce the severity of pouchitis, thereby enhancing the outcome of IPAA surgery even further. Thus, there is a need for multicenter, longitudinal trials of chronic UC patients having undergone IPAA to further investigate the etiology and pathophysiology of pouchitis. The inclusion of patients with FAP, who rarely experience pouchitis, would offer a unique control group and the opportunity to elucidate and define the underlying pathologic sequence that leads to ileal pouch inflammation.

REFERENCES

1. Larson DW, Pemberton JH. Current concepts and controversies in surgery for IBD. *Gastroenterology.* 2004; 126:1611-1619.
2. Kock NG. Intra-abdominal "reservoir" in patients with permanent ileostomy. Preliminary observations on a procedure resulting in fecal "continence" in five ileostomy patients. *Arch Surg.* 1969;99:223-231.
3. Parks AG, Nicholls RJ. Proctocolectomy without ileostomy for ulcerative colitis. *Br Med J.* 1978;2:85-88.
4. Parks AG, Nicholls RJ, Belliveau P. Proctocolectomy with ileal reservoir and anal anastomosis. *Br J Surg.* 1980;67:533-538.
5. Utsunomiya J, Iwama T, Imajo M, et al. Total colectomy, mucosal proctectomy, and ileoanal anastomosis. *Dis Colon Rectum.* 1980;23:459-466.
6. Ravitch MM, Sabiston DL Jr. Anal ileostomy with preservation of the sphincter: a proposed operation in patients requiring total colectomy for benign lesions. *Surg Gynecol Obstet.* 1947;84:1095-1099.
7. Becker JM, Stucchi AF. Proctocolectomy with ileoanal anastomosis. *J Gastrointest Surg.* 2004;8:376-386.
8. Metcalf AM. Elective and emergent operative management of ulcerative colitis. *Surg Clin North Am.* 2007;87:633-641.
9. Onaitis MW, Mantyh C. Ileal pouch-anal anastomosis for ulcerative colitis and familial adenomatous polyposis: historical development and current status. *Ann Surg.* 2003;238:S42-48.
10. Becker JM, Stucchi AF. Inherited colorectal polyposis syndromes. In: Cameron JL, ed. *Current Surgical Therapy,* 8th ed. Philadelphia, PA: Elsevier Mosby; 2004:200-211.
11. Cima RR, Pemberton JH. Surgical indications and procedures in ulcerative colitis. *Curr Treat Options Gastroenterol.* 2004;7: 181-190.
12. Hahnloser D, Pemberton JH, Wolff BG, et al. Results at up to 20 years after ileal pouch-anal anastomosis for chronic ulcerative colitis. *Br J Surg.* 2007;94:333-340.
13. Muir AJ, Edwards LJ, Sanders LL, et al. A prospective evaluation of health-related quality of life after ileal pouch anal anastomosis for ulcerative colitis. *Am J Gastroenterol.* 2001;96:1480-1485.
14. Mahadevan U, Sandborn WJ. Diagnosis and management of pouchitis. *Gastroenterology.* 2003;124:1636-1650.
15. Tremaine WJ. Pouchitis. In: Sartor RB, Sandborn WJ, eds. *Kirsner's Inflammatory Bowel Disease,* 6th ed. New York: Saunders; 2004: 673-681.
16. Kock NG, Darle N, Hulten L, et al. Ileostomy. *Curr Probl Surg.* 1977;14:1-52.
17. Moskowitz RL, Shepherd NA, Nicholls RJ. An assessment of inflammation in the reservoir after restorative proctocolectomy with ileoanal ileal reservoir. *Int J Colorectal Dis.* 1986;1:167-174.
18. Sandborn WJ, Tremaine WJ, Batts KP, et al. Pouchitis after ileal pouch-anal anastomosis: a pouchitis disease activity index. *Mayo Clin Proc.* 1994;69:409-415.
19. Heuschen UA, Autschbach F, Allemeyer EH, et al. Long-term follow-up after ileoanal pouch procedure: algorithm for diagnosis, classification, and management of pouchitis. *Dis Colon Rectum.* 2001;44:487-499.
20. Shen B, Achkar JP, Connor JT, et al. Modified pouchitis disease activity index: a simplified approach to the diagnosis of pouchitis. *Dis Colon Rectum.* 2003;46:748-753.
21. Shen B, Lashner BA. Pouchitis: a spectrum of diseases. *Curr Gastroenterol Rep.* 2005;7:404-411.
22. Shen B, Lashner BA. Diagnosis and treatment of ileal pouch diseases in patients with underlying ulcerative colitis. *Curr Treat Options Gastroenterol.* 2006;9:3-12.
23. Cheifetz A, Itzkowitz S. The diagnosis and treatment of pouchitis in inflammatory bowel disease. *J Clin Gastroenterol.* 2004;38: S44-S50.
24. Sandborn WJ. Pouchitis following ileal pouch-anal anastomosis: Definition, pathogenesis, and treatment. *Gastroenterology.* 1994;107:1856-1860.
25. Aitola P, Matikainen M, Mattila J, et al. Chronic inflammatory changes in the pouch mucosa are associated with cholangitis found on preoperative liver biopsy specimens at restorative proctocolectomy for ulcerative colitis. *Scand J Gastroenterol.* 1998;33:289-293.
26. Schouten WR. Pouchitis. *Mediators Inflamm.* 1998;7:175-181.
27. Lohmuller JL, Pemberton JH, Dozois RR, et al. Pouchitis and extraintestinal manifestations of inflammatory bowel disease after ileal pouch-anal anastomosis. *Ann Surg.* 1990;211:622-627; discussion 627-629.
28. Penna C, Dozois R, Tremaine W, et al. Pouchitis after ileal pouch-anal anastomosis for ulcerative colitis occurs with increased frequency in patients with associated primary sclerosing cholangitis. *Gut.* 1996;38:234-239.
29. Shen B, Achkar JP, Lashner BA, et al. Endoscopic and histologic evaluation together with symptom assessment are required to diagnose pouchitis. *Gastroenterology.* 2001;121:261-267.
30. Stucchi AF, Materne O, Beer E, et al. Evidence for oxidative stress in the etiology of pouchitis. *Gastroenterology.* 1999;116:A1359.
31. Thomas PD, Forbes A, Price AB, et al. Differential expression of cell adhesion molecules within inflamed ileal pouch mucosa: relationship to recruited cell subtypes. *Eur J Gastroenterol Hepatol.* 2002;14:137-144.
32. Shepherd NA, Jass JR, Duval I, et al. Restorative proctocolectomy with ileal reservoir: pathological and histochemical study of mucosal biopsy specimens. *J Clin Pathol.* 1987;40:601-607.
33. Hinojosa J, Bau I, Martinez B, et al. Morphological, histochemical and immunochemical characteristics of the terminal ileum of patients with ulcerative colitis. Relationship with the development of pouchitis. *Gastroenterol Hepatol.* 2000;23:263-268.
34. Gionchetti P, Amadini C, Rizzello F, et al. Diagnosis and treatment of pouchitis. *Best Pract Res Clin Gastroenterol.* 2003;17:75-87.
35. Merrett MN. Ileal pouches: adaptation and inflammation. *Baillieres Clin Gastroenterol.* 1997;11:175-193.
36. Garcia-Armengol J, Hinojosa J, Lledo S, et al. Prospective study of morphologic and functional changes with time in the mucosa of the ileoanal pouch: functional appraisal using transmucosal potential differences. *Dis Colon Rectum.* 1998;41:846-853.
37. Setti Carraro P, Talbot IC, Nicholls RJ. Long-term appraisal of the histological appearances of the ileal reservoir mucosa after restorative proctocolectomy for ulcerative colitis. *Gut.* 1994;35:1721-1727.
38. Apel R, Cohen Z, Andrews CW Jr, et al. Prospective evaluation of early morphological changes in pelvic ileal pouches. *Gastroenterology.* 1994;107:435-443.
39. Lerch MM, Braun J, Harder M, et al. Postoperative adaptation of the small intestine after total colectomy and J-pouch-anal anastomosis. *Dis Colon Rectum.* 1989;32:600-608.
40. de Silva HJ, Millard PR, Kettlewell M, et al. Mucosal characteristics of pelvic ileal pouches. *Gut.* 1991;32:61-65.
41. Hill MJ, Fernandez F. Pouch workshop: bacteriology. *Int J Colorectal Dis.* 1989;4:217.
42. Kuisma J, Nuutinen H, Luukkonen P, et al. Long term metabolic consequences of ileal pouch-anal anastomosis for ulcerative colitis. *Am J Gastroenterol.* 2001;96:3110-3116.
43. Veress B, Reinholt FP, Lindquist K, et al. Long-term histomorphological surveillance of the pelvic ileal pouch: dysplasia develops in a subgroup of patients. *Gastroenterology.* 1995;109:1090-1097.
44. Stallmach A, Moser C, Hero-Gross R, et al. Pattern of mucosal adaptation in acute and chronic pouchitis. *Dis Colon Rectum.* 1999;42:1311-1317.

45. Gullberg K, Stahlberg D, Liljeqvist L, et al. Neoplastic transformation of the pelvic pouch mucosa in patients with ulcerative colitis. *Gastroenterology.* 1997;112:1487-1492.
46. Stahlberg D, Veress B, Tribukait B, et al. Atrophy and neoplastic transformation of the ileal pouch mucosa in patients with ulcerative colitis and primary sclerosing cholangitis: a case control study. *Dis Colon Rectum.* 2003;46:770-778.
47. Fruin AB, El-Zammer O, Stucchi AF, et al. Colonic metaplasia in the ileal pouch is associated with inflammation and is not the result of long-term adaptation. *J Gastrointest Surg.* 2003;7: 246-254.
48. Thompson-Fawcett MW, Marcus V, Redston M, et al. Risk of dysplasia in long-term ileal pouches and pouches with chronic pouchitis. *Gastroenterology.* 2001;121:275-281.
49. Nilubol N, Scherl E, Bub DS, et al. Mucosal dysplasia in ileal pelvic pouches after restorative proctocolectomy. *Dis Colon Rectum.* 2007;50:825-831.
50. Scarpa M, van Koperen PJ, Ubbink DT, et al. Systematic review of dysplasia after restorative proctocolectomy for ulcerative colitis. *Br J Surg.* 2007;94:534-545.
51. Shen B, Achkar JP, Lashner BA, et al. Irritable pouch syndrome: A new category of diagnosis for symptomatic patients with ileal pouch-anal anastomosis. *Am J Gastroenterol.* 2002;97:972-977.
52. Sandborn WJ. Pouchitis in the Kock continent ileostomy and the ileoanal pouch. In: Kirsner JB, ed. *Inflammatory Bowel Disease,* 5th ed. Philadelphia, PA: WB Saunders; 2000:736-747.
53. Shen B, Fazio VW, Remzi FH, et al. Clinical approach to diseases of ileal pouch-anal anastomosis. *Am J Gastroenterol.* 2005;100:2796-2807.
54. Michelassi F, Lee J, Rubin M, et al. Long-term functional results after ileal pouch anal restorative proctocolectomy for ulcerative colitis: a prospective observational study. *Ann Surg.* 2003;238:433-441.
55. Reissman P, Piccirillo M, Ulrich A, et al. Functional results of the double-stapled ileoanal reservoir. *J Am Coll Surg.* 1995;181:444-450.
56. Kuisma J, Jarvinen H, Kahri A, et al. Factors associated with disease activity of pouchitis after surgery for ulcerative colitis. *Scand J Gastroenterol.* 2004;39:544-548.
57. Simchuk EJ, Thirlby RC. Risk factors and true incidence of pouchitis in patients after ileal pouch-anal anastomoses. *World J Surg.* 2000;24:851-856.
58. Farouk R, Pemberton JH, Wolff BG, et al. Functional outcomes after ileal pouch-anal anastomosis for chronic ulcerative colitis. *Ann Surg.* 2000;231:919-926.
59. Fazio VW, Ziv Y, Church JM, et al. Ileal pouch-anal anastomoses complications and function in 1005 patients. *Ann Surg.* 1995;222:120-127.
60. Lehrmann J, Stucchi AF, LaMorte WW, et al. Complications and outcomes after ileal pouch-anal anastomosis (IPAA): a meta-analysis of more than 8300 patients. *Gastroenterology.* 2003;124:A814.
61. Stahlberg D, Gullberg K, Liljeqvist L, et al. Pouchitis following pelvic pouch operation for ulcerative colitis: incidence, cumulative risk, and risk factors. *Dis Colon Rectum.* 1996;39:1012-1018.
62. Meagher AP, Farouk R, Dozois RR, et al. J ileal pouch-anal anastomosis for chronic ulcerative colitis: complications and long-term outcome in 1310 patients. *Br J Surg.* 1998;85:800-803.
63. Hurst RD, Chung TP, Rubin M, et al. The implications of acute pouchitis on the long-term functional results after restorative proctocolectomy. *Inflamm Bowel Dis.* 1998;4:280-284.
64. Heuschen UA, Allemeyer EH, Hinz U, et al. Diagnosing pouchitis: Comparative validation of two scoring systems in routine follow-up. *Dis Colon Rectum.* 2002;45:776-786; discussion 786-788.
65. Keranen U, Luukkonen P, Jarvinen H. Functional results after restorative proctocolectomy complicated by pouchitis. *Dis Colon Rectum.* 1997;40:764-769.
66. Becker JM, Stucchi AF, Bryant DE. How do you treat refractory pouchitis and when do you decide to remove the pouch? *Inflamm Bowel Dis.* 1998;4:167-169; discussion 170-161.
67. Saltzberg SS, DiEdwardo C, Scott TE, et al. Ileal pouch salvage following failed ileal pouch-anal anastomosis. *J Gastrointest Surg.* 1999;3:633-641.
68. Tekkis PP, Heriot AG, Smith JJ, et al. Long-term results of abdominal salvage surgery following restorative proctocolectomy. *Br J Surg.* 2006;93:231-237.
69. Jewell DP, Mortensen NFM. Pouchitis. In: Allan RN, et al, eds. *Inflammatory Bowel Diseases,* 3rd ed. New York: Churchill Livingstone; 1997:803-809.
70. Tiainen J, Matikainen M, Aitola P, et al. Histological and macroscopic changes in the pelvic pouch: long-term follow up after restorative proctocolectomy for ulcerative colitis (UC). *Colorectal Dis.* 2001;3:28-32.
71. Heuschen UA, Hinz U, Allemeyer EH, et al. One- or two-stage procedure for restorative proctocolectomy: rationale for a surgical strategy in ulcerative colitis. *Ann Surg.* 2001;234:788-794.
72. Pace DE, Seshadri PA, Chiasson PM, et al. Early experience with laparoscopic ileal pouch-anal anastomosis for ulcerative colitis. *Surg Laparosc Endosc Percutan Tech.* 2002;12:337-341.
73. Merrett MN, Mortensen N, Kettlewell M, et al. Smoking may prevent pouchitis in patients with restorative proctocolectomy for ulcerative colitis. *Gut.* 1996;38:362-364.
74. Snook JA, Dwyer L, Lee-Elliott C, et al. Smoking benefits celiac sprue and pouchitis: implications for nicotine therapy? *Gastroenterology.* 1997;112:1048-1050.
75. Thomas GA, Rhodes J, Green JT, et al. Role of smoking in inflammatory bowel disease: implications for therapy. *Postgrad Med J.* 2000;76:273-279.
76. Aisenberg J, Wagreich J, Shim J, et al. Perinuclear anti-neutrophil cytoplasmic antibody and refractory pouchitis: a case-control study. *Dig Dis Sci.* 1995;40:1866-1872.
77. Hata K, Watanabe T, Shinozaki M, et al. Patients with extraintestinal manifestations have a higher risk of developing pouchitis in ulcerative colitis: multivariate analysis. *Scand J Gastroenterol.* 2003;38:1055-1058.
78. Andreyev HJ, Kamm MA, Forbes A, et al. Joint symptoms after restorative proctocolectomy in ulcerative colitis and familial polyposis coli. *J Clin Gastroenterol.* 1996;23:35-39.
79. de Silva HJ, de Angelis CP, Soper N, et al. Clinical and functional outcome after restorative proctocolectomy. *Br J Surg.* 1991;78:1039-1044.
80. Yantiss RK, Sapp HL, Farraye FA, et al. Histologic predictors of pouchitis in patients with chronic ulcerative colitis. *Am J Surg Pathol.* 2004;28:999-1006.
81. Schmidt CM, Lazenby AJ, Hendrickson RJ, et al. Preoperative terminal ileal and colonic resection histopathology predicts risk of pouchitis in patients after ileoanal pull-through procedure. *Ann Surg.* 1998;227:654-662; discussion 663-655.
82. Samarasekera DN, Stebbing JF, Kettlewell MG, et al. Outcome of restorative proctocolectomy with ileal reservoir for ulcerative colitis: comparison of distal colitis with more proximal disease. *Gut.* 1996;38:574-577.
83. Gustavsson S, Weiland LH, Kelly KA. Relationship of backwash ileitis to ileal pouchitis after ileal pouch-anal anastomosis. *Dis Colon Rectum.* 1987;30:25-28.
84. Luukkonen P, Jarvinen H, Tanskanen M, et al. Pouchitis–recurrence of the inflammatory bowel disease? *Gut.* 1994;35:243-246.
85. Achkar JP, Al-Haddad M, Lashner B, et al. Differentiating risk factors for acute and chronic pouchitis. *Clin Gastroenterol Hepatol.* 2005;3:60-66.
86. Shen B, Fazio VW, Remzi FH, et al. Effect of withdrawal of nonsteroidal anti-inflammatory drug use on ileal pouch disorders. *Dig Dis Sci.* 2007.

87. Hui T, Landers C, Vasiliauskas E, et al. Serologic responses in indeterminate colitis patients before ileal pouch-anal anastomosis may determine those at risk for continuous pouch inflammation. *Dis Colon Rectum.* 2005;48:1254-1262.
88. Okon A, Dubinsky M, Vasiliauskas EA, et al. Elevated platelet count before ileal pouch-anal anastomosis for ulcerative colitis is associated with the development of chronic pouchitis. *Am Surg.* 2005;71:821-826.
89. Fleshner P, Ippoliti A, Dubinsky M, et al. A prospective multivariate analysis of clinical factors associated with pouchitis after ileal pouch-anal anastomosis. *Clin Gastroenterol Hepatol.* 2007;5:952-958.
90. Remzi FH, Fazio VW, Oncel M, et al. Portal vein thrombi after restorative proctocolectomy. *Surgery.* 2002;132:655-661; discussion 661-652.
91. Ball CG, MacLean AR, Buie WD, et al. Portal vein thrombi after ileal pouch-anal anastomosis: its incidence and association with pouchitis. *Surg Today.* 2007;37:552-557.
92. Shen B, Lashner B. Can we immunogenotypically and immunophenotypically profile patients who are at risk for pouchitis? *Am J Gastroenterol.* 2004;99:442-444.
93. Vecchi M, Gionchetti P, Bianchi MB, et al. p-ANCA and development of pouchitis in ulcerative colitis patients after proctocolectomy and ileoanal pouch anastomosis. *Lancet.* 1994;344:886-887.
94. Shanahan F, Duerr RH, Rotter JI, et al. Neutrophil autoantibodies in ulcerative colitis: familial aggregation and genetic heterogeneity. *Gastroenterology.* 1992;103:456-461.
95. Sandborn WJ, Landers CJ, Tremaine WJ, et al. Antineutrophil cytoplasmic antibody correlates with chronic pouchitis after ileal pouch-anal anastomosis. *Am J Gastroenterol.* 1995;90:740-747.
96. Yang P, Oresland T, Jarnerot G, et al. Perinuclear antineutrophil cytoplasmic antibody in pouchitis after proctocolectomy with ileal pouch-anal anastomosis for ulcerative colitis. *Scand J Gastroenterol.* 1996;31:594-598.
97. Brett PM, Yasuda N, Yiannakou JY, et al. Genetic and immunological markers in pouchitis. *Eur J Gastroenterol Hepatol.* 1996;8:951-955.
98. Esteve M, Mallolas J, Klaassen J, et al. Antineutrophil cytoplasmic antibodies in sera from colectomized ulcerative colitis patients and its relation to the presence of pouchitis. *Gut.* 1996;38:894-898.
99. Yasuda N, Thomas P, Ellis H, et al. Perinuclear anti-neutrophil cytoplasmic antibodies in ulcerative colitis after restorative proctocolectomy do not correlate with the presence of pouchitis. *Scand J Gastroenterol.* 1998;33:509-513.
100. Fleshner PR, Vasiliauskas EA, Kam LY, et al. High level perinuclear antineutrophil cytoplasmic antibody (pANCA) in ulcerative colitis patients before colectomy predicts the development of chronic pouchitis after ileal pouch-anal anastomosis. *Gut.* 2001;49:671-677.
101. Duerr RH, Targan SR, Landers CJ, et al. Neutrophil cytoplasmic antibodies: a link between primary sclerosing cholangitis and ulcerative colitis. *Gastroenterology.* 1991;100:1385-1391.
102. Seibold F, Weber P, Schoning A, et al. Neutrophil antibodies (pANCA) in chronic liver disease and inflammatory bowel disease: Do they react with different antigens? *Eur J Gastroenterol Hepatol.* 1996;8:1095-1100.
103. Stocchi L, Pemberton JH. Pouch and pouchitis. *Gastroenterol Clin North Am.* 2001;30:223-241.
104. Dendrinos KG, Becker JM, Stucchi AF, et al. Anti-*Saccharomyces cerevisiae* antibodies are associated with the development of postoperative fistulas following ileal pouch-anal anastomosis. *J Gastrointest Surg.* 2006;10:1060-1064.
105. Carter MJ, Di Giovine FS, Cox A, et al. The interleukin 1 receptor antagonist gene allele 2 as a predictor of pouchitis following colectomy and IPAA in ulcerative colitis. *Gastroenterology.* 2001;121:805-811.
106. Rogler G, Andus T. Cytokines in inflammatory bowel disease. *World J Surg.* 1998;22:382-389.
107. Andus T, Daig R, Vogl D, et al. Imbalance of the interleukin 1 system in colonic mucosa–association with intestinal inflammation and interleukin 1 receptor antagonist genotype 2. *Gut.* 1997;41:651-657.
108. Geng X, Biancone L, Dai HH, et al. Tropomyosin isoforms in intestinal mucosa: production of autoantibodies to tropomyosin isoforms in ulcerative colitis. *Gastroenterology.* 1998;114:912-922.
109. Biancone L, Palmieri G, Lombardi A, et al. Tropomyosin expression in the ileal pouch: a relationship with the development of pouchitis in ulcerative colitis. *Am J Gastroenterol.* 2003;98:2719-2726.
110. Nicholls RJ, Banerjee AK. Pouchitis: risk factors, etiology, and treatment. *World J Surg.* 1998;22:347-351.
111. Oresland T, Fasth S, Nordgren S, et al. The clinical and functional outcome after restorative proctocolectomy. *Int J Colorectal Dis.* 1989;4:50-56.
112. Becker JM, Becich MJ, Nash SV, et al. Pouchitis-aetiology, pathogenesis, therapy. In: Rachmilewitz D, ed. *Inflammatory Bowel Diseases.* Boston, MA: Kluwer Academic; 1994:276-288.
113. Shebani KO, Stucchi AF, McClung JP, et al. Stasis is associated with ileal J-pouch inflammation and oxidative stress in a rat model of ileal J-pouch anal anastomosis. *Gastroenterology.* 2000;118:A1048.
114. Gosselink MP, Schouten WR, Van Lieshout LM, et al. Eradication of pathogenic bacteria and restoration of normal pouch flora: comparison of metronidazole and ciprofloxacin in the treatment of pouchitis. *Dis Colon Rectum.* 2004;47:1519-1525.
115. de Silva HJ, Millard PR, Soper N, et al. Effects of the faecal stream and stasis on the ileal pouch mucosa. *Gut.* 1991;32:1166-1169.
116. Go PM, van Dieijen-Visser MP, Davies BI, et al. Microbial flora and bile acid metabolism in patients with an ileal reservoir. *Scand J Gastroenterol.* 1988;23:229-236.
117. Ruseler-van Embden JG, Schouten WR, van Lieshout LM. Pouchitis: Result of microbial imbalance? *Gut.* 1994;35:658-664.
118. Nasmyth DG, Godwin PG, Dixon MF, et al. Ileal ecology after pouch-anal anastomosis or ileostomy: a study of mucosal morphology, fecal bacteriology, fecal volatile fatty acids, and their interrelationship. *Gastroenterology.* 1989;96:817-824.
119. Shebani KO, Stucchi AF, Fruin B, et al. Pouchitis in a rat model of ileal J pouch-anal anastomosis. *Inflamm Bowel Dis.* 2002;8:23-34.
120. Onderdonk AB, Dvorak AM, Cisneros RL, et al. Microbiologic assessment of tissue biopsy samples from ileal pouch patients. *J Clin Microbiol.* 1992;30:312-317.
121. McLeod RS, Antonioli D, Cullen J, et al. Histologic and microbiologic features of biopsy samples from patients with normal and inflamed pouches. *Dis Colon Rectum.* 1994;37:26-31.
122. Komanduri S, Gillevet PM, Sikaroodi M, et al. Dysbiosis in pouchitis: evidence of unique microfloral patterns in pouch inflammation. *Clin Gastroenterol Hepatol.* 2007;5:352-360.
123. Gionchetti P, Rizzello F, Helwig U, et al. Prophylaxis of pouchitis onset with probiotic therapy: a double-blind, placebo-controlled trial. *Gastroenterology.* 2003;124:1202-1209.
124. Chapman TM, Plosker GL, Figgitt DP. Spotlight on VSL#3 probiotic mixture in chronic inflammatory bowel diseases. *BioDrugs.* 2007;21:61-63.
125. Roediger WE. The colonic epithelium in ulcerative colitis: an energy-deficiency disease? *Lancet.* 1980;2:712-715.
126. Windmueller HG, Spaeth AE. Identification of ketone bodies and glutamine as the major respiratory fuels in vivo for postabsorptive rat small intestine. *J Biol Chem.* 1978;253:69-76.
127. Alles MS, Katan MB, Salemans JM, et al. Bacterial fermentation of fructooligosaccharides and resistant starch in patients with an ileal pouch-anal anastomosis. *Am J Clin Nutr.* 1997;66:1286-1292.
128. Cook SI, Sellin JH. Review article: short chain fatty acids in health and disease. *Aliment Pharmacol Ther.* 1998;12:499-507.

129. Roediger WE, Moore A. Effect of short-chain fatty acid on sodium absorption in isolated human colon perfused through the vascular bed. *Dig Dis Sci.* 1981;26:100-106.
130. Clausen MR, Tuede M, Mortensen PB. Short-chain fatty acids in pouch contents from patients with and without pouchitis after ileal pouch-anal anastomosis. *Gastroenterology.* 1992;103:1144-1153.
131. Sagar PM, Taylor BA, Godwin P, et al. Acute pouchitis and deficiencies of fuel. *Dis Colon Rectum.* 1995;38:488-493.
132. Den Hoed PT, van Goch JJ, Veen HF, et al. Severe pouchitis successfully treated with short-chain fatty acids [letter]. *Can J Surgery.* 1996;39:168-169.
133. Tonelli F, Dolara P, Batignani G, et al. Effects of short chain fatty acids on mucosal proliferation and inflammation of ileal pouches in patients with ulcerative colitis and familial polyposis. *Dis Colon Rectum.* 1995;38:974-978.
134. Welters CF, Heineman E, Thunnissen FB, et al. Effect of dietary inulin supplementation on inflammation of pouch mucosa in patients with an ileal pouch-anal anastomosis. *Dis Colon Rectum.* 2002;45:621-627.
135. Ehrenfried JA, Chen J, Li J, et al. Glutamine-mediated regulation of heat shock protein expression in intestinal cells. *Surgery.* 1995;118:352-357.
136. Heuschen UA, Allemeyer EH, Hinz U, et al. Glutamine distribution in patients with ulcerative colitis and in patients with familial adenomatous polyposis coli before and after restorative proctocolectomy. *Int J Colorectal Dis.* 2002;17:245-252.
137. Wischmeyer P, Pemberton JH, Phillips SF. Chronic pouchitis after ileal pouch-anal anastomosis: responses to butyrate and glutamine suppositories in a pilot study. *Mayo Clin Proc.* 1993;68:978-981.
138. Salemans JM, Nagengast FM, Tangerman A, et al. Postprandial conjugated and unconjugated serum bile acid levels after proctocolectomy with ileal pouch-anal anastomosis. *Scand J Gastroenterol.* 1993;28:786-790.
139. Christl SU, Scheppach W. Metabolic consequences of total colectomy. *Scand J Gastroenterol Suppl.* 1997;222:20-24.
140. Natori H, Utsunomiya J, Yamamura T, et al. Fecal and stomal bile acid composition after ileostomy or ileoanal anastomosis in patients with chronic ulcerative colitis and adenomatosis coli. *Gastroenterology.* 1992;102:1278-1288.
141. Merrett MN, Owen RW, Jewell DP. Ileal pouch dialysate is cytotoxic to epithelial cell lines, but not to CaCo-2 monolayers. *Eur J Gastroenterol Hepatol.* 1997;9:1219-1226.
142. Breuer NF, Rampton DS, Tammar A, et al. Effect of colonic perfusion with sulfated and nonsulfated bile acids on mucosal structure and function in the rat. *Gastroenterology.* 1983;84:969-977.
143. Simpson R, Alon R, Kobzik L, et al. Neutrophil and nonneutrophil-mediated injury in intestinal ischemia-reperfusion. *Ann Surg.* 1993;218:444-453; discussion 453-454.
144. Keighley MR. ["Pouchitis"; histology]. *Ann Chir.* 1993;47:1029-1033.
145. Perbeck L, Lindquist K, Liljeqvist L. The mucosal blood flow in pelvic pouches in man: a methodologic study of fluorescein flowmetry. *Dis Colon Rectum.* 1985;28:931-936.
146. Sakaguchi M, Hosie K, Tudor R, et al. Mucosal blood flow following restorative proctocolectomy: pouchitis is associated with mucosal ischaemia. *Br J Surg.* 1989;76:1331-1338.
147. Surh S, Kienle P, Weitz J, et al. Monitoring of mucosal blood flow in the ileoanal pouch by measuring the pHi. *Gastroenterol.* 1998;114: A1427.
148. Buffinton GD, Doe WF. Depleted mucosal antioxidant defences in inflammatory bowel disease. *Free Radic Biol Med.* 1995;19:911-918.
149. Levin KE, Pemberton JH, Phillips SF, et al. Role of oxygen free radicals in the etiology of pouchitis. *Dis Colon Rectum.* 1992;35:452-456.
150. Joelsson M, Andersson M, Bark T, et al. Allopurinol as prophylaxis against pouchitis following ileal pouch-anal anastomosis for ulcerative colitis: a randomized placebo-controlled double-blind study. *Scand J Gastroenterol.* 2001;36:1179-1184.
151. Sartor RB. Review article: role of the enteric microflora in the pathogenesis of intestinal inflammation and arthritis. *Aliment Pharmacol Ther.* 1997;11 Suppl 3:17-22; discussion 22-13.
152. Pavlick KP, Laroux FS, Fuseler J, et al. Role of reactive metabolites of oxygen and nitrogen in inflammatory bowel disease. *Free Radic Biol Med.* 2002;33:311-322.
153. Davies NM, Jamali F. Pharmacological protection of NSAID-induced intestinal permeability in the rat: effect of tempo and metronidazole as potential free radical scavengers. *Hum Exp Toxicol.* 1997;16:345-349.
154. Pearson DC, Jourd'Heuil D, Meddings JB. The antioxidant properties of 5-aminosalicyclic acid. *Free Radical Biol Med.* 1996;21:367-373.
155. Gionchetti P, Rizzello F, Venturi A, et al. Long-term efficacy of bismuth carbomer enemas in patients with treatment-resistant chronic pouchitis. *Aliment Pharmacol Ther.* 1997;11:673-678.
156. Tremaine WJ, Sandborn WJ, Kenan ML. Bismuth subsalicylate tablets for chronic antibiotic-resistant pouchitis. *Gastroenterol.* 1998;114:A1101.
157. Bagchi D, Carryl OR, Tran MX, et al. Stress, diet and alcohol-induced oxidative gastrointestinal mucosal injury in rats and protection by bismuth subsalicylate. *J Appl Toxicol.* 1998;18:3-13.
158. Kroesen AJ, John M, Schonfelder G, et al. A possible role of inducible nitric oxide synthase (iNOS) in the pathogenesis of primary pouchitis after ileo-pouch anal anastomosis (IPAA). *Gastroenterology.* 1997;112:A1105.
159. Patel RT, Bain I, Youngs D, et al. Cytokine production in pouchitis is similar to that in ulcerative colitis. *Dis Colon Rectum.* 1995;38:831-837.
160. Boerr LA, Sambuelli AM, Filinger E, et al. Increased mucosal levels of leukotriene B4 in pouchitis: evidence for a persistent inflammatory state. *Eur J Gastroenterol Hepatol.* 1996;8:57-61.
161. Gertner DJ, Rampton DS, Madden MV, et al. Increased leukotriene B4 release from ileal pouch mucosa in ulcerative colitis compared with familial adenomatous polyposis. *Gut.* 1994;35:1429-1432.
162. Bulois P, Tremaine WJ, Maunoury V, et al. Pouchitis is associated with mucosal imbalance between interleukin-8 and interleukin-10. *Inflamm Bowel Dis.* 2000;6:157-164.
163. Helwig U, Gionchetti P, Rizzello F, et al. CXC and CC chemokine expression in inflamed and noninflamed pelvic ileal pouch tissue. *Int J Colorectal Dis.* 2004;19:165-170.
164. Campbell AP, Smithson J, Lewis C, et al. Altered expression of TGF alpha and TGF beta 1 in the mucosa of the functioning pelvic ileal pouch. *J Pathol.* 1996;180:407-414.
165. Boerr L, Sambuelli A, Sugay E, et al. Serum TGF-beta 1 and interferon-gamma levels in ileal-pouch anal anastomosis in ulcerative colitis. *Gastroenterology.* 1998;114:A936.
166. Collins SM. Neural influences in intestinal inflammation. In: Caprilli R, ed. *Inflammatory Bowel Disease: Trigger Factors and Trends in Therapy.* Stuttgart, Germany: F.K. Schattauer; 1997:35-43.
167. O'Connor TM, O'Connell J, O'Brien DI, et al. The role of substance P in inflammatory disease. *J Cell Physiol.* 2004;201:167-180.
168. Gross KJ, Pothoulakis C. Role of neuropeptides in inflammatory bowel disease. *Inflamm Bowel Dis.* 2007;13:918-932.
169. Bernstein CN, Robert ME, Eysselein VE. Rectal substance P concentrations are increased in ulcerative colitis but not in Crohn's disease. *Am J Gastroenterol.* 1993;88:908-913.
170. Goode T, O'Connell J, Anton P, et al. Neurokinin-1 receptor expression in inflammatory bowel disease: molecular quantitation and localisation. *Gut.* 2000;47:387-396.

171. Keranen U, Kiviluoto T, Jarvinen H, et al. Changes in substance P-immunoreactive innervation of human colon associated with ulcerative colitis. *Dig Dis Sci.* 1995;40:2250-2258.
172. Keranen U, Jarvinen H, Kiviluoto T, et al. Substance P- and vasoactive intestinal polypeptide-immunoreactive innervation in normal and inflamed pouches after restorative proctocolectomy for ulcerative colitis. *Dig Dis Sci.* 1996;41:1658-1664.
173. Keranen U, Jarvinen H, Karkkainen P, et al. Substance P–an underlying factor for pouchitis: prospective study of substance P- and vasoactive intestinal polypeptide-immunoreactive innervation and mast cells. *Dig Dis Sci.* 1996;41:1665-1671.
174. Stucchi AF, Shebani KO, Leeman SE, et al. A neurokinin 1 receptor antagonist reduces an ongoing ileal pouch inflammation and the response to a subsequent inflammatory stimulus. *Am J Physiol Gastrointest Liver Physiol.* 2003;285:G1259-G1267.
175. Madden MV, Farthing MJ, Nicholls RJ. Inflammation in ileal reservoirs: "pouchitis." *Gut.* 1990;31:247-249.
176. Brunel M, Penna C, Tiret E, et al. Restorative proctocolectomy for distal ulcerative colitis. *Gut.* 1999;45:542-545.
177. de Silva HJ, Jones M, Prince C, et al. Lymphocyte and macrophage subpopulations in pelvic ileal pouches. *Gut.* 1991;32:1160-1165.
178. Mignon M, Stettler C, Phillips SF. Pouchitis–a poorly understood entity. *Dis Colon Rectum.* 1995;38:100-103.
179. Chaussade S, Denizot Y, Valleur P, et al. Presence of PAF-acether in stool of patients with pouch ileoanal anastomosis and pouchitis. *Gastroenterology.* 1991;100:1509-1514.
180. Hale W, Floch M, Burakoff R, et al. Indeterminate colitis. *J Clin Gastroenterol.* 2004;38:S57.
181. Subramani K, Harpaz N, Bilotta J, et al. Refractory pouchitis: Does it reflect underlying Crohn's disease? *Gut.* 1993;34:1539-1542.
182. Shen B, Fazio VW, Remzi FH, et al. Risk factors for clinical phenotypes of Crohn's disease of the ileal pouch. *Am J Gastroenterol.* 2006;101:2760-2768.
183. Shen B, Fazio VW, Remzi FH, et al. Clinical features and quality of life in patients with different phenotypes of Crohn's disease of the ileal pouch. *Dis Colon Rectum.* 2007.
184. Pardi DS, Sandborn WJ. Systematic review: the management of pouchitis. *Aliment Pharmacol Ther.* 2006;23:1087-1096.
185. Hurst RD, Molinari M, Chung TP, et al. Prospective study of the incidence, timing and treatment of pouchitis in 104 consecutive patients after restorative proctocolectomy. *Arch Surg.* 1996;131:497-500; discussion 501-492.
186. Miner P, Wedel M, Bane B, et al. An enema formulation of alicaforsen, an antisense inhibitor of intercellular adhesion molecule-1, in the treatment of chronic, unremitting pouchitis. *Aliment Pharmacol Ther.* 2004;19:281-286.
187. Mimura T, Rizzello F, Helwig U, et al. Once daily high dose probiotic therapy (VSL#3) for maintaining remission in recurrent or refractory pouchitis. *Gut.* 2004;53:108-114.
188. McLeod RS, Taylor DW, Cohen Z, et al. Single-patient randomised clinical trial. Use in determining optimum treatment for patient with inflammation of Kock continent ileostomy reservoir. *Lancet.* 1986;1:726-728.
189. Madden MV, McIntyre AS, Nicholls RJ. Double-blind crossover trial of metronidazole versus placebo in chronic unremitting pouchitis. *Dig Dis Sci.* 1994;39:1193-1196.
190. Fischer JE, Nussbaum MS, Martin LW, et al. The pull-through procedure: technical factors in influencing outcome, with emphasis on pouchitis. *Surgery.* 1993;114:828-834; discussion 834-835.
191. Shen B, Achkar JP, Lashner BA, et al. A randomized clinical trial of ciprofloxacin and metronidazole to treat acute pouchitis. *Inflamm Bowel Dis.* 2001;7:301-305.
192. Nygaard K, Bergan T, Bjorneklett A, et al. Topical metronidazole treatment in pouchitis. *Scand J Gastroenterol.* 1994;29:462-467.
193. Sambuelli A, Boerr L, Negreira S, et al. Budesonide enema in pouchitis–a double-blind, double-dummy, controlled trial. *Aliment Pharmacol Ther.* 2002;16:27-34.
194. Shen B, Fazio VW, Remzi FH, et al. Comprehensive evaluation of inflammatory and noninflammatory sequelae of ileal pouch-anal anastomoses. *Am J Gastroenterol.* 2005;100:93-101.
195. Mowschenson PM, Critchlow JF, Peppercorn MA. Ileoanal pouch operation: Long-term outcome with or without diverting ileostomy. *Arch Surg.* 2000;135:463-465.
196. Shen B. Diagnosis and treatment of patients with pouchitis. *Drugs.* 2003;63:453-461.
197. Gionchetti P, Rizzello F, Venturi A, et al. Review–antibiotic treatment in inflammatory bowel disease: rifaximin, a new possible approach. *Eur Rev Med Pharmacol Sci.* 1999;3:27-30.
198. Abdelrazeq AS, Kelly SM, Lund JN, et al. Rifaximin-ciprofloxacin combination therapy is effective in chronic active refractory pouchitis. *Colorectal Dis.* 2005;7:182-186.
199. Isaacs KL, Sandler RS, Abreu M, et al. Rifaximin for the treatment of active pouchitis: a randomized, double-blind, placebo-controlled pilot study. *Inflamm Bowel Dis.* 2007.
200. Mimura T, Rizzello F, Helwig U, et al. Four-week open-label trial of metronidazole and ciprofloxacin for the treatment of recurrent or refractory pouchitis. *Aliment Pharmacol Ther.* 2002;16:909-917.
201. Shen B, Fazio VW, Remzi FH, et al. Combined ciprofloxacin and tinidazole therapy in the treatment of chronic refractory pouchitis. *Dis Colon Rectum.* 2007;50:498-508.
202. Tremaine WJ, Sandborn WJ, Wolff BG, et al. Bismuth carbomer foam enemas for active chronic pouchitis: a randomized, double-blind, placebo-controlled trial. *Aliment Pharmacol Ther.* 1997;11:1041-1046.
203. Gionchetti P, Rizzello F, Poggioli G, et al. Oral budesonide in the treatment of chronic refractory pouchitis. *Aliment Pharmacol Ther.* 2007;25:1231-1236.
204. Miglioli M, Barbara L, Di Febo G, et al. Topical administration of 5-aminosalicylic acid: a therapeutic proposal for the treatment of pouchitis. *N Engl J Med.* 1989;320:257.
205. Gionchetti P, Rizzello F, Venturi A, et al. Maintenance treatment of chronic pouchitis: a randomized placebo-controlled, double-blind trial with a new probiotic preparation. *Gastroenterology.* 1998;114:A985.
206. Gosselink MP, Schouten WR, van Lieshout LM, et al. Delay of the first onset of pouchitis by oral intake of the probiotic strain *Lactobacillus rhamnosus* GG. *Dis Colon Rectum.* 2004;47:876-884.
207. Sartor RB. Probiotics in chronic pouchitis: restoring luminal microbial balance. *Gastroenterology.* 2000;119:584-587.
208. Shen B, Shermock KM, Fazio VW, et al. A cost-effectiveness analysis of diagnostic strategies for symptomatic patients with ileal pouch-anal anastomosis. *Am J Gastroenterol.* 2003;98:2460-2467.
209. Thompson-Fawcett MW, Mortensen NJ, Warren BF. "Cuffitis" and inflammatory changes in the columnar cuff, anal transitional zone, and ileal reservoir after stapled pouch-anal anastomosis. *Dis Colon Rectum.* 1999;42:348-355.
210. Shen B, Lashner BA, Bennett AE, et al. Treatment of rectal cuff inflammation (cuffitis) in patients with ulcerative colitis following restorative proctocolectomy and ileal pouch-anal anastomosis. *Am J Gastroenterol.* 2004;99:1527-1531.
211. Mann SD, Pitt J, Springall RG, et al. *Clostridium difficile* infection–An unusual cause of refractory pouchitis: report of a case. *Dis Colon Rectum.* 2003;46:267-270.
212. Fruin AB, Stucchi AF, Becker JM. The incidence and treatment of fungal pouchitis following ileal pouch-anal anastomosis. *Dis Colon Recum.* 2002;45:A50.

213. Pfau PR, Lichtenstein GR. Cytomegalovirus infection as a cause of ileoanal pouchitis. *Dis Colon Rectum.* 2000;43:113-114.
214. Moonka D, Furth EE, MacDermott RP, et al. Pouchitis associated with primary cytomegalovirus infection. *Am J Gastroenterol.* 1998;93:264-266.
215. Munoz-Juarez M, Pemberton JH, Sandborn WJ, et al. Misdiagnosis of specific cytomegalovirus infection of the ileoanal pouch as refractory idiopathic chronic pouchitis: Report of two cases. *Dis Colon Rectum.* 1999;42:117-120.
216. Berrebi W, Chaussade S, Bruhl AL, et al. Treatment of Crohn's disease recurrence after ileoanal anastomosis by azathioprine. *Dig Dis Sci.* 1993;38:1558-1560.
217. Ricart E, Panaccione R, Loftus EV, et al. Successful management of Crohn's disease of the ileoanal pouch with infliximab. *Gastroenterology.* 1999;117:429-432.
218. Colombel JF, Ricart E, Loftus EV Jr, et al. Management of Crohn's disease of the ileoanal pouch with infliximab. *Am J Gastroenterol.* 2003;98:2239-2244.
219. Viscido A, Caprilli R. Development of fistulae in ileo-anal pouch does not necessarily indicate Crohn's disease. *Am J Gastroenterol.* 2004;99:2066-2067; author reply 2067.
220. Viscido A, Kohn A, Papi C, et al. Management of refractory fistulizing pouchitis with infliximab. *Eur Rev Med Pharmacol Sci.* 2004;8:239-246.
221. Parsi MA, Shen B, Achkar JP, et al. Fecal lactoferrin for diagnosis of symptomatic patients with ileal pouch-anal anastomosis. *Gastroenterology.* 2004;126:1280-1286.
222. Phillips MI. Antisense therapeutics: a promise waiting to be fulfilled. *Methods Mol Med.* 2004;106:3-10.
223. Thirlby RC, Kelly R. Pectin and methyl cellulose do not affect intestinal function in patients after ileal pouch-anal anastomosis. *Am J Gastroenterol.* 1997;92:99-102.
224. Ng SC, Arebi N, Kamm MA. Medium-term results of oral tacrolimus treatment in refractory inflammatory bowel disease. *Inflamm Bowel Dis.* 2007;13:129-134.
225. Crema MD, Richarme D, Azizi L, et al. Pouchography, CT, and MRI features of ileal J pouch-anal anastomosis. *AJR Am J Roentgenol.* 2006;187:W594-603.
226. Nadgir RN, Soto JA, Dendrinos K, et al. MRI of complicated pouchitis. *Am J Roentgenol.* 2006;187:W386-391.
227. Calabrese C, Fabbri A, Gionchetti P, et al. Controlled study using wireless capsule endoscopy for the evaluation of the small intestine in chronic refractory pouchitis. *Aliment Pharmacol Ther.* 2007;25:1311-1316.
228. Baixauli J, Delaney CP, Wu JS, et al. Functional outcome and quality of life after repeat ileal pouch-anal anastomosis for complications of ileoanal surgery. *Dis Colon Rectum.* 2004;47:2-11.
229. Dehni N, Remacle G, Dozois RR, et al. Salvage reoperation for complications after ileal pouch-anal anastomosis. *Br J Surg.* 2005;92:748-753.
230. Borjesson L, Oresland T, Hulten L. The failed pelvic pouch: Conversion to a continent ileostomy. *Tech Coloproctol.* 2004;8:102-105.
231. Dean PA, Dozios RR. Surgical options-ileoanal pouch. In: Allan RN, et al, eds. *Inflammatory Bowel Diseases,* 3rd ed. New York: Churchill Livingstone; 1997:761-772.
232. Kennedy ED, Rothwell DM, Cohen Z, et al. Increased experience and surgical technique lead to improved outcome after ileal pouch-anal anastomosis: a population-based study. *Dis Colon Rectum.* 2006;49:958-965.
233. Robb B, Pritts T, Gang G, et al. Quality of life in patients undergoing ileal pouch-anal anastomosis at the University of Cincinnati. *Am J Surg.* 2002;183:353-360.
234. Hait E, Rufo PA. Why good pouches go bad. *Inflamm Bowel Dis.* 2007;13:116-117.
235. Shen B, Fazio VW, Remzi FH, et al. Risk factors for diseases of ileal pouch-anal anastomosis after restorative proctocolectomy for ulcerative colitis. *Clin Gastroenterol Hepatol.* 2006;4:81-89; quiz 82-83.

37

Dietary Manipulations

Oral and Enteral Nutritional Therapy for Ulcerative Colitis

Traci M. Temmen, MD and John L. Rombeau, MD

Malnutrition occurs frequently in patients with inflammatory bowel disease (IBD). Up to 85% of patients hospitalized with exacerbations of IBD have protein-energy malnutrition, while 25% to 50% of hospitalized patients with ulcerative colitis (UC) have hypoalbuminemia.[1] Additionally, 18% to 62% UC patients have experienced significant weight loss.[2] Several nutrient deficiencies are associated with adverse clinical outcomes, thus, extensive investigations are ongoing to identify, prevent, and correct these nutrient deficits.[3] In hospitalized patients, the decision as to whether to feed orally, enterally, or intravenously must often be made. This decision is often based on clinical judgment, especially in the absence of controlled clinical trials. This chapter discusses oral and enteral nutrition and their adjuvant role in the treatment of UC. Dietary supplements, such as fish oil, short-chain fatty acids, and other investigational additives, will also be reviewed. Crohn's disease and the specifics of parenteral nutrition are discussed in sections IV and V and in Chapter 38.

BACKGROUND

Pathogenesis of Malnutrition

In contrast to patients with CD who usually develop malnutrition insidiously, an acute exacerbation of UC often leads to severe cachexia and profound nutrient deficiencies. Multiple factors contribute to malnutrition in these patients, as shown in Table 37-1.

Decreased nutrient intake is a frequent cause of malnutrition in patients with UC. Patients may be anorexic due to the high levels of cytokines, such as IL-1 and TNFα.[1] Sitophobia may be due to the patient's association of food intake with diarrhea and abdominal pain. Drug side effects and altered taste sensation secondary to specific mineral deficiencies (eg, zinc, copper, and nickel) may also contribute to decreased oral intake.

Inadequate intestinal absorption of nutrients often compounds a decreased oral intake. Malabsorption occurs less commonly in patients with UC than in those with CD, due to a lack of inflammation of the small bowel. However, concomitant ileal resections can result in decreased vitamin B12 and bile salt absorption with ileocecal valve resection causing bacterial overgrowth, which may also lead to intestinal nutrient malabsorption.[1]

Increased nutrient losses via protein-losing enteropathies (eg, exudative losses of protein occurring in areas of inflamed and ulcerated intestinal mucosa) and bleeding, combined with increased nutritional requirements secondary to a hypercatabolic state (eg, fever, sepsis) also deplete these patients of necessary nutrients.

Consequences of Malnutrition

The consequences of protein-energy malnutrition in patients with UC are numerous (Table 37-2). Decreased immunocompetency secondary to malnutrition may be important in controlling disease activity.[2] Finally, decreased tolerance to blood loss (a common symptom of UC exacerbations) and decreased functioning of the gastrointestinal tract have also been linked to protein-energy malnutrition.[2]

Lichtenstein GR, ed.
Ulcerative Colitis: The Complete Guide to Medical Management (pp 433-444)

TABLE 37-1

CAUSES OF MALNUTRITION IN PATIENTS WITH ULCERATIVE COLITIS

Decreased nutrient intake
Anorexia, vomiting
Altered taste
Intake-associated pain or discomfort
Intestinal obstruction
Iatrogenic dietary restrictions
Malabsorption
Altered mucosal permeability/inflammation
Diminished absorptive surface
Bacterial overgrowth and bile salt deconjugation
Excessive losses
Protein-losing enteropathy
Bleeding
Increased requirements/hypercatabolic states
Drugs
Corticosteroids
Sulfasalazine
Cholestyramine

TABLE 37-2

CONSEQUENCES OF PROTEIN-ENERGY MALNUTRITION IN ULCERATIVE COLITIS

Primarily related to protein-energy malnutrition
Immunosuppression
Poor wound healing
Intestinal villous atrophy/malabsorption self-perpetuation
Derangement of gut mucosal barrier
Growth failure/delayed sexual maturation
Deficient finding of drugs to plasma proteins
Increased surgical risk
Increased mortality
Modulation of IBD course
Impaired defense against free-radical damage
Changes in poly-unsaturated fatty acid and eicosanoid synthesis
Increased mucosal dysplasia

A detailed discussion of the specific nutrient deficits in IBD is beyond the scope of this chapter; however, the reported prevalence of these deficits is shown in Table 37-3.

Diagnosis of Nutrient Deficiencies

The subjective global assessment (SGA) of nutritional status is the preferred method of diagnosing malnutrition. It includes 3 classifications: generally well-nourished, moderately malnourished, or severely malnourished (Table 37-4). The SGA is based upon nutritionally relevant features of the medical history and physical examination and emphasizes such criteria as body weight loss, dietary intake, gastrointestinal symptoms, functional capacity, disease type, and levels of catabolism. Loss of subcutaneous fat, muscle wasting, dependent edema, and ascites are also included in the SGA. The SGA is indeed subjective, and as such, the clinician's evaluation of the complete clinical picture and assessment of each patient determines its validity and effectiveness.

INDICATIONS FOR NUTRITIONAL SUPPORT IN ULCERATIVE COLITIS

Indications for supplemental nutritional support in patients with UC include moderate to severe protein-energy malnutrition and perioperative conditions. Moderate to severe protein-energy malnutrition is often defined clinically as serum albumin levels less than 3.3 g/dL in the euvolemic state and/or nonvolitional loss of greater than 15% of usual body weight. Perioperative conditions include the preoperative colectomy patient with moderate to severe protein-energy malnutrition and/or the postcolectomy patient who is unable to tolerate adequate oral intake by postoperative day 7.

To our knowledge, no study has definitively outlined the role of enteral feedings in perioperative patients with UC; however, 2 randomized clinical trials have investigated the role of parenteral nutrition alone and parenteral/enteral nutrition in perioperative management of varied surgical patients, including UC, with severe malnutrition. Perioperative parenteral nutrition significantly decreased noninfectious complications in severely malnourished patients in the Veterans Affairs Total

TABLE 37-3

REPORTED PREVALENCE OF NUTRITIONAL DEFICIENCIES IN ULCERATIVE COLITIS

Weight loss	18% to 62%
Hypoalbuminemia	25% to 50%
Intestinal protein loss	ND
Negative nitrogen balance	ND
Anemia	66%
Iron deficiency	81%
Vitamin B12 deficiency	5%
Folic acid deficiency	30% to 40%
Calcium deficiency	ND
Magnesium deficiency	ND
Potassium deficiency	ND
Vitamin A deficiency	NR
Vitamin C deficiency	NR
Vitamin D deficiency	35%
Vitamin K deficiency	NR
Zinc deficiency	ND
Copper deficiency	NR

ND = reported but incidence not described, NR = not reported.

Adapted from Rombeau JL, Afonso JJ. Clinical and scientific basis for nutritional support of patients with inflammatory bowel disease. In: MacDermott RP, Stenson WF, eds. *Inflammatory Bowel Disease*. New York, NY: Elsevier Science Publishing Company, Inc; 1992:527.

Parenteral Nutrition Cooperative Study Group.[4] Mildly malnourished patients placed on parenteral nutrition, however, exhibited a much higher incidence of infectious complications that could not be explained by line sepsis alone. In another study, severely malnourished patients undergoing surgery for either colonic or gastric carcinoma were found to have an increase in septic complications when compared to adequately nourished patients. Supplementing these patients with either parenteral or enteral nutrition eliminated the risk of septic complications.[5] While promising and intuitively sound, it must be noted that neither study was performed primarily on patients with UC, and each study was limited to severely malnourished individuals.

ENTERAL NUTRITION

Enteral Diets

Enteral nutrition support is the provision of nutrients via the gastrointestinal tract, either orally or by tube, in amounts to maintain or replete nutritional reserves of the patients.[6]

Despite their frequent use, the mechanism of actions of enteral diets on the underlying disease process is still unclear. Several hypotheses have been proposed, but it is not known whether enteral nutrition has a direct effect on the gut or if the efficacy of enteral nutrition is due to indirect effects such as improvement in nutritional and immune status.[7]

Indications

Enteral nutrition support via tube feeding should be considered for malnourished patients who are unable to ingest adequate amounts of nutrients and who have an adequately functioning gastrointestinal tract, absence of nausea, vomiting, obstruction, abdominal distension, and severe diarrhea. The advantages of enteral feeding versus parenteral feeding may include a lower cost to the patient, avoidance of complications associated with parenteral feedings (eg, sepsis, pneumothorax, catheter embolism), maintenance of gastrointestinal mucosal integrity, and prevention of bacterial translocation by way of its trophic action intestinal mucosa (which in itself may play a role in the prevention of bacteremia and sepsis).[7] A common clinical dictum is, "When the gut works, use it." Despite initial concerns that enteral feeding would worsen diarrhea, it is usually tolerated even in moderate attacks of UC. In a small prospective, uncontrolled study of 9 patients hospitalized with severe, nonspecific colitis treated with enteral feedings and steroids for 10 days, there was a significant reduction in daily stool weight and frequency when compared with the pretreatment period.[8] This, combined with the lower cost, equal efficacy, and fewer complications than parenteral nutrition, makes enteral nutrition a suitable type of nutritional support in patients with severe attacks of ulcerative colitis.[9]

In our experience, enteral and parenteral feedings are viewed as complementary, not competitive. Most patients with severe UC receive both types of feedings. During the severe flare of UC, parenteral feeding is prescribed with a gradual increase in enteral/oral intake when the pronounced gastrointestinal symptoms begin to subside.

TABLE 37-4

CLASSIFICATION OF NUTRITIONAL STATUS

Criterion	Well-Nourished	Moderately Malnourished	Severely Malnourished
A. Subjective global assessment			
1. Medical history			
a. Body weight change in the past 6 months	Loss <5%	Loss = 5% to 15%	Loss >15%
b. Dietary intake	Balanced diet that meets requirements	60% to 90% of required	<60% of required
c. GI symptoms (vomiting, diarrhea)	No	Intermittent	Daily for >2 weeks
d. Functional capacity	Full capacity	Reduced	Bedridden
2. Physical examination			
a. Edema (ankle, sacral)	No	+	+
b. Ascites	No	+	+
B. Serum albumin level	>3.3 g/dL	3.0 to 3.3 g/dL	<3.0 g/dL

Adapted from Rombeau JL, Afonso JJ. Clinical and scientific basis for nutritional support of patients with inflammatory bowel disease. In: MacDermott RP, Stenson WF, eds. *Inflammatory Bowel Disease.* New York, NY: Elsevier Science Publishing Company, Inc; 1992:528.

TABLE 37-5

CURRENT ADVANCEMENTS IN THE NUTRITIONAL THERAPY OF ULCERATIVE COLITIS

	Purported Effects
Fish oil	Proven effective as adjuvant treatment of active UC
Short-chain fatty acids	Suggested efficacy of topically administered SCFAs in patients with short active episodes of distal UC
Pre-/Probiotics	Proven to prevent acute pouch-itis and prevent flare-ups of chronic pouchitis
Fiber	Suggested efficacy in patients with active UC

Contraindications

Enteral nutrition should be avoided in patients who do not have an adequately functioning gastrointestinal tract. Such conditions include, but are not limited to, small bowel obstruction (distal to the site of enteral feeding initiation), bowel perforation, mid-jejunal fistulas, short bowel syndrome (ie, less than 100 cm of small bowel), upper gastrointestinal hemorrhage, and toxic megacolon.

Enteral Formula Categories

Polymeric Formulas

Polymeric diets, the most often prescribed formula, consist of starches, protein, long-chain and medium-chain triglycerides, vitamins, minerals, and trace elements and require breakdown in the small bowel to dipeptides and tripeptides, free amino acids, and simple sugars. Polymeric formulas require adequate digestive and absorptive capability and are indicated in patients with normal or near-normal gastrointestinal function. There are 2 basic types of polymeric formulas:

- Synthetic formulas are generally used for standard tube feedings. Caloric content generally ranges from 1.0 kcal/mL to 2.0 kcal/mL. The protein content consists of whole protein, generally casein or soy protein sources, providing 12% to 20% of total energy. The carbohydrate source is generally hydrolyzed cornstarch, maltodextrins, corn syrup solids, and/or sucrose, and it generally provides 40% to 90% of total energy. The fat content ranges from less than 10% to more than 50% of total energy; sources are commonly corn or soybean oil. These formulas usually have a low osmolality (300 to 500 mOsm/kg of water). Because a high incidence of lactase deficiency in illness is presumed, lactose is not present in most synthetic enteral formulas.

- Blenderized formulas are a blenderized mixture of meats, fruits, vegetables, nonfat dry milk solids, and added vitamins and minerals. They are available as lactose-free and lactose-containing formulas. Some have a moderate to high viscosity, therefore requiring administration via a larger-bore feeding tube, as well as moderate osmolality. They are usually less expensive than synthetic polymeric diets and are used extensively in developing countries. As the result of variable methods of preparation and composition, these diets are more prone to contamination with enteric pathogens.

Monomeric/Semi-Elemental

These formulas consist of predigested macronutrients and are much more expensive than polymeric formulations. Protein is present either as free amino acids (monomeric) or as amino acids with dipeptides or tripeptides (oligomeric). Carbohydrate sources consist of oligosaccharides, sucrose, or both. Most monomeric diets have low fat content or a high percentage of medium-chain triglycerides. These formulas are also low-residue, hyperosmolar, and usually lactose-free. These diets are reserved for patients with compromised gastrointestinal function, short bowel syndrome, or intolerance to polymeric diets.[10]

Elemental Diets

There is no uniformly acceptable definition of an elemental diet. A truly "elemental" diet is one consisting only of predigested nutrients such as glucose, L-amino acids, free fatty acids, vitamins, and minerals. However, health-care professionals often use the term elemental when referring to a diet consisting of hydrolyzed protein, reduced pancreatic secretions, low residue, and rapid absorption. An even broader definition is often used in the clinical setting when referring to a range of formulas that provide protein as free amino acids to formulas that provide protein as peptides, such as elemental formulas.[11] Historically, elemental diets have been reserved for use in patients with severe malabsorption secondary to decreased luminal or brush-border hydrolysis or decreased surface area for absorption.

In vitro studies have shown no changes in the IL-1ra:IL-1β ratio (an indicator of anti-inflammatory effect) between ileal or colonic biopsies from patients with CD and UC incubated with enteral formulations using free amino acids, oligopeptides, or whole protein as the nitrogen source.[7] These results agreed with those from clinical studies of elemental, oligopeptide, or polymeric enteral diets, which found no difference between diet efficacy and nitrogen source.

To our knowledge, only one well-controlled study compares elemental diet to polymeric diets in UC. In this double-blind study, 43 patients with IBD (24 with UC and 19 with CD) in a mild to moderate state of disease activity were randomized to receive either an elemental diet or a blenderized polymeric diet for 14 days. A significant decrease ($P<0.05$) in disease activity, primarily due to a decrease in the number of bowel movements, was found in the UC patients regardless of the treatment regimen.[12] The appearance of rectal mucosa on sigmoidoscopy and urinary excretion of ^{51}Cr-EDTA (as an expression of leaky bowel mucosa) was not significantly changed between dietary groups.[12] This study is hampered by a small population size, with 4 of 12 UC patients receiving a polymeric diet and 1 of 12 UC patients receiving an elemental diet withdrawing from the study because of diet unpalatability, leaving only 19 patients in the UC group. Still, based on the results of this study in addition to the opinions of many experienced clinicians, it is concluded that a polymeric diet is as effective as an elemental diet in reducing the clinical symptoms of UC, without affecting the basic inflammatory process.

In summary, because of their increased cost, decreased palatability/patient compliance, and unproven efficacy, elemental diets are seldom indicated for patients with UC.

Enteral Nutrition as Primary Therapy in Ulcerative Colitis

In contrast to CD, there is no conclusive evidence to support the use of enteral nutrition as a primary therapy in UC. This observation is supported by retrospective studies that showed a limited role of nutritional support in reducing the likelihood of surgery, shortening the time to achieve clinical remission, or improving UC patients' natural history.[13] A few reports suggest a 30% disease remission rate in hospitalized patients receiving enteral nutrition as primary therapy for UC. This is slightly lower than the 41% rate reported for TPN. However, all of these preliminary studies are limited by small sample sizes, lack of long-term follow-up, and a disparity in the severity of illnesses in the patients selected.[3]

Enteral Nutrition as Adjuvant Therapy in Ulcerative Colitis

Nutritional support (total enteral nutrition, TEN, or TPN) is recommended as an adjunct to steroid therapy in UC patients who are moderately or severely malnourished.[10] UC patients tend to present acutely while still in an adequate state of nourishment, which can rapidly deteriorate if nutrition sufficient to meet the increased needs of the patient is not provided.

The use of TEN in patients with severe UC was investigated in 2 controlled trials in steroid-treated patients, comparing TPN plus bowel rest to oral diet.[11] TPN plus bowel rest did not improve clinical outcome or reduce the need for surgery. Long-term surgery-related complications were not fully evaluated.

The question of which type of nutrient support is better as adjuvant therapy to steroids in severe UC has been examined in a prospective controlled trial of isocaloric and isonitrogenous TPN vs TEN.[9] Clinical remission was achieved in 54% and 50% of patients in TEN and TPN groups, respectively, with a similar number of patients requiring surgery. However, postoperative infection and nutritional support-related complications were significantly more frequent in the TPN group than in the TEN patients. Nutritional assessment showed a greater increase in serum albumin levels in the TEN group than in the TPN group. These results suggest that TEN should be the preferred modality of artificial nutrition in severe UC, unless the previously-mentioned contraindications for enteral feeding are present.

However, is a conventional oral diet nutritionally efficacious in patients with severe UC? One trial comparing TPN vs hospital diet measured total-body nitrogen before and after treatment in a subset of matched patients in each group.[14] A significant decrease in total-body nitrogen was found in patients receiving an oral diet, but not in those receiving TPN. Alternatively, data from retrospective, nonrandomized studies suggest that TEN, but not hospital diet, is able to prevent nutritional derangements in patients with acute attacks of UC.[11] Moreover, TEN is an easy way to achieve an adequate nutrient intake in these patients, who often must be encouraged to eat. Randomized clinical trials comparing TEN versus oral diet are needed to answer this query.[11]

Patients presenting with severe UC often have a high rate of early surgery.[15] Recognition of malnutrition-related complications and the reduced morbidity associated with administration of TPN in the perioperative period has led to increased use of enteral nutritional support in these patients. The American Society for Parenteral and Enteral Nutrition (ASPEN) guidelines recommend that nutritional support be given if 7 to 10 days of postoperative starvation is expected in a previously healthy patient, or 5 to 7 days in a previously malnourished patient, thus including many patients with active UC.

In summary, moderately or severely malnourished patients or those patients likely to undergo surgery and suffering from an acute attack of UC benefit from enteral nutrition as an adjuvant therapy to steroid and other medical treatments. The effect of an isocaloric, isonitrogenous oral diet compared to an enteral diet on clinical outcome in patients with UC is yet to be examined in well-controlled trials (Figure 37-1).

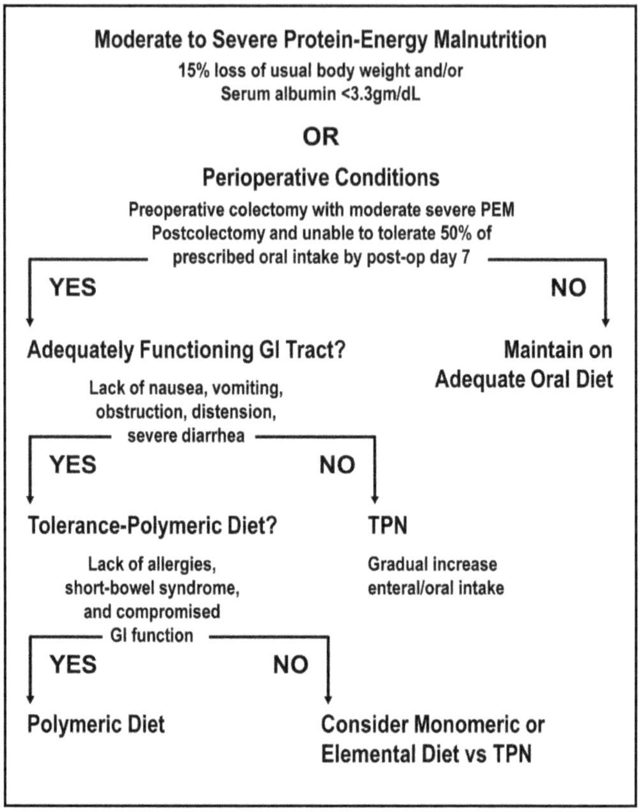

FIGURE 37-1. Decision-making algorithm for nutritional support of patients with ulcerative colitis.

Administration

Continuous Feeding/Delivery

Continuous feedings require that the enteral formula be administered at a controlled rate using a pump over a prescribed length of time. Continuous feedings are indicated for selected critically ill patients, individuals unable to tolerate high-volume feedings, those with malabsorption, or patients at increased risk for aspiration. Feedings may be initiated at full strength in the stomach or at an isotonic strength in the small bowel, at a rate of 10 to 50 mL/hr, and gradually increased as tolerated in increments of 10 to 25 mL/hr to meet the prescribed goal. Strength and volume of feedings should not be increased simultaneously.

Transitional Feedings, Enteral to Oral

Oral intake should begin with liquids and advance to appropriate foods as tolerated depending on the swallowing function of the patient. When oral intake reaches 500 kcal or more, the dosage of tube feedings may be proportionately tapered. The transition from a continuous tube feeding to night tube feeding only or discontinuing tube feeding 1 to 2 hours before meals will often stimulate appetite and shorten the time to adequate oral intake. When oral intake consistently meets or exceeds 60% of the patient's energy requirements and 100% of fluid requirements, discontinuation of tube feedings should be considered.[10]

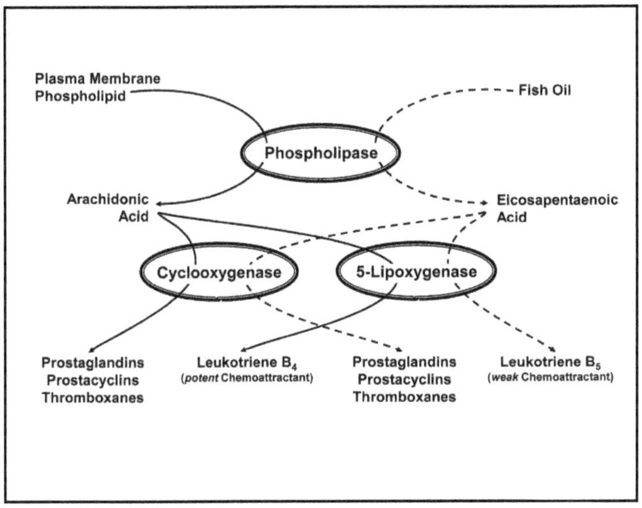

FIGURE 37-2. Phospholipase releases arachidonic acid from the cell membrane. It is converted to prostaglandins, prostacyclins, and thromboxanes by the cyclooxygenase pathway and to leukotriene B_4 by the 5-lipoxygenase pathway. When ingested in large quantities, fish oil is incorporated into the cell membrane of all cells, and it is converted to eicosapentaenoic acid by phospholipase. Eicosapentaenoic acid competes with arachidonic acid at the cyclooxygenase and lipoxygenase level, resulting in decreased leukotriene B_4 (a potent chemoattractant) synthesis and increased leukotriene B_5 (a weak chemoattractant) synthesis. Fish oil supplementation also modulates prostaglandin, prostacyclin, and thromboxane metabolism (not shown), and in high doses has antithrombotic and anti-inflammatory properties.[16] Solid lines indicate eicosanoid synthesis from plasma membrane phospholipid; dashed lines indicate eicosanoid synthesis from fish oil.

FISH OIL

The understanding of eicosanoids and their derivatives in the pathogenesis of inflammation has stimulated interest in nutritionally altering the inflammatory response by modifying tissue fatty acid and phospholipid contents.[16]

The eicosanoid, leukotriene B_4 (LTB_4), is the main neutrophil chemotactant agent in UC. In patients with UC, concentrations of LTB_4 are increased in rectal dialysates and these levels correlate with disease activity.[1] Fish oil, an omega-3 polyunsaturated fatty acid (PUFA), competes with arachidonic acid, an omega-6 PUFA (which accounts for the majority of PUFAs in the Western diet), for prostaglandin and leukotriene synthesis at the cyclooxygenase and lipoxygenase level.[16] Ingestion of fish or fish oil leads to competitive inhibition in the production of LTB_4 with an increase in the less potent proinflammatory leukotriene B_5 (Figure 37-2).[16] Current research is directed at the use of fish oil supplementation in the treatment of UC.

Fish Oil as Primary Therapy in Ulcerative Colitis

To our knowledge, there are no conclusive studies to support the sole use of fish oil as primary therapy for acute UC. Moreover, the current availability of outstanding medications makes it highly unlikely that fish oil would ever be investigated as primary therapy.

Fish Oil as Adjuvant Therapy in Ulcerative Colitis

The use of fish oil as adjuvant therapy in UC is gaining acceptance. In a large prospective, randomized controlled trial, 87 patients with diagnosed UC (restricted to patients who had 2 or more relapses in the previous 3 years) received either 20 mL of fish oil (4.5 g eicosapentaenoic acid) or olive oil placebo, along with conventional treatment with sulfasalazine or mesalazine, and corticosteroids, daily for 1 year.[17] The main endpoint was the relapse rate for all patients achieving stable remission. Remission was defined as patients having no symptoms of active disease, eg, rectal bleeding, loose stools, bowel frequency, or other symptoms; not taking steroids; and having uninflamed rectal mucosa (grade 0 or 1) at sigmoidoscopy after 4 or more weeks. Patients in relapse were defined as those with active symptoms and/or inflamed rectal mucosa (sigmoidoscopic grade 2 or 3). The relapse rate of the subgroup of patients in remission entering the trial was also measured.

This study found that 25% of patients taking fish oil relapsed by 6 months, compared with 40% for olive oil, but at 1 year, the proportions were 42% for fish oil and 48% (NS) for olive oil, respectively. Similarly, patients in remission treated with fish oil tended to spend more time in remission, but these differences were not significant. The median corticosteroid dosage at entry for patients in relapse was 10 mg for both fish oil and olive oil groups. Patients on fish oil, however, had reduced corticosteroid requirements at 1 (5 mg) and 2 months (nil), compared with the olive oil group (8 mg at 1 month and 5 mg at 2 months, $P=0.01$, at both 1 and 2 months).[17]

In another randomized, double-blind, placebo-controlled, crossover trial, 18 patients with active UC were randomized to receive daily treatment with fish oil (3.24 g eicosapentaenoic acid capsules) or vegetable oil (identical, isocaloric capsules) for 4-month treatment periods separated by a 1-month washout, in addition to conventional treatment with prednisone and sulfasalazine. The mean dose of prednisone from the start of the fish oil period to the end of the fish oil period decreased by 53%. As described earlier, this study also reports a significant decrease (with an average change of 43.3 pg/mL) in rectal dialysate levels of LTB_4, improvement in histologic findings (including loss of colonocyte polarity, mucin content of surface epithelium, denudation or erosion, superficial inflammatory cell infiltrate, deep inflammatory cell infiltrate, architectural distortion, and fibrosis), and weight gain in patients treated with fish oil over the control group.[18] The findings of histologic improvement in patients with active UC receiving fish oil vs a control oil were supported in later double-blind studies.[19,20]

In summary, the use of fish oil as adjuvant treatment in active UC reduces corticosteroid requirements, promotes weight gain, decreases rectal dialysate levels of LTB_4, and improves the histologic appearance of rectal mucosal biopsies. However, because of its poor taste, need for multiple daily doses, and relatively recent investigation, fish oil has not yet been widely accepted. Fish oil as adjuvant therapy for patients in remission is yet to be proven.

SHORT-CHAIN FATTY ACIDS

SCFAs, often referred to as "volatile acids," are the 2, 3, and 4 carbon saturated monocarboxylic acids (ie, acetic, propionic, and n-butyric acids) produced in the human colon by bacterial enzymatic breakdown of dietary fiber, undigested starch, and non-absorbed simple carbohydrates. They provide an important energy source for the colon, with butyrate being the preferred energy source, and spare the oxidation of the alternative substrates, glucose and glutamine.[21] SCFA deficiency is associated with colitis in animals and humans, and the mucosal metabolism of these compounds is decreased in UC.[22] SCFAs are metabolized both locally and systemically in the colon. Luminal SCFA stimulates epithelial absorption of sodium (which helps control intracellular pH via a Na^+/H^+ exchanger) and aids in mucosal growth and epithelial proliferation.[21]

During the past decade, many studies have investigated the structural and physiologic effects of SCFA on the colon in various animal species. More recently, important physiologic studies haven been performed in humans. The exogenous administration of SCFA to humans, particularly for those with proctosigmoiditis, has also been investigated.

Effects of SCFAs on NF-κB Activity

NF-κB is a widely expressed transcription factor that plays a central role in regulating the expression of numerous cytokines and cell adhesion molecules involved in immune and inflammatory responses. Due to the possibility of butyrate deficiency in IBD, the effect of butyrate on NF-κB activity in the human HT-29 colonic cell line was investigated.[23] The exposure of HT-29 cells to butyrate eliminated their constitutive NF-κB, p50 dimer activity. This inhibition corresponded with a reduction in p50 dimer activity. Butyrate also suppressed the activation of NF-κB by TNFα and phorbol ester more than 10-fold. These findings suggest that the reduction of colonic inflammation by butyrate may result in part from its influence on NF-κB activation. Moreover, the activity of butyrate apparently involves its ability to inhibit deacetylases.

Effect of SCFAs in Patients W ith Ulcerative Colitis

Clinical trials suggest that topically administered butyrate reduces the severity of inflammation in patients with UC. The potential effects of NF-κB activation in lamina propria macrophages were investigated.[24] Eleven patients with distal UC were treated for up to 8 weeks with butyrate at 100 mM (n = 6) or placebo (n = 5) enemas. At entry and after 4 and 8 weeks, clinical status was noted, and endoscopic and histologic grading of inflammation was performed respectively. Double-staining with antibodies against NF-κB (p65) and CD68 was used to detect NF-κB and macrophages respectively. In control patients, nuclear translocation of NF-κB was detectable in virtually all macrophages. Butyrate treatment for 4 and 8 weeks produced a significant reduction in the number of macrophages being positive for nuclear translocated NF-κB. These findings correlated with a significant decrease in the DAI. It was concluded that the decrease in DAI and mucosal inflammation in butyrate-treated patients is associated with a reduction of NF-κB translocation in lamina propria macrophages. Because the inflammatory process is usually sustained by macrophage-derived cytokines, the anti-inflammatory effects of butyrate may be partly mediated by an inhibition of NF-κB activation in these macrophages.[24]

In a randomized, placebo-controlled trial performed on patients with left-sided UC, 91 patients were treated with SCFA enemas (consisting of sodium acetate, propionate, and butyrate) or placebo enemas (NaCl) upon rising and at bedtime for 6 weeks while oral medication was maintained.[22] Endpoints were the DAI and histological improvements. Although the SCFA-treated patients improved more in each measurement and the decrease in the DAI was almost twice that for placebo, none of the differences in the pre- to post-treatment changes between the groups were statistically significant. While the mean total histology score for the SCFA-treated patients improved slightly during the trial, that for the placebo group worsened; and neither trend was statistically significant. To detect whether baseline characteristic influenced outcome, the relation between a short duration of current colitis attack (≤6 months), baseline disease activity, and gender as compared to treatment response was evaluated. Only short duration of current colitis attack seemed to influence treatment outcome significantly. In conclusion, although SCFA enemas were not of therapeutic value in this controlled trial, the results suggest efficacy in subsets of patients with distal UC, including those with short active episodes.[22]

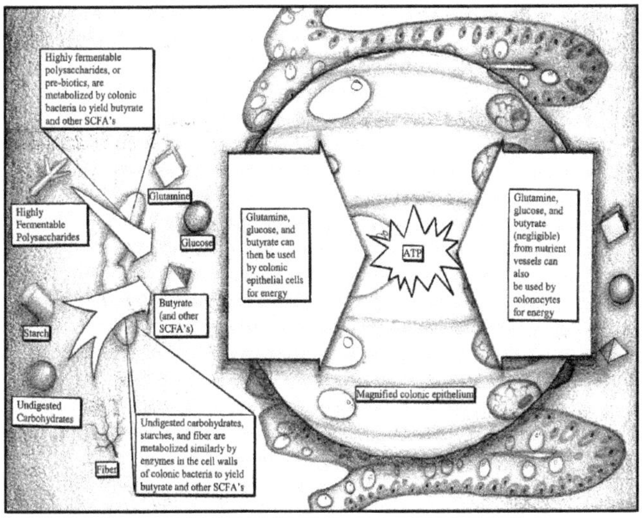

FIGURE 37-3A. Energy metabolism by colonic epithelium. SCFAs, with butyrate as the preferred energy source, are produced in the human colon by bacterial cell wall enzymatic breakdown of dietary fiber, undigested starch, and nonabsorbed simple carbohydrates. SCFAs are also produced in the human colon via colonic bacterial fermentation of prebiotics, undigested, highly-fermentable polysaccharides. Luminal glutamine and glucose are a minor alternative energy source for colonic epithelial cells (left). Glutamine, glucose, and negligible amounts of butyrate circulating in colonic nutrient vessels are an additional source of energy for colonic epithelial cells (right). (Courtesy of John V. Tedesco, DO.)

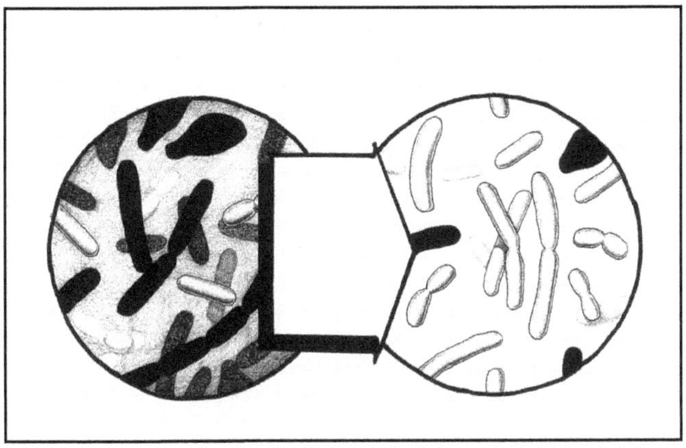

FIGURE 37-3B. Pre- and probiotic effect on colonic bacteria. Colonic administration of both prebiotics, undigested, highly-fermentable polysaccharides, and probiotics, living lactic acid bacteria, increase the number of colonies of lactobacilli and bifidobacteria (white rods) and decrease the number of colonies of harmful clostridia and bacteroides (black rods). (Courtesy of John V. Tedesco, DO.)

FUTURE DIRECTIONS

Future directions in the nutritional treatment of UC include fiber supplementation, pre- and probiotics, butyrate administration, and modulation of the inflammatory cascade (Table 37-5).

BUTYRATE, PRE- AND PROBIOTICS, AND FIBER

Recently, there has been increased evidence to support the treatment of IBD via manipulation of the resident enteric microflora. SCFAs, including butyrate, propionate, and lactate, are generated in the colon as a consequence of bacterial fermentation of dietary fiber and nondigested dietary polysaccharides (Figure 37-3). Along with pre- and probiotics, SCFAs may play a pivotal role in the maintenance of a healthy gut.

Oxidation of butyrate produces acetyl CoA, which is involved in the synthesis of cholesterol and phospholipids, important elements of cell membranes, as well as mucus synthesis. Deficient butyrate oxidation has been described in UC in vivo,[25] which has been attributed to the presence of an excessive number of sulphate-reducing bacteria in the colon. This may jeopardize the important acetyl-CoA-dependent metabolic pathways inducing changes in cell membrane structure and in mucous, which might favor the triggering and perpetuation of the inflammatory process.

It has been shown experimentally that adding some highly fermentable polysaccharides to a fermentation system with human luminal colonic contents and feces increases the number of colonies of lactobacilli and bifidobacteria and decreases those of the harmful clostridia and bacteroides.[26] This is known as the prebiotic effect of fiber. Besides the butyrate enemas discussed earlier, alternative strategies of delivering SCFAs to the inflamed colon are by providing a substrate, a prebiotic, for SCFA production by colonic bacteria. In animal and human studies, ingestion of "resistant" fiber has resulted in an increase in the population of normal luminal bacteria in the colon and an increase in fecal butyrate concentration.[27]

Another method of enhancing the production of colonic SCFA is by the administration of probiotics. Probiotics are living lactic acid bacteria (LAB), which are a heterogeneous group of gram-positive bacteria that normally inhabit the human gastrointestinal tract. Upon ingestion in certain numbers, LAB may improve the health of the colonic mucosa beyond their inherent basic nutrition by competing with pathogens at the intestinal epithelium and enhancing intestinal mucosal secretion.[28]

While controlled clinical trials with probiotics in UC are scarce, two recent double-blind, placebo-controlled trials investigated the use of a probiotic "cocktail" (VSL#3) containing high bacterial concentrations of 4 strains of *Lactobacillus spp.*, 3 strains of *Bifidobacterium*, and 1 strain of *Streptococcus* in UC patients with chronic and acute pouchitis following IPAA. In the first study, 40 UC patients with clinical and endoscopic remission of chronic pouchitis were randomized to receive 6 g of VSL#3 or placebo for nine months.[29] Three patients (15%) in the treatment group had relapses in the 9-month follow-up period, compared with 20 (100%) in the placebo group ($P<0.001$).[29] In the second study, 40 UC patients in the first year following IPAA were randomized to receive either VSL#3 (900 billion bacteria a day) or placebo immediately after ileostomy closure for 1 year.[30] Two (10%) of the treated patients compared with 8 (40%) of the placebo group had an episode of acute pouchitis ($P<0.5$). Additionally, patients in the treatment group reported significant improvement in health-related quality of life as determined by an Inflammatory Bowel Disease Questionnaire score.[30] In summary, the probiotic VSL#3 prevents acute pouchitis, prevents flare-ups of chronic pouchitis, and improves the quality of life of UC patients with IPAA.

Further investigations have looked at new foodstuffs as ways of modulating the inflammatory cascade. A germinated barley product that contains hemicellulose-rich fiber and glutamine-rich protein has been studied by Japanese investigators. It attenuates inflammation in dextran sodium sulfate, trinitrobenzene sulfonic acid (TNBS), and HLA transgenic animal models of colitis.[27] Improvement in clinical and endoscopic indices has been reported in a pilot study of 10 active UC patients with 4 weeks of treatment with germinated barley foodstuff.[25] A lack of significant adverse events and good tolerability were also cited. Furthermore, the fiber may also firm up stool consistency due to its high water-holding capacity and possibly its adsorption of luminal bile salts.[27] An open-label, parallel-group, randomized study of another fiber, plantago ovata seeds, reported equal efficacy to mesalazine in maintaining remission in patients with UC.[27]

CONCLUSION

Malnutrition occurs frequently and rapidly in patients with UC, and it adversely affects the clinical outcome. The SGA is the best method to identify malnourished patients. Those who are moderately or severely malnourished, especially pre- or postoperatively malnourished patients, may benefit from nutritional support. Enteral nutrition is preferred over TPN in UC patients because of its lower cost, equal efficacy, and fewer associated complications. Polymeric diets are preferred because of their increased palatability/patient compliance, decreased cost, and equivalent therapeutic benefits when compared to elemental diets.

New research suggests a role for fish oil as adjuvant therapy in UC as a means to reduce corticosteroid requirements and promote weight gain. Luminal SCFAs, specifically butyrate, have an anti-inflammatory effect on the colonic mucosa and may be effective as adjuvant therapy in patients with short episodes of distal UC. Current research advances include modifying the colonic microflora via administration of dietary fiber and other highly fermentable polysaccharides, along with pre- and probiotics.

REFERENCES

1. Han PD, Burke A, Baldassano RN, Rombeau JL, Lichtenstein GR. Nutrition and inflammatory bowel disease. *Gastroenterol Clin North Am.* 1999;28(2):423-443.
2. Lewis JD, Fisher RL. Nutrition support in inflammatory bowel disease. *Med Clin NA.* 1994;73(6):1443-1456.
3. Rombeau JL, Afonso JJ. Clinical and scientific basis for nutritional support of patients with inflammatory bowel disease. In: MacDermott RP, Stenson WF, eds. *Inflammatory Bowel Disease.* New York, NY: Elsevier Science; 1992:525-553.
4. The Veterans Affairs Total Parenteral Nutrition Cooperative Study Group: perioperative total parenteral nutrition in surgical patients. *N Engl J Med.* 1991;325(8):525-532.
5. Von Meyenfeldt MF, Meijerink WJHJ, Rouflart MMJ, et al. Perioperative nutritional support: a randomized clinical trial. *Clin Nutr.* 1992;11:180-186.
6. ASPEN Board of Directors. Definitions of terms used in ASPEN: guidelines and Standards. *Nutr Clin Pract.* 1995;10:1-3.
7. Aldhous MC, Meister D, Ghosh S. Modification of enteral diets in inflammatory bowel disease. *Proc Nutr Soc.* 2001;60:457-461.
8. Rao SSC, Holdsworth CD, Forrest AWR. Small intestinal absorption and tolerance of enteral nutrition in acute colitis. *Br Med J.* 1987;295:698.
9. Gonzalez-Huix F, Fernandez-Banares F, et al. Enteral versus parenteral nutrition as adjunct therapy in acute ulcerative colitis. *Am J Gastroenterol.* 1993;88(2):227-232.
10. Manual of Clinical Nutrition Management. Enteral nutrition support for adults. www.utmb.edu/food/Manual2003/i/B/B22.html. Accessed April 15, 2004.
11. Gassull MA, Fernandez-Banares F, Cabre E, Esteve-Comas M. Enteral nutrition in inflammatory bowel disease. In: Rombeau JL, Rolandelli RH, eds. *Clinical Nutrition: Enteral and Tube Feeding.* Philadelphia, PA: WB Saunders; 1997:403-416.
12. Larsen PM, Rasmussen D, Ronn B, Munck O, Elmgreen J, Binder V. Elemental diet: a therapeutic approach in chronic inflammatory bowel disease. *J Int Med.* 1989;225:325-331.
13. Wu S, McCraig R. Intense nutritional support in inflammatory bowel disease. *Dig Dis Sci.* 1995;40(4):843-852.
14. Dickinson RJ, Ashton MG, Axon ATR, et al. Controlled trial of intravenous hyperalimentation and total bowel rest as an adjunct to the routine therapy of acute colitis. *Gastroenterology.* 1980;79:1199.
15. Burke A, Lichtenstein GR, Rombeau JL. Nutrition and ulcerative colitis. *Bailliere's Clin Gastroenterol.* 1997;11(1):153-174.
16. Simopoulos AP. Omega-3 fatty acids in inflammation and autoimmune diseases. *J Am Col Nutr.* 2002;21(6):495-505.
17. Hawthorne AB, Daneshmend TK, Hawkey CJ, et al. Treatment of ulcerative colitis with fish oil supplementation: a prospective 12 month randomized controlled trial. *Gut.* 1992;33:922-928.
18. Stenson WF, Cort D, Rodgers J, et al. Dietary supplementation with fish oil in ulcerative colitis. *Ann Int Med.* 1992;116(8):609-614.
19. Almallah YZ, Richardson S, O'Hanrahan T, et al. Distal procto-colitis, natural cytotoxicity, and essential fatty acids. *Am J Gastroenterol.* 1998;93(5):804-809.
20. Almallah YZ, Ewen SW, El-Tahir A, et al. Distal proctocolitis and n-3 polyunsaturated fatty acids (n-3 PUFAs): the mucosal effect *in situ. J Clin Immunol.* 2000;20(1):68-76.

21. Roediger WEW. The place of short-chain fatty acids in colonocyte metabolism in health and ulcerative colitis: the impaired colonocyte barrier. In: Cummings JH, Rombeau JL, Sakata T, eds. *Physiological and Clinical Aspects of Short-Chain Fatty Acids.* Cambridge, UK: Cambridge University Press; 1995:337-351.
22. Breuer RI, Soergel KH, Lashner BA, et al. Short chain fatty acid rectal irrigation for left-sided ulcerative colitis: a randomized, placebo controlled trial. *Gut.* 1997;40(4):485-491.
23. Inan MS, Rasoulpour RJ, Yin L, et al. The luminal short-chain fatty acid butyrate modulates NF-κB activity in a human colonic epithelial cell line. *Gastroenterology.* 2000;118:724-734.
24. Luhrs H, Gerke E, Muller G, et al. Butyrate inhibits NF-κB activation in lamina propria macrophages of patients with ulcerative colitis. *Scand J Gastroenterol.* 2002;4:458-466.
25. Rombeau JL. Investigations of short chain fatty acids in humans. *Clin Nutr.* 2004;1(s):19-23.
26. Cummings JH. Ferementation in the human large intestine: evidence and implications for health. *Lancet.* 1983;1:1206-1209
27. Goh J, O'Morain A. Review article: nutrition and adult inflammatory bowel disease. *Aliment Pharmacol Ther.* 2003;17:307-320.
28. Guslandi M. Probiotics for chronic intestinal disorders. *Am J Gastroenterol.* 2003;98(3):520-521.
29. Gionchetti P, Rizzello F, Venturi A, et al. Oral bacteriotherapy as maintenance treatment in patients with chronic pouchitis: a double-blind, placebo-controlled trial. *Gastroenterology.* 2000;119(2):305-309.
30. Gionchetti P, Rizzello F, Helwig U, et al. Prophylaxis of pouchitis onset with probiotic therapy: a double-blind, placebo-controlled trial. *Gastroenterology.* 2003;124(5):1202-1209.

38

Parenteral Nutrition Use in Ulcerative Colitis

Alan L. Buchman, MD, MSPH

There are very few data concerning the use of parenteral nutrition (PN) either as primary therapy, or as adjunctive therapy in patients with ulcerative colitis (UC). Most reports are open-label case series during which patients received concomitant corticosteroids, and, often, patients with Crohn's colitis were grouped together with those having UC. Reported follow-up was often brief and generally included only the immediate hospitalization; few objective data were presented. Patients were categorized as being in "remission" or showing a "response," although this was often described subjectively in the absence of objective criteria. This chapter will focus on the use of parenteral nutrition in patients with UC.

In 1970, Gimpel and Schilling from the University of Oklahoma reported that 72 days of postoperative TPN improved the nutritional status of a malnourished patient with severe UC who required colectomy but had been unable to eat sufficiently due to multiple postoperative complications.[1] This was the first time TPN had been used in a patient with UC, although it was used primarily for nutritional support, rather than to induce remission. In 1973, Fischer et al described the use of TPN in 4 UC patients who were prescribed complete bowel rest; concomitant medical therapy was not described.[2] Only one-fourth of patients avoided colectomy during that admission. In 1974, Truelove and Jewell described their experience with 49 patients with severe UC in whom a 5-day regimen of PN had been prescribed.[3] Thirty-six of the 49 patients had achieved "remission" by the end of the 5-day course of PN, and, in addition, some patients were described as having a "partial response." All patients received concomitant corticosteroids. Approximately two-thirds of the patients who achieved remission remained symptom-free for an average of 3 years following PN. Subsequently, Truelove's experience in 100 patients was reported, in which 60 achieved remission.[4] In 1976, Dean et al described 5 patients with UC who were provided with PN, but in whom colectomy was still required in 4 out of 5 during the hospitalization.[5] Reilly et al reported a series of 11 patients (including the 4 patients described by Fischer et al[2]), of whom 10 required colectomy during their hospital admission despite the use of PN, although postoperative complications were more frequent in a historic control group that did not receive PN.[6] Most patients were treated with corticosteroids in addition to PN. Fazio reported 1 out of 4 patients who received PN achieved remission during their hospitalization and did not require colectomy.[7] Elson described the University of Chicago experience of 10 patients "refractory" to corticosteroids, in whom 3 had "significant" improvement after a mean of 21 days of PN.[8] These patients were able to avoid colectomy for 5 to 43 months.

Dickinson et al reported the results of one of only 2 prospective, randomized, controlled trials of PN in UC.[9] The study was small and underpowered, although similar outcomes were described in patients who received PN (6/13 achieved remission) without oral food intake and the control group (8/16 achieved remission); there were some long-term remissions in both groups. All patients received corticosteroids. Sitzman et al reported the results of a series of patients who failed oral prednisone (83%) as outpatients and were admitted to the hospital for TPN and IV corticosteroids (91%).[10] Five out of 22 patients were discharged without requirement for colectomy, although only 4 of those achieved long-term remission ranging between 15 and 56 months. McIntyre et al reported the results of the other randomized, controlled trial. Similar to the results reported by Dickinson et al, 6/15 patients with "severe"

Lichtenstein GR, ed.
Ulcerative Colitis: The Complete Guide to Medical Management (pp 445-446)

TABLE 38-1

USE OF PARENTERAL NUTRITION IN PATIENTS WITH ULCERATIVE COLITIS

Study	Remission Rate	Follow-up
Gimpel/Schilling[1]	?	72 days
Truelove/Jewell[3]	60/100	up to 3 yrs
Dean et al[5]	1/5	same admission
Reilly et al[6]	1/10	same admission
Fazio et al[7]	1/4	same admission
Elson et al[8]	3/21	5 to 43 months
Dickinson et al[9]	6/13	same admission
Sitzman et al[10]	5/22 (4/22)	same admission (15 to 56 months)
McIntyre et al[11]	6/15	same admission
Gonzalez-Huix et al[12]	10/20	same admission

UC who were NPO and received PN achieved remission, compared with 7/12 who achieved remission while on an oral diet; all patients received concomitant corticosteroid therapy.[11] Gonzalez-Huix et al randomized patients with severe UC (using the Truelove-Witt criteria) to receive PN or TEN, the latter of which utilized nasoenteric feeding with a polymeric formula.[12] Ten out of 20 patients who received TPN achieved remission compared with 12/22 enterally fed patients.

The use of TPN does not appear to have clinical benefit as a primary means for induction of remission in patients with UC. However, it may be a useful adjunctive therapy when patients have toxic megacolon or are otherwise unable to eat because of severe abdominal cramping. There appears to be no additional benefit from PN itself in patients with UC who are otherwise able to eat or to receive enteral nutritional support.

REFERENCES

1. Gimpel A, Schilling JA. Long-term hyperalimentation in ulcerative colitis. *Oklahoma State Med Assoc J.* 1970;68:371-375.
2. Fischer JE, Foster GS, Abel RM, et al. Hyperalimentation as primary therapy for inflammatory bowel disease. *Am J Surg.* 18973;125:165-175.
3. Truelove SC, Jewell DP. Intensive intravenous regimen for severe attacks of ulcerative colitis. *Lancet.* 1974;i:1067-1070.
4. Truelove SC, Willoughby CP, Lee EG, Kettlewell MG. Further experience in the treatment of severe attacks of ulcerative colitis. *Lancet.* 1978;2:1086-1088.
5. Dean RE, Campos MM, Barrett B. Hyperalimentation in the management of chronic inflammatory intestinal disease. *Dis Colon Rectum.* 1976;19:601-604.
6. Reilly J, Ryan JA, Strole W, Fischer JE. Hyperalimentation in inflammatory bowel disease. *Am J Surg.* 1976;131:192-200.
7. Fazio VW, Kodner I, Jagelman DG, et al. Parenteral nutrition as primary of adjunctive treatment. *Dis Colon Rectum.* 1976;19: 574-578.
8. Elson CO, Layden TJ, Nemchausky BA, et al. An evaluation of total parenteral nutrition in the management of inflammatory bowel disease. *Dig Dis Sci.* 1980;25:42-48.
9. Dickinson RJ, Ashton MG, Axon ATR, et al. Controlled trial of intravenous hyperalimentation and total bowel rest as an adjunct to the routine therapy of acute colitis. *Gastroenterology.* 1980;79:1199-1204.
10. Sitzman JV, Converse RL Jr, Bayless TM. Favorable response to parenteral nutrition and medical therapy in Crohn's colitis. *Gastroenterology.* 1990;99:1647-1652.
11. McIntyre PB, Powell-Tuck J, Wood SR, et al. Controlled trial of bowel rest in the treatment of severe ulcerative colitis. *Gut.* 1986;27:481-485.
12. Gonzalez-Huix F, Fernandez-Banares F, Esteve-Comas M, et al. Enteral versus parenteral nutrition as adjunct therapy in acute ulcerative colitis. *Am J Gastroenterol.* 1993;88:227-232.

39

Maintenance of Remission in Ulcerative Colitis

Kenneth W. Schroeder, MD, PhD and William J. Tremaine, MD

The goals of treatment of ulcerative colitis (UC) are first to reduce the colon inflammation responsible for the gastrointestinal symptoms, and second to establish a medical program that will keep the inflammation in remission so the patient will maintain a normal or near-normal bowel pattern. Maintenance therapy may also reduce the need for surgery for poorly controlled colitis symptoms and could potentially reduce the long-term risk of developing colon carcinoma. Different medications may be required for induction therapy and maintenance therapy. At the time the patient first seeks attention, both induction and maintenance therapy should be considered, and therapy for both phases may be started simultaneously. Some maintenance drugs, such as aminosalicylates, may prove effective for both induction and maintenance of remission, while others, such as some immunomodulatory drugs, require 4 to 8 weeks of use before achieving a therapeutic benefit. The choice of therapies will be determined by such factors as severity of the symptoms, patient allergies or history of drug intolerances, and previous history of response to treatment.

The risk of symptomatic relapse after induction of remission in UC is significant. Studies assessing the efficacy of maintenance therapies show that up to 75% of those receiving placebo will have recurrence of inflammation and symptoms within the first year after induction of remission.[1] However, it is difficult to predict the clinical course for an individual patient. Several factors may give clues about the long-term clinical course in patients with UC:

- The clinical activity in the first 2 years of disease is predictive of the level of activity in the next 5 years, and a prior history of multiple relapses predicts a significant continued risk.[2]
- Patients who have not had a symptomatic relapse for several years are less likely to experience a flare than patients who have had a relapse within the past 12 months.[3]
- At any point in time, one-half of patients are in remission, and 90% have intermittent symptomatic disease.[2]
- There is no consistent pattern of relapse based on the patient's age at disease onset or gender.[4]
- More extensive disease is more likely to lead to surgical intervention, suggesting a greater risk of relapse.[5]
- Patients requiring corticosteroids for induction therapy are more likely to relapse.[6]
- Cigarette smoking does not appear to affect the risk of relapse.[4]
- Initial presentation as distal UC extends proximally to become more extensive disease in at least 10% of cases.[7]

Despite maintenance therapy, one assessment of patients with UC treated with corticosteroids for induction therapy and aminosalicylates for maintenance found a 50% cumulative relapse rate at 1 year, and patients younger than 50 years old were more likely to have a relapse.[4] Hence, maintenance therapy may alter the natural history of UC by reducing recurrence rates, but maintenance therapy will not eliminate all chance of disease recrudescence. Patients to be treated with maintenance therapy will only benefit from such treatment if they are first treated to complete symptomatic remission. For example, treatment with corticosteroids for induction of remission must lead to complete relief of symptoms before tapering the dose, or else it is likely the maintenance therapy will prove ineffective. It

Lichtenstein GR, ed.
Ulcerative Colitis: The Complete Guide to Medical Management (pp 447-464)

TABLE 39-1

AMINOSALICYLATE PREPARATIONS

Preparation	Description	Unit Size	Release Mechanism	Release Location
Prodrugs				
Sulfasalazine (Azulfidine)	5-ASA Sulfapyridine	1 g	Diazo bond cleaved by bacteria	Colon
Olsalazine (Dipentum)	Dimer of 5-ASA	250 mg	Diazo bond cleaved by bacteria	Colon
Balsalazide (Colazide/Colazal)	5-ASA inert carrier	750 mg	Diazo bond cleaved by bacteria	Colon
Targeted Release				
5-ASA (Pentasa)	Ethylcellulose microgranule encapsulation	250 mg 500 mg	Acid and alkaline pH	Small bowel and colon
5-ASA (Asacol)	Eudragit-S coating	400 mg to 800 mg	pH >7	Distal ileum and colon
5-ASA (Salofalk)	Eudragit-L coating	1 g*	pH >6	Distal small bowel and colon
Delayed Release				
5-ASA (Liada)	Coated with a gastro-resistant pH-dependent polymer film	1.2 g	pH >7	Distal small bowel and colon
Extended Release				
5-ASA (Apriso)	Polymer matrix with an enteric coating	0.375 g	pH >6	Distal small bowel and colon
Rectal Delivery				
5-ASA Enema	Enema	4 g	Enema	Distal colon to splenic flexure
5-ASA Suppository	Suppository	500 mg	Suppository	Distal 20 cm of the rectosigmoid colon

*Not available in the United States.

is often appropriate to initiate the maintenance treatment at the same time as the treatment for induction of remission. This chapter will focus on the long-term maintenance options, with emphasis on the aminosalicylates and thiopurine immunomodulatory drugs, for treating patients with UC once the disease has been brought under control.

AMINOSALICYLATES

Aminosalicylates are currently the first-line maintenance therapy for ulcerative colitis, exhibiting both efficacy and safety for many patients. This group of drugs has historically been the mainstay of therapy for both induction and maintenance of remission in UC. There are now several forms of delivery (Table 39-1) of the active ingredient, 5-ASA (mesalamine, mesalazine), to the colon where it acts topically.[8]

PRODRUGS

This class of aminosalicylates combines a carrier molecule with the 5-ASA using a diazo bond. The drug is passed unaffected through the stomach and small bowel,

TABLE 39-2

ADVERSE REACTIONS TO AMINOSALICYLATES

	Dose-Related	Idiosyncratic Reactions	
Reactions that can occur with all 5-ASA drugs		Worsening colitis symptoms Renal toxicity Interstitial nephritis Nephrotic syndrome Pulmonary toxicity Interstitial lung disease Bronchiolitis obliterans Pulmonary granulomatosis Interstitial lung fibrosis Eosinophilic pleural effusion Pericarditis Pancreatitis Hair loss	
Reactions specific to sulfasalazine therapy	Nausea, vomiting* Headache* Malaise* Abdominal pain*	Hypersensitivity rash Male infertility Agranulocytosis Aplastic anemia	Hemolytic anemia Hepatic dysfunction Pulmonary dysfunction Worsening bowel symptoms
Reaction specific to 5-ASA enemas		Sulfite allergy	
Reaction specific to olsalazine	Diarrhea†		

*Primarily related to acetylator phenotype in metabolism of sulfapyridine.

†Caused by the prodrug molecule.

and, when reaching the colon, bacterial diazoreductase cleaves the diazo bond, releasing free 5-ASA and the carrier molecule.

SULFASALAZINE (AZULFIDINE, PHARMACIA & UPJOHN)

This first aminosalicylate was developed by Dr. Nana Svartz of the Karolinska Institute in the late 1930s with the combination of 5-ASA and a sulfa moiety, sulfapyridine, bound by a diazo bond. The 5-ASA constitutes about 40% of sulfasalazine. She reported it was an effective therapy, usually at doses of 4 to 6 g/d, in 75% to 80% of patients with UC.[9] It was first critically assessed in the United States in the early 1950s and was shown to be superior to other sulfa drugs.[10] Sulfasalazine has remained a reliable therapy of UC treatment over the years since then. In 1965, a controlled trial proved the maintenance benefit of the drug.[1] Efficacy was noted with a dose of 4 g/d, but more side effects with this dose led to the recommendation for 2 g/d as a balance between benefit and adverse effects.[11] The drug is available as tablets of 500 mg, and doses of up to 4 g/d, or occasionally up to 6 g/d, may be used.

Studies in the 1970s showed that enteric bacteria cleaved the diazo bond of the sulfasalazine to release the 5-ASA and sulfapyridine in the distal small bowel and colon.[12] Enema studies showed that the clinical benefit from 2 g/d of sulfasalazine can be reproduced by 0.7 g/d of 5-ASA, suggesting this is the active moiety, while 1.3 g/d of sulfapyridine had little effect.[13] Much of the sulfapyridine is absorbed from the colon and appears responsible for many of the adverse effects associated with sulfasalazine. Adverse symptoms with sulfasalazine occur in up to 30% of patients receiving this treatment and are both dose-related (related to acetylator status) and idiosyncratic (Table 39-2). As these adverse effects may limit the usefulness of the drug, alternative delivery systems, including other prodrugs as well as targeted delayed-release preparations, have been developed.

OLSALAZINE (DIPENTUM, PHARMACIA & UPJOHN)

This preparation is a dimer of 5-ASA joined by the diazo bond.[14] The prodrug passes through the small bowel with minimal absorption and is cleaved in the colon by bacterial diazoreductase to free 5-ASA with no residual carrier.[15] Equivalent doses of 5-ASA are delivered by olsalazine and sulfasalazine in a ratio of approximately 1:2.5. Olsalazine is available as 250-mg capsules. FDA approval is for a dose of 1 g/d. Doses of up to 3 g daily have been used for active disease.[16]

In a comparison of 4 g/d of sulfasalazine to 2 g/d of olsalazine for 48 weeks, comparable relapse rates were noted (30.4% versus 26.1%).[17] A 1-year comparison of 2 g/d of sulfasalazine to 1 g/d of olsalazine also showed similar recurrence rates (42.4% versus 46.9%).[18] Similar rates of adverse effects were noted with the 2 drugs in both studies. The primary side effect of olsalazine was diarrhea[19] related to small bowel fluid secretion.[20] This appears to be a dose-related reaction and may be reduced by taking the medication with food.

BALSALAZIDE (COLAZAL, COLAZIDE, SALIX)

This preparation combines 5-ASA with an inert amino acid, 4-amino-benzoyl-alanine, to create a prodrug that releases the 5-ASA in the colon from the carrier, which appears to have no clinical effect.[21] Additionally, the prodrug itself appears to have no systemic effects. Balsalazide consists of 35% 5-ASA and is available as capsules of 750 mg. FDA approval is for a dose of 6.75 g/d.

Maintenance therapy has been assessed at varying doses: 2 g/d versus 4 g/d for 1 year showed less relapse at the higher doses (55 % versus 36%, $P<0.01$),[22] and a comparison of 3 g/d versus 6 g/d for 1 year showed comparable remission rates (77% versus 68%).[23] Withdrawals in 8% to 19% of treated patients related to side effects usually occurred in the first few weeks of treatment and were primarily from gastrointestinal intolerance. When compared to mesalamine preparations, such as Asacol, at comparable doses, remission rates at the end of 12 months were comparable (58%), and adverse events were comparable for the 2 groups.[24] In a 6-month trial, low-dose balsalazide (3.0 g/d) was compared to low-dose 5-ASA, as Salofalk (1.5 g/d), and to high-dose balsalazide (6 g/d). They found comparable remission rates for low-dose balsalazide and 5-ASA (43.8% and 56.8%) and a superior remission rate for higher dose balsalazide (77.5%).[25] Adverse events were uncommon in all treatment groups.

TARGETED RELEASE PREPARATIONS

Unprotected 5-ASA given orally is rapidly absorbed from the proximal small bowel, then acetylated in the liver and excreted into the urine.[26] This virtually eliminates any contact of the drug with the colonic mucosa and prevents any therapeutic benefit from orally administered, unprotected 5-ASA. Several preparations have been developed to delay the release of the drug in the upper gut and deliver the drug more distally. These products are similar in that the drug is coated to delay the release until reaching distal small bowel or proximal colon. Such formulations include Asacol (Procter & Gamble Pharmaceuticals), Pentasa (Ferring-Shire Pharmaceuticals), and Salofalk (Falk). The mechanism of drug delivery is the primary difference between the drugs. Because the active ingredient in all these preparations is 5-ASA, they are discussed by their proprietary name.

ASACOL

This preparation coats 400 mg or 800 mg of 5-ASA with the pH-sensitive acrylic polymer, Eudragit S, which dissolves at pH levels above 6.8.[27] A tablet of Asacol taken orally will pass unaffected through the upper GI tract until reaching the distal ileum or proximal colon, there the sustained pH levels cause the coating to dissolve with release of about 80% of the ingested 5-ASA dose to the colon.[28,29] Asacol is approved by the FDA in doses of 1.6 to 2.4 g/d. Doses up to 4.8 g/d have been used for active disease.[30]

In a maintenance of remission study, a 6-month assessment of Asacol at a dose of 1.6 g/d was compared to placebo with a significantly better rate of remission with Asacol (43% versus 63%, $P=0.017$).[31] In another maintenance trial over 6 months, Asacol at doses of 0.8 g/d was superior to placebo in maintaining remission (58.8% versus 39.7%, $P=0.05$), and Asacol 1.6 g/d was superior to placebo (65.5% versus 39.7%, $P=0.005$).[32] A 1-year study of maintenance effects with a dose of 1.2 g/d of Asacol compared to placebo showed that patients with a short-term remission before entering the study had a significantly reduced rate of relapse with therapy (relapse rates of 49% with placebo and 23% with Asacol, $P=0.035$); though patients who had a history of remission for more than 2 years before study entry had no significant benefit from the addition of Asacol (relapse rates of 18% with Asacol versus 26% with placebo, $P=0.35$).[33]

In a 48-week trial, 0.8 g of Asacol versus 2 g of sulfasalazine and 1.6 g of Asacol versus 4 g of sulfasalazine produced comparable rates of symptomatic relapse. Patients tolerated the Asacol better than the sulfasalazine, however.[34]

PENTASA

This drug contains 250 mg or 500 mg of 5-ASA encapsulated in ethylcellulose microgranules which releases the drug slowly and fairly evenly throughout the small bowel and colon.[35] This system delivers approximately half the dose of 5-ASA to the colon,[36] with the remainder of the 5-ASA absorbed from the small bowel and excreted in the urine. Pentasa is approved by the FDA for use in doses up to 4 g/d.

In a 12-month comparison of Pentasa at 4 g/d to placebo, the remission rate for Pentasa was 64% and 38% for the placebo group (*P*=0.0004). Adverse events were rare, and there was no significant difference in the number of adverse events for those who received active therapy compared to those who received placebo.[37] When 1.5 g/d of Pentasa was compared to 3 g/d of sulfasalazine for maintenance therapy in UC, the rate of remission at 6 months was 63% for Pentasa versus 72% for sulfasalazine, and at 12 months it was 54% for Pentasa and 46% for sulfasalazine. These were not significantly different, suggesting comparable doses of these drugs were of comparable efficacy for maintenance therapy in UC. No adverse events were noted in the 41 patients treated with Pentasa, while of the 31 patients treated with sulfasalazine, 5 had one or more adverse events. In a dose comparison of 1.5 g/d versus 3.0 g/d of Pentasa, there was no significant difference between the rates of remission or adverse events.[38]

SALOFALK

This preparation, not available in the US, coats 500 mg of 5-ASA with Eudragit L, which is a pH-dependent coating dissolving at pH of 6 or higher. Similar to other directed release preparations, this drug is released in the distal small bowel and colon.

LIALDA AND APRISO

Lialda (multimatrix [MMX] mesalamine) is a novel, once-daily, high-strength (1.2-g tablet) formulation of mesalamine, utilizing MMX Multimatrix System technology designed to deliver the active drug throughout the colon. Two studies have shown MMX mesalamine, given either once or twice a day in 2.4 or 4.8 g/d doses, to be more effective than placebo.[39,40] This formulation is currently approved by the FDA for treatment of active UC with a dose of 2.4 to 4.8 g/d. Apriso—a granulated formulation of mesalamine that releases mesalamine at a ph ≥6 and is administered once daily—has recently been approved by the FDA at a dose of 1.5 g/d (for 375-mg capsules).[41,42]

RECTAL PREPARATIONS

Many patients with UC have only distal disease, and topical treatment by suppository or enema directed toward the distal colon may be more effective than oral treatment for these patients. 5-ASA preparations are available as 1-g suppositories and 4-g enemas. In addition, foam preparations of 5-ASA for rectal administration are available in some countries, though not in the US. Suppositories may be used 1 to 3 times daily for induction of remission, and enemas are taken at bedtime. Once in remission, maintenance therapy may also be continued by the rectal approach or orally, or with a combined approach of both oral and rectal therapy. Rectally administered maintenance therapy is given at less frequent intervals than for induction, ranging from once daily to 2 to 3 times per week. Occasionally, the combination of a rectal and an oral drug will prove beneficial.

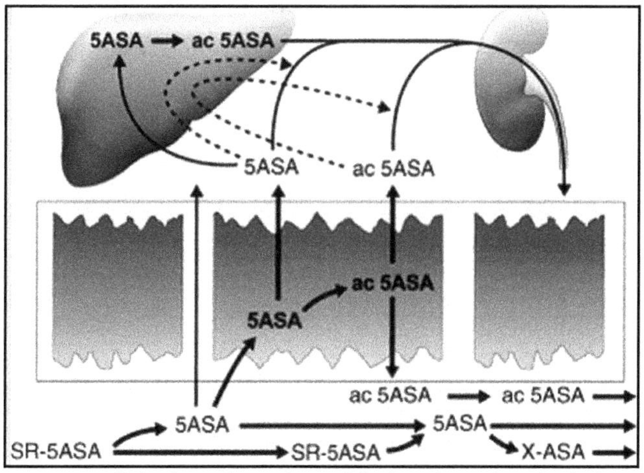

FIGURE 39-1. Elimination pathways of 5-ASA following release of sustained release drug. SR-5-ASA: sustained release 5-ASA; Ac-5-ASA: N-acetyl 5-ASA; 5-ASA: 5-aminosalicylic acid; X-ASA: other metabolites/not defined. (Reprinted with permission from Sandborn WJ, Hanauer SB, Buch A. Comparative pharmacokinetics of equimolar doses of 5-aminosalicylate administered as oral mesalamine (Asacol) and balsalazide: a randomized, single-dose, crossover study in healthy volunteers. *Aliment Pharmacol Ther.* 2004;19:1089-1098.)

5-ASA enemas given 1 g/d or suppositories (3 g weekly to 1.0 g/d) have been shown superior to placebo for maintenance therapy for 1 year, with remission rates of 52% to 92% and an overall pooled OR for maintaining remission of 5.6 (95% CI 3.0-10.5).[43] Dosing studies compared 5-ASA enemas of 2.0 versus 4.0 g daily and found no difference in the response to these doses,[44] though another trial of suppositories comparing 500 mg/d versus twice daily found a higher remission at 12 months with the higher dose (68% versus 90%, *P*=0.03).[45] To date, a dose-response relationship has not been established for rectal preparations in maintenance therapy, and the dosing should be individualized for each patient.

Comparison of oral versus rectal 5-ASA for maintenance of distal colitis found the rectal preparations (enemas given as 4 g/d for 1 week/month, 4 g every 3 days, or 2 g/d) were similar or superior to oral sulfasalazine (2 g/d) or mesalamine (500 mg three times daily) after 6 to 24 months. Their pooled OR for maintaining remission was 2.3 (95% CI 1.1-4.8).[46-48]

PHARMACOKINETICS OF 5-ASA

Regardless of the formulation to deliver the 5-ASA to the bowel, the activity of the drug is directly related to the free luminal 5-ASA molecule, which acts as a topical anti-inflammatory agent (Figure 39-1). Drug released in the small bowel is readily absorbed and taken up in the liver, where it is inactivated by acetylation at the amino group to form N-acetyl-5-ASA and is then excreted into the urine along with a small amount of free, non-acetylated 5-ASA.[49-51] The drug absorbed by the small bowel has no significant anti-inflammatory effect on the colon.

The 5-ASA reaching the colon is absorbed by the colonic mucosal cells where it also undergoes metabolism to N-acetyl-5-ASA. Some of this is absorbed into the blood and excreted into the urine or is secreted back into the lumen and excreted into the feces.[52] There is minimal acetylation of the 5-ASA by bacteria in the colon lumen.[53] The clinical benefit of the 5-ASA is dependent on the level of 5-ASA reaching the colonic mucosa.[54]

Adverse Events From Aminosalicylates

Adverse events associated with aminosalicylate therapy can be associated with either the prodrug preparation, designed to deliver the drug to the colon, or the 5-ASA itself (see Table 39-2). Adverse events from a prodrug will likely mean an alternative delivery system for 5-ASA will be tolerated, while adverse events associated with 5-ASA may limit the dosage of 5-ASA that may be used or may preclude its use entirely.

Prodrug-Associated Adverse Events

Sulfasalazine

Adverse reactions are relatively common and have been noted in up to 30% of patients taking this drug.[55] These fall into 2 categories: dose-related (correlating to acetylator phenotype in metabolizing the sulfapyridine moiety) and non-dose-related or idiosyncratic.[56] Starting at a low dose and slowly increasing the dosage may allow patients with a dose-related adverse reaction to tolerate adequate doses, while the idiosyncratic reactions (including allergy to sulfa compounds) usually precludes use of sulfasalazine entirely. In 80% to 90% of patients who experience adverse reactions to sulfasalazine, other 5-ASA products are tolerated well, suggesting many of the sulfasalazine-associated adverse effects are related to intolerance to sulfapyridine.[57,58] Side effects associated with sulfasalazine worthy of note include pulmonary symptoms[59,60] (same as with 5-ASA); male infertility,[61] which may be reversed with switching to another aminosalicylate[62]; and worsening of colitis symptoms, which may also be caused by other aminosalicylate.[63,64]

Olsalazine

The most common adverse effect from this preparation is diarrhea in 10% to 20% of patients. This appears to be related to prodrug-induced increased small bowel fluid secretion.[65] Starting a low dose and increasing slowly and taking with food may minimize this reaction.

Balsalazide

Adverse reactions to this prodrug are no more common or different from other targeted release drugs, suggesting the carrier molecule is relatively inert.

Targeted Release 5-ASA Preparations

These drugs are primarily different in the mode of drug delivery to the colon, but the final result is the arrival of the 5-ASA in the colonic lumen. Adverse reactions are rare and, in most studies, at no greater level than seen with placebo and usually less common than seen with sulfasalazine.[66] Of particular importance is an increase in colitis-type symptoms, similar to that seen originally with sulfasalazine. Onset is usually within 24 to 48 hours of starting the drug and consists of increasing diarrhea, perhaps with blood, along with cramping abdominal pain, fevers, myalgias, and arthralgias.[64] This is independent of the dose taken and will subside within 24 to 48 hours of stopping the drug. Because this idiosyncratic reaction may occur with any aminosalicylate preparation, it usually precludes use of any other preparation, including rectal products. If a patient in remission is started on an aminosalicylate and experiences a symptomatic flare shortly thereafter, this idiosyncratic reaction should be considered in addition to the possibility of a flare of the colitis itself.

An adverse event that is unique to 5-ASA enemas and does not occur with other forms of 5-ASA therapy is an allergic reaction to sulfites. As 5-ASA is relatively unstable in solution, sulfites are added to prevent decomposition of the 5-ASA moiety. Individuals who are intolerant to sulfites may have an allergic reaction to 5-ASA enemas and yet tolerate oral 5-ASA or 5-ASA suppositories.

Renal toxicity has been a concern because animal studies showed significant renal problems with high doses of 5-ASA,[67,68] though clinical experience has shown the occurrence of renal toxicity with sulfasalazine is relatively rare.[69,70] Additionally, there is evidence that UC may be associated with some underlying renal dysfunction that may be confused with a drug effect.[71] Nonetheless, several case reports have appeared suggesting 5-ASA is capable of inducing significant renal toxicity,[72] and regular monitoring of the serum creatinine and urinary sediment is recommended.[73] While the renal abnormalities may develop after a few days of therapy, these abnormalities are more common after months of therapy. Treatment-related renal abnormalities may resolve with discontinuation of the 5-ASA drug. It is wise to monitor the renal function in a patient with known renal dysfunction who is started on a 5-ASA product at 3- to 6-month intervals for the first year to screen for any deterioration.

Pulmonary toxicity has been described with onset from 5 days to months or years after drug initiation[74] and may be characterized by insidious onset of dyspnea on exertion, dry cough, fever, or pleural effusion. Whether pulmonary toxicity is an idiosyncratic reaction or a dose-related toxicity is controversial.[75] Cessation of the drug will reverse the pulmonary reaction in most cases.

Other adverse effects reported include pericarditis,[76] pancreatitis,[77] hepatitis,[78] and hair loss. These are rare

TABLE 39-3

POSSIBLE MODES OF ACTION OF 5-ASA

Disrupt arachidonic acid metabolism by
Inhibition of 5-lipoxygenase pathway
Inhibition of cyclo-oxygenase pathway
Inhibition of cytokine (IL-1, IL-2, IL-6) generation
Diminish antibody secretion and lymphocyte function
Inhibition of TNFα
Scavenger of reactive oxygen metabolites
Reduce neutrophil/macrophage chemotaxis
Enhance expression of heat shock proteins to protect intestinal epithelium
Inhibition of platelet activation
Inhibition of Nuclear Factor κB

and may become evident only after a prolonged phase of therapy with an aminosalicylate. Some of these effects are reversible if the drug is stopped, and all appear to be dose-independent. Such reactions will preclude further use of any aminosalicylate.

Mechanism of Action of Aminosalicylates

The benefit from aminosalicylates is typically ascribed to the 5-ASA component. In the case of sulfasalazine, there may be some unique anti-inflammatory effects from sulfasalazine, perhaps attributable to the sulfa component or the parent molecule.[79,80] The other prodrugs, olsalazine and balsalazide, have no known anti-inflammatory effects aside from that associated with the 5-ASA.

Possible anti-inflammatory mechanisms of action for 5-ASA are summarized in Table 39-3.[81-83] More than one mechanism of action may be important in the reduction and control of colonic inflammation.

Assessment of Aminosalicylate Therapy for Ulcerative Colitis

In the most recent Cochrane analysis of maintenance therapy with aminosalicylates for UC, 16 studies involving a total of 2479 patients were assessed.[84] Five of these trials were placebo-controlled, and the others were comparisons with sulfasalazine. Aminosalicylates were superior to placebo, but there was a higher degree of therapeutic effectiveness with sulfasalazine, suggesting there may be some benefit from the sulfapyridine moiety not present in the other formulations. Adverse events were somewhat more common with olsalazine than the others, and there was no difference between the adverse effects of the sulfasalazine as compared to the other aminosalicylates.

Another systematic review of 8 placebo-controlled trials of aminosalicylates over intervals of 6 or 12 months, including 3 assessing sulfasalazine, noted a remission rate of 86% with an aminosalicylate compared to a placebo response rate of 38%. The number needed to treat (NNT) for clinical benefit from the aminosalicylate was very favorable at 5 (95% CI 4-8).[85] These studies indicate that the aminosalicylates are highly beneficial for long-term maintenance.

It is less clear which preparation and what dose to use. Choosing a 5-ASA preparation can be confusing with the variety of options available, and proving a dose-response relationship for the 5-ASA preparations in maintenance therapy has been difficult.[86]

Various studies have addressed the delivery of drug to the colon with different preparations[87-91] in order to identify an optimal delivery system. However, as methodologies vary, it is difficult to compare the results of different studies.[92] A recent systematic review assessed the published literature to identify the results in normal volunteers or patients with UC.[93] These authors concluded that the systemic exposure to 5-ASA, as measured by urinary excretion of total active and inactive 5-ASA and fecal excretion of total active and inactive 5-ASA, is comparable for all oral 5-ASA formulations and prodrugs. Therefore, the choice of a 5-ASA preparation should be based on the tolerability of the parent 5-ASA compound and its metabolites, compliance with 5-ASA dose forms and dose schedules, and cost.

Aminosalicylates During Pregnancy

Sulfasalazine, the other 5-ASA prodrugs (olsalazine, balsalazide), and delayed release 5-ASA preparations (Apriso, Asacol, Lialda, Pentasa) all appear to be safe for use during pregnancy and may be continued during nursing of the child. Doses do not need to be modified.[94-96]

Aminosalicylates for Chemoprevention of Cancer in Ulcerative Colitis

Patients with longstanding ulcerative colitis are at increased risk for development of colorectal carcinoma, usually after 8 to 10 years for extensive disease and somewhat later for left-sided disease.[97] Epidemiologic studies have shown that nonsteroidal anti-inflammatory drugs, such as aspirin or sulindac, may reduce the risk of colorectal carcinoma in the normal population. Subsequent studies suggest that continued maintenance therapy with aminosalicylates may help prevent the development of colorectal carcinoma in long-standing UC.[98] In one retrospective comparison of UC patients with cancer to matched UC patients without cancer, sulfasalazine treatment for 3 months appeared to have a protective effect.[99] Continued sulfasalazine therapy, but not intermittent use, was shown to reduce the incidence of colon cancer.[100] In a large retrospective, matched case, controlled study from the UK, UC patients with colorectal carcinoma were compared to patients without cancer: 5-ASA at doses of more than 1.2 g/d was shown to reduce the risk of cancer by 81% (P=0.006), and 5-ASA was the only therapy shown to reduce this risk.[101] In addition, a meta-analysis of observational studies showed that use of 5-ASAs was associated with a reduced risk of colorectal cancer (OR = 0.51).[102] In summary, there is reasonable evidence suggesting a role for the 5-ASAs as a potential chemopreventive agent in patients with long-standing ulcerative colitis.

For a chemopreventive benefit from maintenance therapy, patients must adhere to a long-term regimen, even when they feel well. Recent reports suggest such compliance with continued therapy is relatively poor. A study of 94 patients with at least a 6-month history of clinically quiescent disease, maintained on Asacol, found overall adherence to their maintenance regimen to be about 40%. Nonadherent patients were more likely to be male, unmarried, have left-sided disease, and be on 4 or more prescription medications.[103] A subsequent report from the same medical center on 99 patients on maintenance therapy with Asacol was followed at 6, 12, and 24 months. Symptomatic relapse developed in 12 patients at 6 months, all nonadherent to therapy. Nineteen patients relapsed at 12 months, of whom 13 were nonadherent, and an additional 8 patients relapsed by 24 months, with 6 of the 8 nonadherent.[104] Another study noted that multiple doses per day, full-time employment, and depression increased the chance of nonadherence.[105] These studies point out the important role of patient education on the need for continued use of the maintenance medication and the need for simplified schedules for long-term treatment of UC.

Clinical Use of 5-ASA Maintenance Therapy in Ulcerative Colitis

A 5-ASA drug is usually started as monotherapy or in combination with a corticosteroid. If a corticosteroid is used for induction therapy, this will subsequently be tapered once the symptoms are in remission with continuation of the aminosalicylate for maintenance of remission. After several weeks to months of stable dosing, the aminosalicylate may be slowly reduced to a lower dose in order to simplify the medical regimen and to reduce associated costs. Tapering the dose slowly should make it possible to identify a dose that maintains remission, and below which symptoms recur. Combining oral and rectal preparations may provide additional benefit for some patients who do not maintain remission with oral therapy alone.

IMMUNOMODULATORY DRUGS

Azathioprine/6-Mercaptopurine

Alternative maintenance therapy is needed for those patients in whom 5-ASAs are not effective for maintaining remission. Additionally, patients who have achieved remission with steroids, but have recurrent symptoms when the steroids are reduced or stopped (steroid-dependent), are candidates for maintenance therapy with an immunomodulator such as AZA or 6-MP. AZA (Imuran, Azasan) has been widely used in Europe while 6-MP (Purinethol) has been more commonly used in North America. The initial reports of these agents for treatment of UC first appeared in the 1960s.[106,107]

Pharmacokinetics of Azathioprine/6-Mercaptopurine

AZA is a prodrug rapidly converted into 6-MP by a nonenzymatic nucleophilic attack by sulfhydryl-containing compounds, such as glutathione, as found in erythrocytes and other tissues.[108] AZA is 55% 6-MP by molecular weight, and 88% of the AZA is converted to 6-MP. Thus, a conversion factor of 2.07 is used to convert a dose of 6-MP in milligrams to the equivalent dose of AZA.[109] The 6-MP is competitively metabolized by 3 enzyme systems: xanthine oxidase and thiopurine methyltransferase, which break down the 6-MP to inactive metabolites, and hypoxanthine phosphoribosyltransferase, followed by several other enzymes that convert 6-MP to the active metabolites, the 6-TG nucleotides (Figure 39-2).[110] The 6-TGs act as purine antagonists, which interfere with nucleic acid synthesis and inhibit cell growth.[111] AZA and 6-MP also have immunosuppressive properties by a cytotoxic effect on lymphoid cells.[112] Thiopurine methyltransferase (TPMT) is subject to genetic polymorphism: absent in 0.3%, heterozygous in 11%, and normal in 89% of the population.[113] Thus the TPMT enzyme level may impact the dose of AZA or 6-MP tolerated by a patient.

The half-lives of AZA/6-MP in plasma are short, ranging from 1 to 2 hours, while the half-life of the 6-TG nucleotides is prolonged (3 to 13 days) and the time to reach steady state for these active metabolites can range from 4 days to 3 years.[114,115] This likely explains the clinical observation that prolonged therapy of 1 to 6 months with AZA or 6-MP is usually required for a beneficial therapeutic response.

Adverse Events With Azathioprine/6-Mercaptopurine

Side effects associated with AZA/6-MP treatment can be divided into allergic, which are not dose-related, and nonallergic reactions, which are dose-related (Table 39-4).

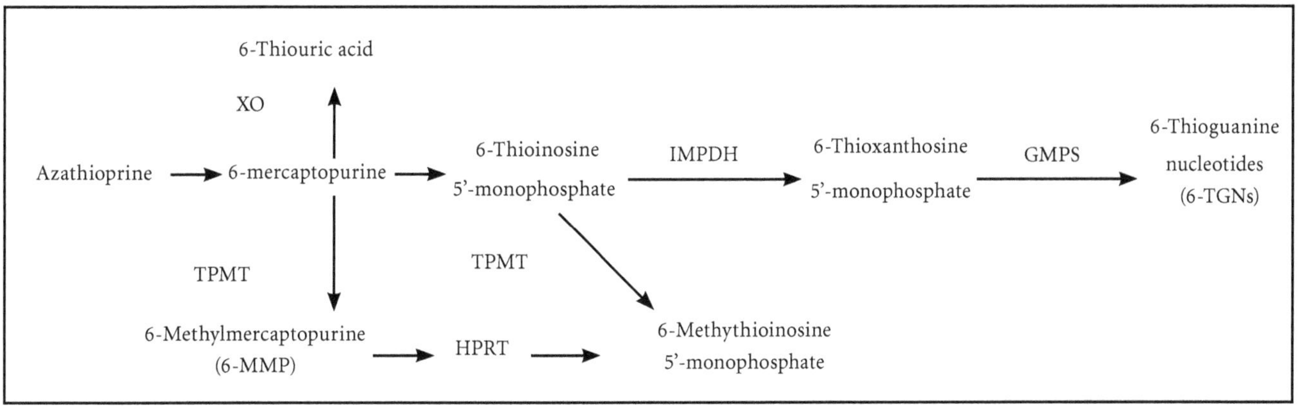

FIGURE 39-2. Metabolism of AZA and 6-MP. XD: xanthine oxidase; HPRT: hypoxanthine phosphoribosyltransferase; TPMT: thiopurine methyltransferase; IMPDH: inosine monophosphate dehydrogenase; GMPS: guanosine monophosphate synthetase. (Reprinted with permission from Su CG, Stein RB, Lewis JD, Lichtenstein GR. Azathioprine or 6-mercaptopurine for inflammatory bowel disease: do risks outweigh benefits? *Dig Liver Dis.* 2000;32:518-531.)

One study of the frequency of side effects with 6-MP has shown an overall incidence of adverse effects in 15% of treated patients. Rates of specific adverse effects included pancreatitis (3%), infection (7%), hepatitis (0.3%), and miscellaneous allergic reactions (2%). This study reported bone marrow depression in 2%.[116] Another report found a risk of bone marrow suppression (primarily leukopenia) of 5% with AZA, which could occur anytime from 2 weeks to 11 years of treatment. Regular monitoring of the complete blood count (CBC) is recommended as long as the patient stays on AZA or 6-MP and could be done every 2 to 4 weeks for the first 2 to 3 months and every 1 to 2 months thereafter.[117] When bone marrow suppression is detected, the drug may be stopped for a few days and restarted at a somewhat lower dose, or the dose may be reduced with continued close monitoring. In a meta-analysis of AZA or 6-MP therapy, the pooled OR for experiencing an adverse event requiring withdrawal from therapy was 5.26 (CI 2.20-12.60) compared to placebo therapy.[118]

Pancreatitis usually develops within 3 to 4 weeks of initiating therapy and resolves quickly once the drug is stopped. If re-challenged after developing pancreatitis, recurrent pancreatitis will develop. This adverse effect will preclude future use of the drug. There are no reports of chronic pancreatitis related to AZA or 6-MP.

Other allergic reactions, such as fever, rash, or arthralgias, will resolve once the drug is stopped but will recur with re-challenge. Symptoms such as nausea, vomiting, and abdominal pain are relatively common but are mild and will often improve with continued therapy. Some patients intolerant of AZA may tolerate 6-MP[119] or vice versa.[120]

Infections have been reported, including disseminated cytomegalovirus, liver abscess, pneumonia, listeria cerebritis, herpes zoster, septic phlebitis with arthritis, viral hepatitis, Q fever, and CMV colitis, and may occur without leukopenia.[110]

TABLE 39-4

ADVERSE REACTIONS TO AZATHIOPRINE/ 6-MERCAPTOPURINE

Allergic Reactions	Nonallergic Reactions
Pancreatitis	Bone marrow suppression
Fever	Leukopenia
Rash	Thrombocytopenia
	Anemia
Arthralgias	
Malaise	Infection
Nausea	Hepatitis
Diarrhea	Malignancy

Abnormal liver-associated tests have been noted in 2% of patients with CD on long-term therapy with AZA.[121] These abnormalities resolved with discontinuation of the therapy. One patient treated for 6 months with 6-MP developed hepatitis, which resolved when the drug was stopped.[116]

Malignancy with long-term AZA/6-MP therapy has been a concern following reports of increased risk of non-Hodgkins lymphoma in patients treated with such therapy for rheumatoid arthritis and solid-organ transplantation.[122,123] Lymphoma has been reported in 3% to 4% of patients with IBD treated with AZA/6-MP, but this was not increased over a control population.[124] Treatment of IBD with AZA/6-MP appears to be associated with a small increased risk of Epstein-Barr virus-positive lymphoma.[125] Patients with UC of longer than 10 years duration are known to be at increased risk of colorectal carcinoma.[126,127]

The chance that AZA/6-MP may increase this risk has been assessed in 86 patients receiving AZA, where 8 cancers were identified; while in 180 patients without AZA therapy, 15 cases were noted.[124] These rates were not significantly different. Another uncontrolled study of 170 patients with UC treated with 6-MP reported 3 patients with bowel cancer and 1 patient with breast cancer.[128]

Drug interactions may be an issue with the use of AZA/6-MP. Allopurinol inhibits xanthine oxidase activity, which may reduce the oxidative metabolism of AZA/6-MP and result in an increased risk of toxic effects with standard doses. Another potential interaction is between AZA/6-MP and 5-ASA. In vitro studies have shown 5-ASA-containing drugs may noncompetitively inhibit recombinant human TPMT activity.[129,130] However, one study failed to demonstrate any effect of concurrent 5-ASA on 6-TG and 6-MMP levels, on clinical response, or on drug-induced toxicity.[118]

Efficacy of Azathioprine/ 6- Mercaptopurine in Maintenance Therapy of Ulcerative Colitis

There are fewer controlled trials assessing the efficacy of AZA in maintenance of UC than in CD.[131] No controlled studies with 6-MP have been published.

The first placebo-controlled maintenance trial of AZA in UC included 80 patients who were treated with AZA at a dose of 1.5 to 2.5 mg/kg/d. There was no benefit of the drug in preventing relapse at 12 months of maintenance therapy.[132] In contrast, a withdrawal trial followed 67 patients with UC (33 continued AZA, 34 received placebo) in remission for 2 months or more and on AZA for 6 months or more, and 12 patients with chronic low-grade or corticosteroid-dependent disease (5 received AZA, 7 placebo).[133] Aminosalicylates were continued in all patients. In the patients in remission, continued AZA (at doses of 50 to 200 mg/d) for 1 year resulted in a relapse rate of 36% compared to 59% in the placebo-treated group ($p = 0.039$). For a subgroup of 54 patients in long-term remission (over 6 months) at entry, continued AZA also resulted in significantly less relapse (31%) than placebo (61%, $p < 0.01$). A 30-year retrospective review of AZA treatment of at least 6 months in 346 patients with UC showed 1, 3, and 5 year remission rates of 95%, 69%, and 55%, respectively.[134] When the AZA was stopped, relapse occurred in 75%, suggesting AZA therapy should be continued on an indefinite basis.

Controlled studies in patients with UC who had been unable to discontinue steroids without worsening of symptoms (steroid-dependent) demonstrated some steroid-sparing effect with the addition of AZA: the first used AZA at 1.5 mg/kg/d (16 patients) versus placebo (14 patients) for 6 months and noted patients on AZA therapy required a significantly lower dose of corticosteroid at the completion of the study.[135] Another report compared AZA therapy at 2.0 to 2.5 mg/kg/d in 24 patients to placebo in 20 patients over 6 months and also resulted in significantly lower doses of corticosteroids in the group receiving the AZA.[136] An uncontrolled report of 34 patients considered steroid-dependent were treated initially with AZA at doses of 2.0 to 2.5 mg/kg. Steroids were discontinued in 70% within 12 months (mean 4.6 months). Adverse events were noted in 38%, requiring withdrawal of AZA in 7 patients and substitution with 6-MP in 4 of these patients for abnormal liver function tests.[137]

The use of 6-MP in 81 patients was found to allow elimination in 48% and reduction of the steroid dose in 13% of the patients who were previously steroid-dependent.[138] Patients were started on a dose of 50 mg/d and advanced as tolerated (based on serial leukocyte counts) to 100 mg/d if needed. A similar study of 105 patients considered steroid-dependent or with chronic refractory symptoms showed that doses of 6-MP of 50 mg/d or higher allowed complete cessation of corticosteroids in 65% and reduced steroids in 24% of treated patients. When the 6-MP was withdrawn in 15 patients who were in remission, relapse occurred in 87%.[139] The benefit in patients with distal UC may, however, be somewhat less than in patients with more extensive disease.[140]

Maximizing the Benefit of Azathioprine/6-Mercaptopurine Therapy

The dose of AZA/6-MP is most safely chosen based on the erythrocyte TPMT enzyme activity and the patient's weight. With a normal TPMT enzyme activity level, initial doses of AZA are 2 to 2.5 mg/kg/d and 6-MP are 1 to 1.5 mg/kg/d. If the TPMT enzyme activity level is below normal and in the range found with heterozygosity of the genes that express the enzyme, then a lower dose of AZA/6-MP should be started. If the patient is homozygote-deficient for TPMT, a situation that occurs in about 0.3% of the population, then AZA and 6-MP should not be used because of the certainty of bone marrow toxicity and cytopenias. Some studies have suggested more benefit from the drug in treatment of CD with doses sufficient to induce leukopenia.[141] However, in one retrospective assessment, treatment for at least 6 months with AZA in 173 patients with IBD, including 77 patients with UC, found neutropenia was not associated with a better response rate. Forty-four patients developed neutropenia. Four of these stopped the drug for severe neutropenia, and 3 developed life-threatening sepsis.[142] Therefore, regular monitoring of the leukocyte count is important to identify leukopenia early and allow adjustment in the dosage, but should not be a therapeutic goal. Macrocytosis is also a common effect of AZA/6-MP therapy but has not been shown to predict clinical benefit. More recently, the monitoring of the erythrocyte 6-TG level has been suggested as a gauge for adjustment of the oral dosage.[143-145] While this marker may explain the lack of response to standard doses in some patients, there is significant overlap between patients who do and do not respond to AZA/6-MP. Thus, for those nonresponsive to standard doses, measurement of this metabolite level may allow safe upward adjustment of drug dosage.

Immunosuppressive Therapy During Pregnancy

AZA and 6-MP are characterized by the FDA as Category D drugs, which are not recommended for use during pregnancy. To avoid the potential risks of the drug to the fetus, therapy can be stopped several months before conception.[146] Use of these drugs at conception by either the father or mother and use of these drugs during pregnancy remains controversial. Some recent reports suggest the use of these medications does not lead to reduced fertility in either fathers or mothers or adverse effects on the fetus,[147-149] while one report showed a risk of birth defects among the children of fathers who took one of these drugs at the time of conception.[150] In patients whose condition may warrant the use of AZA/6-MP through conception and pregnancy, a decision to proceed with treatment should be made by the patient only after the patient and partner have been thoroughly informed of the potential risks of birth defects.

Effect of Azathioprine/6-Mercaptopurine on Risks of Subsequent Surgery

Many UC patients requiring immunosuppressive therapy are candidates for surgical intervention if they fail to respond to therapy or if they elect to proceed with surgery. The issue of surgical complications attributable to preoperative immunomodulatory therapy has been addressed in a review of 209 patients treated with proctocolectomy. They found that preoperative high-dose corticosteroids and severe disease are associated with increased postoperative complications, while preoperative AZA or 6-MP was not associated with increased postoperative complications.[151]

Clinical Use of Azathioprine/6-Mercaptopurine in Maintenance Therapy of Ulcerative Colitis

Current indications for use of AZA/6-MP include a history of 3 or more relapses per year that require corticosteroid therapy, a history of relapse of symptoms with tapering of corticosteroids (steroid-dependence), or a history of symptom relapse within 6 weeks of discontinuing corticosteroid therapy.[152,153] These drugs have a slow onset and require 1 to 6 months for clinical benefit, though initiating an adequate dose at treatment onset will shorten this onset phase.[154] They are not appropriate therapy for induction of remission and must be combined with effective induction therapy, usually with corticosteroids or in some patients with cyclosporine.

When starting AZA/6-MP, an initial assessment of the erythrocyte TPMT will help guide the dosage of medication. For those with a normal TPMT level, AZA can be started at 2.0 to 2.5 mg/kg/d, or 6-MP can be started at 1.0 to 1.5 mg/kg/d. For patients with a reduced TPMT level, a reduced dosage should be started, such as 25 to 50 mg/d of AZA or 25 mg/d of 6-MP. If the TPMT level is not known, then a lower initial dose of AZA or 6-MP should be used, with a gradual increase in the dose over the first 4 weeks of therapy, with weekly monitoring of the CBC. Careful monitoring of the CBC is needed to screen for bone marrow suppression, especially leukopenia, and should be done regularly at intervals of 1 to 2 weeks for the first 2 to 4 months of therapy and continued at 1- to 2-month intervals indefinitely. Liver-associated tests, including the alkaline phosphatase and alanine aminotransferase (ALT), should be checked after 4 to 8 weeks and then periodically as long as the patient continues this medication.

Although it is common for patients to be treated with both aminosalicylates and AZA/6-MP initially, many will be able to discontinue the aminosalicylate.[155] This can be done by slowly tapering the aminosalicylate over several weeks or months with resumption of an increased aminosalicylate dose if symptoms recur. Most patients who are maintained in remission on AZA/6-MP will require prolonged and indefinite treatment.[156]

As with all patients with ulcerative colitis, those receiving immunomodulatory therapy should be monitored regularly for the risk of colorectal neoplasia, as well as health maintenance screening. There is no need to discontinue such therapy in preparation for surgery. Patients should be apprised of the potential risk of such therapy in conjunction with pregnancy, though it is probably not necessary to discontinue the drug if it was clinically warranted to begin such treatment initially.

Other Immunosuppressive Therapy

Methotrexate

Since introduction of methotrexate as therapy for IBD,[157] randomized, controlled studies have documented the benefits from parenteral methotrexate therapy in CD at 25 mg/week[158] for induction and 15 mg/week for long-term maintenance.[159] Studies in maintenance of UC have been less convincing. A randomized, controlled trial in UC used an oral dose of 12.5 mg/week and showed no benefit for induction or maintenance of remission in 67 patients for 9 months.[160] Another randomized, controlled trial assessed induction of remission and maintenance of remission in 34 patients with UC by comparing prednisone plus 6-MP, prednisone plus methotrexate

15 mg/week (not stated if orally or parenterally administered), and prednisone plus 5-ASA for an induction period of 30 weeks followed by a maintenance period of 76 weeks. During the maintenance phase, methotrexate alone was not an effective maintenance therapy as compared to 6-MP treatment.[161] An open-label study of parenteral methotrexate at 12.5 mg/week suggested this was an effective alternative in 10 patients intolerant or nonresponsive to AZA therapy for treatment of steroid-dependent and steroid-resistant UC.[162] A retrospective review of 22 patients with UC and 48 patients with CD were treated with varying doses of methotrexate with a mean dose of 20 mg/week, usually orally. Both groups showed similar rates of relapse.[163] In light of the currently available data, methotrexate cannot be recommended as first-line maintenance therapy.[164] Additional randomized, controlled trials using higher doses should be considered.

Pharmacokinetics-oral ingestion of methotrexate is highly variable as compared to parenteral administration. The drug has a relatively short half-life in the circulation and is metabolized to longer-lived methotrexate polyglutamates, which inhibit dihydrofolate reductase. This interferes with the de-novo synthesis of purines and pyrimidines, the formation of polyamines, and the transmethylation of phospholipids and proteins. The anti-inflammatory activity may result from inhibition of adenosine deaminase and subsequent accumulation of adenosine, which is released into extracellular space where it decreases polymorphonuclear chemotaxis and other inflammatory mediators, such as interleukins and eicosanoids.[165]

Adverse Events

Early toxicity from methotrexate is of a gastrointestinal nature, including nausea, vomiting, diarrhea, and stomatitis. Later toxicity includes liver disease, pancytopenia, and pneumonitis. There appears to be a low risk of malignancy and infections. Methotrexate is contraindicated in women considering pregnancy or during pregnancy because of teratogenicity.

Cyclosporine

Experience with induction therapy in UC, especially for severe symptoms, has shown benefit. Long-term maintenance therapy with cyclosporine is not advised, however, because of nephrotoxicity.[166] Overlap of cyclosporine with a thiopurine drug should serve as a bridge to maintenance treatment with AZA/6-MP.[167]

Infliximab

There is excellent evidence demonstrating efficacy of infliximab in maintenance treatment of UC. Infliximab is approved for reducing signs and symptoms, achieving clinical remission and mucosal healing, and eliminating corticosteroid use in patients with moderate to severe active UC who have had an inadequate response to conventional therapy. The approval was based on 2 randomized, double-blind, placebo-controlled studies (ACT 1 and ACT 2), which evaluated the efficacy of infliximab for induction and maintenance therapy in adults with moderate to severe active UC.[168] The studies showed that patients with moderate to severe active UC treated with infliximab at weeks 0, 2, and 6, and every 8 weeks thereafter, were more likely to have a clinical response at weeks 8, 30, and 54 than those receiving placebo.

NONEFFECTIVE THERAPIES

Corticosteroids

Long-term, low-dose glucocorticosteroids are ineffective for maintenance therapy of ulcerative colitis[169] and put the patient at risk for the sequelae of chronic steroid therapy. Patients who are dependent on low-dose steroid therapy are candidates for immunomodulatory therapy administration.

Nicotine

A single randomized, controlled trial of transdermal nicotine therapy for maintenance of UC assigned 80 patients to receive 15 mg of nicotine versus placebo for 16 hours/d over 6 months. There was no difference in the clinical or endoscopic outcome of these 2 groups, though more adverse effects were noted in those receiving the nicotine patches.[170]

PROBIOTICS

One popular theory of pathogenesis for UC is the abnormal response of the host to endogenous microflora, leading to the concept of modifying the host bacteria in order to downregulate the colon pathologic immune response.[171] Such microorganisms are known as probiotics and are defined as "live nonpathogenic organisms that confer health benefits by improving the microbial balance."[172] Suitable organisms would be of human origin; resist acid and bile; and adhere, colonize, and survive in the human intestine. They must be safe for human use, have clinically validated health effects, and be suitable for commercial production.[173] For treatment of UC, this has led to the use of bacteria, usually lactic acid-producing, such as *lactobacilli*, *bifidobacteria*, and *streptococci*, or yeasts such as *Saccharomyces boulardii*.[174]

An *E. coli* strain, designated Nissle 1917 serotype 06:K5:H1, has been assessed in 3 randomized studies in comparison to 5-ASA preparations. The first assessed maintenance benefit of this *E. coli* strain against 1500 mg/d of 5-ASA and found after 12 weeks relapse occurred in 16% of the *E. coli*-treated group versus 11% of the 5-ASA-treated group. This response rate was not significantly different.[175] Another maintenance study over 1 year in 327 patients compared this *E. coli* strain with 1500 mg/d of 5-ASA and found equivalent rates of relapse (45% versus 36%, respectively).[176] The third study included an induction phase with a maintenance phase of therapy and again suggested a comparable effectiveness of the probiotic and 5-ASA (1200 mg/d).[177] However, a low dose of 5-ASA was used in these studies, raising concern that the probiotic may be inferior to the higher doses of 5-ASA commonly used for maintenance therapy of UC.

VSL#3 is a lyophilized preparation of 4 strains of lactobacilli, 3 strains of bifidobacteria, and 1 strain of *Streptococcus salivarius* subsp. *thermophilus* (VSL Pharmaceuticals, Inc, Ft. Lauderdale, FL) and has been assessed in an open-label maintenance study in 20 patients with UC. These patients were intolerant or allergic to 5-ASA compounds and had a history of at least 2 relapses per year and had experienced a relapse within the previous 3 months. In a 1-year treatment, 15 of the 20 patients remained in remission.[178]

While these reports are promising, additional controlled trials are needed to establish the role for probiotics in maintenance treatment of ulcerative colitis.

MONITORING FOR DRUG SIDE EFFECTS

Most patients with UC will require some form of long-term maintenance therapy to maintain remission. Monitoring of such patients has been assessed and recommendations include the following[179]:

- Baseline measurement for all patients: CBC, serum creatinine, and liver function tests (LFTs), including the serum alkaline phosphatase and the ALT.
- Aminosalicylates: Creatinine at 6 and 12 months of therapy and annually thereafter. For sulfasalazine, a CBC may be considered for monitoring of leukopenia within the first 2 to 3 months of therapy.
- AZA/6-MP: Thiopurine methyltransferase determination at baseline is useful, but optional; a CBC every 2 to 4 weeks for the first 2 to 3 months and then every 1 to 2 months indefinitely.
- Methotrexate: CBC and LFTs should be done every 1 to 3 months.
- Corticosteroids: Bone density testing at initiating therapy and periodically, perhaps at 1- to 3-year intervals, as long as the patient remains on steroid therapy.

REFERENCES

1. Misiewicz JJ, Lennard-Jones JE, Connell AM, et al. Controlled trial of sulphasalazine in maintenance therapy for ulcerative colitis. *Lancet.* 1965;1:185-188.
2. Langholz E, Munkholm P, Davidsen M, et al. Course of ulcerative colitis: analysis of changes in disease activity over years. *Gastroenterology.* 1994;107:3-11.
3. Kamm MA. Review article: maintenance of remission in ulcerative colitis. *Aliment Pharmacol Ther.* 2002;16(Suppl 4):21-24.
4. Moum B, Elbom A, Vatn MH, et al. Clinical course during the first year after diagnosis in ulcerative colitis and Crohn's disease: results of a large, prospective population-based study in southeastern Norway, 1990-93. *Scand J Gastroenterol.* 1997;32:1005-1012.
5. Leijonmarck CE, Persson PG, Hellers G. Factors affecting colectomy rate in ulcerative colitis: an epidemiologic study. *Gut.* 1990;31:329-333.
6. Feagan BG. Maintenance therapy for inflammatory bowel disease. *Am J Gastroenterol.* 2003;98:S6-S17.
7. Meucci G, Vecchi M, Astegiano M, et al. The natural history of ulcerative proctitis: a multicenter, retrospective study. *Am J Gastroenterol.* 2000;95:469-473.
8. Campieri M, Lanfranchi GA, Boschi S, et al. Topical administration of 5-aminosalicylic acid enemas in patients with ulcerative colitis: studies on rectal absorption and excretion. *Gut.* 1985;26:400-405.
9. Svartz N. Sulfasalazine: II. Some notes on the discovery and development of salazopyrin. *Am J Gastroenterol.* 1988;83:497-503.
10. Moertel CG, Bargen JA. A critical analysis of the use of salicylazosulfapyridine in chronic ulcerative colitis. *Ann Intern Med.* 1959;51:879-889.
11. Azad Khan AK, Howes DT, Prris J, et al. Optimum dose of sulphasalazine for maintenance treatment in ulcerative colitis. *Gut.* 1980;21:232-240.
12. Schroder H, Lewkonia RM, Price Evans DA. Metabolism of salicylazosulfapyridine in healthy subjects and in patients with ulcerative colitis: effects of colectomy and of phenobarbital. *Clin Pharmacol Ther.* 1973;14:802-809.
13. Azad Khan AK, Piris J, Truelove SC. An experiment to determine the active therapeutic moiety of sulphasalazine. *Lancet.* 1977;2:892-895.
14. Wadworth AN, Fitton A. Olsalazine: a review of its pharmacodynamic and pharmacokinetic properties, and therapeutic potential in inflammatory bowel disease. *Drugs.* 1991;41:647-664.
15. Campbell DES, Berglindh T. Pharmacology of olsalazine. *Scand J Gastroenterol.* 1988;148(Suppl):7-12.
16. Meyers S, Sachar DB, Present DH, Janowitz HD. Olsalazine sodium in the treatment of ulcerative colitis among patients intolerant of sulfasalazine: a prospective, randomized, placebo-controlled, double-blind, dose-ranging clinical trial. *Gastroenterology.* 1987;93:1255-1262.
17. Rijk MCM, van Leir HJJ, Tongeren JHM, Relapse-preventing effect and safety of sulfasalazine and olsalazine in patients with ulcerative colitis in remission: a prospective, double-blind, randomized multicenter study. *Am J Gastroenterol.* 1992;87:438-442.
18. Kiilerich S, Ladefoged K, Rannem T, et al. Prophylactic effects of olsalazine v sulphasalazine during 12 months maintenance treatment of ulcerative colitis. *Gut.* 1992;33:252-255.
19. Jarnerot G. Clinical tolerance of olsalazine. *Scand J Gastroenterol.* 1988;148(Suppl):21-23.

20. Pamukcu R, Hanauer SB, Chang EB. Effect of disodium azodisalicylate on electrolyte transport in rabbit ileum and colon in vitro: comparison with sulfasalazine and 5-aminosalicylic acid. *Gastroenterology.* 1988;95:975-981.
21. Prakash A, Spencer CM. Balsalazide. *Drugs.* 1998;56:83-89.
22. Giaffer MH, Holdsworth CD, Lennard-Jones JE, et al. Improved maintenance of remission in ulcerative colitis by balsalazide 4 g/d compared with 2 g/d. *Aliment Pharmacol Ther.* 1992;6:479-485.
23. Green JRB, Swan CH, Rowlinson A, et al. Short report: comparison of two doses of balsalazide in maintaining ulcerative colitis in remission over 12 months. *Aliment Pharmacol Ther.* 1992;6:647-652.
24. Green JRB, Gibson JA, Kerr GD, et al. Maintenance of remission of ulcerative colitis: a comparison between balsalazide 3 g daily and mesalazine 1.2 g daily over 12 months. *Aliment Pharmacol Ther.* 1998;12:1207-1216.
25. Kruis W, Schreiber S, Theuer D, et al. Low dose balsalazide (1.5 g twice daily) and mesalazine (0.5 g three times daily) maintained remission of ulcerative colitis but high dose balsalazide (3.0 g twice daily) was superior in preventing relapses. *Gut.* 2001;49:783-789.
26. Nielson OH, Bondesen S. Kinetics of 5-aminosalicylic acid after jejunal instillation in man. *Br J Clin Pharmacol.* 1983;16:738-740.
27. Brogden RN, Sorkin EM. Mesalazine: a review of its pharmacodynamic and pharmacokinetic properties, and therapeutic potential in chronic inflammatory bowel diseases. *Drugs.* 1989;38:500-523.
28. Dew MJ, Ryder REJ, Evans M, et al. Colonic release of 5-aminosalicylic acid from an oral preparation in active ulcerative colitis. *Br J Clin Pharmacol.* 1983;16:185-187.
29. Al Mardini H, Lindsay DC, Deighton CM, et al. Effect of polymer coating on faecal recovery of ingested 5-aminosalicylic acid in patients with ulcerative colitis. *Gut.* 1987;28:1084-1089.
30. Schroeder KW, Tremaine WJ, Ilstrup DM. Coated oral 5-aminosalicylic acid therapy for mildly to moderately active ulcerative colitis: a randomized study. *N Engl J Med.* 1987;317:1625-1629.
31. Hawkey CJ, Dube LM, Rountree LV, et al. A trial of zileuton versus mesalazine or placebo in the maintenance of remission of ulcerative colitis. *Gastroenterology.* 1997;112:718-724.
32. Hanauer S, Sninsky C, Robinson M, et al. An oral preparation of mesalamine as long-term maintenance therapy for ulcerative colitis: a randomized, placebo-controlled trial. *Ann Intern Med.* 1996;124:204-211.
33. Ardiazzone S, Petrillo M, Imbesi V, et al. Is maintenance therapy always necessary for patients with ulcerative colitis in remission? *Aliment Pharmacol Ther.* 1999;13:373-379.
34. Riley SA, Mani V, Goodman MJ, et al. Comparison of delayed-release 5-aminosalicylic acid (mesalazine) and sulfasalazine as maintenance treatment for patients with ulcerative colitis. *Gastroenterology.* 1988;94:1383-1389.
35. Clemett D, Markham A. Prolonged-release mesalazine: a review of its therapeutic potential in ulcerative colitis and Crohn's disease. *Drugs.* 2000;59:929-956.
36. Layer PH, Goebell H, Keller J, et al. Delivery and fate of oral mesalamine microgranules within the human small intestine. *Gastroenterology.* 1995;108:1427-1433.
37. Miner P, Hauauer S, Robinson M, et al. Safety and efficacy of controlled-release mesalamine for maintenance of remission in ulcerative colitis. *Dig Dis Sci.* 1995;40:296-304.
38. Fockens P, Mulder CJJ, Tytgat GNJ, et al. Comparison of the efficacy and safety of 1.5 compared with 3.0 g oral slow-release mesalazine (Pentasa) in the maintenance treatment of ulcerative colitis. *Eur J Gastroenterol Hepatol.* 1995;7:1025-1030.
39. Lichtenstein GR, Kamm MA, Boddu P, et al. Effect of once- or twice daily MMX mesalamine (SPD476) for the induction of remission of mild to moderately active ulcerative colitis. *Clin Gastroenterol Hepatol.* 2007;5:95-102.
40. Kamm MA, Sandborn WJ, Gassull M, et al. Once-daily, high-concentration MMX mesalamine in active ulcerative colitis. *Gastroenterology.* 2007;132:66-75.
41. Lichtenstein G, Merchant K, Shaw A, et al. Once-daily 1.5-g granulated mesalamine effectively maintains remission in patients with ulcerative colitis who switch from different 5-ASA formulations [abstract 1100]. *Am J Gastroenterol.* 2008;13(suppl 1):s429-s430.
42. Kruis W, Kiudelis, Rácz I, et al. Once daily versus three times daily mesalazine granules in active ulcerative colitis: a double-blind, double-dummy, randomised, non-inferiority trial. *Gut.* 2009;58:233-240.
43. Marshall JK, Irvine EJ. Putting rectal 5-amionsalicylic acid in its place: the role in distal ulcerative colitis. *Am J Gastroenterol.* 2000;95:1628-1636.
44. Biddle WL, Greenberger NJ, Swan JT, et al. 5-aminosalicylic acid enemas: effective agent in maintaining remission in left-sided ulcerative colitis. *Gastroenterology.* 1988;94:1075-1079.
45. D'Albasio G, Paoluzi P, Campieri M, et al. Maintenance treatment of ulcerative proctitis with mesalazine suppositories: a double-blind placebo-controlled trial. *Am J Gastroenterol.* 1998;93:799-803.
46. Andreoli A, Spinella S, Levenstein S, et al. 5-ASA enema versus oral sulphasalazine in maintaining remission in ulcerative colitis. *Ital J Gastroenterol.* 1994;26:121-125.
47. D'Albasio G, Trallori G, Ghetti A, et al. Intermittent therapy with high-dose 5-amionsalicylic acid enemas for maintaining remission in ulcerative proctosigmoiditis. *Dis Colon Rectum.* 1990;44:494-497.
48. Mantzaris GH, Hatzis A, Petraki I, et al. Intermittent therapy with high-dose 5-aminosalicylic acid enemas maintains remission in ulcerative proctitis and proctosigmoiditis. *Dis Colon Rectum.* 1994;37:58-62.
49. Binder VS, Halskov E, Hvidberg E, et al. A controlled study of 5-acetoaminosalicylic acid (5-Ac-ASA) as enema in ulcerative colitis. *Scand J Gastroenterol.* 1981;16:1122.
50. Van Hogenzand RA, van Hees PA, van Gorp, et al. Double-blind comparison of 5-aminosalicylic acid and acetyl-5-aminosalicylic acid suppositories in patients with idiopathic proctitis. *Aliment Pharmacol Ther.* 1988;2:33-40.
51. Willoughby CP, Piris J, Truelove SC. The effect of topical N-acetyl-5-amionsalicylic acid in ulcerative colitis. *Scand J Gastroenterol.* 1980;15:715-719.
52. Bondesen S. Intestinal fate of 5-aminosalicylic acid: regional and systemic kinetic studies in relation to inflammatory bowel disease. *Pharmacol Toxicol.* 1997;81:1-28.
53. Allgayer H, Ahnfelt NO, Kruis W, et al. Colonic-N-acetylation of 5-aminosalicylic acid in inflammatory bowel disease. *Gastroenterology.* 1989;97:38-41.
54. Frieri G, Giacomelli R, Pimpo M, et al. Mucosal 5-aminosalicylic acid concentration inversely correlates with severity of colonic inflammation in patients with ulcerative colitis. *Gut.* 2000;47:410-414.
55. Taffet SL, Das KM. Sulphasalazine-adverse effects and desensitization. *Dig Dis Sci.* 1983;28:833-842.
56. Das KM, Eastwood MA, McManus JPA, et al. Adverse reactions during salicylazosulphapyridine therapy and the relation with drug metabolism and acetylator phenotype. *N Engl J Med.* 1973;289:491-495.
57. Sharma BK, Safety profile of the new 5-ASA based compounds. *Can J Gastroenterol.* 1990;4:443-445.
58. Turunen U, Elomaa I, Antitila VJ. et al. Mesalazine tolerance in patients with inflammatory bowel disease and previous intolerance or allergy to sulphasalazine or sulphonamides. *Scand J Gastroenterol.* 1987;22:798-802.

59. Leino R, Liippo K, Ekfors T. Sulphasalazine-induced reversible hypersensitivity pneumonitis and fatal fibrosing alveolitis: report of two cases. *J Intern Med.* 1991;229:553-556.
60. Jones GR, Malone DNS. Sulphasalazine-induced lung disease. *Thorax.* 1972;27:713-717.
61. Birnie GG, McLeod TIF, Watkinson G. Incidence of sulphasalazine-induced male infertility. *Gut.* 1981;22:452-455.
62. Riley SA, LeCarpentier J, Mani V, et al. Sulphasalazine induced seminal abnormalities in ulcerative colitis: results of mesalazine substitution. *Gut.* 1987;28:1008-1012.
63. Schwartz AG, Targan SR, Saxon A, et al. Sulfasalazine-induced exacerbation of ulcerative colitis. *N Engl J Med.* 1982;306:409-412.
64. Sturgeon JB, Bhatia P, Hermans D, et al. Exacerbation of ulcerative colitis with mesalamine. *Gastroenterology.* 1995;108:1889-1893.
65. Mohsen AQM, Mulvey D, Priddle JK, et al. Effects of olsalazine in the jejunum of rat. *Gut.* 1987;28:1474-1477.
66. Loftus EV, Kane SV, Bjorkman D. Systemic review: short-term adverse effects of 5-aminosalicylic acid agents in the treatment of ulcerative colitis. *Aliment Pharmacol Ther.* 2004;19:179-189.
67. Calder IC, Funder CC, Green CR, et al. Nephrotoxic lesions from 5-aminosalicylic acid. *Br Med J.* 1972;1:152-154.
68. Bilyard KG, Joseph EC, Metcalf R. Mesalazine: an overview of key preclinical studies. *Scand J Gastoenterol.* 1990(Suppl);172:175.
69. Birketvedt GS, Berg KJ, Fausa O, et al. Glomerular and tubular renal functions after long-term medication of sulphasalazine, olsalazine, and mesalazine in patients with ulcerative colitis. *Inflamm Bowel Dis.* 2000;6:275-279.
70. Van Staa TP, Travis S, Leufkens HGM, et al. 5-Aminosalicylic acids and the risk of renal disease: a large British epidemiologic study. *Gastroenterology.* 2004;126:1733-1739.
71. Herrlinger KR, Noftz MK, Fellermann K, et al. Minimal renal dysfunction in inflammatory bowel disease is related to disease activity but not to 5-ASA use. *Aliment Pharmacol Ther.* 2001;15:363-369.
72. World MJ, Stevens PE, Ashton MA, Rainford DJ. Mesalazine-associated interstitial nephritis. *Nephrol Dial Transplant.* 1996;11:614-621.
73. Corrigan G, Stevens PE. Review article: interstitial nephritis associated with the use of mesalazine in inflammatory bowel disease. *Aliment Pharmacol Ther.* 2000;14(1):1-6.
74. Bitton A, Peppercorn MA, Hanrahan JP, et al. Mesalamine-induced lung toxicity. *Am J Gastoenterol.* 1996;91:1039-1040.
75. Sossai P, Cappellato MG, Stefani S. Can a drug-induced pulmonary hypersensitivity reaction be dose related: a case with mesalamine. *Mt Sinai J Med.* 2001;68:389-395.
76. Oxentenko AS, Loftus EV, Oh JK, et al. Constrictive pericarditis in chronic ulcerative colitis. *J Clin Gastroenterol.* 2002;34:247-251.
77. Fernandez J, Sala M, Panes J, et al. Acute pancreatitis after long-term 5-aminosalicylic acid therapy. *Am J Gastroenterol.* 1997;92: 2302-2303.
78. Deltenre P, Berson A, Marcellin P, et al. Mesalazine (5-aminosalicylic acid) induced chronic hepatitis. *Gut.* 1999;44:886-888.
79. Gaginella TS, Walsh RE. Sulfasalazine: multiplicity of action. *Dig Dis Sci.* 1992;37:801-812.
80. Wahl C, Liptay S, Adler G, et al. Sulfasalazine: a potent and specific inhibitor of Nuclear Factor Kappa B. *J Clin Invest.* 1998;101:1163-1174.
81. Ireland A, Jewell DP. Mechanism of action of 5-aminosalicylic acid and its derivatives. *Clin Sci.* 1990;78:119-125.
82. Greenfield SM, Punchard NA, Teare JP, et al. Review article: the mode of action of the aminosalicylates in inflammatory bowel disease. *Aliment Pharmacol Ther.* 1993;7:369-383.
83. Kaiser GC, Yan F, Polk DB. Mesalamine blocks tumor necrosis factor growth inhibition and Nuclear Factor B in mouse colonocytes. *Gastroenterology.* 1999;116:602-609.
84. Sutherland L, Roth D, Beck P, et al. Oral 5-aminosalicylic acid for maintenance of remission in ulcerative colitis. *Cochrane Library.* 2002;3:Update Software, Oxford.
85. Bebb JR, Scott BB. Systematic review: how effective are the usual treatments for ulcerative colitis? *Aliment Pharmacol Ther.* 2004;20:143-149.
86. Riley S. What dose of 5-aminosalicylic acid (mesalazine) in ulcerative colitis? *Gut.* 1998;42:761-763.
87. Staerk Laursen L, Stokholm M, Bukhave K, et al. Disposition of 5-aminosalicylic acid by olsalazine and three mesalazine preparations in patients with ulcerative colitis: comparison of intraluminal colonic concentrations, serum values, and urinary excretion. *Gut.* 1990;31:1271-1276.
88. Christensen LA, Fallingborg J, Jacobsen BA, et al. Comparative bioavailability of 5-aminosalicylic acid from a controlled release preparation and an azo-bond preparation. *Aliment Pharmacol Ther.* 1994;8:289-294.
89. Stretch GL, Campbell BJ, Dwarakanath AD, et al. 5-Aminosalicylic acid absorption and metabolism in ulcerative colitis patients receiving maintenance sulphasalazine, olsalazine, or mesalazine. *Aliment Pharmacol Ther.* 1996;10:941-947.
90. Karamanolis DG, Papatheodoridis GV, Xourgias V. Systemic absorption of 5-aminosalicylic acid in patients with inactive ulcerative colitis treated with olsalazine and mesalazine. *Eur J Gastroenterol Hepatol.* 1996;8:1083-1088.
91. Rijk MCM, Van Schaik A, Van Tongeren JHM. Disposition of mesalazine from mesalazine-delivery drugs in patients with inflammatory bowel disease, with and without diarrhea. *Scand J Gastroenterol.* 1992;27:863-868.
92. Sandborn WJ. Editorial. Rational selection of oral 5-aminosalicylate formulations and prodrugs for the treatment of ulcerative colitis. *Am J Gastroenterol.* 2002;97:2939-2941.
93. Sandborn WJ, Hanauer SB. Systemic review: the pharmacokinetic profiles of oral mesalazine formulations and mesalazine pro-drugs used in the management of ulcerative colitis. *Aliment Pharmacol Ther.* 2003;17:29-42.
94. Deav-Citrin O, Park YH, Veerasuntharam G, et al. The safety of mesalamine in human pregnancy: a prospective controlled cohort study. *Gastroenterology.* 1998;114:23-28.
95. Connell WR. Safety of drug therapy for inflammatory bowel disease in pregnant and nursing women. *Inflamm Bowel Dis.* 1996;2:33-47.
96. Habal FM, Hui G, Greenberg GR. Oral 5-aminosalicylic acid for inflammatory bowel disease in pregnancy: safety and clinical course. *Gastroenterology.* 1993;105:1057-1060.
97. Ransohoff DF. Colon cancer in ulcerative colitis. *Gastroenterology.* 1988;94:1089-1091.
98. Eaden J. Review article: the data supporting a role for aminosalicylates in the chemoprevention of colorectal cancer in patients with inflammatory bowel disease. *Aliment Pharmacol Ther.* 2003;18(Suppl. 2):15-21.
99. Pinczowski D, Ekbom A, Baron J, et al. Risk factors for colorectal cancer in patients with ulcerative colitis: a case-control study. *Gastroenterology.* 1994;107:117-120.
100. Moody GA, Jayanthi V, Probert CSJ, et al. Long term therapy with sulphasalazine protects against colorectal cancer in ulcerative colitis: a retrospective study of colorectal cancer risk and compliance with treatment in Leicestershire. *Eur J Gastroenterol Hepatol.* 1996;8:1179-1183.
101. Eaden JA, Abrams K, Ekbom A. et al. Colorectal cancer prevention in ulcerative colitis: a case-control study. *Aliment Pharmacol Ther.* 2000;14:145-153.

102. Velayos FS, Terdiman JP, Walsh JM. Effect of 5-aminosalicylate use on colorectal cancer and dysplasia risk: a systematic review of metaanalysis of observational studies. *Am J Gastroenterol.* 2005;100:1345-1353.
103. Kane SV, Cohen RD, Aikens JE, et al. Prevalence of nonadherence with maintenance mesalamine in quiescent ulcerative colitis. *Am J Gastroenterol.* 2001;96:2929-2933.
104. Kane S, Dezheng H, Aikens J, et al. Medication nonadherence and the outcomes of patients with quiescent ulcerative colitis. *Am J Med.* 2003;114:39-43.
105. Shale MJ, Riley SA. Studies of compliance with delayed-release mesalazine therapy in patients with inflammatory bowel disease. *Aliment Pharmacol Ther.* 2003;18:191-198.
106. Bowen GE, Irons GV, Rhodes JB, et al. Early experiences with azathioprine in ulcerative colitis. *JAMA.* 1966;195:460-464.
107. Bean RHD. The treatment of chronic ulcerative colitis with 6-mercaptopurine. *Med J Aust.* 1962;2:592-593.
108. De Miranda P, Beacham LM, Creagh TH, et al. The metabolic fate of the methylnitroimidazole moiety of azathioprine in the rat. *J Pharmacol Exp Ther.* 1973;187:588-601.
109. Elion GB. The comparative metabolism of imuran and 6-mercaptopurine in man. *Proc Am Assoc Cancer Res.* 1969;10:21.
110. Su CG, Stein RB, Lewis JD, Lichtenstein GR. Azathioprine or 6-mercatopurine for inflammatory bowel disease: do risks outweigh benefits? *Digest Liver Dis.* 2000;32:518-531.
111. Lennard L. The clinical pharmacology of 6-mercaptopurine. *Eur J Clin Pharmacol.* 1992;43:329-339.
112. Brogan M, Hiserodt J, Oliver M, et al. The effect of 6-mercaptopurine on natural killer cell activities in Crohn's disease. *J Clin Immunol.* 1985;5:204-211.
113. Weinshilboum RN, Sladek SL. Mercaptopurine pharmacogenetics: monogenic inheritance of erythrocyte thiopurine methyltransferase activity. *Am J Hum Genet.* 1980;32:651-662.
114. Lennard L, Keen D, Lilleyman JS. Oral 6-mercaptopurine in childhood leukemia: parent drug pharmacokinetics and active metabolite concentrations. *Clin Pharmacol Ther.* 1986;40:287-292.
115. Lennard L, Harrington DI, Wood M, et al. Metabolism of azathioprine to 6-thioguanine nucleotides in patients with pemphigus vulgaris. *Br J Pharmacol.* 1987;23:229-233.
116. Present DH, Meltzer SJ, Krumholz MP, et al. 6-mercatopurine in the management of inflammatory bowel disease: short and long-term toxicity. *Ann Intern Med.* 1989;111:641-649.
117. Connell WR, Kamm MA, Ritchie JK, et al. Bone marrow toxicity caused by azathioprine in inflammatory bowel disease: 27 years experience. *Gut.* 1993;34:1081-1085.
118. Pearson DC, May GR, Fick GH, et al. Azathioprine and 6-mercaptopurine in Crohn's disease: a meta-analysis. *Ann Intern Med.* 1995;122:132-142.
119. Cheng BK, Lichtenstein GR. Are individuals with Crohn's disease who are intolerant to 6-mercaptopurine able to tolerate azathioprine? *Gastroenterology.* 2000;118:A1336.
120. Boulton-Jones JR, Pritchard K, Mahmoud AA. The use of 6-mercaptopurine in patients with inflammatory bowel disease after failure of azathioprine therapy. *Aliment Pharmacol Ther.* 2000;14:1561-1565.
121. Bouhnik Y, Lemann M, Mary JY, et al. Long term follow-up of patients with Crohn's disease treated with azathioprine or 6-mercaptopurine. *Lancet.* 1996;347:215-219.
122. Asten P, Marrett J, Symmons D. Risk of developing certain malignancies is related to duration of immunosuppressive drug exposure in patients with rheumatic disease. *J Rheumatol.* 1999;26:1705-1714.
123. Opelz G, Henderson R. Incidence of non-Hodgkin's lymphoma in kidney and heart transplant recipients. *Lancet.* 1993;342:1514-1516.
124. Connell WR, Kamm MA, Dickson M, et al. Long-term neoplasia risk after azathioprine treatment in inflammatory bowel disease. *Lancet.* 1994;343:1249-1252.
125. Dayharsh GA, Loftus EV, Sandborn WJ, et al. Epstein-Barr virus-positive lymphoma in patients with inflammatory bowel disease treated with azathioprine or 6-mercaptopurine. *Gastroenterology.* 2002;122:72-77.
126. Beaugerie L, Carrat F, Bouvier A, et al. Excess risk of lymphoproliferative disorders (LPD) in inflammatory bowel diseases (IBD): interim results of the Cesame Cohort [abstract 818]. *Gastroenterology.* 2008;134(4 suppl 1):A116.
127. Kandiel A, Fraser AG, Korelitz BI, Brensinger C, Lewis JD. Increased risk of lymphoma among inflammatory bowel disease patients treated with azathioprine and 6-mercaptopurine. *Gut.* 2005;54:1121-1125.
128. Korelitz BI, Mirsky FJ, Fleisher MR, et al. Malignant neoplasms subsequent to treatment of inflammatory bowel disease with 6-mercaptopurine. *Am J Gastroenterol.* 1999;94:3248-3253.
129. Szumlanski CL, Weinshilboum RM. Sulphasalazine inhibition of thiopurine methyltransferase: possible mechanism for interaction with 6-mercaptopurine and azathioprine. *Br J Clin Pharmacol.* 1995;39:456-459.
130. Lewis LD, Benin A, Szumlanski CL, et al. Olsalazine and 6-mercaptopurine related bone marrow suppression: a possible drug-drug interaction. *Clin Pharmacol Ther.* 1997;62:464-475.
131. Dubinsky MC. Azathioprine, 6-mercaptopurine in inflammatory bowel disease: pharmacology, efficacy, and safety. *Clin Gastroenterol Hepatol.* 2004;2:731-743.
132. Jewell DP, Truelove SC. Azathioprine in ulcerative colitis: final report on controlled therapeutic trial. *Br Med J.* 1974;4:627-630.
133. Hawthorne AB, Logan RFA, Hawkey CJ, et al. Randomized controlled trial of azathioprine withdrawal in ulcerative colitis. *Br Med J.* 1992;305:20-22.
134. Fraser AG, Orchard TR, Jewell DP. The efficacy of azathioprine for the treatment of inflammatory bowel disease: a 30 year review. *Gut.* 2002;50:485-489.
135. Rosenberg JL, Wall AJ, Levin B, et al. A controlled trial of azathioprine in the management of chronic ulcerative colitis. *Gastroenterology.* 1975;69:96-99.
136. Kirk AP, Lennard-Jones JE. Controlled trial of azathioprine in chronic ulcerative colitis. *Br Med J.* 1982;284:1291-1292.
137. Lopez-Sanroman A, Bermejo F, Carrera E, et al. Efficacy and safety of thiopurinic immunomodulators (azathioprine and mercaptopurine) in steroid-dependent ulcerative colitis. *Aliment Pharmacol Ther.* 2004;20:161-166.
138. Adler DJ, Korelitz BI. The therapeutic efficacy of 6-mercaptopurine in refractory ulcerative colitis. *Am J Gastroenterol.* 1990;85(6):717-722.
139. George J, Present DH, Pou R, et al. The long-term outcome of ulcerative colitis treated with 6-mercaptopurine. *Am J Gastroenterol.* 1996;91:1711-1714.
140. Falasco G, Zinicola R, Forbes A. Review article: immunosuppressants in distal ulcerative colitis. *Aliment Pharmacol Ther.* 2002;16:181-187.
141. Colonna T, Korelitz BI. The role of leukopenia in the 6-mercaptopurine-induced remission of refractory Crohn's disease. *Am J Gastroenterol.* 1994;89:362-366.
142. Campbell S, Ghosh S. Is neutropenia required for effective maintenance of remission during azathioprine therapy in inflammatory bowel disease? *Eur J Gastroenterol Hepatol.* 2001;13:1073-1076.
143. Cuffari D, Hunt S, Bayless T. Utilization of erythrocyte 6-thioguanine metabolite levels to optimize azathioprine therapy in patients with inflammatory bowel disease. *Gut.* 2001;48:642-646.

144. Dubinsky MC, Lamothe S, Yang HY, et al. Pharmacogenomics and metabolite measurement for 6-mercaptopurine therapy in inflammatory bowel disease. *Gastroenterology.* 2000;118:705-713.
145. Achkar J-P, Stevens T, Easley K, et al. Indicators of clinical response to treatment with 6-mercaptopurine or azathioprine in patients with inflammatory bowel disease. *Inflamm Bowel Dis.* 2004;10:339-345.
146. Korelitz BI. Pregnancy, fertility and inflammatory bowel disease. *Am J Gastroenterol.* 1985;80:365-370.
147. Dejaco C, Mittermaier C, Walter R, et al. Azathioprine treatment and male fertility in inflammatory bowel disease. *Gastroenterology.* 2001;121:1048-1053.
148. Francella A, Dyan A, Bodian C, et al. The safety of 6-mercaptopurine for childbearing patients with inflammatory bowel disease: a retrospective cohort study. *Gastroenterology.* 2003;124:9-17.
149. Moskovitz DN, Bodian C, Chapman ML, et al. The effect on the fetus of medications used to treat pregnant inflammatory bowel-disease patients. *Am J Gastroenterol.* 2004;99:656-661.
150. Rajapakse RO, Korelitz BI, Slantanic J, et al. Outcome of pregnancies when fathers are treated with 6-mercaptopurine for inflammatory bowel disease. *Am J Gastroenterol.* 2000;95:684-688.
151. Mahadevan U, Loftus EV, Tremaine WJ, et al. Azathioprine or 6-mercaptopurine before colectomy for ulcerative colitis is not associated with increased postoperative complications. *Inflamm Bowel Dis.* 2002;8:311-316.
152. Nielsen OH, Vainer B, Rask-Madsen J. Review article: the treatment of inflammatory bowel disease with 6-mercaptopurine or azathioprine. *Aliment Pharmacol Ther.* 2001;15:1699-1708.
153. Sandborn, WJ. A review of immune modifier therapy for inflammatory bowel disease: azathioprine, 6-mercaptopurine, cyclosporine, and methotrexate. *Am J Gastroenterol.* 1996;91:423-433.
154. Sandborn WJ, Tremaine WJ, Wolf DC, et al. Lack of effect of intravenous administration on time to respond to azathioprine for steroid-treated Crohn's disease. *Gastroenterology.* 1999;117:527-535.
155. Campbell S, Ghosh S. Effective maintenance of inflammatory bowel disease remission by azathioprine does not require concurrent 5-aminosalicylate therapy. *Eur J Gastroenterol Hepatol.* 2001;13:1297-1301.
156. McGovern DPB, Travis SPL. Thiopurine therapy: when to start and when to stop. *Eur J Gastroenterol.* 2003;15:219-223.
157. Kozarek RA, Patterson DJ, Gelfand MD, et al. Methotrexate induces clinical and histologic remission in patients with refractory inflammatory bowel disease. *Ann Intern Med.* 1989;110:353-356.
158. Feagan BG, Rochon J, Fedorak RN, et al. Methotrexate for the treatment of Crohn's disease. *N Engl J Med.* 1995;332:292-297.
159. Feagan BG, Fedorak RN, Irvine EJ, et al. A comparison of methotrexate with placebo for the maintenance of Crohn's disease. North America Crohn's Study Group Investigators. *N Engl J Med.* 2000;342:1664-1666.
160. Oren R, Arber N, Odes S, et al. Methotrexate in chronic active ulcerative colitis: a double-blind, randomized, Israel multicenter trial. *Gastroenterology.* 1996;110:1416-1421.
161. Mate-Jimenez J, Hermida C, Cantero-Perona J, et al. 6-Mercaptopurine or methotrexate added to prednisone induces and maintains remission in steroid-dependent inflammatory bowel disease. *Eur J Gastroenterol Hepatol.* 2000;12:1227-1233.
162. Paoluzi OA, Pica R, Marcheggiano A, et al. Azathioprine or methotrexate in the treatment of patients with steroid-dependent or steroid-resistant ulcerative colitis: results of an open-label study on efficacy and tolerability in inducing and maintaining remission. *Aliment Pharmacol Ther.* 2002;16:1751-1759.
163. Fraser AG, Morton D, McGovern D, et al. The efficacy of methotrexate for maintaining remission in inflammatory bowel disease. *Aliment Pharmacol Ther.* 2002;16:693-697.
164. Fraser AG. Methotrexate: first-line or second-line immunomodulator? *Eur J Gastroenterol Hepatol.* 2003;15:225-231.
165. Cronstein BN. The mechanism of action of methotrexate. *Rheum Dis Clin North Am.* 1997;23:739-755.
166. Feutren G, Mihatsch MJ. Risk factors for cyclosporine-induced nephropathy in patients with autoimmune diseases: international kidney biopsy registry of cyclosporine in autoimmune diseases. *N Engl J Med.* 1992;326:1654-1660.
167. Actis GC, Bresso F, Astegiano M, et al. Safety and efficacy of azathioprine in the maintenance of ciclosporin-induced remission of ulcerative colitis. *Aliment Pharmacol Ther.* 2001;15:1307-1311.
168. Rutgeerts P, Sandborn WJ, Feagan BG, et al. Infliximab for induction and maintenance therapy for ulcerative colitis. *N Engl J Med.* 2005;353:2462-2476.
169. Lennard-Jones JE, Misiewicz JJ, Connell AM, et al. Prednisone as maintenance treatment for ulcerative colitis in remission. *Lancet.* 1965;191:188-189.
170. Thomas GAO, Rhodes J, Mani V, et al. Transdermal nicotine as maintenance therapy for ulcerative colitis. *N Engl J Med.* 1995;332:988-992.
171. Shanahan F. Probiotics and inflammatory bowel disease: from fads and fantasy to facts and future. *Br J Nutr.* 2002;88:S5-S9.
172. Fuller R. Probiotics in man and animals. *J Appl Bacteriol.* 1989;66:365-378.
173. Salminen S, Isolauri E, Salminen E. Clinical uses of probiotics for stabilizing the gut mucosal barrier: successful strains and future challenges. *Antoine Van Leeuwenhoek.* 1996;70:347-358.
174. Hart AL, Stagg AJ, Kamm MA. Use of probiotics in the treatment of inflammatory bowel disease. *J Clin Gastroenterol.* 2003;36:111-119.
175. Kruis W, Schutz E, Fric P, et al. Double-blind comparison of an oral *Escherichia coli* preparation and mesalazine in maintaining remission of ulcerative colitis. *Aliment Pharmacol Ther.* 1997;11:853-858.
176. Kruis W, Fric P, Stolte M, et al. Maintenance of remission in ulcerative colitis is equally effective with *Escherichia coli* 1917 and with standard mesalamine (abstract). *Gastroenterology.* 2001;120:680.
177. Rembacken BJ, Snelling AM, Hawkey PM, et al. Non-pathogenic *Escherichia coli* versus mesalazine for treatment of ulcerative colitis: a randomized trial. *Lancet.* 1999;354:635-639.
178. Venturi A, Gionchetti P, Rizzello F, et al. Impact on the composition of the faecal flora by a new probiotic preparation: preliminary data on maintenance treatment of patients with ulcerative colitis. *Aliment Pharmacol Ther.* 1999;13:1103-1108.
179. Cunliffe RN, Scott BB. Review article: monitoring for drug side-effects in inflammatory bowel disease. *Aliment Pharmacol Ther.* 2002;16:647-662.

Financial Disclosures

Dr. Jean-Paul Achkar has not disclosed any relevant financial relationships.

Dr. Pietro G. Andres has not disclosed any relevant financial relationships.

Dr. Leonard Baidoo has not disclosed any relevant financial relationships.

Dr. Robert N. Baldassano has not disclosed any relevant financial relationships.

Dr. James M. Becker has no financial or proprietary interest in the materials presented herein.

Dr. Stephen J. Bickston has not disclosed any relevant financial relationships.

Dr. Wojciech Blonski has no financial or proprietary interest in the materials presented herein.

Dr. Richard S. Bloomfeld has not disclosed any relevant financial relationships.

Dr. Brian P. Bosworth has not disclosed any relevant financial relationships.

Dr. Alan L. Buchman has not disclosed any relevant financial relationships.

Dr. Anne Burke has no financial or proprietary interest in the materials presented herein.

Dr. Massimo Campieri has not disclosed any relevant financial relationships.

Dr. Adam S. Cheifetz has not disclosed any relevant financial relationships.

Dr. Ashish Chawla has not disclosed any relevant financial relationships.

Dr. Robynne Chutkan has not disclosed any relevant financial relationships.

Dr. Russell D. Cohen has not disclosed any relevant financial relationships.

Dr. Carmen Cuffari has not disclosed any relevant financial relationships.

Dr. Eugeni Domènech has not disclosed any relevant financial relationships.

Dr. Marla C. Dubinsky has not disclosed any relevant financial relationships.

Dr. Francis A. Farraye has not disclosed any relevant financial relationships.

Dr. Richard N. Fedorak's research is supported by the Canadian Institute for Health Research and the Crohn's and Colitis Foundation of Canada.

Dr. Lawrence S. Friedman has not disclosed any relevant financial relationships.

Dr. Sonia Friedman has no financial or proprietary interest in the materials presented herein.

Dr. Miguel Gassull has not disclosed any relevant financial relationships.

Dr. Louis R. Ghanem has no financial or proprietary interest in the materials presented herein.

Dr. Jesse A. Green has no financial or proprietary interest in the materials presented herein.

Dr. Douglas B. Haghighi has not disclosed any relevant financial relationships.

Dr. Hans Herfarth has not disclosed any relevant financial relationships.

Dr. Kim L. Isaacs has no financial or proprietary interest in the materials presented herein.

Dr. Vinita Elizabeth Jacob has not disclosed any relevant financial relationships.

Dr. Niraj Jani has no financial or proprietary interest in the materials presented herein.

Dr. Thomas A. Judge has not disclosed any relevant financial relationships.

Dr. Sunanda V. Kane receives research support from and is a consultant for Shire and Proctor and Gamble.

Dr. Jeffry A. Katz has not disclosed any relevant financial relationships.

Dr. Seymour Katz has not disclosed any relevant financial relationships.

Dr. Joshua R. Korzenik has not disclosed any relevant financial relationships.

Dr. David Kotlyar has no financial or proprietary interest in the materials presented herein.

Harrison Lakehomer has not disclosed any relevant financial relationships.

Dr. Bret A. Lashner has not disclosed any relevant financial relationships.

Dr. James D. Lewis has received research funding from Centocor, Takeda, and Shire. He has served as a paid consultant for Millenium, AstraZeneca, GlaxoSmithKline, Elan, Proctor & Gamble, and Amgen.

Dr. Gary Lichtenstein is a consultant for Abbott Corporation, Alaven, Bristol-Myers Squibb, Centocor Orthobiotech, Elan, Ferring, Meda Pharmaceuticals, Millenium Pharmaceuticals, Pfizer Pharmaceuticals, Proctor and Gamble, Prometheus Laboratories Inc, Salix Pharmaceuticals, Santarus, Schering-Plough Corporation, Shire Pharmaceuticals, UCB, Warner Chilcotte, and Wyeth.

Dr. Ming V. Lin has not disclosed any relevant financial relationships.

Dr. Edward V. Loftus Jr has received research support in past 12 months from Procter and Gamble and UCB/Celltech. He was a consultant in the past 12 months for UCB/Celltech, Prometheus Laboratories, Abbott Laboratories.

Dr. Richard P. MacDermott has no financial or proprietary interest in the materials presented herein.

Dr. Karen L. Madsen's research is supported by the Canadian Institute for Health Research, Crohn's and Colitis Foundation of Canada, and the Alberta Heritage Foundation for Medical Research.

Dr. Lloyd Mayer has not disclosed any relevant financial relationships.

Dr. Philip B. Miner Jr has not disclosed any relevant financial relationships.

Dr. Alan C. Moss has no financial or proprietary interest in the materials presented herein.

Dr. Jeffrey W. Nathanson has not disclosed any relevant financial relationships.

Dr. Jaime A. Oviedo has not disclosed any relevant financial relationships.

Dr. Mansour A. Parsi has not disclosed any relevant financial relationships.

Dr. Robert M. Penner's research is supported by the Canadian Institute for Health Research, Crohn's and Colitis Foundation of Canada, and the Alberta Heritage Foundation for Medical Research.

Dr. Robert Pittman has not disclosed any relevant financial relationships.

Dr. Miguel Regueiro has not disclosed any relevant financial relationships.

Dr. John L. Rombeau has no financial or proprietary interest in the materials presented herein.

Dr. Anthony L. Rosa has not disclosed any relevant financial relationships.

Dr. Paul Rutgeerts has not disclosed any relevant financial relationships.

Dr. William J. Sandborn has not disclosed any relevant financial relationships.

Dr. Ellen Scherl has not disclosed any relevant financial relationships.

Dr. Jürgen Schölmerich has not disclosed any relevant financial relationships.

Dr. Kenneth W. Schroeder has not disclosed any relevant financial relationships.

Dr. Corey A. Siegel has not disclosed any relevant financial relationships.

Dr. Kenneth Simpson has not disclosed any relevant financial relationships.

Dr. Antoni Stadnicki has not disclosed any relevant financial relationships.

Dr. Arthur F. Stucchi has no financial or proprietary interest in the materials presented herein.

Dr. Chinyu Su is currently an employee of Pfizer, Inc. She was formerly an employee of and a stockholder in Wyeth, which was acquired by Pfizer, Inc, in October 2009.

Dr. Lloyd Sutherland has not disclosed any relevant financial relationships.

Dr. Traci M. Temmen has no financial or proprietary interest in the materials presented herein.

Dr. Nabil Toubia has not disclosed any relevant financial relationships.

Dr. William J. Tremaine has not disclosed any relevant financial relationships.

Dr. Truc T. Trinh has not disclosed any relevant financial relationships.

Dr. Gert Van Assche has not disclosed any relevant financial relationships.

Dr. Ryan Urquhart Warren has not disclosed any relevant financial relationships.

INDEX

For Product Safety Concerns and Information please contact our EU representative GPSR@taylorandfrancis.com
Taylor & Francis Verlag GmbH, Kaufingerstraße 24, 80331 München, Germany

www.ingramcontent.com/pod-product-compliance
Ingram Content Group UK Ltd.
Pitfield, Milton Keynes, MK11 3LW, UK
UKHW052223190926
475702UK00006B/1178
* 9 7 8 1 5 5 6 4 2 9 4 5 3 *